Jarvis's

HEALTH ASSESSMENT & PHYSICAL EXAMINATION

AUSTRALIAN AND NEW ZEALAND

3RD EDITION

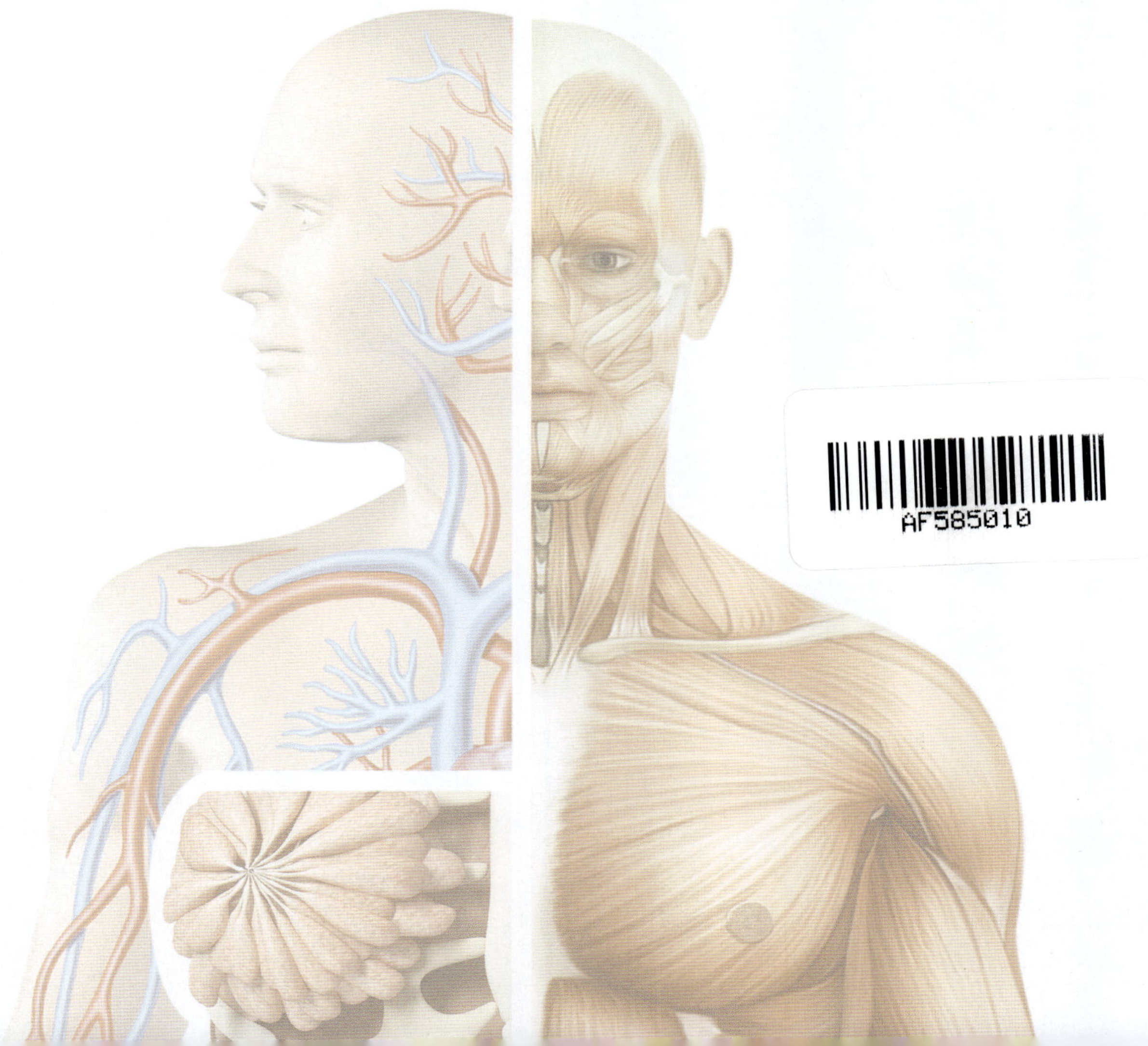

Jarvis's

HEALTH ASSESSMENT & PHYSICAL EXAMINATION

AUSTRALIAN AND NEW ZEALAND 3RD EDITION

Carolyn Jarvis
PhD, APRN, CNP
Professor of Nursing
Illinois Wesleyan University
Bloomington, Illinois
and
Family Nurse Practitioner
Bloomington, Illinois

With Ann Eckhardt
PhD, RN
Associate Professor of Nursing
Illinois Wesleyan University
Bloomington, Illinois

Australian Adapting Editors

Helen Forbes
RN, BAppSc (Adv Nurs)
(La Trobe University),
MEdStudies (Monash University),
PhD (University of Sydney)
Nurse Consultant (Education)
Formerly Associate Professor and Associate Head of School (Teaching & Learning)
School of Nursing & Midwifery,
Deakin University, Melbourne, Victoria

Elizabeth Watt
RN, DipN (College of Nursing Australia),
BAppSc (Adv Nurs) (Lincoln Institute of Health Sciences), MNS (La Trobe University),
Cert Prom Cont, FACN
Nurse Consultant (Education),
Formerly Course Coordinator Master of Nursing (Urological & Continence) Course
School of Nursing & Midwifery, La Trobe University,
Melbourne Campus, Melbourne, Victoria

Original illustrations by Pat Thomas, CM, FAMI
East Troy, Wisconsin

Assessment photographs by Kevin Strandberg
Professor of Art, Illinois Wesleyan University, Bloomington, Illinois

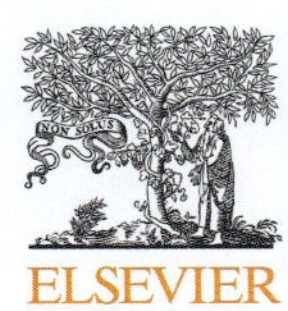

ELSEVIER

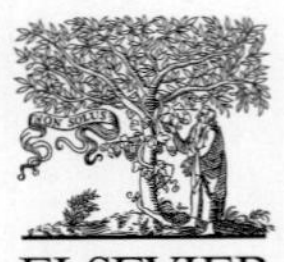

ELSEVIER
Elsevier Australia. ACN 001 002 357
(a division of Reed International Books Australia Pty Ltd)
Tower 1, 475 Victoria Avenue, Chatswood, NSW 2067

ISBN: 978-0-323-51080-6

This adaptation of Physical Examination and Health Assessment, 8th edition by Carolyn Jarvis with Ann Eckhardt, was undertaken by Elsevier Australia and is published by arrangement with Elsevier Inc.

Jarvis's Health Assessment & Physical Examination; 3rd edition

ISBN: 978-0-7295-4337-8

Reprinted 2021

Notice

The adaptation has been undertaken by Elsevier Australia at its sole responsibility. Practitioners and researchers must always rely on their own experience and knowledge in evaluating and using any information, methods, compounds or experiments described herein. Because of rapid advances in the medical sciences, in particular, independent verification of diagnoses and drug dosages should be made. To the fullest extent of the law, no responsibility is assumed by Elsevier, authors, editors or contributors in relation to the adaptation or for any injury and/or damage to persons or property as a matter of products liability, negligence or otherwise, or from any use or operation of any methods, products, instructions, or ideas contained in the material herein.

National Library of Australia Cataloguing-in-Publication Data

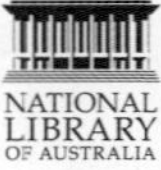

A catalogue record for this book is available from the National Library of Australia

Senior Content Strategist: Libby Houston
Content Project Manager: Shruti Raj
Edited by Kathryn Mason Pak
Proofread by Tim Learner
Cover and design by Lisa Petroff
Index by Innodata Indexing
Typeset by GW India
Printed in China by 1010 Printing International Limited

Last digit is the print number: 9 8 7 6 5 4 3 2

Contents

Text features

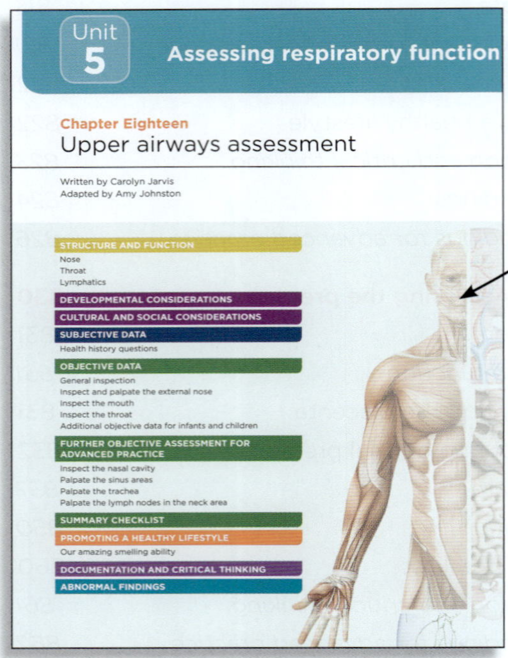
Unit 5 Assessing respiratory function

Chapter Eighteen
Upper airways assessment

Written by Carolyn Jarvis
Adapted by Amy Johnston

STRUCTURE AND FUNCTION
Nose
Throat
Lymphatics
DEVELOPMENTAL CONSIDERATIONS
CULTURAL AND SOCIAL CONSIDERATIONS
SUBJECTIVE DATA
Health history questions
OBJECTIVE DATA
General inspection
Inspect and palpate the external nose
Inspect the mouth
Inspect the throat
Additional objective data for infants and children
FURTHER OBJECTIVE ASSESSMENT FOR ADVANCED PRACTICE
Inspect the nasal cavity
Palpate the sinus areas
Palpate the trachea
Palpate the lymph nodes in the neck area
SUMMARY CHECKLIST
PROMOTING A HEALTHY LIFESTYLE
Our amazing smelling ability
DOCUMENTATION AND CRITICAL THINKING
ABNORMAL FINDINGS

Colour-coded structure

All health assessment chapters (Chapters 11–29) provide a clearly identified colour-coded structure to define the five major sections of health assessment

Easy navigation tabs

Highlight the section within each chapter

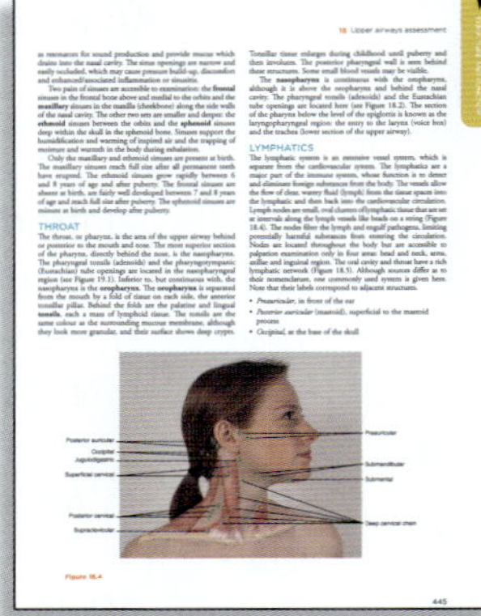

18 Upper airways assessment

STRUCTURE AND FUNCTION

Tonsillar tissue enlarges during childhood until puberty and then involutes. The posterior pharyngeal wall is seen behind these structures. Some small blood vessels may be visible.

The **nasopharynx** is continuous with the oropharynx, although it is above the oropharynx and behind the nasal cavity. The pharyngeal tonsils (adenoids) and the Eustachian tube openings are located here (see Figure 18.2). The section of the pharynx below the level of the epiglottis is known as the laryngopharyngeal region: the entry to the larynx (voice box) and the trachea (lower section of the upper airway).

LYMPHATICS

The lymphatic system is an extensive vessel system, which is separate from the cardiovascular system. The lymphatics are a major part of the immune system, whose function is to detect and eliminate foreign substances from the body. The vessels allow the flow of clear, watery fluid (lymph) from the tissue spaces into the lymphatic and then back into the cardiovascular circulation. Lymph nodes are small, oval clusters of lymphatic tissue that are set

Clinical Case Studies

Highlight health assessment techniques across a range of clinical situations

Clear headings

User-friendly design makes the text easy to use

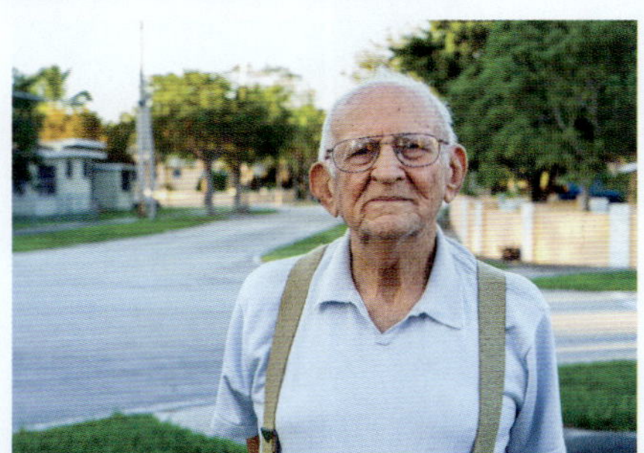
Documentation and critical thinking

FOCUSED ASSESSMENT: CLINICAL CASE STUDY

Subjective
Mr Williams is currently stating that he … the bus stop'. This is despite being re… place and person.

Objective
Mental status: Dressed in hospital gow… he appears alert with appropriate eye … intently to history. Speech is slow, requ… and voice tone is very soft. Verbal cont… place and time.
Eye opening in response to speech.
Motor: Obeying commands. Right han… right arm drifts, right leg weak. Spastic… and leg muscles, limited range of motio… motion

The upper sections of the trachea (subglottic region) tend to be proportionally narrower in young children with a very vascular and loosely attached mucosal lining. This increases the risks of partial and even total occlusion of the airway with infection and inflammation, particularly associated with high risk conditions such as epiglottitis.

The pregnant woman
Nasal stuffiness and epistaxis may occur during pregnancy because of increased vascularity in the upper respiratory tract. The gums may be hyperaemic and softened, and may bleed with normal toothbrushing.

Late adulthood (65+ years)
A gradual loss of subcutaneous fat starts during later middle adult years, making the nose appear more prominent in some people. The nasal hairs grow coarser and stiffer and may not filter the air as well. The hairs may protrude and cause itching and sneezing. Many older people clip these hairs, thinking them unsightly, but this practice may increase the risk of infection and airway irritation. Olfaction, or the sense of smell, may diminish for many reasons, including underlying neurodegenerative disorders.

Highly illustrated

Full colour illustrations show detailed anatomy and physiology, and demonstrate physical examination techniques and abnormal findings

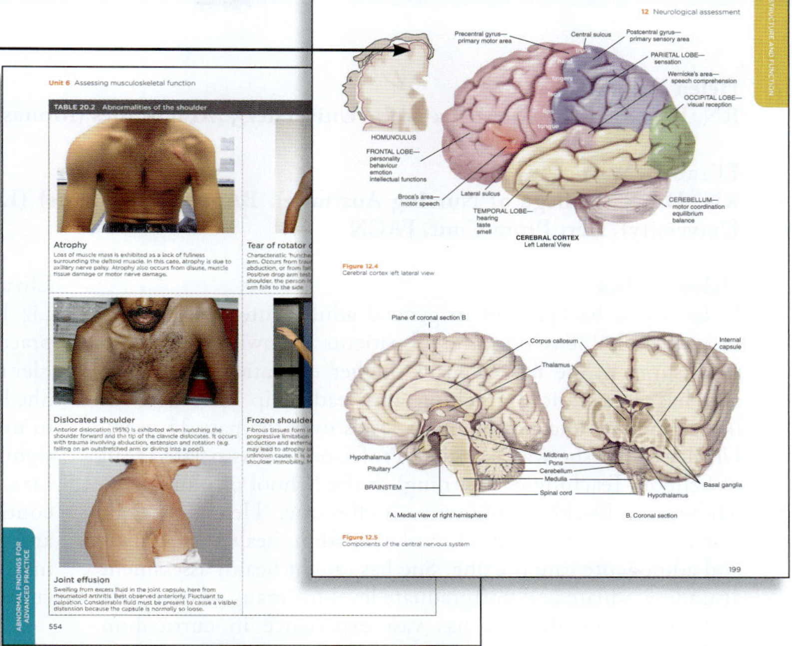

Cultural and social considerations

Highlights specific cultural and social considerations relevant to the Australian and New Zealand context

CULTURAL AND SOCIAL CONSIDERATIONS

The major modifiable risk factors for heart disease and stroke are high blood pressure, smoking, high cholesterol levels, obesity, physical inactivity and diabetes. In addition, for some women, the use of oral contraceptives and postmenopausal hormones is a risk factor.

Hypertension. Hypertension causes heart disease by decreasing vascular compliance which results in stiff, inelastic blood vessels and initiates endothelial injury. This process causes a cascade of events accelerating the development of atherosclerosis (Tortora & Derrickson 2019). Untreated hypertension risks damage to heart, main blood vessels, heart valves, brain and kidneys and can cause cardiac arrhythmias including atrial fibrillation (Kjeldsen 2018). The most current report identified 34% of Australians have

Summary checklist

Provides quick overview of subjective and objective data collection to reinforce learning

Promoting a healthy lifestyle

Provides Health Promotion information for key health concerns

Developmental considerations

Highlight the needs of specific age groups

DEVELOPMENTAL CONSIDERATIONS

Infants and children

The fetal heart functions early; it begins to beat at the end of 3 weeks' gestation. The lungs are nonfunctional, but the fetal circulation compensates for this (Figure 17.13). Oxygenation

Summary Checklist

CARDIAC ASSESSMENT

Subjective data

1. Presenting concern
2. Chest pain
3. Dyspnoea
4. Orthopnoea
5. Cough
6. Fatigue
7. Cyanosis or pallor
8. Oedema
9. Nocturia
10. Past cardiac history
11. Family cardiac history
12. Health and lifestyle management

Objective Data

1. General inspection
2. Identify relevant surface lan
3. Inspect and palpate neck v
4. Inspect and palpate the pra
5. Auscultation of apical (mitr
6. Laboratory studies

PROMOTING A HEALTHY LIFESTYLE

WOMEN AND HEART ATTACKS

When someone complains of chest pain or pain radiating down the left arm, almost everyone thinks heart attack. After all, these are the symptoms that typically occur. Aren't they? Well, yes and no. They are the most 'typical' symptoms men get, but not women. For women, the symptoms can be quite different or atypical. These 'atypical' symptoms may be one of the reasons that more women than men are dying from heart disease these days.

Women are more likely to feel angina as a hot or cold burning sensation, or even as a tenderness to touch, in their back, shoulders, arms or jaw. They often have no chest discomfort or pain at all. Women's symptoms of heart attacks frequently include nausea, vomiting, indigestion, shortness of breath or extreme fatigue but, again, no chest pain. All of these symptoms are easy to attribute to something else other than the heart and are often ignored. Scientific evidence now shows that women tend to minimise their symptoms of cardiac disease. However, part of this may be due to a lack of awareness.

Women's not so 'atypical' symptoms of cardiovascular disease or a heart attack include:

- Pain, discomfort, deep ache, pressure or

- Breathlessness or inabil breath—with or without waking up
- Clammy sweating and c refer to as a 'cold sweat
- Anxiety—feelings of imp unusual nervousness
- Oedema or swelling, us legs
- Nausea and indigestion
- Sleep disturbance
- Unusual fatigue or weak

Cardiovascular disease is death in women. Women and pay attention to the seek immediate care if t resources have up to dat about heart disease

The Heart Foundation (A heartfoundation.org.au/ heart-disease

The Heart Foundation (N www.heartfoundation.or and-heart-disease

Health Assessment Videos

The enhanced eBook features the following videos:

Abdominal Assessment
Respiratory Assessment
Cardiac Assessment
Neurological Assessment
Vital Signs (electronic)
Vital Signs (manual)

hyperthyroidism, anaemia), the apical impulse increases in amplitude and duration

Auscultation of the apical (mitral) area

In most situations, the generalist registered nurse will only need to perform the skil

About the Australian adapting editors

Helen Forbes
RN, BAppSc (Adv Nurs) (La Trobe University), MEdStudies (Monash University), PhD (University of Sydney)

Elizabeth Watt
RN, DipN (College of Nursing Australia), BAppSc (Adv Nurs) (Lincoln Institute of Health Sciences), MNS (La Trobe University), Cert Prom Cont, FACN

Helen Forbes
Helen has a background in general adult acute care nursing as well as a focus on care of patients following head and neck surgery. She has extensive higher education experience and has held various teaching and leadership roles at both undergraduate and postgraduate levels over the past 35 years. Until recently she was Associate Professor and Associate Head of School (Teaching & Learning) at the School of Nursing & Midwifery, Deakin University, Melbourne. Helen's current teaching interests include clinical education, health assessment and adult acute care nursing. She has taught health assessment at undergraduate and postgraduate level for many years locally and internationally. She has vast experience in curriculum design and development in nursing education. Helen is now a Nurse Education Consultant.

Elizabeth Watt
Liz has a background in adult acute care nursing and has practiced in both hospital and community-based midwifery. Her main clinical focus is in urological and continence nursing. She has over 30 years' experience in higher education, teaching in undergraduate and postgraduate nursing programs. She has significant experience in curriculum design and development. Liz's current teaching interests include urological and continence nursing, health assessment, adult acute care nursing and clinical education. She has taught health assessment at undergraduate and postgraduate level for many years. Liz is currently working as a nurse consultant (education).

About the US author

Carolyn Jarvis received her PhD from the University of Illinois at Chicago, with a research interest in the physiologic effect of alcohol on the cardiovascular system; her MSN from Loyola University (Chicago); and her BSN cum laude from the University of Iowa. She is Professor, School of Nursing at Illinois Wesleyan University, where she teaches Health Assessment, Pathophysiology, and Pharmacology. Dr Jarvis has taught physical assessment and critical care nursing at Rush University (Chicago), the University of Missouri (Columbia), and the University of Illinois (Urbana). Her current research interest concerns alcohol-interactive medications, and she includes Honors students in this research.

In 2016, Illinois Wesleyan University honored Dr Jarvis for her contributions to the ever-changing field of nursing with the dedication of the Jarvis Center for Nursing Excellence. The Jarvis Center for Nursing Excellence equips students with laboratory and simulation learning so that they may pursue their nursing career with the same commitment as Dr Jarvis.

Dr Jarvis is the Student Senate Professor of the Year (2017) and was honored to give remarks at commencement. She is a recipient of the University of Missouri's Superior Teaching Award; has taught physical assessment to thousands of baccalaureate students, graduate students, and nursing professionals; has held 150 continuing education seminars; and is the author of numerous articles and textbook contributions.

Dr Jarvis has maintained a clinical practice in advanced practice roles—first as a cardiovascular clinical specialist in various critical care settings and as a certified family nurse practitioner in primary care. During the last 12 years, her enthusiasm has focused on Spanish language skills to provide healthcare in rural Guatemala and at the Community Health Care Clinic in Bloomington. Dr Jarvis has been instrumental in developing a synchronous teaching program for Illinois Wesleyan students both in Barcelona, Spain, and at the home campus.

Australian and New Zealand contributors

Josh Allen
RN, BN, BN(Hons), GradDipNurPrac(Critical Care), GradCertHEd
Lecturer in Nursing
School of Nursing and Midwifery
Faculty of Health
Deakin University, Melbourne
Victoria, Australia

Mari Botti
PhD, PostGradDip(Psych), BA, DipNsg
Alfred Deakin Professor
School of Nursing and Midwifery
Faculty of Health
Deakin University, Geelong
Victoria, Australia

Rhonda Brown
PhD, MSocSci, PostGradCommHlth, PostGradFamilyTherapy, GradCertHigherEd, RN
Conjoint Clinical Associate Professor
School of Nursing and Midwifery
Deakin University, Geelong
Victoria, Australia

Trish Burton
DipAppSc, BSc, BAppSc, MEd, PhD, FCNA
Senior Lecturer, Nursing, College of Health and Biomedicine
Victoria University
Victoria, Australia

Rebecca Corbett
RPN, MANP
Psychiatric Nurse Consultant
Mental Health, Drugs and Alcohol Education Team
Barwon Health
Victoria, Australia

Bronwyn Coulton
MN(NPrac), GDipNurs(CritCare), BNurs, RN, NP
Neurovascular Stroke Nurse Practitioner
Clinical Trial Coordinator
Neurosciences Department
Monash Health, Clayton
Victoria, Australia

Leonie Cox
PhD, GradCert (Higher Education), RN
Senior Lecturer,
School of Nursing,
Queensland University of Technology,
Kelvin Grove, Brisbane
Queensland, Australia

Helen Forbes
RN, BAppSc (Adv Nurs) (La Trobe University), MEdStudies (Monash University), PhD (University of Sydney)
Nurse Consultant (Education)
Formerly Associate Professor and Associate Head of School (Teaching & Learning)
School of Nursing & Midwifery,
Deakin University, Melbourne,
Victoria, Australia

Nicki Hartney
RN, RM, MProfEd&Trng (Deakin)
Lecturer, School of Nursing and Midwifery
Deakin University, Geelong
Victoria, Australia

Amy N. B. Johnston
PhD, MEd, GradCert(Adult Ed), BSc(hons), BN
Conjoint Senior Research Fellow,
Department of Emergency Medicine—Princess Alexandra Hospital and
School of Nursing, Midwifery and Social Work
University of Queensland, Woolloongabba Queensland, Australia

David M. Lee
DrPH MPH GradDip(CCRN, Emerg/Trauma) BAppSc DipAppSc(Nsg)
Nurse Practitioner (Primary Health)/Epidemiologist
Melbourne
Victoria, Australia

Jennifer Lillibridge
MSN, PhD
Professor Emerita, School of Nursing
California State University, Chico
California, USA

Maria Murphy
PhD, PGDip (critical care), PG Cert (TT+L), BN, Dip App Sci (Nurs).
Lecturer in Nursing -Teaching & Research
La Trobe University
Victoria, Australia

Elizabeth Pascoe
PhD, MSc (Nursing), BSc (Hons), Dip (Education)
Program Director, Continuing Professional Development Program
La Trobe University, Bundoora,
Victoria, Australia

Frances Pearce
RN, MSc Ortho, MPET(Deakin)
Nurse Educator
Austin Health, Melbourne
Victoria, Australia

Sue Sharrad
PhD, B.Ed, CCRN, Grad Dip. (Intensive Care), M.Ng
Nurse Consultant Parkinson's Disease
Rural Support Service
Barossa Hills Fleurieu Local Health Network
South Australia, Australia

Chris Taua
PhD, MN, PostGradCert(MH), CertAdTch, DipN, CertDD, FNZCMHN
Director/Senior Consultant
Pumahara Consultants
North Canterbury
New Zealand

Rebecca Thornton
PhD, MNSc, DipEd, DipPaeds, RN, BN
Lecturer of Nursing,
Deakin University, Burwood
Victoria, Australia

Elizabeth Watt
RN, DipN (College of Nursing Australia), BAppSc (Adv Nurs) (Lincoln Institute of Health Sciences), MNS (La Trobe University), Cert Prom Cont, FACN
Nurse Consultant (Education), Formerly Course Coordinator
Master of Nursing (Urological & Continence) Course
La Trobe University/School of Nursing & Midwifery,
La Trobe University, Melbourne Campus, Victoria.

Amanda Wylie
RN, BN, MN, GCert Nursing (Clinical Education), GCert Ophthalmic Nursing

Contributors to US edition

CHAPTER CONTRIBUTOR
Lydia Bertschi
DNP, APRN, ACNP-BC
The co-contributor for Chapter 22 (Abdomen), Dr. Bertschi is an Assistant Professor at Illinois Wesleyan University School of Nursing and a nurse practitioner in the intensive care unit at UnityPoint Health—Methodist.

ASSESSMENT PHOTOGRAPHERS
Chandi Kessler
BSN, RN
Chandi is a former Intensive Care Unit nurse and is an award-winning professional photographer. Chandi specializes in newborn and family photography in and around Central Illinois.

Kevin Strandberg
Kevin is a Professor of Art Emeritus at Illinois Wesleyan University in Bloomington, Illinois. He has contributed to several editions of *Physical Examination & Health Assessment.*

INSTRUCTOR AND STUDENT ANCILLARIES
Case Studies
Melissa M. Vander Stucken
MSN, RN
Clinical Assistant Professor
School of Nursing
Sam Houston State University
Huntsville, Texas

Key Points
Joanna Cain
BSN, BA, RN
President and Founder
Auctorial Pursuits, Inc.
Boulder, Colorado

PowerPoint Presentations
Daryle Wane
PhD, ARNP, FNP-BC
BSN Program Director—Professor of Nursing
Department of Nursing and Health Programs
Pasco-Hernando State College
New Port Richey, Florida

Review Questions
Kelly K. Zinn
PhD, RN
Associate Professor
School of Nursing
Sam Houston State University
Huntsville, Texas

TEACH for Nurses
Jennifer Duke
Freelancer
St. Louis, Missouri

Test Bank
Heidi Monroe
MSN, RN-BC, CAPA
Assistant Professor of Nursing
NCLEX-RN Coordinator
Bellin College
Green Bay, Wisconsin

Test Bank Review
Kelly K. Zinn
PhD, RN
Associate Professor
School of Nursing
Sam Houston State University
Huntsville, Texas

Australian and New Zealand reviewers

James Bonnamy
MNurs, GradCertHPE, BNurs(Hons), BNurs, RN, MACN, MANZBA
Clinical Nurse Specialist, Victorian Adult Burns Service, The Alfred Hospital
Lecturer, Monash Nursing and Midwifery, Monash University
Victoria, Australia

Kolleen Miller-Rosser
EN., RN., Grad Dip (Paediatrics). MSN, Graduate Certificate Academic Practice, PhD
Teaching Scholar
Southern Cross University
New South Wales, Australia

Dr. Zaneta Smith
RN, BN, PGDip (Clin Prac), MNurs (Clin Prac with Distinction), Cert IV Business, PhD, FACORN
Senior Lecturer Nursing/Master of Nursing Practice Course Coordinator
Faculty of Medicine & Health
University of New England
Armidale, NSW, Australia

Penny Coogan
RN, BNSc, GradDipNurPrac (Emergency), MN (NP)
Lecturer in Nursing
College of Healthcare Sciences; James Cook University
Townsville, Queensland, Australia

Melissa Slattery RN
MNg (Cwk), BNg, BHlthSc, DipNg
Academic Manager (VET) and Head of Discipline for Nursing,
EQUALS International
Adelaide, Australia

N'Tonya Surynt
RN/RM Grad Cert Clin Ed
Midwifery Clinical Facilitator
Flinders Medical Centre, Adelaide, Australia

Evan Plowman
RN, MN, GradCertCritCareNur(ICU), BN/BPara
Lecturer in Nursing, School of Nursing, Midwifery$ Indigenous Health
Faculty of Science, Charles Sturt University
Wagga Wagga, NSW, Australia

Preface

Health assessment is central to nursing practice. By practising and developing the knowledge and skills of health assessment you will develop confidence and competence in understanding and responding to each person's situation. You need to listen to the cues from the person as these will guide and direct your questioning and physical examination. Whether you are an undergraduate nursing student, a newly qualified registered nurse or an experienced nurse seeking to advance your practice, this book holds the content you need to develop and refine your health assessment skills.

As a learner you should use this text in conjunction with videos for self-directed learning and active participation in formal on-campus skills development sessions and clinical placements. You need to be continuously reflecting on your learning and on the feedback provided by your learning facilitators and clinicians to refine your health assessment skills and knowledge. The third edition of this text is contextualised to suit the Australian and New Zealand healthcare environments. We hope this text will become an invaluable part of your professional library and we look forward to ongoing feedback from you, our readers.

NEW TO THE THIRD AUSTRALIAN AND NEW ZEALAND EDITION

The third ANZ edition of *Jarvis's Health Assessment & Physical Examination* has been fully revised and updated for the Australian and New Zealand contexts and structured to enhance learning for undergraduate and postgraduate students, Nurse Practitioner candidates and clinicians.

Each chapter begins with an overview highlighting the importance and relevance of the given topics to nursing practice. The introductory chapter describes the purpose of health assessment in nursing practice and how it contributes to a multidisciplinary health assessment. All spelling, terminology, measurements, cultural and social considerations, and clinical procedures reflect the Australian and New Zealand contexts. In addition, you will find:

- Updated contents to assist the reader to understand the relevance of the health assessment areas to the functional status of the person.
- Updated chapters are provided on *Screening for family violence* and *Substance abuse assessment.*
- The context of health for Aboriginal and Torres Strait Islander people and Māori and Pacific Islander people is extensively explored.
- Fully revised *Mental health assessment chapter*
- A new chapter, *Using health assessment in clinical practice,* focuses on the critical role that health assessment plays in the quality and safety of healthcare. This chapter discusses the important role of monitoring patient progress and identifying indicators of physiological deterioration and deterioration in mental state. Clinical case studies are provided to challenge the reader to apply knowledge of health assessment techniques and clinical reasoning in the planning and conduct of focused health assessments.
- *Clearly identified health assessment skills* in each chapter for beginning and advanced nursing practice.
- *Revised clinical case studies* in each chapter which illustrate documentation and critical thinking related to the chapter focus.

DUAL FOCUS AS TEXT AND REFERENCE

Jarvis's Health Assessment & Physical Examination is a **text for beginning students of health assessment** as well as a **text and reference for advanced practitioners**. The chapter progression and format permit this scope without sacrificing one use for the other.

Chapters 1 to 4 focus on **approaches and contexts of health assessment in nursing**, including critical thinking, considerations for stages of development across the life span and cultural safety.

Chapters 5 and 6 focus on **Screening for family violence and abuse** and **Substance abuse**.

Chapters 7 to 10 focus on **health assessment tools and techniques**, including the health interview and health history, physical assessment techniques, general survey and vital signs.

Chapters 11 to 29 focus on the **key areas for health assessment** which are organised around functional areas relevant to nursing practice. **Each of these chapters has eight major sections:** Structure and Function, Developmental Considerations and Cultural and Social Considerations, Subjective Data (history), Objective Data (procedures and normal findings/abnormal findings and clinical alerts), Promoting Healthy Lifestyles, Documentation and Critical Thinking, and Abnormal Findings.

The nursing student can review anatomy and physiology and learn the skills, normal findings and common variations for generally healthy people and selected abnormal findings in the Objective Data sections. They will also be prompted to report and refer clinically significant abnormal findings. The advanced practice nurse or Nurse Practitioner candidate will be able to review anatomy and physiology and fundamental health assessment skills, while focusing on the more complex knowledge and skills required for specialty nursing practice. Students can also study the extensive pathology illustrations and detailed text in the Abnormal Findings sections.

- Chapter 30 is focused on **utilising health assessment in practice.** The important role of monitoring patient progress and identifying indicators of physiological deterioration and deterioration in mental state are discussed.

CONCEPTUAL APPROACH

Jarvis's Health Assessment & Physical Examination reflects a commitment to:

- **Person-centred care**, in the focus on the person as a whole, both in wellness needs and illness needs, as well as their perceptions of their health and the impact of health issues on their quality of life.

- **Health promotion and disease prevention**, in the health history questions that elicit health and lifestyle management, the age-specific charts for periodic health examinations, and the Promotion of a Healthy Lifestyle.
- Interacting with the person as an **active participant in healthcare**, by encouraging discussion of their experience of their current situation and health and lifestyle management.
- **Cultural and social considerations** that affect health, including the social determinants of health and illness.
- The individual **across the life span**, supported by the belief that a person's state of health must be considered in light of the person's developmental stage. Chapter 3 presents a baseline of developmental tasks and topics expected for each age grouping, and subsequent chapters integrate relevant developmental content. Developmental anatomy, modifications of history taking and physical examination technique, and expected findings are given for infants and children, adolescents, pregnant women, and older adults.

APPROACH TO LEARNING HEALTH ASSESSMENT

This text has been designed to reflect clinical practice in the Australian and New Zealand context. There has been much debate in the nursing literature about the extent of health assessment skills required by registered nurses and therefore which skills need to be taught in undergraduate nursing curricula. Research by Birks et al (2013)[1] and Birks et al (2014)[2] found that Australian registered nurses are not utilising many of the physical assessment skills being taught in undergraduate nursing programs, nor does their role require these skills. On the other hand, undergraduate health assessment subjects are often crowded with content that students are never likely to practise in the clinical setting. More recently, there has been pressure for course designers to remove health assessment as a discreet unit and instead integrate assessment skills into other units. There is potential for health assessment skill development to get lost. This textbook has been designed to separate those skills that all registered nurses require from those required by nurses in specialty areas of practice. It is hoped that this will make it easy for course developers, subject coordinators, and nursing students to focus on the critical knowledge and skills required for RN practice.

FEATURES FROM THE SECOND EDITION

Jarvis's Health Assessment & Physical Examination is built on the strengths of the previous two editions and is designed to engage and enhance student learning:

- The **two-column format** begins in the Subjective Data section, where the running column provides assessment guidelines and clinical significance and clinical alerts. In the Objective Data section, the running column highlights procedures and normal findings and abnormal findings and clinical alerts.
- **Subjective Data** section (Health history) is detailed in each chapter, including questions that elicit the person's perception of their health and the impact of health problems on their quality of life. In addition, health and lifestyle management activities are highlighted.
- **Objective Data** section (Techniques and sequence of physical examination) is clear, orderly, and easy to follow. Hundreds of examination illustrations are linked directly with the text to demonstrate the techniques in a step-by-step format.
- **Abnormal Findings** tables organise and expand on material in the Objective Data section. The format of these extensive collections of pathology and original illustrations helps students recognise, sort, and describe abnormal findings.
- **Developmental approach** in each chapter is focused on the adult, then age-specific content for the infant, child, adolescent, pregnant woman, and older adult so that students can learn common variations and approaches for all age groups.
- Stunning **full-colour art** shows detailed human anatomy, physiology, examination techniques and abnormal findings.
- **Summary checklists** towards the end of each chapter provide a quick overview of the main areas of subjective and objective data collection.
- **Focused assessment/clinical case studies** of commonly encountered situations show the application of assessment techniques and critical thinking for people of different ages and in differing clinical situations.
- **User-friendly design and use of colour** make the book easy to use. Frequent subheadings and instructional headings assist in easy retrieval of material.

SUPPLEMENTS

- The *EVOLVE Website* (located at http://evolve.elsevier.com/AU/Forbes/assessment) provides facilitators with PowerPoints and Test Banks for each of the 30 chapters, along with an Image Collection. Students have access to Multiple Choice Review Questions, Health Assessment Videos and WebLinks—in effect, a comprehensive online resource that takes advantage of the dynamic nature of electronic content and online delivery.
- Six videos demonstrating core health assessment techniques are available online to complement the text and support student learning.

ACKNOWLEDGMENTS

We would like to acknowledge the people who made the third Australian and New Zealand edition of this text possible:

- Libby Houston (Senior Content Strategist) for her support and leadership in the development of the supporting vidoes.
- Kathryn Mason Pak (Editor) for her editorial skills.
- Shruti Raj (Content Project Manager) for her efforts in transforming the manuscript into a textbook.

1 Birks M, Cant R, James A et al: The use of physical assessment skills by registered nurses in Australia: issues for nursing education, Collegian, 20(1):27-33, 2013.

2 Birks M, James A, Chung C, Cant R, Davis J. The teaching of physical assessment skills in pre-registration nursing programmes in Australia: Issues for nursing education. Collegian. 2014. 21(3):245-53.

We would also like to thank our families for allowing us to take over our respective dining room tables, computers, and study over the past two and a half years. In the final stages of the textbook we have all been challenged by the requirements for periods of lockdown and social distancing during the COVID-19 pandemic. We thank our families and friends for their support, encouragement and for the endless cups of tea.

We would like to dedicate this edition to the nursing students and registered nurses who will use this text to develop their clinical skills. We encourage you to continually strive to develop and refine your health assessment skills. Your efforts will contribute to improving the person's experience and the overall quality and safety of nursing care.

To nursing curriculum designers, we encourage you to prioritise health assessment knowledge and skill development by ensuring a strong focus, particularly in undergraduate curricula. To the nursing lecturers, we thank you for your continuing motivation and encouragement of student learning in this critical area of nursing practice.

The publisher and editors would also like to thank each of the chapter authors and reviewers who ensured the relevance, accuracy and strong clinical application of the content. In this new edition we would also like to acknowledge past contributors and reviewers who provided a strong foundation on which we could build.

Helen Forbes
Elizabeth Watt

Contents

Approaches and contexts of health assessment in nursing

Unit 1

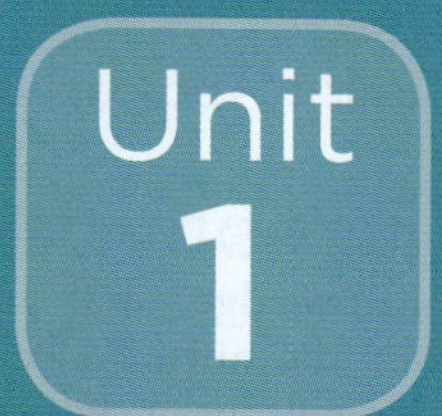

Chapter One

The context and frameworks of health assessment

Adapted by Helen Forbes and Elizabeth Watt

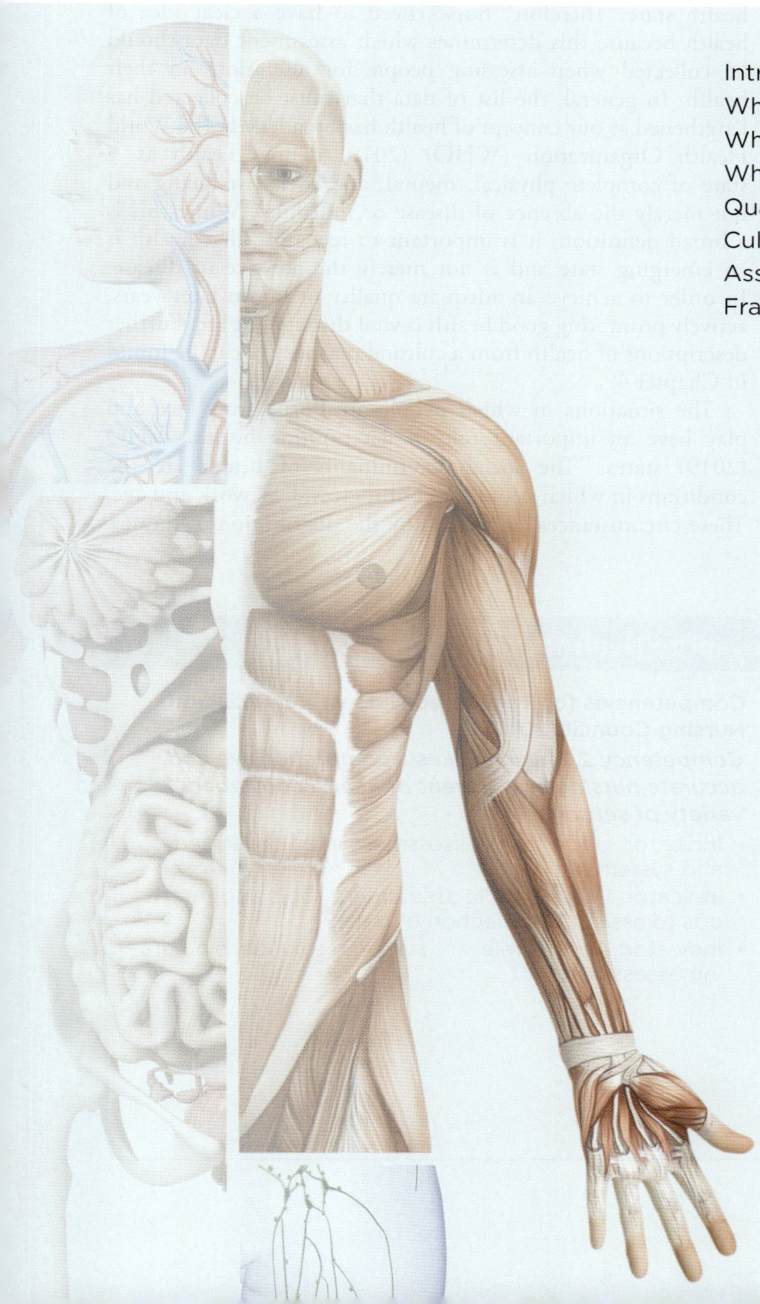

Introduction
What is health assessment?
What is health?
What is nursing?
Quality and safety in healthcare
Cultural and social considerations
Assessment approaches for different situations
Frameworks for assessment

INTRODUCTION

Knowledge, skill and a professional approach are essential for the nurse to be able to provide healthcare for a person. Knowledge or skill on their own is not enough, however. Nurses must be able to anticipate the problems or health issues that the person may have and relate them to known medical diagnoses or in situations where a medical diagnosis has not yet been established. Nurses also have an important role in identifying changes over time to the person's health state. Knowledge of health and underpinning health sciences are fundamental to the identification of health issues.

Nurses have a range of health assessment frameworks to choose from depending on the situation. Use of the most appropriate health assessment framework ensures that all of the relevant information is identified. The nurse focuses on exploring the symptoms the person is reporting, the impact of the symptoms on day-to-day function and any possible risks that the person may have in relation to their symptoms and altered function. Once all of the person's problems are identified (symptoms, risk and altered function) the nurse then proceeds to identify health outcomes and prioritise and plan care. In this chapter, you will be introduced to health assessment, the concept of health, models of health, the concept of nursing, quality and safety in health care, lifespan and social and cultural considerations, approaches to health assessment in different situations and frameworks for health assessment.

WHAT IS HEALTH ASSESSMENT?

Assessment is the collection of data about an individual's health state. Throughout this text, you will be studying the techniques of collecting and analysing **subjective data** (i.e. what the person *says* about themself during history taking) and **objective data** (i.e. what you as the health professional *observe* by inspecting, percussing, palpating and auscultating during the physical examination). Together with the patient's record and laboratory studies, these elements form the **database** of the assessment of the person's health.

The nurse makes a clinical judgement or diagnosis about the individual's health state. This diagnosis is based on the data collected by the nurse by asking the person questions (subjective data), conducting a physical examination and taking any relevant measurements (objective data). The problems (diagnoses) identified may be related to the person's symptoms (subjective data) or alterations in function and/or risks for further health issues. Thus, the purpose of a health assessment is to make a clinical judgement or diagnosis by identifying the person's actual or potential health problems. Knowledge and skill in health assessment is a requirement of the Nursing and Midwifery Board of Australia and the Nursing Council of New Zealand for Registered Nurse registration. See Box 1.1.

Because all healthcare treatments and decisions are based on the data gathered during assessment, it is paramount that the assessment be factual and complete, providing the foundation for clinical decision making. Chapter 2 provides more detail about the process of clinical decision making that requires critical thinking and health assessment.

WHAT IS HEALTH?

Assessment is the collection of data about an individual's health state. Therefore, nurses need to have a clear idea of health because this determines which assessment data should be collected when assessing people for alterations in their health. In general, the list of data that must be collected has lengthened as our concept of health has broadened. The World Health Organization (WHO) (2019) defines health as 'a state of complete physical, mental, and social wellbeing and not merely the absence of disease or infirmity'. While this is a broad definition, it is important to recognise that health is an emerging state and is not merely the absence of disease. In order to achieve an adequate quality of life in later years, actively promoting good health is vital throughout life. Further descriptions of health from a cultural perspective can be found in Chapter 4.

The situations in which people are born, grow, live and play have an important role in determining health. WHO (2019) states: 'The social determinants of health are the conditions in which people are born, grow, live, work and age. These circumstances are shaped by the distribution of money,

BOX 1.1 Nursing Registration Requirements Relevant to Health Assessment

Nursing and Midwifery Board of Australia, Registered Nurse Standards for Practice (2016)

Standard 4: Comprehensively conducts assessments.

RNs accurately conduct comprehensive and systematic assessments. They analyse information and data and communicate outcomes as the basis for practice.

The RN:

- 4.1 conducts assessments that are holistic as well as culturally appropriate
- 4.2 uses a range of assessment techniques to systematically collect relevant and accurate information and data to inform practice
- 4.3 works in partnership to determine factors that affect, or potentially affect, the health and wellbeing of people and populations to determine priorities for action and/or for referral, and
- 4.4 assesses the resources available to inform planning.

Competencies for Registered Nurses, New Zealand Nursing Council (2016)

Competency 2.2: Undertakes a comprehensive and accurate nursing assessment of health consumers in a variety of settings.

- Indicator: Undertakes assessment in an organised and systematic way.
- Indicator: Uses suitable assessment tools and methods to assist the collection of data.
- Indicator: Applies relevant research to underpin nursing assessment.

power and resources at global, national and local levels. The social determinants of health are mostly responsible for health inequities—the unfair and avoidable differences in health status seen within and between countries.'

Therefore, conducting health assessment on a person requires acknowledgment of both the social and the environmental context in which they live. For example, consider the discharge needs of a homeless young male patient following a motorcycle accident. How could his wound care and nutritional needs be managed in the community context if he has no fixed address?

Models of health

The **social model of health** acknowledges the effect of social, economic, cultural and political factors and conditions on a person's state of health and wellbeing. Use of the model aims to improve health outcomes, prevent and reduce illness and address the inequalities and disadvantage that exist within the community. Community healthcare, as a part of primary healthcare, is informed by the values and principles supported in the Alma-Ata Declaration on Primary Health Care (WHO 1978) and the Ottawa Charter for Health Promotion (WHO 1986).

The social model of health recognises:

- The social, economic and environmental determinants of health and illness
- The importance of health promotion and disease prevention
- The importance of community participation in decision making
- The importance of working with sectors outside the health sector
- That equity is an important outcome of health service intervention.

The **biomedical model** of western tradition views health as the absence of disease. Health and disease are opposites, extremes on a linear continuum. Disease is caused by specific agents or pathogens. Thus, the biomedical focus is the diagnosis and treatment of those pathogens and the curing of disease. Assessment factors are a list of biophysical symptoms and signs. The person is certified as healthy when these symptoms and signs have been eliminated. When disease does exist, medical diagnosis is worded to identify and explain the cause of disease.

The accurate diagnosis and treatment of illness is an important part of healthcare but the medical model has limiting boundaries. The public's concept of health has expanded since the 1950s. Now we view health in a wider context. We have an increasing interest in lifestyle, personal habits, exercise and nutrition, and the social and natural environment. **Wellness** is a dynamic process, a move towards optimal functioning. Different levels of wellness exist, with optimal health described as 'high-level wellness'. Wellness is a direction of progress. Healthcare professionals serve to maximise the person's potential, and to assist the person to grow towards high-level wellness.

Consideration of the whole person is the essence of **holistic health**. Holistic health views the mind, body and spirit as interdependent and functioning as a whole within the environment. Health depends on all these factors working together. The basis of disease is multifaceted, originating both from within the person and from the external environment. Thus, the treatment of disease requires the services of numerous providers.

A natural progression to **health promotion** and disease prevention now rounds out our concept of health. The leading causes of death among Australians and New Zealanders aged 65 years and over are related to ischaemic heart disease, dementia, Alzheimer's disease, cerebrovascular disease, lung cancer or chronic obstructive pulmonary disease (Australian Institute of Health and Welfare 2018, and Ministry of Health, New Zealand 2018). Many of these chronic conditions can be modified by changes to lifestyle. Health promotion is focused on public policy change, counselling and support to motivate people to improve their health. Policy changes in recent times has focused on reduction of smoking and alcohol and drug use, encouraging activity and exercise, healthy eating, safety in the home and on the road and safe sexual practices. Health promotion is a much broader concept than disease prevention. Health promotion was defined in the Ottawa Charter for Health Promotion (WHO 1986) and includes building public health policy, creating supportive environments for healthy living, strengthening community action, developing personal knowledge and skills and reorienting the healthcare system (Talbot & Verrinder 2018). There is further discussion of varying cultural conceptualisations of health in Chapter 4.

WHAT IS NURSING?

The International Council of Nurses (ICN) states that nursing includes 'autonomous and collaborative care of individuals of all ages, families, groups and communities, sick or well and in all settings. Nursing includes the promotion of health, prevention of illness, and the care of ill, disabled and dying people. Advocacy, promotion of a safe environment, research, participation in shaping health policy and in-patient and health systems management, and education are also key nursing roles' (ICN 2019). This implies that the nursing approach to healthcare is holistic in nature and therefore health assessment should reflect that philosophy with its focus on the whole person and their context.

There is a range of clinical contexts in which you may work as a nurse. These include community health settings, mental healthcare, acute and critical care contexts, remote and rural settings, rehabilitation or residential aged care. The nature of the context will usually determine the type and focus of health assessment required. In the community, you may focus on assessing an individual, a family or a community and be interested in gathering information about wellness as opposed to illness. In an acute setting, whether it is in a critical care or more general ward area, your focus will differ depending on the health status of the person. Patient problems may vary across the treatment trajectory, which means that you will need to time and focus your health assessment accordingly.

In the provision of care, nurses and midwives are ethically responsible and accountable to the recipient of care (ICN 2012). From an ethical point of view, it is expected that nurses and midwives will respect, promote, protect and uphold the rights of people either receiving care or providing healthcare. The nursing and midwifery codes of ethics outline minimum national standards of conduct that members of the professions are expected to uphold. These codes inform the community of the standards of professional conduct it can expect nurses and midwives to uphold and provide the consumer, regulatory, employing and professional bodies with a basis for evaluating their professional conduct. The Nursing and Midwifery Board of Australia and Nursing Council of New Zealand codes of professional conduct provide guidelines about expected behaviour of nurses and midwives. Nurses and midwives are expected to conduct their practice using exemplary standards of behaviour. In summary, it is expected that each professional will be safe and competent and practise in accordance with the standards of nursing and the broader health system. Nurses must conduct their practice according to laws relevant to nursing. Nurses and midwives are also legally responsible for their practice and answerable to the relevant professional registering body: the Nursing and Midwifery Board of Australia or the Nursing Council of New Zealand. All nurses and midwives in Australia and New Zealand must meet the professional standards in a range of domains, one of which relates to the conduct of comprehensive and systematic nursing health assessment (Nursing and Midwifery Board of Australia 2016, Nursing Council of New Zealand 2016). Nurse Practitioners also have legal requirements to meet in their specialist area related to advanced health assessment (Nursing and Midwifery Board of Australia 2014, Nursing Council of New Zealand 2012). See the bibliography for references to the relevant codes of ethics and professional conduct for nurses and midwives and professional standards in Australia and New Zealand.

QUALITY AND SAFETY IN HEALTHCARE

Once a person accesses the healthcare system for treatment of illness, a number of factors pose potential risk for harm. Examples include increasing age, comorbidity and the increasing use of complex technology, the use of numerous and complex interventions during an episode of illness, movement between community and hospital health sectors giving rise to possible duplication of, or gaps in care and/or communication breakdown. The Australian Charter of Healthcare Rights and the New Zealand Code of Rights describe the rights of patients and other people using the Australian or New Zealand health systems. One of the principles of these Charters is the recognition that every person has the right to the highest standard of care (Australian Commission on Safety and Quality in Health Care (ACSQHC) 2019, New Zealand Health and Disability Commissioner 2019). While the solutions to decreasing risk to the person are complex, improving the use, availability and communication of health information is critical to the provision of high quality and safe care (ACSQHC 2019, Quality and Safety Commission New Zealand 2020). Quality and safe care of people requires that nurses assess in order to determine care needs. Assessment is conducted in collaboration with the patient and the multidisciplinary healthcare team to achieve positive goals and health outcomes for the recipient of care.

Life span considerations

It is important to consider health assessment from a life cycle approach, no matter what clinical context you are working in. First, you must be familiar with the usual and expected developmental tasks for each age group (Chapter 3). This alerts you to which physical, psychosocial, cognitive and behavioural tasks are important for each person. For example, if you are assessing a six-year-old child with asthma, your approach will need to take into account the developmental tasks for that child's age group which include mastering skills that will be needed later as an adult, building self-esteem and a positive self-concept, adopting moral standards and taking a place in a peer group. This knowledge will guide how you approach the collection of subjective and objective data. The data from the physical examination is more accurate when you consider age-specific information about anatomy, method of examination, normal findings and abnormal findings. For example, an average normal respiratory rate for a six-year-old child is 21–26 breaths per minute.

CULTURAL AND SOCIAL CONSIDERATIONS

The population of Australia is in excess of 25 million; New Zealand is approximately 5 million. Both New Zealand and Australia are countries that are ethnically and culturally diverse. Cultural and social considerations are critical to health assessment: there is an introduction to these concepts in Chapter 4 and the concepts are emphasised throughout the text as they relate to specific chapters.

ASSESSMENT APPROACHES FOR DIFFERENT SITUATIONS

The approach you take to health assessment will depend on the context of care and the reason for the assessment. In many situations, assessment is guided by a pre-printed form, for example, an admission assessment and risk identification form. However, this should not restrict you from seeking additional information relevant to the person's situation and needs.

Comprehensive health assessment

A comprehensive health assessment is performed at a person's first entry in an outpatient setting or initial admission to the hospital.

A comprehensive health assessment includes a complete health history (Chapter 8) and relevant physical examination. It describes the current and past health state and forms a baseline against which all future changes can be measured. It yields the first cues to actual and potential health problems.

In community health or domiciliary care settings, the nurse is usually the first health professional to see the person and has primary responsibility for monitoring the person's healthcare. In the community setting, the comprehensive health assessment could also be conducted on a well person with the purpose of focusing on health maintenance and health promotion. In acute care settings, the comprehensive health assessment is performed on admission to the hospital. Often, the person has completed a standard pre-printed health history form prior to admission. Part of the admission assessment would then be focused on clarifying and validating the information with the person and extending the health history where needed. In an admission assessment, you will go on to collect additional information on the person's perception/impact of illness, functional ability and impact on activities of daily living, health maintenance activities, coping patterns and health goals. An important outcome of a comprehensive assessment is to identify potential risk factors which may impact on the person's hospitalisation or discharge.

Often a comprehensive assessment is also performed when a person moves from one area of a hospital to another, for example, from intensive care to a ward, or from a ward to a rehabilitation facility. This serves as a summary of the person's health state at that time, and gives the next group of clinicians a new baseline on which future assessment and care decisions can be made.

Focused (episodic) assessment

Focused assessment is for a limited or short-term problem. Here, you complete a focused assessment, which is smaller in scope than the comprehensive health assessment. It concerns mainly one problem, one cue or one body system. The cue could be something that the person has told you ('I feel very nauseated' or 'I feel like I need to go to the toilet all the time') or can be a sign that you observe—the person appears to be in pain, or the urine output is less per hour than expected. Focused assessment is used in all settings—hospital, primary care or long-term care. For example, 2 days following surgery, a hospitalised person suddenly has a congested cough, shortness of breath and fatigue. The history and examination is focused primarily on the respiratory and cardiovascular systems.

Ongoing assessment

In ongoing assessment the status of any identified problems should be evaluated at regular and appropriate intervals. For example, in the acute care setting, assessment of the person following a surgical procedure, or frequent neurological observations (neuro obs) in the person who has an actual or potential change in conscious state. In a primary care setting the assessment may be related to, for example, ongoing monitoring of an asthma or diabetes plan. In this situation, your assessment focuses on determining if any change in health state has occurred, whether an intervention is effective and how the person is managing their health. This type of assessment is used in all settings to follow up short-term or chronic health problems.

Primary survey

Primary survey is conducted in emergency and non-emergency situations. In the emergency situation, patient assessment must be rapid and focused and often conducted concurrent with life-saving measures in order to identify and manage impending or actual life threats for the person. A systematic approach using ABCDE is used (Table 1.1).

Primary survey in a non-emergency clinical setting

When you take over the care of a person at the beginning of a shift it is important to do a primary survey which includes airway, breathing, circulation, level of consciousness and environment.

The following example is focused on hospitalised people and their immediate environment. Assessment may include:

- Airway, breathing, circulation, level of consciousness
- Location of emergency equipment and readiness to function
- Check IV fluids, medications and/or gastric feeding that is in progress (syringe drivers, other pumps and drains) to make sure that the correct solution is being infused at the prescribed rate (check against the medical orders)
- IV site is clean, covered and not inflamed or swollen
- Oxygen is being delivered at the right rate and flow
- Oxygen and suction equipment is available at the bedside and functioning correctly
- Drains or drainage equipment are functioning correctly; noting the amount of drainage at the time of the assessment
- Appearance and location of surgical and other wounds
- Urinary catheters are draining correctly, and that the system is intact; noting the amount and colour of urine in the drainage bag at the time of the assessment.

Primary survey in a domiciliary setting

When working in a domiciliary environment the primary survey often includes elements listed in the acute care setting above but in addition the home environment is surveyed for actual or potential risks to the person or yourself.

- Access to the home
- State of the home—cleanliness, tidiness, presence of rubbish, etc.
- Safety—presence of animals, trip hazards, electrical hazards, weapons
- Assess availability of running water for handwashing, availability of a clean area to put equipment for procedures.

The following table provides a quick summary of the main points for each of the assessment approaches (Table 1.2).

TABLE 1.1 Summary of primary survey (A, B, C, D, E)

A= airway	Ask the person their name and listen carefully for air movement. If they speak then the airway is considered to be patent
B= breathing	Is the person breathing without effort? Observe rate, depth and symmetry of breathing and use of accessory muscles
C= circulation	Palpate the radial or carotid pulse for rate, strength and rhythm. Also check capillary refill time, skin colour and survey for obvious bleeding
D= disability	Assess level of conscious state
E= exposure and environment	Exposure of the body may need to be done sequentially, uncovering one body area at a time to maintain patient dignity and temperature control. The environment should be checked to ensure the person is not in danger of further trauma

TABLE 1.2 Summary of assessment approaches

COMPREHENSIVE ASSESSMENT	FOCUSED ASSESSMENT	ONGOING ASSESSMENT	PRIMARY SURVEY
• Performed at a person's first entry to the health setting • Includes complete health history and physical examination • Yields first clues to actual and potential health problems and risks during hospitalisation • May include use of a pre-printed form • Forms a baseline for future assessments • Usually performed by the first health professional to see the person on admission	• Used for limited or short term problems • Concerns one health problem, one cue or one body system • Used in all settings • History and physical examination focuses on the relevant body system • Informs impact on function and risks to the person	• Assessment is performed at regular intervals, e.g. two hourly neuro observations • Related to a specific health problem, e.g. acute/chronic • Determines change in health state or effectiveness of an intervention • Used in all settings	• Conducted in emergency and non-emergency situations • In emergency situations ABCDE is used—see Table 1.1 • In non-emergency situations, i.e. start of a shift ABC, level of consciousness and environment survey

FRAMEWORKS FOR ASSESSMENT

There are several frameworks to guide health assessment. These frameworks guide the sequence of data collection, and to some extent the type of data that is collected. The head-to-toe and body systems approaches tend to be medically rather than nursing focused and are commonly used in acute care settings. The functional health approach is used in acute, subacute, rehabilitation and community nursing settings. This approach is more focused on the whole person, and aims to explore the impact of health issues on the person and their daily activities and to identify potential health risks. However, a body systems approach is evident in the functional approach and should not be seen as a separate framework. The content in this text book has been arranged as a combination of functional and body systems approaches.

Regardless of the approach you choose, you need to include important aspects of the person's health status that are relevant to nursing practice, such as interpersonal relationships and resources, values and beliefs, coping and stress management, and sleep and rest (see Chapter 8 for details). These aspects of health assessment are often overlooked in the head-to-toe and body systems approaches and can lead to fragmented care and poor discharge planning.

Functional approach

Subjective data—the health history

Collect the history, complete or limited, as relevant to the person's specific health concerns. Always start with asking the person and/or their carer about their presenting concern or the reason for their hospitalisation (if relevant). Each area being assessed includes the impact of the health issues on the whole person, such as interpersonal relationships and resources, values and beliefs, coping and stress management, and sleep and rest (see Chapter 8 for details).

Objective data—physical examination, measurement and specimen screening

- While obtaining the history and throughout the assessment, note the person's general appearance.
- To further assess change in function or risk for change you will draw on information from relevant chapters identified in the table below.
- In addition to the areas for assessment outlined in Table 1.3, you may also need to consider screening for family violence and abuse (Chapter 5) and/or substance abuse (Chapter 6).

TABLE 1.3 Areas for assessment: functional approach

AREAS FOR ASSESSMENT	RELEVANT CHAPTER/S
General survey, measurement and vital signs	10
Mental health, neurological and sensory function	11, 12, 13, 14, 15
Cardiovascular function (peripheral vascular and cardiac)	16, 17
Respiratory function (upper and lower airways)	18, 19
Musculoskeletal function	20
Nutritional and metabolic function (nutrition, metabolic, skin, hair and nails)	21, 22
Urinary and bowel function (abdominal, urinary and bowel)	23, 24, 25
Sexuality and reproductive function	26, 27, 28, 29

Body systems approach

Subjective data—the health history

Collect the history, complete or limited, as relevant to the person's specific health concerns. Always start with asking the person and/or their carer about their presenting concern or the reason for their hospitalisation (if relevant). Includes psychosocial assessment such as their perception of their health status, interpersonal relationships and resources, values and beliefs, coping and stress management and sleep and rest.

Objective data—physical examination

- While obtaining the history and throughout the assessment, note the person's general appearance.
- To further assess change in function or risk for change you will draw on information from relevant chapters identified in the table below.
- In addition to the areas for assessment outlined in Table 1.4, you may also need to consider screening for family violence and abuse (Chapter 5) and/or substance abuse (Chapter 6).

Head-to-toe approach

Subjective data—the health history

- Collect the history, complete or limited, as relevant to the person's specific health concerns. Always start with asking the person and/or their carer about their presenting concern or the reason for their hospitalisation (if relevant).

Objective data—physical examination

- While obtaining the history and throughout the assessment, note the person's general appearance.
- To further assess change in function or risk for change you will draw on information from relevant chapters identified in the table below
- There is a risk with taking only a head to toe approach to assessment that conclusions drawn tend to be medically focused rather nursing focused. You will need to keep this in mind as you approach your assessment.
- In addition to the areas for assessment outlined in Table 1.5, you may also need to consider screening for family violence and abuse (Chapter 5) and/or substance abuse (Chapter 6).

TABLE 1.4 Areas for assessment: body systems approach

AREAS FOR ASSESSMENT	RELEVANT CHAPTER/S
General survey, vital signs	10
Neurological	12, 13, 14, 15
Mental health	11
Cardiovascular system	16, 17
Respiratory system	18, 19
Gastrointestinal system	21, 23, 25
Endocrine system	21
Renal/bladder	23, 24
Skin, hair, nails	22
Musculoskeletal	20
Reproductive system	26, 27, 28, 29
Ears	15
Eyes	14

TABLE 1.5 Areas for assessment: Head-to-toe assessment

AREAS FOR ASSESSMENT	RELEVANT CHAPTER/S
General appearance	10
Measurement of height and weight	10
Vital signs	10
Nutritional assessment (including skin, hair and nails)	21, 22
Head (including eyes, ears, mouth and throat)	12, 14, 15, 18, 21
Upper extremities (musculoskeletal, peripheral, vascular)	16, 20
Neurological assessment	12
Mental health	11
Chest posterior and lateral (inspection, palpation and auscultation of breath sounds)	17, 19
Chest anterior (inspection, palpation and auscultation of breath sounds)	17, 19
Breasts	28
Heart (inspection, palpation and auscultation of apical rate and rhythm)	17
Abdomen (including bowel function)	23, 25
Anus, rectum, prostate	23, 24, 25, 27
Genito-urinary (external genitalia, urinary function)	24, 26, 27
Lower extremities (musculoskeletal, peripheral vascular)	16, 20

BIBLIOGRAPHY

Australian Institute of Health and Welfare. Australia's health 2018. Australia's health series no. 16. AUS 221. Canberra: AIHW; 2018. Available at: https://www.aihw.gov.au/reports/australias-health/australias-health-2018/contents/table-of-contents.

Australian Bureau of Statistics. Population clock. 2019. Available at: http://www.abs.gov.au/ausstats/abs@.nsf/web+pages/population+clock?opendocument.

Australian Commission on Quality and Safety in Health Care. Australian Charter of Healthcare Rights. 2nd ed. 2019. Available at: https://www.safetyandquality.gov.au/sites/default/files/2019-06/Charter%20of%20Healthcare%20Rights%20A4%20poster%20ACCESSIBLE%20pdf.pdf.

International Council of Nurses. Nursing definitions. 2019. Available at: https://www.icn.ch/nursing-policy/nursing-definitions.

International Council of Nurses. The ICN code of ethics for nurses. Geneva: ICN; 2012. Available at: https://www.icn.ch/sites/default/files/inline-files/2012_ICN_Codeofethicsfornurses_%20eng.pdf.

Ministry of Health, New Zealand. Major causes of death. 2018. Available at: https://www.health.govt.nz/our-work/populations/maori-health/tatau-kahukura-maori-health-statistics/nga-mana-hauora-tutohu-health-status-indicators/major-causes-death.

New Zealand College of Midwives. Code of ethics. n.d. Available: https://www.midwife.org.nz/midwives/professional-standards/philosophy-and-code-of-ethics/.

New Zealand Health Quality and Safety Commission. 2019. Available at: https://www.hqsc.govt.nz.

New Zealand Health and Disability Commissioner. Statement of intent 2017–2021. 2019. Available at: www.hqsc.govt.nz/about-the-commission/.

New Zealand Health and Disability Commissioner. Code of health & disability services: Consumers' rights. 2019. Available at: https://www.hdc.org.nz/your-rights/about-the-code/code-of-health-and-disability-services-consumers-rights/.

Nursing and Midwifery Board of Australia. Nurse Practitioner standards for practice. 2014. Available at: www.nursingmidwiferyboard.gov.au/Codes-Guidelines-Statements/Codes-Guidelines.aspx.

Nursing and Midwifery Board of Australia. Registered nurse standards for practice. 2016. Available at: https://www.nursingmidwiferyboard.gov.au/codes-guidelines-statements/professional-standards.aspx.

Nursing and Midwifery Board of Australia. Code of conduct for nurses. 2018. Available at: https://www.nursingmidwiferyboard.gov.au/codes-guidelines-statements/professional-standards.aspx.

Nursing and Midwifery Board of Australia. Midwife standards for practice. 2018. Available at: https://www.nursingmidwiferyboard.gov.au/Codes-Guidelines-Statements/Codes-Guidelines.aspx.

Nursing Council of New Zealand. Competencies for Registered Nurses. 2016. Available at: https://www.nursingcouncil.org.nz/Public/Nursing/Standards_and_guidelines/NCNZ/nursing-section/Standards_and_guidelines_for_nurses.aspx?hkey=9fc06ae7-a853-4d10-b5fe-992cd44ba3de

Nursing Council of New Zealand: Competencies for the Nurse practitioner scope of practice. 2017. Available at: https://www.nursingcouncil.org.nz/Public/Nursing/Scopes_of_practice/Nurse_practitioner/NCNZ/nursing-section/Nurse_practitioner.aspx.

Quality and Safety Commission New Zealand. New Zealand Government. 2020. Available at: https://www.hqsc.govt.nz.

Stats New Zealand. Population. 2019. Available at: https://www.stats.govt.nz/topics/population.

Talbot L, Verrinder G. Promoting health: the primary health care approach. 6th ed. Sydney: Elsevier; 2018.

World Health Organization (WHO). Social determinants of health. 2019. Available at: https://www.who.int/social_determinants/sdh_definition/en/.

World Health Organization (WHO). Constitution of the World Health Organization: principles 2019. 2019. Available at: https://www.who.int/about/mission/en/.

World Health Organization (WHO). Universal health coverage. 2019. Available at: https://www.who.int/news-room/fact-sheets/detail/universal-health-coverage-(uhc).

World Health Organization (WHO). Ottawa charter for health promotion,1986. 2019. Available at: www.who.int/healthpromotion/conferences/previous/ottawa/en/.

World Health Organization (WHO). Declaration of Alma-Ata. 1978. Available at: https://www.who.int/publications/almaata_declaration_en.pdf.

Websites

Australian Commission on Safety and Quality in Health Care. www.safetyandquality.gov.au

Australian Health Practitioner Regulation Agency. www.ahpra.gov.au

Health Quality and Safety Commission New Zealand. www.hqsc.govt.nz

Nursing Council of New Zealand. www.nursingcouncil.org.nz

Nursing and Midwifery Board of Australia. www.nursingmidwiferyboard.gov.au

Chapter Two

Critical thinking in health assessment

Written by Carolyn Jarvis and Ann Eckhardt
Adapted by Helen Forbes

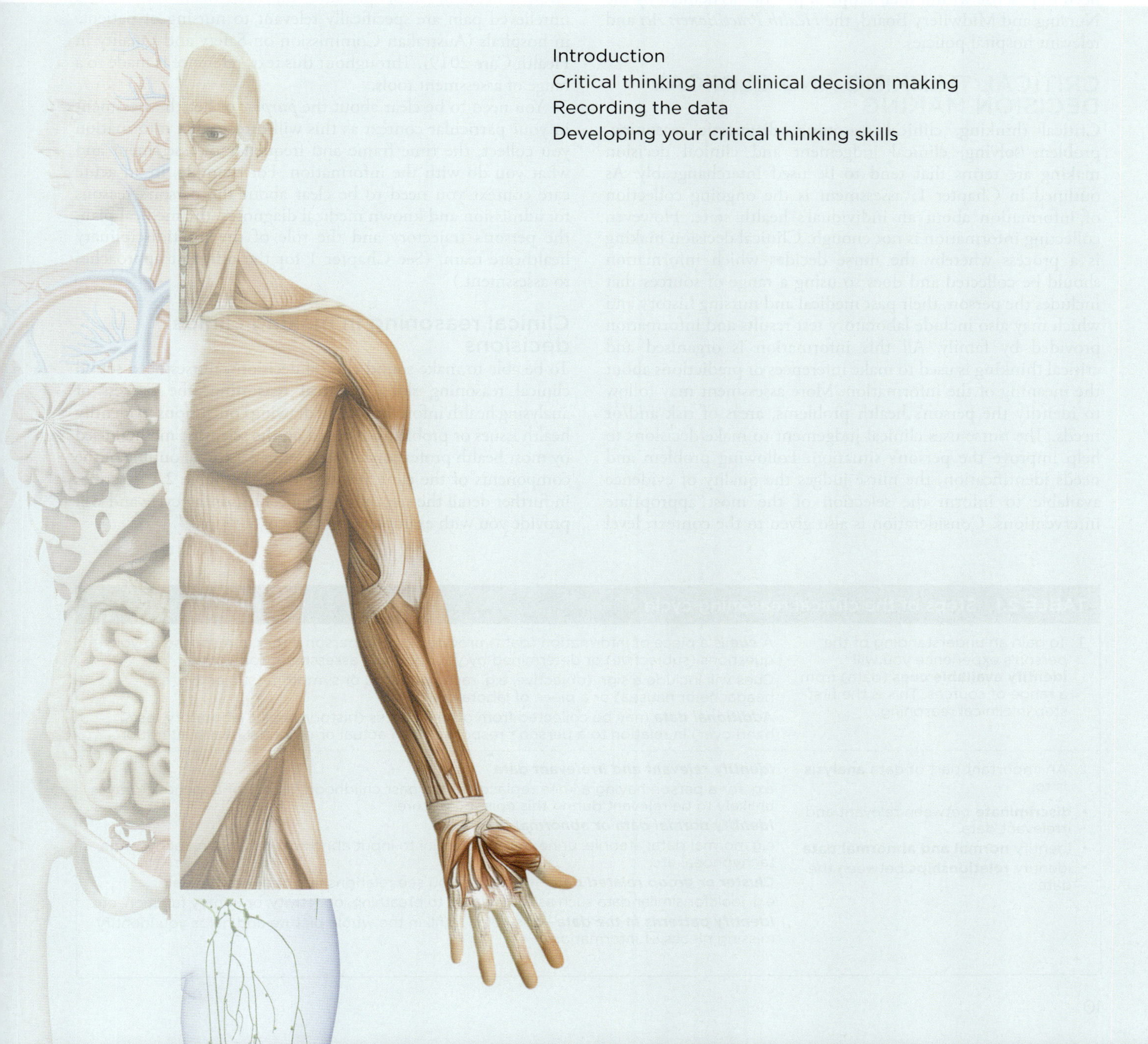

INTRODUCTION

The registered nurse provides evidence-based nursing care for people of varying ages, experiencing physical or mental illness in a range of clinical contexts. Nursing care is aimed at promoting and maintaining health and preventing illness; that is, it is focused on health outcomes. Nurses work collaboratively with healthcare team members to help the person/family/community meet their health outcomes. Regardless of role or context of care, nurses are responsible and accountable for making clinical decisions as part of their role in nursing care (Nursing and Midwifery Board of Australia 2016, Nursing Council of New Zealand 2016). In addition, nurses need understanding of the roles of the different health professionals who will be involved in the care of the person (e.g. nurse, surgeon and other medical staff, physiotherapist, occupational therapist, speech therapist, diabetes educator, stomal therapist, dietitian, pharmacist, social worker) and the collaborative health outcomes. Nurses also need to practise within their scope of practice as defined by the Nursing and Midwifery Board, the *Health Practitioners Act* and relevant hospital policies.

CRITICAL THINKING AND CLINICAL DECISION MAKING

Critical thinking, clinical reasoning, diagnostic reasoning, problem solving, clinical judgement and clinical decision making are terms that tend to be used interchangeably. As outlined in Chapter 1, assessment is the ongoing collection of information about an individual's health state. However, collecting information is not enough. Clinical decision making is a process whereby the nurse decides which information should be collected and does so using a range of sources that includes the person, their past medical and nursing history and which may also include laboratory test results and information provided by family. All this information is organised and critical thinking is used to make inferences or predictions about the meaning of the information. More assessment may follow to identify the person's health problems, areas of risk and/or needs. The nurse uses clinical judgement to make decisions to help improve the person's situation. Following problem and needs identification, the nurse judges the quality of evidence available to inform the selection of the most appropriate interventions. Consideration is also given to the context, level of evidence, availability of resources, preference of the person and level of expertise of the nurse. Finally, the effectiveness of nursing interventions is evaluated in terms of achievement or non-achievement of health outcomes.

Clinical decision making is a continuous process commencing on the first encounter with the person and continues as the nurse plans and implements care and evaluates the person's responses to interventions. Whether the person's situation is stable or rapidly changing, the nurse's decisions affect health outcomes. Clinical decision making is underpinned by the nurse's knowledge and level of experience. To ensure the effectiveness and appropriateness of clinical decisions there are a number of clinical tools, clinical guidelines, hospital/agency policies and protocols and best practice resources available to support the nurse's clinical decision making. Use of these resources will ensure the safety of all people. There are a number of indicators of quality and safe care of which the incidence of medication error, infection, falls, pressure injuries, malnutrition and unrelieved pain are specifically relevant to nursing of patients in hospitals (Australian Commission on Safety and Quality in Health Care 2019). Throughout this text, reference is made to a range of assessment tools.

You need to be clear about the *purpose* of health assessment in your particular context as this will direct what information you collect, the time frame and frequency of assessment and what you do with the information. For example, in an acute care context you need to be clear about the person's reasons for admission and known medical diagnoses, the medical plan, the person's trajectory and the role of the multidisciplinary healthcare team. (See Chapter 1 for the different approaches to assessment.)

Clinical reasoning in making clinical decisions

To be able to make sound clinical decisions, nurses need sound clinical reasoning skills. **Clinical reasoning**, the process of analysing health information and drawing conclusions to identify health issues or problems, is based on the scientific method used by most health professionals. See Figure 2.1 for an outline of the components of the clinical reasoning cycle. Table 2.1 describes in further detail the steps of the clinical reasoning cycle and will provide you with examples of each step.

TABLE 2.1 Steps of the clinical reasoning cycle

1. To gain an understanding of the person's experience you will **identify available cues** (data) from a range of sources. This is the first step in clinical reasoning.	A ***cue*** is a piece of information (data) provided by the person either in response to your questions (subjective) or determined by your physical assessment (objective). Cues will include a sign (objective, e.g. rash or cough) or symptom (subjective, e.g. headache or nausea) or a piece of laboratory data. ***Additional data*** may be collected from other sources (history, family, laboratory tests, hand over) in relation to a person's response to an actual or potential health alteration.
2. An important part of data **analysis** is to: • **discriminate** between relevant and irrelevant data. • identify **normal and abnormal data** • identify **relationships** between the data	***Identify relevant and irrelevant data*** e.g. for a person having a knee replacement, a past childhood history of appendectomy is unlikely to be relevant during this episode of care ***Identify normal data or abnormal data*** e.g. normal data: afebrile, urine output is equal to input abnormal data: pain, tachycardia, tachypnoea, etc. ***Cluster or group related data***—this helps you see relationships between the data e.g. look for similar data such as that related to breathing, or activity, or urinary function, etc. ***Identify patterns in the data***—this helps to fill in the whole picture and helps you identify missing pieces of information

TABLE 2.1 Steps of the clinical reasoning cycle—cont'd

3. Draw conclusions **by making inferences/predictions/hypotheses*** about the data by interpreting, validating and testing. (*Note that different nursing textbooks have a preference for one or the other of these terms)	***Interpret*** the data by formulating inferences*, predictions or forming hypotheses. An ***inference/prediction or hypothesis*** is a tentative explanation for a cue or a set of cues that can be used as a basis for further investigation, e.g. patient hasn't opened bowels for 4 days. This triggers you to think about possible constipation. ***Draw on your clinical knowledge*** and ask what do you think might be going on? You know that when a person hasn't been moving about, taking opioid pain medications or not eating a normal diet they are at risk of constipation. ***Validate*** or check the accuracy and reliability of your inferences/hypotheses/predictions by gathering more information to *test* the tentative inferences/prediction/hypotheses. Continuing the above example, you would ask further questions about normal bowel patterns, dietary intake, exercise, activity and medications and perform an abdominal assessment to confirm constipation.
4. A **nursing diagnosis** is a statement of an actual or potential patient problem/health issue that registered nurses are licensed to treat as part of their scope of practice. The statement is identified by analysing the data/cues.	Assessment is aimed at ***diagnosing actual and potential (risk) health problems***. ***Actual problems/diagnoses:*** existing problems that are amenable to independent nursing interventions, e.g. constipation related to immobility and opioid medication. ***Potential health problems/diagnoses:*** problems that an individual does not currently have but is particularly vulnerable to developing, e.g. risk of pressure injury related to immobility.
5. **Goals** of care are determined	***Goals*** should be person-centred, achievable and measurable and have a suitable timeframe, e.g. the person will have a bowel movement within 24 hours. The person will resume a normal bowel movement (Bristol 3–4) within 3 days.
6. **Interventions** selected that are person centred and evidence-based	***Nursing interventions*** are selected to meet each of the identified problems and goals. Following the previous example, if constipation was confirmed on assessment, the interventions would focus on addressing the specific factors that have caused the problem, e.g. increasing fluid intake, mobility and dietary fibre.
7. **Outcomes** of interventions are evaluated	***Evaluation*** is ongoing and is aimed at the achievement of the patient goals, e.g. has the person had a bowel movement within 24 hours that is soft and easily evacuated?

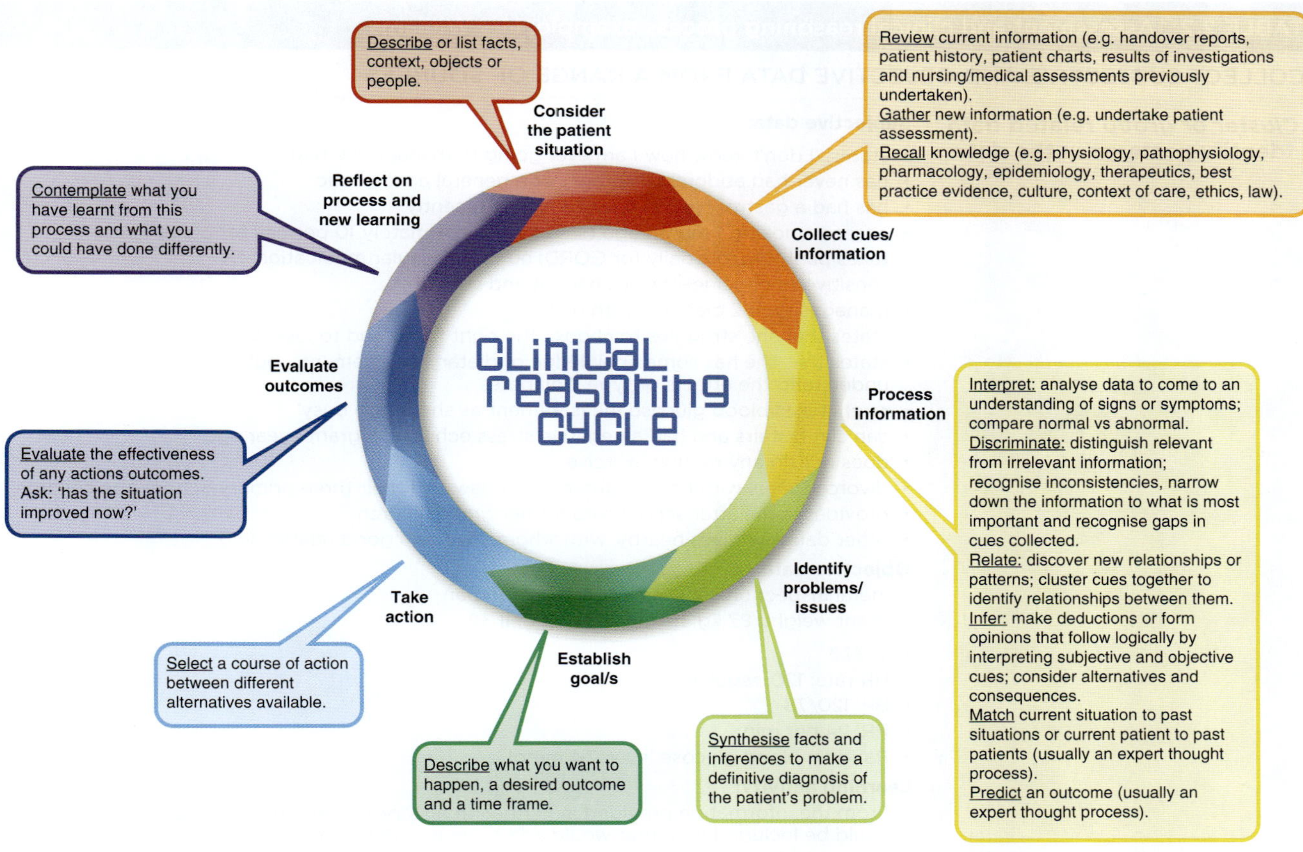

Figure 2.1
Clinical reasoning cycle.

A clinical example is provided to further exemplify the clinical reasoning and clinical decision making cycle as described in Table 2.1 and Figure 2.1 (Levett-Jones 2018).

Mrs Williams' health history

Mrs Sarah Williams, aged 66 years, works part-time as a sales assistant. She will be admitted to hospital next week for a low anterior bowel resection and formation of a loop ileostomy for adenocarcinoma of the rectum. Her daughter accompanies her. Her past medical history includes:

- Peptic ulcer disease—*Helicobacter pylori*—identified three years ago. Treated and she has no current symptoms
- Gastro-oesophageal reflux disorder (GORD)—managed on 40 mg pantoprazole daily
- Transient ischaemic attack (TIA) three years ago
- Type 2 diabetes—diet controlled
- She has had two normal pregnancies and births.

Context

You are the nurse who conducts the preoperative assessment in the pre-admission clinic one week before the surgery.

From your reading of Mrs Williams' health history you discover the following information:

One month ago, Mrs Williams was referred to the hospital by her local general practitioner for investigation of rectal discomfort and a positive faecal occult blood test (identified by the national bowel screening program). A colonoscopy revealed the presence of a tumour in the rectum, which was biopsied. Visually, the surgeon determined that it was likely to be adenocarcinoma. Histology confirmed the diagnosis. Subsequently, Mrs Williams was booked in for a low anterior bowel resection to be performed next week. As part of the preoperative assessment she had an ECG, full blood examination and chest X-ray before admission to hospital. Most results were within normal limits; however, her random blood glucose level was 7.9 mmol.

Assessment

You conduct an assessment of Mrs Williams which is detailed in Table 2.2 below.

From this assessment you can see that Mrs Williams has several actual and potential health problems, but at the time of the assessment she is not in any acute discomfort. The aim of the assessment is to:

- identify any significant issues that could impact during and after surgery;
- take the opportunity to provide information about the surgical procedure and what to expect postoperatively;
- and begin the discharge plan.

The nurse in this context would *not* be in a position to fully evaluate Mrs Williams' nutritional status, management of her type 2 diabetes or begin the education process about stoma care. The plan would be to refer to specialist nurses or other clinicians for more comprehensive assessment and care planning.

TABLE 2.2 Assessment and clinical reasoning process example: Mrs Williams

COLLECT SUBJECTIVE AND OBJECTIVE DATA FROM A RANGE OF SOURCES	
***Cluster or group* related data** **Identify patterns in the data**	**Subjective data:** • states, 'I don't know how I am ever going to manage the bag' • has never had abdominal surgery or a general anaesthetic • has had a gastroscopy and colonoscopy recently • ceased smoking 1 month ago (smoked approximately 10 per day for 30 years) • takes pantoprazole daily for GORD; no other regular medication • sensitive to codeine—causes nausea and vomiting • manages type 2 diabetes with diet • states that she struggles to choose the right foods and to lose weight • states that she has some knowledge of dietary requirements, but doesn't really understand the effects of type 2 diabetes • rarely takes blood glucose measurement as she is 'too busy' • can climb stairs and had a negative stress echocardiogram 1 year ago • does not do any regular exercise • divorced, lives with her daughter, son-in-law and their three primary-school-age children • provides some after school care for her grandchildren • other daughter lives nearby, with whom she has a good relationship **Objective data:** General Inspection: Obese middle aged woman Current weight: 87 kg; height 164 cm; BMI 32 • T: 37.3 • HR rate: 120, regular • BP: 120/75 • RR: 24 per min • Random blood glucose level: 7.4 mmoL **Learning activity:** • From the information provided in her health history, is there further objective data that could be included here that would add to your understanding of Mrs Williams' situation? • The subjective data has been grouped. Where will you insert the objective data into the groupings above?

TABLE 2.2 Assessment and clinical reasoning process example: Mrs Williams—cont'd

***Interpret* the data by formulating inferences, predictions or forming hypotheses**	**Key issues:** History of smoking, nutrition/exercise imbalance, expressed fear and anxiety about having surgery and ileostomy bag, poor diabetes management. **Strengths:** Exercise tolerance is adequate for her daily activities Family support **Recall of knowledge:** Your knowledge about the following will help you to make inferences/hypotheses/ predictions from the available data: These may include: • impact of obesity and type 2 diabetes on health in general and potential risks in the perioperative period *(risk for elevated blood glucose levels)* • risk of chest infection in smokers following abdominal surgical procedures and general anaesthesia (*risk for infection*) You also know that: • it is normal for a person to feel anxious about forthcoming surgery, the possibility of a cancer diagnosis and the need to manage an ileostomy bag and stoma (*anxiety*). • managing an ileostomy bag brings with it an impact on self-concept, body image and a need to refocus many activities of daily living (*risk for altered self-image; knowledge deficit*) • adequate preparation of the person for surgery, pain management and other aspects of postoperative care are important (*knowledge deficit*).
***Validate* or check the accuracy and reliability of your inferences/hypotheses/ predictions by gathering more information to *test* the tentative inferences/ hypotheses/predictions**	You will then collect more information to validate your inferences/hypotheses/predictions by collecting more information. Is her increased heart rate due to the stress of admission and prospective surgery? Is it related to obesity? You will need to get more information about Mrs Williams' diet and her activity and exercise patterns. What additional questions and objective data will you collect? Mrs Williams' daughter may be able to clarify some information, if necessary. Physical examination data can be compared to findings of other health professionals and data from diagnostic tests if needed.
NURSING DIAGNOSES/PATIENT PROBLEMS	
Actual potential (risk) health problems	**Actual nursing diagnoses/patient problems:** • Fear and anxiety related to upcoming surgery, new cancer diagnosis and ileostomy • Knowledge deficit: management of type 2 diabetes • Alteration in nutritional status: more than body requirements • Knowledge deficit: management of ileostomy • Knowledge deficit: surgical procedure and usual postoperative care **Potential (risk) nursing diagnoses/patient problems:** • risk for unstable postoperative blood glucose levels related to stress response • risk for chest infection related to surgery and recent smoking history • risk for postoperative pain related to surgical incision
GOAL STATEMENTS	
Goals statements are: **• person-centred,** **• achievable,** **• measurable and** **• have a suitable timeframe**	**Mrs Williams will:** • be knowledgeable about surgical procedure, anaesthesia, typical postoperative care and recovery including pain management using a PCA, tubes, intravenous access, urinary catheter, etc., prior to surgery • have postoperative pain <4/10 at all times • have postoperative blood glucose levels between 3.0 and 7.7 mmol/L at all times • will not develop a chest infection in the postoperative phase as demonstrated by effective deep breathing and coughing techniques and effective pain management • will be knowledgeable and confident with managing an ileostomy bag within five days postoperative • be knowledgeable about management of type 2 diabetes, including dietary requirements and activity and exercise requirements

Collaborative patient problems

The clinical reasoning process detailed above is one which is used by nurses to identify actual and potential patient problems and then plan and evaluate care. Collaborative problems are those in which the approach to treatment involves multiple disciplines. For example, Mrs Williams has several medical diagnoses (type 2 diabetes, bowel cancer and gastro-oesophageal reflux disorder. It is the medical practitioner's responsibility to diagnose and prescribe the treatments for these conditions. The nurse, the medical practitioner and other allied health team members work together in managing the care of Mrs Williams during hospitalisation and after discharge. However, the nurse is also focused on managing specific nursing-related patient problems as described above (see Table 2.1).

RECORDING THE DATA

Throughout the text we will give examples of how to record health assessment data. As you develop more knowledge and skills you will become more efficient and accurate in your documentation. Always record the data from the history and physical examination as you conduct the assessment, but in such a way that does not get in the way of your communication with the person. The documentation of your findings should be systematic, comprehensive and detailed. This includes charting *relevant* normal or abnormal findings. The selected assessment framework as described in Chapter 1 will guide your documentation.

Electronic health records

The use of technology at the bedside extends far beyond the standard equipment. An increasing number of hospitals and clinics use a basic or a comprehensive electronic health record system. The electronic health record replaces the paper health record, placing all relevant patient information in an easily accessible electronic system. The functions typically include clinical notes, medication charts, fluid balance and observation charts, consultation and referral requests, laboratory and diagnostic imaging requests and results and discharge summaries from all health professionals.

Electronic health records allow all providers, regardless of geographic location, to access the health information, place orders and receive timely patient status updates. No longer does a provider have to be on the clinical unit to retrieve test results, vital signs or the most recent nurse's or doctor's note. Well-designed electronic health records can notify providers of potential medication interactions, dosage adjustments for use in relevant situations and additional required testing (e.g. laboratory tests). Nurses can benefit from electronic health records use in medication administration through the use of barcode scanners, which identify both the patient and the medication. Checklists built into electronic health records can help clinicians identify healthcare-associated infections or patients at risk for these infections. Although no system is perfect, well-designed electronic health records can increase patient safety when successfully integrated into the workflow of a clinic or hospital. As electronic health records use becomes the standard of care, more research is needed to determine the specific factors that contribute to patient safety and increased quality of care.

In Australia, MyHealth Record (Australian Government, Australian Digital Health Agency 2019) was introduced to the Australian public and is aimed at providing personal health information available to nominated health professionals such as GPs, specialists and pharmacists. The information includes:

- a shared health summary (overview of health)
- reports of tests and scans
- current medications
- discharge plan
- referral letters as relevant.

The general Australian public has had the opportunity to opt in or opt out of this arrangement. Discussions are underway in New Zealand to implement a digital health strategy (Ministry of Health, New Zealand 2017). The Australian MyHealth Record is a separate platform from the electronic health records of health services.

DEVELOPING YOUR CRITICAL THINKING SKILLS

All healthcare treatments and decisions are based on the information you gather during assessment, and therefore it is important that your assessment be factual and complete. The way in which nurses make clinical decisions depends on level and extent of experience. The *novice* nurse usually has extensive knowledge but needs to develop the ability to apply that knowledge; they may have little experience with specified populations and use rules to guide practice (Benner 2009, Jewell 2013). It takes time, perhaps two to three years in similar clinical situations, to achieve *proficiency*, where the nurse sees actions in the context of goals or daily plans for the people they care for. With more time and experience, the *proficient* nurse understands a person's situation as a whole rather than as a list of tasks. This nurse sees long-term goals for the person and how today's nursing actions apply to the point the nurse wants the person to be in, say, six weeks. Finally, it seems that *expert* nurses jump over the steps and arrive at a clinical decision or judgement in one leap. The expert nurse has an intuitive grasp of a clinical situation and zeroes in on the accurate solution (Benner et al 1997).

The way to move from novice to expert practitioner is through the use of critical thinking. We all start as novices who need the familiarity of clear-cut rules to guide actions. Critical thinking is the means by which we learn to assess and modify, if indicated, before acting. Critical thinking is required for sound diagnostic reasoning and clinical judgement. During your career, you will need to sort through vast amounts of data and information in order to make sound judgements to manage care of the person. This data will be dynamic, unpredictable and ever-changing. There will not be any one protocol you can memorise that will apply to every situation. This is true particularly with expert nurses in critical care or emergency situations in which a person's health status changes rapidly and accurate decisions are paramount. The stakes are high, and nursing autonomy is strong. In these cases, the expert focuses on the person's responses and prevents complications through anticipation and vigilant monitoring (Hoffman et al 2009). The expert has well-developed observational skills and trusts their physical assessment skills, even if this conflicts with technologically driven data.

To be an effective critical thinker, the following attributes are needed:

Holistic and contextual perspective: the whole person is considered, as well as their entire situation including background, relationships and environment

Creativity: capable of generating, discovering or restructuring ideas and being able to imagine other options

Inquisitiveness: careful questioning and investigation of a range of possibilities

Perseverance: dedication to trying to understand the person's situation

Intuition: recognition of patterns based on past experiences

Flexibility: ability to adapt thinking and behaviours

Academic integrity: use of processes that are honest and truthful, even if the results are contrary to one's beliefs and assumptions

Reflexivity: thoughtful review of assumptions, thinking and approaches to ensure understanding

Confidence: belief in one's abilities

Open-mindedness: open and sensitive to other views.

(Adapted from Levett-Jones 2018).

BIBLIOGRAPHY

Australian Commission on Safety and Quality in Health Care. Indicators of safety and quality. 2019. Available at: https://www.safetyandquality.gov.au/our-work/indicators-measurement-and-reporting.

Australian Government, Australian Digital Health Agency. My health record. 2019. Available at: https://www.myhealthrecord.gov.au/.

Benner P. From novice to expert—excellence and power in clinical nursing practice. Upper Saddle River, NJ: Prentice Hall; 2001.

Benner P, Tanner CA, Chesla CA. Becoming an expert nurse. Am J Nurs 1997;97(6):16BBB–DDD.

Benner P, Tanner CA, Chesla CA. Expertise in nursing practice: caring, clinical judgement and ethics. New York, NY: Springer; 2009.

Hoffman KA, Aitken LM, Duffield C. A comparison of novice and expert nurses' cue collection during clinical decision-making: Verbal protocol analysis. Int J Nurs Stud 2009;46(10):1335–44.

Jewell A. Supporting the novice nurse to fly: a literature review. Nurse Educ Pract 2013;13(4):323–7.

Levett-Jones T, editor. Clinical reasoning: learning to think like a nurse. 2nd ed. Frenchs Forest, NSW: Pearson Australia; 2018.

Ministry of Health, New Zealand. Digital Health 2020. 2017. Available at: https://www.health.govt.nz/our-work/digital-health/digital-health-2020.

Nursing and Midwifery Board of Australia. Registered nurse s tandards for practice. 2016. Available at: https://www.nursingmidwiferyboard.gov.au/codes-guidelines-statements/professional-standards.aspx.

Nursing Council of New Zealand. Competencies for registered nurses. 2016. Available at: http://www.nursingcouncil.org.nz/Nurses/Scopes-of-practice/Registered-nurse.

Tanner CA. Thinking like a nurse: a research-based model of clinical judgement in nursing. J Nurs Educ 2006;45(6):204–11.

Websites

Australian Commission on Quality and Safety in Health Care: www.safetyandquality.gov.au/

Nursing Council of New Zealand: www.nursingcouncil.org.nz

Chapter Three

Developmental tasks across the life span

Written by Carolyn Jarvis
Adapted by Rebecca Thornton

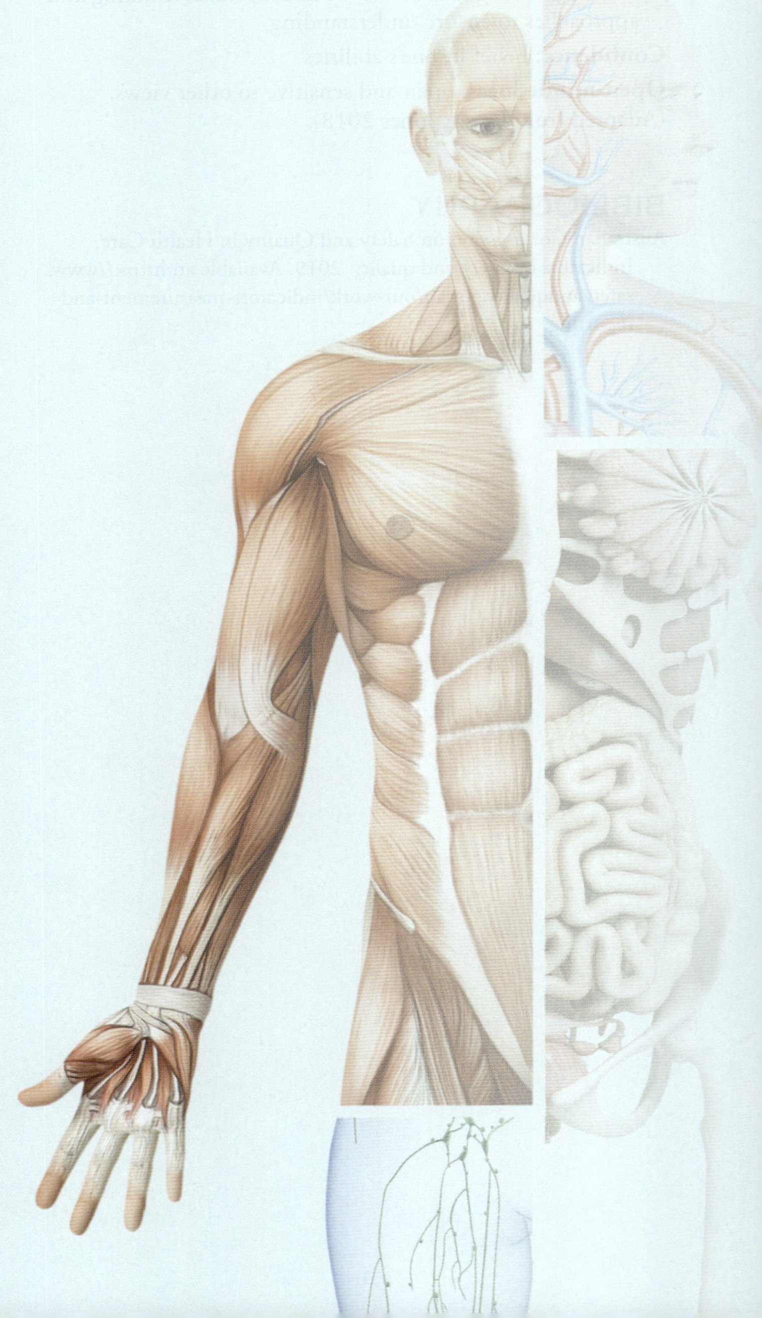

INTRODUCTION

As described in Chapter 1, the focus of this text is on the collection of subjective and objective data about the individual, in order to construct a **database**. This database can be used to identify and promote health-related strengths, and to identify and manage health concerns. However, this data needs to be considered in the context of the individual's development. Understanding the developmental tasks which become relevant at different stages in the life span enables us to appreciate the individual as a whole.

Consider Lachlan, a 15-year-old who was diagnosed with type 1 diabetes at the age of five. Your initial interview reveals several concerns: Lachlan has been experiencing worsening glycaemic control, with frequent episodes of hyperglycaemia. His parents also state that he has become increasingly withdrawn and moody over the past few months. Lachlan's parents explain that he has recently been diagnosed with mild depression by the family's general practitioner.

The management of Lachlan's diabetes will be influenced by his current mental state, as there is a significant relationship between symptoms of depression and poor self-management of diabetes (Gonzalez et al 2016). At the same time, Lachlan's chronic health condition may impact on his ability to achieve developmental tasks which are typical for adolescents. For example, Lachlan may have trouble developing a sense of independence if he is reliant on his parents for medical care, or have difficulty forming close relationships with peers if he is constantly missing school due to illness. In particular, Lachlan may feel that his condition and its treatment makes him 'different' from his peers, during a stage of development where fitting in and being 'normal' is prized (Babler & Strickland 2015). Working with Lachlan and his parents to address both the physical and psychosocial aspects of his condition is crucial. Consider: what interventions could you implement with Lachlan which might support him in meeting the developmental tasks of adolescence? Would these interventions be different in a young adult presenting with the same symptoms?

Growth can be conceptualised as an increase in the size and complexity of the physical being, while development extends beyond maturation of physical systems, and includes changes to social, emotional and cognitive functioning. The following sections will explore growth and development to provide a picture of the individual across the life span. Physical, psychosocial, cognitive and behavioural development will be examined at each developmental stage. These stages are:

1. Infancy (birth to 1 year)
2. Early childhood: Toddler (1 to 3 years)
3. Early childhood: Preschooler (3 to 5 or 6 years)
4. School-aged child (6 to 10 or 11 years)
5. Preadolescence (10 to 12 or 13 years)
6. Adolescence (12 or 13 to 19 years)
7. Early adulthood (20 to 40 years)
8. Middle adulthood (40 to 64 years)
9. Late adulthood (65+ years).

INFANCY (BIRTH TO 1 YEAR)

The first year of life represents the most dramatic and rapid period of growth and development. The infant changes from a totally dependent being into a person who interacts with the environment and forms close relationships with other people (Figure 3.1).

Physical development

Weight, length and head circumference reflect physical growth and are sensitive indicators of the infant's general health. The average healthy term infant weighs 3.4 kg, with 95% of full-term infants ranging from 2.5 to 4.6 kg (World Health

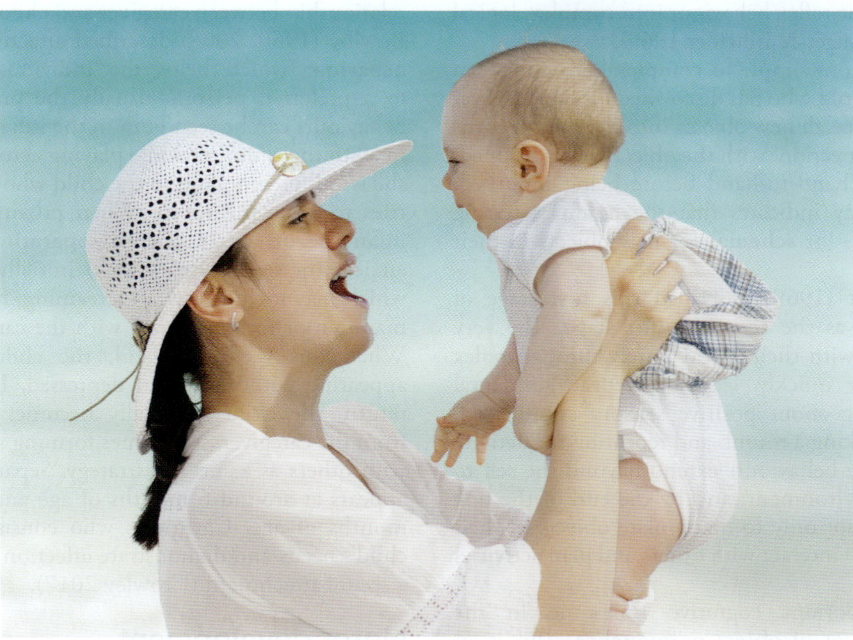

Figure 3.1

Organization (WHO) 2014). In the first few days of life, most infants lose weight while excess extracellular fluid is lost and feeding is established (Ringer 2018); however, this weight is typically regained by day 10 of life. Growth spurts result in doubling of birth weight by 4 to 6 months and tripling of birth weight by 1 year. Length increases 50% by 1 year.

Head circumference also increases rapidly across the first year, signifying an increase in brain size. At birth, the average head circumference is 35 cm, with about 95% of infants within the range of 32.6 to 37.2 cm (WHO 2014). Nutrition in this period is particularly critical, as brain development during infancy is in part regulated by the availability of both macro and key micronutrients (Cusick & Georgieff 2016).

Of all the organ systems, the central nervous system undergoes the most dramatic changes during infancy. Protective reflexes, such as cough, sneeze and gag are present at birth and persist throughout life. However, maturation of the brain allows primitive reflexes, such as grasping, to be suppressed by the developing cerebral cortex. In the healthy infant, the appearance and extinction of primitive reflexes follows a predictable sequence (Chapter 12). Vision also develops rapidly across the first years of life; infants have poor visual acuity at birth (about 20/400) as their macula are immature (Dobson & Teller 1978). By 3 months of age, the typically developing infant is able to fix on an object and follow its movement, and visual acuity improves rapidly across the first year of life.

Cognitive development

Cognition refers to our ability to think; our ability to attend to information, develop concepts, apply reason and to remember past experiences (Shute & Slee 2015). Jean Piaget (1896–1980) described stages of cognitive development in the growing child. Each stage represents new ways of thinking and behaving. According to Piaget's theory of cognitive development, each stage is the foundation for the next, and the next stage builds on the stage before it. Piaget believed that a child's thinking develops progressively from simple reflex behaviour into complex, logical and abstract thought (Piaget & Inhelder 1969).

This development from simple to complex behaviours can be seen in the 6-month-old who has discovered his hands. Over time, the instinct to place all new objects into the mouth turns into a more detailed inspection, with the object being dropped, picked up and passed hand-to-hand before being mouthed. This more complex play indicates that the infant is testing their conceptual models (or **schema**) for new objects in their environment.

Piaget and Inhelder (1969) described this first stage of cognitive development as the **sensorimotor** stage. The very young infant interacts with their world purely through reflex actions; however, they quickly learn to repeat accidental behaviours which bring about positive sensory stimulation, such as accidentally sucking a thumb and repeating the activity for pleasure. Soon these behaviours extend beyond the self to include the external environment, and by the end of the first year the infant is able not only to manipulate objects in their environment, but also to interact with others and plan activities to attain specific goals.

A particularly important cognitive milestone in the infant is the development of **object permanence**. This is an understanding that objects out of sight continue to exist. At about 7–8 months of age, infants will start to look for objects which are hidden while they watch. For example, a child of this age will drop their spoon over the edge of the highchair and then look over the edge to see where it went, but will give up their search unless the spoon is spotted immediately. By 9 months, the infant will continue searching for a hidden object, indicating that they understand the object still exists, even though it cannot be seen. At the same time, the infant is learning that they are an individual separate to others and to the objects in their environment.

While Piaget's theory provides a useful framework for understanding the development of thought, more recent research indicates that Piaget may have underestimated the cognitive capacity of infants. For example, even young infants appear surprised and look longer at unexpected events, such as the unanticipated disappearance or appearance of an object (Bremner et al 2017), indicating they have already developed some understanding of the rules that govern their physical world.

Psychosocial development

Erik Erikson (1902–1994) was concerned with the growth of the **ego**, the conscious, organised, rational part of the personality. Erikson (1995) conceptualised a series of eight ego qualities which emerge due to 'crises' during critical periods of development. Erikson claimed the first psychosocial crisis the infant experiences is **trust vs mistrust**. The infant is completely dependent on the outside world to meet their basic needs, including food, warmth and comfort. When these basic needs are consistently met by a responsive caregiver, the infant learns that the world is a safe and reliable place. Conversely, if the primary caregivers are poorly attuned to the needs of the infant, or if care is unreliable, the infant learns to mistrust themselves and others. Perhaps most importantly, Erikson stressed that it is the quality of the parent–child relationship that enables the infant to develop a sense of trust, and ultimately to view the world as a benign and welcoming place.

Another developmental theory which emphasises the relationship between caregiver and child is **attachment theory**. Bowlby (1960, 2008) described attachment behaviour as any behaviour which helps the individual maintain proximity to a preferred person—usually the primary caregiver. These behaviours can be seen both in the infant who visually 'checks-in' with their mother while playing across the room to confirm she is still present, and in the child who clings when the parent tries to leave the room. When proximity is threatened, the infant begins to experience **separation anxiety**. Separation anxiety (or separation distress) initially appears with protest, which may include crying, screaming, following or clinging to maintain or regain contact with the caregiver (Bowlby 1960). When this is unsuccessful, the child experiences despair, appearing withdrawn and depressed. If the caregiver fails to return, the child eventually becomes emotionally detached from the caregiver, sometimes forming superficial relationships with others as a survival strategy. Separation anxiety typically appears at around 6 months of age and peaks at around 8–9 months of age. Caregivers who consistently respond to the child's needs and demonstrate affection help the child develop a secure attachment (Crowley 2017).

Motor development

As described by Feldman (2016), motor function across the first year of life transitions from reflexive responses to the environment, to purposeful, functional movements. **Gross motor skills** include gaining control of the head and trunk, learning to sit, to crawl, to stand and eventually to walk. The pattern of development of these skills is predictable, following the pattern of myelination of the spinal and peripheral nerves; development occurs from the centre of the body to the extremities (proximodistal development), and from the head to the toes (cephalocaudal development).

Infants are born with rudimentary head control, enabling them to turn their head to the side when lying prone to avoid suffocation. However, at birth, this head control is underdeveloped, resulting in significant head lag when the infant is pulled from a lying position into a sitting position. Head control develops rapidly, however; by 3 months the typically developing infant can raise their head and shoulders from a prone position, and use their arms to support this posture. By 4 months, head lag is minimal when the infant is pulled into a sitting position, and by 6–7 months, head and trunk control are sufficient to allow the infant to sit independently (Figure 3.2).

Gross motor function continues to develop rapidly across the first year. By 7 months, most infants will start to crawl, and will show an interest in exploring their environment. By 8 months, the typically developing infant is able to pull themselves into a standing position, and stand while holding an object for support. Soon after, the infant begins to 'cruise'—walking upright while holding onto furniture or caregivers—and this leads to independent walking by about 12 months of age (Figure 3.3).

The development of **fine motor skills** involves using the hands and fingers for prehension, or the act of grasping. The infant is born with a grasp reflex which fades at 2 months of age and is absent at 3 months of age. This extinction of the grasp reflex allows the infant to begin deliberately gripping and releasing objects. The voluntary two-handed grasp is present at 4 to 5 months. Further refinement of fine motor function occurs between 6 and 12 months, with a crude pincer grasp evident at around 7 or 8 months, followed by a neat pincer grasp at around 10 months (Figure 3.4). During this time, the infant is absorbed with picking up small items and these are frequently conveyed straight to the child's mouth. By 11 months, the infant can place small objects into a container and remove them again and by 13 months they can stack two blocks to build a tower.

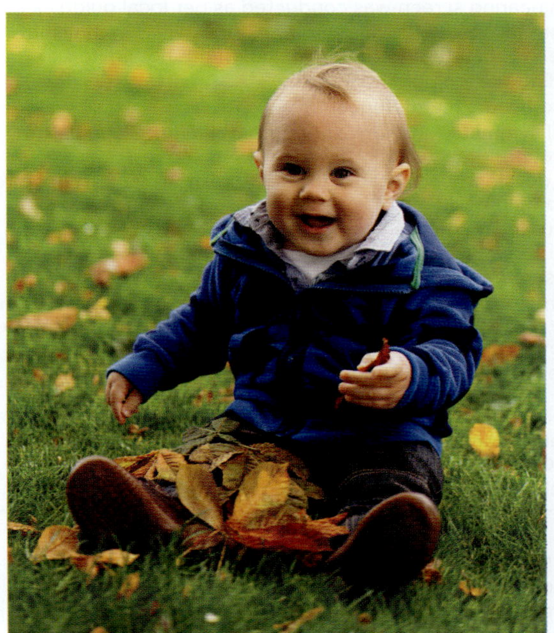

Figure 3.2

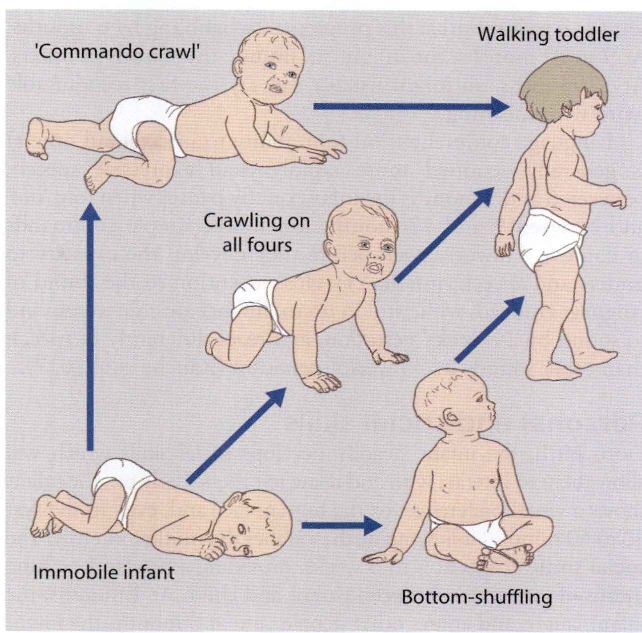

Figure 3.3

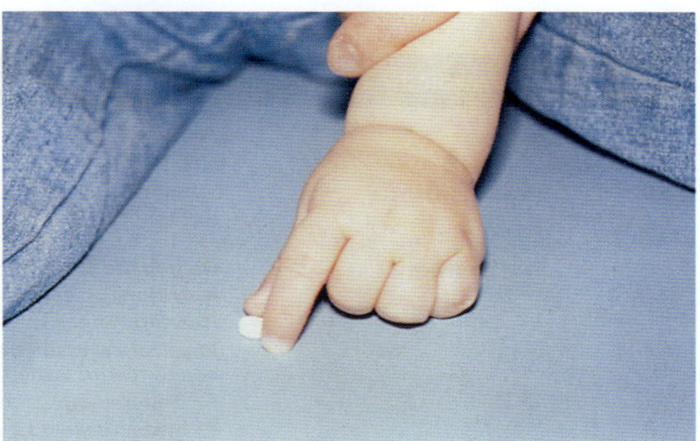

Figure 3.4

Language skills

The newborn relies on crying as their primary form of verbal communication. Indeed, crying is an extremely adaptive behaviour, creating physical and attentional arousal in caregivers designed to mobilise them into responding to the infant's needs (Dudek et al 2016). From crying in early infancy, vocal sounds build rapidly: the infant coos when they awaken or when someone talks to them at 2 to 4 months and laughs out loud at 3 to 4 months; this progresses to babbling by 6 months. At 9 to 10 months, the infant can imitate the sounds of others. At 12 months, an infant usually can say the first recognisable word with meaning.

Language comprehension (our ability to understand others) is generally acquired more rapidly than expressive speech; between 6 and 9 months the infant briefly pauses when told 'no!' and between 9 and 12 months can follow simple commands in context. However, well before they develop the capacity to understand speech, infants pay close attention to the sound of language. Indeed, while still in utero, infants are able to respond to sound by 24 weeks' gestation, and react differently to speech than other sounds by 35 weeks' gestation (Zauche et al 2017).

Personal and social skills

From birth, the infant steadily develops social skills which will allow them to interact with and relate to others. Early on, the infant shows a visual preference for the human face and, even in the first 30 to 60 minutes following birth, watches the mother intently. The **social smile** erupts at 6 to 8 weeks, providing a new and exciting means of interaction between parent and child. At 4 months, the infant laughs and enjoys other people, and at 6 months the infant will extend their arms to the parent to be picked up.

With development of the neurological system, the infant's imitations become increasingly complex; by 7 months the infant can copy simple actions, at 9 months they imitate sounds and at 10 months they begin to engage in social behaviours such as waving or games such as peek-a-boo. At 11 months, the infant can help with feeding and dressing and follows simple directions. Emotional expression develops across the first year, and by 12 months the infant can give a hug or kiss and demonstrate jealousy, fear or anger.

Another key aspect of social interaction which develops towards the end of the first year is called **joint attention**. Initially, the infant is able to follow another person's pointing to regard an object in the environment. By 9 to 12 months, the infant uses pointing and gaze to direct the attention of others; a skill known as declarative (or protodeclarative) pointing. This behaviour represents a significant leap in social awareness. Declarative pointing indicates that the infant is gradually becoming aware that their view of the world is different to that of others; this will later serve as a basis for the child's **theory of mind**—an understanding that one's own thoughts and awareness are separate from that of other people (Sodian & Kristen-Antonow 2015).

Periodic health check of the infant

Tables 3.1 and 3.2 outline important aspects of well-child checks occurring in the neonatal period and the first 12 months of life. Note the aspects of screening at birth, the immunisation

TABLE 3.1 Periodic health check: neonate (0–28 days)

	AUSTRALIA	NEW ZEALAND
Immunisations	Vitamin K Hepatitis B (H-B-Vax II Paediatric)	n/a
Assessment	***Diagnostic testing:*** Metabolic screening (newborn screen) 48–72 hours of life ***Nutrition:*** Discuss method of feeding and provide breastfeeding support if applicable ***Hearing:*** Check that newborn hearing screen was conducted as per local guidelines ***Physical assessment:*** Complete the child health assessment as outlined in the child health record issued by the relevant state or territory, including but not limited to: • General appearance including skin colour and integrity • Measure weight, length and head circumference • Observe head shape, facial symmetry and formation of facial features; palpate fontanelles; check that palate is intact; elicit red reflexes • Examine neurological and developmental status, including responsiveness, posture and tone; examine spine for anomalies • Assess cardiovascular status including auscultation of heart sounds and palpation of femoral pulse • Examine umbilicus and ensure normal healing • Examine hips, limbs for symmetry and length, joints for normal range of movement, hands (including presence of palmar creases and number of digits), feet (for talipes and number of digits). See Chapter 20 for further information • Examine perianal structures for congenital anomalies; check that testes are descended in males	
Psychosocial support	• Identify family strengths, elicit concerns and promote parental confidence, competence and mental health • Discuss any developmental questions or concerns that parents may have	
Safety and preventive care	***Discuss:*** • Non-accidental injury and reinforce that parents should never shake their infant • Risks to infant from passive smoking • Use of appropriate restraints in motor vehicles • Safe sleeping and recommendations for prevention of sudden and unexplained death in infancy • Infant CPR	

TABLE 3.1 Periodic health check: neonate (0–28 days)—cont'd

INTERVENTIONS FOR HIGH-RISK POPULATIONS	
Premature or low-birth-weight infants	Check haemoglobin and haematocrit
Infants in low income families	Check haemoglobin and haematocrit
Aboriginal and Torres Strait Islanders	Check haemoglobin and haematocrit

Adapted from: Royal Australian College of General Practitioners, 2018, Ministry of Health, New Zealand Government, 2018; Queensland Health, Queensland Government, 2019.

TABLE 3.2 Periodic health check: infant

	AUSTRALIA	NEW ZEALAND
Immunisations	***2 and 4 months:*** Diphtheria, tetanus, pertussis (whooping cough), hepatitis B, polio, *Haemophilus influenzae* type b (Hib) (Infanrix hexa) Pneumococcal (Prevnar 13) Rotavirus (Rotarix) ***6 months:*** Diphtheria, tetanus, pertussis (whooping cough), hepatitis B, polio, *Haemophilus influenzae* type b (Hib) (Infanrix hexa) ***12 months:*** Meningococcal ACWY (Nimenrix) Measles, mumps, rubella (MMR II or Priorix) Pneumococcal (Prevnar 13) High-risk groups: Hepatitis A (Vaqta Paediatric)	***6 weeks, 3 months and 5 months:*** Diphtheria, tetanus, pertussis, polio, hepatitis B, *Haemophilus influenzae* type b (Infanrix-Hexa); pneumococcal (SYNFLORIX®); rotavirus
Assessment	***Nutrition:*** Discuss method of feeding and provide breastfeeding support if applicable; discuss introduction of solids from 4–6 months; highlight potential for iron deficiency ***Development:*** Explore developmental progress (e.g. parents' evaluation of developmental status (PEDS) assessment) ***Hearing and vision:*** conduct hearing and vision screening ***Physical assessment (2, 4 and 6 months):*** • Note general appearance including skin colour and integrity; head symmetry • Measure weight, length and head circumference and record on centile charts • Examine neurological and developmental status, including responsiveness and tone • Assess cardiovascular status including femoral pulse (for radio-femoral delay) • Examine umbilicus • Examine perianal structures and hips • Evaluate oral health/tooth eruption, palate and frenulum ***Physical assessment (12 months):*** • Measure weight, length and head circumference and record on centile charts • Assess head symmetry • Check for visual fixing and following, test corneal light reflex • Evaluate oral health/tooth eruption	
Psychosocial support	• Assess quality of parent–child interactions • Identify family strengths, elicit concerns and promote parental confidence, competence and mental health	
Safety and preventive care	***Discuss:*** • Non-accidental injury and reinforce that parents should never shake their infant • Risks to infant from passive smoking and UV exposure • Risk to infant from home environment (e.g. water temperature, bath safety, choking hazards, burns prevention) • Safe sleeping and SIDS prevention; strategies for settling the infant • Car restraints • Play and promotion of normal development (promote secure attachment and positive interaction) • Infant CPR	

Continued

TABLE 3.2 Periodic health check: infant—cont'd

INTERVENTIONS FOR HIGH-RISK POPULATIONS	
Aboriginal and Torres Strait Islander	Consider hepatitis A and pneumococcal vaccine
Infants with chronic health conditions	Consider pneumococcal and influenza (flu) vaccines

Adapted from: Royal Australian College of General Practitioners, 2018; Ministry of Health, New Zealand Government, 2018; Queensland Health, Queensland Government, 2019.

schedule and the parent counselling items regarding diet and injury prevention. Note also that these tables are not intended to be a complete list of all the steps that *should* be included in the examination checkup. Instead, the table lists preventive services that have been studied and shown to be clinically effective (Royal Australian College of General Practitioners (RACGP) 2018).

EARLY CHILDHOOD, TODDLER (1 TO 3 YEARS)

Achievement of milestones across the first year of life establish a basis for future development. Gross and fine motor development enable interaction with the world (Figure 3.5), while the toddler's developing cognitive and social skills demand perpetual stimulation. Children of this age are constantly investigating their environment, while using their caregivers as a secure base for exploration.

Developmental tasks of this next stage include:

1. Differentiating self from others, particularly the mother
2. Tolerating separation from mother or parent
3. Withstanding delayed gratification
4. Controlling bodily functions
5. Acquiring socially acceptable behaviour
6. Acquiring verbal communication
7. Interacting with others in a more empathic way (i.e. understanding another person's emotional state).

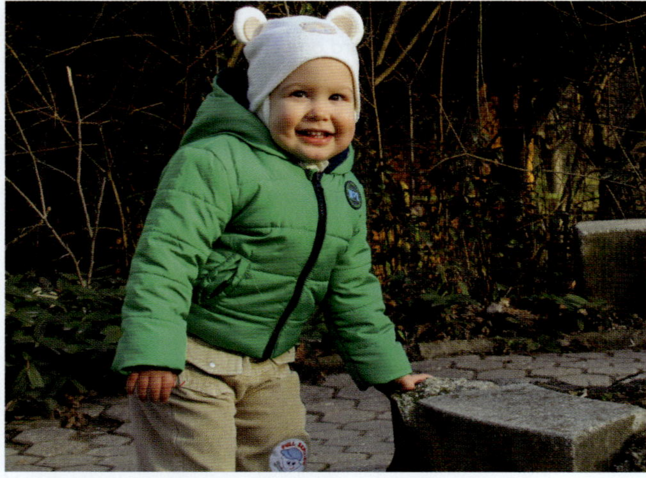

Figure 3.5

Physical development

The velocity of growth slows in the toddler, with children typically gaining 2.5 kg in weight and 12 cm in height across the second year of life (WHO 2014). Increases in head circumference also slow in the second and third year of life. Physical changes enable the child to master increasingly complex skills; for example, with the eruption of molars, the child is able to learn to chew. While maturation of physical systems will be discussed throughout this text, it is important to consider the interplay between neurological development and the achievement of developmental milestones. For example, increasing maturation of the cerebral cortex enables the development of comprehensible speech and meaningful language. Similarly, myelination of the spinal cord is almost complete by the end of the second year, facilitating motor development and resulting in increasingly coordinated movement.

Cognitive development

During the second year, the toddler is still considered to be in Piaget's **sensorimotor period** (Crowley 2017). Between 12 and 18 months, the child increasingly engages in experiments, using trial-and-error to reach a goal. For example, a toddler who is struggling to reach a desired toy at the bottom of their toybox may try numerous methods to reach it, including taking out all of the toys one by one, overturning the box or climbing in to retrieve the toy. While this exploration is an important part of the child's learning, toddlers have limited awareness of risk, so careful supervision is important to ensure safety.

The concept of **object permanence** is now fully developed (Piaget & Cook 1954); the toddler will seek objects even when they did not see them hidden, and will search in multiple locations if the desired object is not discovered initially.

Between 18 and 24 months, the child begins to develop **mental representation** for external events (Crowley 2017). Mental representation allows the toddler to think through actions before undertaking them and to solve basic problems. While limited by egocentrism and rigidity of thought, these mental representations become increasingly organised and complex over time, and will eventually form the basis of the child's understanding of cause and effect.

Psychosocial development

Autonomy is the aim of all activity for the toddler. Newly developed motor skills allow for independent actions such as walking and exploring, as well as involvement with self-care activities such as feeding and dressing. Simultaneously, the child is developing language which allows for the expression of needs and desires. As a result, toddlers will typically demand independence, and will become frustrated if others try to do things for them. Between the ages of 12 and 18 months, the toddler begins to venture away from the parent to explore their environment, but uses the parent as a 'secure base' to which they return for reassurance and protection.

Autonomy versus shame and doubt (1 to 3 years)

This quest for autonomy characterises the psychological conflict of Erikson's second stage (Erikson 1995). The toddler wants to be autonomous and to govern their own body and experiences. They want to apply newly attained skills to explore the world. However, the toddler has not yet attained any sense of discrimination or judgement. The parent must attempt to balance the toddler's desire to explore with the need to protect them from danger, or from experiences which would overwhelm their available coping mechanisms. According to Erikson, overly permissive or controlling parenting can result in the child developing a sense of shame and doubt in their ability to act within the world. Conversely, this conflict is resolved favourably when the parent is patient, provides guidance and holds reasonable expectations with regard to the child's current abilities and attention span.

Motor skills development

The primary motor skill acquired during toddlerhood is walking. By 12 to 15 months, most toddlers are walking independently (WHO Multicentre Growth Reference Study Group 2006), although they typically exhibit a wide-based gait which provides greater stability. By 18 months, the typical toddler is able to run, but trips and stumbles frequently. By 2 years of age, most toddlers can walk up and down stairs and run without falling, and by 30 months, they are able to balance briefly on one foot, or jump with both feet.

Fine motor development progresses rapidly in the toddler. By 12 months of age, the toddler should exhibit a well-developed pincer grasp, enabling them to pick up and manipulate small objects. By 15 months, most toddlers can hold a pencil and scribble; by the age of 2 years, their dexterity allows them to reproduce a vertical line following a demonstration.

Language skills

The toddler's vocabulary expands rapidly from a few distinct words at around 1 year of age to an average of 200 words by their second birthday. In addition, speech becomes increasingly complex, with the 2-year-old learning to combine words into simple two-word phrases, such as 'we go' and 'all gone'. This **telegraphic speech** typically includes a noun and a verb, and includes only words with concrete meaning (Crowley 2017). By the age of 3 years, most children are consistently using three-word phrases. Receptive language skills remain more advanced than expressive skills; toddlers are typically able to comprehend a two-part command without cues, such as 'pick up your shoes and bring them here', by 18 to 24 months.

Personal and social skills

From around the age of 2 years, the child begins to appreciate that certain actions are acceptable while others are not. Kohlberg (1984) argued that children at this age develop a sense of right and wrong through punishment or praise; an action is good if the child is rewarded for it, and bad if the child is punished. He labelled this a 'punishment/obedience' orientation. Children of this age require firm and consistent boundaries in order to determine right from wrong.

Tantrums are a common form of expression in this age group and often stem from a frustrated urge to be independent. Because the young child has not yet developed coping mechanisms to manage these frustrations, they find expression through physical resistance and aggression. Similarly, negativism is common in the toddler age group—all requests and suggestions are met with a firm and defiant 'NO!' This is closely related to the toddler's growing need for independence and individuality. Providing limited choices, rather than asking open-ended questions, may help provide boundaries for the toddler, while providing them with a sense of control that supports their growing autonomy.

Closely related to negativism in this age group is ritualism. Toddlers typically want things done in a consistent way, and any change in a routine or habit can be distressing. A consistent routine reassures the child that the world is predictable and orderly. Awareness of this developmental norm helps parents to anticipate and understand the toddler's strong reaction to anything which threatens an established routine, such as the arrival of a sibling or the need for hospitalisation.

Toddlers engage in parallel play with peers. Parallel play occurs when the toddler plays alongside another child; the two children may subtly observe each other, but don't engage in shared activity. Imitation in play is apparent in this age group as well; in particular, toddlers frequently imitate parent activities, such as sweeping the floor or cooking. As mental representations become more robust, play becomes increasingly imaginative.

Periodic health check of the toddler

Table 3.3 outlines key aspects of the periodic health examination for the toddler.

EARLY CHILDHOOD, PRESCHOOL (3 TO 5 OR 6 YEARS)

Successful achievement of the developmental tasks of toddlerhood allow the preschool child to build on their new-found autonomy to develop a sense of initiative. The social world of the young child is also expanding and preschoolers begin to develop relationships with people in addition to primary caregivers. While still predominantly egocentric, the preschooler is becoming increasingly aware of the needs, thoughts and feelings of others.

Developmental tasks for the preschool-aged child include:

1. Realising separateness as an individual
2. Identifying gender role and its functions
3. Developing a conscience
4. Developing a sense of initiative
5. Interacting with others in socially acceptable ways
6. Growing use of language for social interaction
7. Developing readiness for school.

Physical development

While the major organ systems are relatively mature by 4 to 5 years of age, the musculoskeletal system is still rapidly developing throughout early childhood. In order to develop strength, coordination and balance, the young child needs space and time to engage in physical play. Similarly, refinement

TABLE 3.3 Periodic health check: young child

	AUSTRALIA	NEW ZEALAND
Immunisations	***18 months:*** *Haemophilus influenzae type b (Hib) (ActHIB)* Measles, mumps, rubella, varicella (chickenpox) (Priorix Tetra or ProQuad) Diphtheria, tetanus, pertussis (whooping cough) (Infanrix or Tripacel) High-risk groups: Hepatitis A (Vaqta Paediatric) ***4 years:*** Diphtheria, tetanus, pertussis (whooping cough), polio (Infanrix IPV or Quadracel) High-risk groups: Pneumococcal (Pneumovax 23)	***15 months:*** *Haemophilus influenzae type b (Act-HIB)* Measles/mumps/rubella (M-M-R® II) Pneumococcal (SYNFLORIX®) ***4 years:*** Diphtheria/tetanus/pertussis/polio (INFANRIX™-IPV) Measles/mumps/rubella (M-M-R® II)
Assessment	***Nutrition:*** Discuss nutritional intake and needs; emphasise importance of physical activity ***Development:*** Explore developmental progress (e.g. PEDS assessment) Evaluate communication ***Physical assessment (2 years):*** • Measure weight, length and head circumference and record on centile charts • Evaluate gait • Evaluate oral health and dentition • Evaluate vison and hearing ***Physical assessment (3–4 years):*** • Measure height and weight (plot and interpret growth curve/calculate BMI) • Evaluate oral health (teeth and gums) • Discuss toileting • Discuss allergies • Conduct vision and hearing screening	
Psychosocial support	***Discuss:*** • Emerging behavioural or emotional problems • Identify family strengths, elicit concerns and promote parental confidence, competence and mental health	
Safety and preventive care	***Discuss:*** • Injury prevention (e.g. water safety, burns, falls, poisoning, car restraints, helmets) • Sun protection • Sleeping and eating • Regular dental visits • Social and emotional wellbeing • CPR in children • Promoting development (limit screen time <1 hour a day. talking and reading to the child)	
INTERVENTIONS FOR HIGH-RISK GROUPS		
Children with chronic health conditions	Influenza vaccine and pneumococcal polysaccharide (23vPPV)	

Adapted from: Royal Australian College of General Practitioners, 2018; Ministry of Health, New Zealand Government, 2018; Queensland Health, Queensland Government, 2019.

of fine-motor skills requires practice through activities such as drawing or manipulation of small toys. During the preschool years, the child's proportions become more adult-like, with the limbs lengthening and the posture becoming more upright. The rate of growth continues at a slower pace and the average child gains about 2 kg in weight and 7 cm in height per year (WHO 2014).

Cognitive development

Piaget and Inhelder's (1969) **preoperational stage** begins at around 2 years of age and extends until 7 or 8 years of age. One of the distinguishing features of this stage is the use of **symbolic** thought; the child is now able to use symbols to represent people, objects and events. The symbolic function is revealed in child's play, as in delayed imitation. This means a child can witness an event, form a mental representation of it and imitate it later in the absence of the model. For example, a young child may see their mother talking on the phone and later mimic this conversation by talking into a remote control or other similarly shaped object. However, the preschooler's thought processes are still very concrete and literal, and they are only able to focus on one aspect of a problem at a time (this is known as **centration**). For example, a child in this stage of development may be able to correctly classify the family pet as a dog, but will not recognise that their pet also fits into the broader category of 'animal'.

Additionally, thought during this period is often intuitive rather than logical, which can lead the preschooler to make faulty assumptions regarding cause and effect. Magical thinking is also common in this period of development, and the preschooler can have difficulty distinguishing wishes or stories from real-life events. In particular, children of this age may believe they have caused events to occur by wishing for them, or may connect two unrelated events because they occurred close together in time. Anthropomorphising is part of magical thinking—that is, attributing human characteristics such as thoughts, feelings and sensations to inanimate objects. This can be seen in the young child who packs teddy into a bag for an outing and leaves his head sticking out 'so he can see'.

Piaget and Inhelder (1969) also claimed that children in the preoperational stage are **egocentric**. The egocentric child cannot see another's point of view, and assumes that others see things the way that they do. However, more recent research suggests that 4-year-olds can develop **theory of mind** (the understanding that others may have different thoughts or beliefs) and it is development of theory of mind which sets the stage for development of empathy later in childhood (Brown et al 2017).

Psychosocial development

According to Erikson (1963), the young child experiences a crisis involving **initiative versus guilt**. Increasing physical and cognitive abilities give rise to new levels of energy and determination. Young children 'attack' new tasks with enthusiasm and are able not only to plan their efforts, but also to persist in the face of frustrations. When the parent encourages and reassures the child (while protecting them from harm), the child learns self-assertion, spontaneity, self-sufficiency, direction and purpose. But if the parent ridicules, punishes or prevents the child from following through on tasks that could be done, the child feels guilty not only for their actions, but also for their thoughts and plans, hindering creativity and initiative.

Another important aspect of psychosocial development in the preschooler is **identification of gender roles**. Around 3 years of age, children develop knowledge of their own gender (i.e. gender identity), although they may start using gender labels (i.e. 'boy' or 'girl') at an earlier age. Between 3 and 5 years, the preschooler develops stereotypes regarding acceptable activities (e.g. girls play with dolls), physical features (e.g. boys have short hair) and occupational roles (e.g. men are firefighters) connected with gender. These stereotypes tend to be fairly inflexible until middle childhood, when the child develops an understanding that gender roles are socially dictated; however, gender stereotypes tend to persist in some form into adulthood (Feldman 2016).

Motor skills development

Skills such as running, jumping and climbing are well established by 3 years of age and continue to become increasingly well coordinated. Skills such as hopping on one foot indicate the development of increasing control and balance; most children are able to accomplish this between 3 and 4 years of age. By 5 years, most children possess adequate gross motor control to enjoy games such as skipping and activities such as skating and swimming.

Fine motor control also becomes increasingly refined during this period. The scribbles of the toddler are replaced by recognisable drawings by the age of 4 to 5 years. The typically developing 5-year-old can string beads, use scissors proficiently and is able to manipulate buttons and zippers to dress and undress independently.

Language skills

Between 3 and 4 years of age, the child uses 3 to 4-word telegraphic sentences containing only essential words. Grammar in this age is developing and the child may use simplified grammatical forms. By 5 to 6 years, the sentences are 6 to 8 words long, and grammar is well developed. The typically developing 3-year-old has a vocabulary of around 1000 words, and this will more than triple by the time they are ready to start primary school.

The preschooler talks incessantly, often to themselves rather than to others. Piaget (1975) described this pattern of speech as egocentric. However, it appears that this **private speech** is in fact a problem-solving tool which assists children to think through problems and manage their behaviour (Feldman 2016). Children around the age of 4 chatter to themselves constantly; this fades to muttering in early school years, but re-emerges as a coping strategy when the child encounters unfamiliar or stressful situations.

Personal and social skills

Socially, the preschooler's world is expanding (Figure 3.6). Fear of separation and anxiety around strangers diminishes, and children of this age are generally able to tolerate brief separations from parents to visit peers or attend preschool. With their growing social regard, preschoolers increasingly engage in **cooperative play** with each other (Crowley 2017). This means that they play the same game and interact with each other as part of their play. The child's imagination runs rampant, and this is evident in the games that they choose. Preschoolers love to dress up and imitate the behaviours of their parents or other adult models, such as nurses, doctors, media heroes, firefighters or police officers. This imaginative play has the potential to enhance learning, but also acts as an emotional outlet through which children can work through conflicts or fears.

With regard to moral development, children progress from a 'punishment/obedience' orientation in toddlerhood, towards an individualistic orientation at around 4 years of

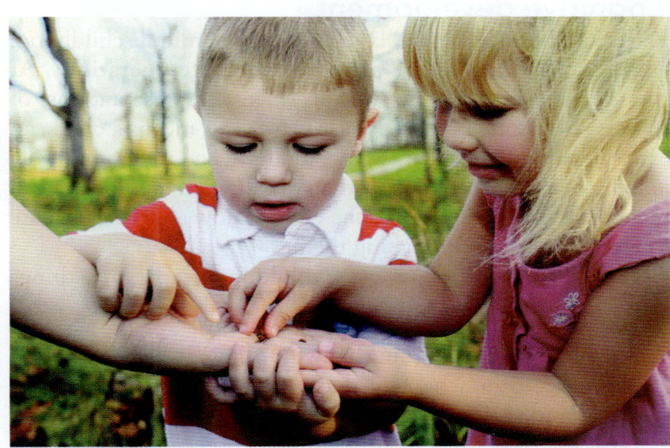

Figure 3.6

age (Kohlberg 1984). Children in the pre-conventional stage of moral development are motivated to follow rules to benefit themselves, and behave well towards others to ensure reciprocal gains, rather than out of a sense of true 'right' or 'wrong'. For a child at this level of moral reasoning, it is right to behave nicely towards others so that they will behave nicely towards you.

Periodic health check of the young child

Table 3.3 outlines important aspects of well-child checks occurring in early childhood. In this age group, non-intentional injuries are a leading cause of morbidity and mortality, therefore health teaching with families focuses on identifying and managing possible risks.

MIDDLE CHILDHOOD, SCHOOL-AGED CHILD (6 TO 10 OR 11 YEARS)

Early development of trust and a sense of initiative enables the child to enter primary school and develop a sense of themselves as worthwhile individuals, as well as a part of a larger community.

Developmental tasks for the school-aged child include:

1. Mastering skills that will be needed later as an adult
2. Winning approval from other adults and peers
3. Building self-esteem and a positive self-concept
4. Taking a place in a peer group
5. Adopting moral standards.

Physical development

The growth of the school-aged child is typically steady, with most children gaining around 2–3 kg per year and growing around 6 cm per year. The physical appearance of the school-aged child is relatively slimmer than that of the younger child because of the older child's proportionately longer legs, diminishing body fat and lower centre of gravity. Deciduous (or 'baby') teeth are lost at around 6 years of age, and new adult dentition erupts. Bones continue to ossify during these years, and bone replaces cartilage. Muscles are stronger and more developed, though not yet fully mature. Neuromuscular control is more refined. All of these changes enable the school-aged child to engage in complex physical tasks requiring strength, agility and coordination.

Cognitive development

Piaget and Inhelder (1969) labels the stage of middle childhood, ages 7 to 11 years, as the period of **concrete operations**. At this age, the child can use symbols (mental representations) of objects and events in more logical ways. This means a child can experience mentally what they would have had to do physically before. For example, rather than needing to demonstrate a manoeuvre in a video game, the child is now able to articulate the steps without undertaking them.

Armed with the ability to use thinking to experience things or events, the school-aged child can:

- Use numbers. While counting with numbers begins in preschool years, the school-aged child has the combinational skill to add and subtract, multiply and divide.
- Read. By using printed symbols (words) for objects and events, the child can process a significant amount of information. Also, reading fosters independence in learning.
- Serialise. While this begins in preschool years, the school-aged child can order objects by an increasing or decreasing scale, such as according to number size (smallest to largest) or weight (lightest to heaviest).
- Classify. This is the ability to sort objects by something they have in common. While young children can do this, the school-aged child is able to organise a hierarchy of classes and subclasses. This can be seen in the school-aged child's penchant for collections: rocks, shells, novelty cards, cars and dolls. A child spends many hours sorting the collections, and the logic of the classification system gets more complex as the child grows.
- Understand conservation principles. Understanding conservation of matter is the ability to see that mass or quantity stays constant even though shape or position is transformed. For example, the child who can conserve sees that two equal amounts of water remain the same even if one is poured into a glass with a different shape.

However, there are limitations to the school-aged child's cognitive abilities. While they are able to reason through problems that have a physical basis, they struggle to understand more abstract concepts. In this sense, school-aged children often learn best through practical demonstrations and hands-on experiences.

Psychosocial development

Erikson labelled the psychosocial crisis facing the school-aged child **industry versus inferiority**. During this stage of development, the child's energy is focused on achievement and accomplishment. The approval and esteem of people outside the immediate family takes on greater importance, and the child takes pride in attempting new tasks and carrying them through to completion. Play and fantasy begin to give way to the mastery of tasks that the child will eventually need to compete in an adult world. The child 'learns to win recognition by producing things' (Erikson 1995). Real achievement at this stage builds a feeling of confidence, competence and industry. The child is rewarded by their own inner sense of satisfaction in achieving a skill and, more importantly at this age, by external rewards such as approval from teachers, parents and peers in the form of marks, praise or gifts. Problems arise when the child feels inferior. If the child believes that they cannot measure up to society's expectations, they lose confidence in their abilities and may cease to gain satisfaction from their efforts. While it is not possible for children to master every skill they encounter, it is important for caregivers to balance these weaker skills with opportunities for the child to excel in other areas.

During middle childhood, it is important to belong to a peer group. The peer group is a key socialising agent, and group solidarity is enhanced by secret codes or strict rules. The child conforms to group rules because acceptance is paramount. The child eventually begins to prefer peer group activities to activities with the parents.

Motor skills development

Fine motor dexterity continues to improve in the school-aged child. Writing becomes smaller and more controlled and hand–eye coordination reaches its peak at around 8 years of age for most children. Gross motor skills are well established and movements become increasingly graceful. All these refinements ready the school child for pursuit of activities requiring fine motor skills, such as writing, drawing, needlework, small model building and playing instruments, and gross motor activities, such as running, skipping, throwing, jumping, bike-riding and swimming (Figure 3.7).

Language skills

Language development in the school-aged child shifts in focus from language acquisition to more nuanced expression. At around 8 years of age, children are capable of giving precise definitions to terms and by age 10 they are able to articulate their thoughts and understand another person's perspective in conversation. School-aged children are able to appreciate increasingly subtle humour and may express sarcasm.

Personal and social skills

The school-aged child exhibits an increasing need to socialise with peers of the same gender, and peer acceptance is increasingly important as the school-aged child moves towards adolescence. Initially, the child may have a large peer group, although by around 9 or 10 years of age, closer relationships have generally developed with one or more 'best friends'. More broadly, the value of social relationships emerges as the child sees the benefits of working in an organised group. Children learn to divide labour and to cooperate to achieve a common goal.

From a moral perspective, school-aged children are increasingly able to follow rules, but are motivated to do the right thing to ensure others think well of them. Kohlberg (1984) termed this form of moral reasoning a 'nice girl' or 'nice boy' orientation. By the time the child is approaching preadolescence, they start to appreciate the need for social order, and the need for rules to keep systems working effectively. This form of moral reasoning is often dependent on outside reinforcement; however, the school-aged child will typically follow the rules or do the 'right' thing if they know they are being monitored, but this may not persist if the child is left to their own devices.

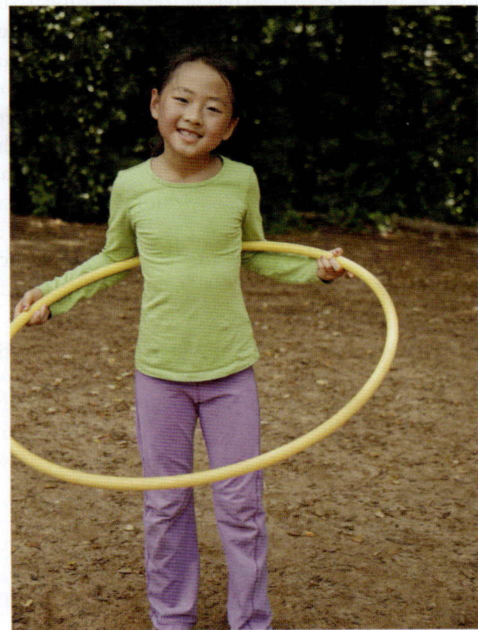

Figure 3.7

Periodic health check of the middle/school-aged child

Table 3.3 outlines important aspects of well-child checks during middle childhood.

PREADOLESCENCE (10 OR 11 TO 12 OR 13 YEARS)

Preadolescence begins at around 10 to 11 years of age and ends with puberty. Although this stage is still part of childhood, children in this group have common skills and interests that set them apart (Figure 3.8). A child may be at one level physically and intellectually but at another level socially. Additionally, development can differ significantly between children of the same age during preadolescence.

Physical development

Growth and development differs significantly between genders during this stage. On average, girls begin their growth spurt at around 10 years of age and growth reaches its maximum velocity at around 12, while boys typically begin their growth spurt at around 12 and reach peak growth velocity at approximately 14 years of age. Weight gain during this period is predominantly caused by an increase in muscle mass; however, care is needed to ensure that the adolescent's diet provides sufficient energy and adequate nutrients while maintaining weight within the healthy weight range. This is especially important as adolescents who are obese stand an 80% chance of being obese in adulthood (Feldman 2016).

Attainment of secondary sexual characteristics also varies widely between individuals of the same age. At the age of 10, some girls will still have the proportions and characteristics of children, while others have begun their growth spurt and show signs of early breast development and growth of pubic hair. Over time, the breasts enlarge, areolae darken and menarche occurs. Physical size among 11-year-old boys is fairly uniform. At 12 years, boys show a wider range of growth. Most demonstrate the onset of secondary sex characteristics with initial genital growth, appearance of pubic hair and the occurrence of erections and nocturnal emissions.

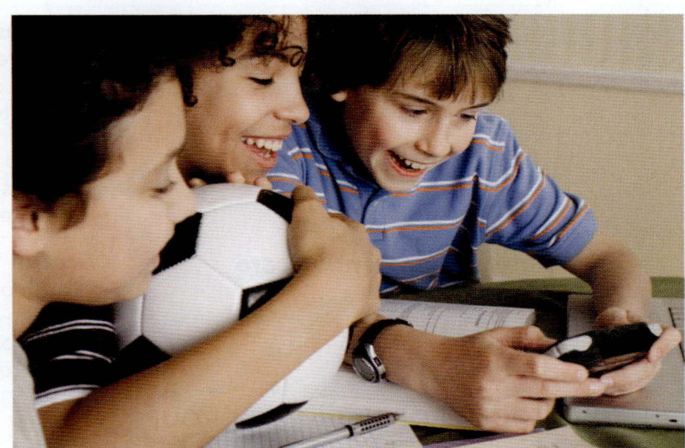

Figure 3.8

Cognitive development

According to Piaget and Inhelder (1969), children in this age group are beginning to transition from concrete operations, in which the focus is on what is occurring in the present and limited to what currently exists, to formal operations, in which the future can be considered and abstract thought becomes possible. Formal operations will be discussed in the following section.

Psychosocial development

Parent–child relationships frequently become strained during preadolescence, as the child begins to drift away from the family unit, placing increasing value on peer relationships. While parents continue to set standards and values, the child begins to challenge authority and to reject these standards. This stage of development is marked by ambivalence towards one's family; there is an increasing desire for independence which conflicts with a continuing need for support and boundaries to feel secure.

Preadolescents demonstrate strong social interest outside of the family. There is strong identification with the peer group through a small clique or a larger, more loosely organised crowd formation. Girls and boys tend to stay within their own gender group. The clique has an exclusive membership, and one is privileged to belong; the code of the clique is important, with rules for dressing, speaking and behaving in common (Meadows 2018). The child merges their own identity with that of the peer group. The child begins to substitute conformity with the family to that with the peers because they need the security of a temporary identity before formulating a clear sense of self.

Despite the fact that peer groupings are composed of the same gender, some preadolescents show an emerging interest in mixed groups, an interest that will flourish in adolescence.

Periodic health check of the older child

Table 3.4 outlines important aspects of well-child checks occurring in middle childhood and preadolescence. Unintentional injury remains a leading cause of morbidity and mortality throughout childhood and into adolescence, so harm minimisation strategies are an important part of health teaching.

ADOLESCENCE (12 OR 13 TO 19 YEARS)

Adolescence is a transition stage between childhood and adulthood (Figure 3.9). Beginning at puberty and extending through the teenage years, the most important task of adolescence is the **search for identity**—now the adolescent must form a personal identity that is more than just the sum of childhood experiences. This search for identity is the motive behind all the other tasks of the period:

1. Searching for one's identity
2. Appreciating one's achievements
3. Growing independent from parents
4. Forming close relationships with peers
5. Developing analytical thinking
6. Evolving one's own value system
7. Developing a sexual identity
8. Beginning to choose a career.

Physical development

Adolescence begins with puberty. Puberty is a time of dramatic physiological change. It includes the growth spurt—rapid growth in height, weight and muscular development; development of primary and secondary sex characteristics; and maturation of the reproductive organs. Preoccupation with appearance and the body is characteristic during early adolescence. The young person is constantly comparing themselves with close friends and peers, as well as to standards of attractiveness gleaned through exposure to the media.

Physical health is typically good during adolescence; illnesses of childhood are behind the young person and illnesses associated with ageing are not yet a concern. However, adolescence is associated with an increase in risk-taking behaviours which pose a threat to wellbeing. Poor decision making may result in accidental injury, injury through violence, abuse of alcohol and other drugs or unprotected sexual activity leading to sexually transmitted infections (STIs) or unplanned pregnancy. In

TABLE 3.4 Periodic health check: older child

Immunisations	N/a
Assessment	***Physical assessment:*** • Measure weight and height (plot and interpret growth curve and calculate BMI) • Dental check—encourage regular dental screening • Evaluate vision and hearing
Psychosocial support	• Anticipate and explore potential emotional and behavioural problems • Discuss school performance • Explore family functioning and family environment
Safety and preventive care	***Discuss:*** • Nutritional requirements and physical activity • Parent–child relationships and interaction • Injury prevention (e.g. car restraints, safe play, bicycle safety) • Sun protection
INTERVENTIONS FOR HIGH-RISK GROUPS	
Children with chronic health conditions	Influenza vaccine

Adapted from: Royal Australian College of General Practitioners, 2018; Ministry of Health, New Zealand Government, 2018; Queensland Health, Queensland Government, 2019.

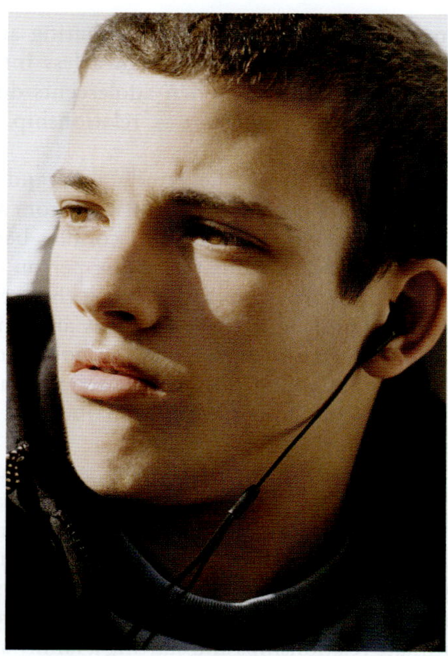

Figure 3.9

particular, early initiation of risk-taking behaviours has been linked with negative outcomes which persist into adulthood. For example, a recent Australian study demonstrated that weekly drinking in people younger than 17 was associated with a two- to threefold increase in high-risk behaviours in adulthood, including binge-drinking and alcohol dependence (Silins et al 2018).

Cognitive development

Adolescence corresponds to Piaget's fourth stage, in which the person develops the capacity for **formal operations**; the ability to develop abstract thinking, deal with hypothetical situations and make logical conclusions from reviewing evidence (Piaget 1965). Once the young person enters formal operations, thinking is no longer confined to the concrete or the real but encompasses all that is possible. Abstract thinking is liberating. The young person is no longer limited to the present but can consider the lessons of the past and the possibilities of the future. They can imagine hypotheses, then set up experiments to test them. They learn to use logic and solve problems by methodically eliminating each possibility one by one. This opens the doors to new academic achievements such as mastering advanced mathematical concepts.

This analytical thinking extends to values. Developing personal values is a part of the young person's search for identity. They no longer passively accept the values of parents or institutions but can reason through their inconsistencies and recognise injustices. The adolescent is sensitive to hypocrisy and notes when an adult professes a value and then acts counter to it. According to Kohlberg (1984), some young people are capable of post-conventional reasoning, the mature form of moral thought. The young person who achieves this level of reasoning has an internalised moral code, rather than relying on external definitions of right or wrong. However, it must be noted that not all individuals will reach this phase of moral development, and many continue to define right and wrong through rules and consequences throughout adulthood.

Psychosocial development

According to Erikson (1995), adolescents experience a crisis of identity versus role confusion; the young person is focused on 'what they appear to be in the eyes of others as compared with what they feel they are'. In this search for identity, young people often form cliques; wear fad clothing; and follow singers, movie stars or charismatic heroes in an attempt to siphon identity from them. Falling in love also feeds the quest for personal identity; the young person projects their own qualities onto another person and tries to understand them as they are reflected back by the loved one. If the young person successfully negotiates this crisis, they are left with a stable sense of self, whereas young people who struggle to develop their sense of identity may be left feeling unsure about themselves and their place in the world, resulting in feelings of isolation and anxiety.

Risk-taking is another way in which young people test their emerging identity. Risk-taking behaviours are argued to be a normative aspect of development, with large scale international studies demonstrating a consistent trend towards increased 'sensation seeking' behaviours peaking at around 19 years of age and then declining; simultaneously, young people developed increasing self-regulation which reached a steady state at between 23 and 26 years of age (Steinberg et al 2018). While risk-taking can be seen to be a typical part of adolescent psychosocial development, some risky behaviours, such as experimentation with alcohol and other drugs, high-risk sexual activity and unsafe driving practices, have significant implications for health and wellbeing (Figure 3.10).

Given the major psychosocial and physiological transitions associated with adolescence, young people are also particularly

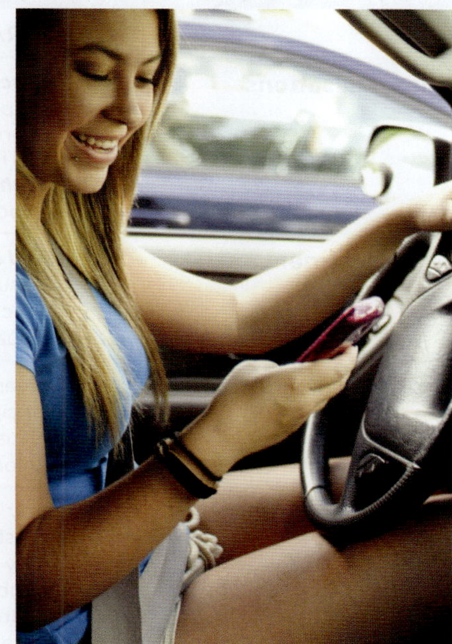

Figure 3.10

vulnerable to mental health problems. Young people with mental health disorders may experience stigma, isolation and discrimination, and are at increased risk of self-harming behaviour and suicide. Indeed, suicide has been identified as the leading cause of death among Australian adolescents and young adults (ABS 2019). In addition to mental health conditions, social and environmental factors may intensify or moderate risk for self-harm or suicide. Factors such as bullying or difficult family relationships increase risk, as does an unsupportive environment for young people who identify as lesbian, gay, bisexual or transgender (Shain 2016). Conversely, connections between the young person and supports such as peers, school and their parents have been shown to be protective (Shain 2016).

Behavioural development

As previously discussed, the search for identity is all-consuming for young people, and this guides many of the behavioural changes which occur during adolescence. While the young person may identify with their family less, they do not yet have a strong sense of their own identity. One strategy many adolescents use to cope with this transition is to immerse themselves in a peer group. Within their peer group, the young person can test out a variety of social roles and receive validation and support from others.

While belonging to a peer group is vital to the psychosocial wellbeing of the young person, developing close friendships is also important to personal identity. In preadolescence, experiencing a relationship with a best friend is valuable in teaching intimacy, trust and regard for another person. These lessons prepare the young person to develop future close relationships. Finding a girlfriend or boyfriend enables the adolescent to learn their own sex role identity. In many settings, group dating (multiple couples sharing an activity) is the norm at first. This may represent a less intimidating situation than paired dating. When adolescents do pair off, the healthy goal is a monogamous relationship involving affection and fidelity.

Gradual separation from the family unit and adopting personal responsibility is part of the transition from adolescent to adult. This is frequently a source of conflict between the young person and parent; while the young person outwardly expresses the need for freedom and control, they still require support from the family unit both practically and emotionally. The struggle for parents is often in setting boundaries which are respectful of the young person's burgeoning autonomy, while providing enough stability to maintain a sense of security.

Defining the end of adolescence is highly dependent on context and culture. In many cultures, there are rituals or rites of passage which mark the transition from child to adult, often coinciding with puberty and physical maturation. Conversely, in many western cultures, traditional markers of the transition into adulthood such as moving away from home, forming intimate relationships and starting a family are steadily occurring later in the individual's life span, for a variety of social and economic reasons. This makes it harder to determine when adolescence ends and adulthood begins.

Periodic health check in the adolescent

Adolescents should undertake periodic general checks as well as health promotion. Health promotion information should include skin self-examination, breast self-examination or testicular self-examination, substance use, contraception and STI risk reduction. See Table 3.5 for a summary of the adolescent periodic health check.

TABLE 3.5 Periodic health check: adolescent

	AUSTRALIA	NEW ZEALAND
Immunisations	***10–15 (school programs)*** Human papillomavirus (HPV) (GARDASIL®) Diphtheria, tetanus, pertussis (whooping cough) (BOOSTRIX™) ***15+ High risk groups*** Pneumococcal (Pneumovax 23)	Tetanus/diphtheria/pertussis (BOOSTRIX™) ***Girls only:*** human papillomavirus (GARDASIL®)
Assessment	***Physical assessment:*** • Measure weight and height (plot and interpret growth curve and calculate BMI) • STI screening if sexually active • Evaluate oral health	
Psychosocial support	• Screen for major depressive disorders • Anticipate and explore potential emotional and behavioural problems • Discuss school performance • Explore family functioning and family environment	
Safety and preventive care	***Discuss:*** • Breast/testicular self-examination • Injury prevention—harm minimisation strategies and assess for risky behaviours • Possible effects of alcohol and other drug use • Nutrition and physical activity • Sexual health education (contraception and safer sex practices) • Skin examination—sun protection	

TABLE 3.5 Periodic health check: adolescent—cont'd

INTERVENTIONS FOR HIGH-RISK GROUPS	
Aboriginal and Torres Strait Islander	Influenza (flu) and consider pneumococcal vaccines
High-risk sexual behaviours	STI screening including gonorrhoea, human immunodeficiency virus (HIV) and syphilis
Known illicit drug use	Screen for HIV; hepatitis A vaccine Education regarding blood-borne virus prevention
Individuals with a chronic health condition	Influenza and pneumococcal vaccines

Adapted from: Royal Australian College of General Practitioners, 2018; Ministry of Health, New Zealand Government, 2018; Queensland Health, Queensland Government, 2019.

EARLY ADULTHOOD (20 TO 40 YEARS)

The young adult is concerned with emancipation from their parents and building an independent lifestyle. Developmental tasks during this phase of the life span include:

1. Growing independent from the parents' home and care
2. Establishing a career or vocation
3. Forming an intimate bond with another and choosing a mate
4. Learning to cooperate in an intimate relationship
5. Setting up and managing one's own household
6. Making friends and establishing a social group
7. Assuming civic responsibility and becoming a citizen in the community
8. Beginning a parenting role
9. Forming a meaningful philosophy of life.

Physical development

Physical growth, in terms of height, weight and maturation of organ systems, is generally complete by early adulthood. The epiphyses of the long bones typically fuse in the early twenties, and motor coordination and strength peak between the ages of 20 and 30 (Beckett & Taylor 2019). Maximal bone mass is achieved by 35 years of age (Polan & Taylor 2018). Since growth has finished, nutritional needs are dictated by maintenance and repair requirements and on activity levels. If activity decreases from its level during adolescence, kilojoules must be reduced. Sensible nutrition is a major problem for many adults; being overweight and obesity are at epidemic levels in Australia (AIHW 2019). The diet should be high in fruits, vegetables and lean proteins but all too often it is high in sugar, salt and fat. A sedentary lifestyle contributes to both increases in body mass index and associated health risks. However, more adults are learning that frequent steady exercise maintains weight, muscle strength and joint flexibility; builds heart and lung capacity; and reduces stress (Figure 3.11). Table 3.6 lists these and other preventive counselling measures to address during healthcare visits.

Cognitive development

Intellectual and cognitive skills reach a peak during early adulthood. During adolescence, the young person achieves formal operations, and develops the capacity for abstract thought (Piaget 1965). While the young adult retains this capability, their thinking is qualitatively different. Indeed, some theorists have proposed the term 'post-formal' operations to capture this subtle but important distinction (Sinnott et al 2016). These theorists claim that the young adult's growing experience allows them to view problems in a less egocentric way, integrating multiple perspectives in order to arrive at a solution. This gives the young adult more sophisticated problem-solving capabilities and expands their potential for creative thinking.

Education continues for many young adults, from formal courses in a university or technical and further education (TAFE) environment to on-the-job training and continuing education classes. Usually, this education is designed to prepare the individual for employment. Work is an important factor in the young adult's life because it is tied closely with the individual's sense of identity (Polan & Taylor 2018). A person with job satisfaction feels challenged, rewarded and fulfilled, whereas the individual who is frustrated with work may begin to experience diminished self-worth. Those who are unable

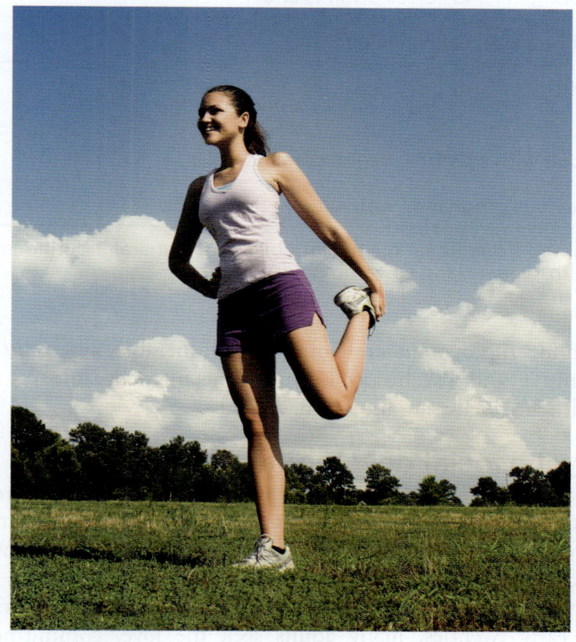

Figure 3.11

TABLE 3.6 Periodic health check: young adult and middle adult

	AUSTRALIA	NEW ZEALAND
Immunisations	***Pregnant women:*** Influenza Pertussis (whooping cough) (BOOSTRIX™ or Adacel) ***High risk groups:*** Pneumococcal (Pneumovax 23)	***45 years:*** diphtheria/tetanus (ADT™ Booster)
Assessment	***20–40 years:*** • Measure BMI and waist circumference or waist-to-hip ratio • Record blood pressure • Measure fasting lipids (from 35 years in high-risk groups) • Evaluate risk factors relating to smoking, alcohol, nutrition and activity • Assess for type 2 diabetes (from 19 years in Aboriginal and Torres Strait Islander peoples) • Sexual health screening • Preconceptual care and breast cancer and cervical screening for women ***40–65 years:*** • Measure BMI and waist circumference or waist-to-hip ratio • Record blood pressure • Measure fasting lipids • Evaluate risk factors relating to smoking, alcohol, nutrition and activity • Assess for type 2 diabetes • Calculate absolute cardiovascular risk (from 35 years in high-risk groups) • Pre-conceptual care, cervical screening test and breast cancer screening for women • Colorectal cancer screening (from 50 years) • Assess risk for osteoporosis (from 45 years in women and 50 in men)	
Psychosocial support	• Assess depression risk	
Safety and preventive care	***Discuss:*** • Nutrition and physical activity guidelines • Sexual health and STI prevention • Substance use including alcohol, tobacco and illicit drugs • Sun protection	

INTERVENTIONS FOR HIGH-RISK POPULATIONS	
Aboriginal and Torres Strait Islander	Influenza (flu) and consider pneumococcal
High-risk sexual behaviours	STI screening including gonorrhoea, HIV and syphilis
History of illicit drug use	Screen for HIV; hepatitis A vaccine Education regarding blood-borne virus prevention
Adult with a chronic health condition	Influenza vaccine and pneumococcal
Previous pregnancy with neural tube defect	Folic acid supplementation

Adapted from: Royal Australian College of General Practitioners, 2018; Ministry of Health, New Zealand Government, 2018; Queensland Health, Queensland Government, 2019.

to find employment are potentially vulnerable, not only to cognitive and psychosocial issues, but financial impacts on health and wellbeing more broadly.

Psychosocial development

Erikson's sixth stage covers the first years of early adulthood, from 20 to 24 years. He believed the major psychological conflict to be resolved is that of **intimacy versus isolation** (Erikson 1995). Once self-identity is established after adolescence, it can be merged with another's in an intimate relationship. During the early twenties, many adults seek the love, commitment and intimacy of an intense, lasting relationship. This mature relationship includes mutual trust, cooperation, sharing of feelings and goals and complete acceptance of the other person. Although Erikson had a heterosexual union in mind, this intimacy could be satisfied through a same sex relationship or through a bond with a cause or an institution.

Erikson believed that without a secure personal identity, a person cannot form a love relationship. The result is that the person becomes isolated, withdrawn and lonely. Such issues with psychosocial development may result in attempts to fill the void with transient or casual sexual relationships. Erikson proposes that these do not meet the needs of the individual, exacerbating feelings of loneliness. However, not all young adults desire or seek marriage or family, finding fulfilment in their career or delaying child-rearing until later in life.

It has been proposed that individuals in their twenties may be in a period of 'emerging adulthood', representing a newly defined stage of development (Wood et al 2017). As pressures such as housing affordability, limited employment opportunities for young people and the rising cost of education have come to bear, more young adults are choosing to stay in the family home for a prolonged period, and therefore may adopt the responsibilities and independence central to early adulthood later than previous generations.

In contrast to the twenties, an individual's thirties are typically characterised by 'settling down', and a search for order and stability. Part of this settling down may include having children. For those young adults who do choose to start a family, parenting raises a new series of developmental tasks to be accomplished. On discovering a pregnancy, both positive and negative emotions may be experienced. If this was a planned conception, there may be feelings of excitement and a strong desire to be the perfect parent; however, this may be counterbalanced with concerns about one's parenting ability, and the impact that child-rearing will have on lifestyle, career and other commitments. Having children also results in a major readjustment to roles within an intimate relationship. Decisions about work and parenting leave may need to be made, and parental preferences regarding care at home may need to be weighed against financial and workplace obligations.

Periodic health check in the young adult

Table 3.6 outlines the periodic health check for the young adult.

MIDDLE ADULTHOOD (40 TO 65 YEARS)

The primary focus of middle adulthood is developing meaningful life structures. Developmental tasks during this stage of the life span include:

1. Accepting and adjusting to the physical changes of middle age
2. Reviewing and redirecting career goals
3. Achieving desired performance in career
4. Developing hobby and leisure activities
5. Adjusting to ageing parents
6. Helping adolescent children in their search for identity
7. Accepting and relating to the spouse as a person
8. Coping with an empty nest at home.

Physical development

During middle adulthood, the function of organ systems is typically stable, with only small deceases in respiratory reserve and cardiac function. There may be some changes to the person's vision, with presbyopia (decreasing near vision accommodation) becoming more prevalent (Polan & Taylor 2018). Many of the physical changes occurring during this period are to do with appearance, with thinning and greying of hair and a loss of skin elasticity becoming increasingly evident. These physical signs of ageing, combined with occasional news of a peer's illness or death, may lead those in middle adulthood to contemplate their own mortality.

In the late forties and early fifties, females experience menopause, the decreasing frequency and finally the cessation of menstruation. There is decreased production of the female hormones oestrogen and progesterone which brings attendant symptoms such as atrophy of reproductive organs, vasomotor disturbances and mood swings (Chapter 26). Although men do not have such an abrupt halt to reproductive ability, they experience a decrease in the production of testosterone, which causes decreased sperm and semen production.

During this stage of the life span, a decrease in lean muscle mass and bone density occurs, particularly if there is a decline in physical activity, while adipose tissue increases and tends to accumulate around the abdomen or hips. This increase in adiposity is a risk factor for cardiovascular disease including hypertension, disorders of glucose metabolism and musculoskeletal dysfunction such as arthritis and back pain. It is important to note that while body mass index (BMI) is a commonly used measure of adiposity, waist-to-hip ratio (WHR) has been shown to have a causal association with both cardiovascular disease and type 2 diabetes (Emdin et al 2017). As such, there is strong evidence for including these measures in the assessment of health risk in adults. According to the Australian Institute of Health and Welfare (AIHW), mortality in people aged 45–64 is frequently a result of chronic disease. In recent years, cardiovascular disease and dementia have been predominant causes of death for both men and women (AIHW 2018).

Cognitive development

Intelligence levels remain generally constant during middle adulthood. Intelligence is further enhanced by the knowledge that comes with life experience, self-confidence, a sense of humour and flexibility. The middle-aged adult is interested in how new knowledge is applied, not just in learning for learning's sake. Cognitively, the middle-aged adult may require more time to assimilate new knowledge; however, once learned, they have more accurate recall than younger age groups.

Psychosocial development

Erikson (1995) argued that the most important task for personality development is resolution of the conflict of generativity versus stagnation. Erikson believed that during the middle years, adults have an urge to contribute to the next generation. This need can be fulfilled either by actively engaging in child rearing (Figure 3.12) or by producing something to

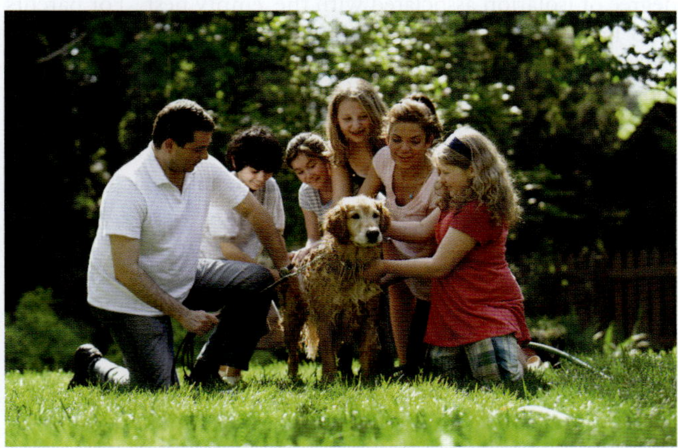

Figure 3.12

pass on to the next generation. Thus, middle-aged adults may focus on child rearing or engage in other creative, socially useful work. Generativity may also include developing a career, managing a household or fostering close relationships.

The middle-aged adult needs to be needed, to leave something behind and to leave their mark on the world. Generativity is associated with sharing, giving, contributing to the growth of others. If this conflict is not successfully negotiated, the individual experiences stagnation, turning their attention inwardly and becoming self-absorbed and potentially experiencing a loss of meaning and connectedness.

Mid-life transition occurs between the ages of 40 and 45 years. As with the re-evaluation which occurs at around 30 years of age, this mid-life appraisal includes questions about direction and purpose. The person may confront the reality that not all life goals will be met, while others require adjustment. For women, one aspect of the mid-life transition is consideration of the approaching biological boundary of childbearing. For those who set aside childbearing in earlier adulthood, a review of options may occur at this point; indeed, this review occurs even in women who are satisfied with their family size and structure. The mid-life transition often also incorporates a review of career goals and changes in career direction.

Another important aspect of psychosocial development in middle adulthood is the maintenance of positive self-image. However, this can be difficult in cultures which place value on looking and acting young. When the individual attempts to deny ageing or has trouble viewing themselves as middle-aged, they may experience difficulty making necessary lifestyle adjustments and depression can result. Sometimes this denial of ageing can lead to a 'mid-life crisis', in which the individual engages in behaviours which are out of character (Polan & Taylor 2018). Alternatively, the reflection associated with middle adulthood can bring about new insights regarding the individual's past experiences and sense of self.

Family also contributes to this adjustment; a supportive intimate relationship or strong connections with children may promote adaptation, while challenges such as divorce or separation or caring for ageing parents may impact on psychosocial function in a negative way. The middle-aged adult may also be supporting their own adolescent children as they strive for greater independence and control. Finally, once children leave home, the middle-aged adult may experience a degree of isolation associated with the 'empty nest'. For parents who have focused vast amounts of time and energy on their children, this transition may challenge the parent's identity and sense of purpose. Parents may also experience a change to their intimate relationships once children have moved away from home. Some struggle to adjust to being a 'couple' again, while others revel in the increased freedom and intimacy that this phase of development can bring.

Periodic health check of the middle adult

Table 3.6 outlines the periodic health check for the middle adult.

LATE ADULTHOOD (65+ YEARS)

Developmental tasks during this stage of the life span include:

1. Adjusting to changes in physical strength and health
2. Forming a new family role as a parent-in-law and/or grand-parent
3. Affiliating with one's age group
4. Adjusting to retirement and reduced income
5. Developing postretirement activities that enhance self-worth and usefulness
6. Arranging satisfactory housing
7. Adjusting to the death of spouse, family members and friends
8. Conducting a life review
9. Preparing for the inevitability of one's own death.

Physical development

Ageing is a normal physiological process, although its mechanism is not fully understood. While ageing can be associated with an increase in health problems, each individual ages differently. Indeed, differences in personal attitudes, health behaviours, physical activity, genetics and the occurrence of physical illness mean that one individual at 80 years may be more vigorous and have a better subjective sense of wellbeing than another at the same age (Polan & Taylor 2018).

Typical processes which occur as part of ageing include loss of total body water and bone mass. Within the cardiovascular system, structural changes over time lead to thickening and stiffening of arterial walls, increasing blood pressure and compromising blood flow to the cardiac muscle. Hypertension is a common finding in the older adult, and the proportion of adults experiencing uncontrolled hypertension increases with age, peaking at around 53% for adults aged 85 years and older. Chronic illnesses are increasingly common in this age group, while recovery from illness or injury may be prolonged. All of these issues mean that the older adult may be a more frequent consumer of healthcare than other age groups.

Cognitive development

Ageing does not have a predictable effect on intelligence. Intellectual function depends on various factors, such as motivation, interest, sensory impairment, educational level, general health, social concerns and involvement in community activities or stimulating leisure activities. How we solve problems also tends to change with age. While younger adults tend to rely primarily on 'fluid' reasoning ability (the ability to adapt mental operations to new tasks) to solve everyday problems, older adults retain and even build on their 'crystalised' abilities (those formed from accumulated experiences and knowledge of the world) (Chen et al 2017). Older adults may experience a decline in memory function, especially in terms of storage and retrieval of short-term memories; however, many older adults retain strong recall of long-term memories.

Psychosocial development

The adult over 65 has frequently stepped off centre stage both in formal employment and in the family. For some, this can be traumatic because it means a loss of recognition and authority. But now the person can direct energy inwards. When financially and socially secure, the older adult can pursue activities which hold personal significance for them. The person creates a new balance with society; they are less interested in society's extrinsic rewards and more interested in using inner resources (Figure 3.13).

However, retirement can be a difficult period for some older adults, particularly if their sense of identity is closely tied to their

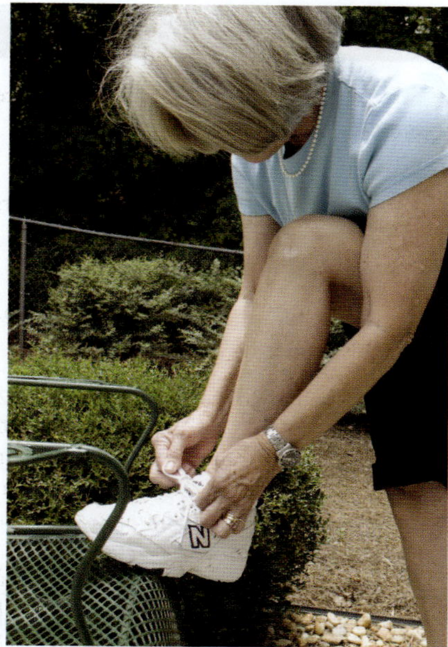

Figure 3.13

work. There is also a loss of social contact through co-workers, and potentially a decrease in intellectual stimulation and activity if the job was relatively demanding. For this reason, it is important to develop postretirement activities that enhance self-worth and give a feeling of usefulness. These activities may include developing a new 'semi-retired' career, or a hobby, sport interest or community service activity. For other older adults, this may include assisting with the care of grandchildren. The transition to retirement is eased if these activities are well in place before the last formal day on the job.

Loss of income associated with retirement and the potential for altered living arrangements may also impact on the psycho-social wellbeing of the older adult. There may be a significant drop in income and even those who own their own home may become overwhelmed with increasing costs of living on a fixed pension or superannuation benefit. Living arrangements may also need to change depending on financial circumstances and the need for support with day-to-day living. While some cultures incorporate their elders into the family home and view them as an active part of the family unit, this is less common in western cultures. This may leave the older adult with difficult choices to make about moving into a retirement village or aged care facility.

One important task of late adulthood is performing a life review. Older adults have completed much of their life's work. Their contribution to society and to their own immortality is reaching a conclusion (Levinson et al 1986). The life review is a cataloguing of life events, a considering of one's successes and failures with the perspective of age. According to Erikson, the key psychological conflict for the older adult is one of **ego integrity versus despair**. When the older adult negotiates this conflict successfully, they are able to review life events, experiences and relationships. Engaging in life review can help older adults to find meaning and value in their life experiences, and this has been found to improve subjective wellbeing (Robinson & Murphy-Nugen 2018). Conversely, an individual who struggles to find integration may be left with a sense of despair, resentment, futility, hopelessness and a fear of death. However, a successful outcome completes a cycle. The contented older adult who does not fear death serves as a role model for younger adults.

Periodic health check for the adult over 65 years

Table 3.7 outlines the periodic health check for late adulthood.

CULTURAL AND SOCIAL CONSIDERATIONS

Much of the developmental content of this chapter is informed by the findings of research and experience with people from

TABLE 3.7 Periodic health check: late adulthood (65+)

	AUSTRALIA	NEW ZEALAND
Immunisations	Influenza (flu); pneumococcal herpes zoster (Zostavax)	Influenza (flu); diphtheria/tetanus (ADT™ Booster)
Assessment	***Physical assessment:*** • Measure BMI and waist circumference or waist-to-hip ratio • Record blood pressure • Measure fasting lipids • Evaluate risk factors relating to smoking, alcohol, nutrition and activity • Assess for type 2 diabetes • Calculate absolute cardiovascular risk • Pap screen or cervical screening test and breast cancer screening for women (to age 69) • Colorectal cancer screening • Assess risk for osteoporosis • Assess vision and hearing • Assess falls risk • Assess risk for dementia	
Psychosocial support	• Discuss issues with memory • Discuss social supports and social activities • Assess for mood and depression	

Continued

TABLE 3.7 Periodic health check: late adult (65+)—cont'd

	AUSTRALIA	NEW ZEALAND
Safety and preventive care	*Discuss:* • Falls prevention strategies • Nutrition and physical activity guidelines • Medication safety • Sun protection	
INTERVENTIONS FOR HIGH-RISK POPULATIONS		
Individuals living in care	Hepatitis A vaccine; hepatitis B vaccine	
Aboriginal and Torres Strait Islander	Influenza (flu) and consider pneumococcal polysaccharide (23vPPV)	
High-risk sexual behaviours	STI screening including gonorrhoea, HIV and syphilis	
History of illicit drug use	Screen for HIV; hepatitis A vaccine Education regarding blood-borne virus prevention	
Adult with a chronic health condition	Influenza vaccine and pneumococcal polysaccharide (23vPPV)	

Adapted from: Royal Australian College of General Practitioners, 2018; Ministry of Health, New Zealand Government, 2018; Queensland Health, Queensland Government, 2019.

cultures which are dominant in high-income countries. Given the rate of demographic change, it is imperative to consult with cultural brokers and/or patient advocates from the person's cultural heritage who have a deeper understanding of the expected norms of the various developmental tasks.

The immunisation protocols from other nations differ from those of Australia and careful examination of health records must be undertaken when engaging with individuals who have received care outside of Australia. When assessments are conducted, competent interpreters must be used.

Social factors also play a significant role in development and health across the life span. The role of socioeconomic status as a determinant for health and wellbeing has been well explored, in infants and children (Goldfeld et al 2017, Moore et al 2015) and extending from childhood into adult life (Evans 2016). Interventions that promote socioeconomic equity and limit childhood adversity have been demonstrated to improve a host of health-related benefits including increased adult income, educational attainment and improved health biomarkers (Black et al 2017).

Socioeconomic disadvantage experienced in adulthood may also have a significant effect on morbidity and mortality and, in particular, on the rates of potentially harmful health behaviours (Mehta et al 2015). Such information is helpful in designing effective health policy and providing valuable support to vulnerable populations.

DEVELOPMENTAL SCREENING TOOLS

Parent's evaluation of developmental status (PEDS)

Age: Birth to 8 years
Time required: 2–5 min
Author: F. P. Glascoe
Available from: www.pedstest.com

PEDS is a developmental screening tool designed to elicit parents' concerns about their child's development across a range of domains, including fine and gross motor function, receptive and expressive language, behaviour and social and emotional skills (Glascoe 2011). The tool is designed to ensure early identification of developmental risk factors and signs of delay and to prompt further investigation where needed. As described by the Centre for Community Child Health (Royal Children's Hospital (RCH) 2019), one of the potential weaknesses of traditional developmental screening tools is that they are typically performed in isolation, without due consideration of the child's sociocultural context, and without soliciting systematic input from parents who have extensive insight into their child's behaviour and abilities. The Centre also highlights that involving parents actively in screening may improve accuracy as well as making families more likely to follow recommendations (RCH 2019).

PEDS relies on responses from parents to 10 specific questions, which can be administered either as a written questionnaire or as an interview with the health provider. The tool includes suggested scoring, with a response algorithm which provides recommendations ranging from referral for detailed assessment, use of additional screening measures or education and reassurance depending on the concerns expressed and the age of the child.

The PEDS tool is well validated (Glascoe 2013), demonstrating strong sensitivity and specificity (Glascoe 2011). A systematic review including 37 studies across 12 countries indicates that about 14% of parents identified concerns regarding their child's development when the PEDS tool was used, and that these concerns were more likely in children experiencing biological and psychosocial adversity (Woolfenden et al 2013). Benefits of this tool include its simplicity, meaning that providers require minimal training; the assessment package includes a reference guide, which is used to interpret results. Its brevity also means that it is feasible to include in brief healthcare interactions.

Adult life stress measures

Some tools are available that attempt to quantify the impact of life change on a person's health. They are based on the assumption that a relationship exists between daily life stress and a person's susceptibility to physical and psychological problems. Many of the life change events are the developmental tasks discussed earlier in the chapter.

The hassles and uplifts scale

Age range: adult
Author: DeLongis

This is a 53-item self-administered questionnaire whose purpose is to assess day-to-day stress (Table 3.8). Take this test yourself just before you go to bed one day. Consider each item on the list and circle a number on the left-hand side regarding how much of a hassle the item was for you that day. On the right-hand side, circle a number regarding how much of an uplift the same item was for you that day. Total scores are obtained by summing across ratings given to all items.

Relatively minor but frequently experienced stresses, termed *Hassles* in this tool, have been found to correlate strongly with negative health status. DeLongis et al (1988) found a significant relationship between daily stress and concurrent or later occurrence of physical health problems, such as flu, sore throat, headaches and backaches. There was great individual variation, however, with one-third of the respondents reporting a somewhat improved health and mood with increased stress levels. Regarding daily stress and psychological disturbance, they found that individuals with unsupportive social relationships and low self-esteem had a greater risk of psychological and somatic health problems, both on their stressful days and following their stressful days, than did individuals with positive social networks and high self-esteem (DeLongis et al 1988).

TABLE 3.8 The hassles and uplifts scale

HASSLES are irritants—things that annoy or bother you; they can make you upset or angry. UPLIFTS are events that make you feel good; they can make you joyful, glad or satisfied. Some hassles and uplifts occur on a fairly regular basis and others are relatively rare. Some have only a slight effect; others have a strong effect.		
This questionnaire lists things that can be hassles and uplifts in day-to-day life. You will find that during the course of a day some of these things will have been only a hassle for you and some will have been only an uplift. *Others will have been both a hassle AND an uplift.*		
DIRECTIONS: Please think about how much of a hassle and how much of an uplift each item was for you today. Please indicate on the left-hand side of the page (under 'HASSLES') how much of a hassle the item was by circling the appropriate number. Then indicate on the right-hand side of the page (under 'UPLIFTS') how much of an uplift it was for you by circling the appropriate number.		
Remember, circle one number on the left-hand side of the page *and* one number on the right-hand side of the page for *each* item.		
PLEASE FILL OUT THIS QUESTIONNAIRE JUST BEFORE YOU GO TO BED.		
After you complete the scale you are encouraged to use the information as a baseline to consider how psychosocial and lifestyle factors influence your wellbeing over time.		
HASSLES AND UPLIFTS SCALE		
How much of a hassle was this item for you today?		**How much of an uplift was this item for you today?**
HASSLES		**UPLIFTS**
0 = None or not applicable		0 = None or not applicable
1 = Somewhat		1 = Somewhat
2 = Quite a bit		2 = Quite a bit
3 = A great deal		3 = A great deal
DIRECTIONS: Please circle one number on the left-hand side and one number on the right-hand side for each item.		
0 1 2 3	1. Your child(ren)	0 1 2 3
0 1 2 3	2. Your parents or parents-in-law	0 1 2 3
0 1 2 3	3. Other relative(s)	0 1 2 3
0 1 2 3	4. Your spouse	0 1 2 3
0 1 2 3	5. Time spent with family	0 1 2 3
0 1 2 3	6. Health or wellbeing of a family member	0 1 2 3
0 1 2 3	7. Sex	0 1 2 3
0 1 2 3	8. Intimacy	0 1 2 3
0 1 2 3	9. Family-related obligations	0 1 2 3

Continued

TABLE 3.8 The hassles and uplifts scale—cont'd

0 1 2 3	10. Your friend(s)	0 1 2 3
0 1 2 3	11. Fellow workers	0 1 2 3
0 1 2 3	12. Clients, customers, patients, etc	0 1 2 3
0 1 2 3	13. Your supervisor or employer	0 1 2 3
0 1 2 3	14. The nature of your work	0 1 2 3
0 1 2 3	15. Your work load	0 1 2 3
0 1 2 3	16. Your job security	0 1 2 3
0 1 2 3	17. Meeting deadlines or goals on the job	0 1 2 3
0 1 2 3	18. Enough money for necessities (e.g. food, clothing, housing, healthcare, taxes, insurance)	0 1 2 3
0 1 2 3	19. Enough money for education	0 1 2 3
0 1 2 3	20. Enough money for emergencies	0 1 2 3
0 1 2 3	21. Enough money for extras (e.g. entertainment, recreation, holidays)	0 1 2 3
0 1 2 3	22. Financial care for someone who doesn't live with you	0 1 2 3
0 1 2 3	23. Investments	0 1 2 3
0 1 2 3	24. Your smoking	0 1 2 3
0 1 2 3	25. Your drinking	0 1 2 3
0 1 2 3	26. Mood-altering drugs	0 1 2 3
0 1 2 3	27. Your physical appearance	0 1 2 3
0 1 2 3	28. Contraception	0 1 2 3
0 1 2 3	29. Exercise(s)	0 1 2 3
0 1 2 3	30. Your medical care	0 1 2 3
0 1 2 3	31. Your health	0 1 2 3
0 1 2 3	32. Your physical abilities	0 1 2 3
0 1 2 3	33. The weather	0 1 2 3
0 1 2 3	34. News events	0 1 2 3
0 1 2 3	35. Your environment (e.g. quality of air, noise level, greenery)	0 1 2 3
0 1 2 3	36. Political or social issues	0 1 2 3
0 1 2 3	37. Your neighbourhood (e.g. neighbours, setting)	0 1 2 3
0 1 2 3	38. Conserving (gas, electricity, water, petrol, etc)	0 1 2 3
0 1 2 3	39. Pets	0 1 2 3
0 1 2 3	40. Cooking	0 1 2 3
0 1 2 3	41. Housework	0 1 2 3
0 1 2 3	42. Home repairs	0 1 2 3
0 1 2 3	43. Garden work	0 1 2 3
0 1 2 3	44. Car maintenance	0 1 2 3
0 1 2 3	45. Taking care of paperwork (e.g. paying bills, filling out forms)	0 1 2 3
0 1 2 3	46. Home entertainment (e.g. TV, music, reading)	0 1 2 3

TABLE 3.8 The hassles and uplifts scale—cont'd		
0 1 2 3	47. Amount of free time	0 1 2 3
0 1 2 3	48. Recreation and entertainment outside the home (e.g. movies, sports, eating out, walking)	0 1 2 3
0 1 2 3	49. Eating (at home)	0 1 2 3
0 1 2 3	50. Religious or community organisations	0 1 2 3
0 1 2 3	51. Legal matters	0 1 2 3
0 1 2 3	52. Being organised	0 1 2 3
0 1 2 3	53. Social commitments	0 1 2 3

DeLongis A, Folkman S, Lazarus RS: The impact of daily stress on health and mood: psychological and social resources as mediators, *Journal of Personality and Social Psychology*, 54(3):486-495, 1988. ©1988 by the American Psychological Association. Used with permission. No further reproduction or distribution is permitted without written permission of the American Psychological Association.

BIBLIOGRAPHY

Australian Bureau of Statistics (ABS). 3303.0 - Causes of Death, Australia, 2018. Australian Bureau of Statistics; 2019. Available at: https://www.abs.gov.au/ausstats/abs@.nsf/Lookup/by%20Subject/3303.0~2018~Main%20Features~Intentional%20self-harm,%20key%20characteristics~3.

Australian Government, Department of Health. National immunisation program schedule. 2019. Available at: https://beta.health.gov.au/health-topics/immunisation/immunisation-throughout-life/national-immunisation-program-schedule.

Australian Institute of Health and Welfare. Deaths in Australia [Internet]. 2018. Available at: https://www.aihw.gov.au/reports/life-expectancy-death/deaths-in-australia/contents/leading-causes-of-death.

Australian Institute of Health and Welfare. Overwight and obesity. Australian Institute of Health and Welfare; 2019. Available at: https://www.aihw.gov.au/reports/overweight-obesity/a-picture-of-overweight-and-obesity-in-australia/contents/table-of-contents.

Babler E, Strickland CJ. Normalizing: adolescent experiences living with type 1 diabetes. Diabetes Educ 2015;41(3):351–60.

Beckett C, Taylor H. Human growth and development. 3rd ed. Melbourne: Sage; 2019.

Black MM, Walker SP, Fernald LCH, et al. Early childhood development coming of age: science through the life course. Lancet 2017;389(10064):77–90.

Bowlby EJM. Loss-Sadness and depression: attachment and loss, vol. 3. New York: Random House; 2008.

Bowlby J. Separation anxiety. Br J Psychiatry 1960;XLI:89–113.

Bremner JG, Slater AM, Hayes RA, et al. Young infants' visual fixation patterns in addition and subtraction tasks support an object tracking account. J Exp Child Psychol 2017;162:199–208. Available at: http://dx.doi.org/10.1016/j.jecp.2017.05.007.

Brown MMI, Thibodeau RB, Pierucci JM, et al. Supporting the development of empathy: the role of theory of mind and fantasy orientation. Soc Dev 2017;26(4):951–64.

Chen X, Hertzog C, Park DC. Cognitive predictors of everyday problem solving across the lifespan. Gerontology 2017;63(4):372–84.

Crowley K. Child development: a practical introduction. 2nd ed. Thousand Oaks, CA: Sage Publications Inc; 2017.

Cusick SE, Georgieff MK. The role of nutrition in brain development: the golden opportunity of the 'First 1000 Days.' J Pediatr 2016;175:16–21.

DeLongis A, Folkman S, Lazarus RS. The impact of daily stress on health and mood: psychological and social resources as mediators. J Pers Soc Psychol 1988;54(3):486–95.

Dobson V, Teller DY. Visual acuity in human infants: a review and comparison of behavioral and electrophysiological studies. Vision Res 1978;18(11):1469–83.

Dudek J, Faress A, Bornstein MH, et al. Infant cries rattle adult cognition. PLoS One 2016;11(5):1–17.

Emdin CA, Khera AV, Natarajan P, et al. Genetic association of waist-to-hip ratio with cardiometabolic traits, type 2 diabetes, and coronary heart disease. JAMA 2017;317(6):626–34.

Erikson EH. Childhood and society. London: Random House; 1963 & 1995.

Evans GW. Childhood poverty and adult psychological well-being. Proc Natl Acad Sci U S A 2016;113(52):14949–52.

Feldman RS. Child development. 7th ed. Boston: Pearson Education Inc; 2016.

Glascoe FP, Marks KP. Detecting children with developmental-behavioral problems: the value of collaborating with parents in early detection. Psychol Test Assess Model 2011;53(2):258–79.

Glascoe FP. Collaborating with parents: using parents' evaluation of developmental status (PEDS) to detect and address developmental and behavioral problems. 2nd ed. Nolensville, TN: PEDSTest.com, LLC; 2013.

Goldfeld S, O'Connor M, Cloney D, et al. Understanding child disadvantage from a social determinants perspective. J Epidemiol Community Health 2017;72(3):223–9.

Gonzalez JS, Tanenbaum ML, Commissariat PV. Psychosocial factors in medication adherence and diabetes self-management: implications for research and practice. Am Psychol 2016;71(7):539–51.

Kohlberg L. The psychology of moral development. New York: Harper & Row; 1984.

Lawrence D, Hafekost J, Johnson SE, et al. Key findings from the second Australian Child and Adolescent Survey of Mental Health and Wellbeing. Aust N Z J Psychiatry 2016;50(9):876–86.

Levinson DJ. The seasons of a man's life. 2nd ed. New York: Ballantine; 1986.

Meadows, S. Understanding Child Development: Psychological Perspectives and Applications. 2nd ed. New York: Routledge; 2018.

Mehta NK, House JS, Elliott MR. Dynamics of health behaviours and socioeconomic differences in mortality in the USA. J Epidemiol Community Health 2015;69(5):416–22.

Ministry of Health, New Zealand Government. Child Health 2018. Available at: https://www.health.govt.nz/our-work/life-stages/child-health.

Moore TG, McDonald M, Carlon L, et al. Early childhood development and the social determinants of health inequities. Health Promot Int 2015;30:ii102–ii115.

Piaget J. The stages of the intellectual development of the child. Educational psychology in context: Readings for future teachers. 1965;63(4):98–106.

Piaget J. The construction of reality in the child. New York: Ballantine; 1975.

Piaget J, Cook M. The development of object concept. In: The construction of reality in the child. New York, NY: Basic Books; 1954. pp. 3–96.

Piaget J, Inhelder B. The psychology of the child. New York: Basic Books; 1969.

Polan E, Taylor D. Journey across the lifespan: Human development and health promotion (E-Book). Philadelphia, PA: USA; 2018. pp. 183–94.

Queensland Health, Queensland Government. Personal Health Record. [Internet]. 2018. Available at: https://www.childrens.health.qld.gov.au/chq/information-for-families/personal-health-record

Queensland Health, Queensland Government. *Primary Clinical Care Manual -10th ed. 2019. Available:* https://www.publications.qld.gov.au/dataset/primary-clinical-care-manual-10th-edition

Ringer S. Fluid and electrolyte therapy in newborns. In: Abrams SA, Mattoo TK, editors. UpToDate, [Internet]. Waltham, MA: UpToDate Inc; 2018 [updated 2018, March 13; Cited 2019, March 8] Available at: https://www.uptodate.com/contents/fluid-and-electrolyte-therapy-in-newborns#H275993503.

Robinson JT, Murphy-Nugen AB. It makes you keep trying: Life review writing for older adults. J Gerontol Soc Work 2018;61(2):171–92. Available at: https://doi.org/10.1080/01634372.2018.1427645.

Royal Australian College of General Practitioners (RACGP). Guidelines for preventive activities in general practice [Internet]. 9th ed. Melbourne, Australia: 2018. Available at: https://www.racgp.org.au/clinical-resources/clinical-guidelines/key-racgp-guidelines/red-book

Royal Children's Hospital (RCH). Parents' Evaluation of Developmental Status (PEDS). [Internet]. Melbourne, Australia: Updated 2019. Available at: https://www.rch.org.au/ccch/peds/.

Shain B. Suicide and suicide attempts in adolescents. Pediatrics 2016;138(1):e20161420.

Shute RH, Slee PT. Child development : theories and critical perspectives. International Texts in Developmental Psychology. Hoboken, NJ: Taylor & Francis; 2015 [cited 2019 Mar 7].

Silins E, Horwood LJ, Najman JM, et al. Adverse adult consequences of different alcohol use patterns in adolescence: an integrative analysis of data to age 30 years from four Australasian cohorts. Addiction 2018;113(10):1811–25.

Sinnott J, Hilton S, Wood M, et al. Does motivation affect emerging adults' intelligence and complex postformal problem solving? J Adult Dev 2016;23(2):69–78.

Sodian B, Kristen-Antonow S. Declarative joint attention as a foundation of theory of mind. Dev Psychol 2015;51(9): 1190–200.

Steinberg L, Icenogle G, Shulman EP, et al. Around the world, adolescence is a time of heightened sensation seeking and immature self-regulation. Dev Sci 2018;21(2):1–13.

Wood D, Crapnell T, Lau L, et al. Handbook of life course health development. In: Halfon N, Forrest CB, Lerner RM, et al. editors. Handbook of life course health development. Cham, Switzerland: Springer; 2017. pp. 123–43.

Woolfenden S, Goldfeld S, Raman S, et al. Inequity in child health: the importance of early childhood development. J Paediatr Child Health 2013;49(9):E365–9.

World Health Organization (WHO). WHO child growth standards. Geneva, Switzerland: WHO; 2014. Available at: www.who.int/childgrowth/standards/en/.

WHO Multicentre Growth Reference Study Group. WHO Motor Development Study: Windows of achievement for six gross motor development milestones. Acta Paediatr 2006;450:86–95.

Zauche LH, Mahoney AED, Thul TA, et al. The power of language nutrition for children's brain development, health, and future academic achievement. J Pediatr Health Care 2017;31(4): 493–503.

Chapter Four
Cultural safety

Written by Leonie Cox and Chris Taua

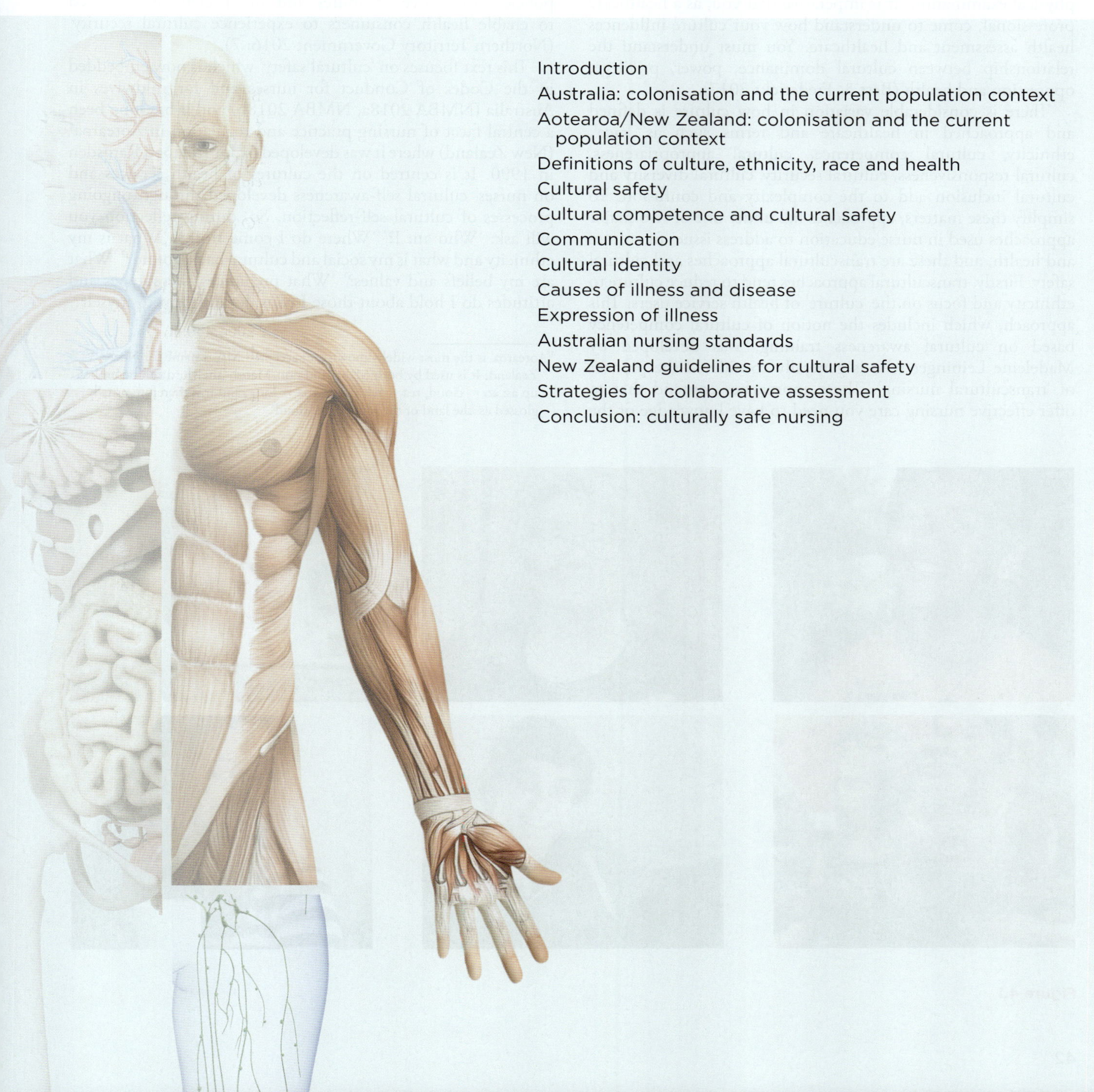

INTRODUCTION

Over the course of your nursing professional education, you will study human developmental tasks and much about human health across the life span. You will learn to conduct numerous assessments, such as a complete health history, mental health assessments (e.g. psychosocial history, mental status, suicide risk), nutritional assessments, pain assessments and physical examinations. There are many factors that influence health; for example, personal, social and political history, environment, government policy and practice, racism, gender, gender identity, age, class and other sociocultural circumstances (Figure 4.1). However, depending on your reactions to the person seeking your care, there may be wide variations in the information you gather in these assessments and in the findings of the physical examination. It is imperative that you, as a healthcare professional, come to understand how your culture influences health assessment and healthcare. You must understand the relationship between cultural dominance, power, privilege, oppression and health (Best & Fredericks 2017).

There is considerable variation in how culture is defined and approached in healthcare and terms such as 'race', ethnicity, cultural competence, cultural appropriateness, cultural responsiveness, cultural security, cultural diversity and cultural inclusion add to the complexity and confusion. To simplify these matters, approaches fall under one of two major approaches used in nurse education to address issues of culture and health, and these are transcultural approaches and cultural safety. Firstly, transcultural approaches tend to reduce culture to ethnicity and focus on the 'culture' of health service users. This approach, which includes the notion of cultural competency based on cultural awareness training, was developed by Madeleine Leininger who is generally considered the pioneer of 'transcultural nursing'. These approaches contend that to offer effective nursing care you need to have knowledge of the cultural heritage, language requirements and culturally based health and illness beliefs and practices of the people for whom you are caring. Cultural responsiveness also falls under this approach (Northern Territory Government 2016).

In this chapter, our focus is not on the culture of others, as we agree with the Australian national review of Multicultural Nurse Education in 2001 which reported that Leininger's work was 'criticised as being too focused on the culture of the "other": presenting cultures as static and deterministic' (Department of Education, Science & Training 2001). Cultural capability, yet another framework, has aspects of a transcultural approach but like cultural safety, it works with issues of power, discrimination and oppression (Bennett 2013). Another related model is cultural security which 'refers to the embedded structures, policies, workforce attributes and other elements required to enable health consumers to experience cultural security' (Northern Territory Government 2016: 7).

This text focuses on 'cultural safety' which is now embedded in the Codes of Conduct for nurses and for midwives in Australia (NMBA 2018a, NMBA 2018b) and it has long been a central facet of nursing practice and regulation in Aotearoa[1] (New Zealand) where it was developed by Dr Irihapeti Ramsden in 1990. It is centred on the cultures of health services and on nurses' cultural self-awareness developed through ongoing processes of cultural self-reflection. So, during reflection you will ask: 'Who am I?' 'Where do I come from?' 'What is my ethnicity and what is my social and cultural background?' 'What are my beliefs and values?' 'What prejudices, stereotypes and attitudes do I hold about those I consider different to myself?'

[1]'Aotearoa' is the most widely known and accepted Māori name for New Zealand. It is used by both Māori and non-Māori. The word can be broken up as: ao = cloud, tea = white and roa = long, and it is therefore usually glossed as 'the land of the long white cloud'.

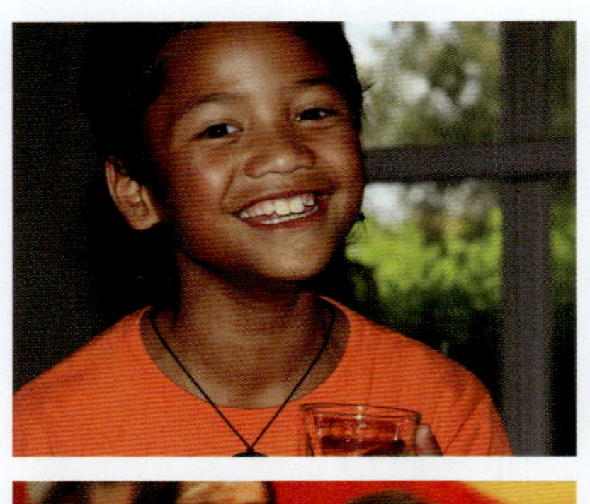
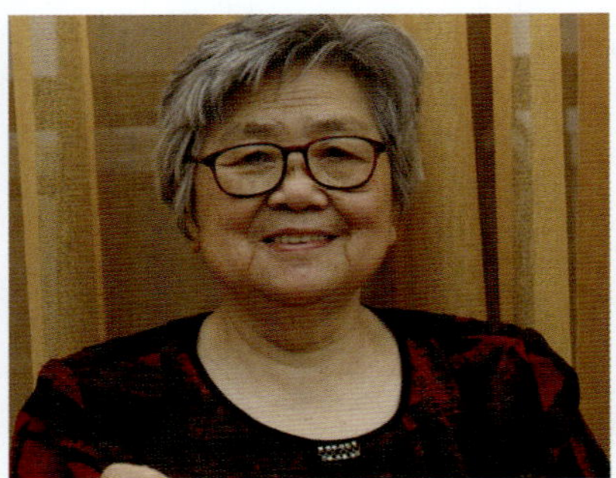
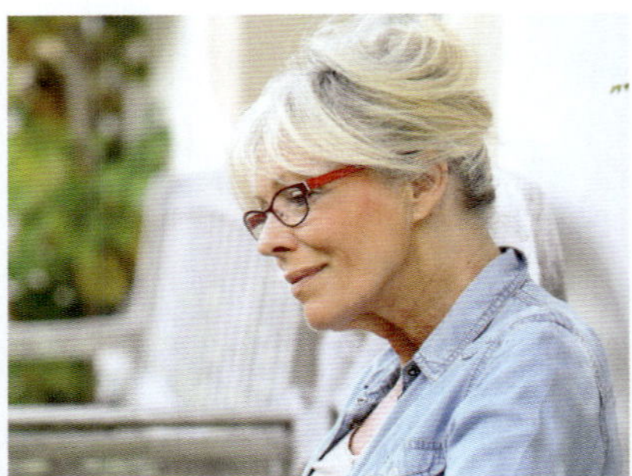
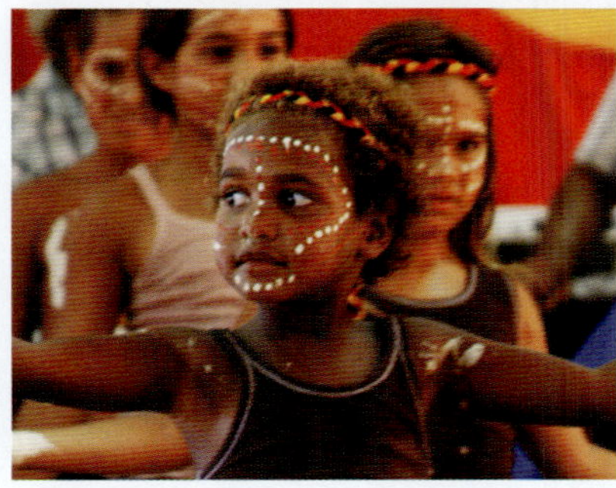
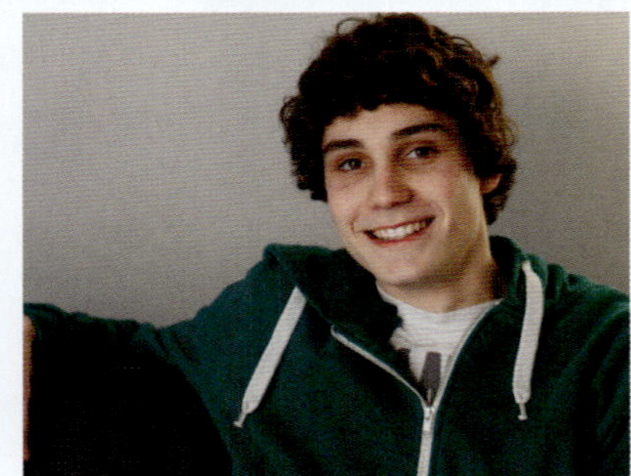
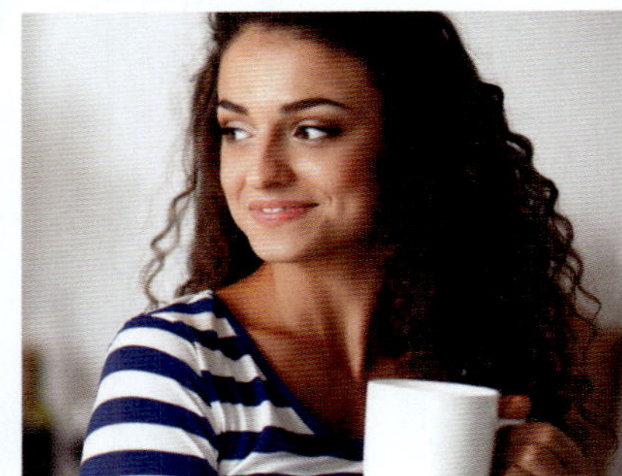

Figure 4.1

'How might my cultural identity impact on this person?' 'Have I really listened to how this person experiences pain or have I made assumptions about them, what they are saying or their behaviour?' So cultural safety is not about cultural practices of service users but is about how institutions treat people differently. A focus on the current social crisis in healthcare for groups such as immigrants and Indigenous[2] people in political terms is a central feature of providing culturally safe care, so you will also need to become knowledgeable about the history of your country and how it functions socially and politically to impact on the health of those in your care. A comment from an Australian Indigenous student following a unit on cultural safety in a Bachelor of Nursing Program reveals these concerns:

> The best aspect of this unit for me was having a subject that I understand and can relate to being Indigenous. We have come a long way from not being citizens in our own country and all the rest of it to have my people fight for rights and it is a huge thing for me as a Murri to see my people and culture be recognised and educating mainstream Australians about it because it obviously needs to be done.

The purpose of this chapter is to: introduce the population contexts of Australia and Aotearoa/New Zealand; consider the relationship between health and culture in Australian and Aotearoa/New Zealand demographic contexts; define culture, race, ethnicity and health; consider ideas of cultural competence and cultural safety; describe the position on Indigenous issues and cultural assessment of the Nursing and Midwifery Board of Australia and the Nursing Council of New Zealand; discuss the steps to cultural safety and strategies to achieve it; and describe methods for cultural considerations in health assessment.

AUSTRALIA: COLONISATION AND THE CURRENT POPULATION CONTEXT

Given the history of colonisation in Australia, the population is comprised of First Nations peoples, descendants of European colonisers and more recent migrants. Before discussing more fully how culture and healthcare interact it is important for nurses planning to work in Australia to understand the context of their work in terms of the populations they will be serving. This is true for both international and domestic nurses. In Cox's experience (Cox 2007), the former often have little understanding of Australian populations and their histories and the latter have variable levels of historical knowledge and a mix of attitudes towards various population groups. Some people carry entrenched and unexamined attitudes towards Indigenous Australians, mainstream[3] Australians or migrants. In the case of attitudes towards Indigenous Australians, these may in part be due to their lack of experience and exposure to specific Indigenous contexts, or to their lack of knowledge about Indigenous history, as reflected in this comment from a student:

> I was surprised to see the number of students that had never had any interaction with Indigenous Australians or travelled outside their birth city. It was good to see them able to discuss their own culture and learn of the suffering still inflicted on Indigenous persons. I later saw it as a relevant topic to those students.

Most people, however, are well aware that Australia is now a multicultural society, but what is perhaps less well known is that before the British began the colonisation of Australia in 1788, some 500 Indigenous language groups had lived here for up to 80,000 years (Clarkson et al 2017, Cox & Taua 2017). Further, Indigenous people were not the aimless wandering nomads so often depicted. Pascoe (2014:121–2) notes: 'these journals revealed a much more complicated Aboriginal economy than the primitive hunter–gatherer lifestyle we had been told … Hunter–gatherer societies forage and hunt for food and do not employ agricultural methods or build permanent dwellings; they are nomadic … I came across repeated references to building dams and wells, planting, irrigating and harvesting seed, preserving the surplus and storing it in houses, sheds or secure vessels, creating elaborate cemeteries and manipulating the landscape'. Indigenous people lived in well-defined socioeconomic, political, land-owning units as Cox and Taua note (Cox & Taua 2017). From the perspective of Indigenous people then, the 200-odd years since colonisation is but a moment in their overall history. This point is important because it explains why it is that Indigenous Australians consider themselves to be First Nations or Status People; that is, it is why they have specific and enduring rights in Australia.

Many non-Indigenous Australians lack knowledge of or refuse to accept Australia's black history and either support or are unaware of the state's ongoing discriminatory approaches towards Indigenous people. Author Cox has, over the past 13 years, taught Australian history and contemporary issues in an undergraduate program to several thousand students. Countless discussions show that many see colonisation as a single event that occurred over 200 years ago and find it difficult to understand why it is that 'historical' issues remain fresh for Indigenous people. In Australia, colonisation is an ongoing process and it continues to be played out in government approaches to Indigenous people forming what is called neocolonialism.[4] Unlike the situation in Aotearoa/New Zealand (see below), the colonisation of Australia was enacted under the legal fiction of terra nullius (empty land) which, in the minds of the newcomers, morally justified the takeover of the land with its subsequent impact on Indigenous peoples. The war over land saw thousands of Indigenous people die in retaliatory massacres by the colonists while restricted access to food sources and the imposition of an incoming population resulted in starvation, neglect and introduced diseases. Many Indigenous people still see themselves in a state of war that continues to be unrecognised and undeclared by the state.

[2]The term 'Indigenous' is used in this chapter for brevity; however, it should be noted that Indigenous people of mainland Australia and the Torres Strait Islands comprise many different groups with language group names and other terms that they use to refer to themselves. Indigenous people also use terms to refer to themselves that are roughly based on state boundaries: New South Wales: Koori, Goorie, Koorie, Coorie, Murri; Victoria: Koorie; South Australia: Nunga, Nyungar, Nyoongah; Western Australia: Nyungar, Nyoongar; Northern Territory: Yolngu (Top End); Anangu (Central); Queensland: Murri; Tasmania: Palawa, Koori. The term 'Aboriginal and Torres Strait Islanders' tends to be used most often but remember that both the Torres Strait Island context and the mainland context are informed by locally specific cultural and historical backgrounds and are extremely diverse. The term may also be used to refer to Māori who identify as Indigenous to Aotearoa/NZ.

[3]'Mainstream' is used to refer to members of the dominant culture in Australia.

[4]See, for example, the Northern Territory Emergency Response 2007 and the Stronger Futures Legislation that extended until 2022 (Perche 2017).

To this day, Australian governments do not afford Indigenous people the dignity of truly recognising them as the original owners with whom the negotiation of a treaty and reparation for war crimes should properly be held and finalised.

Further, it was said of the Australian Indigenous cultures and the incoming colonisers that it would be hard to find more differing understandings of the world and humans' place in it than those held by the original owners and the newcomers. For Indigenous peoples, country (place) was and is the source of identity and the basis of their cosmological understandings of the universe; for the newcomers, it was merely a resource to be exploited. The current crisis in Indigenous health that we see today is profoundly related to dispossession and removal from kin and country and related traditions, including language and ceremonial (religious) life, which often reduced Indigenous people to the status of slaves and fringe dwellers in their own land during the nineteenth and twentieth centuries. Many were deterred from hunting and gathering traditional foods as they saw their countrymen and women shot, poisoned or harassed if they attempted to access lands that they had been using for thousands of years. Instead, Indigenous people were forced to live on poor quality rations such as white flour, sugar and the fatty remains of meat unwanted by whites. Substances such as tea, tobacco and alcohol were introduced as a form of 'payment' for the menial work performed, entrapping the residents into cycles of addiction to sugar, alcohol and tobacco that we see today in the often-repeated poor population health status of Indigenous Australians.

The 20th century brought complex legislative frameworks in all states and territories that attempted to control every aspect of the lives of Indigenous people, first under the banner of 'protection' since the authorities assumed that Aboriginal people would 'die out'. As in Aotearoa/New Zealand, the authorities were concerned about increasing numbers of those they conceived of as 'mixed-race'[5] children and they set about developing policy and practice to remove 'fair-skinned' children from their Aboriginal parents and kinship groups: those now generally known in Australia as 'the Stolen Generations' following a national enquiry into the removal of Indigenous children from their families (see Human Rights and Equal Opportunity Commission (HREOC) 1997). When the state came to terms with the fact of continued Aboriginal existence, the policy changed to assimilation where the goal was to train the Stolen Generations, and Indigenous people more generally, to live like whites. In these complex processes, families were fragmented by institutionalisation on government or mission reserves and reformatory schools and by marginalisation from the workforce, education and health services (HREOC 1996, 1997, Kidd 1997, Reynolds 1982, Rintoul 1993). Indeed, health services were involved in some of these processes. The result is that since health services are largely run by governments, attending them is often resisted, as the experiences are bound up in fear and a lack of trust towards health services (Cox 2007, Forsyth 2007, Best & Fredericks 2017). Historical processes, such as deeming petty misdemeanours a crime under the special laws on missions and reserves, also saw the widespread criminalisation of Indigenous populations that we still see today in the overrepresentation of Indigenous people at all levels of the criminal justice system (Russell & Cuneen 2018).

Although in the late 1970s the special laws in the states and territories for Indigenous Australians began to be changed, the ideal of true self-determination is difficult to achieve without a treaty or proper political representation. Space does not permit us to discuss Native Title and Land Rights here and the ongoing struggles for people to be recognised in these processes, given the many different contexts in which they live. Students are referred to Ritter (2009) for further information on these topics. The federal government finally made a national apology to Indigenous Australians in 2008; however, adequate concrete compensation has never been realised.

It is also important to understand that Aboriginality or Indigenous identity is not about skin colour but is about relationships. As Gee et al (2014:59) state: 'Family and kinship systems have always been central to the functioning of traditional and contemporary Aboriginal and Torres Strait Islander societies. These systems are complex and diverse and serve to maintain interconnectedness through cultural ties and reciprocal relationships'. Because of the lack of trust and reciprocal relationships between mainstream health services and Indigenous Australians, the latter began to set up their own primary healthcare services from the 1970s. These are known as Aboriginal Medical Services and their peak body, the National Aboriginal Community Controlled Health Organisation (NACCHO), supports the nationally accepted means of determining Aboriginality. The means of determining has three parts and all are needed for Aboriginality to be recognised: descent (the individual can prove that a parent is of Aboriginal or Torres Strait Islander descent); self-identification (the individual identifies as an Aboriginal or Torres Strait Islander); and community recognition (the individual is accepted as such by the Aboriginal or Torres Strait Islander community) (NACCHO 2007).

In 2016, the Australian Bureau of Statistics (ABS) estimated that there were 649,200 Indigenous Australians, being 2.8% of the population. Ninety-one per cent of the Indigenous population identified as Aboriginal, 5% identified as Torres Strait Islander and 4.1% identified as both. The median age of Indigenous people is 23 compared to 38 for the non-Indigenous population. In 2016, 35% of all Aboriginal and Torres Strait Islander people lived in major cities and 20% lived in rural areas with a total of 81% living in non-remote areas, while the proportion of Indigenous people rises the more remote the area (ABS 2016b).

Another important factor for you as professional nurses is that more than one in five Australians was born overseas which means that you, your colleagues and those seeking your services will come from a range of ethnic, national and cultural backgrounds and have variable social positions as Australian born, as migrants or as someone with experiences of seeking refuge or asylum. According to the ABS 2019 the proportion of the population born overseas changed from 27% to 29% of the total population. Nevertheless, those born in England continue to be the largest group of overseas born residents (4.0% of the total population) (ABS 2019).

Since communication is central to nursing care it is important that you understand that there is a multiplicity of languages in Australia. One in ten spoke an Indigenous language at home

[5]The concept of race (a social construction) is discussed later in this chapter.

and 150 Indigenous languages were spoken in 2016 (ABS 2016a). Sixteen per cent of the total Australian population did not speak English at home. The 2016 Census (ABS 2016c) 'shows that two-thirds (67%) of the Australian population were born in Australia. Nearly half (49%) of Australians had either been born overseas (first generation Australian) or one or both parents had been born overseas (second generation Australian). In 2016, there were over 300 separately identified languages spoken in Australian homes. More than one-fifth (21%) of Australians spoke a language other than English at home. After English, the next most common languages spoken at home were Mandarin, Arabic, Cantonese and Vietnamese. Tasmania had the highest rate of people speaking only English at home (88%), while the Northern Territory had the lowest rate at 58%. The 2016 census shows Australia's religious diversity with Christianity remaining the most commonly reported religion (52.1% of the population). The Islamic population with 2.6% of the total population was the second largest religion, closely followed by Buddhism (2.4%) (ABS 2016b). Something that many Indigenous and mainstream Australians have in common is religion, as 73% of Indigenous Australians who answered the question about religion in the census were of a Christian denomination (ABS 2006).[6]

AOTEAROA/NEW ZEALAND: COLONISATION AND THE CURRENT POPULATION CONTEXT

Most people living in Aotearoa/New Zealand know something of the history of the land, in as much as Māori settled Aotearoa/New Zealand from the Pacific over 1000 years before European explorers started arriving. Pre-European contact saw Māori as a people deeply connected to the land and natural world around them (Consedine & Consedine 2001). Their societal life structures were based on kinship and tribal affiliations; laws were based on custom. When the British began their antipodean colonising they initially opted for the larger continent of Australia and it was the sealers and whalers who set up temporary residence in New Zealand. Eventually, settlers arrived and by the early 1800s the population of Europeans was believed to be around 2000. Numbers of Māori at that time were estimated to be around 125,000 (Waitangi Tribunal n.d.).

In 1838, the British sought to annex Aotearoa/New Zealand due to numerous unscrupulous purchases of Māori land and the lawlessness that had arisen among the people. On 6 February 1840, a treaty was drafted (the Treaty of Waitangi) and signed by the English and approximately 45 Māori Rangatira (chiefs). In addition, a Māori text of the treaty (Te Tiriti O Waitangi hereinafter referred to as Te Tiriti) was taken to northern parts of the country and copies were sent to other areas of the land to obtain additional Māori signatures. In signing Te Tiriti, the chiefs are believed to have yielded their sovereignty to the Queen of England in exchange for the Queen's protection and the granting to Māori the same citizenship rights, privileges and duties enjoyed by the citizens of England. Te Tiriti also guaranteed Māori possession of their land; however, with a stipulation they could sell their land only to the Crown. Te Tiriti was to recognise New Zealand at that time as one nation but two peoples: Māori and non-Māori, mainly European settlers and their descendants. There has been a great deal of debate over the ensuing years about translations between the two versions which were not fully correct and therefore interpreted differently by many of the Māori chiefs who originally signed Te Tiriti.

Initial reading of Te Tiriti seemed to promise benefits for both sides, but when more and more settlers arrived, they wanted to buy land. If Māori did not wish to sell, conflict would eventuate. Many lost their lives in the wars that erupted. But it was not only the wars that eroded the Māori population; it was also the diseases introduced by the Europeans to which Māori had little or no natural immunity. Loss of land also saw many living in poor conditions in makeshift camps with poor sanitation. By 1900, the Māori population had dropped to an estimated 45,000 (Consedine & Consedine 2001) and Māori were seen by the settlers to be a 'disappearing race'. Their tikanga (general behaviour guidelines for daily life and interaction in Māori culture, commonly based on experience and learning that has been handed down through generations) was also being eroded.

The intent and provisions of the Treaty of Waitangi were largely ignored until the 1970s, when legislation was introduced requiring statutory bodies and government to undertake their responsibilities in a manner consistent with the founding promises of the treaty. In 1975, the Waitangi Tribunal (see www.waitangi-tribunal.govt.nz/) was established to consider claims by Māori against the Crown regarding breaches of principles of the treaty and to make recommendations to the government to provide recompense. Since 1985, the tribunal has been able to consider acts and omissions by the Crown dating back to 1840. This has provided Māori with an important means to have their grievances against the actions of past governments investigated. Aside from these actions and grievances, attention and awareness is now also on the aforementioned health and social disparities, and there is a focus on improving the health and social status of Māori while recognising and respecting all aspects of cultural being.

The legacy from those early years is a society with 'major ethnic and cultural disparities in health status and most other markers of Indigenous wellbeing' (Kearns et al 2009). As well as alienation from land, Māori experienced impacts on their language (te reo) as a first language and their cultural way of being, their tikanga. They are overrepresented in nearly all negative social and health statistics; for example, unemployment, poverty, housing, income, education, youth suicide rates and general health and wellbeing. Kearns et al (2009:124) suggest that the processes of colonisation such as that which Māori experienced resulted in the 'denigration, marginalisation and alienation' of the very essence of their culture. Consedine and Consedine (2001:218) suggest that as a result of this colonisation '… the infrastructure of New Zealand society is structured to deliver white privilege. Only the exotic features of Māori culture were encouraged, where they benefited the country in areas such as tourism and sport'.

While the majority of early settlers were British, since that period people have arrived from Europe as well as Asia. In the second half of last century, following the world wars, a significant migration of people from the Pacific began (Khawaja et al 2007). The population of Pacific peoples in New

[6] We have so far been unable to locate more recent statistics on this matter.

Zealand grew quite rapidly during the late 1960s and early 1970s and caused a great deal of racial tension at times with both Māori and non-Māori groups. An important aspect of reducing this tension and ultimately accepting Pacific groups was the formation of partnerships with various community groups and activities as well as an increase in intermarriage. By the late 1990s, a large proportion of Pacific people were born in New Zealand and increasingly their children were also of Māori and other ethnic descent. The other major population group to appear was from Asia. Arrival of Asian groups actually predates the Pacific groups although in much smaller numbers. Many arrived in the late 19th century during gold rush days. Later in the 20th century, the number of different Asian groups increased dramatically and at the 2006 census they had exceeded the Pacific groups in population numbers. Much more recently, refugees and other settlers from Africa and the Middle East have arrived.

The diverse generations born and arriving in New Zealand since the first colonial settlers have afforded opportunities for miscegenation (a very old term referring to the process by which children are born to parents who were assumed to be of different 'races') of New Zealand's population groups (Khawaja et al 2007). As suggested earlier, although colonial thinking was that Māori would eventually disappear or be absorbed into the European population, this assumption has been discredited. However, it is this thinking that firmly influenced the collection of official statistics for much of the 20th century. Khawaja et al (2007) refer to the routine assignment of 'ethnic grouping on the basis of ancestry (degree of blood), with little or no regard to lifestyle, culture or beliefs'. As we discuss further below, these concerns also characterised the Australian situation.

The census of 2018 revealed that in a population of almost 4.7 million people, 74% identified themselves as being of European ethnicity, 16.5% Māori, with the remainder being Asian (15.1%), Pacific Islander (8.1%), Middle Eastern, Latin American, African (1.5%) and other (1.2%) (Stats New Zealand 2020). The apparent anomaly in these figures is caused by people identifying with more than one ethnic group. Because people can identify with more than one ethnicity, the total number of ethnic responses may be greater than the number of people. Consequently, understanding ethnicity is important, and having a mutual understanding of this might be even more important. This is, however, not so simple and later in this chapter we explore the ideology of ethnicity.

Suffice to say in summary that Indigenous groups have their own structural, institutional and interpersonal philosophies and practices from which they operate. Nonetheless, colonised societies such as Aotearoa/New Zealand and Australia develop to fit the lifestyle, values, priorities and beliefs of the incoming dominant cultures and so the culture of the colonisers becomes the norm in society's main institutions such as health, education, welfare, corrections, the media and so on. It is this kind of sometimes hidden but always present cultural dominance and unexamined privilege that the practice of cultural safety, discussed below, seeks to overcome. For example, in Australia, the National Health and Hospitals Reform Commission (NHHRC) (2008) noted that 'Generally, the health system delivers services in a way that is better suited to the needs of the broader population rather than the particular needs of Aboriginal and Torres Strait Islander people'. Given the preventable deaths and poor health outcomes Indigenous Australians continue to experience in the Australian Health Care System, there is no reason to think this has changed in the ensuing years (National Justice Project n.d., NACCHO 2019). Just consider the case of Ms Dhu (Fogliani 2016, 2018) who died in police custody after being taken in for unpaid fines, or that of Gurrumul Yunupingu (Davidson 2016), an internationally renowned singer whose internal bleeding was neglected for 8 hours by health professionals who made misguided assumptions that alcohol was the cause of his ill health, or that of Naomi Williams (Zhou 2019), who was pregnant and sent home 18 times after seeking help before dying from a treatable infection.

DEFINITIONS OF CULTURE, ETHNICITY, RACE AND HEALTH

Before we can begin to consider cultural issues as they relate to professional nursing practice, we need to be clear about what we mean by the various terms used in this context. The common terms used include culture, ethnicity, race and health. While there are numerous definitions of these terms, we have taken a constructionist view referring to the notion that humans create ideas about culture, ethnicity, race and health. That is, such concepts do not just appear from nature but are constructed by humans to serve certain purposes at certain times, so cultural safety is underpinned by the theory of social constructionism (Ramsden 2002).

Culture

Some definitions of culture focus on material culture: art, dress, artifacts and so on, while others focus on the capacity of humans to symbolise their world and experience through, for example, language, religion and kinship. Many definitions discuss cultures as 'bounded wholes' where members share systematised/patterned values and beliefs. We particularly like the definition in Kluckhohn and Kelly (1945:63) as it indicates the **importance of history** for our cultural identity and it is clear that culture is created and acts as a **potential** guide to action: 'By culture we mean all those historically created designs for living, explicit and implicit, rational, irrational, and nonrational, which exist at any given time as potential guides for the behavior of men … culture is constantly being created and lost'. Such definitions can be contrasted with other versions which suggest that cultures are unvarying, bounded canons of beliefs and practices that all members of a society embrace to an equal degree.

Our view of culture is grounded in the idea that cultures are dynamic and adapt to new circumstances and that they are learned, that is, one is **born into a culture, not born with culture**. Further, we assume that culture is strategic since we emphasise or de-emphasise aspects of our culture depending on current needs and circumstances. So, we are less interested in Culture (for example, high art or classical artistic traditions) and more interested in culture as the everyday meanings and motivations in peoples' lived experience, how they make sense of life experiences such as illness and explain it to themselves. That is to say, in cultural safety, culture is in the interaction between **worldviews** (values, beliefs, etc.) and **lifeworlds** (everyday life and the context in which it is experienced).

Further, for our purposes, culture includes but is not just about ethnicity and customs such as food, dress and religion, beliefs and values; it addresses differences in socioeconomic status, age, gender, gender identity, sexual orientation, ethnic origin, citizenship/migrant/refugee status, religious beliefs, values, disability and power relations (Ramsden 2002). It is crucial that you are able to distinguish ethnicity from culture. To do this, think about the culture of nursing or policing, for example, which have nothing to do with ethnicity, food and so on but are about ways of doing things, thinking about things and understanding things. Does this mean all nurses do and think the same thing when faced with a particular situation or set of circumstances? NO! Culture is always learned, dynamic, changing and strategic. It is negotiated and expressed and understood differently by individuals who identify with a particular cultural group. So it follows from the above that we often have multiple cultural identities where we might identify primarily as a woman, or as a mother, or as a feminist, or as a footballer, or as LGQBTI+, or as a nurse and as a working class Australian with English or some other ethnicity. Our culture influences the many tiny and significant decisions we make in everyday life that then determine what actions we take. Part of your challenge is to bring your cultural assumptions to mind, so you can understand why you act the way you do, particularly in your professional life as a nurse. We discuss cultural assumptions further below.

Ethnicity

In current usage, the term ethnicity is generally used to refer to the ethnic group or groups a person identifies with or feels they belong to. It is also now recognised that individuals may identify with more than one ethnic group. As indicated above, ethnicity can be part of culture but is not the same thing as culture. Ethnicity refers to socially constructed group identification or belonging based on familial descent (kinship) and history and traditions in language, food, dress and so on. In multicultural Australia—with Aboriginal people and Torres Strait Islanders being the Indigenous population—non-Indigenous Australians are still reluctant to speak of ethnicity and ethnic differences in relation to their own identities. Many New Zealanders and Australians no longer feel any links to the cultures to which their ancestors belonged but do not have a well-established or well-recognised alternative ethnic identity, either. An example of this is the term 'New Zealand European' often used on data collection sheets; there are now many generations of New Zealanders who feel no linkage to their European ancestors and express a reluctance to note this term in relation to their ethnicity (Statistics New Zealand 2013). People in this situation may say things like 'I don't have an ethnic identity', 'I am a New Zealander' or 'I'm just Australian'. At the beginning of a unit on cultural safety, Bachelor of Nursing students were asked to tell the group about their cultural and ethnic identity. Consider this comment by a student of European descent in her reflection: 'Learning about cultural safety was great! Never actually sat down and thought about my own personal culture before. Very rewarding!'

This way of thinking, that culture and ethnicity is only about 'others', stems from the fact that many non-Indigenous Australians come from generations of people born in Australia, a country with a long tradition of seeing ethnicity and culture as belonging solely to 'people of colour' or to 'the others from elsewhere' not realising that, ethnically speaking, this includes them. We only have to reflect on the term 'culturally and linguistically diverse' background; commonly rendered as CALD in government policies in Australia. It is a catch-all phrase to describe immigrants and implies that culture and diversity belong to immigrants, not to 'us'. An Australian internet search using CALD will yield many hits that make this point evident. Further, newcomers are expected to assimilate into the mainstream culture, as is particularly evident in the process of becoming an Australian citizen, when it is necessary to sit a citizenship test (see www.citizenship.gov.au/).

Early thinking in both Australia and Aotearoa/New Zealand around ethnicity was related to biological lineage only. To take the Aotearoa/New Zealand example, if your father was 'full Māori' and your mother non-Māori, you were considered by default ethnically 'half-Māori' regardless of your cultural beliefs, upbringing or cultural affiliations. A similar concept used in Australia was 'half-caste' to refer to someone with a parent who the state deemed to be a 'full-blood Aborigine' and a parent who the state deemed to be white; the term, along with related terms such as 'quarter-caste' and 'octoroon', are considered highly insulting to Indigenous Australians who recognise them as a form of identity policing that seeks to control who can and cannot identify as Aboriginal and to reduce cultural identity to base biological ancestry (Bond 2014). Interestingly, these terms are never applied to white people, revealing an underlying assumption about the purity of white ancestral lines which of course is nonsense, particularly as there is no such entity as different biological races, a point we turn to below.

Race

Race is commonly perceived by many as a way to identify differences not only in skin colour and physical attributes but also in language, nationality and religion. According to Rapport and Overing (2007), the idea of race became strong in the Middle Ages as a result of travel lore from ancient Greece and Rome. As they say, 'the imagery of the brutish giant—the naked, cannibalistic, Wildman … caught the imagination of medieval Europe'. These images were applied to European lower classes and 'such "inferiorisation" of excluded others became a constant throughout the development of European thought' (Rapport & Overing 2007). In the 1940s, scientists began to realise that the 'racial atlas' of humans did not match what was being learnt about human genetics (Montagu 1962). That is, there are no significant genetic variations within the human species to justify some kind of grouping of 'races'. Although the concept of race insists there is some genetic significance that creates variations in skin colour, we know that race has no scientific merit outside of this sociological classification.

However, as Jablonski (2013:1) cautions:

> Today one of the biggest concerns is the reinvention of clinical concepts of race, based on inaccurate generalizations about the susceptibility of people to certain disease risks. If clinical constituencies redefine and repackage the races as real biological entities, then we face a new era of scientific racism no less frightening than the first. Clinical authorities hold a sanctified place in American society and are capable of creating a new

reality of labeled races that will be widely believed and promulgated because it is 'for the good'.

The idea that race is a social construct is becoming more widespread, but that doesn't diminish scientific racism as a real concept in the minds of many people who want to believe in it. Nor does it lessen the lived experience of racism today. Racist beliefs, anchored in the scientific racism of a bygone era, persist today but are mostly hidden because it is socially and politically unacceptable to air them.

This type of race thinking is sometimes called 'scientific racism' despite there being no scientific basis to these ideas. In fact, Templeton argues that more similarity is found between Europeans and sub-Saharan Africans and between Europeans and Melanesians than between Africans and Melanesians despite the similarities in appearance of the latter groups (Templeton 1998, 2002, 2007). Templeton (2013:262) concludes:

> Much of the recent scientific literature on human evolution portrays human populations as separate branches on an evolutionary tree. A tree-like structure among humans has been falsified whenever tested, so this practice is scientifically indefensible. It is also socially irresponsible as these pictorial representations of human evolution have more impact on the general public than nuanced phrases in the text of a scientific paper. Humans have much genetic diversity, but the vast majority of this diversity reflects individual uniqueness and not race.

Nonetheless, race categories are often used to justify the exploitation of one group by another. So, just like the concepts of health and culture, race is a **social construct** and, since there are no distinct evolutionary lineages among humanity, there is no biological basis for race, as in evolutionary terms all humans are modern humans and there is only one human race, genetically speaking. Believers in scientific racism see health inequality as natural and inevitable and engage in 'blame the victim' thinking that sufferers 'brought it all on themselves'. Such claims are then used to justify and perpetuate structural inequality when we know that social marginality is the result of specific policies, laws, historical events and cultural contexts.

Historically, the concept of race was used to support claims by Europeans that they were superior to all other people and so had the right to control other people and to take their land, as happened in Australia and New Zealand. This assumed superiority of some groups over others is also called 'social Darwinism', a theory advanced by Herbert Spencer who applied biological evolutionary theory to social life (see Box 4.1) and linked it to ideas such as the Great Chain of Being (see Box 4.2) (Jeynes 2011). Because dominant cultures are so used to thinking in terms of race, it is hard for many to accept that the variation in how humans look can be understood in terms of genetic adaptation to environments and to familial descent and is not evidence of the existence of discrete races of humans. Racism then is treating people, not on the basis of shared humanity but on the basis of assumed 'race'.

Finally, there is one more issue concerning race that some readers may find confusing. In a strategic reversal and rejection of inferiorisation, belonging to an Australian Aboriginal 'race' is a source of pride amongst Indigenous Australians. These circumstances are hardly surprising given that Indigenous Australians have been distinguished, categorised and subordinated since colonisation because of notions that they were a separate (and inferior) race and, like many non-Indigenous Australians, many believe that there is a biological basis to race. When someone identifies as a particular race based on history, nationality and geography, their right to reclaim this social construct and use it in this way to identify and differentiate themselves can only be legitimate. Clearly, there are differences between people in terms of culture, ancestry and language and different nationalities depending on where one has full citizenship rights. There are differences, too, in opportunity and social experience, all of which contribute to differences in health, which we turn to now.

BOX 4.1 Race Overview

Historically, the concept of 'race' was used to say some people were inferior to others

- At first, women were considered to be inferior to men, then 'people of colour' were placed lower than white women and so on. See Box 4.2

'Social Darwinism' applies biological evolution to the evolution of societies; linked to the idea that white people are superior

- 'Whites' claim that they are destined or have the right to rule over others
- At their worst, ideas of the superiority of white people led to Hitler's fanatical eugenics and justified all forms of imperialism, as happened in the European settlement of Australia and the accompanying concept of terra nullius.

BOX 4.2 The So-Called Great Chain of Being and its Misguided Social Hierarchy

Great Chain of Being

- God
- Angels
- Demons
- Man
- Woman
- Animals
- Plants
- Minerals

Misguided racial hierarchy

- Anglo Saxons/Europeans
- Asians
- Africans
- Aborigines

Health

Willis and Shandell (2011) discuss the development of notions such as 'health', demonstrating that concepts we take as givens are constructed by humans. For our purposes, it is important that you understand that *health is not just about the absence of disease* as it may be defined in western medical terms but is about the whole person within their life context. This contextual aspect is captured in the following definition which was articulated in the development of Aboriginal and Torres Strait Islander health policy:

> (Health) 'means not just the physical wellbeing of an individual but refers to the social, emotional and cultural wellbeing of the whole Community in which each individual is able to achieve their full potential as a human being thereby bringing about

the total wellbeing of their Community. It is a whole of life view and includes the cyclical concept of life–death–life'. (Department of Aboriginal Affairs, 1989: x)

For Māori, 'health' is also realised through an understanding of various holistic health models. One commonly used model, Te Whare Tapa Wha, is known as the 'four cornerstones of health'. This approach compares health to the four walls of a house (a Whare), in which all four walls are necessary to ensure strength and symmetry (Durie 1994). It can be applied to any health issue affecting Māori from physical to psychological wellbeing. Looking after all aspects of wellbeing (the four walls) are **taha wairua** (spiritual), **taha hinengaro** (mental and emotional), **taha tinana** (physical) and **taha whanau** (family) considerations. Together all four are necessary and when in balance, they represent 'best health'. Accordingly, if any one of these components is deficient this may impact negatively on a person's health or, metaphorically speaking, affect the integrity of the house (Durie & Te Kingi 1997). Interestingly, Ramsden clarified that the four walls symbolised in Durie's model do not constitute an ancient whakatauki (reference point or maxim) since the model was initially constructed for nursing to 'assist in healing the division between biomedicine and an integrated approach to human care' (Ramsden 2002). Ramsden argued that this rather individualistic model did not consider social determinants such as education, unemployment, racism and powerlessness issues that are vitally connected to health. However, the model has prevailed and still informs Māori health policy. It is the framework for Māori and Iwi health and disability service providers and clinicians (Pitama et al 2007). What is important is that, when using this model, nurses think beyond the individual and see them within the whole context of their life and the impacts that broader social issues have on health.

Another holistic model used in Aotearoa/New Zealand is the Fonofale model created by Karl Pulotu-Endemann, a Samoan mental health nurse living and working in Aotearoa/New Zealand. The Fonofale presents a similar metaphor of a house (fale in Samoan) to that of Te Whare Tapa Wha in incorporating the concepts of spiritual, physical, mental wellbeing of an individual in the posts of the fale (a meeting house), the fourth post is unspecified and named 'other' and it is where the individual decides what is important to them (e.g. gender, sexual orientation, age, social class) (Figure 4.2). The fale is encapsulated in a circle where the concepts of environment, time and context are placed around outside the notions of culture and family (Pulotu-Endemann 2001). These terms are there to remind us that each of these interacts to produce change.

When health is understood from a western traditional biological model, the attention is on treating disease and symptoms with drugs and/or surgery. Today, nurses are taught

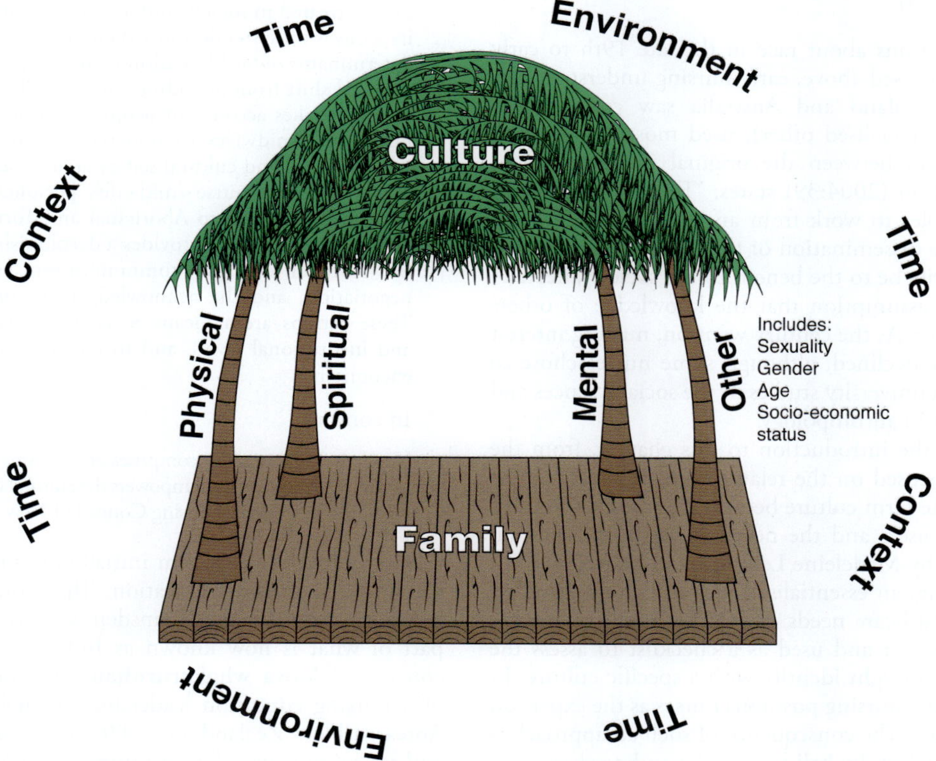

Figure 4.2
The Fonofale model.

to care for people within a holistic model, in which the focus is on finding the underlying cause of the symptoms and making lifestyle changes that are conducive to health. There is a strong emphasis on personal responsibility: the person is encouraged to be an active participant in their healthcare plan. The person, therefore, is the authority on their body and becomes the expert in caring for themselves. Mainstream holistic healthcare is similar to the Indigenous models previously discussed in acknowledging that all people have physical, intellectual, psychological, social, emotional and spiritual needs. The neglect of any of these areas may reduce the ability to withstand the effects of stress and ill health. However, when healthcare or health promotion is individualistic, it can result in blaming people in terms of their 'lifestyle'. Focusing solely on the behaviour of individuals denies the impact of social determinants and unhelpfully assumes that everyone has the same access to the conditions necessary to promote, create or maintain health.

Nevertheless, the relationship between the person and the healthcare professional is cooperative and complementary today compared to previous eras where patients were just expected to do as they were told. Such shifts in the relationship between nurses and patients can be enhanced by the model of cultural safety which also recognises that, not only might we all be culturally different, but also that society treats us differently, that there are social determinants of health. It is these dynamics that cultural safety seeks to address.

CULTURAL SAFETY

> Maa te matatau, ka tau te whiringa—with awareness comes choice (Clear 2008:4).

In keeping with notions about race in the late 19th to early 20th century as discussed above, early nursing understandings in Aotearoa/New Zealand and Australia saw culture as a racialised term (the racialised other), used mostly to refer to superficial differences between the original inhabitants and colonisers. Richardson (2004:39) states: 'There is a tendency for colonising peoples to work from an ethic of beneficence, to presume that the dissemination of their cultural norms and beliefs will necessarily be to the benefit to the society affected', with an associated assumption that the knowledge of others was therefore inferior. As the century went on, nursing interest in culture generally declined, although some nurses chose to explore it further in university studies in the social sciences and humanities, such as in anthropology.

As indicated in the introduction to this chapter, from the 1970s, interest refocused on the relationships between nurses and patients and the term culture became important to nurses and health service users and the new ideology, 'transcultural nursing', authored by Madeleine Leininger, was developed. In transcultural nursing, an essentialised idea of culture assumed culturally based healthcare needs of specific minority groups. These were to be learnt and used as a checklist to assess the needs of people who might identify with a specific culture. In this way, transcultural nursing positions nurses as the expert on the culture of 'others'. The consequence of such an approach is perhaps best summed up by bell hooks (the author chooses to not capitalise their name):

> No need to hear your voice when I can talk about you better than you can speak about yourself… Only tell me about your pain. I want to know your story. And then I will tell it back to you in a new way. Tell it back to you in such a way that it becomes mine, my own. Re-writing you I write myself anew. I am still author, authority. I am still colonizer, the speaking subject and you are now the center of my talk (bell hooks, 1990:208).

The key point is that the unique experience of the person becomes cannibalised by the nurse and the person is expected to behave according to stereotypical attributes that outsiders have deemed as 'typical' of their particular group according to these idealist notions of the group's culture. The transcultural model was not fully embraced in New Zealand or Australia, although the second author of this text can recall her nursing student days in Aotearoa when she was directed to visit various cultural (religious) sites to interview key leaders and ask them what their particular beliefs were around healthcare practices. She then had to write a report describing particular health preferences for these groups. An assumption made then was that, having undertaken this exercise, the nurse would know how to work with any person from that group if they come into hospital. However, we do not accept this argument. In this text, we focus on holism: students are facilitated to develop cultural self-awareness and to assess and respond to the biological, psychological and social needs of specific people and not to expect them to be idealised representatives of any cultural label or identity. The transition to culturally safe nursing from this point seems much simpler.

The NMBA (2018:15) defines cultural safety as:

> A philsophy of practice that is about how a health professional does something, not [just] what they do. It is about how people are treated in society, not about their diversity as such, so its focus is on systemic and structural issues and on the social determinants of health. Cultural safety represents a key philosophical shift from providing care regardless of difference, to care that takes account of people's unique needs. It requires nurses and midwives to undertake an ongoing process of self-reflection and cultural self-awareness, and an ackowledgment of how a nurse's/midwife's personal culture impacts on care. In relation to Aboriginal and Torres Strait Islander health, cultural safety provides a decolonising model of practice based on dialogue, communication, power sharing and negotiation, and the acknowledgement of white privilege. These actions are a means to challenge racism at personal and institutional levels, and to establish trust in healthcare encounters.

In contrast:

> Unsafe cultural practice comprises any nursing practice which diminishes, demeans or disempowers the cultural identity and wellbeing of the individual (Nursing Council of New Zealand, 2011:7).

Cultural safety is a term initially unique to Aotearoa/New Zealand and nursing education. The pioneer of the concept is Māori nurse Irihapeti Ramsden, so it is considered to form part of what is now known as Indigenous knowledges. The concept of **kawa whakaruruhau** (cultural safety) arose out of a nursing education leadership hui held in Christchurch, Aotearoa/New Zealand in 1989 in response to recruitment and retention issues of Māori nurses. The National Health and Hospitals Reform Commission guidelines were initially written by Ramsden in 1991 and further developed by a council committee and Ramsden. By 1992, the Nursing Council of

New Zealand (NCNZ) had adopted the following definition of cultural safety:

> The effective nursing practice of a person or family from another culture, and is determined by that person or family. Culture includes, but is not restricted to, age or generation; gender; sexual orientation; occupation and socioeconomic status; ethnic origin or migrant experience; religious or spiritual belief; and disability. The nurse delivering the nursing service will have undertaken a process of reflection on his or her own cultural identity and will recognise the impact that his or her personal culture has on his or her professional practice. Unsafe cultural practice comprises any action which diminishes, demeans or disempowers the cultural identity and wellbeing of an individual (Nursing Council of New Zealand, 2011:8).

Cultural safety relates to the experience of the recipient of a healthcare service. It provides health services' users with the power to comment on practices and contribute to the achievement of positive health outcomes and experiences. By this process, the meaning and experience of a person's illness is validated rather than challenged by biomedical understandings, and people retain the ability to provide feedback on any negative experiences. The process inherent in cultural safety education includes exploring the culture of nursing, recognising the impact that personal culture has on professional practice and the subsequent power relationship between nurses and the consumers of nursing care (NCNZ 2011). Cultural safety then '... contends that people are so diverse that teaching simple ritual and custom stereotypes, rigidifies ideas of culture and does not allow for human diversity (nurse or patient), nor does it take into account historical effects and socio-economic status' (Ramsden 1992, cited in Ramsden 2002:110). See Ramsden's explanation in Box 4.3.

Following the model of 'cultural safety', we support the position that describing the practices, beliefs and values of diverse population groups in nurse education should not occur, as this fosters an ideology of sameness and an erroneous assumption that culture is a simplistic concept which can be captured in lists of things to remember and do. It is this checklist mentality that is intrinsic to transcultural nursing. Think about yourself being the recipient of nursing care. What do you need the nurse to know about you? Will that be the same as the person in the bed next to you who may share your cultural identity and come from the same ethnic group as you and be the same age and gender as you?

BOX 4.3 Ramsden's Explanation (2002)

Cultural safety is based in a postmodern, transformed and multilayered meaning of culture as diffuse and individually subjective. It is concerned with power and resources, including information, its distribution in societies and the outcomes of information management. Cultural safety is deeply concerned with the effect of unequal resource distribution on nursing practice and patient wellbeing. Its primary concern is with the notion of the nurse as a bearer of his or her own culture and attitudes, and consciously or unconsciously exercised power.

What if there are two Vietnamese people in hospital? What if both identify as Vietnamese but one grew up in Australia and one in Vietnam? What if one happens to also identify as gay? What happens if one is a male and one a female? What happens if the male is 50 years old and very well off, but the woman is 16 years old from a poor family? Are their needs the same because they both identify as Vietnamese? We stress that each person is an individual with many unique ways of being. Therefore, the underpinning philosophy of cultural safety is that each person should be nursed 'regardful of all that makes them unique', encompassing the cultural, emotional, social, economic and political contexts in which they live (Ramsden 1993, 2002). Ramsden talks here about the nurse as a bearer of culture. She maintains that nurses must understand their own culture in order to fully respond to the culture of others.

Cultural safety in contrast with transcultural nursing is summed up well by this newly graduated registered nurse in Aotearoa/New Zealand reflecting on her own cultural safety education and initial puzzlement that she wasn't learning about specific cultures. She said in her summary of the course:

> I can remember finding the concepts quite confusing initially. I think it was because I had trouble distinguishing them from a more transcultural perspective, as I thought it was concerned with learning about specific cultural differences and applying those in practice to various groups (i.e. Māori, Muslims, etc.). My understanding of cultural safety now is about knowing my own assumptions and being mindful about how this might impact on interactions. ... On the whole though, cultural safety prevents us taking a one-size-fits-all approach to care (Helen A. 2010).

Self-reflexivity and self-awareness

As indicated in the definition of cultural safety above, the first step of the process is undertaking a process of self-reflection on one's own cultural identity and on social status, privilege and overall life experiences. It is by acknowledging and knowing our own beliefs, attitudes, assumptions, biases and values, and respecting that the beliefs and values of others are equally legitimate, that we minimise the impact of cultural dominance in healthcare. To truly understand how to relate to others, you must first understand yourself; this requires personal self-reflection and self-critique of the various personal, historical and social influences that impact on you. Students often find this process of self-awareness highly rewarding, as is shown in this student's comment: 'The personal reflection that was common in this unit opened a side of myself that I had never ventured to, made me really think where I had come from, etc'.

In Box 4.4 below are some guidelines to help you become culturally self-aware.

The misunderstandings

Many individuals when they first come across the term cultural safety immediately think about 'race' and ethnicity—of others! Common statements heard are 'when I nurse people, I don't see colour; we're all equal'; and 'I treat everyone the same'. The problem with this thinking is that treating everyone the same is a denial of inequality. If colour does not matter, then why are there so many disadvantages or even entitlements that go with skin colour or with a family's cultural membership? An individual's culture of origin and colour does matter in a culturally unsafe

BOX 4.4 Strategies for Self-Awareness

Think about the cultural group/s that you identify with.

- List them.
- What is your way of living within your group/s? (Think about age or generation, gender, gender identity, sexual orientation, occupation and socio-economic status, ethnic origin or migrant experience, citizenship or refugee status, religious or spiritual belief, and disability).
- Are there different groups within these areas that you can identify with?
- Think about the people, things and places that have socialised you.
- Who and what had impacts on you as you grew up (e.g. family, school, peers, environment, the mass media, popular culture, social media, politics, society in general/laws/policies/public health; national events/national celebrations; international events; global events)?
- What did you learn from these areas regarding healthcare practices?
- What experiences shaped you?
- Did you grow up with enough (love, food, friends, money, etc)?
- What values did you learn from your family?
- Were these the same as values held by your peers/teachers/friends/others?
- Do you hold the same values today as you did when you were growing up?
- Which values guide your decision making and how you see the world?
- Are values something that will affect your practice as a nurse?
- What customs/traditions do you and your families have around events such as births, birthdays, deaths, weddings, graduations?
- Are there certain cultural celebrations that your family participates in, e.g. Chinese New Year, Christmas, Ramadan?
- What types of food do you eat?
- What are your beliefs about the big questions in life? For example, how did the world get here? How did I get here? What is my purpose?
- Where did these beliefs come from? Are they changeable?
- What attitudes do you hold about people you see as different to yourself?
- Are there particular groups of people that you hold prejudices towards?
- How do these prejudices make you feel?
- Do you feel these prejudices are justified? What values are these based on?
- What could you do to change your prejudices?

world as it brings different privileges, assumptions and varying levels of influence over health outcomes. Consider this story by nurse academic Professor Margaret Pharris (2008:10):

> Upon arrival at the ED, I took a report from an excellent White nurse. She and a very fine White physician had both been caring for two young women who happened to arrive to the ED at the same time… both presented with 9 out of 10 flank pain, indicative of kidney stones. After receiving report, I went to assess the patients. The first… a White woman, was lying on a[n] ED bed dressed in a patient gown and wrapped in a warm blanket. She had received a significant amount of morphine… The second… a Black woman, was in a fetal position in the procto room, was still in her street clothes, and had received nothing for pain… it hit me that I might not have noticed this inequality had I not come directly from the dialogue about racism and healthcare. I wondered how much else I was missing.

The power you have as a nurse in a healthcare relationship is well illustrated here and often is about your proximity to the dominant cultures of the country you are in. As relayed earlier, such issues have not gone away as Australia has a National Justice Project (n.d.) that is investigating instances of racial profiling, discrimination and negligence experienced in the Australian Health Care System by First Nations Australians and some other marginalised groups. Health inequality and what could be considered criminal neglect such as in the cases of Ms Dhu, Naomi Williams and Gurrumul Yunupingu cited earlier, is directly related to the decisions nurses and other health professionals make when working with Aboriginal people and Torres Strait Islanders. That is, these unnecessary and tragic outcomes result from the culture of healthcare professionals, not from that of Aboriginal people and Torres Strait Islanders or any other service user. **It is circumstances such as these that make cultural safety a necessary approach in nursing care.**

Biculturalism was a key element of the postcolonial theory of cultural safety; biculturalism originally referred to the relationship between Māori and the colonising state—the Crown—gesturing to the inherent imbalance of power involved (Ramsden 2002). The concept has evolved somewhat to refer to interpersonal encounters in clinical practice which always involve at least two cultures; the culture of the nurse and the culture of the person being served. These interactions of course take place within the cultures of professions, services and institutions. The recognition that these multi-faceted cultural dimensions influence healthcare is in contrast to transcultural nursing that does not recognise the power differences inherent in its assumption that health service users are exotic, and that nurses and health systems are somehow free of culture. Furthermore, people have different abilities to exert control and influence in situations or relationships, especially in healthcare contexts that are inherently disempowering for service users who must rely on health service staff for their most intimate and basic needs. Imbalanced power relations also characterise our social, economic and political structures and institutions, with power and control usually being vested in members of dominant groups. See also Box 4.5 below.

Cultural safety education

The purpose of cultural safety in nursing education is not about the description of practices, beliefs and values of ethnic groups. As we now know, learning other peoples' rituals, customs and practices can be misleading and does not address the complexity of human behaviours and social realities. The assumption that cultures are simplistic in nature can lead to a checklist approach by health professionals, which negates the contingent, strategic, contextual and dynamic nature of culture. Cultural safety education is focused on the knowledge and understanding of the self, professions, institutions, history and power structures of society. To practice cultural safety nurses must understand their own culture, the sociopolitical context they are working in and the theory of power relations (Box 4.5 and Figure 4.3). Cultural safety education facilitates the ongoing process of reflection enabling clarification of values, beliefs and assumptions and how these sit with educational accreditation and with professional regulation, codes and standards. It gives a theoretical underpinning to professional nursing practice, introduces sociological approaches to health and health service, provides tools and a language to think with and so deepens the capacity for critical thinking on the part of nursing graduates.

BOX 4.5 The Process Towards Achieving Cultural Safety in Nursing Practice

- Know your own journey and accept that your way of knowing and doing things is not the only way
- Practice cultural humility—never assume you know
- Show respect—ask permission
- Engage community accompaniment—find allies, contact cultural advisors
- Always be respectful and collaborative
- Remember that therapeutic nursing practice is grounded in relationships
- Be aware of your timing. Ask yourself 'Is this the right time to be offering this particular form of service?'
- Focus on family-centred care when possible
- Remember the best solutions are found through collaborative problem solving rather than expert/authority
- Every situation should be reciprocal and mutual
- Be aware that old and new forms of colonialism deplete cultures, communities and roles for families
- Think about informed consent and what you may need to do to ensure it is understood
- Do not demean, disempower or diminish others' choices

In everyday work, cultural safety is underpinned by communication and recognition of the diversity in worldviews and lifeworlds (both within and between cultural groups including nurses' own). The impact of colonisation and ongoing marginalisation of minority groups or of those who choose to live differently to the expectations of the dominant culture creates diversity in lifeworlds—the context of life as it is experienced. As Ramsden put it: 'In the future it must be the patient who makes the final statement about the quality of care which they receive. Creating ways in which this commentary may happen is the next step in the cultural safety journey' (Ramsden 2002:181). This step remains a challenge in the implementation of cultural safety to date.

CULTURAL COMPETENCE VS. CULTURAL SAFETY

A new graduate nurse reflecting on her experience of learning about cultural safety as a student describes a clinical situation which helped her make sense of her learning and which nicely articulates the problem with the idea of cultural competency, the 'other' centred approach of transculturalism.

> Our cultural safety education was awesome; I just went to an in-service session at [hospital] a few weeks ago about cultural competency, and a lot of the stuff we were taught in nursing

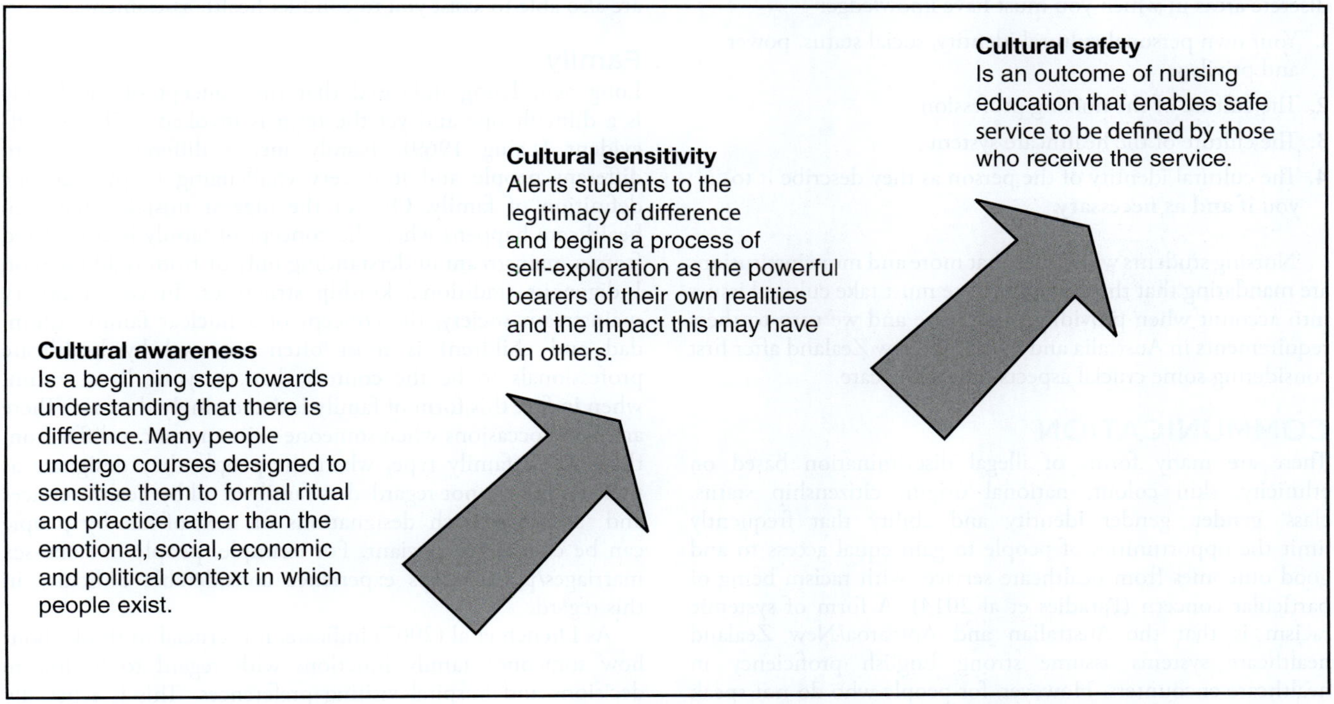

Figure 4.3
The process towards achieving cultural safety in nursing practice.

> school was in there. Cultural awareness is a massive aspect of my nursing … the best point I took from it all was to take cues from the patient/service user. If I'm not sure, I ask the service user directly … they know their own culture best. I recently had a patient with a 'Buddhist outlook on life'; I offered to access some support for him, but he declined stating that he doesn't practise; he just shares some of the same views. So it would have been inappropriate to access that support for him, however it was appropriate to ask. Another person might have the same view AND want to access spiritual support … I also think the biggest thing to cultural safety is being aware of my own culture. I'm working on this all the time and exploring it during my supervision (G Yates 2010).

As we indicated at the beginning of this chapter, there are many terms used to describe approaches to matters of culture and nursing care. Here we've focused on the approach of cultural safety. Many students come to courses on culture expecting to learn all about other cultures. The first author recalls a student who, after doing a unit of study on cultural safety, complained, 'I don't even know what that headdress that Muslims wear is called!' This, of course, brings us to the very crux of the matter: there are various and complex dimensions to head, face and body coverings with different words, meanings and applications amongst the many cultural and linguistic groups who wear them. With so many different cultures and so much variation within culture, it is actually quite impossible to expect students to learn about the diverse cultures that they'll encounter in their work. As Warren (2009) argues, generalising approaches to cultural competence conceptualises cultures as bounded wholes that exist out there to be learned, rather than appreciating culture as a broad, dynamic, relational concept as used in cultural safety.

Becoming culturally safe is not a one-lesson program but rather a lifetime journey of study and learning. There are several discrete areas in which you must have knowledge:

1. Your own personal cultural identity, social status, power and privilege
2. The culture of the nursing profession
3. The culture of the healthcare system
4. The cultural identity of the person as they describe it to you **if and as necessary.**

Nursing students will notice that more and more institutions are mandating that those who practise must take cultural issues into account when providing healthcare and we turn to these requirements in Australia and Aotearoa/New Zealand after first considering some crucial aspects of nursing care.

COMMUNICATION

There are many forms of illegal discrimination based on ethnicity, skin colour, national origin, citizenship status, class, gender, gender identity and ability that frequently limit the opportunities of people to gain equal access to and good outcomes from healthcare services with racism being of particular concern (Paradies et al 2014). A form of systemic racism is that the Australian and Aotearoa/New Zealand healthcare systems assume strong English proficiency in healthcare encounters. However, for people who do not speak English or for whom it is a second or third language, seeking care in healthcare settings such as hospitals, nursing homes, clinics, day care centres and mental health centres, language is a considerable barrier. As we saw in the section on population statistics, for each context there is a remarkable variety of languages used as a first language in Australia.

Those for whom English is not a first language experience barriers due to the system doing all its business in English. If there are challenges in speaking, reading, writing and understanding English the result is limited access to critical public health, hospital and other medical and social services to which all Australians are legally entitled. Many health and social service programs provide information about their services in English only. When persons whose first language is not English seek healthcare at hospitals or medical clinics in Australia and Aotearoa/New Zealand, they are frequently faced with receptionists, nurses and doctors who speak English only. These language barriers severely limit the ability to gain access to these services and to participate in programs. In addition, the language barrier often results in the denial of medical care or social services, delays in the receipt of such care and services or the provision of care and services on the basis of inaccurate or incomplete information. For example, with regard to medication, if a person who has a minimal understanding of English is not given clear, understandable instructions regarding their medication, adherence to or incorrect dosage may be a problem. Services denied, delayed or provided under such circumstances could have serious consequences for both users and providers of healthcare.

Chapter 7 describes in more detail how to communicate with people for whom English may be their second, third or fourth language or not in their lexicon at all, how to interact with interpreters and what services are available when no interpreter is available. It is vital that interpreters be present to not only serve to verbally translate the conversation but who are also able to assist you to conduct health assessments.

Family

Long ago, Laing indicated that the concept of the family is a difficult one and yet the term is invoked as if it is self-evident (Laing 1969). Family means different things to different people and it is very challenging to provide one definition of family. One of the biggest mistakes made in healthcare happens when the concept of family is considered from a mainstream understanding only or from rigid takes on Indigenous traditional kinship structures. In contemporary mainstream society, the concept of a nuclear family (mum, dad and children) is most often assumed by healthcare professionals to be the context that everyone lives within, when in fact this form of family is decreasingly the case. There are many occasions when someone's circumstances differ from the nuclear family type, when the people they designate as their family are not regarded as family at all by health services and, at times, such designations of next-of-kin by people can be considered deviant. For example, people in same-sex marriages/partnerships experience considerable difficulty in this regard.

As Drench et al (2007) indicate, it is crucial to think about how someone's family functions with regard to healthcare decisions and hospital visiting preferences. This is especially important for Indigenous people who may designate next-of-kin and family relatedness in ways that are unfamiliar to nurses whose knowledge base is grounded in the assumptions made by the cultures of medicine and nursing. These nurses focus their care decisions on individuals and, for many, the idea of traditional marriage and the notion of blood relatedness as the only acceptable conditions to name someone as next-of-kin is entrenched.

Consider the following scenario: A young Indigenous man was admitted to a metropolitan intensive care unit (ICU) following a serious suicide attempt. His mother rang author Cox (a non-Indigenous person) and requested that she go to the ICU to visit him. At the hospital ward, staff insisted that only close family could be allowed in to see the man. The problem was that the man's close family was several hundred kilometres away. An Indigenous health worker was at the ICU and knew of the first author's longterm relationship with the family and convinced the nurses that she should be allowed to visit. When the young man was moved to a general ward he introduced the author to the doctor as 'my sister'.

We encourage you to bring to mind through reflection your assumptions about family and then to think very differently about family to encompass varied circumstances. We know that in Australia and Aotearoa/New Zealand families are diverse, so it is important we understand how to ensure family is considered in a person's healthcare, according to the context they describe. Historically, due to government policy of the day, many Indigenous people were raised in institutions or with white families, and so consider the people with whom they were reared as family (HREOC 1997). Sadly, this is still true today due to the vast overrepresentation of Indigenous children in child removal practices (Australian Institute of Family Studies 2017). Think about who you include when you talk about your family. You might live with people you regard as family even though they are not blood relatives. Who can correctly say who someone's next-of-kin is? It might be the birth family or those who raised the person or perhaps the family they have created with a partner. There are numerous possibilities. How will you support same-sex relationships and struggles to have partners accepted as spouses and next-of-kin? How about those situations in which children have two mothers or two fathers? Think about people with longstanding estrangement from their families due to institutionalisation, imprisonment and other factors. There are times when the person may want staff members contacted because they are their significant others, rather than their birth families.

Making assumptions in this area of nursing care can bring significant distress for people. As nurses we must be aware that our cultural assumptions are just that—they are not universal ways of being. We need to be alert to different ways of understanding the world and social institutions such as the family, or the support networks that constitute family for many. In sum, the concept of family and who is important and who can make decisions for someone can be decided only by individuals in the context of their particular circumstances.

CULTURAL IDENTITY

Our identities as cultural beings are not only based on being born into a particular cultural milieu but are strongly related to our experiences as we go through life. Just as all members of a single family are not exactly the same and in fact may hold quite different beliefs and values to their parents and siblings, those who identify as belonging to a particular culture do not experience or express that cultural identity in the same way. In line with the broad definition of culture used in cultural safety, aspects of a person's cultural identity are influenced by their ethnicity, their gender and gender identity, their socioeconomic status, their ability or disability, their education and their status within society as members of either dominant or minority groups. In addition, many people socialised in cultures in which traditional healthcare resources are used, such as in some Indigenous communities, may prefer to use this type of care even when residing in a mainstream cultural setting with mainstream healthcare resources available. It is therefore not possible to teach you all the cultural dimensions that shape a person's worldview and create their lifeworld, as these will be unique to each individual. However, it is important that you understand that differences exist and are legitimate and that you know your own cultural identity and the assumptions that underlie it.

Spirituality and religion; philosophy and secularity

One possible component of a person's cultural identity is their religion or spirituality, but nurses must be mindful that many people hold an atheist and secularist philosophy and will not appreciate discussions of religion or spirituality. This point is especially relevant for those nurses who hold strong religious or spiritual beliefs themselves, as at times they may not appreciate how distressing it is to non-religious people to have these issues raised. Nonetheless, spiritual or religious factors are important to many people, but these dimensions are often overlooked in health assessment and this could be a particular problem for a secularist nurse who is indifferent to spiritual matters. If religion or spirituality is an integral component of a person's culture, their beliefs may influence their explanation of the cause(s) of illness, perception of its severity and choice of healer(s). In times of crisis, such as serious illness and impending death, religion and spirituality may be a source of consolation for the person and for their family. Religious or spiritual leaders may exert considerable influence on the person's decision making concerning acceptable medical and surgical treatment, choice of healer(s) and other aspects of the illness.

Religion and spirituality and a secular position play a most significant role in the ways people practise their healthcare. There are countless health-related behaviours promoted by nearly all religions or spiritualities and by rationalist secularity. The following list presents selected examples: ceremonies and rituals, meditating, exercising and maintaining physical fitness, getting enough sleep, being vaccinated, being willing to have the body examined, undertaking a pilgrimage for health reasons, telling the truth about how you feel, maintaining family viability, hoping for recovery, coping with stress, undergoing genetic screening and counselling, being able to live with a disability and caring for children (Levin 2001).

One's philosophy then, be it religious/spiritual or secular, gives a frame of reference and a perspective with which to organise information about health. Beliefs vis-à-vis health can constitute a system of health practices that are meaningful to the person. In healthcare settings, you will frequently encounter people who are searching for a spiritual meaning to help explain their illnesses or disabilities. Some healthcare providers find spiritual assessment difficult because of the abstract and personal nature of the topic, or due to their own secular position, whereas others feel quite comfortable discussing spiritual matters. Comfort with and mindfulness of your own beliefs is the foundation to effective assessment of the needs of others, including the ability to assess **whether or not a person requires a discussion of such matters.**

The concept and experience of time

Inherent in human socialisation are particular approaches to time. Bruce (2007) discusses alternative concepts of time. Western cultures, medicine and nursing are based on notions of historical time, which is conceived of as linear with a past, a present and a future; here, time is a resource that is going to run out at the end of life (Bruce 2007). So nurses and health systems are especially concerned with tasks and goals focused on 'now' and the future is perceived as vague or unpredictable. However, there are alternative concepts of time such as that time is circular, as evident in various religious traditions, so that life and death are interdependent and constitute a neverending cycle rather than coming to an abrupt end as in linear time. This idea is evident in the Indigenous definition of health quoted earlier (NAHSWP 1989).

These circumstances have implications for nursing care. As Bruce (2007:152) explains:

> If time is primarily understood as a resource that is running out and must be managed effectively, then nursing actions may be guided by values of efficiency and management in assisting families to use their precious time in the best way possible. A role for nurses becomes one of assisting patients to better understand what they need to do in preparing to die and using the remaining time wisely and effectively.

As this author argues, such an approach may prevent a person fully experiencing the now as they are rushed from one thing to the next. Bruce also clarifies that time is both a concept and an experience and that our perceptions of time shift depending on what is happening. We all know this from our own experience. As Bruce puts it, we are familiar with 'feeling the spaciousness of "free time" or the taut constriction of "running out" of time, the symmetry of "being timely", or the paradox of going beyond time' (2007:154). Thus, one of the major areas in which cultural conflicts between nursing culture and service users occur is the failure to understand that there is more than one way to perceive and experience time.

Further, the way people value time differently may impact on the way they assess priorities to do with their healthcare. There could be problems with keeping appointments, adhering to medication regimens or differing priorities where family business may take precedence over appointments and the use of resources on personal health. It is important that nurses seek to understand what is happening in people's lives [the lifeworld] to limit a sense of frustration and to prevent applying a nurse's own uncritical perceptions, values, assumptions and judgements to people's health and illness behaviours.

CAUSES OF ILLNESS AND DISEASE

Disease causation may be viewed in a number of ways, including biomedical, naturalistic or holistic, magico-religious and sociological perspectives or some combination of these.

Biomedical

The view that dominates health systems in Australia and Aotearoa/New Zealand is called the **biomedical** or **scientific** theory of illness causation. It is based on the assumption that all events in life have a cause and effect, that the human body functions more or less mechanically (i.e. the functioning of the human body is analogous to the functioning of a car), that all life can be reduced or divided into smaller parts (e.g. the reduction of the human person into body, mind and spirit) and that all of reality can be observed and measured (e.g. intelligence tests and psychometric measures of behaviour). Among the biomedical explanations for disease is the germ theory, which posits that microscopic organisms such as bacteria and viruses are responsible for specific disease conditions. Most educational programs for doctors, nurses and other healthcare providers embrace the biomedical or scientific theories that explain the causes of both physical and psychological illnesses. When people come to hospital they may react to this environment with various stages of culture shock, that is, a state of disorientation or an inability to respond to the behaviour of a different cultural group (in this case the culture of nurses and doctors) because of its sudden strangeness, unfamiliarity and incompatibility with their perceptions and expectations.

Naturalistic

Another way in which people explain the cause of illness is from a **naturalistic** or **holistic** perspective: the belief that human life is only one aspect of nature and is a part of the general order of the cosmos. People with this perspective may believe that the forces of nature must be kept in natural balance or harmony. The naturalistic perspective posits that the laws of nature create imbalances, chaos and disease. People embracing the naturalistic view may use metaphors such as the 'healing power of nature', and they may call the earth 'Mother'.

Magico-religious

Another major way in which people explain the causation of illness is from a **magico-religious** perspective. The basic premise is that the world is seen as an arena in which supernatural forces dominate. The fate of the world and those in it depends on the action of supernatural forces for good or evil.

Sociological

Sociological understandings of health and illness consider health and illness in their historical and social context and consider the social determinants of health which are beyond the capacity of single individuals to control, e.g. patterned inequality impacting on specific populations such as poverty, racism and other forms of discrimination, housing, employment, education and so on (Willis & Shandell 2011).

The variety of healing beliefs and practices used by the many populations found in Australia and Aotearoa/New Zealand far exceeds the limitations of this chapter. It is important, however, that you are aware of the existence of various practices and recognise that, in addition to folk practices, traditional practices such as Rongoa Māori (Māori healing) (Ministry of Health 2018), traditional Chinese medicine and Ayurveda are used along with many other complementary healing practices such as herbalism, homeopathy and acupuncture to name just a few.

Of course, it is possible to have a combination of worldviews, and many people are likely to offer more than one explanation for the cause of their illness. As a profession, nursing largely embraces the scientific/biomedical worldview, but some other aspects are gaining popularity, including techniques for management of chronic pain, such as acupuncture, herbal therapies, hypnosis, therapeutic touch and biofeedback. For cultural safety it is imperative that nurses engage in power sharing and be prepared to both listen to and respect how people understand and choose to treat their own illnesses.

EXPRESSION OF ILLNESS

Expression of pain

To illustrate the manner in which symptom expression may reflect our cultural background, let's use an extensively studied symptom—pain. Pain is a universally recognised phenomenon and it is an important aspect of assessment for people of various ages. Pain is a very private, subjective experience that is greatly influenced by our sociocultural background. Expectations, manifestations and management of pain are all embedded in sociocultural contexts. The definition of pain, like that of health or illness, is socially and culturally informed. The word pain is derived from the Greek word for penalty, which helps explain the long association between pain and punishment in Judeo-Christian thought. The meaning of painful stimuli, the way we define our situation and the impact of personal experience all help determine the experience of pain.

Some cross-cultural research has been done on pain with the acknowledgment that it may be perceived as a multidimensional experience. For example, Fenwick (2006) did work on the experience of pain amongst Central Australian Indigenous people. Pain has been found to be a highly personal experience, depending on cultural learning, the meaning of the situation and other factors unique to the person. Sussex (2016) observes that: 'Many things contribute to how we experience and express pain. Gender, age, education, socioeconomic status, the relative power of the participants in the conversation, and whether the person in pain is speaking in their mother tongue or another language all affect a person's experience of pain. Each of these factors can have a crucial impact on how we communicate about pain, and how we understand pain communication from others'.

Therefore, pain should be explored not only in consideration of the physical or psychological experience but also its social, spiritual and cultural perceptions. Silent suffering has been identified as the most valued response to pain by healthcare professionals probably based on the stoicism of the English stiff upper lip since western medicine and nursing arose from English culture. The majority of nurses are socialised to believe that in virtually any situation, self-control is better than open displays of strong feelings and such ideas lead to many poor outcomes and even death when assumptions are made by nurses and doctors about the veracity of someone's pain. They may be denied pain relief or treatment, as in some cases being investigated by the National Justice Project.

Disease prevalence

It is well known that neither health nor disease are distributed equally among segments of the population. For several generations, the mainstream population in Australia and Aotearoa/New Zealand has enjoyed improved health status. There continues to be major disparity in deaths and illnesses experienced by Indigenous people and other minority groups. Historically produced and currently reproduced poverty, lack of employment opportunities, poor housing, low levels of education and other socially marginalising issues such as **scientific, institutional and personal racism on the part of health services and society generally play a central role in health disparities.**

AUSTRALIAN NURSING STANDARDS

In 2016 the NMBA released the updated Registered Nurse Standards. On p. 1, it is stated:

> Registered nurse (RN) practice is person-centred and evidence-based with preventative, curative, formative, supportive, restorative and palliative elements. RNs work in therapeutic and professional relationships with individuals, as well as with families, groups and communities. These people may be healthy and with a range of abilities, or have health issues related to physical or mental illness and/or health challenges. These challenges may be posed by physical, psychiatric, developmental and/or intellectual disabilities.
>
> The Australian community has a rich mixture of cultural and linguistic diversity, and the *Registered nurse standards for practice* are to be read in this context. RNs recognise the importance of history and culture to health and wellbeing. This practice reflects particular understanding of the impact of colonisation on the cultural, social and spiritual lives of Aboriginal and Torres Strait Islander peoples, which has contributed to significant health inequity in Australia.

Of particular relevance are the following dimensions (NMBA 2016:3). A registered nurse:

> 1.3 respects all cultures and experiences, which includes responding to the role of family and community that underpin the health of Aboriginal and Torres Strait Islander peoples and people of other cultures
> 2.2 communicates effectively, and is respectful of a person's dignity, culture, values, beliefs and rights

- The NMBA (2018:8) Code of conduct for nurses specifies cultural safety:

> **3.1 Aboriginal and/or Torres Strait Islander peoples' health**
>
> Australia has always been a culturally and linguistically diverse nation. Aboriginal and/or Torres Strait Islander peoples have inhabited and cared for the land as the first peoples of Australia for millennia, and their histories and cultures have uniquely shaped our nation. Understanding and acknowledging historic factors such as colonisation and its impact on Aboriginal and/or Torres Strait Islander peoples' health helps inform care. In particular, Aboriginal and/or Torres Strait Islander peoples bear the burden of gross social, cultural and health inequality. In supporting the health of Aboriginal and/or Torres Strait Islander peoples, nurses must:
>
> **a.** provide care that is holistic, free of bias and racism, challenges belief based upon assumption and is culturally safe and respectful for Aboriginal and/or Torres Strait Islander peoples
> **b.** advocate for an act to facilitate access to quality and culturally safe health services for Aboriginal and/or Torres Strait Islander peoples, and
> **c.** recognise the importance of family, community, partnershop and collaboration in the healthcare decision-making of Aboriginal and/or Torres Strait Islander peoples, for both prevention strategies and care delivery.

See the National Aboriginal and/or Torres Strait Islander Health Plan 2013–2023.

See also Congress of Aboriginal and/or Torres Strait Islander Nurses and Midwives.

3.2 Culturally safe and respectful practice

Culturally safe and respectful practice requires having knowledge of how a nurse's own culture, values, attitudes, assumptions and beliefs influence their interactions with people and families, the community and colleagues. To ensure culturally safe and respectful practice, nurses must:

- **a.** understand that only the person and/or their family can determine whether or not care is culturally safe and respectful
- **b.** respect diverse cultures, beliefs, gender identities, sexualities and experiences of people, including among team members
- **c.** acknowledge the social, economic, cultural, historic and behavioural factors influencing health, at the individual, community and population levels
- **d.** adopt practices that respect diversity, avoid bias, discrimination and racism, and challenge belief based upon assumption (for example, based on gender, disability, race, ethnicity, religion, sexuality, age or political beliefs)
- **e.** support an inclusive environment for the safety and security of the individual person and their family and/or significant others, and
- **f.** create a positive, culturally safe work environment through role modelling, and supporting the rights, dignity and safety of others, including people and colleagues.

NEW ZEALAND GUIDELINES FOR CULTURAL SAFETY

Registered nurses are required to demonstrate competency specific to cultural safety to achieve initial registration, and subsequently in order to maintain a practising certificate from the Nursing Council of New Zealand (NCNZ). The following principles (Box 4.6) underpin cultural safety education (NCNZ 2011).

The NCNZ (2011) also stipulates the expected outcome of nursing education in New Zealand; that registered nurses are to

BOX 4.6 Nursing Council of New Zealand

Principle one

Cultural safety aims to improve the health status of New Zealanders and applies to all relationships through:

1.1 an emphasis on health gains and positive health outcomes

1.2 nurses acknowledging the beliefs and practices of those who differ from them. For example, this may be by: age or generation, gender, sexual orientation, occupation and socioeconomic status, ethnic origin or migrant experience, religious or spiritual belief, disability.

Principle two

Cultural safety aims to enhance the delivery of health and disability services through a culturally safe nursing workforce by:

2.1 identifying the power relationship between the service provider and the people who use the service. The nurse accepts and works alongside others after undergoing a careful process of institutional and personal analysis of power relationships

2.2 empowering the users of the service. People should be able to express degrees of perceived risk or safety. For example, someone who feels unsafe may not be able to take full advantage of a primary healthcare service offered and may subsequently require expensive and possibly dramatic secondary or tertiary intervention

2.3 preparing nurses to understand the diversity within their own cultural reality and the impact of that on any person who differs in any way from themselves

2.4 applying social science concepts that underpin the art of nursing practice. Nursing practice is more than carrying out tasks. It is about relating and responding effectively to people with diverse needs in a way that the people who use the service can define as safe.

Principle three

Cultural safety is broad in its application:

3.1 recognising inequalities within healthcare interactions that represent the microcosm of inequalities in health that have prevailed throughout history and within our nation more generally

3.2 addressing the cause and effect relationship of history, political, social, and employment status, housing, education, gender and personal experience upon people who use nursing services

3.3 accepting the legitimacy of difference and diversity in human behaviour and social structure

3.4 accepting that the attitudes and beliefs, policies and practices of health and disability service providers can act as barriers to service access

3.5 concerning quality improvement in service delivery and consumer rights.

Principle four

Cultural safety has a close focus on:

4.1 understanding the impact of the nurse as a bearer of his/her own culture, history, attitudes and life experiences and the response other people make to these factors

4.2 challenging nurses to examine their practice carefully, recognising the power relationship in nursing is biased toward the provider of the health and disability service

4.3 balancing the power relationships in the practice of nursing so that every consumer receives an effective service

4.4 preparing nurses to resolve any tension between the cultures of nursing and the people using the services

4.5 understanding that such power imbalances can be examined, negotiated and changed to provide equitable, effective, efficient and acceptable service delivery, which minimises risk to people who might otherwise be alienated from the service.

The full document Guidelines for cultural safety, the Treaty of Waitangi, and Māori health in nursing education and practice (amended and reprinted). Wellington: Nursing Council of New Zealand; 2011) is available at: www.nursingcouncil.org.nz/content/download/721/2871/file/Guidelines%20for%20cultural%20safety,%20the%20Treaty%20of%20Waitangi,%20and%20Maori%20health%20in%20nursing%20education%20and%20practice.pdf 'practise in a culturally safe manner, as defined by the recipients of their care'. They require that the nursing student will:

a. examine their own realities and the attitudes they bring to each new person they encounter in their practice;
b. evaluate the impact that historical, political and social processes have on the health of all people; and
c. demonstrate flexibility in their relationships with people who are different from themselves.

STRATEGIES FOR COLLABORATIVE ASSESSMENT

The first author of this chapter was alerted to the difficulties students in Australian nursing contexts have when it comes to appreciating the need for cultural assessment. Students often marked 'not applicable' beside an item that asked whether cultural considerations had been included in their care on an assessment form used in a clinical practicum. This was because students do not appreciate that every encounter has cultural elements, even if the person has the same personal cultural identity as the nurse; they would include the item only if the person was seen as an 'ethnic' other. Cultural safety, however, teaches that all encounters are bicultural as they include the culture of the nurse (with aspects of their identity drawn from the culture of nursing and their personal cultural identity) and the culture of the person. As Warren (2009) notes: '… information is not gained by specifically cultural questions and this is also an important tenet of cultural safety'. One tool for assessment is the LEARN model (Box 4.7).

Various authors warn of the problem of trying to teach, learn or assess cultural generalities (Warren 2009, Drench et al 2007) and instead refer to the work of medical anthropologist Arthur Kleinman who, rather than focusing on cultural generalisations, offers questions to elicit what he calls the 'client's explanatory framework'. To help you elicit information of relevance to the person we suggest the questions in Box 4.8 designed by Kleinman (1980).

In Box 4.9 we offer some additional questions.

In Box 4.10 there is the basis for all care of people from any background whatsoever.

BOX 4.7 The LEARN Model

L = Listen to the person's comments
E = Explain your interpretations of what you think they said and clarify if the interpretation is correct or needs to be changed
A = Acknowledge the importance of what the person is saying and what it means to them
R = Recommend strategies and collaborate with the person to develop interventions that include the cultural perspectives of the client
N = Negotiate and collaborate with the person and their significant others (e.g. family) to provide culturally safe care

Adapted from Berlin E, Fowkes W: A teaching framework for cross-cultural healthcare, *The Western Journal of Medicine*, 139(6):934–8, 1982. www.ncbi.nlm.nih.gov/pmc/articles/PMC1011028/pdf/westjmed00196-0164.pdf
Also cited in Warren BJ: Teaching the fluid process of cultural competence at the graduate level: a constructionist approach. In Bosher SD, Pharris MD (eds): *Transforming nurse education: the culturally inclusive environment*, New York, 2009, Springer.

BOX 4.8 Kleinman's Explanatory Framework

1. What do you call your problem? What name does it have?
2. What do you think caused your problem?
3. Why do you think it started when it did?
4. What does your sickness do to you? How does it work?
5. How severe is it? Will it have a short or a long course?
6. What do you fear most about your sickness?
7. What are the chief problems your sickness has caused?
8. What kind of treatment do you think you should receive? What are the most important results you hope to receive from the treatment?

BOX 4.9 Health Beliefs and Practices Assessment

1. How do you define health?
2. How do you rate your health?
3. Describe your illness to me.
4. What do you believe caused the illness?
5. How do you keep yourself from getting sick and what home remedies do you use?

BOX 4.10 Guide for Care

Preparing

Discover and understand your own social position, ethnicity, cultural values, biases, health beliefs and practices and those of the profession you belong to and the organisation/service you work for.

R.E.S.P.E.C.T.

Realise that you MUST know and understand your heritage
Examine people within the context of their cultural and social position
Select questions that are not complex and do not ask questions rapidly
Pace questions throughout any health assessment or health service encounter
Encourage people to discuss the meanings of health and illness with you
Check for the people's understanding and acceptance of recommendations
Touch can be therapeutic but you must respect people's personal preferences and boundaries—manners are a vital component of the relationships in healthcare

CONCLUSION: CULTURALLY SAFE NURSING

In your professional nurse education, you are now learning the contemporary scientific meanings of health and illness, but such knowledge is just one part of the art of nursing care. There are several steps that we must take in the lifelong practice of cultural safety. The integration of this knowledge into day-to-day practice will take time because many practitioners in the healthcare system are hesitant to adopt new ideas. Culturally safe nursing practice does not come instantly, certainly not after reading a chapter or several chapters or books on this specialised area. It is complex and multifaceted, and many facets change over time. It is confronting for many people to discuss issues such as racism, ageism, homophobia and various other biases, preconceptions and prejudices about specific ethnic, religious, sexual or socioeconomic groups. We have to admit and challenge our socialisation into these damaging ways of perceiving people. It is hard and yet rewarding to practise deep self-reflection on our family's background, social position and traditional beliefs and practices. It can be harder still to contemplate systemic racism and marginalisation arising from systems that are set up ostensibly to help and serve the public.

The first step in understanding the healthcare needs of others is to understand our own social position and cultural values, beliefs, attitudes and practices. The second step is to identify the meaning of health to the other person, being open to their interpretations, being flexible and aiming for the professional acquisition of trust.

Third, we must understand the culture of the healthcare delivery system, how it works, what it does, the meanings of various procedures and the costs and consequences to the public and to us as nurses. Fourth, we must be knowledgeable about the social backgrounds of people including experiences of immigration, racism, socioeconomic status, ageing and so forth. Fifth, we must be aware if English is not understood and of the resources available to help with interpreting.

This chapter is about developing a deep understanding that each person and nurse has their own reality, that these multiple realities are socially constructed and that they are informed by, but not reducible to, culture. **A central aim of this chapter is to change the way you see yourself and the world around you so you can impact positively on the power relations between nurses and service users and between service users and health services.** Further, we aim to establish an appreciation that there is as much variation within cultures as there is between cultures. Health contexts such as hospitals and the health professions such as nursing and medicine also have their own cultures. Your challenge is to work within these systems without diminishing, demeaning or disempowering any person (see Box 4.11).

We urge you to remember the many aspects of human experience connected to cultural safety: culture, ethnicity, religion, socialisation, population diversity, immigration, religion, demographic change, globalisation, health and illness, modern and traditional beliefs and practices, sociopolitical issues, education, sanitation, housing and infrastructure. The bibliography includes various books and selected websites to link you to further introductory material related to this content.

In concluding, we refer you to the reflections of eminent medical anthropologist Professor Arthur Kleinman which arose from his own experience of caring for his wife of 40 years who developed a debilitating neurological disorder. He sums up perfectly the enduring need for self-awareness in caring professions such as nursing:

> In my view, what is needed is reform of the very culture of contemporary biomedicine. We must train students and practitioners in critical self-reflection on that which limits their care-giving; in strategies and techniques aimed at opening a space for the moral acts of care-giving; and in the most concrete and practical acts of assistance, so that they never forget what care-giving actually means (Kleinman, 2009).

BOX 4.11 Cultural Safety Summary

- Cultural safety involves recognising nurses as the bearers of our own personal culture and that of the nursing profession and organisation
- Cultural safety is applicable in any context since all people have culture(s) and workplaces and professions also have cultures; it is not only relevant to Indigenous populations, although it is a form of Indigenous knowledge
- Cultural safety is achieved through a process of self-reflection and developing self-awareness on the part of nurses, other health professionals and organisations
- Cultural safety sees culture as learned, dynamic and strategic
- The definition of personal culture used in cultural safety includes dimensions such as ethnicity, age, sex, gender identity, class, education, attitudes and political, philosophical and religious beliefs
- Cultural safety requires that, as nurses, we are respectful of our colleagues' and service users' nationality, history and social experiences
- Cultural safety is in contrast to transcultural nursing care; cultural safety encourages nurses to deliver service with respect to people's' diverse experiences and needs
- Culturally safe care empowers people because it reinforces the idea that each person's knowledge and reality is valid and valuable. It facilitates open communication and allows people to voice concerns about nursing care that they may deem unsafe
- Cultural safety is political because it attempts to change health professionals' attitudes about their power relationships with service users and it actively promotes power sharing and negotiation. This is true also at organisational levels
- Cultural safety does not focus on how people are different to dominant cultures and norms but how they are treated in society
- Care may be deemed culturally unsafe if the person seeking service feels diminished, demeaned or disempowered or directly or indirectly dissuaded from accessing necessary care

BIBLIOGRAPHY

Australian Bureau of Statistics. Australia's population by country of birth. 2011a. Available at: www.abs.gov.au/ausstats/abs@.nsf/Products/84074889D69E738CCA257A5A00120A69?opendocument.

Australian Bureau of Statistics. Census shows growing Aboriginal and Torres Strait Islander population. 2016a. Available at: https://www.abs.gov.au/ausstats/abs@.nsf/MediaRealesesByCatalogue/02D50FAA9987D6B7CA25814800087E03.

Australian Bureau of Statistics. 2071.0 - Census of Population and Housing: Reflecting Australia - 2016b. Available at: https://www.abs.gov.au/ausstats/abs@.nsf/Lookup/by%20Subject/2071.0~2016~Main%20Features~About%20this%20Release~9999

Australian Bureau of Statistics. 2016 Census: Multicultural. 2016c. Available at: https://www.abs.gov.au/ausstats/abs@.nsf/lookup/Media%20Release3

Australian Bureau of Statistics. Migration, Australia, 2017-18, Number. 3412.0. 2019. Available at: https://www.abs.gov.au/ausstats/abs@.nsf/Latestproducts/3412.0Main%20Features22017–18

Australian Institute of Family Studies. The Family Matters Report 2017: Measuring trends to turn the tide on the over-representation of Aboriginal and Torres Strait Islander children in out-of-home care in Australia. 2017. Available at: https://aifs.gov.au/cfca/2018/05/07/growing-over-representation-aboriginal-and-torres-strait-islander-children-care.

Bennett J. Training mental health professionals in cultural capability: sustainability of knowledge and skills. Int J Cult Ment Health 2013;6(1):72—80.

Best O, Fredericks B. Yatdjuligin: Aboriginal and Torres Strait Islander nursing and midwifery care. Melbourne: Cambridge University Press; 2017.

Bond C. Andrew Bolt isn't a racist, but ... The Drum 25 March, 2014. Available at: www.abc.net.au/news/2014-03-25/andrew-bolt-isnt-a-racist-but/5344286.

Bruce A. Time(lessness): Buddhist perspectives and end-of-life. Nurs Philos 2007;8(3):151–7.

Clarkson C, Jacobs Z, Marwick B, et al. Human occupation of northern Australia by 65,000 years ago. Nature 2017;547(7663):306–10. doi:10.1038/nature22968.

Clear G. A re-examination of cultural safety: a national imperative (editorial). Nurs Prax N Z 2008;24(2):2–4.

Consedine R, Consedine J. Healing our history: the challenge of the Treaty of Waitangi. Auckland: Penguin; 2001.

Cox L. Fear, trust and Aborigines: the historical experience of state institutions and current encounters in the health system. Health History 2007;9(2):70–92.

Cox L, Taua C. Socio-cultural considerations and nursing practice. In Crisp J, Taylor C, Douglas C, et al, editors. Potter and Perry's fundamentals of nursing. 5th ed. Chatswood, NSW: Elsevier; 2017.

Davidson H. Gurrumul hospital row highlights Indigenous health obstacles. Guardian 2016. Available at: https://www.theguardian.com/music/2016/apr/14/race-row-rages-on-over-gurrumul-hospital-ordeal?CMP=share_btn_link.

Department of Education, Science and Training. National review of nurse education: multicultural nursing education, 2001. Canberra: Commonwealth of Australia; 2001.

Drench M, Cassidy Noonan A, Sharby N, et al. Psychosocial aspects of healthcare. Upper Saddle River, NJ: Prentice-Hall; 2007.

Durie M. Whaiora: Māori health development. New Zealand: Oxford University Press; 1994.

Durie MH, Te Kingi KR. A framework for measuring Māori mental health outcomes. A report prepared for the Ministry of Health. Palmerston North, New Zealand: Department of Māori Studies, Massey University; 1997.

Fenwick C. Assessing pain across the cultural gap: central Australian Indigenous peoples pain assessment. Contemp Nurse 2006;22(2): 218–27.

Fogliani R. Record of investigation into death of Ms Dhu. Coroner's Court of Western Australia; 2016. Available at: http://www.coronerscourt.wa.gov.au/_files/dhu%20finding.pdf.

Fogliani R. Inquest into the death of Ms Dhu. Coroner's Court of Western Australia; 2018. Available at: http://www.coronerscourt.wa.gov.au/I/inquest_into_the_death_of_ms_dhu.aspx?uid=1644-2151-2753-9965.

Forsyth S. Telling stories: nurses, politics and Aboriginal Australians, c.1900–1980s. Contemp Nurse 2007;24(1):33–44.

Gee G, Dudgeon P, Schultz C, et al. Aboriginal and Torres Strait Islander social and emotional wellbeing. In: Dudgeon P, Milroy H, Walker R, editors. Working together: Aboriginal and Torres Strait Islander mental health and wellbeing principles and practice. Canberra: Commonwealth of Australia; 2014.

hooks b. Choosing the margin as a space of radical openness. In: Yearning: race, gender, and cultural politics. Boston: South End Press; 1990. pp. 203–9.

Human Rights and Equal Opportunity Commission. Indigenous deaths in custody 1989–1996. Sydney: Commonwealth of Australia; 1996.

Human Rights and Equal Opportunity Commission. Bringing them home: a guide to the findings and recommendations of the National Inquiry into the Separation of Aboriginal and Torres Strait Islander Children from their Families. Sydney: Commonwealth of Australia; 1997.

Jablonski N. What is it about skin color? 2013. Available at: https://www.theroot.com/what-is-it-about-skin-color-1790895168

Jeynes WH. Race, racism, and Darwinism. EUS 2011;43:535.

Kearns R, Moewaka-Barnes H, McCreanor T. Placing racism in public health: a perspective from Aotearoa/New Zealand. GeoJournal 2009;74:123–9.

Khawaja M, Boddington B, Didham R. Growing ethnic diversity in New Zealand and its implications for measuring differentials in fertility and mortality. Wellington: Statistics New Zealand; 2007.

Kidd R. The way we civilise: Aboriginal affairs – the untold story. St Lucia, QLD: University of Queensland Press; 1997.

Kleinman A. Patients and healers in the context of culture: an exploration of the borderland between anthropology, medicine, and psychiatry. Berkeley, CA, 1980, University of California Press.

Kleinman A. Care-giving and the moral impoverishment of medicine. Project Syndicate; 2009. Available at: www.project-syndicate.org/commentary/kleinman1/English.

Kluckhohn C, Kelly H. The concept of culture. In: Linton R, editor. The science of man in the world culture. New York: Columbia University Press; 1945.

Laing RD. The politics of the family and other essays. Middlesex, UK: Penguin; 1969.

Levin J. God, faith and health: exploring the spirituality-healing connection. New York: John Wiley; 2001.

Ministry of Health. Rongoā Māori: Traditional Māori healing. 2018. Available at: https://www.health.govt.nz/our-work/populations/maori-health/rongoa-maori-traditional-maori-healing.

Montagu A. The concept of race. Am Anthropol 1962;64(5):919–28. Available at: www.americanethnography.com/article.php?id=36.

National Aboriginal Community Controlled Health Organisation. Aboriginality. 2007. Available at: www.naccho.org.au/aboriginal-health/definitions/.

National Aboriginal Community Controlled Health Organisation. The State of Aboriginal Health. 2019. Available at: https://www.naccho.org.au/about/aboriginal-health/the-state-of-aboriginal-health/.

National Aboriginal Health Strategy Working Party. The national Aboriginal health strategy. An evaluation report. Canberra: Department of Aboriginal Affairs; 1989.

National Health and Hospitals Reform Commission. A healthier future for all Australians. 2008. Available at: https://apo.org.au/node/2223

National Justice Project. Aboriginal Health Justice Project. n.d. Available at: https://justice.org.au/what-we-do/#aboriginal-health

Northern Territory Government. Northern Territory Health Aboriginal Cultural Security Framework 2016– 2026. Northern Territory Government; 2016. Available at: https://digitallibrary.health.nt.gov.au/prodjspui/bitstream/10137/730/8/Northern%20Territory%20Health%20Aboriginal%20Cultural%20Security%20Framework%202016-2026.pdf.

Nursing and Midwifery Board of Australia. Registered nurse standards for practice. 2016. Available at: http://www.nursingmidwiferyboard.gov.au/Codes-Guidelines-Statements/Professional-standards.aspx.

Nursing and Midwifery Board of Australia. Code of conduct for nurses. 2018a. Available at: https://www.nursingmidwiferyboard.gov.au/Codes-Guidelines-Statements/Professional-standards.aspx

Nursing and Midwifery Board of Australia. Code of conduct for midwives. 2018b. Available at: https://www.nursingmidwiferyboard.gov.au/Codes-Guidelines-Statements/Professional-standards.aspx

Nursing Council of New Zealand. Guidelines for cultural safety, the Treaty of Waitangi, and Māori health in nursing education and practice. Te whakarite i ngā mahi tapuhi kia tiakina ai te haumaru ā-iwi Regulating nursing practice to protect public safety. Wellington: Nursing Council of New Zealand; 2011.

Paradies Y, Truong M, Priest N. A systematic review of the extent and measurement of healthcare provider racism. J Gen Intern Med 2014;29:364. Available at: https://doi-org.ezp01.library.qut.edu.au/10.1007/s11606-013-2583-1.

Pascoe B. Dark Emu: Black seeds agriculture or accident? Broome, Australia: Magabala Books; 2014. ProQuest Ebook Central. Available at: https://ebookcentral.proquest.com/lib/qut/detail.action?docID=1675076.

Perche D. Ten years on, it's time we learned the lessons from the failed Northern Territory Intervention. The Conversation; 2017. Available at: http://theconversation.com/ten-years-on-its-time-we-learned-the-lessons-from-the-failed-northern-territory-intervention-79198.

Pharris MD. Inclusivity: attending to who is in the center. In: Bosher SD, Pharris MD, editors. Transforming nursing education: the culturally inclusive environment. New York: Springer; 2008. ProQuest Ebook Central. Available at: https://ebookcentral.proquest.com/lib/qut/detail.action?docID=423421.

Pitama S, Robertson P, Cram F, et al. Meihana model: a clinical assessment framework. NZ J Psychol 2007;36(3):118–125.

Pulotu-Endemann FK. Fonofale model of health. 2001. Available at: https://d3n8a8pro7vhmx.cloudfront.net/actionpoint/pages/437/attachments/original/1534408956/Fonofalemodelexplanation.pdf?1534408956

Ramsden I. Kawa Whakaruruhau: guidelines for nursing and midwifery education. Wellington: Nursing Council of New Zealand; 1992.

Ramsden I. Kawa Whakaruruhau: cultural safety in nursing education in Aotearoa (New Zealand). Nurs Prax N Z 1993;8(3):4–10.

Ramsden I. Cultural safety and nursing education in Aotearoa and Te Waipounamu. Unpublished PhD thesis. Victoria University of Wellington, New Zealand; 2002.

Rapport N, Overing J. Social and cultural anthropology: the key concepts. London: Routledge; 2007.

Reynolds H. The other side of the frontier: aboriginal resistance to the European invasion of Australia. Ringwood, VIC: Pelican; 1982.

Richardson S. Aotearoa/New Zealand nursing: from eugenics to cultural safety. Nurs Inq 2004;11(4):35–42.

Rintoul S. The wailing: a national black oral history. Port Melbourne: William Heinemann; 1993.

Ritter D. Contesting native title: from controversy to consensus in the struggle over Indigenous land rights. Sydney: Allen & Unwin; 2009.

Russell S, Cuneen C. As Indigenous incarceration rates keep rising, justice reinvestment offers a solution. The Conversation; 2018. Available at: http://theconversation.com/as-indigenous-incarceration-rates-keep-rising-justice-reinvestment-offers-a-solution-107610.

Statistics New Zealand. 2013 Quick stats. 2013. Available at: http://archive.stats.govt.nz/Census/2013-census/profile-and-summary-reports/quickstats-culture-identity.aspx

Statistics New Zealand. 2018 Census place summaries New Zealand. Available at: https://www.stats.govt.nz/tools/2018-census-place-summaries/new-zealand#population-counts

Sussex R. How different cultures experience and talk about pain. The Conversation; 2016. Available at: https://bodyinmind.org/cultures-pain/.

Templeton AR. Human races: a genetic and evolutionary perspective. American Anthropologist 1998;100(3):632–50.

Templeton AR. The genetic and evolutionary significance of human races. In: Fish J, editor: Race and intelligence: separating science from myth. Mahwah, NJ: Lawrence Erlbaum; 2002.

Templeton AR. Genetics and recent human evolution, Evolution 2007;61(7):1507–19.

Templeton AR. Biological Races in Humans. Stud Hist Philos Biol Biomed Sci Part C 2013;44(3):262–71. Available at: https://doi.org/10.1016/j.shpsc.2013.04.010.

Waitangi Tribunal Te ropu whakamana I Te Tiriti O Waitangi. Treaty of Waitangi. n.d. Available at: www.justice.govt.nz/tribunals/waitangi-tribunal.

Warren BJ. Teaching the fluid process of cultural competence at the graduate level: a constructionist approach. In: Bosher SD, Pharris MD, editors. Transforming nurse education: the culturally inclusive environment. New York: Springer; 2009.

Willis K, Shandell E. Society, culture and health: an introduction to sociology for nurses. 2nd ed. Melbourne VIC: Oxford University Press; 2011.

Zhou N. Naomi Williams's inquest: pregnant woman sent home too quickly, expert says. Guardian 2019. Available at: https://www.theguardian.com/australia-news/2019/mar/13/naomi-williams-inquest-pregnant-woman-sent-home-too-quickly-expert-says.

Websites

Australian Nursing and Midwifery Accreditation Council: www.anmc.org.au

Careers New Zealand for an interactive diagram of Te Whare Tapa Wha Model: www.careers.govt.nz/educators-practitioners/career-practice/career-theory-models/te-whare-tapa-wha/Indigenous health status: www.healthinfonet.ecu.edu.au/health-facts

National Aboriginal Community Controlled Health Organisation (NACCHO): www.naccho.org.au

National Council of Māori Nurses: www.Māorihealth.co.nz

New Zealand History online: www.nzhistory.net.nz/politics/treaty-of-waitangi

Nursing Council of New Zealand: www.nursingcouncil.org.nz

Chapter Five

Screening for family violence and abuse

Adapted by Rhonda Brown

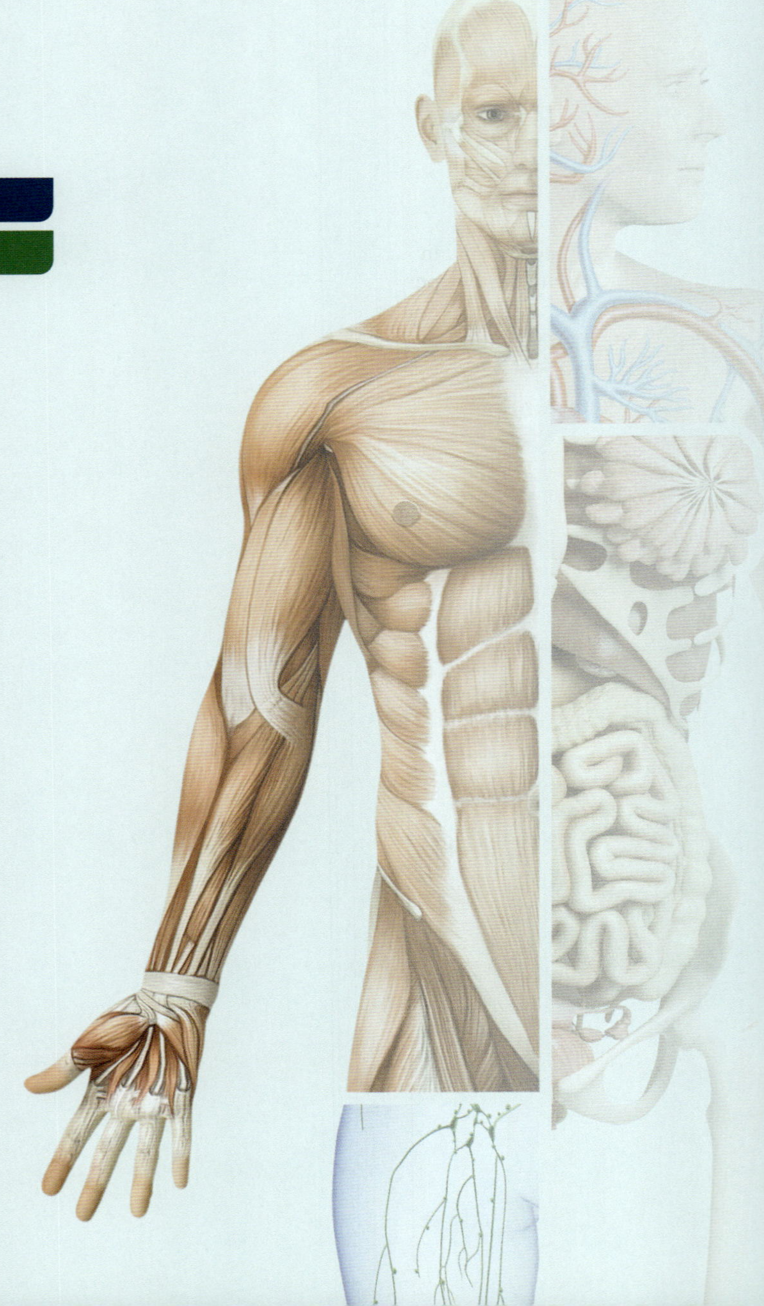

INTRODUCTION

Family violence is a significant determinant of health and health professionals have an important role in identifying individuals and families in their care who may be affected. Major nursing and medical organisations such as the Australian Nursing & Midwifery Federation (ANMF), New Zealand Nurses Organisation (NZNO), the Australian Medical Association (AMA) and the Royal Australian College of General Practitioners (RACGP) support the need for healthcare professionals to recognise, assess and respond to family violence. Nurses are often the first point of contact within the healthcare system for individuals and families affected by family violence and are therefore ideally situated to facilitate disclosure, assess needs and assist with access to relevant assistance and support.

TERMINOLOGY AND KEY CONCEPTS

Family violence defined

'Family violence' refers to violent behaviours directed towards a person, perpetrated by a family member, who may be a current or former intimate partner. It also includes acts of violence between an adult and a child or between siblings. The term family violence is now more commonly used in place of 'domestic violence' recognising the broader implications of violence perpetrated by family members. The term family violence is preferred by Aboriginal and Torres Strait Islander peoples as it covers extended family and kinship relationships (Australian Institute of Health and Welfare (AIHW) 2018).

Family violence is an ongoing pattern of behaviour aimed at controlling another person, for example by using behaviour which is violent and threatening or coercive that causes another family member to be fearful. In most cases, the violent behaviour is part of a range of tactics to exercise power and control over women and children (AIHW 2019a). There is a range of behaviours associated with family violence (see Table 5.1).

Intimate partner violence defined

Intimate partner violence is defined as any behaviour within an intimate relationship that causes physical, psychological, emotional or sexual harm. This includes:

- physical aggression such as hitting, kicking and beating
- psychological violence such as intimidation and constant humiliation
- forced intercourse and other sexual coercion
- various controlling behaviours such as isolation from family and friends, monitoring movements, financial control and restricting access to services (World Health Organization (WHO) 2017).

The lifetime prevalence of violent acts within intimate relationships is comparable for women and men, but repeated coercive, sexual or severe physical violence is perpetrated largely against women by men (WHO 2017). Intimate partner violence also occurs in same-sex relationships but much of the research to date has focused on heterosexual relationships.

Child abuse and neglect defined

Child abuse and neglect occurs when the behaviour of a parent, caregiver, other adult or older adolescent is outside the norms

TABLE 5.1 Behaviours associated with family violence

Emotional abuse	Any behaviour that deliberately undermines a person's confidence or self-esteem including intimidation, belittling, humiliation, repeated criticism, blaming and threatening, not allowing an individual to express their own feelings and thoughts, not allowing privacy and silence and withdrawing as a means of abuse
Verbal abuse	Screaming, shouting, name calling, put downs, sarcasm, ridicule and continual criticism in public or private
Social abuse	Isolation from family and friends, social networks and supports, continually putting friends and family down, being physically and verbally abusive in social settings, preventing contact with people who speak the same language or come from the same culture
Psychological abuse	Reckless driving, destroying possessions, abuse of pets in front of family members, making threats regarding custody of any children, threatening to harm children, asserting that the police and justice system will not assist
Economic abuse	Denying access to money. Withholding financial support needed for reasonable living expenses for an individual or children in their care when these family members are financially dependent. Making significant decisions without consultation, selling an individual's possessions without consent or incurring debt in their name
Spiritual abuse	Ridiculing or putting down another's beliefs or culture. Preventing participation in or belonging to a group or activity that is important to the person's spiritual or religious beliefs. Using religion or spiritual beliefs to justify other forms of abuse
Physical abuse	Physical abuse and aggression such as slapping, pushing, spitting, choking, punching or kicking; use of weapons including objects; locking the victim out of the house; sleep and food deprivation; destroying possessions
Sexual abuse	Forced or unwanted sex, unwanted sexual touching, unwanted sexual advances or harassment, coercion to perform unwanted sexual acts or to have sex with others, sexual exploitation, including taking photos without consent

Source: Department of Human Services, Victoria: *Family violence risk assessment and risk management framework and practice guidelines*. Melbourne, 2012, Victorian Government.

of conduct and entails a substantial risk of causing physical, emotional or psychological harm to a child or young person (Australian Institute of Family Studies (AIFS) 2018). Such behaviours may be intentional or unintentional and include exposing a child to violence, intimate partner violence, sexual abuse or exploitation which results in actual or potential harm to a child's health, development or dignity. Child abuse and neglect occurs within the context of a relationship of responsibility, trust or power (AIFS 2018). Child abuse occurs when a child hears or witnesses family violence. For categories of child abuse see Table 5.2.

Definitions of child maltreatment are defined by cultural values and beliefs; what may be acceptable in one culture may not be in another. All states and territories in Australia have legislation to protect children from abuse and neglect and it is mandatory for nurses to report suspected child abuse to the appropriate authorities. However, legislative definitions of abuse or what constitutes abuse or maltreatment differ from state to state. Nurses are advised to familiarise themselves with the legislation in their state. It is not currently mandatory to report child abuse in New Zealand but practitioners who identify or suspect child abuse are advised to report it to an appropriate statutory authority such as the police or a child, youth or family service (Ministry of Health New Zealand 2018).

Elder abuse and neglect defined

Elder abuse is a serious and complex problem that affects many vulnerable older people and may occur in different settings including the privacy of the person's home, residential care or hospital. The World Health Organization defines elder abuse as 'a single or repeated act, or lack of appropriate action, occurring within any caring relationship in which there is an expectation of trust' (WHO 2018). The prevalence of elder abuse has been estimated to be 2–14% (Pillemer et al 2016). However, the true extent of elder abuse is likely to be underestimated, remains largely invisible and the number of those affected will rise with the rapidly growing older population (Pillemer et al 2016). Elder abuse can occur within an intimate partner relationship, adult child and parent relationship and within other caregiving relationships including within institutional care. There are many forms of elder abuse including physical, sexual, psychological, emotional, harassment, financial and material, abandonment, neglect and serious loss of dignity and respect (WHO 2018, Gallione et al 2017). See categories of elder abuse further defined in Table 5.3.

One of the most common types of elder abuse is financial abuse, and women are twice as likely to be abused as men (Yon et al 2017). The term financial abuse is used when the family member (or carer) deprives the older person of sufficient

TABLE 5.2 Categories of child abuse

Physical abuse	Any non-accidental physical act inflicted upon a child by a person having the care of the child that caused physical injury, including hitting, shaking, throwing, burning and biting
Emotional and psychological abuse	Any act by a person having the care of children that results in the child suffering any kind of significant emotional deprivation or trauma. For example, constant criticism, teasing, ignoring, yelling and rejection. Also includes the effects on children of exposure to family violence
Sexual abuse	Any act by a person having care of a child that exposes the child to, or involves the child in, sexual processes and activities beyond their understanding or contrary to accepted community standards
Neglect	Any serious act or omission by a person having the care of a child that, within the bounds of cultural tradition, constitutes a failure to provide conditions that are essential for healthy physical and emotional development. This includes when a child's basic needs for food, housing, healthcare and warm clothing are not met. Leaving children without adequate supervision for their age is also a form of neglect

Source: Australian Institute of Family Studies (AIFS). Child abuse and neglect statistics CFCA Resource Sheet – June 2017. [Available from https://aifs.gov.au/cfca/publications/child-abuse-and-neglect-statistics]

TABLE 5.3 Definitions of elder abuse

Physical abuse	Infliction of physical pain, injury or force, including medication abuse (deliberate or accidental misuse of medication and prescriptions that sedate or result in harm to the older person) and inappropriate use of restraint or confinement that causes pain or bodily harm
Sexual abuse	Any forced, coerced or exploitive sexual behaviour or threats imposed on an individual, including sexual acts imposed on a person unable to give consent, or sexual activity that an adult lacking mental capacity is unable to understand
Psychological abuse	Any behaviour that causes anguish, stress or fear, including verbal abuse, intimidation, harassment, damage to property, threats of physical or sexual abuse and the removal of decision-making powers
Financial/material abuse	Illegal or improper exploitation and/or use of funds or other resources, including financial abuse, occurring when a person who has been given ordinary or enduring power of attorney abuses their powers and fails to operate in the best interests of the older person. Failure to use the assets of the elderly person to provide services needed by the elderly person

Source: Glasgow K, Fanslow JL: *Family violence intervention guidelines: elder abuse and neglect*. Wellington, 2006, Ministry of Health, New Zealand.

financial resources to fulfil their basic needs (Australian Securities and Investment Commission (ASIC) 2019). Another area of abuse that has also been identified is the abuse of power of attorney. This type of abuse occurs when a person given enduring power of attorney fails to operate in the best interests of an older person (ASIC 2019). Risk factors for elder abuse include functional dependence or physical disability, cognitive impairment including dementia, poor mental health, social isolation and low socioeconomic status (WHO 2018). Elder neglect may be intentional (active neglect) or unintentional (passive neglect) caused by a carer's own condition or inadequate knowledge. Neglect occurs when another person fails to meet the physical and emotional needs of an older person (WHO 2018).

HEALTH EFFECTS OF FAMILY VIOLENCE

Intimate partner violence

Intimate partner violence is a global health problem associated with serious public health consequences. It has been found that there is a significant association between lifetime experience of partner violence and poor mental and physical health outcomes (VicHealth 2017). In Australia, since the age of 15, 1 in 6 women and 1 in 16 men have experienced physical and/or sexual violence by a current or previous partner (AIHW 2019a). Men were more likely to have experienced violence from strangers (35%) compared with women who were more likely to have known their abuser (35%). While both women and men experience violence, overwhelmingly sexual assault, domestic and family violence is perpetrated by men against women and children (ABS 2017, AIHW 2018).

Research has found intimate partner violence rates in same-sex relationships are similar if not higher than opposite-sex relationships and that the violence can be bi-directional (Longobardi & Badenes-Ribera 2017). Contributing factors include internalised homophobia, stigma, degree of 'outness', social constraints and discrimination based on sexual orientation (Longobardi & Badenes-Ribera 2017). These factors are also likely to contribute to a reluctance to disclose intimate partner violence. However, the number of family violence reports to police is rising according to AIHW (2019a) report.

Of the women who reported physical violence from a current or previous partner, 68% stated their children had been present at the time (ABS 2017). Indigenous women, women with disabilities, pregnant women, women and men who experienced abuse or witnessed violence as children, younger women and those experiencing financial hardship experience high rates of violence (AIHW 2018). Australian Indigenous women are 32 times more likely to experience family violence and sustain serious injury requiring hospitalisation, and 10 times more likely to die due to family violence than non-Indigenous women (AIHW 2018). In New Zealand, Māori women are twice as likely to experience current partner violence than the national average (Ministry of Justice, New Zealand 2018). Family violence is also a significant contributing factor to homelessness among Australian women (AIHW 2018).

In 2015–16 the cost of violence against women and their children in Australia was estimated to be $22 billion (AIHW 2018). This includes the cost of pain and suffering, health, productivity and administration related to violence against women. Intimate partner violence has been found to be a leading contributor to death, disability and illness in women aged between 15 and 44 years and is responsible for more disease burden than many wellknown risk factors such as high tobacco use, high cholesterol and illicit drug use with wide-ranging and persistent effects on physical and mental health (VicHealth 2017, AIHW 2018). Those who experience family violence are also more likely to need to take time off work and have an increased cycling in and out of homelessness (AIHW 2018).

It is likely that women who have been abused will need to access healthcare. Physical injury is the most obvious and immediate health problem including fractures, bruising and lacerations. Those women who have experienced severe physical violence are more likely to have told someone than those with less severe injuries. Intimate partner violence causes more illness, disability and deaths than any other risk factor for women aged 25–34 years (AIHW 2019a). They are also at greater risk of developing a range of psychological and mental health problems including stress, anxiety, depression, phobias, posttraumatic stress disorder (PTSD), unexplained somatic complaints, suicidal ideation and problems with alcohol and substance abuse (WHO 2017).

Abuse during pregnancy is also a significant health problem, with serious consequences for both the pregnant woman (e.g. depression and substance abuse) and the infant (e.g. low birth weight and increased risk of child abuse) (AIHW 2018).

Women who have been abused will have need of healthcare services either for regular check-ups or for treatment for one of the longterm health problems described above. Because many women who have been abused are not yet ready to seek help, healthcare providers are extremely important as an early point of contact with the opportunity to provide support. Early identification of the signs of abuse may stop the pattern of violence and longterm health problems avoided or minimised. Barriers to disclosure include women themselves feeling shame, and/or minimising or normalising the abuse (AIHW 2018). There is also evidence that healthcare providers are reluctant to ask clients about the possibility of abuse. Barriers to asking include lack of time, lack of confidence and limited resources (Soh et al 2018).

In addition, nurses and midwives should be alert for the conditions particularly associated with intimate partner violence and sexual abuse, including gynaecological problems (especially sexually transmitted infections (STIs), pelvic pain, complaints of sexual dysfunction, antepartum haemorrhage, unwanted pregnancy and pregnancy in very young girls), chronic irritable bowel syndrome, back pain, depression and symptoms of PTSD (especially problems sleeping, anxiety and 'panic' attacks). When these problems occur, and especially when they persist, a thorough and repeated assessment for family violence is needed.

Child abuse

Child abuse is also a significant global health issue with far-reaching consequences (see Box 5.1). Child abuse is defined as abuse or maltreatment of children under the age of 18 years and includes physical and/or emotional ill-treatment, sexual abuse, neglect, negligence and commercial or other exploitation, which results in actual or potential harm to the child's health, survival, development or dignity in the context

Box 5.1 Health Consequences of Child Abuse

Disruption of early brain development
- Extreme stress can impair development of nervous and immune system

Risk of behavioural, physical and mental health problems:
- depression
- smoking
- obesity
- alcohol and drug misuse
- high-risk sexual behaviour
- unintended pregnancy
- perpetrating or being a victim of violence

These factors can contribute to:
- heart disease
- cancer
- suicide
- sexually transmitted infections

Economic impact including cost of:
- healthcare
- child welfare
- longer term health costs

Source: World Health Organization (WHO). *Child maltreatment: Key Facts; 2016* [Available from: https://www.who.int/news-room/fact-sheets/detail/child-maltreatment]

of a relationship of responsibility, trust or power (WHO 2016). Exposure to and witnessing intimate partner violence is also increasingly recognised as abuse.

In Australia, 1 in 6 women and 1 in 10 men had been sexually and/or physically assaulted before the age of 15 (ABS 2017, AIHW 2018). Aboriginal and Torres Strait Islander children were almost seven times as likely to be the subject of substantiated abuse and neglect as non-Indigenous children (AIHW 2018). The economic cost of child protection services in Australia is estimated to be $5.2 billion (AIFS 2018). Australian Indigenous children are overrepresented in child protection service, at eight times the rate of non-Indigenous children (AIHW 2019). Of children referred to children protection services in Australia, girls have a higher rate of sustained sexual abuse than boys (11% vs 7%), with boys having a slightly higher rate of sustained neglect and physical abuse (AIHW 2019b). There are many factors that contribute to child abuse and neglect. Risk factors include personal, family, community and social factors:

Child characteristics

Being under 4 years old
Having special needs, crying persistently or having physical disability
Being unwanted, or failing to fulfil the expectations of parents

Family characteristics

Family breakdown
Violence between family members, including intimate partner abuse
Unstable family environment when the composition of the household changes frequently
A breakdown of support in child-rearing from extended family members
Being isolated in the community or lacking a support network

Parental characteristics

Having been mistreated themselves as a child
Experiencing financial difficulties
Low self-esteem, poor control of impulses, difficulty coping with stress
Physical, developmental or mental health problems of a family member
Displays of antisocial behaviour
Misusing alcohol and drugs

Community and societal factors

Gender and social inequality
Lack of adequate housing or family support services
High levels of unemployment
Inequities related to gender and income
Social and cultural norms that promote or glorify violence towards others, that demand rigid gender roles or diminish the status of the child in parent–child relationships
Social, economic, health and education policies that lead to poor living standards or to socioeconomic inequality

(Adapted from WHO 2016).

The risk of abuse decreases as age increases, that is, younger children are at higher risk. For example, of the substantiated cases of harm or risk to children in Australia, 17.2 in 1000 were infants (below 1 year), 9 in 1000 were aged 1–4 years and 4.1 in 1000 were aged 15–17 years (AIHW 2019b). However, relying on reported cases of abuse can be misleading, as many cases of child abuse and neglect go unreported and many cases may never be disclosed (Mathews et al 2016). The immediate consequences of child abuse can include a spectrum of physical injuries such as bruises, fractures and lacerations, and can involve more severe injury such as shaken baby syndrome. More severe forms of abuse can lead to death or longterm physical and mental disability. Children experiencing violence or neglect may exhibit diminished executive functioning and cognitive skills, poor mental or emotional health, attachment and social difficulties, posttraumatic stress and behavioural consequences such as unhealthy sexual practices, substance misuse and future perpetration of maltreatment (Child Welfare Information Gateway 2019).

Elder abuse and neglect

Elder abuse can occur in community settings or within institutional settings (WHO 2018). Elder abuse can have severe physical consequences including pain, discomfort and life-threatening injuries and is associated with increased risk of premature morbidity and mortality and long-lasting psychological consequences (WHO 2018).

Caregivers may themselves be dependent on the older person for their own emotional and financial support, be it sharing housing, or may be struggling with their own mental health or substance abuse challenges and frailty (Pillemer et al 2016). Frailty can impact on their capacity and judgement as a carer. The carer's intentions may be good; however, the older person in their care may experience profound unintentional neglect or other forms of abuse. While unintentional neglect is usually not viewed as a crime, it is still a serious problem that needs to be addressed.

While some older women have been in abusive relationships for decades, others are experiencing physical and sexual violence for the first time from normally non-abusive partners who themselves are afflicted with behaviour-altering neurological illness (e.g. Alzheimer's disease, organic brain syndromes). An older woman who has been abused in a longterm abusive relationship may be trying to outlive her abuser, whereas the newly abused older woman may be reluctant to disclose because of embarrassment, shame and fear that her partner will be institutionalised.

Older people are also vulnerable to abuse from other family members and caretakers. Assessment of physical abuse and/or neglect in the cognitively impaired person is much more complicated. Physical findings that are inconsistent with the history provided by the patient, family member or caregiver are significant red flags of possible abuse and neglect. Older people may be reluctant to disclose abuse or neglect because they are scared or fear they will be relocated to a different institution or nursing home; they are dependent on or have a co-dependent relationship with their abuser and fear the abuse will get worse or that they will be abandoned.

CULTURAL AND SOCIAL CONSIDERATIONS

Family violence crosses all cultures, religions and socioeconomic circumstances. There may be different interpretations of what constitutes abuse in different cultures (Glasgow & Fanslow 2006); for example, the right of parents to discipline their children using physical force such as slapping or hitting; rites of passage rituals that result in physical injury. Also, definitions of abuse may include disrespect, dishonour and/or ignoring needs of the person (Glasgow & Fanslow 2006). Further, some health treatments such as 'cupping' used in Chinese medicine, involving application of pressure to cups placed on the skin, can leave bruising from the rim of the cups that might be misinterpreted when examined by the untrained person. Therefore, it is important for nurses to take into account the individual and family's cultural context and religious beliefs when assessing and responding to family violence.

Not all persons of the same gender, sexuality, family, ethnicity or culture will share the same attitudes, values or beliefs. The needs of persons of culturally and linguistically diverse backgrounds will also differ for a range of reasons including cultural and religious beliefs, level of education, language skills and fluency, family relationships, length of time since migration, prescribed gender roles, social networks, economic circumstance, lack of understanding of Australian laws and beliefs and attitudes towards family violence. Differences across cultures may affect disclosure because of fear of religious beliefs, need to protect the family name, fear of stigmatising their entire community and fear of reprisal, for example, social exclusion, death threats and honour killings (Sawrikar & Katz 2017).

It is important to seek advice from other professionals with expertise and understanding of different cultural and religious beliefs and, if possible, to include them in the interview. An interpreter should also be considered if an individual's first language is other than English. However, it is also important to be aware of the potential sensitivities associated with disclosure in the presence of a person from the same cultural or religious background. While beliefs and interpretations about violence may differ across cultures, this is not an excuse for violence. Being equipped with knowledge of different cultural and religious beliefs will assist the nurse to approach a family violence assessment in a culturally appropriate and sensitive way.

ASSESSING FOR FAMILY VIOLENCE AND ABUSE

There are many points at which individuals and families experiencing family violence enter the healthcare system which provides health professionals many opportunities to support the person or family to access much needed services. However, this relies on health professionals being able to identify family violence and assess needs (Victorian Government 2019). Individuals and families should be able to expect professional and compassionate care and that the complexity of their needs regarding abusive situations will be taken into account. Even if a woman chooses not to follow up with referral or take any other action at that first point of contact, if she has received a sensitive and appropriate response, it is more likely she will seek assistance at a later stage.

Nurses are often the first point of contact and therefore have an important role in identifying and responding to family violence. Nurses are in an ideal position to facilitate disclosure about abuse and to respond in a supportive, appropriate and timely manner while respecting privacy and the individual's right to make their own decisions (Australian Nursing & Midwifery Federation 2016). Screening for family violence as part of routine assessment and care can assist in the identification of women and children at risk; however, any assessment must be done within a context of effective systems of support, with the capacity to protect family members following disclosure. There is increasing support for routine screening of all women presenting to health services. However, the efficacy of this practice remains contentious, particularly if health professionals do not fully appreciate the complexities of family violence and consequences of disclosure for women and their children or their responsibilities as health professionals. Even when health professionals have knowledge and screening skills, women may choose not to disclose abuse for a variety of reasons including shame and fear of consequences (Miller & McCaw 2019). Others have also found use of short structured screening tools do not promote disclosure or detail of women's experiences. However, discussions about parenting, safety and health relationships have been found to be more helpful (Jack et al 2017). Women who themselves have experienced family violence value opportunities to be asked about their experiences in a safe and private setting (Miller & McCaw 2019).

In New Zealand, the Ministry of Justice (2017) proposed a three-step approach to screening, assessing and managing family violence risk. The first step is screening or routine enquiry, which involves enquiring about personal history and history of family violence in a way that helps the individual feel comfortable enough to disclose their experience. The goal is to identify those at risk who need further assessment and potentially interventions. Second is risk assessment which is usually a longer and more detailed process to learn more about someone's views, behaviours, circumstances and interactions to be able to determine the risk of harm to themselves and other family members. Finally, risk management includes safety planning to remove, reduce or mitigate the risks to minimise harm and maximise safety (Ministry of Justice 2017). Risk management involves helping the person access appropriate support. Screening should therefore be followed by risk assessment and risk management if screening is to be effective in preventing harm and breaking the cycle of family violence.

Before asking questions about family violence, nurses should be aware of the complexities of family violence, the implications of asking questions about family violence and women's disclosure. While the gender of the nurse does not necessarily affect disclosure, nurses should be sensitive to the possibility that the person may have a preference. Nurses should also have a good understanding of resources to assist a person experiencing violence, potential referral options and ask if the person has a gender preference of the practitioner to whom they are being referred.

Subjective data

Given the high incidence of family violence in Australia and New Zealand, there is an argument that every person should be screened at each interaction with the healthcare system. However, the collection of information needs to be done sensitively and within a context of support. This section is divided into three parts to guide subjective data collection related to intimate partner violence, child abuse and elder abuse and neglect.

Prior to undertaking an assessment of a person who you suspect has been abused, read the contents of Table 5.4 and Box 5.2.

TABLE 5.4 Approaches to assessment and disclosure about abuse

Before disclosure or asking questions about violence:	Immediate response to disclosure:
Knowledge of community services and appropriate referral options	Be nonjudgemental, compassionate, supportive, believe what you are being told
Create a welcoming, supportive non-threatening environment	Acknowledge the complexity of the problem, and respect the woman's unique concerns and decisions
Provide assurance of privacy, safety and confidentiality	Respect the woman's wishes and do not pressure her into making any decisions
Be alert to the signs of abuse and raise the possibility	Validate the experience, challenge assumptions and provide encouragement
Build rapport using both verbal and non-verbal communication skills to develop trust	Be nonjudgemental if a woman does not follow up referrals immediately
Be compassionate, supportive and respectful when the topic of domestic violence is raised	Put the needs identified by the woman first and help to ensure that social and psychological needs are met
Be nonjudgemental, compassionate and caring when questioning about abuse	Respond to any concerns about safety
Be confident and comfortable asking about domestic violence	Take time to listen, provide information and offer referrals to specialist help
Do not pressure women to disclose abuse: simply raising the topic can be helpful	
Ensure that the environment is private and confidential, and provide time.	

Source: Hegarty K, Taft A, Feder G. Violence between intimate partners: working with the whole family, *British Medical Journal*, 337:a839, 2008.

Box 5.2 Responding to Disclosure of Family Violence

- Ensure privacy—away from public areas, partners, carers, family
- Listen attentively and without judgement
- Demonstrate cultural awareness and sensitivity
- Affirm the client's decision to disclose
- Provide reassurance—they are not to blame, they have a right to feel safe, there is help available
- Ensure confidentiality if an adult
- If client is a child, you will need information about who the perpetrator is and to follow policy and mandatory reporting requirements in your institution and state
- Assess immediate and longer term safety—do they currently feel safe, are they safe to return home, are children or others at risk?
- Be aware of your own feelings and reaction to the disclosure, abuse, violence
- Consult with colleagues and others with family violence expertise
- Provide information and referral to support services—family services, domestic violence and sexual assault services, counselling, support groups, refuge and emergency accommodation, police
- Assist to develop a safety plan—who can assist, where can they go if they cannot return home, who can they call if they need support?
- Document the outcome of assessment and intervention

Intimate partner violence

1. Starting the discussion
2. Opening the discussion about personal safety
3. Screening tools
4. Probing questions about intimate partner violence
5. Past history of abuse

Child abuse and neglect

1. Developmental stage
2. Psychological history
3. Social circumstances
4. Past health history
5. Further questions for the older child

Elder abuse and vulnerable person's abuse

1. Screening for intimate partner violence in older people
2. Screening for possible elder abuse and neglect
3. Opening the discussion about elder abuse and neglect
4. Suggested questions

ASSESSMENT GUIDELINES	CLINICAL SIGNIFICANCE AND CLINICAL ALERTS
1. Intimate partner violence	
Starting the discussion: To alert the woman that questions about family violence are coming and to reassure her that she is not being singled out the following statements are suggested. • Because family violence is so common in our community, we are asking all women the following questions	**Possible presentations:** *Psychological* Insomnia, depression; suicidal ideation; anxiety symptoms and panic disorder; somatoform disorder; posttraumatic stress disorder; eating disorders; drug and alcohol misuse *Physical* Obvious injuries, especially to the head and neck or multiple areas; bruises in various stages of healing; injuries from sexual assault; sexually transmitted diseases; chronic pelvic pain; chronic abdominal pain; chronic headaches; chronic back pain; numbness and tingling from injuries; lethargy (Feder et al 2009).
Opening the discussion about personal safety When asking questions about violence it is important for the nurse to first listen to, then validate, the woman's experiences. A woman may not be ready to take action but having her experience validated and feelings acknowledged by a compassionate nurse can help facilitate the first steps towards change. Nurses may feel more comfortable introducing questions about violence if the following approach to questioning is adopted. To facilitate disclosure, nurses should consider using a 'funnelling' technique, which involves starting with indirect questions such as: • How are things at home? and moving towards more direct questions such as • Do you ever feel unsafe at home? • I am concerned about your health condition; is there any chance that stress at home is contributing to your health problems?'	It is appropriate for you to show your concern about the degree of violence. Important messages to convey during the assessment are that the abuse is not the woman's fault; you are concerned about what is happening and there is help available. It is also important to convey that there are several potential health problems associated with family violence for both the woman and her children and this is why you are concerned and asking about her experience.
Screening tools The opportunity for screening for intimate partner violence presents itself each time the nurse has an interaction with a woman; however, there are some presentations that may strongly suggest experience of violence. Awareness of such signs and symptoms should alert the nurse to the possibility of violence. If intimate partner violence is suspected, it is appropriate to undertake an assessment. A number of tools to screen for intimate partner abuse are available. The 'HARK questionnaire' focuses on four key areas of enquiry—humiliation, being afraid, sexual assault and physical violence (Sohal et al 2007). • H: HUMILIATION Within the last year, have you been humiliated or emotionally abused in other ways by your partner or your ex-partner? • A: AFRAID Within the last year, have you been afraid of your partner or ex-partner? • R: RAPE Within the last year, have you been raped or forced to have any kind of sexual activity by your partner or ex-partner? • K: KICK Within the last year, have you been kicked, hit, slapped or otherwise physically hurt by your partner or ex-partner?	All survivors of violence should be given a mental status examination, with particular attention to the most frequent mental health problems associated with violence: depression, suicidality, PTSD, substance abuse and anxiety. Chapter 11 gives direction for conducting this part of the assessment.

SUBJECTIVE DATA

ASSESSMENT GUIDELINES	CLINICAL SIGNIFICANCE AND CLINICAL ALERTS
Probing questions about intimate partner violence If a woman answers yes to any of your questions about violence, you should consider moving to a more detailed collection of subjective data to better understand the woman's circumstances and to assess her and her children's safety. It is important to validate the woman's experience. Some possible ways to validate her disclosure would be to make statements such as: • Everybody deserves to feel safe at home. • You don't deserve to be hit or hurt. It is not your fault. • I am concerned about your safety and wellbeing. • You are not alone. I will help you to get help. • Whatever you decide. Help is available. • You are not to blame. Abuse is common and happens in all kinds of relationships. It tends to continue. • Abuse can affect your health and your children's health in many ways (Hegarty et al 2008).	
Even if the woman minimises the level of abuse such as it is 'only emotional' or 'not that bad' or 'we just fight a lot', more may be revealed as you gently assess the situation. Further enquiry should be made about: • the length of time of the abuse, • whether it is still occurring, • the severity of the abuse and • the impact on the woman and her children. A good way to start is by asking the woman • Tell me about this abuse in your relationship.	This type of assessment is like 'peeling layers of an onion' when more is uncovered as the assessment continues. A woman is not 'in denial' if she minimises the abuse; it is not uncommon for this response to accompany the experience of trauma from violence.
Past history of abuse It is important to also assess and document prior abuse, including: • prior intimate partner violence, • childhood physical and sexual abuse and • prior sexual assaults of all kinds (stranger, date, intimate partner) and • traumatic injuries.	It is important to determine the impact on the person's current health condition. For example, a woman may have experienced prior episodes of head trauma, which may be related to chronic but subtle neurological symptoms and problems.
2. Assessing for child abuse and neglect	
The aim of collecting subjective data for suspected child abuse and neglect is to paint a picture of the child's world which includes the child's developmental level, psychological function and the social circumstances in which they live (Royal Children's Hospital Melbourne (RCH) 2019a). Because the nurse may not be able to directly observe the child's motor and cognitive milestones during the history taking, it is important to ask the caretakers directly.	Nurses who suspect child abuse or neglect should involve other members of the healthcare team (medical practitioners, social workers, counsellors) as screening and assessment processes are complex and there are serious implications for the child and their family. There are also requirements for a notification to be made (mandatory reporting) to child protection authorities. If a notification is to be made, the team should gather and document the evidence carefully before proceeding. If abuse and neglect go unchecked, the implications and risks for the child and perhaps other family members are serious.

ASSESSMENT GUIDELINES	CLINICAL SIGNIFICANCE AND CLINICAL ALERTS
Developmental stage Ask the parent or caregiver questions about the child's stage of development (see Chapter 3). For example: • Is your child crawling, pulling to stand or walking? • language development • toilet training	Consider if the child could have suffered the injury that is being reported based on their developmental level. For example, the history that a 3-week-old child rolled off a bed causing injury is not developmentally plausible.
Psychological functioning Assessment should include assessment of the child's past patterns of behaviour and current behavioural problems (RCH, 2019a). See Chapter 3. • Observe the interaction between the child and parent or care giver and enquire about this relationship. • Observe the care giver's pattern of behaviour Ask the parent or care giver: • What is it like caring for your child? • Are you experiencing any difficulties getting your child to bed? • Have you noticed any changes in behaviour or mood? • How is school/kindergarten going?	Observation of the parent or caregiver while collecting subjective data from the child gives you the opportunity to consider the caregiver's capacity to parent the child and can provide evidence of attachment to the child.
Social circumstances In order to obtain a picture of the child's work, parents or caregivers are asked questions about (RCH 2019a): • Family relationships. See Chapter 8 • Current members of the household • Arrangements when parents are separated • Child care arrangements If indicated: • Parenting practices • Family routines • Parent's history • Family history For older children • School activities • Extracurricular activities • Friendships and peer relationships • Drug and alcohol use • Sexual relationships For adolescents, see Chapter 8 HEEADSSS assessment	
Past health history • Has the child had previous hospitalisations, injuries? • Do they suffer from any chronic medical conditions? • Does the child take any medication that may cause easy bruising? • Does the child have a history of repeated visits to the hospital? • Was there a delay in seeking care for anything other than a minor injury?	In addition, being alert to non-physical signs and symptoms including: • depression • emotional disturbance • sleep problems • fear • adjustment problems • school attendance issues and behavioural problems

ASSESSMENT GUIDELINES	CLINICAL SIGNIFICANCE AND CLINICAL ALERTS
Further questionning for the older child If the child is verbal or is older, interviewing and taking a history from the child can add additional information. Open-ended questions using age-appropriate language and familiar words are important when taking a history from a child. When potential abuse is suspected, prompting questions can help nurses gather important information that can be used when making a referral for a more comprehensive assessment. Questions may include: • Do you feel safe at home? • Has anyone touched you in a way you don't like? • Is there anyone at home (or elsewhere) who makes you feel scared? • I notice you have a bruise here, how did that happen? • Can you tell me more about that? • You seem upset (angry) when I asked about that?	This should be done away from the parents or caregiver (RCH 2019b). *Clinical alert:* Consultation with other team members and referral to a health professional experienced with interviewing children who are suspected to have experienced abuse will ensure a more comprehensive and accurate assessment. It is important to consider the history from the child in the context of the whole assessment and examination of the child. Children older than 11 years of age can generally be expected to provide a history at the level of most adults.
3. Assessing for elder and vulnerable person abuse and neglect	
Screening for intimate partner violence in older people Screening for intimate partner violence in older people is the same as screening among younger women and similar questions can be used. However, you may modify the introductory statement as follows: • Because domestic violence has such serious health consequences we are asking women of all ages the following questions	There is no mandatory reporting of elder abuse in either Australia or New Zealand as yet; however, there are policies and systems set up so complaints about elder abuse can be investigated. For example, in Australia under the *Aged Care Act 1997* there is a Charter of Residents Rights and Responsibilities, which states explicitly that people living in aged care homes have the right to be treated with dignity and respect and to live without exploitation, abuse or neglect. If anyone suspects elder abuse, they are able to make a complaint via an aged care complaints investigation scheme.
Screening for possible elder abuse and neglect This screening can be more complicated than screening for intimate partner violence. Older people can present for healthcare with few or multiple health, physical and cognitive challenges. The assessment should include a thorough medical and surgical history, current medications and psychosocial assessment. See Chapter 8.	While it is essential to assess and screen for potential signs of abuse, it is also important to differentiate signs and symptoms of elder abuse from normal signs of ageing (Pickens et al 2011). Unexplained bruising, skin tears, long-bone and multiple fractures should raise suspicion of physical abuse.
Opening the discussion about elder abuse and neglect When assessing the older person, it is useful to start with indirect questions, then move to a more direct inquiry if abuse is suspected. A suggested beginning is: • Can you tell me what happened? and • What do you remember about how the injury occurred?	In the case of those who rely on care from others in aged care facilities or in their home, it is important to include caregivers in your assessment.

ASSESSMENT GUIDELINES	CLINICAL SIGNIFICANCE AND CLINICAL ALERTS
Suggested questions for assessing older people Begin with initial questions such as: • Describe your typical day. • What time do you get up in the morning and what activities might you do? • Are you happy at home/in residential care? • Who helps you with your day-to-day activities? • Do you feel you are getting enough help? • Are you and your (partner/husband/wife/son/daughter/caregiver) managing with the resources you have? Where there are high risk factors or signs and symptoms to indicate possible abuse, the following open-ended questions can be asked: • Are you afraid of anyone at home? • Has anyone ever locked you in a room or locked you in your house? • Has anyone at home ever pushed you, hit you or hurt you? • Has anyone demanded money from you? • Has anyone persuaded you to sign any documents even though it was not in your best interests? • Has anyone ever failed to help you take care of yourself when you needed help? • Does anyone scold or threaten you? Questions that should be asked of the caregiver: • How has your life changed since becoming the primary caregiver? • Have you been able to talk to someone about the changes in your life since becoming a caregiver? • Are you aware of what resources and practical help are available to help you? If it is suspected that the caregiver is the abuser they should be interviewed alone. The following questions can be asked: • Do you feel that (older person receiving care) expects too much from you? • Do you feel that because of the time you spend with (older person receiving care) you don't have enough time to do things you would like to do? • Are you tired of taking care of (older person receiving care)? • Have you ever felt like physically hurting (older person receiving care)? (Conrad et al 2013, Standards New Zealand 2006)	

OBJECTIVE DATA

Objective data

Important components of objective data collection for suspected abuse includes general survey of the person, inspection and palpation. When the examination reveals physical findings that could be associated with physical or sexual abuse, knowledge and use of accurate terminology is essential in all documentation. See Table 5.5. It is important that a structured process is undertaken when approaching examination of people who may have been abused. Detailed and accurate documentation is critical and should include the use of diagrams for recording skin marks and injuries. Consultation with senior members of the health team is essential. If sexual abuse or assault is suspected or reported, a specialist healthcare team will take over the assessment of the person, collection of forensic evidence and care. It is important that the person does not change their clothes or wash any body part until seen by this specialist team. You are advised to check your local health service policies and procedures for details about expected processes.

PROCEDURES AND NORMAL FINDINGS	ABNORMAL FINDINGS AND CLINICAL ALERTS
General Survey	
See Chapter 8 for details	
Inspection of skin	
Inspect skin for: • bruises • abrasions • burns • handprints from grabbing or slapping • bite marks • lacerations There are multiple factors that contribute to bruising other than physical abuse. For example, an older person may bruise more readily or more severely than younger people. Medications and abnormal blood values related to medication side effects and underlying haematological disorders can result in ease of bruising or the formation of ecchymoses. Common medications that increase risk for bruising or bleeding complications include, but are not limited to: aspirin, clopidogrel, heparin, ibuprofen, any of the non-steroidal anti-inflammatory drugs, prednisone, valproic acid and warfarin. It is common for toddlers and children to sustain bruising on the knees, anterior shins and the forehead, but bruising on the feet, face, trunk, buttocks, posterior legs and arms are less likely to be accidental and therefore should be viewed with suspicion as they are indicators of abuse. A new bruise is usually red and will often develop a purple or purple-blue appearance 12–36 hours after blunt-force trauma. The colour of bruises generally progresses from purple-blue to bluish-green to greenish-brown to brownish-yellow before fading away. It is important to document any bruising in children whether or not there is a history of accidental trauma. The forensic terminology used in documentation of intimate partner violence and elder abuse also applies to children. See Table 5.5.	See also Chapter 22. Many inflicted injuries may not be reported by the person or their care giver making careful inspection necessary. Significant injuries can be hidden under clothing, nappies, socks and under long hair. Accidental bruising in healthy, active people is common, yet the presence of bruises on an infant has significance in further assessing a child for abuse (RCH 2019b). Any bruise that takes the shape of an object should be cause for concern, as belts, electric cords and kitchen utensils (e.g. wooden spoons or spatulas) are common instruments of physical abuse. Bruising found in children who are not yet mobile should also raise concern and prompt further assessment for potential other injuries including fractures and intracranial injury.
Inspection and palpation of muscles and joints	
Inspection and palpation Any suspicious areas that might indicate a fracture or dislocation of joints. See Chapter 20.	Physical signs of abuse include fractures and dislocations.

TABLE 5.5 Forensic terminology

Abrasion	A wound caused by rubbing the skin or mucous membrane
Avulsion	The tearing away of a structure or part
Bruise	Superficial discolouration due to haemorrhage into the tissues from ruptured blood vessels beneath the skin surface, without the skin itself being broken; also called a contusion
Contusion	A bruise; injury to tissues without breakage of skin; blood from broken blood vessels accumulates, producing pain, swelling, tenderness
Cut	See incision
Ecchymosis	A haemorrhagic spot or blotch, larger than petechiae, in the skin or mucous membrane, forming a non-elevated, rounded or irregular, blue or purplish patch.
Haematoma	A localised collection of extravasated blood, usually clotted in an organ, space or tissue
Haemorrhage	The escape of blood from a ruptured vessel, which can be external, internal and/or into the skin or other organ
Incision	A cut or wound made by a sharp instrument; the act of cutting
Laceration	The act of tearing or splitting; a wound produced by the tearing and/or splitting of body tissue, usually from blunt impact over a bony surface
Lesion	A broad term referring to any pathological or traumatic disruption of tissue
Patterned injury	An injury caused by an object that leaves a distinct pattern on the skin and/or organ (e.g. being whipped with an extension cord) or an injury caused by a unique mechanism of injury (e.g. immersion burns to the hands (glove burn) or feet (sock burns)
Pattern of injuries	Injuries, usually bruises and fractures, in various stages of healing
Petechiae	Minute, pinpoint, non-raised, perfectly round, purplish-red spots caused by intradermal or submucous haemorrhage, which later turn blue or yellow
Puncture	The act of piercing or penetrating with a pointed object or instrument
Stab wound	A penetrating, sharp, cutting injury that is deeper than it is wide
Traumatic alopecia	Loss of hair from pulling and yanking or by other traumatic means
Wound	A general term referring to a bodily injury caused by physical means

Adapted from Miller BF, Keane CB, O'Toole M. *Miller-Keane encyclopedia & dictionary of medicine, nursing, & allied health.* 7th edn. Philadelphia: Saunders, 2005; Sheridan DJ. Treating survivors of intimate partner abuse: forensic identification and documentation. In: Olshaker JS, Jackson MC, Smock WS, eds. *Forensic emergency medicine.* Philadelphia: Lippincott Williams & Wilkins, 2001; Taft A, O'Doherty L, Hegarty K et al: 2013 Screening women for intimate partner violence in healthcare settings, *Cochrane Database Syst. Rev.*, 30(4), CD007007.

DOCUMENTATION

Documentation of intimate partner violence, child and elder abuse must include detailed, nonbiased progress notes and the use of injury maps and photographic documentation in the health record. Written documentation of histories of intimate partner violence and elder abuse needs to be verbatim, in the words of the person, but within reason. It is clinically unrealistic to document verbatim every statement made by an abused person. However, it is critical to document exceptionally poignant statements made by the victim that identify the reported perpetrator and severe threats of harm made by that person. Other aspects of the abuse history, including reports of past abusive incidents, can be paraphrased with the use of partial direct quotations.

When quoting or paraphrasing the history, do not sanitise the words reportedly heard by the victim. Verbatim documentation of the reported perpetrator's threats interlaced with curses and expletives can be extremely useful in future legal proceedings. Also, be careful to use the exact terms a person who has been abused uses to describe sexual organs or sexually assaultive behaviours.

Photographic and/or video documentation of injuries are invaluable and are undertaken by specialist photographers or medical staff (RCH 2019c). Prior written consent to take photographs is obtained by a medical practitioner from a competent adult. If the person is unconscious or cognitively impaired, the taking of photographs without consent is generally viewed as ethically sound since it is a noninvasive, painless intervention that has high potential to help a suspected abuse victim.

When documenting the history and physical findings of child abuse and neglect, use the words the child has given to describe how their injury occurred. Remember that there is a possibility that the abuser may be accompanying the child. If the child is nonverbal, use statements from caregivers. It is important to know your employer/institutional protocol for obtaining a history in cases of suspected child abuse. Some protocols may delay a full interview until it can be done by an expert in child abuse.

BIBLIOGRAPHY

Australian Bureau of Statistics. Personal Safety Survey 2016. ABS cat. no. 4906.0. Canberra: Australian Bureau of Statistics; 2017. Available at: https://www.abs.gov.au/ausstats/abs@.nsf/mf/4906.0.

Australian Institute of Family Studies. Child abuse and neglect statistics CFCA Resource Sheet. June 2017. Available at: https://aifs.gov.au/cfca/publications/child-abuse-and-neglect-statistics.

Australian Institute of Family Studies. Reporting child abuse and neglect: information for service providers. 2018. Available at: https://aifs.gov.au/cfca/publications/cfca-resource-sheet/reporting-child-abuse-and-neglect.

Australian Institute of Health and Welfare. Family, domestic and sexual violence in Australia 2018. Cat. no. FDV 2. Canberra: Australian Institute of Health and Welfare; 2018.

Australian Institute of Health and Welfare. Family, domestic and sexual violence in Australia: continuing the national story 2019. Cat. no. FDV 3. Canberra: AIHW; 2019a. Available at: https://www.aihw.gov.au/getmedia/b0037b2d-a651-4abf-9f7b-00a85e3de528/aihw-fdv3-FDSV-in-Australia-2019.pdf.aspx?inline=true.

Australian Institute of Health and Welfare. Child protection Australia: 2017–18. Child welfare series no. 70. Cat. no. CWS 65. Canberra: AIHW; 2019b.

Australian Nursing & Midwifery Federation. Position statement: domestic violence. Melbourne: Australian Nursing & Midwifery Federation; 2016. Available at: http://anmf.org.au/documents/policies/PS_Domestic_violence.pdf.

Australian Securities and Investment Commission. Financial abuse. 2019. Available at: https://www.moneysmart.gov.au/life-events-and-you/families/financial-abuse.

Child Welfare Information Gateway. Longterm consequences of child abuse and neglect. Washington, DC: U.S. Department of Health and Human Services, Administration for Children and Families, Children's Bureau; 2019.

Conrad KJ, Iris M, Riley BB, et al. Developing end-user criteria and a prototype for an elder abuse assessment system. Final Technical Report. February 2013. Available at: https://www.ncjrs.gov/pdffiles1/nij/grants/241390.pdf.

Department of Human Services, Victoria. Family violence risk assessment and risk management framework and practice. Melbourne: Victorian Government; 2012.

Feder G, Ramsay J, Dunne D, et al. How far does screening women for domestic (partner) violence in different healthcare settings meet criteria for a screening programme? Systematic reviews of nine UK National Screening Committee criteria. Health Technol Assess 2009;13:iii–iv, xi–xiii, 1–113, 37–347.

Gallione C, Dal Molin A, Cristina FVB, et al. Screening tools for identification of elder abuse: a systematic review. J Clin Nurs 2017;26(15–16):2154–76.

Glasgow K, Fanslow JL. Family violence intervention guidelines: elder abuse and neglect. Wellington: Ministry of Health; 2006.

Hegarty K, Taft A, Feder G. Violence between intimate partners: working with the whole family. BMJ 2008;337:a839.

Jack SM, Ford-Gilboe M, Davidov D et al. Identification and assessment of intimate partner violence in nurse home visitation. J Clin Nurs 2017;26(15–16):2215–28.

Longobardi C, Badenes-Ribera L. Intimate partner violence in same-sex relationships and the role of sexual minority stressors: a systematic review of the past 10 years. J Child Fam Stud 2017;26(8):2039–49.

Mathews BP, Walsh KM, Dunne MP, et al. Scoping study for research into the prevalence of child abuse in Australia: Final report. Prepared for the Royal Commission into Institutional Responses to Child Sexual Abuse. Sydney: Social Policy Research Centre (SPRC Report 13/16) , UNSW Australia in partnership with Australian Institute of Family Studies, Queensland University of Technology and the Australian Centre for Child Protection (University of South Australia); 2016. Available at: https://www.childabuseroyalcommission.gov.au/sites/default/files/research_report_-_scoping_study_for_research_into_prevalence_of_child_sexual_abuse_in_australia_-_causes.pdf.

Miller E, McCaw B. Intimate partner violence. N Engl J Med 380(9):850–7.

Ministry of Health, New Zealand. Family violence questions and answers. 2018. Available at: https://www.health.govt.nz/our-work/preventative-health-wellness/family-violence/family-violence-questions-and-answers#mandatory.

Ministry of Justice, New Zealand. Family violence risk assessment and management framework: a common approach to screening, assessing and managing risk. Wellington: New Zealand Government; 2017.

Ministry of Justice, New Zealand. New Zealand crime and victims survey: Help creates safer communities. Wellington: Ministry of Justice, New Zealand Government; 2018.

New Zealand Standard. Screening, risk assessment and intervention for family violence including child abuse and neglect. New Zealand: Standards Council; 2006. Provided permission by Standards New Zealand under license, 001155.

Pickens S, Halphen J, Dyer C. Elder mistreatment in the long-term care setting. Ann Longterm Care 2011;19(8):30–5. Available at: www.annalsoflongtermcare.com/article/elder-mistreatment-long-term-care-setting.

Pillemer K, Burnes D, Riffin C, et al. Elder abuse: global situation, risk factors, and prevention strategies. Gerontologist 2016;56(Suppl. 2):194–205.

Royal Children's Hospital Melbourne. Psychosocial assessments in forensic paediatric medicine. 2019a. Available at: https://www.rch.org.au/vfpms/guidelines/psychological-assessments-in-forensic-paediatric-medicine/.

Royal Children's Hospital Melbourne. Engaging with and assessing the adolescent patient. 2019b. Available at: https://www.rch.org.au/clinicalguide/guideline_index/Engaging_with_and_assessing_the_adolescent_patient/.

Royal Children's Hospital Melbourne. Video and photographic documentation. 2019c. Available at: https://www.rch.org.au/vfpms/guidelines/guidelines-for-video-documentation-of-genital-examinations/.

Sawrikar P, Katz I. Barriers to disclosing child sexual abuse (CSA) in ethnic minority communities: a review of the literature and implications for practice in Australia. Child Youth Serv Rev 2017;83:302–15. doi:10.1016/j.childyouth.2017.11.011.

Soh HJ, Grigg J, Gurvich C, et al. Family violence: an insight into perspectives and practices of Australian health practitioners. J Interpers Violence 2018. Available at: https://doi.org/10.1177/0886260518760609.

Sohal H, Eldridge S, Feder G. The sensitivity and specificity of four questions (HARK) to identify intimate partner violence: a diagnostic accuracy study in general practice. BMC Fam Pract 2007;8(1):49.

Taft A, O'Doherty L, Hegarty K, et al. Screening women for intimate partner violence in healthcare settings, Cochrane Database Syst Rev 2013;30(4):CD007007. doi:10.1002/14651858.CD007007.

VicHealth. Violence against women in Australia: an overview of research and approaches to primary prevention. Carlton South: Victorian Health Promotion Foundation; 2017.

Victorian Government. Family safety Victoria. 2019. Available at: Available at: https://www.vic.gov.au/familyviolence.html.

World Health Organization. Child maltreatment: key facts. 2016. Available at: https://www.who.int/news-room/fact-sheets/detail/child-maltreatment.

World Health Organization. Violence against women. Geneva: World Health Organisation; 2017. Available at: https://www.who.int/news-room/fact-sheets/detail/violence-against-women.

World Health Organization. Elder abuse fact sheet. 2018. Available at: https://www.who.int/news-room/fact-sheets/detail/elder-abuse.

Yon Y, Mikton CR, Gassoumis Z, et al. Elder abuse prevalence in community settings: a systematic review and meta-analysis. Lancet Global Health 2017;5(2):E147–56. Available at: https://doi.org/10.1016/S2214-109X(17)30006-2.

Websites

Australia

1800RESPECT – National sexual assault, domestic family violence, counselling service: https://www.1800respect.org.au

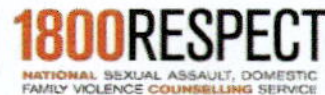

Australian Government, Department of Human Services: https://www.humanservices.gov.au/individuals/subjects/family-and-domestic-violence

Kids Helpline: https://kidshelpline.com.au

Lifeline (Australia): https://www.lifeline.org.au/Get-Help/Facts—-Information/Domestic-Abuse-and-Family-Violence

MensLine Australia: https://mensline.org.au

Reach out.com (Australia): https://au.reachout.com/articles/sexual-assault-support

White Ribbon Australia: https://www.whiteribbon.org.au

New Zealand

Family violence: Its not OK (NZ): http://www.areyouok.org.nz

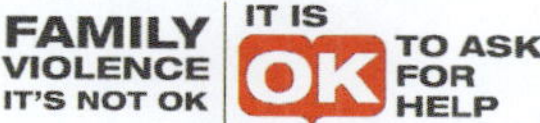

Kidsline NZ: http://www.kidsline.org.nz/Home_312.aspx

New Zealand Government, Domestic or family violence: https://www.govt.nz/browse/law-crime-and-justice/abuse-harassment-domestic-violence/domestic-or-family-violence/

Victims Information – For people affected by sexual violence (NZ): https://sexualviolence.victimsinfo.govt.nz

White Ribbon New Zealand: https://whiteribbon.org.nz

Chapter Six
Screening for substance abuse

Written by Carolyn Jarvis
Adapted by Jennifer Lillibridge

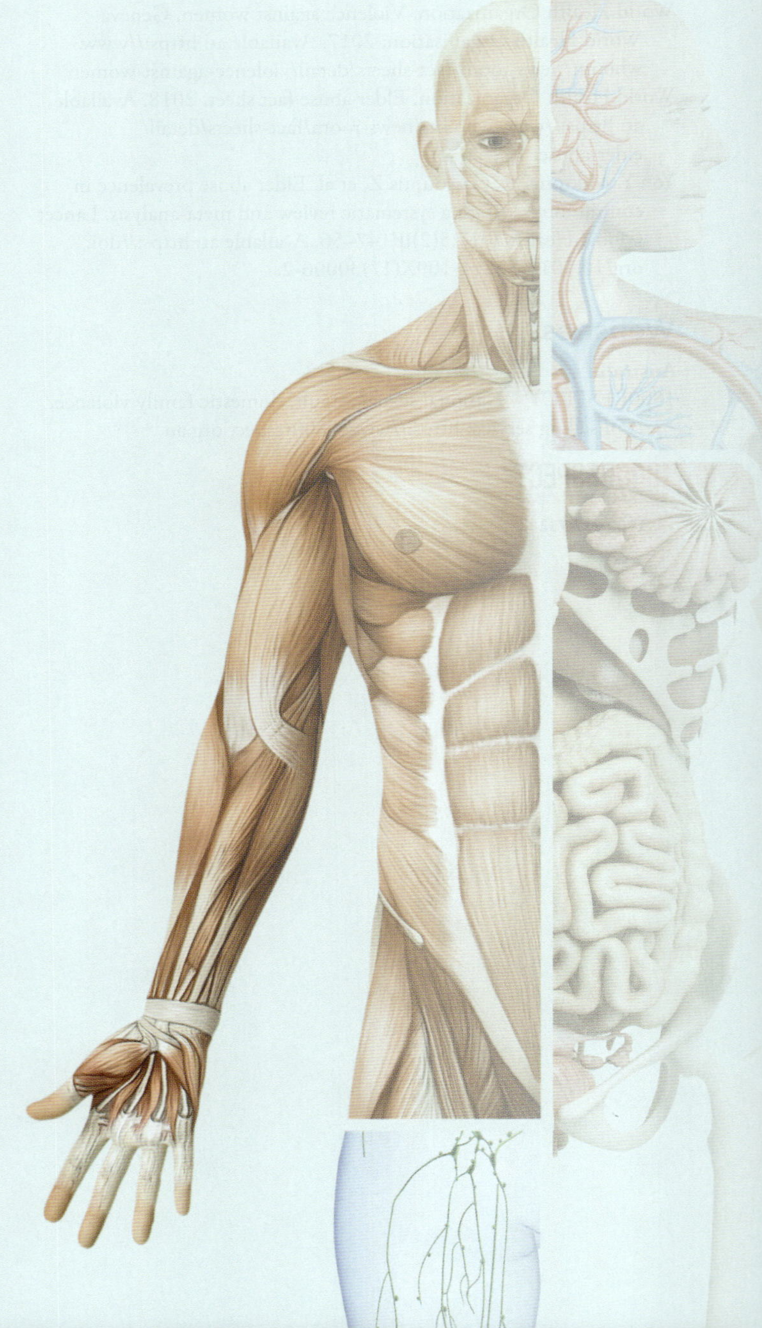

INTRODUCTION

Tobacco smoking, harmful consumption of alcohol and illicit drug use are significant health issues and a disease burden in the Australian and New Zealand communities. According to the Australian Institute of Health and Welfare (AIHW 2020), in addition to harmful consumption of alcohol and tobacco smoking, 'illicit drug use' includes:

- Illegal drugs—use of a drug that is prohibited from manufacture, sale, possession or use in Australia or New Zealand. For example, cannabis (non-medical use), cocaine, heroin, amphetamine-type stimulants.
- Pharmaceutical drugs—drugs that are available from a pharmacy, over the counter or on prescription, which may be subject to misuse (when used for purposes, or in quantities other than for the medical purposes for which they were originally prescribed). For example, opioid-based pain relief medications, opioid substitution therapies, benzodiazepines and steroids.
- Other psychoactive substances—legal or illegal used in a harmful way. For example, synthetic cannabis and other synthetic drugs or inhalants such as petrol, paint or glue.

Many people that nurses routinely interact with may have underlying harmful substance use issues even if these are not the primary reasons for seeking healthcare. The person may not perceive that their substance use is harmful to their health. This chapter provides background and an overview of issues associated with substance abuse that underpin any health assessment. It could be argued that a component of nurses' responsibility relates to the prevention of harmful use of alcohol and or drugs. Therefore, initial contact, regardless of the reason for the health visit, is an opportunity for the nurse to determine if a problem exists or is suspected and, if so, to take necessary action to assist the individual seeking additional specialised healthcare. This chapter focuses on alcohol and illicit drug use, as the issues related to the health effects of smoking have been covered in most other chapters. All people who are current tobacco smokers who come into contact with a health professional should be offered advice on quitting smoking.

ALCOHOL USE AND ABUSE

Results from the 2016 National Drug Strategy Household Survey indicate that 77% of Australians aged 14 years or older had consumed at least one glass of alcohol in the previous 12 months and 5.9% drank daily. While these figures are worrying, the proportion of Australians aged 14 or over who consumed alcohol at a risky level declined from 2013 to 2016, single-occasion risky (binge) drinking behaviours remained stable. Survey data suggest there is evidence of positive changing drinking behaviours in teenagers. Eighty-two per cent of teenagers abstained from drinking in 2016; an increase from 72% in 2013. Another indication of changing drinking behaviour is one in two drinkers took action to reduce their alcohol intake in 2016, citing health-related concerns (AIHW 2016a).

In the most recent published survey, 74% of Aboriginal and Torres Strait Islander people aged 18 years and over reported they had consumed alcohol in the past year. The proportion of male to female alcohol consumption was 81% for males and 69% for females (Australian Bureau of Statistics (ABS) 2019). Although Aboriginal and Torres Strait Islander people aged 15 years and over are more likely than non-Indigenous people to have exceeded the alcohol consumption threshold for single occasion risk, the incidence is decreasing (ABS 2019).

New Zealand statistics reflect similar drinking habits to those in Australia. In 2017–2018 (Ministry of Health NZ 2018a), most adults in New Zealand had consumed alcohol in the past 12 months (79%). As in Australia, a decline is noted with fewer than in 2006–2007 (84%); decreases in past-year drinking were generally seen across all age groups, but particularly among 15–17-year-olds. Among people who had consumed alcohol in the past 12 months ('past-year drinkers'), one in five (19.8%) had hazardous drinking patterns. Māori people have similar rates of past-year drinking as the total population, but had higher rates of hazardous drinking; 31.7% in 2017–2018 (Ministry of Health NZ 2018b). However, rates of hazardous drinking among Māori adults have decreased (Ministry of Health NZ 2018b). Amphetamine use data is also collected in Ministry of Health surveys. The percentage of amphetamine use in adults has remained stable since 2010–2011 at 0.9–1.1% (Ministry of Health NZ 2016).

Morbidity and mortality data reflect the adverse consequences of excessive alcohol use. Australian alcohol-related deaths on the roads has declined since the 1980s. While these data are encouraging, road deaths as of 19 May 2019 were 128, compared to 83 for 2018 (Transport Accident Commission (TAC) 2019). The proportion of drivers and motorcycle riders killed with a blood–alcohol content (BAC) greater than 0.05 g/100 mL decreased from 38% in 1987 to 19% in 2016 (TAC 2016).

The prevalence of alcohol-related emergency department (ED) visits in Australia and New Zealand has, on average, been reported at one in eight presentations in Australia and one in seven in New Zealand (Egerton-Warburton et al 2018).

Although alcohol consumption is common, it carries the risk of adverse health and social consequences related to its intoxicating, toxic and dependence-producing properties. Approximately 3.3 million deaths every year (5.9% of all deaths worldwide) can be attributed to alcohol. It is considered the third leading risk factor for poor health globally. While there are numerous chronic and acute health effects, the harmful effects of alcohol use can be linked to many social, mental and emotional consequences (World Medical Association 2017). Furthermore, harmful drinking among young people and women is an increasing concern in many countries.

Alcohol consumption is a causal factor in more than 200 disease and injury conditions. Drinking alcohol is associated with a risk of developing health problems such as mental and behavioural disorders, including alcohol dependence, major noncommunicable diseases such as liver cirrhosis, some cancers and cardiovascular diseases, as well as injuries resulting from violence and road trauma. The latest causal relationships are those between alcohol consumption and the incidence of infectious diseases such as tuberculosis, as well as the course of HIV/AIDS. Alcohol consumption by an expectant mother may cause fetal alcohol syndrome and preterm birth complications (World Health Organisation (WHO) 2018). In addition, while it has been known for some time that alcohol increases cancer risk, more recent findings now demonstrate 'convincing' evidence of mouth and throat cancers (larynx and pharynx), oesophageal cancer, breast (postmenopausal), colorectal (in men) and a 'probable' cause of breast (premenopausal), liver and colorectal cancers (in women). Statistics show that even small amounts of alcohol increase risk, but the more you drink, the greater the risk (LoConte et al 2017, World Cancer Research Fund/American Institute for Cancer Research 2017).

There is no safe drinking threshold for cancer risk. Up to one alcoholic drink per day increases risk of breast cancer by 7%, and as drinking levels increase so does the risk of developing breast cancer (Cancer Australia: Australian Government 2019). While the mechanism remains complex, the probable association is that alcohol interferes with oestrogen levels, which affect breast tissue or oestrogen receptors directly. The impact may vary depending on a woman's age (adolescent, pre or postmenopausal) (LoConte et al 2018, Rehm et al 2019).

Alcohol has multiple effects on the heart. It has been generally accepted that moderate drinking (above 1–2 drinks per day) for both men and women is linked to hypertension. However, recent reporting of meta analyses of light or moderate alcohol consumption (≤1 drink/day for women and 1–2 drinks/day for men) continue to be associated with a lower risk of coronary artery disease, heart failure and stroke (O'Keefe et al 2018). Heavy drinking, more than four drinks per day, has been associated with reversible hypertension, atrial fibrillation, non-ischaemic dilated cardiomyopathy and both haemorrhagic and ischaemic stroke (O'Keefe et al 2018).

What is a standard drink?

A standard drink in Australia and New Zealand is any drink that contains 10 g of alcohol. One standard drink always contains the same amount of alcohol regardless of container size or alcohol type, for example beer, wine or spirits. Figure 6.1 represents standard drink equivalents (Australian Government Department of Health and Ageing 2019a). The number of standard drinks in alcoholic beverages is shown on the label of the container.

Alcohol withdrawal

The signs and symptoms of alcohol withdrawal may be grouped into three major classes—autonomic hyperactivity, gastrointestinal changes and cognitive and perceptual changes—and may feature uncomplicated or complicated withdrawal. Table 6.1 will assist in assessing signs and symptoms if alcohol withdrawal is suspected (Manning et al 2018). Early assessment and intervention are critical for appropriate management of symptoms.

ILLICIT DRUG USE

Types of illicit drugs used in Australia include amphetamines, cannabis, cocaine, ecstasy, hallucinogens, heroin, inhalants, pharmaceuticals and steroids. The most recent Australian Institute of Health and Welfare (AIHW) survey reports the four most common illicit drugs are cannabis, misuse of pharmaceuticals, cocaine and ecstasy. Some of the more vulnerable population groups identified as more likely to use illicit drugs are Indigenous Australians, people living in remote and very remote areas and people engaged with the criminal justice system (AIHW 2020). Symptoms and signs of illicit drug withdrawal are varied depending on the drug or drugs that have been used, time since use, amount of drug and the stage of withdrawal. Please refer to Manning et al (2018) or another suitable professional source.

Pharmaceutical drug misuse

Pharmaceutical drug misuse in Australia ranks highly among other forms of illicit drug misuse. In 2016, approximately 3.1 million people (or 16%) in Australia aged 14 years or older had illicitly used drugs in the previous 12 months, an increase from previous years (AIHW 2016b). Use was highest in the 20–29 age group, but in the previous 15 years illicit drug use also increased in the 40–50 age group (AIHW 2016b). Opioid analgesics and benzodiazepines are the most widely prescribed and commonly misused classes of pharmaceutical drugs in Australia (Monheit et al 2016). Monheit et al report that the number of Pharmaceutical Benefits Scheme (PBS) opioid and benzodiazepine prescriptions written between 2010 and 2015 more than doubled (2,104,477 to 4,405,382). Another prescription medication on the rise in Australia for misuse is Pregabalin (trade name Lyrica). While it is not a first line treatment for neuropathic pain, Pregabalin is the seventh most expensive PBS expenditure and the risk of self-poisoning and death are increasing (Murnion & Conigrave 2019).

The misuse of prescription drugs has a huge impact not only on health and safety but also on burdens to the emergency department system. In Victoria alone, pharmaceutical drugs contributed to 80% of overdose deaths from 2009 to 2015 (Monheit et al 2016). In an effort to address the growing problem of misuse of pharmaceuticals, the state of Victoria implemented the SafeScript program, which rolled out state-wide online on 1 April 2019. SafeScripts is a clinical tool to provide additional information about a person's use of high-risk medications that goes beyond a single pharmacy visit. Pharmacists can access the prescription history of patients in real time with this program. The SafeScripts program includes 'all Schedule 8 medications and other high-risk medicines such as benzodiazepines, zolpidem or zopiclone, quetiapine and codeine' (Victorian State Government 2019:para 3). A pilot program of SafeScripts was initiated in Western Victoria in 2018. These data revealed over 7000 instances of people at increased risk and in excess of 4000 alerts sent to pharmacists and General Practitioners (GPs) about people who had visited multiple general practices and pharmacies. These initial data highlight the value of a program that identifies people in need of additional services to manage pain, mental health issues and drug dependence.

Amphetamines

Within the illicit drug type of amphetamines (amphetamine-type stimulants (ATS)), methamphetamine use in the form of 'ice' warrants specific consideration. It is encouraging to note that overall use of methamphetamine decreased according to the AIHW 2016 survey data. However, there was a change in the main form in which it was used; use of crystal methamphetamine (ice) increased from 22% in 2010 to 57% in 2016, thus continuing to be a significant problem, both socially and criminally (AIHW 2016c). Rural communities in Australia have been especially hard hit by the use of ATS, specifically ice. The social, as well as health and safety, issues related to ATS mean that if addiction or abuse is suspected, a thorough in-depth assessment and possibly a referral to a specialist practitioner is of utmost importance. Consistent with Australia, the most frequently used amphetamine in New Zealand in the past year was methamphetamine in the form of ice. In 2015–2016, 1.1% of adults (16 years and older)

WHAT ARE STANDARD DRINKS?
Standard drinks are a way to measure how much alcohol you drink. Drinks come in different sizes and some are stronger than others. They have different amounts of alcohol in them. A standard drink is always equal to 10 g of alcohol.
The information below details the approximate number of standard drinks in different types and serves of alcohol.

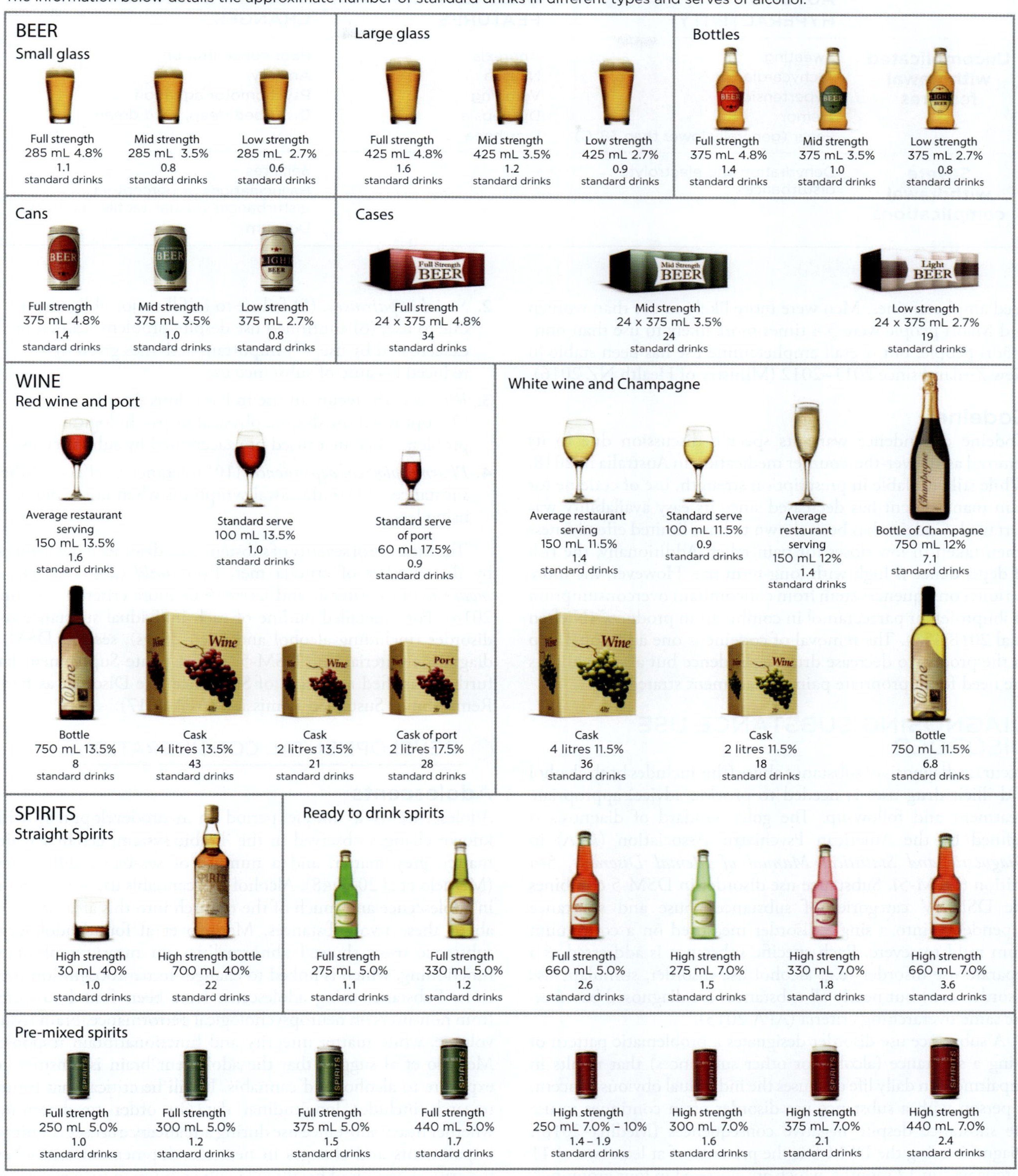

Figure 6.1
Don't lose your standards.
Australian Government, Department of Health. Standard drinks guide. 2019. Available: https://www.health.gov.au/health-topics/alcohol/about-alcohol/standard-drinks-guide?utm_source=alcohol.gov.au&utm_medium=redirect&utm_campaign=digital_transformation&utm_content=%2Finternet%2Falcohol%2Fpublishing.nsf%2FContent%2Fdrinksguide-cnt

TABLE 6.1 Features of alcohol withdrawal

	AUTONOMIC HYPERACTIVITY	GASTROINTESTINAL FEATURES	COGNITIVE AND PERCEPTUAL CHANGES
Uncomplicated withdrawal features	Sweating Tachycardia Hypertension Tremor Fever (generally lower than 38°C)	Anorexia Nausea Vomiting Dyspepsia Diarrhoea	Poor concentration Anxiety Psychomotor agitation Disturbed sleep, vivid dreams
Severe withdrawal complications	Dehydration and electrolyte disturbances	-	Seizures Hallucinations or perceptual disturbances (visual, tactile, auditory) Delirium

used amphetamines. Men were more likely to use than women and Māori people were 3.4 times more likely to use than non-Māori people, but overall amphetamine use has been stable in New Zealand since 2011–2012 (Ministry of Health NZ 2016).

Codeine

Codeine dependence warrants specific discussion due to its removal as an over-the-counter medication in Australia in 2018. While still available in prescription strength, use of codeine for pain management has decreased since its easy availability was curtailed. Codeine has been shown to have limited effectiveness when taken in low doses for pain relief. Additionally, the risk of dependence is high with long-term use. However, the more 'serious consequences stem from concomitant overconsumption of ibuprofen or paracetamol in combination products' (Nielsen et al 2018:451). The removal of codeine is one additional step in the process to decrease drug dependence but also highlights the need for appropriate pain management strategies.

DIAGNOSING SUBSTANCE USE DISORDER

Accurate diagnosis of substance abuse (this includes both alcohol and illicit drug use) is needed to provide advice, appropriate treatment and follow-up. The gold standard of diagnosis is defined by the American Psychiatric Association (APA) in *Diagnostic and Statistical Manual of Mental Disorders*, 5th edition (DSM-5). Substance use disorder in DSM-5 combines the DSM-IV categories of substance abuse and substance dependence into a single disorder measured on a continuum from mild to severe. Each specific substance is addressed as a separate use disorder (e.g. alcohol use disorder, stimulant use disorder, etc.) but nearly all substances are diagnosed based on the same overarching criteria (APA 2013).

A substance use disorder designates a problematic pattern of using a substance (alcohol or other substances) that results in impairment in daily life or causes the individual obvious concern. A person with a substance use disorder often continues to use the substance despite negative consequences (Medina 2018). Diagnosis using the DSM-5 is the presence of at least two of 11 criteria within 12 months, which are clustered in four groupings.

1. *Impaired control:* (1) consuming more or for longer than intended, (2) unsuccessful efforts to stop or cut down use, (3) spending a great deal of time obtaining, using or recovering from use, (4) craving for substance
2. *Social impairment:* (5) failure to fulfill major obligations due to use, (6) continued use despite problems caused or exacerbated by use, (7) important activities given up or reduced because of substance use
3. *Risky use:* (8) recurrent use in hazardous situations, (9) continued use despite physical or psychological problems that are caused or exacerbated by substance use
4. *Pharmacological dependence:* (10) tolerance to effects of the substance, (11) withdrawal symptoms when not using or using less.

The measure of severity of substance use disorder is determined by the number of criteria met, from *mild* (2–3 criteria) to *moderate* (4–5 criteria) and *severe* (6 or more criteria) (Medina 2018). For a detailed outline of each individual substance use disorder (including alcohol and illicit drugs), see the DSM-5 diagnostic criteria. The DSM-5 2017 Update Supplement has further classified remission of Substance Use Disorder as Early Remission or Sustained Remission (APA 2017).

DEVELOPMENTAL CONSIDERATIONS

Adolescents

Adolescence is a unique period in neurodevelopment with known changes observed in the 'limbic system, cerebral white matter, grey matter, and a number of sex-based differences' (Meruelo et al 2017:48). Alcohol and cannabis use are common in adolescence and much of the research into this area has been about these two substances. Meruelo et al found adolescent substance users showed abnormalities on measures of brain functioning, which is linked to changes in neurocognition over time. Substance-using adolescents have been found to differ from non-users on neuropsychological performance, brain tissue volume, white matter integrity and functional brain response. Meruelo et al suggest that the adolescent brain is sensitive to exposure to alcohol and cannabis. It will be critical that future research includes longitudinal data in order to determine whether heavy substance use during adolescence causes cognitive impairments and changes in neurodevelopment, if and when the critical periods of heightened vulnerability to such effects are and if observed abnormalities remit with reduced use.

The well validated CRAFFT 2.1 screening tool (Table 6.2) (Knight 2018) can be administered to adolescents aged 12–21 and includes questions about both drug and alcohol use. The six key words represented by the acronym are Car, Relax, Alone,

TABLE 6.2 Assessing alcohol consumption in adolescents using CRAFFT-2.1 questionnaire

The CRAFFT-II Questionnaire - SBIRT in Schools

DURING THE PAST 12 MONTHS, ON HOW MANY DAYS DID YOU ...

	Question	
1	Drink more than a few sips of beer, wine or any drink containing alcohol?	PUT 0 IF NO USE
2	Use any marijuana (for example, weed, oil or hash by smoking, vaping or in food) or 'synthetic marijuana' (for example 'K2' or 'Spice')?	PUT 0 IF NO USE
3	Use a prescription medication or pill that was NOT prescribed to you or MORE than was prescribed to you (for example, prescription pain pills or ADHD medications)?	PUT 0 IF NO USE
4	Use anything else to get high (for example, other illegal drugs, over-the-counter medications and things that you sniff, huff or vape)?	PUT 0 IF NO USE
C	Have you ever ridden in a CAR driven by someone (including yourself) who was 'high' or had been using alcohol or drugs?	YES NO

STOP If no days of use, then STOP here.

If any days of use, ASK ALL CRAFFT ?s BELOW.

	Question	
R	Do you ever use alcohol or drugs to RELAX, feel better about yourself or fit in?	YES NO
A	Do you ever use alcohol or drugs while you are by yourself, or ALONE?	YES NO
F	Do you ever FORGET things you did while using alcohol or drugs?	YES NO
F	Do your FAMILY or FRIENDS ever tell you that you should cut down on your drinking or drug use?	YES NO
T	Have you ever found yourself in TROUBLE while you were using alcohol or drugs?	YES NO

Reproduced with permission from the Center for Adolescent Substance Abuse Research (CeASAR), Boston Children's Hospital. For more information and versions in other languages, see www.masbirt.org/schools/translations

Forget, Friends and Trouble. The topic areas represented in the CRAFFT 2.1 screening tool can be used by the nurse as talking points to engage an adolescent in a discussion about substance use behaviours.

The pregnant woman

The dangers of alcohol use to the growing fetus during pregnancy are well known. Alcohol easily crosses the placenta, which exposes the baby to similar concentrations of alcohol as the mother. The harmful effects of alcohol on the fetus include impaired development of the fetal nervous system, including the brain, and diminished nourishment of the growing baby. Problems that may occur in the fetus exposed to alcohol before birth include increased risk for miscarriage, stillbirth, low birth weight and birth defects, as well as brain damage (Australian Government Department of Health 2018). Fetal Alcohol Spectrum Disorder (FASD) is the term used to 'describe the lifelong physical and/or neurodevelopmental impairments that can result from fetal alcohol exposure' (NOFASD Australia 2018:para 1). This terminology describes a spectrum on which Fetal Alcohol Syndrome is the most severe form of the disorder. A national strategic plan has been developed to reduce the incidence and impact of FASD in Australia (Australian Government, Department of Health 2019b).

Alcohol is not the only substance harmful to the growing fetus. Licit and illicit drug use can lead to neonatal abstinence syndrome (NAS), which is characterised by hyperactivity of the central and autonomic nervous systems (Reddy et al 2017, Safer Care Victoria 2019).

The AUDIT-C (Australian Government Department of Health 2019c) screening tool can be used to identify women at risk of harmful alcohol or drug use during pregnancy (Table 6.3). A score of 3 or more is considered high risk, indicating the need for a referral. All recommendations for pregnant women and nursing mothers are to abstain from any alcohol or drug intake as any amount can be harmful.

Older adults

Older adults have 'unique health circumstances such as pain, co-morbidities and social circumstances such as isolation' (AIHW 2018a:para 2). It is well known that numerous characteristics of older adults can increase the risk of alcohol use. Liver metabolism and kidney function are decreased, which increases the bioavailability of alcohol in the blood for longer time periods. Ageing people lose muscle mass; less tissue to which the alcohol can be distributed means an increased alcohol concentration in the blood. Due to the frequent presence of comorbidities, the older person may be on multiple medications, which can interact adversely with alcohol. Drinking alcohol increases risk for falls, depression and gastrointestinal problems.

Risky behaviour involving both alcohol and drugs in several older age groups was identified in the 2016 AIHW Survey. The most likely older adult cohort to exceed lifetime risk guidelines for alcohol use were females in the 50s age group and males in the 55–64 age group. Single occasion risky drinking five days a week or more was seen in people in the 60s age group (AIHW 2016a). When compared with younger age groups that previously engaged in more risky drinking behaviours, females in their 50s were the most likely age group to exceed national guidelines for lifetime risk by consuming more than two standard drinks per day. People in the 50s age group have one of the lowest incidences of illicit drug use. However, this group has seen the greatest rise in illicit drug use since 2001. This finding is attributed to an increase in use of cannabis and misuse of pharmaceuticals (AIHW 2016b).

The SMAST-G (Table 6.4) is an assessment tool that can be used to screen older adults for alcohol or drug use (The Regents of the University of Michigan 1991).

ASSESSMENT APPROACHES

Establishing rapport

People come in contact with health professionals for a variety of reasons relating to their health needs. It is common to believe there is no need to mention alcohol or drug use if it is considered unrelated to the reason for the health contact. By maintaining an empathic, nonjudgemental attitude, the nurse can highlight the importance of conducting an alcohol and drug assessment (examples are the screening tools presented in this chapter) as part of a general health assessment for all people over the age of 14 years. It is therefore worthwhile to include alcohol and drug use within a general assessment routine, even if problems are not suspected.

Subjective data

These types of questions or use of screening tools then become a normal part of routine assessment questions. Throughout each of the chapters of this book questions have been included

TABLE 6.3 Assessing alcohol consumption in pregnancy using AUDIT-C

1. How often do you have a drink containing alcohol?
2. How many standard drinks of alcohol do you drink on a typical day when you are drinking?
3. How often do you have 6 or more drinks on one occasion?

AUDIT-C SCORE	0	1	2	3	4
Question 1	Never	Monthly or less	2 - 4 times per month	2 - 3 times per week	4 + times per week
Question 2	1 - 2	3 - 4	5 - 6	7 - 9	10 +
Question 3	Never	Less than monthly	Monthly	Weekly	Daily or almost daily
SCORING GUIDE (Total points)					
3 or greater = increased risk					

https://ndarc.med.unsw.edu.au/sites/default/files/ndarc/resources/Quick%20Guide%20Identifying%20women%20at%20risk.pdf

TABLE 6.4 SMAST-G alcohol screening tool for the older adult

QUESTIONS ARE ANSWERED WITH YES (1) OR NO (0)
1. When talking with others, do you ever underestimate how much you drink?
2. After a few drinks, have you sometimes not eaten or skipped a meal because you didn't feel hungry?
3. Does having a few drinks help decrease your shakiness or tremors?
4. Does alcohol sometimes make it hard for you to remember parts of the day or night?
5. Do you usually take a drink to relax or calm your nerves?
6. Do you drink to take your mind off your problems?
7. Have you ever increased your drinking after experiencing a loss in your life?
8. Has a doctor or nurse ever said they were worried or concerned about your drinking?
9. Have you ever made rules to manage your drinking?
10. When you feel lonely, does having a drink help?
TOTAL SMAST-G SCORE (0–10) ____________
SCORING: 2 OR MORE 'YES' RESPONSES IS INDICATIVE OF AN ALCOHOL PROBLEM.

in the 'health and lifestyle maintenance' section to prompt you to include screening questions related to tobacco, drug and alcohol use. Examples of specific questions are included in Chapter 8: The health history.

Objective data – use of screening tools

Screening instruments are useful to help identify problem alcohol or drug use that requires a more thorough focused assessment. Multiple alcohol screening instruments that target specific populations, such as women, pregnant women and the older adult have been provided in this chapter. There are less well established/validated instruments for illicit drug use or nonmedical use of prescription medications. However, the DAST-10 Questionnaire (Table 6.5) is an established screening tool that can be used if there are concerns about illicit drug use, as it relates only to drug use, excluding questions about alcohol and tobacco. It is accompanied by a scoring guide that will assist the nurse to determine if further assessment or referral is needed.

The AUDIT (Table 6.6) is an example of a widely used generic to any age group alcohol screening questionnaire that can be used in a variety of settings (Babor et al 2001). The AUDIT helps detect both less severe alcohol problems (hazardous and harmful drinking) and alcohol abuse and dependence disorders. The AUDIT is sensitive to current, as opposed to past, alcohol problems. While there are specific age-related screening tools, the AUDIT is also relevant for adolescents and older adults. The AUDIT covers three domains: alcohol consumption (questions 1 to 3); drinking behaviour or dependence (questions 4 to 6); and adverse consequences from alcohol (questions 7 to 10). An AUDIT score of 8 points for men or 4 points for women, adolescents and those older than 60 years indicates hazardous alcohol consumption, prompting a referral to a substance abuse specialist.

Assessment outcomes

It is not normally the responsibility of the nurse who initially identifies a substance use problem to formulate a treatment plan; however, it is the nurse's responsibility to initiate the referral process and know whom to contact. Most hospitals or community settings will have identified alcohol and drug (or mental health) experts who can be contacted if a problem is suspected. Your assessment should provide enough information to determine if such a referral is needed.

TABLE 6.5 General screening for drug abuse using DAST-10

THESE QUESTIONS REFER TO THE PAST 12 MONTHS.	NO	YES
1. Have you used drugs other than those required for medical reasons?	0	1
2. Do you abuse more than one drug at a time?	0	1
3. Are you always able to stop using drugs when you want to? (If you never use drugs, answer 'Yes'.)	1	0
4. Have you had 'blackouts' or 'flashbacks' as a result of drug use?	0	1
5. Do you ever feel bad or guilty about your drug use? (If you never use drugs, choose 'No'.)	0	1
6. Does your spouse (or parents) ever complain about your involvement with drugs?	0	1
7. Have you neglected your family because of your use of drugs?	0	1
8. Have you engaged in illegal activities in order to obtain drugs?	0	1
9. Have you ever experienced withdrawal symptoms (felt sick) when you stopped taking drugs?	0	1
10. Have you had medical problems as a result of your drug use (e.g. memory loss, hepatitis, convulsions, bleeding, etc.)?	0	1
DAST-10 SCORE	**DEGREE OF PROBLEMS RELATED TO DRUG ABUSE**	**SUGGESTED ACTION**
0	No problems reported	None at this time
1–2	Low level	Monitor, re-assess at a later date
3–5	Moderate level	Further investigation
6–8	Substantial level	Intensive assessment
9–10	Severe level	Intensive assessment

Skinner HA. The Drug Abuse Screening Test. Addictive Behavior 1982;7(4);363–71.

TABLE 6.6 The alcohol use disorders identification test—AUDIT

QUESTIONS	0	1	2	3	4
1. How often do you have a drink containing alcohol?	Never	Monthly or less	2-4 times a month	2-3 times a week	4 or more times a week
2. How many drinks containing alcohol do you have on a typical day when you are drinking?	1 or 2	3 or 4	5 or 6	7 to 9	10 or more
3. How often do you have 6 or more drinks on one occasion?	Never	Less than monthly	Monthly	Weekly	Daily or almost daily
4. How often during the last year have you found that you were not able to stop drinking once you had started?	Never	Less than monthly	Monthly	Weekly	Daily or almost daily
5. How often during the last year have you failed to do what was normally expected of you because of drinking?	Never	Less than monthly	Monthly	Weekly	Daily or almost daily
6. How often during the last year have you needed a first drink in the morning to get yourself going after a heavy drinking session?	Never	Less than monthly	Monthly	Weekly	Daily or almost daily
7. How often during the last year have you had a feeling of guilt or remorse after drinking?	Never	Less than monthly	Monthly	Weekly	Daily or almost daily
8. How often during the last year have you been unable to remember what happened the night before because of your drinking?	Never	Less than monthly	Monthly	Weekly	Daily or almost daily
9. Have you or someone else been injured because of your drinking?	No		Yes, but not in the last year		Yes, during the last year
10. Has a relative, friend, doctor or other healthcare worker been concerned about your drinking or suggested that you cut down?	No		Yes, but not in the last year		Yes, during the last year
					Total

BIBLIOGRAPHY

American Psychiatric Association (APA). Diagnostic and statistical manual of mental disorders. 5th ed. Washington, DC: APA; 2013.

American Psychiatric Association (APA). Supplement to diagnostic and statistical manual of mental disorders. 5th ed. American Psychiatric Association Publishing; 2017. Available at: https://psychiatryonline.org/pb-assets/dsm/update/DSM5Update_October2017.pdf.

Australian Bureau of Statistics. National Aboriginal and Torres Strait Islander Health Survey, 2018-19. ABS cat. no. 4715.0. Canberra: ABS; 2019. Available at: https://www.abs.gov.au/AUSSTATS/abs@.nsf/Latestproducts/4715.0Main%20Features12018-19?opendocument&tabname=Summary&prodno=4715.0&issue=2018-19&num=&view=.

Australian Government Department of Health. Information you might not know about alcohol and pregnancy. 2018. Available at: http://www.alcohol.gov.au/internet/alcohol/publishing.nsf/Content/wwtk-cons-leaflet.

Australian Government Department of Health and Ageing. Don't lose your standards. 2019a. Available at: http://www.alcohol.gov.au/internet/alcohol/publishing.nsf/Content/C6738D5F231CC231CA25767200820337/$File/young.pdf.

Australian Government Department of Health. Reducing Fetal Alcohol Spectrum Disorder (FASD) in Australia. 2019b. Available at: https://beta.health.gov.au/resources/publications/national-fetal-alcohol-spectrum-disorder-fasd-strategic-action-plan-2018-2028.

Australian Government Department of Health. Assessing alcohol consumption in pregnancy using AUDIT-C. 2019c. Available at: https://beta.health.gov.au/resources/publications/assessing-alcohol-consumption-in-pregnancy-using-audit-c.

Australian Institute of Health and Welfare (AIHW). Alcohol use – National Drug Strategy Household Survey 2016 key findings. 2016a. Available at: https://www.aihw.gov.au/reports/illicit-use-of-drugs/ndshs-2016-key-findings/contents/alcohol-use.

Australian Institute of Health and Welfare (AIHW). Illicit use of drugs – NDSHS 2016 key findings. 2016b. Available at: https://www.aihw.gov.au/reports/illicit-use-of-drugs/ndshs-2016-key-findings/contents/illicit-use-of-drugs.

Australian Institute of Health and Welfare (AIHW). Australian Drug Strategy Household Survey – 2016. Detailed findings. 2016c. Available at: https://www.aihw.gov.au/reports/illicit-use-of-drugs/ndshs-2016-detailed/contents/table-of-contents.

Australian Institute of Health and Welfare (AIHW). Alcohol, tobacco and other drugs in Australia. Canberra: Australian Institute of Health and Welfare; 2020. Available at: https://www.aihw.gov.au/reports/alcohol/alcohol-tobacco-other-drugs-australia.

Babor TF, Higgins-Biddle JC, Saunders JB, et al. AUDIT: Alcohol Use Disorders Identification Test guidelines for use in primary care. 2nd ed. Geneva: World Health Organisation, Department of Mental Health and Substance Dependence; 2001.

Cancer Australia: Australian Government. Breast cancer risk factors. 2019. Available at: https://breastcancerriskfactors.gov.au/risk-factors/lifestyle-factors.

The Drug Abuse Screening Test (DAST-10). Available at: https://med.dartmouth-hitchcock.org/documents/DAST-10-drug-abuse-screening-test.pdf.

Egerton-Warburton D, Gosbell A, Wadsworth A, et al. A point-prevalence survey of alcohol-related presentations to Australasian emergency departments. Aust N Z J Public Health 2018;42(2):218.

Knight JR. CRAFFT II Questionnaire. Boston, MA: Center for Adolescent Substance Abuse Research (CeASAR) Boston Children's Hospital; 2018. Available at: https://www.masbirt.org/sites/www.masbirt.org/files/School%20SBIRT/CRAFFT/English_CRAFFT-II_2018.pdf.

LoConte NK, Brewster AM, Kaur JS, et al. Alcohol and cancer: a statement of the American Society of Clinical Oncology. J Clin Oncol 2018;36(1):83–93.

Manning V, Arunogiri S, Frei M, et al. Alcohol and other drug withdrawal: practice guidelines. 3rd ed. Richmond, Victoria: Turning Point; 2018. Available at: https://www.turningpoint.org.au/sites/default/files/inline-files/Alcohol-and-Drug-Withdrawal-Guidelines-2018.pdf.

Medina J. Symptoms of substance use disorders. Psych Central 2018. Available at: https://psychcentral.com/disorders/addictions/substance-use-disorder-symptoms/.

Meruelo AD, Castro N, Cota CI, et al. Cannabis and alcohol use, and the developing brain. Behav Brain Res 2017;325(Pt A):44–50.

Ministry of Health NZ. New Zealand Health Survey 2016 – Amphetamine use 2015/16. 2016. Available at: https://www.health.govt.nz/publication/amphetamine-use-2015-16-new-zealand-health-survey.

Ministry of Health NZ. Hazardous drinking. 2018a. Available at: https://minhealthnz.shinyapps.io/nz-health-survey-2017-18-annual-data-explorer/_w_38d56904/#!/key-indicators.

Ministry of Health NZ. Self-rated health. 2018b. Available at: https://minhealthnz.shinyapps.io/nz-health-survey-2017-18-annual-data-explorer/_w_38d56904/#!/explore-topics.

Monheit B, Pietrzak D, Hocking S. Prescription drug abuse – A timely update. Aust Fam Physician 2016;45(12):862–6.

Murnion B, Conigrave KM. Pregabalin misuse: the next wave of prescription medication problems. MJA 2019;210(2):72–3.

Nielsen S, MacDonald T, Johnson JL. Identifying and treating codeine dependence: a systematic review. MJA 2018;208(10):451–61.

NOFASD Australia. Fetal alcohol syndrome disorder. 2018. Available at: https://www.nofasd.org.au/alcohol-and-pregnancy/what-is-fasd/.

O'Keefe EL, DiNicolantonio JJ, O'Keefe JH, et al. Alcohol and CV health: Jekyll and Hyde j-curves. Prog Cardiovasc Dis 2018;61(1):68–75.

Reddy UM, Davis JM, Ren Z, et al. Opioid Use in Pregnancy, Neonatal Abstinence Syndrome, and Childhood Outcomes Workshop Invited Speakers. Opioid use in pregnancy, neonatal abstinence syndrome, and childhood outcomes: executive summary of a joint workshop. Obstet Gynecol 2017;130(1):10–28.

The Regents of the University of Michigan. Short Michigan Alcoholism Screening Test–Geriatric Version (SMAST-G). 1991. Available at: https://consultgeri.org/try-this/general-assessment/issue-17.pdf.

Rehm J, Soerjomataram I, Ferreira-Borges C, et al. Does alcohol use affect cancer risk? Current Nutrition Reports 2019;20:1–8.

Safer Care Victoria. Victorian agency for health information. 2019. Available at: https://bettersafercare.vic.gov.au/resources/clinical-guidance/maternity-and-newborn/substance-use-during-pregnancy-care-of-the-mother-and-newborn.

Transport Accident Commission (TAC) Victoria. Drink driving statistics. 2016. Available at: http://www.tac.vic.gov.au/road-safety/statistics/summaries/drink-driving-statistics.

Transport Accident Commission (TAC) Victoria. Statistics: lives lost year to date. 2019. Available at: http://www.tac.vic.gov.au/road-safety/statistics/lives-lost-year-to-date.

Victorian State Government. SafeScript. 2019. Available at: https://www2.health.vic.gov.au/public-health/drugs-and-poisons/safe-script/about-safescript.

World Cancer Research Fund/American Institute for Cancer Research: Continuous Update Project. Breast cancer. London: WCRF International; 2017. Available at: https://www.wcrf.org/dietandcancer/breast-cancer.

World Health Organisation (WHO). Alcohol: key facts. Geneva: World Health Organisation; 2018. Available at: https://www.who.int/news-room/fact-sheets/detail/alcohol.

World Medical Association. WMA declaration on alcohol. Ferney-Voltaire, France: World Medical Association, Inc; 2017. Available at: https://www.wma.net/policies-post/wma-declaration-on-alcohol/.

Health assessment tools and techniques

Unit 2

Chapter Seven

The health assessment interview

Written by Carolyn Jarvis and Ann Eckhardt
Adapted by Elizabeth Pascoe

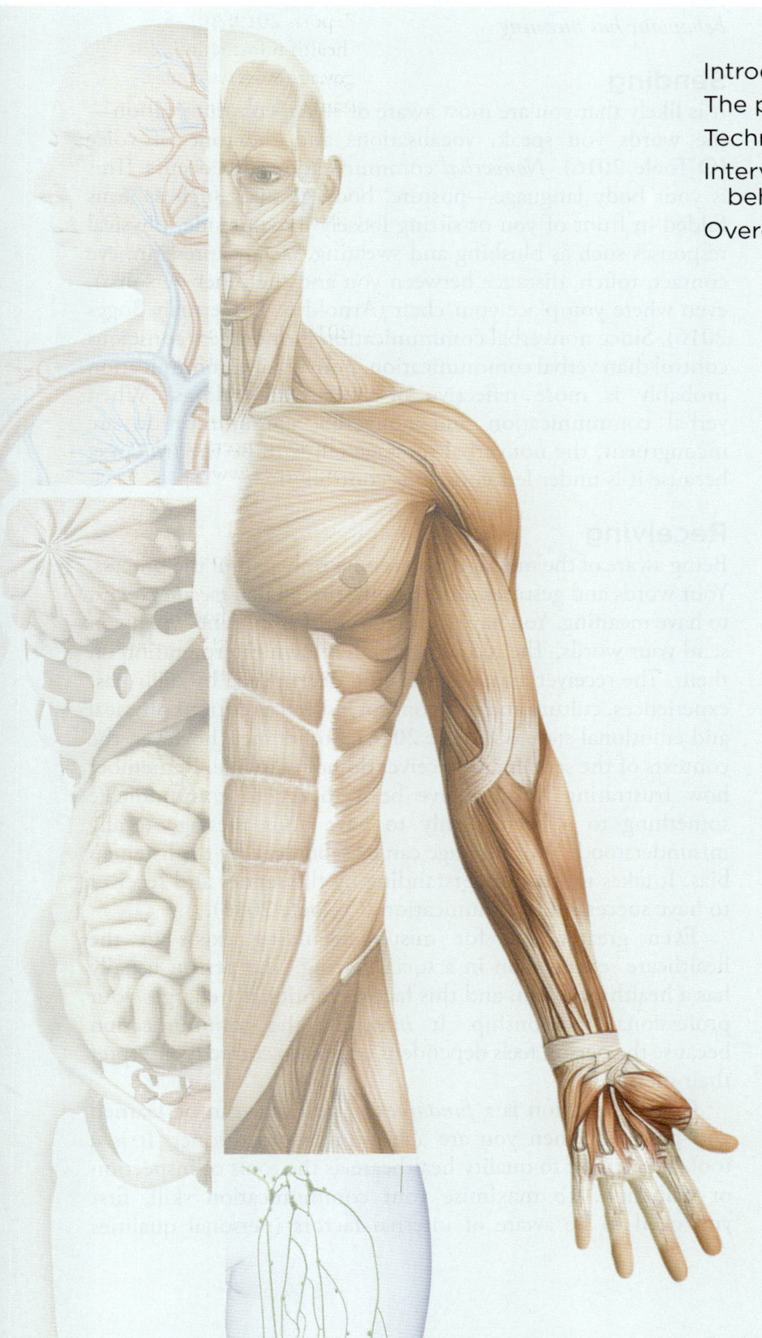

Introduction

The process of communication

Techniques of communication

Interviewing people with special needs and challenging behaviours

Overcoming communication barriers

INTRODUCTION

The health assessment interview is a meeting between you and the person seeking healthcare. The goal is to record a complete person-centred health history. The health history is important in beginning to identify the person's health strengths and problems and as a bridge to the next step in data collection, the physical examination.

The primary purpose of the health assessment interview is to gather **subjective data** from the person—what the person tells you about themself. The health assessment interview is the first and really the most important part of data collection. The interview gives the person permission and the opportunity to tell you what *they* perceive their health state to be. Once people enter the healthcare system, they may relinquish some control. At the interview, however, the person is still in charge. The starting point for the health assessment interview is for you to acknowledge and accept that the person is the most knowledgeable person when it comes to their own health state. Remember that the individual knows everything about their own health state, and you know nothing. Your skill in interviewing is to elicit all the necessary information about the person's health status and to build rapport for a successful working relationship. A successful health interview comprises your ability to:

1. Establish rapport and trust so the person feels accepted and thus free to share all their relevant health history.
2. Gather complete and accurate information about the person's health state, including the description and chronology of any past and present symptoms and illnesses.
3. Educate the person about their health state so that they can participate in identifying potential and actual health issues.
4. Build rapport for a continuing therapeutic relationship; this rapport facilitates future diagnoses, planning and treatment.
5. Begin educating for health promotion and disease prevention.

Consider the health interview as being similar to forming a contract between you and the person. A contract consists of spoken or unspoken rules for behaviour. In this case, the contract concerns what the person needs and expects from healthcare and what you, the health professional, have to offer. Your mutual goal is optimal health outcomes. The contract requires you to:

- Establish the time and place of the interview and subsequent physical examination
- Introduce yourself and provide a brief explanation of your role
- Explain the purpose of the interview
- Identify time parameters for the interview and subsequent physical examination
- Explain the requirements of the person
- Establish the presence of any other people (e.g. the person's family, other health professionals, students)
- Consider confidentiality and to what extent it may be limited.

Although the person may already know some of this information through telephone contact with receptionists or the admitting office, the remaining points need to be stated clearly at the outset. Any confusion could produce resentment and anger, rather than the openness and trust you need to facilitate the interview.

THE PROCESS OF COMMUNICATION

The vehicle that carries you and the person through the interview is communication. Communication is exchanging information so that each person clearly understands the other, i.e. mutual understanding (O'Toole 2016). If you do not understand each other, you have not conveyed a shared meaning and effective communication has **not** occurred.

It is challenging to teach the skill of interviewing because initially health professionals may think little needs to be learned. They assume that if they can talk and hear, they can communicate. But much more than talking and hearing is necessary. Communication includes all behaviour, conscious and unconscious, verbal and nonverbal (O'Toole 2016). *All behaviour has meaning.*

Sending

It is likely that you are most aware of *verbal* communication—the words you speak, vocalisations and the tone of voice (O'Toole 2016). *Nonverbal* communication also occurs. This is your body language—posture, body gestures such as arms folded in front of you or sitting loosely by your side, physical responses such as blushing and sweating, facial expression, eye contact, touch, distance between you and the other person(s), even where you place your chair (Arnold & Underman Boggs 2016). Since nonverbal communication is under less conscious control than verbal communication, nonverbal communication probably is more reflective of your true feelings. When verbal communication and nonverbal communication are incongruent, the nonverbal message tends to be the true one, because it is under less conscious control.

Receiving

Being aware of the messages you send is only part of the process. Your words and gestures must be interpreted in a *specific context* to have meaning. You have a specific context in mind when you send your words. The receiver puts their own interpretation on them. The receiver attaches meaning determined by their past experiences, culture and self-concept, as well as current physical and emotional state (O'Toole 2016). Sometimes, however, the contexts of the sender and receiver do not coincide. Remember how frustrating it may have been to try to communicate something to a friend, only to have your message totally misunderstood? Your message can be sabotaged by the listener's bias. It takes mutual understanding by the sender and receiver to have successful communication (O'Toole 2016).

Even greater risk for misunderstanding exists in the healthcare setting than in a social setting. The person usually has a health problem, and this factor emotionally charges your professional relationship. It *intensifies* the communication because the person feels dependent on you to correctly interpret their messages.

Communication is a *fundamental skill* that can be learned and polished when you are a beginning practitioner. It is a tool, as intrinsic to quality healthcare as the tools of inspection or palpation. To maximise your communication skill, first you need to be aware of internal factors (personal qualities and abilities) and external factors (environmental and other issues) and their influence. Central to the ability to be aware of internal and external factors and their impact is self-awareness (O'Toole 2016). Self-awareness enables us to enhance self-understanding. Greater self-understanding leads to increased control of thought and behaviour—internal and external factors (O'Toole 2016). This then leads to positive interactions and effective communication.

Internal factors (personal qualities and abilities)

Internal factors are those particular to the nurse, i.e. what you bring into the interview. Cultivate the three inner factors of liking others, empathy and the ability to listen.

Liking others. One essential factor for a nurse's 'goodness of fit' into a helping profession is a genuine liking of other people. This means a generally optimistic view of people: an assumption of their strengths and a tolerance for their weaknesses. An atmosphere of warmth and caring is necessary. The person must feel that they are accepted unconditionally.

The respect for other people extends to respect for their own control over their health. Your goal is *not* to make the person dependent on you, but to help them to be increasingly responsible for themselves. You wish to promote their growth. You have the healthcare resources to offer. The person must choose how to apply those resources to their own life.

Empathy. Empathy means viewing the world from the other person's inner frame of reference while remaining yourself. Empathy means recognising and accepting the other person's feelings without criticism. It is described as 'feeling with the person rather than feeling like the person'. It does not mean you become lost in the other person at the expense of your own self. If this occurred, you would cease to be helpful. Rather, it is to *understand with* the person how *they* perceive their world.

The ability to listen. Listening is not a passive role in the communication process; it is active and demanding. Listening requires your complete attention. You cannot be preoccupied with your own needs or the needs of other people, or you will miss something important with this interview. For the time of this interview, no one is more important than this person. This person's needs are your sole concern.

Active listening is the route to understanding. You cannot be thinking of what you are going to say as soon as the person stops for breath. Listen to *what* the person says. The story may not come out in the order you would ask it or will record it later. Let the person talk from their own outline; nearly everything that is said will be relevant. Listen to *the way* a person tells the story, such as difficulty with language, impaired memory, the tone of the person's voice, and even to what the person is leaving out.

External factors (environmental and other issues)

Preparation of the physical setting where the interview is to occur is essential. The setting may be in a hospital room, an examination room in an office or clinic or in the person's home (where you will have less control). In any location, optimal conditions are important to have a smooth interview. Therefore, preparation of the physical setting must include attention to the following elements:

Ensure privacy. Aim for geographic privacy—a private room in the hospital, clinic, office or home. This may involve asking an ambulatory roommate to step out for a while or finding an unoccupied room or an empty lounge. If geographic privacy is not available, 'psychological privacy' by curtained partitions may suffice as long as the person feels sure no one can overhear the conversation or interrupt.

Refuse interruptions. Most people resent interruptions except in cases of an emergency. Inform any support staff of your interview and ask that they not interrupt you during this time. Discourage other health professionals from interrupting you with *their* need for access to the person. You need to concentrate and to establish rapport. An interruption can destroy in seconds what you have spent many minutes building up.

Physical environment

- Set the room temperature at a comfortable level.
- Provide sufficient lighting so that you can see each other clearly. Avoid facing the person directly towards a strong light where they must squint as if on stage.
- Reduce noise. Multiple stimuli are confusing. Turn off the television, radio and any unnecessary equipment.
- Place the distance between you and the person at 1 to 1.5 m (twice arm's length). If you place the person any closer, you may invade their private space and you may create anxiety. If you place the person further away, you seem distant and aloof. (See Cultural and Social Considerations below for more information.)
- Arrange equal-status seating. Both you and the person should be comfortably seated, at eye level. Avoid facing them across a desk or table because that feels like a barrier. Placing the chairs at 90 degrees is good because it allows the person either to face you or to look straight ahead from time to time (Figure 7.1). Most important, avoid standing. Standing does two things: (1) it communicates your haste and (2) it assumes superiority. Standing makes you loom

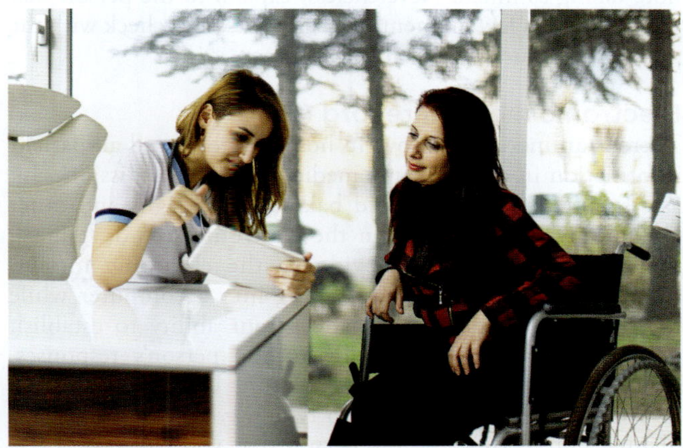

Figure 7.1
Equal-status seating.

over the person as an authority figure. When you are sitting, the person feels some control in the setting.

- Arrange a face-to-face position when interviewing the hospitalised person. If the person is in bed they should not have to stare at the ceiling, because this causes them to lose the visual message of your communication.

Dress

- The person should remain in their own clothes except in the case of an emergency.
- Your appearance and clothing should be appropriate to the setting and should meet conventional professional standards including conservative clothing, a name tag and neat hair. Avoid extremes.

Note-taking

Some use of history forms and note-taking may be unavoidable. When you sit down later to record the interview, you cannot rely completely on memory to furnish details of previous hospitalisations or the review of body systems, for example. But be aware that note-taking during the interview has disadvantages:

- It breaks eye contact too often.
- It shifts your attention away from the person, diminishing their sense of importance.
- It can interrupt the person's narrative flow. You may say 'Please slow down; I'm not getting it all'. Or, the person may see you recording furiously, and in an effort to please you, adjust their tempo to your writing. Either way, the person's natural mode of expression is lost.
- It impedes your observation of the person's nonverbal behaviour.
- It is threatening to the person during the discussion of sensitive issues (e.g. amount of alcohol and drug use, number of sexual partners or incidence of physical abuse).

So keep note-taking to a minimum, and try to focus your attention on the person. Any recording you do should be secondary to the dialogue and should not interfere with the person's spontaneity. With experience, you will not rely on note-taking as much. Nevertheless, explain to the person that you may take a few moments to make notes and check with the person that your interpretation is correct.

Electronic medical record (EMR)

There is an increasing move in hospitals to record all patient information in an electronic medical record. Admission, risk assessment, medication, fluid balance, vital signs and other charts can be located within the electronic record. Clinical progress notes are also moving to the electronic format. As with written note-taking, typing into a computer while interviewing the person can affect your ability to establish rapport and to listen carefully to the person's responses. Try to keep your focus on the person. Use natural pauses in the interview to take time to type in your notes. As with manual note taking, tell the person that you will take a few moments to make notes and check with the person that your interpretation is correct.

TECHNIQUES OF COMMUNICATION

Introducing the interview

The person is here, and you are ready for the health assessment interview. If you are nervous about how to begin, remember to keep the beginning short. Probably they are nervous too, and anxious to start. Address the person, using their surname, and shake hands if that seems comfortable and is culturally appropriate. Introduce yourself and state your role in the organisation (if you are a student, say so). If you are gathering a complete health history, give the reason for this interview:

> 'Mrs Tran, I would like to talk about your illness that caused you to come to the hospital.'
>
> 'Ms Taft, I want to ask you some questions about your health so that we can identify what is keeping you healthy and explore any problems.'
>
> 'Mr Craig, I want to ask you some questions about your health and your usual daily activities so that we can plan your care here in the hospital.'

If the person is in the hospital, more than one health team member may be collecting a health history. Some people are apt to feel exasperated because they believe they are repeating the same thing unless you give a reason for this interview.

After this brief introduction, ask an open-ended question (see below) then let the person proceed. You do not need friendly small talk to build rapport. This is not a social visit; the person has some concern to talk about and wants to get on with it. You will build rapport best by letting them discuss the concern early.

The working phase

The working phase is the data-gathering phase. Verbal skills for this phase include your questions to the person and your responses to what they say. Two types of questions exist: open-ended and closed. Each type has a different place and function in the interview.

Open-ended questions

The **open-ended** question asks for narrative information. It states the topic to be discussed but only in **general** terms. Use it to begin the interview, to introduce a new section of questions and whenever the person introduces a new topic.

> 'Tell me how I can help you.'
>
> 'What brings you to the hospital?'
>
> 'Tell me why you have come here today.'
>
> 'How have you been getting along?'
>
> 'You mentioned shortness of breath. Tell me more about that.'
>
> 'How have you been feeling since your last appointment?'

The open-ended question is unbiased; it leaves the person free to answer in any way. This question encourages the person to respond in paragraphs and to give a spontaneous account in any order chosen. It lets the person express themself fully.

As the person answers, stop and *listen.* What usually happens is that they may answer with a short phrase or sentence, pause and then look at you expecting some direction as to how to go on. What you do next is the key to the interview. If you pose new questions on other topics, you may lose much of the initial story. Instead, respond to the first statement with 'Tell me about it', or 'Anything else?' or merely look acutely interested. The person will then tell the story.

TABLE 7.1 Comparison of open-ended and closed questions

OPEN-ENDED	DIRECT, CLOSED
Use for narrative information	Use for specific information
Calls for long paragraph answers	Calls for short one- or two-word answers
Elicits feelings, opinions, ideas	Elicits cold facts
Builds and enhances rapport	Limits rapport and leaves interaction neutral

Closed or direct questions

Closed or **direct** questions ask for specific information. They elicit a short, one- or two-word answer, a yes or no or a forced choice. Where the open-ended question allows the person to have free rein, the direct question limits their answer (Table 7.1).

Use the direct questions after the person's opening narrative to fill in any details they left out. Also use direct questions when you need many specific facts, such as when asking about past health problems or during the review of systems. You need direct questions to speed up the interview. Asking all open-ended questions would be unwieldy and may take hours. But be careful not to overuse closed questions. Follow these guidelines:

1. Ask only one direct question at a time. Avoid bombarding the person with long lists: 'Have you ever had pain, double vision, watering or redness in the eyes?' Avoid double-barrelled questions, such as 'Do you exercise and follow a diet for your weight?' The person will not know which question to answer. And if the person answers 'yes', you will not know which question the person has answered.
2. Choose language the person understands. Avoid using complicated medical terminology, for example 'How many times do you void per day?' may not be understood. You need to assess the person's level of understanding of medical terminology.

Responses—assisting the narrative

You have asked the first open-ended question, and the person answers. As the person talks, your role is to encourage free expression but not let the person wander off course. Your responses help the teller amplify the story.

Some people seek healthcare for short-term or relatively simple needs. Their history is direct and uncomplicated; for these people, two responses (facilitation and silence) may be all you need to get a complete picture. Other people have a complex story, a long history of a chronic condition or accompanying emotions. Additional responses help you gather data without cutting them off.

There are nine types of verbal responses in all. The first five responses (facilitation, silence, reflection, empathy, clarification) involve your *reactions* to the facts or feelings the person has communicated. Your response focuses on the person's frame of reference. Your own frame of reference does not enter into the response. In the remaining four responses (confrontation, interpretation, explanation, summary), you start to express *your own* thoughts and feelings. The frame of reference shifts from the person's perspective to yours. In the first five responses, the person leads; in the last four responses, you lead.

The person's frame of reference

Facilitation. These responses encourage the person to say more, to continue with the story ('mm-hmm, go on, continue, uh-huh'). Also called general leads, these responses show the person you are interested and will listen further. Simply maintaining eye contact, shifting forwards in your seat with increased attention, nodding 'Yes' or using your hand to gesture 'Yes, go on, I'm with you' encourages the person to continue talking.

Silence. Silence is golden after open-ended questions. Your silent attentiveness communicates that the person has time to think, to organise what they wish to say without interruption from you. This 'thinking silence' is the one health professionals interrupt most often. The interruption destroys the person's train of thought. The person is often interrupted because silence is uncomfortable to beginning nurses. They feel responsible for keeping the dialogue going and feel at fault if it stops. But silence has advantages. One advantage is letting the person collect their thoughts. Also, silence gives you a chance to observe the person unobtrusively and to note nonverbal cues. Finally, silence gives you time to plan your next approach.

Reflection. This response echoes the person's words. Reflection is repeating part of what the person has just said. In this example, it focuses further attention on a specific phrase and helps the person continue in their own way:

> Patient: I'm here because of my water. It was cutting off.
> Response: It was cutting off?
> Patient: Yes, yesterday it took me 30 minutes to pass my water. Finally, I got a tiny stream, but then it just closed off.

Reflection also can help express feeling behind a person's words. The feeling is already in the statement. You focus on it and encourage the person to elaborate:

> Patient: It's so hard having to stay flat on my back in the hospital with this pregnancy. I have two more little ones at home. I'm so worried they are not getting the care they need.
> Response: You feel worried and anxious about your children?

Think of yourself as a mirror reflecting the person's words or feelings. This helps the person to elaborate on the problem.

Empathy. A physical symptom, condition or illness often has accompanying emotions. Many people have trouble expressing these feelings, perhaps because of confusion or embarrassment. In the second reflecting example above, the person had already stated her feeling and you echoed it. But in the first example, he has not said it yet. An empathic response recognises a feeling and puts it into words. It names the feeling and allows the expression of it. When the empathic response is used, the person feels accepted and can deal with the feeling openly.

> Patient (sarcastically): This is just great. I have my own business, I direct 20 employees every day, and now here I am having to call you for every little thing.
> Response: It must be hard—one day having so much control, and now feeling dependent on someone else.

Your response does not cut off further communication as would happen by giving false reassurance ('Oh, you'll be back to work in no time'). Also, it does not deny the feeling and indicate that it is not justified ('Now I don't do *every*thing for you. Why, you are feeding yourself'). An empathic response recognises the feeling, accepts it and allows the person to express it without embarrassment. It strengthens rapport. The person feels understood, which by itself is therapeutic, because it opens the isolation of illness. Other empathic responses are, 'This must be very hard for you', or placing your hand lightly on the person's forearm—if culturally appropriate (Figure 7.2).

Clarification. Clarify what a person means when their word choice is ambiguous or confusing; for example, 'Tell me what you mean by tired blood'. You can also use clarification to summarise the person's words or simplify them to make them clearer. Confirm with the person that you are on the right track: you are asking for agreement, and the person can confirm or deny your understanding.

> Response: Now as I understand you, this heaviness in your chest comes when you mow the lawn or climb stairs, and it goes away when you stop doing those things. Is that correct?
>
> Patient: Yes, that's pretty much it.

Your frame of reference

In these four responses, confrontation, interpretation, explanation and summary, the frame of reference shifts from the person's perspective to yours. These responses now include your own thoughts and feelings. Use these four responses judiciously. If you use them too often, you take over at the person's expense.

Confrontation. In the case of confrontation, you have observed a certain action, feeling or statement and you now focus the person's attention on it. You give your honest feedback about what you see or feel. This may focus on a discrepancy: 'You say it doesn't hurt, but when I touch you here, you grimace'. Or, it may focus on the person's affect: 'You look sad' or 'You sound angry'. Or, you may confront the person when you notice parts of the story are inconsistent: 'Earlier you said you were laying off alcohol and just now you said you had a few drinks after work'.

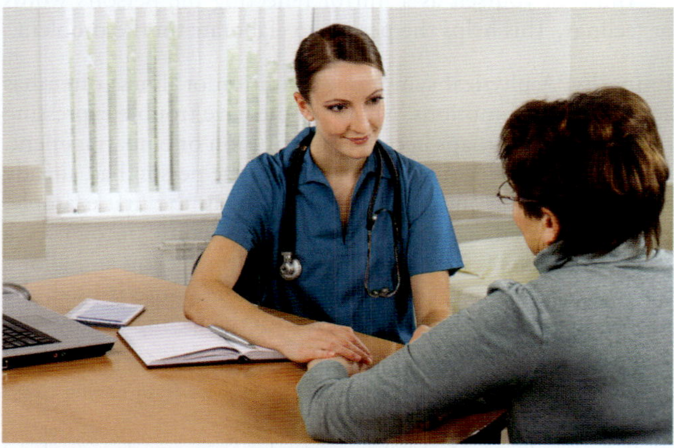

Figure 7.2

Interpretation. Interpretation is based on your inference or conclusion. It links events, makes associations or implies cause: 'It seems that every time you feel the stomach pain, you have had some kind of stress in your life'. Interpretation also ascribes feelings and helps the person understand their own feelings in relation to the verbal message.

> Patient: I have decided I don't want to take any more treatments. But I can't seem to tell my doctor that. Every time she comes in, I tighten up and can't say anything.
>
> Response: Could it be that you're afraid of her reaction?

You do run a risk of making the wrong inference. If this is the case, the person will correct it. But even if the inference is corrected, interpretation helps to prompt further discussion of the topic.

Explanation. With these statements, you inform the person. You share factual and objective information. This may be for orientation to the agency setting: 'Your dinner comes at 5:30 pm'. Or, it may be to explain cause: 'The reason you cannot eat or drink before your blood test is that the food will change the test results'.

Summary. This is a final review of what you understand the person has said. It condenses the facts and presents a summation of how you perceive the health problem or need. The summary provides an opportunity for the person to agree with or correct your understanding and perception. Both you and the person should participate. When the summary occurs at the end of the interview, it signals that termination of the interview is imminent.

Ten traps of interviewing

The verbal skills discussed above are productive and enhance the interview. Now take time to consider nonproductive, defeating verbal messages, or *traps*. It is easy to fall into these traps because you are anxious to help. The danger is that they restrict the person's response. The following traps are obstacles to obtaining complete data and to establishing rapport.

1. Providing false assurance or reassurance. A woman says, 'Oh, I just know this lump is going to turn out to be cancer'. What happens inside you? The automatic response of many clinicians is to say, 'Now don't worry; I'm sure you will be all right'. This 'courage builder' relieves *your* anxiety and gives you the false sense of having provided comfort. But for the woman it actually closes off communication. It trivialises her anxiety and effectively denies any further talk of it. (Also, it promises something that may not happen—that is, she may *not* be all right.) Consider instead these responses:

> 'You are really worried about the lump, aren't you?'
>
> 'It must be hard to wait for the biopsy results.'

These responses acknowledge the feeling and open the door for more communication. A genuine, valid form of reassurance does exist. You *can* reassure the person that you are listening, that you understand, that you have hope for them and that you will take good care of them.

> Patient: I feel so lost here since they transferred me to the medical centre. No one comes to see me. No one here cares what happens to me.
>
> Response: I care what happens to you. I am here today, and I want you to know that I'll be here all week.

This type of reassurance makes a commitment to the person and it can have a powerful impact.

2. Giving unwanted advice. Know when to give advice and when to avoid giving it. Often, people seek healthcare because they want your professional advice and information on the management of a health problem: 'My child has chickenpox; how should I take care of him?' This is a straightforward request for information you have that the parent needs. You respond by giving a health prescription, a therapeutic plan based on your knowledge and experience.

In other situations, advice is different; it is based on a hunch or feeling. It is your personal opinion. Consider the woman who has just left a meeting with her consultant physician: 'Dr Kline just told me my only chance of getting pregnant is to have an operation. I just don't know. What would you do?' Does the woman really want your advice? If you answer, 'If I were you, I'd …' then you would be making a mistake. You are not her. If you give your answer, you have shifted the accountability for decision making from her to you. She has not worked out her own solution. She has learned nothing about herself.

Does the woman really want to know what you would do? Probably not. Instead, a better response is reflection:

Response: Have an operation?

Woman: Yes, and I'm terrified of being put to sleep. What if I don't wake up?

Now you know her *real* concern and can help her deal with it. She will have grown in the process and may be better equipped to meet her next decision.

When asked for advice, other preferred responses are:

'What are the pros and cons of [this choice] for you?'

'What concerns do you have?'

'What is holding you back?'

Although it is quicker just to give advice, take the time to involve the person in the problem-solving process. When a person participates, they are more likely to learn and to change behaviour.

3. Using authority. 'Your doctor/nurse knows best' is a response that promotes dependency and inferiority. A better approach is to avoid using authority. Although you and the person cannot have equality of professional skill and experience, you do have equally worthy roles in the health process, each respecting the other.

4. Using avoidance language. People use euphemisms such as 'passed on' to avoid reality or to hide their feelings. They think if they just say the word 'death', it might really happen. So, to protect themselves, they evade the issue. Although it seems this will make them comfortable with potentially fearful topics, it does not. Not talking about the fear does not make it go away; it just suppresses the fear and makes it even more frightening. Using direct language is the best way to deal with frightening topics.

5. Engaging in distancing. Distancing is the use of impersonal speech to put space between a threat and the self: 'My friend has a problem; she is afraid she …' or 'There is a lump in the left breast'. By using 'the' instead of 'my', the woman can deny any association with her diseased breast and protect herself from it. Health professionals use distancing, too, to soften reality. This does not work because it communicates to the other person that you also are afraid of the procedure. The use of blunt specific terms is actually preferable to defuse anxiety.

6. Using professional jargon. What is called a myocardial infarction in the health profession is called a heart attack by most laypeople. Use of jargon sounds exclusionary and paternalistic. You need to adjust your vocabulary to the person but avoid sounding condescending.

If a person uses medical jargon, do not assume they always know the correct meaning. For example, some people think 'hypertensive' means that they are very tense. As a result, they take their medication only when feeling stressed and not when they feel relaxed. This misinformation must be corrected. They need to understand that hypertension is a chronic condition that needs consistent medication to avoid side effects. On the other hand, you do not need to feel that it is a moral imperative to correct all misstatements (e.g. when a person says 'prostrate' for prostate gland).

7. Using leading or biased questions. Asking a man, 'You don't smoke, do you? implies that one answer is 'better' than another. If the person wants to please you, either he is forced to answer in a way corresponding to your values or he feels guilty when he must admit the other answer. He risks your disapproval. And if he feels dependent on you for care, the last thing he wants to do is alienate you.

8. Talking too much. Some nurses positively associate helpfulness with verbal productivity. If the air has been thick with their oratory and advice, these nurses leave thinking they have met the person's needs. Just the opposite is true. Anxious to please the nurse, the person lets the professional talk at the expense of their need to express themselves. A good rule for every interviewer is to *listen more than you talk.*

9. Interrupting. Often, when you think you know what the person will say, you interrupt and cut the person off. This does not show that you are clever. Rather, it signals that you are impatient or bored with the interview.

A related trap is preoccupation with yourself by thinking of your next remark while the person is talking. As the person speaks, you are thinking about what to say next. Thus, you cannot fully understand what the person says. You are so preoccupied with your own role as the interviewer that you are not really listening. Aim for a second of silence between the person's statement and your next response.

10. Using 'why' questions. A young child asks, 'Why does the moon look like the end of my fingernail?' The motive behind this question is an innocent search for information. This is quite different from that of an adult's 'why' question, such as 'Why were you so late for your appointment?' The adult's use of why questions usually implies blame and condemnation; it puts the person on the defensive.

Consider your use of why questions in the healthcare setting. 'Why did you take so much medication?' Or, let's say you ask a man who has just come to the emergency department, 'Why did you wait so long before coming to the hospital?' The only possible answer to a why question is 'because …' and the man may not know the answer. He may not have worked it out. You sound whining, accusatory and judgemental. And the man now must produce an excuse to rationalise his own behaviour. To avoid this trap, say: 'I see you started to have chest pains early in the day. What was happening between the time the pains started and the time you came to the emergency department?'

Nonverbal skills

There are five types of nonverbal behaviours that convey information about the person: (1) *vocal cues* such as pitch, tone and quality of voice, including moaning, crying and groaning; (2) *action cues* such as posture, facial expression and gestures; (3) *object cues* such as clothes, jewellery and hair styles; (4) *use of personal and territorial space* in interpersonal transactions and care of belongings; and (5) *touch* which involves the use of personal space and action (Stein-Parbury 2018). Unless you make an effort to understand the person's nonverbal behaviour, you may overlook important information such as that conveyed by facial expressions, silence, eye contact, touch and other body language. Communication patterns vary widely even for such conventional social behaviours as smiling and handshaking.

Learn to listen with your eyes as well as with your ears. Nonverbal messages are very important in establishing rapport and in conveying information, especially about feelings. Nonverbal messages provide clues to understanding feelings. When nonverbal and verbal messages are congruent, the verbal is reinforced. When they are incongruent, the nonverbal message tends to be the true one, because it is under less conscious control.

Physical appearance. In his seminal work *The Stress of Life*, Hans Selye (1984) reports his interest in the body's total response to stress began as a student. Unbiased as yet by medical knowledge, he noted that some patients just 'looked sick', even though they did not exhibit the specific characteristic signs that would lead to a precise medical diagnosis. Such people simply felt and looked ill or feverish. The same view can work for you. Inattention to dressing or grooming suggests the person is too sick to maintain self-care or has an emotional dysfunction such as depression. Choice of clothing also sends a message, projecting such varied images as role (student, worker or professional) or attitude (casual, suggestive or rebellious).

Your own appearance sends a message to the person. Professional dress varies among organisations and settings. Depending on the setting, the use of a professional uniform may create a positive stereotype (comfort, expertise or ease of identification) or a negative stereotype (distance, authority or formality). Whatever your personal choice in clothing or grooming, the aim should be to convey a competent, professional image.

Posture. Note the person's position. An open position with extension of large muscle groups shows relaxation, physical comfort and a willingness to share information. A closed position with arms and legs crossed looks defensive and anxious. Note any change in posture. If a person in a relaxed position suddenly tenses, it suggests discomfort with the new topic.

Your own calm, relaxed posture creates a feeling of warmth and trust and conveys an interest in the person. Standing and hastily filling out a history form with periodic peeks at your watch communicates that you are busy with many more important things than interviewing this person. Even when your time is limited, appear calm and unhurried. Sit down, adopt an open and relaxed posture even if it is only for a few minutes, and look as if nothing else matters except this person.

Gestures. Gestures send messages. For example, nodding or an open turning out of the hand shows acceptance, attention or agreement. A wringing of the hands often indicates anxiety. Pointing a finger occurs with anger and vehemence. Also, hand gestures can reinforce a person's description of pain. When a crushing substernal chest pain is described, the person often holds the hand twisted into a fist in front of the sternum. Or, pain that is bright and sharply localised may be shown by pointing one finger to the exact spot: 'It hurts right here'.

Facial expression. The face reflects a wide variety of relevant emotions and conditions. The expression may look alert, relaxed and interested or it may look anxious, angry and suspicious. Physical conditions such as pain or shortness of breath also show in the expression.

Your own expression should reflect a professional who is attentive, sincere and interested in the person. Any expression of boredom, distraction, disgust, criticism or disbelief is picked up by the other person, and rapport will dissolve.

Eye contact. Lack of eye contact suggests that the person is shy, withdrawn, confused, bored, intimidated, apathetic or depressed. This applies to the nurse as well. You should aim to maintain eye contact, but do not 'stare down' the person. Do not have a fixed, penetrating look but rather an easy gaze towards the person's eyes, with occasional glances away. Nevertheless, remember that in some cultures, little or no eye contact is a sign of respect.

Voice. Beside the spoken words, meaning comes through the tone and volume of voice, the intensity and rate of speech, the pitch and any pauses. These are just as important as words in conveying meaning. For example, the tone of a person's voice may show sarcasm, disbelief, sympathy or hostility. An anxious person often speaks in a loud, fast voice. A whining voice is similar; it has a high-pitched wavering quality and long, drawn-out syllables. A soft voice may indicate shyness or fear. A hearing-impaired person may use a loud voice.

Even the use of pauses conveys meaning. When your question is easy and straightforward, a person's long unexpected pause indicates the person is taking time to think of an answer. This may raise some doubt as to the integrity of the answer. However, it also may be that what you consider a straightforward question is not perceived as such. A long pause before a response may indicate that you need to check that your question has been understood. Unusually frequent and long pauses, when combined with speech that is slow and monotonous and a weak breathy voice, may suggest depression.

Touch. Without doubt, touching is a necessary component of a comprehensive assessment. From a cultural perspective, however, you are urged to give careful consideration to issues concerning touch. While recognising the benefits reported by many in establishing rapport through touch, physical contact conveys various meanings. The meaning of physical touch is influenced by the person's age, gender, cultural background, past experience and current setting. The meaning of touch is easily misinterpreted. In most western cultures, physical touch is reserved for expressions of love and affection or for

TABLE 7.2 Nonverbal behaviours of the interviewer

POSITIVE	NEGATIVE
Appropriate professional appearance	Appearance objectionable to person
Equal-status seating	Standing
Close proximity to person	Sitting behind desk, far away, turned away
Relaxed open posture	Tense posture
Leaning slightly towards person	Slouched back
Occasional facilitating gestures	Critical or distracting gestures: pointing finger, clenched fist, finger-tapping, foot-swinging, looking at watch
Facial animation, interest	Bland expression, yawning, tight mouth
Appropriate smiling	Frowning, lip biting
Appropriate eye contact	Shifty, avoiding eye contact, focusing on notes
Moderate tone of voice	Strident, high-pitched tone
Moderate rate of speech	Rate too slow or too fast
Appropriate touch	Too frequent or inappropriate touch

rigidly defined acts of greeting. Do not use touch during the interview unless you know the person well and are sure how it will be interpreted. When appropriate, touch communicates effectively, such as a touch of the hand or arm to signal empathy.

In summary, an interviewer's nonverbal messages that are productive and enhancing to the relationship are those that show attentiveness and unconditional acceptance. Defeating, nonproductive nonverbal behaviours are those of inattentiveness, authority and superiority (Table 7.2).

Closing the interview

The session should end gracefully. An abrupt or awkward closing can destroy rapport and leave the person with a negative impression of the whole interview. To ease into the closing, ask the person:

> 'Is there anything else you would like to mention?'
> 'Are there any questions you would like to ask?'
> 'Are there any other areas I should have asked about?'

This gives the person the final opportunity for self-expression. Then, to indicate that closing is imminent, say something like 'Our interview is just about over'. No new topic should be introduced now. This is a good time to give your summary of what you have learned during the interview. It should include positive health aspects, any health problems that have been identified, any plans for action or an explanation of the following physical examination. As you part from the person, thank them for the time spent and for their cooperation.

DEVELOPMENTAL CONSIDERATIONS

Family-centred practice

When your patient is a child, you must build rapport with two people—the child and the accompanying parent or caregiver. Greet both by name, but with a younger child (1 to 6 years old), focus more on the caregiver. By ignoring the child temporarily, you allow the child to size you up from a safe distance. The child can observe your interaction with the caregiver, see that the caregiver accepts and likes you, and relax (Figure 7.3).

Begin by interviewing the caregiver and child together. Refer to the child by name—not as 'the baby'. Refer to the caregiver by name. Also, be clear when identifying the caregiver. The mother's present husband may not necessarily be the child's father. Instead of asking about 'your husband's health', ask 'Is Joan's father in good health?'

If any sensitive topics arise (e.g. the caregiver's troubled relationship or the child's problems at school or with peers), explore them later when the caregiver is alone. Depending on the child's age, provide toys, picture books and colouring books to occupy the child as you and the caregiver talk. This frees the caregiver to concentrate on the history. Also, it indicates the child's level of attention span or independent

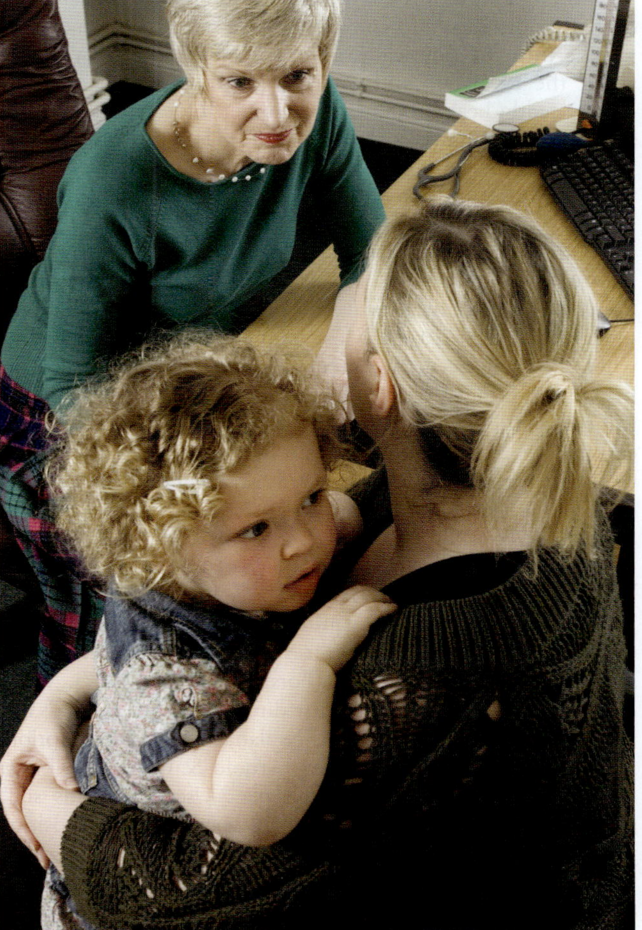

Figure 7.3

play. Through the interview, be alert to ways the caregiver and child interact.

For younger children, the parent or caregiver will provide all or most of the history. Thus, you are collecting the child's health data from the caregiver's frame of reference. Usually, this viewpoint is reliable because most caregivers have the child's wellbeing as a priority and see cooperation with you as a way to enhance this wellbeing. But the possibilities exist for caregiver bias. Bias can occur when caregivers are asked to describe the child's achievements, or whenever their own parenting ability seems called into question. For example, if you say, 'His fever was 39.5°C and you did not bring him in?' you are implying a lack of parenting skill. This puts the caregiver on the defensive and increases anxiety. Instead, use open-ended questions that increase description and defuse threat, such as 'What happened when the fever went up?'

A parent or caregiver with more than one child has more than one set of data to remember. Be patient as the caregiver sorts through their memory to pull out facts of developmental milestones or past history. A comprehensive history may be lacking if the child is accompanied by a family friend or day care provider instead of the parent.

In collecting developmental data, avoid being judgemental about the age of achievement of certain milestones. Parents are understandably proud of their child's achievements and are sensitive to inferences that these milestones may occur late.

Although most of your communication is with the caregiver, do not ignore the child completely. You need to make contact to ease into the physical examination later. Begin by asking about the toys the child is playing with or about a special doll or teddy bear brought from home: 'Does your doll have a name?' or 'What can your truck do?' Stoop down to meet the child at their eye level. Adult size can be overwhelming to young children and can emphasise their smallness.

The infant (1–12 months)

Because the infant uses the senses to receive information, nonverbal communication is the primary method (Arnold & Underman Boggs 2016). Most infants look calm and relaxed when all their needs are met, and they cry when they are frightened, hungry, tired or uncomfortable. They respond best to firm, gentle handling and a quiet, calm voice. Your voice is comforting, even though they do not understand the words. Older infants have anxiety towards strangers. They are more cooperative when the caregiver is kept in view (Kennedy-Sheldon & Foust 2014).

The toddler (12 months to 3 years)

Toddlers have not yet acquired the ability to effectively communicate verbally. They use expressive non-verbal and simple verbal communication (Forster & Fraser 2017). When communicating with toddlers, use direct simple commands and familiar terms (O'Toole 2016). Explanations and descriptions need to be repeated several times (Arnold & Underman Boggs 2016). Establish rapport through play. Use visual aids such as dolls to assist explanations. Where possible, either position yourself down to the child's level, or raise them (if it is safe) to your level (O'Toole 2016). Toddlers and young children are frightened by quick or grandiose gestures. Do not try to maintain eye contact; this feels threatening to a small child. Use a quiet, measured voice and choose simple words in your speech.

The preschooler (3–5 years)

A 3–5-year-old is egocentric. They see the world mostly from their own point of view. Everything revolves around them. It may not work to cite the example of another child's behaviour to get the child to cooperate. It has no meaning. Only the child's own experience is relevant.

Preschoolers' communication is direct, concrete, literal and set in the present. Avoid expressions such as 'climbing the walls', because they are easily misinterpreted by young children. Use short, simple sentences with a concrete explanation. Take time to give a short, simple explanation for any unfamiliar equipment that will be used on the child and allow them to handle the equipment. Preschoolers can have *animistic* thinking about unfamiliar objects. They may imagine that unfamiliar inanimate objects can come alive and have human characteristics (e.g. that a blood pressure cuff can wake up and bite or pinch). Parental proximity is still important for this age group (Forster & Fraser 2017).

The school-age child (6–12 years)

A child 6–12 years old can tolerate and understand others' viewpoints. This child is more objective and realistic. They want to know functional aspects—how things work and why things are done.

Children of this age group have the verbal ability to add important data to the history. Interview the parent and child together, but when a presenting symptom or sign exists ask the child about it first, and then gather data from the parent. For the well child seeking a checkup, pose questions about school, friends or activities directly to the child (Arnold & Underman Boggs 2016).

The pre-adolescent/adolescent (12–19 years)

Adolescents want to be adults, but they do not have the cognitive ability yet to achieve their goal. They are between two stages. Sometimes they are capable of mature actions, and other times they fall back on childhood response patterns, especially in times of stress. You cannot treat adolescents as children, yet you cannot overcompensate and assume that their communication style, learning ability and motivation are consistently at an adult level.

Adolescents value their peers. They crave acceptance and sameness with their peers. They may think no adult can understand them and will act with aloof contempt, answering only in monosyllables. Others make eye contact and tell you what they think you want to hear, but inside they are thinking, 'You'll never know the full story about me'.

This knowledge about adolescents is apt to paralyse you in communicating with them. However, successful communication is possible and rewarding. The guidelines are simple.

The first consideration is your attitude, which must be one of respect. Respect is the most important thing you can communicate to the adolescent. The adolescent needs to feel validated as a human being, to be accepted and worthy.

Second, your communication must be totally honest. The adolescent's intuition is highly tuned and can detect phoniness or when information is withheld. Always give them the truth. Play it straight or you will lose them. They will cooperate if they understand your rationale.

Stay in character. Avoid using language that is absurd for your age or professional role. It is helpful to understand some of the jargon used by adolescents, but you cannot use those words yourself simply to try to bond with the adolescent. Do not try to be their peer. You are not, and they will not accept you as such.

Use icebreakers. Focus first on the adolescent, not on the problem. Although an adult just wants to get on with it and talk about the health concern immediately, the adolescent responds best when the focus is on them as a person. Show an interest in the adolescent. Ask open, friendly questions about school, activities, hobbies and friends. Refrain from asking questions about parents and family for now—these issues can be emotionally charged during adolescence.

Do not assume adolescents know *anything* about a health interview or a physical examination. Explain every step and give the rationale. They need direction. They will cooperate when they know the reason for the questions or actions. Encourage their questions. Adolescents are afraid they will sound 'dumb' if they ask a question to which they assume everybody else knows the answer.

Keep your questions short and simple. 'Why are you here?' sounds brazen to you, but it is effective with the adolescent. Be prepared for the adolescent who does *not* know why they are there. Some adolescents are pushed into coming to the examination by a parent.

The communication responses described for the adult need to be reconsidered when talking with the adolescent. Silent periods are usually best avoided. Giving adolescents a little time to collect their thoughts is acceptable, but a silence for other reasons is threatening. Also, avoid reflection. If you use reflection, the adolescent is likely to answer, 'What?' They just do not have the cognitive skills to respond to that indirect mode of questioning. Also, adolescents are more sensitive to nonverbal communication than are adults. Be aware of your expressions and gestures. They are also more sensitive to any comment they take to mean criticism from you and will withdraw.

Later in the interview, after you have developed rapport with the adolescent, you can address the topics that are emotionally charged, including alcohol and drug use, sexual behaviours, suicidal thoughts and depression. Adolescents will assume that health professionals have similar values and standards of behaviour as most of the other authority figures in their lives, and they may be reluctant to share this information. You can assure them that your questions are not intended to be curious or intrusive but cover topics that are important for most teens and on which you have relevant health information to share.

If confidential material is uncovered during the interview, consider what can remain confidential and what you feel you must share for the wellbeing of the adolescent. State laws vary about confidentiality with minors and, in some states, parents are not notified about, for example, birth control prescriptions or treatment for sexually transmitted infections (STIs). However, if the adolescent talks about an abusive home situation, state that you must share this information with other health professionals for their own protection. Ask the adolescent, 'Do you have a problem with that?' and then talk it through. Tell the adolescent, 'You will have to trust that I will handle this information professionally and in your best interest'.

Finally, take every opportunity for positive reinforcement. Praise every action regarding healthy lifestyle choices: 'That's great that you don't smoke. You get lots of gold stars in my book for staying off the cigarettes. It's great for your heart, it will save you lots of money that you can use on other things and your skin won't be wrinkled when you get older'.

The person over 65 years

Older adults are often treated as if they represent a single cohort; however, there are huge differences in their life experiences and capabilities. Because people are living longer, the term older adult has been broken down into three age cohorts: young-old (65–74 years), middle-old (75–84 years) and oldest-old (85 years and older) (Moody & Sasser 2018).

The person over 65 has the developmental task of finding the meaning of life and the purpose of their own existence and adjusting to the inevitability of death. Some people have developed comfortable and satisfying answers and greet you with a calm demeanour and self-assurance. Be alert for the occasional person who sounds hopeless and despairing about life at present and in the future. Symptoms of illness are even more frightening when they mean physical limitation or threaten independence.

Interviewing older people requires many of the same skills required for interviewing younger adults. However, attention must be paid to the numerous factors that influence communication, such as the presence of multiple chronic conditions, sensory deficits and cognitive limitations. Age-related changes to cognition in healthy older adults are minimal and should not require major modifications in communication, although mental processing and reaction time may be slow (Moody & Sasser 2018). However, if you have any concerns about a person's cognitive capacity, it is prudent to perform a mental status assessment early in the interview to avoid obtaining questionable data (Arnold & Underman Boggs 2016). The mini-mental state examination (Folstein et al 1975) and the clock drawing test are useful assessment tools (Arnold & Underman Boggs 2016).

Establish rapport by always addressing the person by their last name (e.g. 'Hello, Mr Choi'; 'Good morning, Mrs Smith'). Some older adults resent being called by their first name by younger persons, and almost all cringe at the ignominious 'Grandma' or 'Pop'. To avoid undermining rapport, ask the older person what they would like to be called. Treat them as an equal (O'Toole 2016). Use open-ended questions first followed by focused questions. Ask one question at a time. Provide information in small segments. Acknowledge feelings and emotions. Pay attention to sensory deficits such as hearing and visual impairment (Arnold & Underman Boggs 2016).

It is important to adjust the pace of the interview to the age of the person. People over 65 have a great amount of background material to sort through, and this takes some time. Some older adults may need a longer response time to interpret the question and process their answer. Avoid trying to hurry them along.

Consider physical limitations when planning the interview. Frail older adults and sick people may fatigue earlier and may require the interview be broken up into shorter segments. When the person is hearing impaired, face them directly so that your mouth and face are fully visible. Do not shout; it does not help and actually distorts speech. Placing a hand on the arm or shoulder is an empathic message which communicates that you empathise with the person and want to understand their health issue.

INTERVIEWING PEOPLE WITH SPECIAL NEEDS AND CHALLENGING BEHAVIOURS

Hearing-impaired people

Although many people will tell you in advance that they have a hearing deficit, others must be recognised by clues, such as staring at your mouth and face, not attending unless looking at you or speaking in a voice unusually loud or with guttural or garbled sounds. The deaf person may be familiar with some equipment in the hospital or office setting or may have had previous experience with healthcare settings. But without full communication, the hearing-impaired person is sure to feel isolated and anxious. Ask what their preferred way is to communicate—by hearing aid, adjusting the volume of your voice, signing, lip reading or writing (Kennedy-Sheldon & Foust 2014).

A complete health history requires a sign language interpreter. Since most healthcare professionals are not proficient in signing, try to find an interpreter through a social service agency or the person's own social network. You may use family members but be aware that they sometimes edit for the person. Use the same guidelines as for the bilingual interpreter. If the person prefers lip reading, be sure to face them squarely and have good lighting on your face. Do not exaggerate your lip movements because this distorts your words. Similarly, shouting distorts the reception of a hearing aid the person may wear. Articulate clearly and speak in a steady pace using a moderate and even tone. Supplement your voice with appropriate hand gestures. Nonverbal cues are important adjuncts because the lip reader understands at best only 50% of your speech when relying solely on vision. Be sure the person understands your questions. Many hearing-impaired people nod 'yes' just to be friendly and cooperative but really do not understand (Kennedy-Sheldon & Foust 2014).

Written communication is efficient in sections such as past health history or review of symptoms. Nevertheless, appreciate that the syntax of the person's written words will read normally if the hearing impairment occurred after speech patterns developed. If the deafness occurred before speech patterns developed, the written syntax follows that of signing, which is different from that of English.

Vision-impaired person

Because people with vision impairment have a limited or no ability to read information or see non-verbal gestures, posture and body language, they rely on the spoken word. There is a tendency for those communicating with a vision-impaired person to speak loudly and to over enunciate. Unless the person has a hearing impairment as well, tone of voice and speed of delivery should be the same as if you were talking to a non-vision-impaired person (O'Toole 2016). Because the vision-impaired person may struggle to see you or even not see you at all, it is important to alert them when you approach and when you are leaving. Remember to ask other personnel to introduce themselves to the vision-impaired person when they enter and leave a room. Continue to use everyday verbal and body language because they affect tone and meaning, which provides additional information to the visually-impaired person (O'Toole 2016).

Aphasic person

Because language is our basic way of communicating with the world, speech and language deficits can cause considerable distress to the person experiencing aphasia. Aphasia can manifest in several ways: (1) expressive or motor aphasia where words cannot be expressed or formed; (2) receptive or sensory aphasia where language is not understood; and (3) global aphasia which includes both expressive and receptive deficits (Kennedy-Sheldon & Foust 2014). While communication strategies with the aphasic person should attend to the type of presenting aphasia, it should be recognised that there is a high likelihood that the aphasic person's efforts to communicate will be frustrating. In order to minimise actual and potential distress experienced by the aphasic person in their efforts to communicate, allow ample time for them to formulate thoughts and receive information. Show patience and perseverance and keep trying to understand. Avoid responding with frustration (O'Toole 2016). Ensure that you focus on their abilities and their communication preferences. Use of alternative communication methods such as picture boards can be used to supplement or replace verbal communication. Because of the effort involved in communicating, avoid prolonged conversations with the aphasic person. Keep conversations short and to the point. Always remember to acknowledge the aphasic person's efforts (Kennedy-Sheldon & Foust 2014).

Acutely ill people

An emergency demands your prompt action. You must combine questioning with physical examination skills to determine lifesaving actions. Although life support measures may be paramount, still try to ask the person relevant questions as much as possible and provide reassurance. The acutely ill person is likely to be anxious and fearful. They need to be assured that the nurse is taking action. Subjective data are crucial to determine the cause and course of the emergency. Abbreviate your questioning. Identify the main area of distress and direct your questions to them. Gather information from the person's notes and other health professionals rather than repeatedly asking the same questions. If you are unsure about the accuracy of information provided, make statements and ask for verification through non-verbal responses such as head or other body movements (O'Toole 2016). Family or friends can provide important data.

A hospitalised person with a critical or severe illness is usually too weak, too short of breath or in too much pain to talk. First attend to the comfort of the person. Then establish a priority; find out immediately what parts of the health history are the most relevant. Explore the first concern the person mentions. Begin to use closed, direct questions earlier.

People under the influence of illicit substances or alcohol

It is common for persons under the influence of alcohol or other mood-altering drugs to be admitted to a hospital; all these drugs affect the central nervous system, increasing the risk for accidents and injuries. Also, chronic use creates complex medical problems that require increasing care.

Many substance abusers are poly-drug abusers. You may be faced with a wide range of problem behaviours due to current influence. Alcohol, opioids (e.g. heroin) and central nervous system stimulants (e.g. cocaine, ecstasy, methamphetamines) can cause an intense high, agitation and paranoid behaviour. Hallucinogens cause bizarre, inappropriate, sometimes even violent behaviour accompanied by superhuman strength and insensitivity to pain.

When interviewing a person currently under the influence of alcohol or illicit drugs, ask simple and direct questions. Take care to make your manner and questions nonthreatening. Avoid confrontation at this point. Further, avoid any display of scolding or disgust, because this person may become belligerent. One priority is to find out the time of the person's last drink and how much they drank at this episode, as well as the name and number of other drugs taken. This information will help assess any withdrawal patterns. For your own protection, be aware of hospital security or other personnel who could be called on for assistance.

Once they are no longer under the direct influence of alcohol or illicit substances, the person should be assessed for the extent of the problem and the meaning of the problem for them and their family. Initially you will encounter denial and increased defensiveness; special interview techniques are needed. Further discussion related to assessment of people who have a substance abuse problem can be found in Chapter 6.

Responding to challenging behaviours

Personal questions

Occasionally, people will ask you questions about *your* personal life or opinions, such as 'Are you married?', 'Do you have children?' or 'Do you smoke?' You do not need to answer every question. You may supply brief information when you feel it is appropriate but be sensitive to the possibility that there may be a motive behind the personal questions such as loneliness or anxiety. Try directing your response back to the person's frame of reference. You might say something like, 'No, I don't have children; I wonder if your question is related to how I can help you care for little Jamie?'

Sexually aggressive people

On some occasions, personal questions extend to flirtatious compliments, seductive innuendo or advances. Some people experience serious or chronic illness as a threat to their self-esteem and sexual adequacy. This creates anxiety that makes them act in sexually aggressive ways.

Your response must make it clear that you are a health professional who can best care for the person by maintaining a professional relationship. At the same time, you should communicate that you accept the person and you understand the person's need to be self-assertive but that you cannot tolerate sexual advances. This may be difficult, considering that the person's words or gestures may have left you shocked, embarrassed or angry. Your feelings are normal. You need to set appropriate verbal boundaries by saying, 'I am uncomfortable when you talk to me that way; please don't.' A further response that would open communication is: 'I wonder if the way you're feeling now relates to your illness or to being in the hospital?'

Crying

A novice nurse may feel overwhelmed when a person starts crying. But crying is actually a big relief to a person. Health problems come with powerful emotions. Worries about illness, death or loss take a great amount of energy to keep bottled up inside. When you say something that 'makes the person cry', do not think you have hurt the person. You have just hit on a topic that is important. Do not go on to a new topic. Just let the person cry and express their feelings fully. You can offer a tissue and wait until the crying subsides to talk. The person will regain control soon.

Sometimes the person looks as if they are on the verge of tears but is trying hard to suppress them. Again, instead of moving on to something new, acknowledge the expression by saying, 'You look sad.' Do not worry that you will open an uncontrollable floodgate. The person may cry but will be relieved, and you will have gained insight to a serious concern.

Anger

Occasionally you will try to interview a person who is already angry. Try not to personalise this anger; usually it does not relate to you. The person is showing aggression in response to their own feelings of anxiety or helplessness. Do ask about the anger and hear the person out. Deal with the angry feelings before you ask anything else.

Threat of violence

The healthcare setting is not immune to violent behaviour. An individual may act with such angry gestures that you feel a threat to your personal safety. Other red flag behaviours of a potentially disruptive person include fist clenching, pacing back and forth, a vacant stare, confusion, statements out of touch with reality, statements that do not make sense, a history of recent drug use (alcohol, recreational drugs) or perhaps even a recent history of intense bereavement (loss of spouse, loss of job). Trust your instincts. If you sense any suspicious or threatening behaviour, act immediately to defuse the situation. Demonstrate a sincere desire to help. Listen and offer to work with the threatening person to solve the problem. Do not raise your own voice or try to argue with them. Allow the person to set the pace to tell their story. Respond with patience and understanding. Empathise with the person but not necessarily their sentiments. Act calmly and talk to the person in a gentle voice. Behave in an unhurried way.

Leave the examining room door open and position yourself between the person and the door. Seek assistance promptly if the situation is escalating. Within the hospital setting, there is usually a pre-established protocol for managing threats of violence. A prearranged sign or signal is used to alert colleagues to summon security for assistance. In the community setting, systems such as emergency pager or mobile alerts may be used to summon help.

Remember that the most important goal is your personal safety, so avoid taking any risks (Hallet 2018, O'Toole 2016).

Anxiety

Finally, take it for granted that nearly all sick people have some anxiety. This is a normal response to being sick. It makes some people aggressive and others dependent. Remember that the person is not reacting as typically as when they are healthy. Acknowledging the person's situation, appearing unhurried and taking the time to listen to the person's concerns can help diffuse some of the anxiety. For further information on assessment of anxiety, please refer to Chapter 11.

CULTURAL AND SOCIAL CONSIDERATIONS

Chapter 4 provides a comprehensive overview on cultural safety in nursing practice. The issues identified in Box 4.5 (The process towards achieving cultural safety in nursing practice) should be used to inform and guide culturally appropriate communication. The following section examines specific cultural considerations around communicating.

When two people come from different cultural backgrounds, the probability of miscommunication increases. Verbal and nonverbal communications are influenced by the cultural background of the healthcare professional and the person (Figure 7.4). In Australia, information that assists in minimising the risk of miscommunication between the healthcare professional and the person is freely available from the Centre for Culture, Ethnicity and Health (CEH). The information sheets 'Cultural considerations in health assessment' and 'Speaking with clients who have low English proficiency' is located on their website at www.ceh.org.au under 'Knowledge Hub' (CEH 2018a–d). The documents highlight issues associated with a health assessment interview and ways to facilitate effective communication with people of limited English proficiency (CEH 2018a). Effective communication among Australia's First Nation's people is based on a community-centred model as opposed to a person-centred model (O'Toole 2016). Community leaders, community Elders and Indigenous Health Workers play an important role in facilitating culturally respectful communication (O'Toole 2016). There are resources available to assist health professionals to communicate more effectively with Māori people in New Zealand (Ministry of Health 2017).

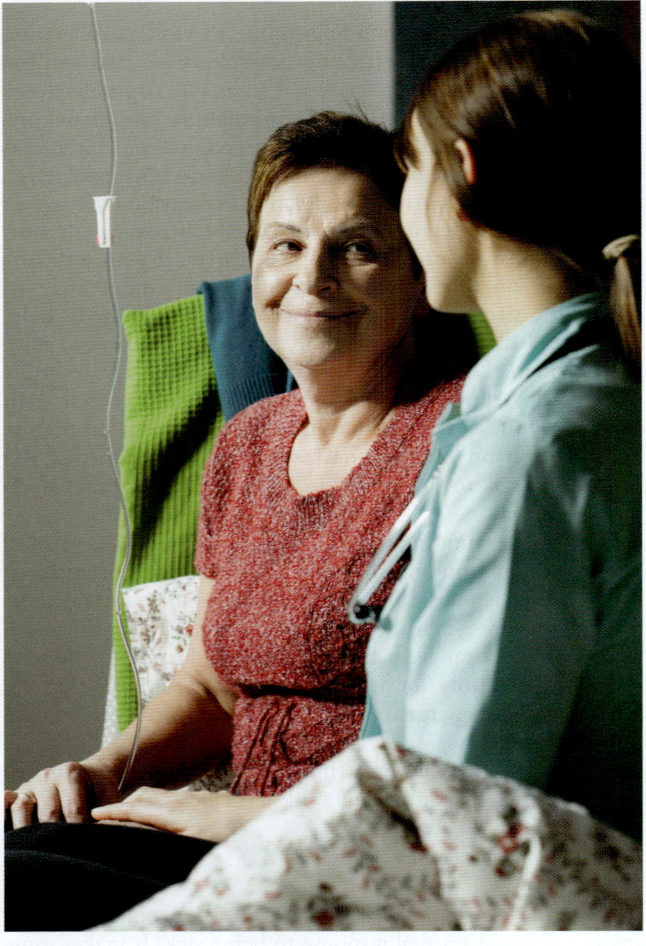

Figure 7.4
Source: Hall E: Proxemics: the study of man's spatial relations. In Galdston I (ed.): *Man's image in medicine and anthropology.* New York, 1963, International University Press, pp. 109–120.

People with limited English proficiency must be provided with an interpreter who is **not** a family member or friend. It is essential to establish whether interpreter services are required. A simple way of establishing this need is to ask the question, 'Would you like an interpreter?' A flash card or cue card can be used to ask the question in the person's preferred language. The Australian Institute of Interpreters and Translators Incorporated (AUSIT) offers practical advice on communication processes and working with interpreters (AUSIT 2019a, 2019b). In New Zealand, Te Tari Matawaki Office of Ethnic Communities offer culturally appropriate resources (Office of Ethnic Communities 2019).

At the completion of the interview at which an interpreter is used, carefully document that the person and family fully understand what is happening to them; what their diagnosis and the implications of this diagnosis are; what procedures, diagnostic and therapeutic, are going to be done; how the procedures will be done and what they mean; how medications are to be taken and when; and the prognosis derived from the given problem(s). The interpreter will also give nurses and other healthcare workers tools and advice on continuing communication with the person and their family (CEH 2018b, 2018c; Raising Children Network 2014).

Etiquette

Etiquette refers to the conventional code of good manners that governs behaviour. For some people, there is a high value placed on developing interpersonal relationships and getting to know about a person's family, personal concerns and interests before they allow you to gather personal and intimate information on their health history and to conduct a physical examination. Recognising that time constraints frequently affect the social interchange expected by some individuals, you should strive to incorporate the person's needs with the health history data categories. For example, using a conversational tone of voice, you might begin the health history by inquiring about the person's family members and their health. An effective way of ensuring that you capture all the important information about the person in a timely manner is by using a structured assessment tool. Issues that should be considered when conducting health assessments with people from migrant and refugee backgrounds are provided in the CEH information sheet 'Cultural considerations in health assessment' (CEH 2018d).

You should be prepared for the converse when conducting a health interview; that is, some individuals may want to interview *you.* They may ask questions about your family, marital status, salary, home address, telephone number and so forth. Remember that you aren't obliged to answer questions that you deem too personal and you always have the right to protect your personal safety. For example, you are **never** to provide your home address, email or telephone number. Rather, you should provide the person with the hospital, clinic or organisation's business number.

When meeting a person for the first time, it is important to be professional in your approach. Another aspect of etiquette concerns the use of *names* and *titles*. In order to ensure that a mutually respectful relationship is established, you should introduce yourself and indicate to the person how you prefer to be called—that is, by first name, last name and/or title. You should elicit the same information from the person because this enables you to address them in a manner that is appropriate and could spare you considerable embarrassment. Everyone likes to be called by their correct name. You must be certain that you know the person's name and pronounce it correctly. Avoid being unduly casual or familiar. For example, refrain from routinely using the person's first name before you have been invited to do so. The same guidelines should be followed when addressing the family members and other visitors. It is suggested to greet the person, 'Hello, Mr or Mrs or Ms …, my name is …'. The common use of 'you guys' and other colloquialisms must be eradicated. Among Chinese, Vietnamese and many other Asian groups, the family or surname is written and spoken first, followed by the first or given name. This is exactly the opposite of most European-Australian naming systems. If you are in doubt, be sure to ask the person or a significant other if they are unable to respond due to their condition.

Space and distance

Spatial distance is significant throughout the interview and physical examination with appropriate distance zones varies widely. Summarised in Table 7.3 are the four distance zones identified for the functional use of space.

TABLE 7.3 Functional use of space

ZONE	REMARKS
Intimate zone (0–0.5 m)	Visual distortion occurs Best for assessing breath and other body odours
Personal distance (0.5–1 m)	Perceived as an extension of the self; similar to a bubble Voice is moderate Body odours not apparent No visual distortion Much of the physical assessment occurs at this distance
Social distance (1–4 m)	Used for impersonal business transactions Perceptual information much less detailed Much of the interview occurs at this distance
Public distance (4 m+)	Interaction with others impersonal Speaker's voice must be projected Subtle facial expressions imperceptible

Cultural considerations on gender, sexuality and sexual orientation

Should you determine that gender differences are important to the person, you might try strategies such as offering to have a third person present. If a family member or friend has accompanied the person, you might inquire whether they would like that person to be present during the history and/or physical examination. It is not unusual for a female to request examination by a female rather than a male and vice versa. Modesty is another issue and it is imperative to ensure that the person is carefully draped at all times, that curtains are closed and, when possible, doors should also be closed. A room must not be entered without knocking first and announcing yourself. It is also important for nurses to not assume that heterosexuality is the norm.

You also need to be aware of making the assumption that the person identifies as heterosexual, lesbian, gay, bisexual or a particular gender. Simple approaches can improve your communication with all people and help you avoid making inappropriate assumptions:

- Use the word 'partner' rather than 'husband' or 'wife' until you determine the person's preferences for these terms.
- Ask the same questions of a homosexual couple as a hetero-sexual couple.
- Don't make assumptions about a person's sexual orientation based on appearance.

Language is important in conveying acceptance of the person; therefore, it is important to understand commonly used terminology related to gender identity and sexuality. More information and guidelines about communicating effectively about sexuality and sexual function are supplied in Chapters 26 and 27.

OVERCOMING COMMUNICATION BARRIERS

Healthcare providers tend to have stereotypical expectations of people's behaviour during the interview and physical examination. In general, we expect behaviour to consist of undemanding compliance, an attitude of respect for the healthcare provider and cooperation with requested behaviour throughout the examination. Although the person may ask a few questions for the purpose of clarification, slight deference to recognised authority figures (i.e. healthcare providers) is expected.

Working with an interpreter

In the most recent dataset, 81% of Australians aged 5 years and over spoke only English, while 2% did not speak English at all; this included both longer-standing migrants and recent arrivals (Australian Bureau of Statistics (ABS) 2014). Almost 4 million people in Australia did not speak the English language at home. Speakers of Indigenous languages numbered 50,000 and comprised 1.7% of all non-English speakers. In New Zealand, the official languages are English, Māori and New Zealand Sign Language (Statistics New Zealand 2014). English is spoken by 96.14%; Māori is spoken by 3.73% of New Zealanders (Statistics New Zealand 2014).

One of the greatest challenges in cross-cultural communication occurs when you and the person speak different languages (Figure 7.5). After assessing the language skills of non-English-

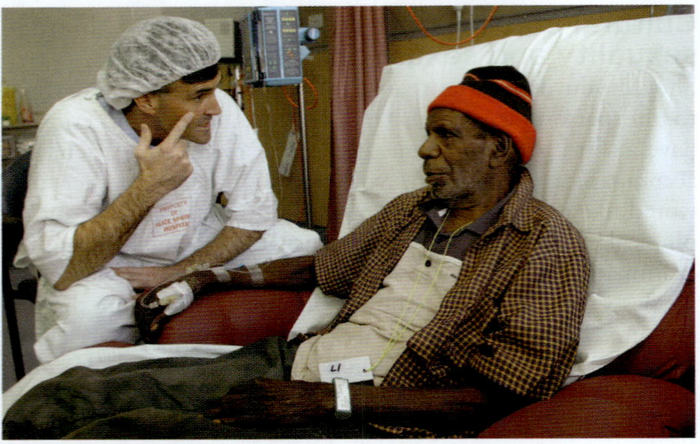

Figure 7.5

speaking people, you may find yourself in one of two situations: trying to communicate effectively through an interpreter or trying to communicate effectively when there is no interpreter.

Interviewing the non-English-speaking person requires a bilingual interpreter for full communication. Even the person from another culture or country who has a basic command of English (those for whom English is a second language) may need an interpreter when faced with the anxiety-provoking situation of entering a hospital, describing a strange symptom or discussing sensitive topics such as those related to reproductive or urological concerns.

It is tempting to ask a relative, friend or even another person to interpret because they are readily available and probably would like to help. This is disadvantageous because it violates confidentiality. Furthermore, the friend or relative, although fluent in ordinary language usage, is likely to be unfamiliar with medical terminology, hospital or clinic procedures and medical ethics.

Whenever possible, work with a bilingual team member or a trained medical interpreter. They know interpreting techniques, have a healthcare background and understand patients' rights. Although interpreters are trained to remain neutral, they can influence both the content of information exchanged and the nature of the interaction. Many trained medical interpreters are members of the linguistic community they serve. While this is largely beneficial, it has limitations. For example, interpreters often know details of the person's circumstances before the interview begins. Although acceptance of a code of ethics governing confidentiality and conflicts of interest is part of the training interpreters receive, discord may arise when they relate information that the person has not volunteered to the nurse.

Although you will be in charge of the focus and flow of the interview, view yourself and the interpreter as a team. Ask the interpreter to meet the person beforehand to establish rapport. Allow more time for this interview. With the third person repeating everything, it can take considerably longer than interviewing English-speaking people. You need to focus on priority data (CEH 2018a–d).

There are two styles of interpreting—line-by-line and summarising. Translating line-by-line takes more time, but it ensures accuracy. Use this style for most of the interview. Both you and the person should speak only a sentence or two, and then allow the interpreter some time. Use simple language yourself, not medical jargon that the interpreter must simplify before it can be translated. Summary translation progresses faster and is useful for teaching relatively simple health techniques with which the interpreter is already familiar. Be alert for nonverbal cues as the person talks. These cues can give valuable data. A good interpreter also notes nonverbal messages and passes them on to you. Summarised in Table 7.4 are suggestions for the selection and use of an interpreter. Table 7.5 summarises some suggestions for overcoming language barriers.

TABLE 7.4 Use of an interpreter

CHOOSING AN INTERPRETER
• Before locating an interpreter, identify the language the person speaks at home. Be aware that it may differ from the language spoken publicly. • Whenever possible, use a *professional* interpreter, preferably one who knows medical terminology. • Be aware of gender differences between interpreter and the person. In general, the same gender is preferred. • Be aware of age differences between interpreter and the person.
STRATEGIES FOR EFFECTIVE USE OF AN INTERPRETER
• Plan what you want to say ahead of time. Meet privately with the interpreter before the interview. • Ask the interpreter to provide a line-by-line verbatim account of the conversation. Ask for a detailed interpretation when provided with brief summaries of longer exchanges between interpreter and the person. • Be patient. When using an interpreter, interviews often take two to three times longer. • Longer-than-expected explanatory exchanges are often required to convey the meaning of words such as *stress, depression, allergy, preventive medicine* and *physiotherapy* because there may not be comparable terms in the language the person understands. • When discussing diagnostic tests such as mammograms, magnetic resonance imaging (MRIs), computed tomography (CT) scans, or those involving body fluids such as blood, urine, stool, spinal fluid or saliva, be sure to clarify the nature of the test to the interpreter. Indicate the purpose of the test, exactly what will happen to the person, approximately how long the test will take, whether the procedure is invasive or noninvasive and what part(s) of the body will be tested. • Avoid ambiguous statements and questions. • Avoid abstract expressions, idioms, similes, metaphors and medical jargon. • To ensure confidentiality and privacy, avoid using children or strangers as interpreters.

Using the health assessment interview as an opportunity for health teaching

The time you have with the person during a health assessment interview provides a perfect opportunity to identify areas where the person needs more information, or where misconceptions need to be corrected. An important part of your assessment at this time is determining if the person understands everything

TABLE 7.5 Overcoming language barriers

1	Be polite and formal.
2	Pronounce names correctly. Use proper titles of respect, such as 'Mr', 'Mrs', 'Ms', 'Dr'. Greet the person using the last or complete name. Gesture to yourself and say your name. Offer a handshake or nod. Smile.
3	Proceed in an unhurried manner. Pay attention to any effort by the person or family to communicate.
4	Speak in a low, moderate voice. Avoid talking loudly. Remember that there is a tendency to raise the volume and pitch of your voice when the listener appears not to understand. The listener may perceive that you are shouting and/or angry.
5	Use any words that you might know in the person's language. This indicates that you are aware of and respect their culture.
6	Use simple words, such as 'pain' instead of 'discomfort'. Avoid medical jargon, idioms and slang. Avoid using contractions (e.g. don't, can't, won't). Use nouns repeatedly instead of pronouns. *Example:* Do not say: 'He has been taking his medicine, hasn't he?' Do say: 'Does Juan take medicine?'
7	Mime words and simple actions while you verbalise them.
8	Give instructions in the proper sequence. *Example:* Do not say: 'Before you rinse the bottle, sterilise it.' Do say: 'First wash the bottle. Second, rinse the bottle.'
9	Discuss one topic at a time. Avoid using conjunctions. *Example:* Do not say: 'Are you cold and in pain?' Do say: 'Are you cold (while miming)? Are you in pain?'
10	Validate if the person understands by having them repeat instructions, demonstrate the procedure or act out the meaning.
11	Write out several short sentences in English and determine the person's ability to read them.
12	Obtain phrase books from a library or bookstore, make or purchase flash cards, contact hospitals for a list of interpreters and use both a formal and an informal network to locate a suitable interpreter.

you say. Several decades ago, the concept of health literacy was introduced because it was clear that people did not always understand the health information provided (Sand-Jecklin et al 2017). Health literacy is about how people understand information about health and healthcare, and how they apply that information to their lives, use it to make decisions and act on it (Australian Commission on Safety and Quality in Health Care (ACSQHC) 2014). Health literacy is important because it shapes people's health and the safety and quality of healthcare (ACSQHC 2014). The Australian Commission on Safety and Quality in Health Care also makes the point that another important component of health literacy is the health literacy environment; that is, the infrastructure, policies, materials, people and relationships within healthcare environments which impact on the way in which a person can access, understand and apply health-related information and services. A person can have adequate literacy and not have adequate health literacy. In Australia, several factors are linked to health literacy capability including personal health, country of birth, language first spoken and age (ACSQHC 2014). It is estimated that 59% of Australians (15–74 years) have poor health literacy skills, which means that they may not be able to determine the correct amount of medicine to give a child or adult from information printed on the package (ACSQHC 2014). People over 50 years of age are likely to have lower health literacy levels than those 49 years or younger (ACSQHC 2014). Similar figures are found in the New Zealand population with 56.2% of adult New Zealanders (16–65 years of age) having poor health literacy skills with high levels of Māori people (4 out of 5 males and 3 out of 5 females) having poor health literacy (Ministry of Health 2017).

Health literacy encompasses a variety of factors beyond basic reading, including the ability to use quantitative (numeric) information and to understand and remember verbal instructions. People with low health literacy struggle to navigate the healthcare system and may not be able to understand or follow instructions because of a misunderstanding. Low health literacy has been associated with increased rates of hospitalisation and greater use of emergency care; lower use of health screening and influenza vaccination; poorer ability to take medications appropriately; poorer ability to interpret labels and health messages; poorer knowledge about personal health issues; poor overall health among older people; and higher risk of death in older people (ACSQHC 2014). There are several factors that can impact a person's individual health literacy including age, education level, disability, culture, their first language being other than English, gender, being Aboriginal or Torres Strait Islander (ACSQHC 2014) or Māori (Ministry of Health 2017).

Tools for determining literacy

As a clinician, you are in a good position to assess and improve the health literacy of your clients. There is a wide variety of tools to measure health literacy—some more challenging than others. Table 7.6 presents three commonly used screening tools.

Each of the tools can be used in the clinical setting. A single-item literacy screener has been suggested, but with only marginal effectiveness. Some clinics simply ask standardised questions such as, 'Do you have any limitations in learning?' or 'What is the last grade level completed?' instead of requiring a specific assessment tool.

Health teaching

As a clinician, there are steps you can take to ensure that your clients understand the information you are providing. Although completing a health literacy screener gives you objective data and can help you determine the appropriate level of information, most clients (regardless of literacy level) want to be provided with simple, easy-to-understand instructions; therefore, the practice of giving all clients simple instructions at a lower reading level is acceptable. When discussing medical information with clients, keep it simple, use short sentences and words containing no more than two syllables (when possible), limit the number of messages you are giving the client, be

TABLE 7.6 Tools for assessing health literacy

TOOL	DESCRIPTION	EXAMPLE QUESTIONS
Test of Functional Health Literacy (TOFHLA) (Parker et al 1995)	• Designed for use in research • Measures reading comprehension and numeracy • Uses actual client instructions and forms • Takes approximately 22 min	Do not eat ______________ a. appointment b. walk-in c. breakfast d. clinic
Rapid Estimate of Adult Literacy in Medicine (REALM) (Davis et al 1993)	• Designed for use in clinical setting • Person reads 66 medical terms aloud • Score based on number of words read and pronounced correctly • Takes 2–3 min to administer	Words include: flu, smear, stress, gallbladder, inflammatory, diagnosis, potassium
Newest Vital Sign (NVS) (Weiss et al 2005)	• Assesses numeracy and comprehension • Uses nutrition label that clients must read and interpret • Total of six questions related to label provided • Takes approximately 3 min	Give client the nutrition label and ask: • If you eat the entire container, how many calories will you eat? • If you usually eat 2500 calories in a day, what percentage of your daily value of calories will you be eating if you eat one serving?

sure to tell the person what they will gain by following your instructions, present only needed information, focus on the client, use the active voice and avoid jargon. Although you may think using complex terms and sentences makes you sound more professional or smarter, it can confuse the client. You are better off speaking to them as you would to a friend, using a conversational structure that includes time for them to ask questions. A few examples follow:

Say: Feel for lumps about the size of a pea.
Don't say: Feel for lumps about 5 to 6 mm.

Say: Birth control
Don't say: Contraception

Say: Mad cow disease
Don't say: Bovine spongiform encephalitis

Say: Place your hand palm up.
Don't say: Supinate your hand.

Say: Cook chicken until it is no longer pink.
Don't say: Cook chicken to an internal temperature of 75°C.

Written materials

When preparing or using written materials, make sure to assess the appropriateness of the materials. Most client education materials are created at a reading level that is not suitable for the majority of clients. Written materials should be at the grade 5 reading level or below. Reading level can be determined with a variety of formulas that use a number of syllables per word and complexity of sentences to determine reading level. Materials should be in at least 12-point font, avoid all capital letters, use headings and subheadings, use bullet points and limit medical jargon. Pictures are often used in written materials, but you must be careful to select appropriate graphics.

Teach back

Although ensuring appropriate verbal and written communication is important, one of the easiest things you can do when teaching a client is to use the teach back approach. Teach back is simple and free. It allows you to assess whether the person understands and to immediately correct misconceptions. Many healthcare professionals ask, 'Do you understand?' or 'Do you have any questions?' throughout the teaching sessions. Just because your client has no questions and indicates understanding with a nod does not mean that they actually understand the information. Using teach back encourages the client to repeat in their own words what you have just said. This verbal discussion allows you to assess the understanding and may open the door for the client to ask questions.

BIBLIOGRAPHY

Arnold EC, Underman Boggs K. Interpersonal relationships: professional communication skills for nurses. 7th ed. St Louis: Elsevier; 2016.

Australian Bureau of Statistics (ABS). Program for the international assessment of adult competencies, Australia, 2011–12. 4228.0, 2014 [Accessed 10.06.2019]. Available at: www.abs.gov.au/ausstats/abs@.nsf/Latestproducts/4228.0Main%20Features202011-12?opendocument&tabname=Summary&prodno=4228.0&issue=2011-12&num=&view=.

Australian Commission on Safety and Quality in Health Care (ACSQHC). Health literacy: taking action to improve safety and quality. Sydney: ACSQHC; 2014 [Accessed 10.06.2019]. Available at: www.safetyandquality.gov.au/wp-content/uploads/2014/08/Health-Literacy-Taking-action-to-improve-safety-and-quality.pdf.

Australian Institute of Interpreters and Translators Incorporated (AUSIT). Guidelines for health professionals working with an Interpreter. 2019a. Available at: https://ausit.org/AUSIT/About/Ethics___Conduct/Get_It_Right/AUSIT/About/What_We_Stand_For_-_Get_It_Right.aspx.

Australian Institute of Interpreters and Translators Incorporated (AUSIT). Getting it right interpreting. 2019b. Available at: https://ausit.org/AUSIT/About/Ethics___Conduct/Get_It_Right/AUSIT/About/What_We_Stand_For_-_Get_It_Right.aspx.

Centre for Culture, Ethnicity and Health (CEH). Speaking with clients who have a low English proficiency. 2018a [Accessed 10.06.2019]. Available at: https://www.ceh.org.au/knowledge-hub?_sf_s=Speaking%20with%20clients%20who%20have%20a%20low.

Centre for Culture, Ethnicity and Health (CEH). Communication via an interpreter. 2018b [Accessed 10.06.2019]. Available at: https://www.ceh.org.au/?s=Communication+via+an+interpreter.

Centre for Culture, Ethnicity and Health (CEH). Debriefing with an interpreter. 2018c [Accessed 10.06.2019]. Available at: https://www.ceh.org.au/?s=Communication+via+an+interpreter.

Centre for Culture, Ethnicity and Health (CEH). Cultural considerations in health assessment. 2018d [Accessed 10.06.2019]. Available at: https://www.ceh.org.au/?s=%27Cultural+considerations+in+health+assessment%27.

Davis TC, Long SW, Jackson RH, et al. Rapid estimate of adult literacy in medicine: a shortened screening instrument. Fam Med 1993;25:391–5.

Folstein MF, Folstein SE, McHugh PR. Mini-mental state: a practical method for grading the cognitive states of patients for the clinician. J Psych Res 1975;12(3):189–98.

Forster E, Fraser J. Paediatric nursing skills for Australian nurses. Sydney, Australia: Cambridge University Press; 2017.

Hallet N. Preventing and managing challenging behavior. Nurs Stand 2018;32(26):51–62. doi: 10.7748/ns2018e10969.

Kennedy-Sheldon L, Foust JB. Communication for nurses. Talking with patients. 3rd ed. Sudbury, MA: Jones & Bartlett; 2014.

Ministry of Health. Manaū Hauora: Māori health models – Te Whare Tapa Whā. Wellington: Ministry of Health. 2017 [Accessed 10.06.2019]. Available at: https://www.health.govt.nz/our-work/populations/maori-health/maori-health-models/maori-health-models-te-whare-tapa-wha.

Moody HR, Sasser JR. Aging: concepts and controversies. 9th ed. Los Angeles: Sage Publication Inc.; 2018.

Office of Ethnic Communities. Te Tari Matawaki, 2019 [Accessed 10.06.2019]. Available at: www.ethniccommunities.govt.nz.

O'Toole G. Communication—core interpersonal skills for health professionals. Sydney: Churchill Livingstone; 2016.

Parker RM, Baker DW, Williams MV, et al. The test of functional health literacy in adults: a new instrument for measuring patients' health literacy skills. J Gen Intern Med 1995;10:537–54.

Raising Children Network. The Australian parenting website: Professionals working with Interpreters – tips for working with Interpreters, Australian Government Department of Social Services. 2014 [Accessed 10.06.2019]. Available at: https://raisingchildren.net.au/for-professionals/working-with-parents/cultural-diversity/working-with-interpreters.

Sand-Jecklin K, Daniels CS, Lucke-Wold N. Incorporating health literacy screening into patients' health assessment. Clin Nurs Res 2017;26(2):176–90. doi:10.1177/1054773815619592.

Selye H. The stress of life. Revised ed. New York: McGraw-Hill; 1984.

Statistics New Zealand. Language, 2014 [Accessed 10.06.2019]. Available at: www.stats.govt.nz/browse_for_stats/people_and_communities/Language.aspx.

Stein-Parbury J. Patient and person: interpersonal skills in nursing. 6th ed. Chatswood, NSW: Elsevier Australia; 2018.

Weiss BD, Mays MZ, Martz W, et al. Quick assessment of literacy in primary care. The newest vital sign. Ann of Fam Med 2005;3:514–22.

Chapter Eight

The health history

Written by Carolyn Jarvis

Adapted by Helen Forbes and Elizabeth Watt

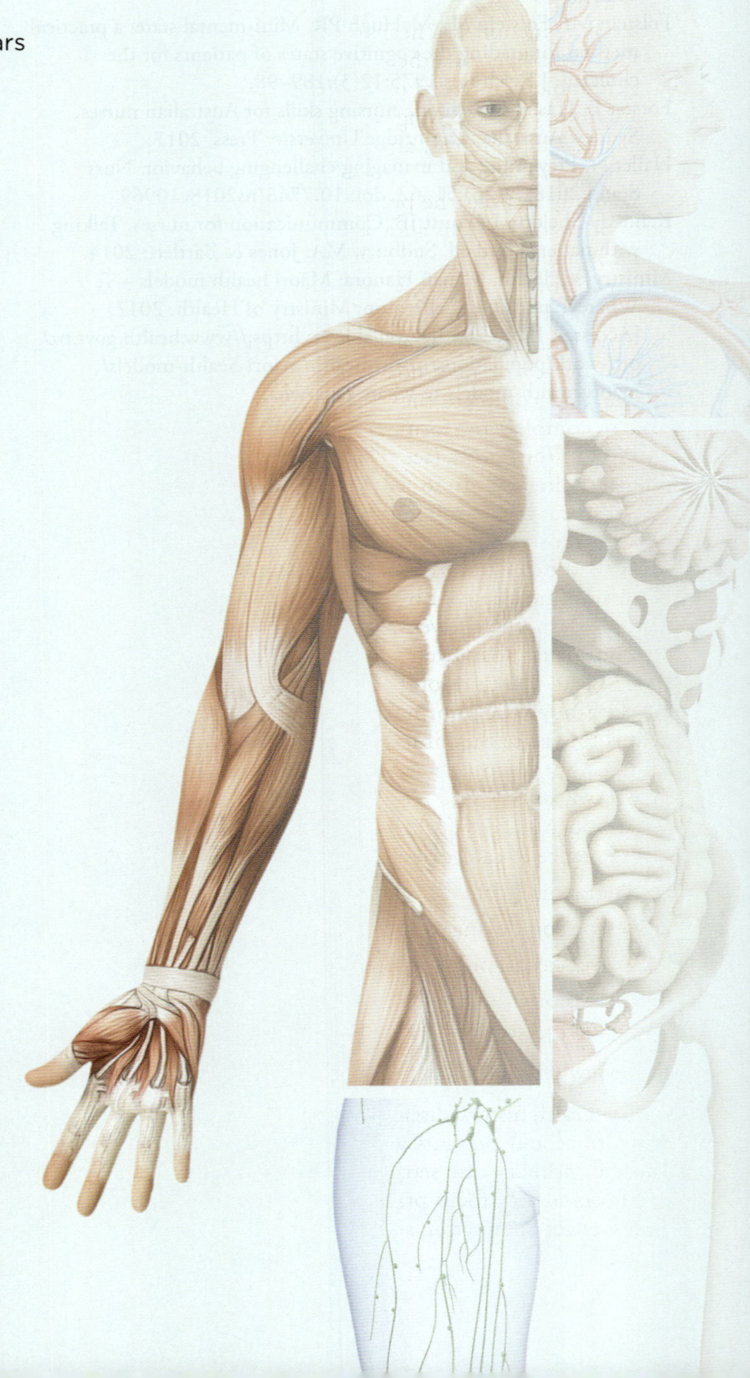

INTRODUCTION

The purpose of the health history is to collect information from the person, their carer or significant other's point of view (subjective data). The health history provides a guide for the nurse as to what needs to be focused on when collecting objective data. The data from the health history are combined with the **objective data** from the physical examination and diagnostic studies to describe the person's current health situation. This information is used to make a clinical judgement or a nursing diagnosis about the state of health of the individual.

The following health history framework provides a complete picture of the person's past and present health. It describes the individual as a whole and how the person interacts with the environment. It also records health strengths and coping skills. The history should recognise and affirm what the person is doing to help stay well. For the well person, the history is used to assess their lifestyle, including such factors as exercise, diet, risk reduction and health promotion behaviours.

For the ill person, the health history includes a detailed and chronological record of the health problem(s). For all, the health history is a screening tool for abnormal symptoms, health problems and concerns, and it records ways of responding to the health problems.

In many settings the person fills out an admission history form or checklist. This allows the person ample time to recall and consider such items as key health events and relevant family history. However, these forms assume that the person has a good understanding of written English and health literacy. You may become aware that the person has poor health literacy or may not have the capacity of the English language to complete the forms. In that case the nurse will need to complete the forms using information provided by the person and/or family (see Chapter 7 for further information on health literacy). In some situations the nurse completes the health history at the time the person is admitted to the ward or unit. However, the health history may also be completed prior to the person arriving at the hospital at a formal pre-admission interview, or by the person completing the printed history form themselves prior to admission. In a hospital setting this is most often completed as part of the admission process. At the time of admission the nurse should always check through the information with the person and clarify the details to ensure the information is accurate and complete. It is important to note that the health interview is conducted in such a way as to ensure the person's privacy.

Although history forms vary, most contain information in this sequence of categories:

1. Biographical data
2. Reason for seeking care
3. Present health or history of present illness
4. Past history
5. Family history
6. Review of symptoms, function and risk.

The health history discussed in the following section follows this format and presents a generic database for all clinicians. Those in primary care settings may use all of it, whereas those in a hospital may focus primarily on the history of the present illness, effect on function and possible risks related to the reason for admission and its treatment. Each chapter in this textbook details specific areas for subjective data collection relevant to the particular area being assessed.

The following information provides an overview of the health history including biographical data, the reasons for seeking care, past history, history of present illness and review of symptoms (including analysis of symptoms), function and risk.

THE HEALTH HISTORY—THE ADULT AND THE ADULT AGED 65 YEARS AND OVER

Before you begin any health assessment, it is important for safety reasons that approved patient identifiers are used to confirm the identity of the person (Australian Commission on Safety and Quality in Health Care 2019a). The approved identifiers include: the person's name (family and given names), date of birth, gender, address, medical record number or an individual healthcare identifier, for example a Medicare number. It is recommended that at least three identifiers are used prior to any procedure, service or care activity. It is important to note that bed or room number should not be used as they are not unique to an individual person because of the likelihood of bed or room changes.

Biographical data

The biographical data set includes the person's name, address and phone number, age and birth date, gender, marital status, religion, first language spoken (and other languages) including Indigenous status, occupation, both usual and present (an illness or disability may have prompted change in occupation), and next of kin name and contact details. In some circumstances, the person's nominated medical power of attorney (if any) is also recorded. The name and address of the person's usual general practitioner is recorded. Often this information is collected and prepared on an admission form by an administrator prior to the person arriving at the ward or unit. The nurse should recheck the validity of the recorded information.

Source of history

1. Record who furnishes the information—usually the person themself, although the source may be a relative or friend.
2. Judge how reliable the informant seems and how willing they are to communicate. A reliable person always gives the same answers, even when questions are rephrased or are repeated later in the interview.
3. Note any special circumstances, such as the need for an interpreter or the need for a nominated spokesperson to speak for the person who is unable to speak for themself, e.g. a person with dementia. Another possibility to consider is that, in some circumstances, a person may have nominated a specific spokesperson through medical power of attorney.

Reason for seeking care

This is a brief spontaneous statement in the person's own words that describes the reason for seeking healthcare. The reason(s) is often a symptom(s) or change in function that is considered by the person to be troublesome. A **symptom** is a subjective abnormal sensation that the person is experiencing, e.g. nausea. Whatever the person says as the reason for seeking care is recorded, enclosed in quotation marks to indicate the person's exact words. For example:

'Chest pain' for 2 hours.
'Earache and unsettled all night.'
'Pain in tummy for 2 days. It is getting worse.'

A **sign** is an objective abnormality that the examiner identifies on physical examination or in laboratory reports, e.g. crackles on ausculation of the person's lungs.

The reason for seeking care is not a diagnostic statement. Avoid translating it into the terms of a medical diagnosis. For example, Mr Jones reports shortness of breath. You consider writing 'emphysema'. Even if he is known to have emphysema from previous visits, it is not the chronic emphysema that prompted *this visit*, but rather the 'increasing shortness of breath' for 4 hours.

Some people try to self-diagnose based on similar signs and symptoms in their relatives or friends, or based on conditions they know they have. Rather than record a woman's statement that she has 'strep throat', ask her what symptoms she has that make her think this is present and record those symptoms.

Occasionally, a person may list many reasons for seeking care. The most important reason to the person may not necessarily be the one stated first. Try to focus on which is the most pressing concern by asking the person which one prompted them to seek help now.

Person's perception of present state of health or health concern

In this section you are trying to ascertain how the person perceives or describes their usual level of health. For people seeking healthcare for illness, this section is a chronological record of the reason for seeking care, from the time the symptom first started until now. Isolate each reason for care identified by the person and say, for example, 'Please tell me all about your headache, from the time it started until the time you came to the hospital'. If the concern started months or years ago, record what occurred during that time and find out why the person is seeking care now.

As the person talks, do not jump to conclusions and bias the story by adding your opinion. Collect all the data by asking the person what the problem is and what they think is the reason for the problem.

Healthcare workers often use a mnemonic to organise questions. A mnemonic ensures that you remember all the points when analysing symptoms such as nausea, constipation, or incontinence.

COLDSPA

The COLDSPA mnemonic is commonly used and includes these seven critical characteristics.

C: Character. This calls for specific description of the symptom using terms such as burning, sharp, dull, aching, gnawing, throbbing, shooting, vice-like. Use similes: does blood in the stool look like sticky tar? Does blood in vomitus look like coffee grounds? Find out the meaning of the symptom by asking how it affects daily activities and quality of life. Also ask directly, 'What do you think it means?' This is crucial because it alerts you to potential anxiety if the person thinks the symptom may be ominous.

O: Onset/timing. When did the symptom first appear? Give the specific date and time, or state specifically how long ago the symptom started prior to arrival at the hospital. 'The pain started yesterday' will not mean much when you return to read the record in the future. If intermittent, what is the frequency? Was it steady (constant) or did it come and go during that time?

L: Location. Be specific; ask the person to point to the location. If the problem is pain, note the precise site. 'Head pain' is vague, whereas descriptions such as 'pain behind the eyes', 'jaw pain' and 'occipital pain' are more precise and are diagnostically significant. Is the pain localised to this site or radiating? Is the pain superficial or deep?

D: Duration. How long did the symptom last? Was it constant or intermittent? Did it resolve completely and reappear later?

S: Severity. Attempt to quantify the symptom such as 'profuse menstrual flow soaking five pads per hour'. How bad is it (on a scale of 1 to 10)? What impact has the symptom had on your daily activities? Then the person might say, 'I was so sick I was doubled up and couldn't move', or 'I was able to go to work, but then I came home and went to bed'.

P: Pattern. What makes the symptom worse? Is it aggravated by weather, activity, food, medication, standing, bent over, fatigue, time of day, season and so on? What relieves it (e.g. rest, medication or ice pack)? What is the effect of any treatment? Ask, 'What have you tried?' or 'What seems to help?' Where was the person or what was the person doing when the symptom started? What brings it on? For example, 'Did you notice the chest pain after mowing the lawn, or did the pain start by itself?

A: Associated factors. Is this primary symptom associated with any others (e.g. urinary frequency and burning associated with fever and chills)? Review the body system related to this symptom now rather than wait for the physical assessment.

PQRSTU

PQRSTU is another example of a mnemonic which is useful for analysing a person's experience of pain:

P: Provocative or Palliative. What brings it on? What were you doing when you first noticed it? What makes it better? Worse?

Q: Quality or Quantity. How does it look, feel, sound? How intense/severe is it?

R: Region or Radiation. Where is it? Does it spread anywhere?

S: Severity scale. How bad is it (on a scale of 1 to 10)? Is it getting better, worse or staying the same?

T: Timing. Onset—exactly when did it first occur? Duration—how long did it last? Frequency—how often does it occur?

U: Understand patient's perception of the problem. What do you think it means?

Symptom measurement tools

There are validated tools available to assess symptoms in detail, for example, assessment of pain (see Chapter 13), depression (see Chapter 11) and distress. The distress thermometer was originally developed in 1998 (Roth et al 1998) and is a self-report screening tool for measuring psychological distress in cancer patients. There is an 11-point scale, ranging from 0 (no distress) to 10 (extreme distress). See Figure 8.1 below. The distress thermometer has been validated internationally in different age groups, settings and cancer types. It is quick and easy to implement and has become a useful screening tool for distress.

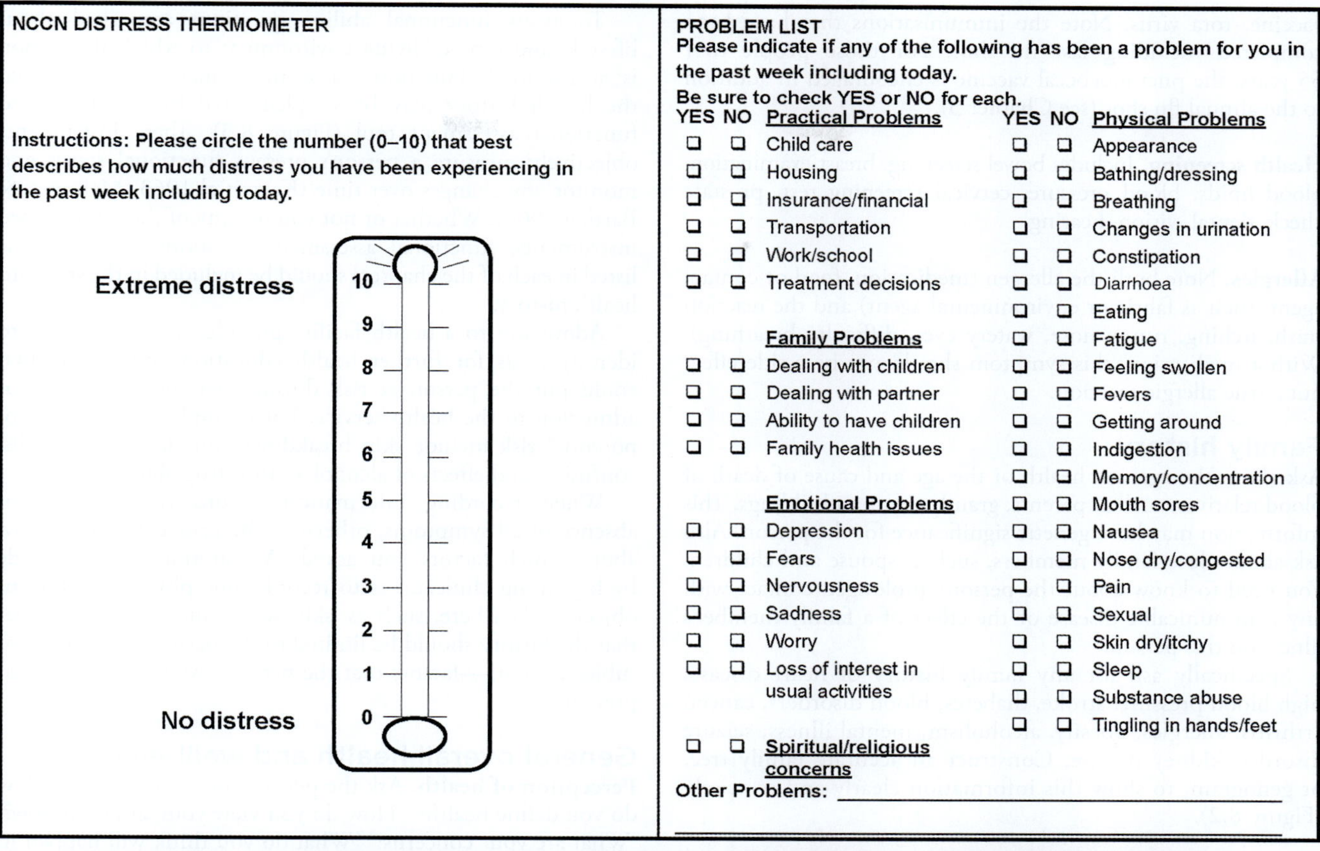

NCCN DISTRESS THERMOMETER

Instructions: Please circle the number (0–10) that best describes how much distress you have been experiencing in the past week including today.

Extreme distress 10

9

8

7

6

5

4

3

2

1

No distress 0

PROBLEM LIST

Please indicate if any of the following has been a problem for you in the past week including today.

Be sure to check YES or NO for each.

YES	NO	Practical Problems
❑	❑	Child care
❑	❑	Housing
❑	❑	Insurance/financial
❑	❑	Transportation
❑	❑	Work/school
❑	❑	Treatment decisions
		Family Problems
❑	❑	Dealing with children
❑	❑	Dealing with partner
❑	❑	Ability to have children
❑	❑	Family health issues
		Emotional Problems
❑	❑	Depression
❑	❑	Fears
❑	❑	Nervousness
❑	❑	Sadness
❑	❑	Worry
❑	❑	Loss of interest in usual activities
❑	❑	Spiritual/religious concerns

YES	NO	Physical Problems
❑	❑	Appearance
❑	❑	Bathing/dressing
❑	❑	Breathing
❑	❑	Changes in urination
❑	❑	Constipation
❑	❑	Diarrhoea
❑	❑	Eating
❑	❑	Fatigue
❑	❑	Feeling swollen
❑	❑	Fevers
❑	❑	Getting around
❑	❑	Indigestion
❑	❑	Memory/concentration
❑	❑	Mouth sores
❑	❑	Nausea
❑	❑	Nose dry/congested
❑	❑	Pain
❑	❑	Sexual
❑	❑	Skin dry/itchy
❑	❑	Sleep
❑	❑	Substance abuse
❑	❑	Tingling in hands/feet

Other Problems: ______________________

Figure 8.1
Distress thermometer.

Past health

Details about past health will depend on the situation and the context. See the following list of key aspects, which may or may not be required information.

Past health events may have residual effects on the current health state. Also, the previous experience with illness may give clues as to how the person responds to illness and to the significance of illness for the person.

Childhood illnesses. Ask about serious childhood illnesses that may have consequences for the person in later years , for example, measles, mumps, rubella, chickenpox, pertussis, poliomyelitis (all uncommon currently because of immunisation), rheumatic fever and scarlet fever.

Accidents or injuries. Motor vehicle accidents, fractures, joint injury, penetrating wounds, head injuries (especially if associated with unconsciousness) and burns.

Serious or chronic illnesses. For example, diabetes, hypertension, heart disease, cancer and seizure disorder.

Hospitalisations. Reason for hospitalisation, name of hospital, how the condition was treated, how long the person was hospitalised and name of the medical practitioner.

Surgical procedures. Type of surgery, date, name of the surgeon, name of hospital and how the person recovered.

Obstetric history. Number of pregnancies, number of deliveries in which the fetus reached full term, number of preterm pregnancies (preterm), number of incomplete pregnancies (miscarriage or termination of pregnancy) and number of children (living). For each complete pregnancy, note the mother's health during the pregnancy; labour and birthing; sex, weight and condition of each infant; and postpartum health.

Immunisations. The following immunisations are on the Australian and New Zealand National Immunisation program schedules. These include: Measles–mumps–rubella, polio, diphtheria–pertussis–tetanus, hepatitis B, human papillomavirus, *Haemophilus influenzae* type b, pneumococcal vaccine, rota virus. Note the immunisations that have been completed including last flu shot. For those people over 65 years, the pneumococcal vaccine is encouraged in addition to the annual flu shot (see Chapter 3).

Health screening. Includes bowel screening, breast examination, blood lipids, blood pressure, cervical screening test, prostate check, dental, vision, hearing.

Allergies. Note both the allergen (medication, food or contact agent, such as fabric or environmental agent) and the reaction (rash, itching, runny nose, watery eyes, difficulty breathing). With a medication, this symptom should not be a side effect but a true allergic reaction.

Family history

Ask about the age and health or the age and cause of death of blood relatives, such as parents, grandparents and siblings. This information may have genetic significance for the person. Also ask about close family members, such as spouse and children. You need to know about the person's prolonged contact with any communicable disease or the effect of a family member's illness on this person.

Specifically ask for any family history of heart disease, high blood pressure, stroke, diabetes, blood disorders, cancer, arthritis, allergies, obesity, alcoholism, mental illness, seizure disorder, kidney disease. Construct an accurate family tree, or genogram, to show this information clearly and concisely (Figure 8.2).

Review of symptoms, function and risks

The purposes of this section are (1) to evaluate the past and present health state of the person, (2) to double check in case any significant data were omitted in the present illness section, (3) to evaluate health promotion practices and (4) to identify symptoms and potential health risks. The items within each section are not inclusive, and only the most common symptoms are listed. If the present illness section covered one body system, you do not need to repeat all the data here. For example, if the reason for seeking care is earache, the present illness section describes most of the symptoms listed for the auditory system. Just ask now what was not asked in the 'present illness' section.

Another area of review is to determine the effect of illness and symptoms on the person's functional ability. Functional assessment measures a person's self-care ability in the areas of general health; activities of daily living, such as bathing, dressing, toileting, eating, walking; or those needed for independent living, such as housekeeping, shopping, cooking, doing laundry, using the telephone, managing finances; nutrition; social relationships and resources; self-concept and coping; and home environment. For example, alterations in cardiovascular, respiratory and/or musculoskeletal health may impact on a person's ability to be active and participate in daily living activities. See Units 4–6 for details. Similarly, alterations in mental status, neurological and sensory function (Unit 3), nutrition and metabolic function (Unit 7), urinary and bowel elimination (Unit 8), sexuality and reproductive function (Unit 9) can also impact on the person's ability to perform their daily activities and participate in exercise and leisure activities. Within each of these areas, the focus is on eliciting the nature of the effect and how it relates to the person's quality of life.

To assess functional ability, questions are asked about lifestyle and type of living environment to which the person is accustomed. Functional assessment may also mean that the health history may be supplemented by a standardised functional assessment tool (Figure 8.3). These instruments objectively measure a person's present functional status and monitor any changes over time (Katz et al 1963, Mahoney & Barthel 1965). Whether or not you use any of these formalised instruments, functional assessment questions such as those listed in each of the chapters should be included in the standard health history.

Admission to a health facility provides an opportunity to identify areas for further health education and factors that could put the person at risk during their hospitalisation or admission to the health service. For example, known areas of potential risk include skin breakdown, unrelieved pain, falls, confusion and effects of alcohol and/or drug abuse.

When recording information, record the presence or absence of all symptoms, otherwise the reader does not know about which factors you asked. A common mistake made by beginning clinicians is to record some physical finding or objective data here, such as 'skin warm and dry'. Remember that the history should be limited to the person's statements or subjective data—factors that the person says were or were not present.

General overall health and wellbeing

Perception of health. Ask the person questions such as: 'How do you define health?' 'How do you view your situation now?' 'What are your concerns?' 'What do you think will happen in the future?' 'What are your health goals?' 'What do you expect from us as nurses, medical practitioners (or other healthcare professionals)?'

Interpersonal relationships/resources. Education level achieved and current employment. For example: 'How would you describe your role in the family?' 'How would you say you get along with family, friends and co-workers?' Ask about support systems composed of family and significant others: 'To whom could you go for support with a problem at work, with your health or a personal problem?' Include contact with spouse, siblings, parents, children, friends, organisations and workplace: 'Is time spent alone pleasurable and relaxing, or isolating?' 'What hobbies do you have?' 'What effect will your current illness/hospitalisation have on your relationships and roles?'

Values and beliefs/spiritual resources. Cultural and ethnic background and practices, as well as religious/spiritual beliefs, values and practices. For example: 'Do you identify with any specific cultural group?' 'In your culture are there some health practices that are important to you?' 'Does religious faith or spirituality play an important part in your life? Do you consider yourself to be a religious or spiritual person?' 'How does your religious faith or spirituality influence the way you think about your health or the way you care for yourself?' 'Are you a part of any religious or spiritual community or congregation?' 'Would you like me to address any religious or spiritual issues or concerns with you?' 'What effect will your current illness/hospitalisation have on your capacity to practise your religion?'

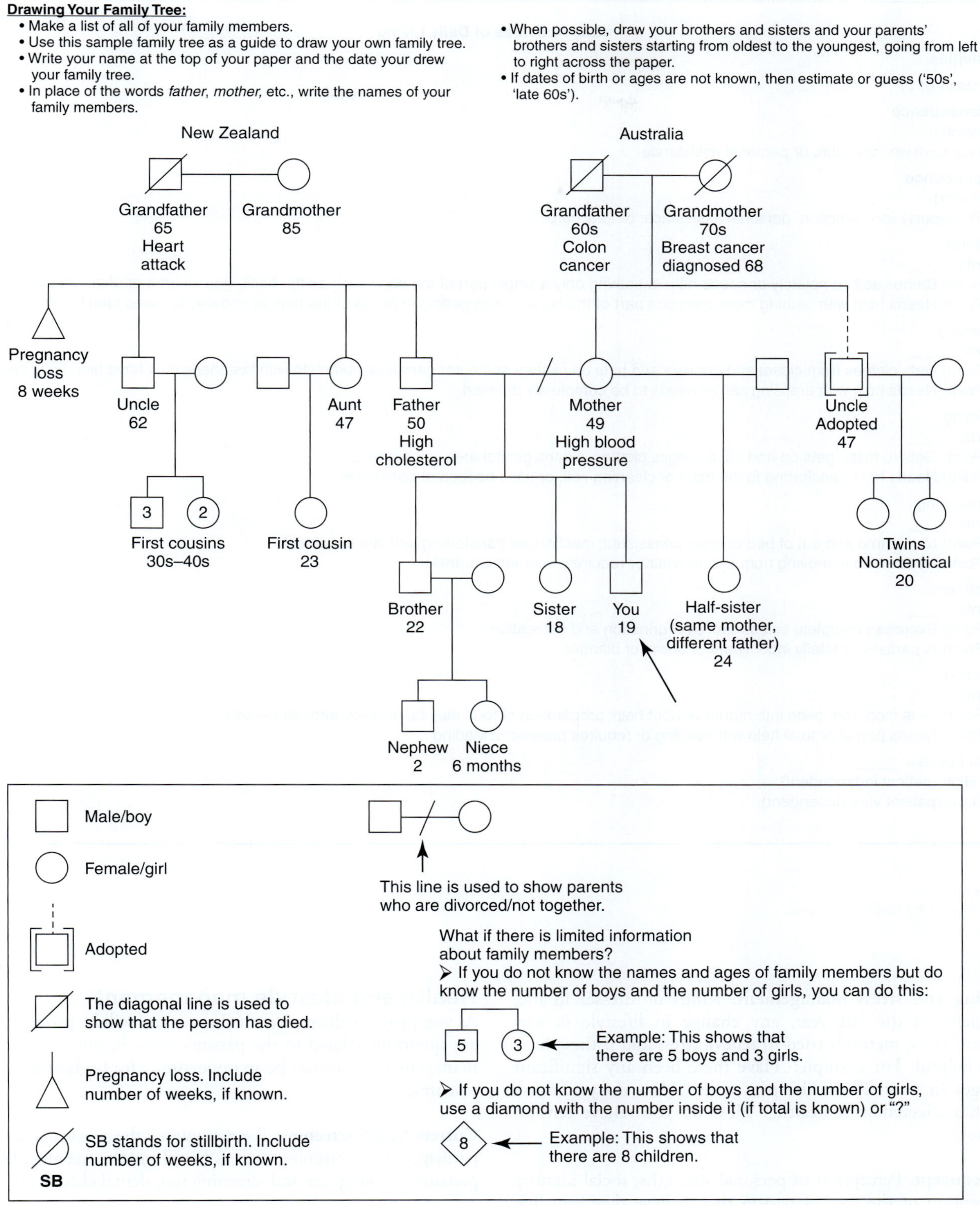
Drawing Your Family Tree:
• Make a list of all of your family members.
• Use this sample family tree as a guide to draw your own family tree.
• Write your name at the top of your paper and the date your drew your family tree.
• In place of the words father, mother, etc., write the names of your family members.
• When possible, draw your brothers and sisters and your parents' brothers and sisters starting from oldest to the youngest, going from left to right across the paper.
• If dates of birth or ages are not known, then estimate or guess ('50s', 'late 60s').
New Zealand
Grandfather 65 Heart attack
Grandmother 85
Australia
Grandfather 60s Colon cancer
Grandmother 70s Breast cancer diagnosed 68
Pregnancy loss 8 weeks
Uncle 62
Aunt 47
Father 50 High cholesterol
Mother 49 High blood pressure
Uncle Adopted 47
3
2
First cousins 30s–40s
First cousin 23
Twins Nonidentical 20
Brother 22
Sister 18
You 19
Half-sister (same mother, different father) 24
Nephew 2
Niece 6 months
Male/boy
Female/girl
Adopted
The diagonal line is used to show that the person has died.
Pregnancy loss. Include number of weeks, if known.
SB stands for stillbirth. Include number of weeks, if known.
SB
This line is used to show parents who are divorced/not together.
What if there is limited information about family members?
➤ If you do not know the names and ages of family members but do know the number of boys and the number of girls, you can do this:
5
3
Example: This shows that there are 5 boys and 3 girls.
➤ If you do not know the number of boys and the number of girls, use a diamond with the number inside it (if total is known) or "?"
8
Example: This shows that there are 8 children.

Figure 8.2
Genogram or family tree.

Katz Activities of Daily Living

Activities

Points (1 or 0)

Independence
(1 Point)
NO supervision, direction, or personal assistance

Dependence
(0 Points)
WITH supervision, direction, personal assistance, or total care

Bathing
Points _____
(1 Point) Bathes self completely or needs help in bathing only a single part of the body such as the back, genital area or disabled extremity
(0 Point) Needs help with bathing more than one part of the body or with getting in or out of the bath or shower; requires total bathing

Dressing
Points _____
(1 Point) Gets clothes from closet and drawers and puts on clothes and outer garments complete with fasteners; may have help tying shoes
(0 Point) Needs help with dressing self or needs to be completely dressed

Toileting
Points _____
(1 Point) Gets to toilet, gets on and off, arranges clothes, cleans genital area without help
(0 Point) Needs help transferring to the toilet or cleaning self, or uses bedpan or commode

Transferring
Points _____
(1 Point) Moves into and out of bed or chair unassisted; mechanical transferring aids are acceptable
(0 Point) Needs help in moving from bed to chair or requires a complete transfer

Continence
Points _____
(1 Point) Exercises complete self-control over urination and defecation
(0 Point) Is partially or totally incontinent of bowel or bladder

Feeding
Points _____
(1 Point) Gets food from plate into mouth without help; preparation of food may be done by another person
(0 Point) Needs partial or total help with feeding or requires parenteral feeding

Total Points = _____
6 = High (patient independent)
0 = Low (patient very dependent)

Figure 8.3
Katz Activities of Daily Living.

Coping and stress management. Kinds of stresses in life, especially in the last year, any change in lifestyle or any current stress, methods tried to relieve stress and if these have been helpful. For example: 'Have there been any significant changes in your life in the past year?' 'How do you think this has affected your health?' 'How do you relieve tension or stress?'

Self-concept. Perception of personal strengths, social identity (perception of the sort of person they believe they are), life values and beliefs and body image. For example: 'What is it about your present situation that is most worrying for you?'

Sleep/rest. Sleep patterns, daytime naps, any sleep aids used. For example: 'What time do you usually go to sleep?' 'When do you normally wake up?' 'Do you have difficulty getting to sleep?' 'If so, how do you manage that?'

Health and lifestyle management

As you progress through each chapter you will be prompted to ask questions related to the person's usual health and lifestyle management. This may be an opportunity for beginning health teaching.

Current health screening. For example ask the person about their participation in screening such as bowel cancer screening, blood pressure checking, cervical screening test, dental checks, etc.

Current medications. Nurses have an important role in medication reconciliation. This is a process where an accurate list of the person's medications must be obtained and verified as part of the admission process. Medications include all over-the-counter medicines and complementary or traditional therapies. Ask specifically about vitamins, oral contraceptives, aspirin, sedatives and antacids, because many people do not consider these to be medications. Efforts are made to match the medicines that should be prescribed to those that are actually prescribed. Explanations for any changes are documented. Particular care must be taken when a person is transferred from one healthcare environment to another.

For each medication, record the name, purpose and daily schedule and ask 'How often do you take it each day?' 'What is it for?' and 'How long have you been taking it?' Does the person have a system to remember to take the medicine? Does medicine seem to work? Are there any side effects? If so, does the person feel like skipping medicine because of them? Also consider the following issues:

- Some people take a large number of medications, prescribed by different medical practitioners.
- Is cost a problem? When the person is unable to afford a medication, they may decrease the dosage, take one pill instead of two or not refill the empty bottle immediately.
- Is travelling to the pharmacy to refill a prescription a problem?
- Has the person ever shared medications with neighbours or friends? Some establish 'lay referral' networks by comparing symptoms and thus medications.

Tobacco, alcohol and illicit drugs. 'Do you smoke cigarettes (pipe)?' 'At what age did you start?' 'How many packs do you smoke per day?' 'How many years have you smoked?' Record the number of packs smoked per day (PPD) and duration, e.g. 1 PPD × 5 years. Then ask, 'Have you ever tried to quit?' and 'How did it go?' to introduce plans about smoking cessation. 'How long since you quit smoking?'

Healthcare professionals often fail to question about alcohol unless problems are obvious. Be alert, then, to early signs of hazardous alcohol use. Ask whether the person drinks alcohol. If yes, ask specific questions about the amount and frequency of alcohol use: 'When was your last drink of alcohol?' 'How much did you drink that time?' 'What do you drink?' 'Out of the last 30 days, about how many days would you say that you drank alcohol?' 'Have you ever had a drinking problem?' 'Any history of alcohol treatment?' 'Involvement in recovery activities?' 'History of family member with problem drinking?'

Ask specifically about illicit drugs such as marijuana, cocaine, crack cocaine, amphetamines and methamphetamines. Indicate frequency of use and how usage has affected work or family. Refer to Chapter 6 for more information about substance abuse.

Environment/hazards. Housing and neighbourhood (living alone, knowledge of neighbours), safety of area, adequate heat and utilities, access to transportation and involvement in community services. Note environmental health, including hazards in workplace, hazards at home, use of seat belts, geographical or occupational exposures and travel or residence in other countries, including time spent overseas.

Occupational health. Ask the person to describe their job. Ever worked with any health hazard, such as asbestos, inhalants, chemicals or repetitive motion? Wear any protective equipment? Any work programs in place that monitor exposure? Aware of any health problems now that may be related to work exposure? Note the timing of the reason for seeking care and whether it may be related to work or home activities such as hobbies, job titles or exposure history. Finally, ask the person what they like or dislike about the job.

THE HEALTH HISTORY—THE CHILD

The health history is adapted to include information specific for the age and developmental stage of the child (e.g. the mother's health during pregnancy, labour and birthing and the perinatal period). Note that the developmental history and nutritional data are listed as separate sections because of their importance for current health.

Biographical data

Include the child's name, nickname, address and phone number, parents' names and work numbers, child's age and birth date, birthplace, gender and information on other children and family members at home.

Source of history

1. Person providing information and relation to child
2. Your impression of reliability of information
3. Any special circumstances, e.g. the use of an interpreter.

Reason for seeking care

Record the parent's spontaneous statement. Reasons for health problems may be initiated by the child, parent or by a third party such as the school teacher. Parent concerns about the health of their child must be taken seriously and thoroughly investigated. The parent's intuitive sense of a problem is often very accurate. Even if proved otherwise, this factor gives you an idea of the parent's area of concern.

Present health or history of present illness

Include a statement about the usual health of the child and any common health problems or major health concerns.

Describe any presenting symptom or sign, using the same format as for the adult. Some additional considerations include:

- Severity of pain: 'How do you know the child is in pain (e.g. pulling at ears alerts parent to ear pain)?' Note effect of pain on usual behaviour (e.g. does it stop the child from playing?).
- Associated factors, such as relation to activity, eating and body position.
- Parent's coping ability and reaction of other family members to child's symptoms or illness.

Past health

Prenatal status (if relevant). What was the mother's health during pregnancy? Were there any complications (bleeding, excessive nausea and vomiting, unusual weight gain, high blood pressure, swelling of hands and feet, infections—rubella or sexually transmitted diseases—falls)? During what month were diet and medications prescribed and/or taken during pregnancy (dose and duration)? Record the mother's use of alcohol, street drugs or cigarettes and any scans taken during pregnancy.

Start with an open-ended question: 'Tell me about your pregnancy'. If she questions the relevancy of the statement, mention that these questions are important to gain a complete picture of the child's health.

Labour and birthing (if relevant). Gravidity (number of times a female is or has been pregnant) and parity (viable pregnancies over 20 weeks' gestation), duration of the pregnancy, name of the hospital, course and duration of labour, use of anaesthesia, type of birth (vertex, breech, caesarean section), birth weight, Apgar scores, onset of breathing, any cyanosis, need for resuscitation and use of special equipment or procedures.

Postnatal status. In the neonatal stage, were there any health problems requiring hospitalisation? Length of hospital stay, neonatal jaundice, whether the baby was discharged with the mother, whether the baby was breast or bottle fed, weight gain, any feeding problems, colic, diarrhoea, patterns of crying and sleeping and the mother's perception of her physical and mental health postpartum.

Childhood illnesses. Age and any illnesses such as tonsil, ear, adenoidal infections. Measles, mumps, rubella, chickenpox, and pertussis are uncommon because of immunisation.

Serious accidents or injuries. Age of occurrence, extent of injury, how the child was treated and complications of motor vehicle accidents, falls, head injuries, fractures, burns and poisonings.

Serious or chronic illness, surgery or hospitalisations. Illnesses, e.g. seizure disorders, asthma, pneumonia, diabetes, renal disorders, allergies (see section below), rheumatic fever, scarlet fever (especially for rural and remote communities), age of onset, reason for hospitalisation, age at admission, name of surgeon or primary care providers, name of hospital, duration of stay, how child reacted to hospitalisation and any complications. (If child reacted poorly, they may be afraid now and will need special preparation for the examination that is to follow.)

Immunisations. Age when administered, date administered and any reactions following immunisations. See Chapter 3 for immunisation schedules.

Allergies or food intolerances. Any medications, foods, contact agents and environmental agents to which the child is allergic, and reaction to allergen. Note allergic reactions particularly common in childhood, such as hay fever, insect hypersensitivity, eczema and urticaria. Note if the child has had a past anaphylactic reaction and whether they carry an Epipen.

Developmental history

The child's growth and development may need to be assessed in detail. See Chapter 3.

Psychosocial history

It is important to get a sense of the child as a person, their usual home environment and the people who care for them. This will provide a baseline for assessing that the child is coping with the current health situation and will assist in person-centred care planning for the child and their family. Matters and Ross (2018) outline the following areas:

- Behavioural history includes unusual behaviours, altered patterns of sleep and toileting problems such as bedwetting
- Social development and interactions, for example for the school aged child, consider school performance, in the context of vision, hearing, speech, gross and fine motor function and social interactions
- Describe a typical day in the life of this child including physical activity, food and diet, living conditions and family life
- Relationships within the family including communication, family support, alternative care arrangements, for example child care, foster care. Does the child spend time between family members?
- Effect of illness on the child and family.

Family history

In some circumstances, a detailed family history may be required. Drawing a family tree for the child, including siblings, parents and grandparents, may be a useful strategy. Give the age, health or age and cause of death of each. Ask specifically for the family history of heart disease, high blood pressure, diabetes, blood disorders, cancer, arthritis, allergies, obesity, cystic fibrosis, alcoholism, mental illness, seizure disorder, kidney disease, developmental disability, learning disabilities, birth defects and sudden infant death. (Avoid making assumptions about the structure of the family. Rather than assume, be sure to ask a parent to clarify the family structure.)

General overall health and wellbeing

As with the adult, changes in any of the areas of the body will impact on function and give rise to symptoms and risks, which need to be investigated in detail. For details of assessment of each of the areas of the body see the relevant units in the text.

THE HEALTH HISTORY—THE ADOLESCENT

As with the child, the health history is adapted to include information specific for the age and developmental stage of the adolescent which is aimed to maximise communication. The **HEEADSSS** method of interviewing focuses on assessment of the **H**ome environment, **E**ducation and employment, **E**ating, peer-related **A**ctivities, **D**rugs, **S**exuality, **S**uicide/depression and **S**afety from injury and violence (Figure 8.4). The tool minimises adolescent stress because it moves from expected and less threatening questions to those that are more personal. The tool presents the questions in three colours: green questions are considered essential to explore with every adolescent; blue are important for you to ask if time permits; red questions delve more deeply if the situation demands it. Parents should not be present during a HEEADSSS assessment. Ask the young person if they would prefer to be assessed without a parent present. The other areas for health history can be adapted from the adult section described above.

The HEEADSSS Psychosocial Interview for Adolescents

Home
Who lives with you? Where do you live? Do you have your own room?
What are relationships like at home?
To whom are you closest at home?
To whom can you talk at home?
Is there anyone new at home? Has someone left recently?
Have you moved recently?
Have you ever had to live away from home? (Why?)
Have you ever run away? (Why?)
Is there any physical violence at home?

Education and Employment
What are your favourite subjects at school? Your least favourite subjects?
How are your grades? Any recent changes? Any dramatic changes in the past?
Have you changed schools in the past few years?
What are your future education/employment plans/goals?
Are you working? Where? How much?
Tell me about your friends at school.
Is your school a safe place? (Why?)
Have you ever had to repeat a class? Have you ever had to repeat a grade?
Have you ever been suspended? Expelled? Have you ever considered dropping out?
How well do you get along with the people at school? Work?
Have your responsibilities at work increased?
Do you feel connected to your school? Do you feel as if you belong?
Are there adults at school you feel you could talk to about something important? (Who?)

Eating
What do you like and not like about your body?
Have there been any recent changes in your weight?
Have you dieted in the past year? How? How often?
Have you done anything else to try to manage your weight?
How much exercise do you get in an average day? Week?
What do you think would be a healthy diet? How does that compare with your current eating patterns?
Do you worry about your weight? How often?
Do you eat in front of the TV? Computer?
Does it ever seem as though your eating is out of control?
Have you ever made yourself throw up on purpose to control your weight?
Have you ever taken diet pills?
What would it be like if you gained (lost) 5 kilos?

Activities
What do you and your friends do for fun? (with whom, where, and when?)
What do you and your family do for fun? (with whom, where, and when?)
Do you participate in any sports or other activities?
Do you regularly attend a church group, club or other organised activity?
Do you have any hobbies?
Do you read for fun? (What?)
How much TV do you watch in a week? How about video games?
What music do you like to listen to?

Drugs
Do any of your friends use tobacco? Alcohol? Other drugs?
Does anyone in your family use tobacco? Alcohol? Other drugs?
Do you use tobacco? Alcohol? Other drugs?
Is there any history of alcohol or drug problems in your family?
Do you ever drink or use drugs when you're alone?
(Assess frequency, intensity, patterns of use or abuse, and how youth obtains or pays for drugs, alcohol or tobacco.)

Sexuality
Have you ever been in a romantic relationship?
Tell me about the people that you've dated. *OR* Tell me about your sex life.
Have any of your relationships ever been sexual relationships?
Are your sexual activities enjoyable?
What does the term 'safer sex' mean to you?
Are you interested in boys? Girls? Both?
Have you ever been forced or pressured into doing something sexual that you didn't want to do?
Have you ever been touched sexually in a way that you didn't want?
Have you ever been raped, on a date or any other time?
How many sexual partners have you had altogether?
Have you ever been pregnant or worried that you may be pregnant? (females)
Have you ever made someone pregnant or worried that that might have happened? (males)
What are you using for birth control? Are you satisfied with your method?
Do you use condoms every time you have intercourse?
Does anything ever get in the way of always using a condom?
Have you ever had a sexually transmitted infection (STI) or worried that you had an STI?

Suicide and Depression
Do you feel sad or down more than usual? Do you find yourself crying more than usual?
Are you 'bored' all the time?
Are you having trouble getting to sleep?
Have you thought a lot about hurting yourself or someone else?
Does it seem that you've lost interest in things that you used to really enjoy?
Do you find yourself spending less and less time with friends?
Would you rather just be by yourself most of the time?
Have you ever tried to kill yourself?
Have you ever had to hurt yourself (by cutting yourself, for example) to calm down or feel better?
Have you started using alcohol or drugs to help you relax, calm down or feel better?

Safety (Savagery)
Have you ever been seriously injured? (How?) How about anyone else you know?
Do you always wear a seatbelt in the car?
Have you ever ridden with a driver who was drunk or high? When? How often?
Do you use safety equipment for sports and/or other physical activities (e.g. helmets for biking or skateboarding)?
Is there any violence in your home? Does the violence ever get physical?
Is there a lot of violence at your school? In your neighbourhood? Among your friends?
Have you ever been physically or sexually abused? Have you ever been raped, on a date or at any other time? (If not asked previously)
Have you ever been in a car or motorcycle accident? (What happened?)
Have you ever been picked on or bullied? Is that still a problem?
Have you been in physical fights in school or your neighbourhood? Are you still getting into fights?
Have you ever felt that you had to carry a knife, gun or other weapon to protect yourself? Do you still feel that way?

Green = essential questions
Blue = as time permits
Red = optional or when situation requires

Figure 8.4
The HEEADSSS psychosocial interview for adolescents.

BIBLIOGRAPHY

Australian Commission on Safety and Quality in Health Care. Falls prevention. Sydney: ACSQHC; 2015. Available at: https://www.safetyandquality.gov.au/our-work/falls-prevention/—:.

Australian Commission on Safety and Quality in Health Care. Communicating for Safety. Sydney: ACSQHC; 2019a. Available at: https://www.c4sportal.safetyandquality.gov.au/.

Australian Commission on Safety and Quality in Health Care. Medication safety. Sydney: ACSQHC; 2019b. Available at: https://www.safetyandquality.gov.au/our-work/medication-safety/.

Australian Government Department of Health. Immunisation, 2019. Available at: www.health.gov.au/internet/immunise/publishing.nsf/Content/Handbook-home.

Crossen, K. Missed opportunities for adolescent friendly care in hospital. J Paediatr Child Health December 2017;53(12):1176-9. doi:10.1111/jpc.13626

Katz S, Ford AB, Moskowitz RW, et al. Studies of illness in the aged. The index of ADL; a standardized measure of biological and psychosocial function. JAMA 1963;185:914–19.

Mahoney FI, Barthel DW. Functional evaluation: the Barthel Index. Md Med 1965;14:61–5.

Matters, J, Ross, B. The paediatric history and examination. In: Talley NJ, O'Connor S, editors. Talley and O'Connor's clinical examination: a guide to specialty examinations. 8th ed. Chatswood: Elsevier; 2018. pp. 619–83.

Ministry of Health New Zealand. Immunisation handbook. Wellington: Ministry of Health New Zealand; 2017. Available at: https://www.health.govt.nz/publication/immunisation-handbook-2017.

Roth AJ, Kornblith AB, Batel-Copel L, et al. Rapid screening for psychologic distress in men with prostate carcinoma: a pilot study. Cancer 1998;82(10):1904–8.

Royal Children's Hospital. Engaging with and assessing the adolescent patient. 2019. Available at: https://www.rch.org.au/clinicalguide/guideline_index/Engaging_with_and_assessing_the_adolescent_patient/.

Taylor A, Broadbent M, Wallis M, et al. The use of functional and cognitive assessment in the emergency department to inform decision making: A scoping review. Australas Emerg Care 2018;21:13–22.

Chapter Nine

Physical assessment techniques

Written by Carolyn Jarvis
Adapted by Elizabeth Watt

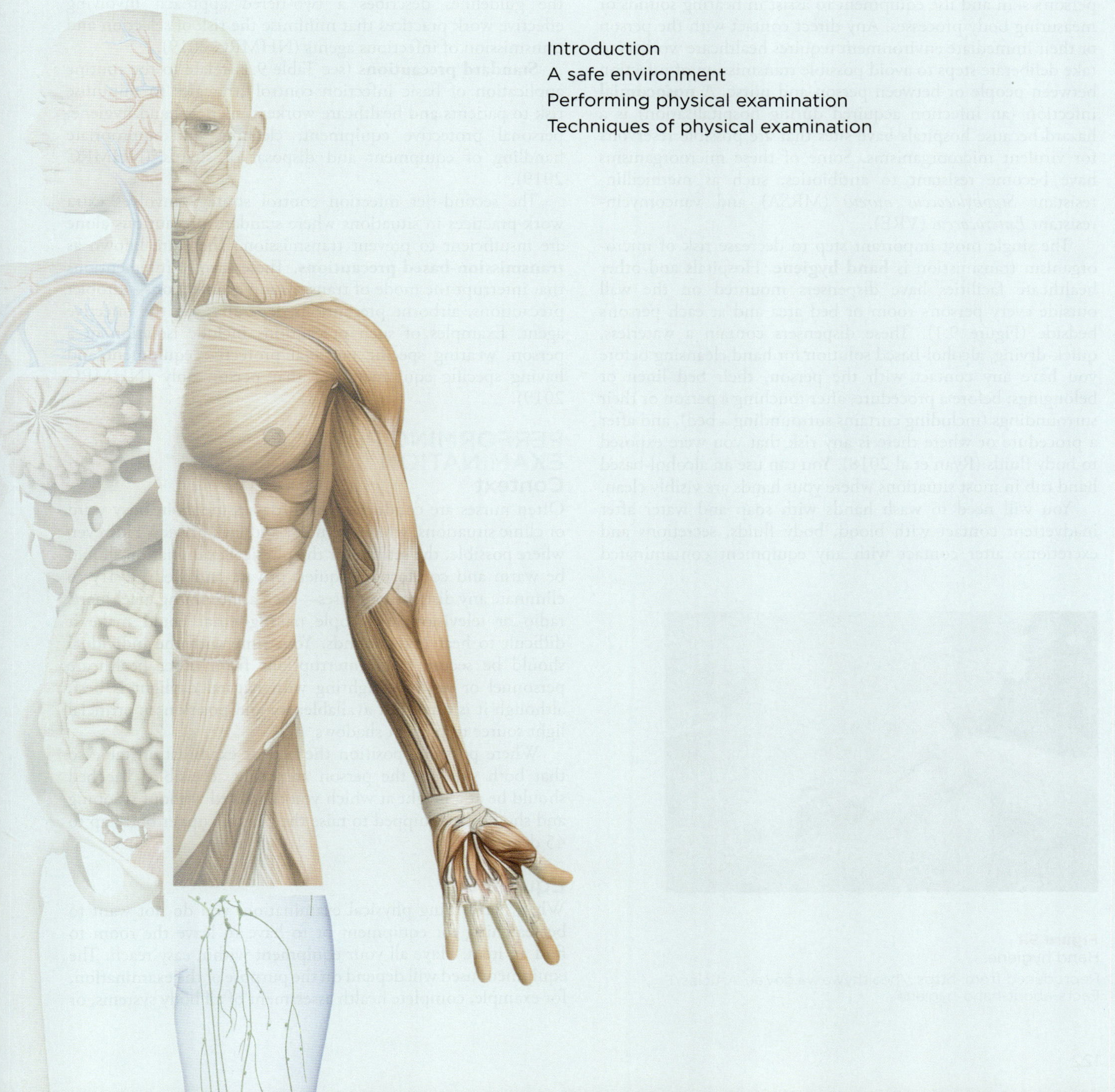

INTRODUCTION

The health history described in the preceding chapter provides **subjective** data for health assessment; the individual's perception of their current health state and their past health history. In this chapter we describe the physical examination techniques that are used to assess all body systems. The data you obtain from physical examination, along with specimen screening and assessment findings obtained from other healthcare team members, including blood tests and diagnostic imaging form the **objective** dataset. You will use your senses—sight, smell, touch and hearing—to gather health assessment data during a physical examination.

A SAFE ENVIRONMENT

Physical examination requires the examiner to touch the person's skin and use equipment to assist in hearing sounds or measuring body processes. Any direct contact with the person or their immediate environment requires healthcare workers to take deliberate steps to avoid possible transmission of infection between people or between person and nurse. A **nosocomial** infection (an infection acquired during hospitalisation) is a hazard because hospitals have sites that are possible reservoirs for virulent microorganisms. Some of these microorganisms have become resistant to antibiotics, such as methicillin-resistant *Staphylococcus aureus* (MRSA) and vancomycin-resistant *Enterococcus* (VRE).

The single most important step to decrease risk of micro-organism transmission is **hand hygiene**. Hospitals and other healthcare facilities have dispensers mounted on the wall outside every person's room or bed area and at each person's bedside (Figure 9.1). These dispensers contain a waterless, quick-drying, alcohol-based solution for hand cleansing before you have any contact with the person, their bed linen or belongings; before a procedure, after touching a person or their surroundings (including curtains surrounding a bed), and after a procedure or where there is any risk that you were exposed to body fluids (Ryan et al 2018). You can use an alcohol-based hand rub in most situations where your hands are visibly clean.

You will need to wash hands with soap and water after inadvertent contact with blood, body fluids, secretions and excretions; after contact with any equipment contaminated with body fluid; or when gloves have not been worn when caring for a patient who has *Clostridium difficile* (*C. difficile*), as the *C. difficile* spores are not killed by the hand hygiene solutions (Ryan et al 2018). See the websites of Hand Hygiene Australia for up-to-date information about hand hygiene practices and an online learning package.

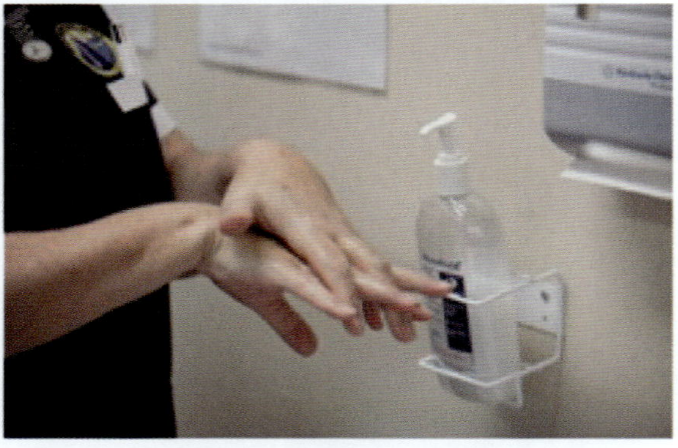

Figure 9.1
Hand hygiene.
Reproduced from: https://healthywa.wa.gov.au/Articles/F_I/Facts-about-hand-hygiene

Wear disposable gloves when the potential exists for contact with any body fluids (e.g. blood, urine, faeces, mucous membranes, drainage, open skin lesions). However, routine hand hygiene should always be performed before putting on gloves and following removal of gloves (National Health and Medical Research Council (NHMRC) 2019).

The Australian Guidelines for the Prevention and Control of Infection in Health Care (2019) describe important aspects of infection prevention and control. A significant part of the guidelines describes a two-tiered approach involving effective work practices that minimise the risk of selection and transmission of infectious agents (NHMRC 2019).

Standard precautions (see Table 9.1) relate to the routine application of basic infection control strategies to minimise risk to patients and healthcare workers, such as hand hygiene, personal protective equipment, cleaning and appropriate handling of equipment and disposal of sharps (NHMRC 2019).

The second-tier infection control strategy involves extra work practices in situations where standard precautions alone are insufficient to prevent transmission. These are known as **transmission-based precautions**. These involve interventions that interrupt the mode of transmission of infections—droplet precautions, airborne precautions depending on the infective agent. Examples of such precautions include isolation of a person, wearing specific personal protective equipment and having specific equipment for that person only (NHMRC 2019).

PERFORMING PHYSICAL EXAMINATION

Context

Often nurses are conducting health assessments in busy ward or clinic situations, which are noisy and lack privacy. However, where possible, the setting for the physical examination should be warm and comfortable, quiet, private and well lit. Try to eliminate any distracting noises—such as humming machinery, radio or television, or people talking—that could make it difficult to hear body sounds. Your time with the individual should be secure from interruptions from other healthcare personnel or visitors. Lighting with natural daylight is best, although it is often not available; try and position an artificial light source to prevent shadows.

Where possible, position the bed or examination table so that both sides of the person are easily accessible. The bed should be at a height at which you can stand without stooping and should be equipped to raise the person's upper body up to 45 degrees.

Equipment

When performing physical examination, you do not want to be searching for equipment or to have to leave the room to find an item. Have all your equipment within easy reach. The equipment used will depend on the purpose of the examination, for example, complete health assessment of all body systems, or

TABLE 9.1 Standard and transmission-based infection control precautions relevant to health assessment

Please note: The information in this table has been adapted from the Australian Guidelines for the Prevention and Control of Infection in Healthcare (NHMRC 2019). Only the information specifically relevant to health assessment has been included. For the complete guidelines document see the bibliography at the end of the chapter. Similar information is available on the Health Quality and Safety Commission New Zealand website: www.hqsc.govt.nz/our-programmes/infection-prevention-and-control/

STANDARD PRECAUTIONS

Standard precautions must be used regardless of known or suspected pathogens being transmitted via the contact, droplet or airborne route.

Hand Hygiene

1. Hand hygiene must be performed before and after every episode of contact. This includes the '5 moments of hand hygiene':
   - before touching a person
   - before a procedure
   - after a procedure or body substance exposure risk
   - after touching a person
   - after touching the person's surroundings.

2. Hand hygiene should also be performed:
   - when arriving at or leaving the clinical environment
   - before and after eating/handling food/drinks
   - before and after using a computer keyboard, tablet or mobile device in a clinical area
   - before putting on gloves and after the removal of gloves
   - after visiting the toilet
   - after blowing/wiping/touching the nose or mouth
   - after handling laundry/equipment/waste.

3. Use alcohol-based hand rubs that contain between 60% and 80% v/v ethanol or equivalent for routine hand hygiene.

4. If hands are visibly soiled, hand hygiene should be performed using soap and water.

5. Hand hygiene for *Clostridium difficile* and non-enveloped viruses such as norovirus should be performed as follows:
   - If gloves have not been worn, if gloves have been breached or if there is visible contamination of the hands despite glove use, use soap and water to facilitate the mechanical removal of spores. After washing, hands should be dried thoroughly with a single-use towel.
   - If gloves have been worn, a lower density of contamination of the hands would be expected and alcohol-based hand rub remains the agent of choice for hand hygiene.

Personal protective equipment

1. Masks/face shields and eye protection should be worn during procedures that generate splashes or sprays of blood and body substances into the face and eyes.

2. Aprons or gowns should:
   - be appropriate to the task being undertaken
   - be worn for a single procedure or episode of care and removed in the area where the episode of care takes place
   - should be removed after use in the area where the episode of care takes place.

3. Single-use, fit for purpose gloves are worn for:
   - each invasive procedure
   - contact with sterile sites and non-intact skin or mucous membranes
   - any activity that has been assessed as carrying a risk of exposure to blood and body substances.

4. Hand hygiene should be performed before putting on gloves and after the removal of gloves.

5. Gloves must be changed between patients and after every episode of individual patient care.

Use and management of sharps, safety engineered devices and medication vials

1. Appropriate use of devices (single-use items such as blood glucose monitoring lancets/needles)
   - Use for one patient only and for one occasion only.
   - Dispose of item immediately into an approved sharps container at the point-of-use.
   - Sharps containers must not be filled above the mark that indicates the maximum fill level.

Routine environmental cleaning

1. Cleaning of shared clinical equipment (e.g. trolleys, stethoscopes, axillary temperature monitoring probes, blood pressure cuffs, etc.)
   - Shared clinical equipment should be cleaned with detergent solution after each use.
   - Disposable equipment, including thermometers and blood pressure cuffs, should be used when caring for people requiring contact precautions (e.g. those with *C. difficile*)

2. Management of blood or other body substance spills
   Strategies for decontaminating spills of blood and other body substances (e.g. vomit, urine) differ based on the setting in which they occur and the volume of the spill (a spill kit should be available in the clinical area); in general:
   - use personal protective equipment
   - healthcare workers can manage small spills by cleaning with detergent solution
   - for spills containing large amounts of blood or other body substances, workers should contain and confine the spill by:
     - removing visible organic matter with absorbent material (e.g. disposable paper towels)
     - removing any broken glass or sharp material with forceps
     - soaking up excess liquid using an absorbent clumping agent (e.g. absorbent granules).
   - Hand hygiene should be performed after the clean up.

Respiratory hygiene and cough etiquette

1. Anyone with signs and symptoms of a respiratory infection, regardless of the cause, should follow or be instructed to follow respiratory hygiene and cough etiquette as follows:
   - cover the nose/mouth with disposable single-use tissues when coughing, sneezing, wiping and blowing noses
   - use tissues to contain respiratory secretions
   - dispose of tissues in the nearest waste receptacle or bin after use
   - if no tissues are available, cough or sneeze into the inner elbow rather than the hand

(Continued)

TABLE 9.1 Standard and transmission-based infection control precautions relevant to health assessment—cont'd

- practice hand hygiene after contact with respiratory secretions and contaminated objects/materials
- keep contaminated hands away from the mucous membranes of the mouth, eyes and nose
- in healthcare facilities, patients with symptoms of respiratory infections should sit as far away from others as possible. If available, healthcare facilities may place these patients in a separate area while waiting for care
- healthcare workers with viral respiratory tract infections should remain at home until their symptoms have resolved.

TRANSMISSION-BASED PRECAUTIONS

Transmission-based precautions are used **in addition** to standard precautions, where the suspected or confirmed presence of infectious agents represents an increased risk of transmission by the contact, droplet or airborne routes.

Contact precautions

Direct transmission—infectious agents are transferred from one person to another person without a contaminated intermediate object or person. For example, blood or other body substances from an infectious person may come into contact with a mucous membrane or breaks in the skin of another person.

Indirect transmission—involves the transfer of an infectious agent through a contaminated intermediate object (fomite) or person. For example, contaminated hands of healthcare workers, contaminated clothing or environmental surfaces.

1. When working with people who require contact precautions:
   - perform hand hygiene
   - put on gloves and gown upon entry to the patient-care area
   - ensure that clothing and skin do not contact potentially contaminated environmental surfaces
   - remove gown and gloves and perform hand hygiene before leaving the patient-care area
   - keep patient notes outside the room
   - keep patient bedside charts outside the room
   - disinfect hands upon leaving the room and after writing in the chart or entering the information in an electronic health record
   - keep doors closed where safe to do so (this may not be possible for patients requiring high visualisation)
   - make sure rooms are clearly signed
   - patient-dedicated equipment or single-use patient-care equipment to be used for patients on contact precautions.

Droplet precautions

In addition to standard precautions, implement droplet precautions for patients known or suspected to be infected with agents transmitted by respiratory droplets that are generated by a person when coughing, sneezing or talking.

1. Hand hygiene as described in the standard precautions section above.
2. Use personal protective equipment (including a surgical mask) when entering a patient-care environment (and hand hygiene before putting on the mask and following removal of the mask).
3. Where possible, patients who require droplet precautions should be placed in a single-occupancy room.

Airborne precautions

In addition to standard precautions, implement airborne precautions for patients known or suspected to be infected with infectious agents transmitted person-to-person by the airborne route (e.g. measles, chickenpox (varicella) and *Mycobacterium tuberculosis*).

1. Standard precautions, including respiratory hygiene and cough etiquette.
2. Wear a correctly fitted P2 respirator when entering the patient-care area when an airborne-transmissible infectious agent is known or suspected to be present.
3. Minimise exposure of other patients and staff members to the infectious agent.

Multi-resistant organisms and outbreak situations

Multi-resistant organisms include methicillin-resistant *Staphylococcus aureus* (MRSA), vancomycin-resistant *Enterococcus* (VRE), and multi-resistant Gram-negative bacteria (MRGN).

1. Applying standard precautions, including hand hygiene, is the most effective measure to prevent and control the spread of multi-resistant organisms.
2. Applying transmission-based and contact-based precautions should be considered for all patients colonised or infected with a multi-resistant organism, including:
   - performing hand hygiene and putting on gloves and gowns before entering the patient-care area
   - using patient-dedicated or single-use noncritical patient-care equipment
   - using a single-patient room or, if unavailable, cohorting patients with the same strain of MRO in designated patient-care areas (upon approval from the healthcare facility's Infection Control Team)
   - ensuring consistent cleaning and disinfection of surfaces in close proximity to the patient and those likely to be touched by the patient and healthcare workers.

the focus of a specific area for assessment (focused neurological assessment). Each chapter outlines the specific equipment required. The equipment is described as it comes into use throughout the text.

In a situation where you will be using several pieces of equipment during the physical examination, designate a 'clean' versus a 'used' area for handling of your equipment. In a ward or clinic setting, use a dressing trolley; the top surface for the clean equipment and the bottom shelf for the used equipment surface. A waste bag or container can be attached for disposal of single use equipment such as tongue blades and gloves.

Establishing rapport and gaining consent

You need to make every contact with the person effective, as it can set the tone for the relationship you have with the person in the future and the person's experience of healthcare. Effective communication between healthcare workers and the recipient of care is fundamental to person-centred care and patient safety. Good communication fosters relationships, encourages a two-way exchange of information, engages the person in decision-making and care planning and helps to manage uncertainty and complexity (ACSQHC 2016). An important start to effective communication is introducing yourself to the person with your name and your position (clinical nurse, nursing student, etc.). See also Chapter 7.

You also need to make sure that the person understands the purpose of the physical examination and the types and extent of examination that will be performed. Be detailed about what you are going to be doing and that you will stop if they ask you to. Make sure that you express yourself in a way that the person understands. The person cannot give you informed consent unless they understand the purpose and extent of the examination. In some circumstances, the person may prefer to have another person (another health professional, a friend or family member) present during the examination. Note this in the person's medical record. In all other cases, additional family or friends should be asked to wait outside until the examination is completed.

General approach

Consider your emotional state and that of the person being examined. The person is usually anxious because of the anticipation of being examined by a stranger and the unknown outcome of the examination. If anxiety can be reduced, the person will feel more comfortable and the data gathered will more closely describe the person's natural state. Anxiety can be reduced by an examiner who is confident and self-assured, as well as considerate and unhurried.

You have to feel comfortable with your psychomotor skills before you can absorb what you are actually seeing or hearing in a 'real' person. This comes with practice under the guidance of an experienced mentor in a simulated situation, in an atmosphere in which it is acceptable to make mistakes and to ask questions. The person should 'act like a patient' so that you can deal with the 'real' situation while still in a safe setting. After you feel comfortable with the skills simulation/laboratory setting, you will be ready to undertake a health assessment on a person who is seeking healthcare.

TECHNIQUES OF PHYSICAL EXAMINATION

The techniques required for physical examination are **inspection** (looking), **palpation** (feeling), **percussion** (tapping) and **auscultation** (listening). They are performed systematically, one at a time, and usually in this order with the exception of abdominal assessment—see Chapter 23. Table 9.2 summarises the four physical examination techniques.

TABLE 9.2 Summary of commonly used physical assessment techniques

TECHNIQUE	APPROACH	ASSESSMENT FOCUS	NOTES
Inspection: Detailed and purposive observation	• General survey • Detailed inspection of each body part/area—see each chapter for full description	• Physical appearance (age, sex, level of consciousness, skin colour, face, overall appearance) • Body structure (stature, nutrition, symmetry, posture) • Mobility (gait, range of motion) • Behaviour (facial expression, mood and affect, speech, speech pattern, personal hygiene)	Compare each side of the body, determine symmetry
Palpation: Use of touch Compare both sides of the body Use of slow and systematic movements	• Surface palpation (for example, a joint)	• Texture • Temperature • Moisture Presence of: • tenderness or pain • crepitation of joints • swelling	The dorsa (backs) of hands and fingers Fingertips
	• Light palpation (only used in abdominal examination)	Presence of: • tenderness or pain • lumps or masses (e.g. faecal loading, distended urinary bladder) • swelling • vibration or pulsation	Base of fingers (metacarpophalangeal joints) Ulnar surface of the hand—best for vibration.
Percussion: Tapping the person's skin and underlying structures with short, sharp strokes	• Indirect (most commonly used in abdominal examination)	• Signalling the density (air, fluid or solid) of a structure by a characteristic note • Detecting a mass or structure if it is fairly superficial (e.g. a distended bladder above the symphysis pubis)	The striking hand contacts the stationary hand fixed on the person's skin Sound described as: resonant, hyper-resonant, tympany, dull or flat (see Table 9.3)
Auscultation: Listening to sounds produced by the body usually with a stethoscope	• systematic sequence • compare both sides of the body	• bowel sounds • breath sounds • heart sounds	Use diaphragm of the stethoscope Avoid listening over clothing

Inspection

Inspection is concentrated observation. It is close, careful scrutiny, first of the person as a whole (**general inspection**) and then of each body system/area (**detailed inspection**). Inspection begins the moment you first meet the person and develop a 'general survey' (specific data to consider for the general survey are presented in the following chapter). Inspection is always the first assessment technique you will use during physical examination. You can begin your general survey of the person while you are talking with them about their health history. Then, as you move through each relevant body system/area you will also begin with a detailed inspection (an outline of the areas for inspection will be presented in each chapter). A detailed inspection takes time and yields a surprising amount of data.

Learn to use each person as their own control and compare the right and left sides of the body. The two sides are nearly symmetrical. Inspection requires good lighting and adequate exposure of the body part being assessed. In some circumstances, you need to use equipment (e.g. an otoscope, penlight torch) to enhance your own sense of vision.

Palpation

Palpation involves the use of touch during physical examination and usually follows detailed inspection of the particular body part or area. Palpation is used to assess: texture, temperature, moisture, organ location and size, as well as any swelling, vibration or pulsation, rigidity, crepitation of joints, presence of lumps or masses and presence of tenderness or pain. Different parts of the hands are best suited for assessing different factors. See Table 9.2.

Practice note: You should always attend to hand hygiene before touching the person and at the end of the physical examination (NHMRC 2019). It is not necessary to use gloves every time you perform a palpation technique. Throughout the subsequent chapters you will be prompted about when it is necessary to use gloves. You should be guided by standard infection control precautions (see Table 9.1) and hospital or healthcare agency policy.

Your palpation technique should be slow and systematic. A person stiffens when touched suddenly, making it difficult for you to feel very much. Use a calm, gentle approach and inform the person about what you are going to do to them. Warm your hands by rubbing them together or holding them under warm water. Identify any tender areas and palpate them last.

There are three palpation techniques: surface palpation, light palpation and bimanual palpation.

- **Surface palpation** involves the use of the gentle pressure from the finger pads of your dominant hand. You need to place the flattened finger pads onto the skin surface (keeping the fingers together) and apply gentle pressure to the body surface (approximately 1–2 cm deep, depending on the part of the body being assessed) while moving the fingers in a gentle, slow, circular motion. Move the hand and cover the entire surface to be examined, noting the findings as you progress. Always start with surface palpation to detect surface characteristics. For example, you would use surface palpation to assess swelling, crepitation, range of movement and pain in an injured joint.
- **Light palpation** follows surface palpation and is usually only performed as part of abdominal assessment. The technique for light palpation is similar to surface palpation; however, the skin surface is more deeply depressed with the fingers. The actual depth of light palpation is largely dependent on the amount of abdominal fat the person has. For a person with a normal body mass index, you may only need to palpate to a depth of 2.5 cm to evaluate abdominal contents, whereas for a person who is obese you may have to palpate to a depth of 5 cm to be able to evaluate abdominal contents. When light palpation is needed (as for abdominal examination), intermittent pressure is better than one long continuous palpation. You should not progress from surface to light palpation when the person complains of pain or when traumatic abdominal injury is suspected, as you could cause further pain or even injury to the person. You should always refer the person to a medical practitioner when you detect significant abdominal pain or discomfort on light palpation.
- **Bimanual palpation** requires the use of both of your hands to envelop or capture certain body parts or organs—such as the spleen, liver, kidneys, uterus, ovaries—for more precise examination of the size, shape. This technique is usually only performed by nurses working in advanced practice roles.

Percussion

Percussion involves tapping the person's skin with short, sharp strokes to assess underlying structures. The strokes yield a palpable vibration and a characteristic sound that depicts the location, size and density of the underlying structure or organ.

Percussion has the following uses:

- Mapping out the **location** and **size** of an organ or structure by exploring where the percussion note changes between the borders of an organ and the adjacent structures
- Signalling the **density** (air, fluid or solid) of a structure by a characteristic note
- Detecting an abnormal mass if it is fairly superficial, a distended urinary bladder or faecal loading; the percussion vibrations penetrate about 5 cm deep—a deeper mass would give no change in percussion
- Eliciting pain if the underlying structure is inflamed, as with maxillary sinus areas or over a kidney
- Eliciting a deep tendon reflex using the percussion hammer.

Two methods of percussion can be used—**direct** and **indirect**. The technique of direct percussion involves the striking hand directly contacting the body wall producing a sound. However, indirect percussion is the technique most commonly used in a nursing health assessment and involves the use of both hands, most commonly in abdominal assessment. The striking hand contacts the stationary hand fixed on the person's skin. This yields a sound and a subtle vibration. The procedure of indirect percussion is as follows.

The stationary hand

Hyperextend the middle finger (sometimes called the pleximeter) and/or index finger of your non-dominant hand and place the distal portion, the phalanx and distal interphalangeal joint, *firmly* against the person's skin, for example over the abdominal skin. Avoid the person's ribs and scapulae. Percussing over a bone yields no data because it always sounds 'dull'. Lift the rest of the stationary hand (finger tips, other fingers, thumb

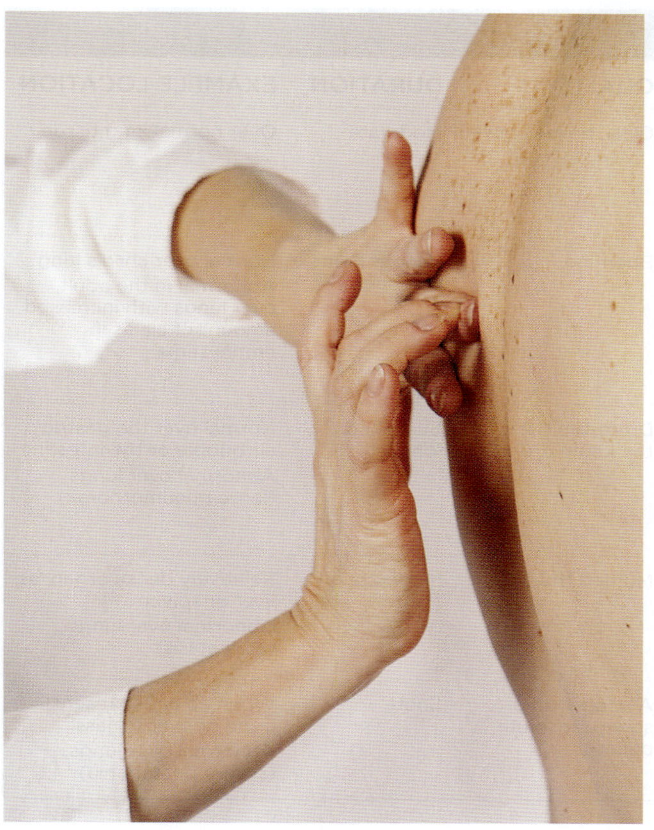

Figure 9.2

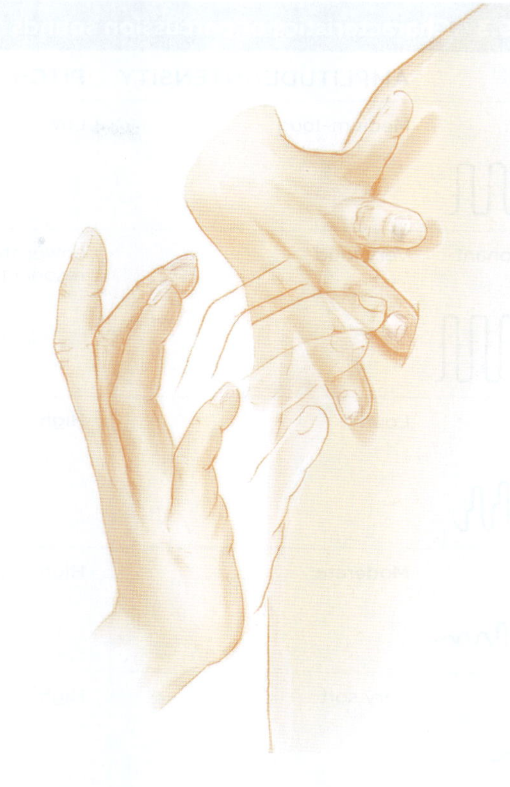

Figure 9.3

and heel of the hand) up off the person's skin (Figure 9.2). Otherwise the resting hand will dampen off the produced vibrations, just as a drummer uses the hand to halt a drum roll.

The striking hand

Use the middle finger of your dominant hand as the *striking finger* (sometimes called the plexor) (Figure 9.3). Hold your forearm close to the skin surface, with your upper arm and shoulder steady. Scan your muscles to make sure they are steady but not rigid. The action is all in the wrist, and it *must* be relaxed. Spread your fingers, move from the wrist in a hammer-like motion and bounce your middle finger off the stationary one. Aim for just behind the nail bed or at the distal interphalangeal joint; the goal is to hit the portion of the finger that is pushing the hardest into the skin surface. Flex the striking finger so that its tip, not the finger pad, makes contact. It hits directly at right angles to the stationary finger.

Percuss two times in this location using even, staccato blows. Lift the striking finger off quickly; a resting finger damps off vibrations. Then move to a new body location and repeat, keeping your technique even. The force of the blow determines the loudness of the note. You do not need a very loud sound; use just enough force to achieve a clear note. The thickness of the person's body wall will be a factor. You will need a stronger percussion stroke for people with obese or very muscular body walls.

Percussion can be an awkward technique for beginning examiners. You may feel surprised and embarrassed if your striking finger misses your stationary hand completely. It will hurt if your nails are too long. As with all new skills, refinement follows practice. After a few weeks your hand placement becomes precise and feels natural, and your ears learn to perceive the subtle difference in percussion notes.

Production of sound

All sound results from vibration of some structure (Figure 9.4). Percussing over a body structure causes vibrations that produce characteristic waves and are heard as 'notes' (see Table 9.3). Each of the five percussion notes is differentiated by the following components:

1. **Amplitude** (or intensity), a loud or soft sound. The louder the sound, the greater the amplitude. Loudness depends on the force of the blow and the structure's ability to vibrate.
2. **Pitch** (or frequency), the number of vibrations per second, written as 'cps', or cycles per second. More rapid vibrations

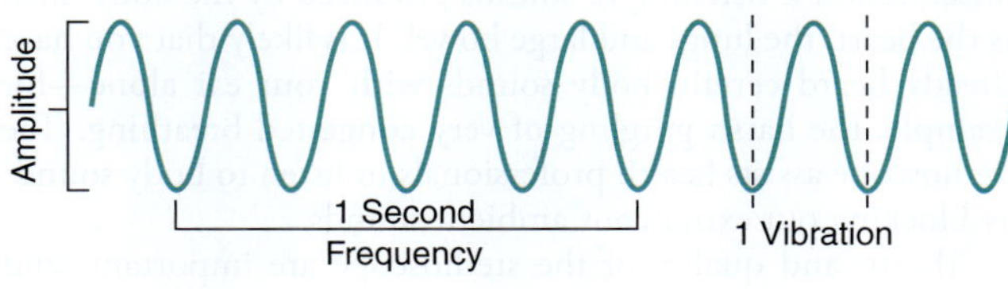

Figure 9.4
Sound wave.

TABLE 9.3 Characteristics of percussion sounds

SOUND	AMPLITUDE/INTENSITY	PITCH	QUALITY	DURATION	EXAMPLE LOCATION
Resonant	Medium–loud	Low	Clear, hollow	Moderate	Over normal lung tissue
Hyperresonant	Very loud	Lower than resonant	Booming	Longer than resonant	Normal over child's lung Abnormal in the adult, over lungs with increased amount of air, as in emphysema
Tympany	Loud	High	Drum-like (like the kettle drum)	Sustained longest	Normal over the gastric air bubble or the intestine Abnormal over lungs (large pneumothorax)
Dull	Moderate	High	Muffled thud	Moderate	Relatively dense organ, as liver or spleen Abnormal over lungs (atelectasis)
Flat	Very soft	High	A dead stop of sound, absolute dullness	Short	When no air is present, bone or over a mass Abnormal over lungs (severe pneumonia)

produce a high-pitched tone; slower vibrations yield a low-pitched tone.

3. **Quality** (timbre), a subjective difference due to a sound's distinctive overtones. A pure tone is a sound of one frequency. Variations within a sound wave produce overtones. Overtones allow you to distinguish a C on a piano from a C on a violin.
4. **Duration**, the length of time the note lingers.

A basic principle is that a structure with relatively more air (such as the lungs) produces a louder, deeper and longer sound because it vibrates freely, whereas a denser, more solid structure (such as the liver) gives a softer, higher, shorter sound because it does not vibrate as easily. Although Table 9.3 describes five 'normal' percussion notes, variations occur in clinical practice. The quality of the percussion note will be affected by the thickness of the body wall. The skill of recognising the various percussion sounds takes repeated practice.

Auscultation

Auscultation is listening to sounds produced by the body, such as the heart, the lungs and large bowel. It is likely that you have already heard certain body sounds with your ear alone—for example, the harsh gurgling of very congested breathing. The stethoscope assists health professionals to listen to body sounds by blocking out extraneous ambient sounds.

The fit and quality of the stethoscope are important, and you are advised to purchase a quality instrument for your own personal use. The slope of the earpiece should point forward towards your nose. This matches the natural slope of your ear canal and efficiently blocks out environmental sound. If necessary, twist the earpieces to parallel the slope of your ear canals. The earpieces should fit snugly, but if they hurt, they are inserted too far. Adjust the tension and experiment with different rubber or plastic earplugs to achieve the most comfort. The tubing should be of thick material, with an internal diameter of 4 mm, and about 36 to 46 cm long. Longer tubing may distort the sound.

Choose a stethoscope with two endpieces—a diaphragm and a bell (Figure 9.5). You will use the **diaphragm** most often because its flat edge is best for high-pitched sounds—breath, bowel and normal heart sounds. Hold the diaphragm firmly against the person's skin—firm enough to leave a slight ring afterwards. The **bell** endpiece has a deep, hollow cup-like shape. It is best for soft, low-pitched sounds such as extra heart sounds or murmurs. Hold it lightly against the person's skin—just enough that it forms a perfect seal. Any harder causes the person's skin to act as a diaphragm, obliterating the low-pitched sounds.

Some stethoscopes have one endpiece with a 'tunable diaphragm'. This enables you to listen to both low and high frequency sounds without rotation of the endpiece. For low frequency sounds (traditional bell mode) hold the endpiece very lightly on the skin; for high frequency sounds (traditional diaphragm mode) press the diaphragm or bell firmly on the skin.

Before you can evaluate body sounds, you should attempt to eliminate or reduce ambient noise from the environment:

- Any extra room noise can produce a 'roaring' in your stethoscope, so the room should be as quiet as possible.

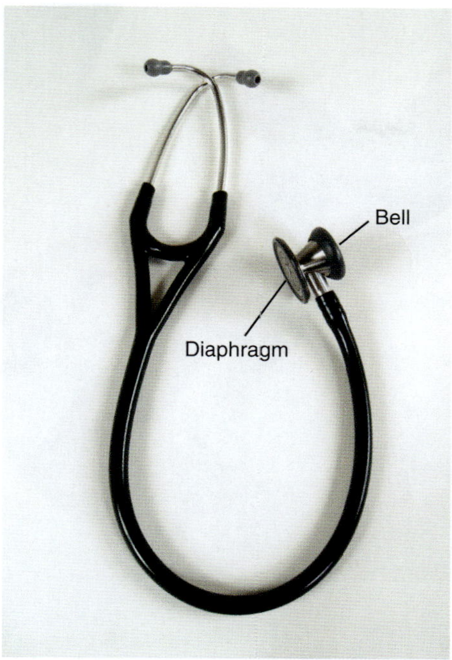

Figure 9.5
Stethoscope diaphragm (front) and bell (back).

- When the diaphragm is placed on, for example, a man's hairy chest, you may hear a crackling sound that mimics an abnormal breath sound called *crackles*. Try to avoid the hairy areas as much as possible to reduce the artifact sounds.
- Never listen through clothing. Where possible ask the person to remove clothing. In situations where this is not possible you will need to place the stethoscope under the clothing to listen but take care that no clothing rubs on the stethoscope.
- Finally, avoid creating your own artifact sounds, such as breathing on the tubing or the 'thump' from bumping the tubing together.

Practice note:

- The diaphragm and bell of the stethoscope must be cleaned before and after use with a disposable disinfectant wipe (NHMRC 2019).
- Warm the stethoscope by rubbing it in your palm before placing it on the person's skin.

Auscultation is a skill that is difficult to master. First you must learn to recognise the wide range of normal sounds. Once you can recognise normal sounds, you can distinguish the abnormal sounds and 'extra' sounds. Be aware that in some body locations you may hear more than one sound; this can be confusing. You will need to listen selectively to only one thing at a time. As you listen, ask yourself: 'What am I *actually hearing*? ... What *should* I be hearing at this spot?'

Beginning objective data collection

The extent and focus of the physical examination is dependent on the purpose and context of the assessment. In most situations, the extent and focus of the physical examination is directed by the person's presenting signs and symptoms. Regardless of the purpose of the assessment, begin by measuring the person's temperature, heart rate, respirations, oxygen saturation and blood pressure (Chapter 10) and pain (Chapter 13). All of these are familiar, relatively nonthreatening actions; they will gradually accustom the person to the examination process. Make sure you perform hand hygiene in the person's presence, before you start the examination. Explain each step in the examination and how the person can cooperate. Encourage the person to ask questions. Keep your own movements slow, methodical and deliberate.

As you proceed through the examination, avoid distractions and concentrate on one step at a time. The sequence of the steps may differ depending on the extent of the assessment, the age of the person and your own preference. Organise the steps so the person does not change positions too often and watch out for the person tiring. Providing rest breaks might be necessary for very sick or frail older people. Although proper exposure is necessary, use additional drapes to maintain the person's privacy and to prevent chilling.

Do not hesitate to write out the examination sequence and refer to it as you proceed. The person will accept this as quite natural if you explain you are making brief notations to ensure accuracy. Many healthcare organisations use a printed form. You will find that you will glance at the form less and less as you gain experience. Even with a form, you sometimes may forget a step in the examination. When you realise this, perform the manoeuvre in the next logical place in the sequence.

As you proceed through the examination, occasionally offer some brief teaching about the person's body. For example, you might say, 'Everyone has two sounds for each heartbeat, something like this—lub-dub. Your own heart beats sound normal'. Do not do this with every single step, or you will be hard pressed to make a comment when you do come across an abnormality. But some sharing of information builds rapport and increases the person's confidence in you as an examiner. It also gives the person a little more control in a situation in which it is easy to feel completely helpless.

At some point, you will want to linger in one location to concentrate on some complicated findings. To avoid anxiety, tell the person, for example, 'I always listen to bowel sounds on a number of places on the abdomen. Just because I am listening a long time does not necessarily mean anything is wrong with you'. And it follows that sometimes you *will* discover a finding that may be abnormal and you want another examiner to double-check. You need to give the person some information, yet you should not alarm the person unnecessarily. Say something like, 'I do not have a complete assessment of your abdomen. I want Ms Wright to listen, too'.

At the end of the examination, summarise your findings and share the necessary information with the person. Thank the person for the time spent. In a hospital setting, advise the person of what is scheduled next. Before you leave a hospitalised person, lower the bed; make the person comfortable and safe; put the call bell within reach; and return the bedside table, television or any equipment to the way it was originally. Perform hand hygiene before leaving the person's bed area.

DEVELOPMENTAL CONSIDERATIONS

Children are different from adults. Their difference in size is obvious. Their bodies grow in a predictable pattern that is assessed during the physical examination. However, their behaviour is also different. Behaviour grows and develops through predictable stages, just as the body does. Each examiner needs to know the expected emotional and cognitive features of these stages and to perform the physical examination based on developmental principles (Duderstadt 2019).

With all children, the goal is to increase their comfort in the setting. This approach reveals their natural state as much as possible and will give them a more positive memory of healthcare providers. Remember that a 'routine' examination is anything but routine to the child. You can increase their comfort by attending to the following developmental principles and approaches. The *order* of the developmental stages is more meaningful than the exact chronological age. Each child is an individual and will not fit exactly into one category. For example, if your efforts to 'play games' with the preschooler are rebuffed, modify your approach to the security measures used with the toddler.

Parents are an important part of the assessment process. Listening carefully to parents' concerns can alert you to possible health issues. Establishing rapport with parents is also important as they can assist in the examination process (for example comforting and holding the child) and in gaining the trust of the child. You are also observing the interaction between the child and the parent, including eye contact, verbal communication, family dynamics, family connectedness and approach to problem solving (Duderstadt 2019).

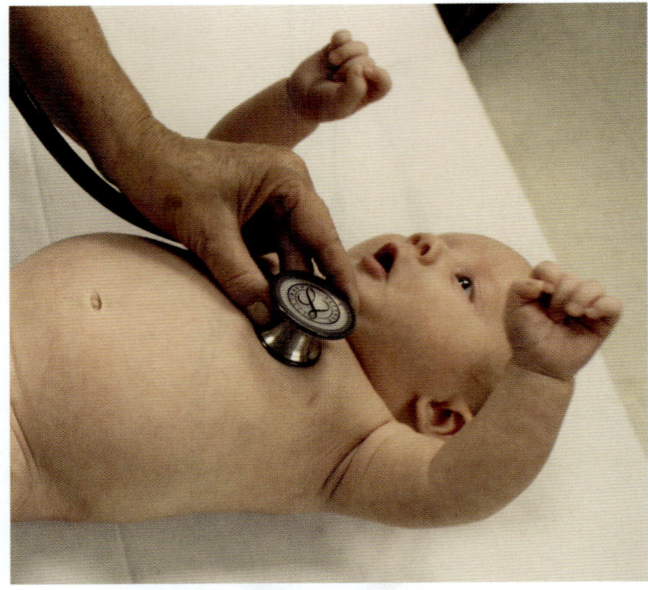

Figure 9.6
Baby and stethoscope.

The infant (birth to 1 year)

Erikson (1998) defines the major task of infancy as establishing trust. An infant is completely dependent on the parent for their basic needs. If these needs are met promptly and consistently, the infant feels secure and learns to trust others.

Position

- The parent/guardian should always be present for the child's feeling of security.
- Place the neonate or young infant flat on a padded examination table (Figure 9.6). The infant may also be held against the parent's chest if necessary.
- Once the baby can sit without support (around 6 months), as much of the examination as possible should be performed while the infant is in the parent's lap.
- By 9 to 12 months, the infant is acutely aware of the surroundings. Anything outside the infant's range of vision is 'lost', so the parent must be in full view.

Preparation

- Timing should be 1–2 hour after feeding, when the baby is not too drowsy or too hungry.
- Maintain a warm environment. A neonate may require an overhead radiant heater.
- Have the parent remove outer clothing when necessary.
- Perform hand hygiene before touching the infant.
- An infant does not mind being touched, but make sure your hands and stethoscope endpiece are warm.
- Use a soft, crooning voice during the examination; the baby responds more to the feeling in the tone of the voice than to what is actually said.
- An infant likes eye contact; lock eyes from time to time.
- Smile; a baby prefers a smiling face to a frowning one. Take time to play.
- Keep movements smooth and deliberate, not jerky.
- Offer brightly coloured toys for a distraction.

Sequence (depends on the purpose of the examination)

- Seize the opportunity with a sleeping baby to listen to heart, lung and abdomen sounds first.
- Perform least distressing steps first. Save the invasive steps of examination of the eyes, ears, nose and throat until last.
- Elicit the Moro or 'startle' reflex at the *end* of the examination because it may cause the baby to cry.

Early childhood: The toddler (1–3 years)

This is Erikson's stage of developing autonomy. However, the need to explore the world and be independent is in conflict with the basic dependency on the parent. This often results in frustration and negativism. The toddler may be difficult to examine; do not take this personally. Since they are acutely aware of the new environment, the toddler may be frightened and cling to the parent. Also, the toddler is likely to be afraid of invasive procedures and dislikes being restrained (Figure 9.7).

Position

- The toddler should be sitting up on the parent's lap for all of the examination. When the toddler must be supine (as in the abdominal examination), move chairs to sit knee-to-knee with the parent. Have the toddler lie in the parent's lap with the toddler's legs in your lap.

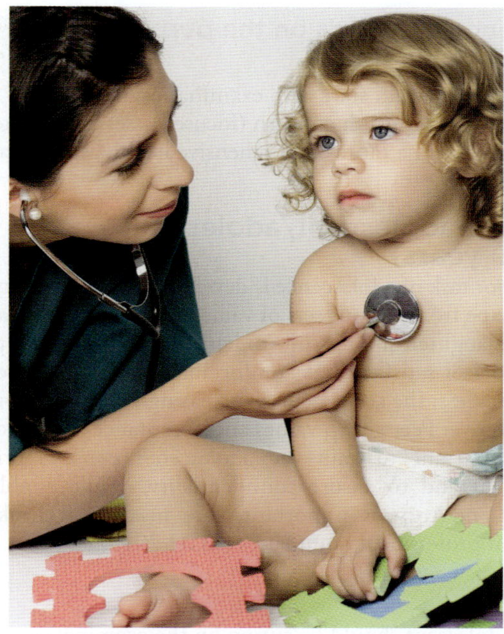

Figure 9.7

- Enlist the aid of a cooperative parent to help position the toddler during invasive procedures. The child's legs can be captured between the parent's. An arm of the parent can encircle the child's head, holding it against the chest, and the other arm can hold the child's arms.

Preparation

- Children 1 or 2 years of age can understand symbols, so a security object, such as a special blanket or teddy bear, is helpful.
- Begin by greeting the child and the accompanying parent by name, but with a child 1 to 6 years old, focus more on the parent. By essentially 'ignoring' the child at first, you allow the child to adjust gradually and to size you up from a safe distance. Then turn your attention gradually to the child, at first to a toy or object the child is holding, or perhaps to compliment clothing or the hair. If the child is ready, you will note these signals: eye contact with you, smiling, talking with you or accepting a toy or a piece of equipment.
- A 2-year-old child does not like to take off their clothes; have the parent undress the child one part at a time.
- Children 1 or 2 years of age like to say 'No'. Do not offer a choice when there really is none. Avoid saying, 'May I listen to your heart now?' When the 1- or 2-year-old child says 'No', and you go ahead and do it anyway, you lose trust. Instead, use clear firm instructions, in a tone that expects cooperation, 'Now it is time for you to lie down so I can check your tummy'.
- Also, 1- or 2-year-old children like to make choices. When possible, enhance autonomy by offering the *limited option*: 'Shall I listen to your heart next, or your tummy?'
- Demonstrate the procedures on the parent, a teddy or doll if needed.
- Praise the child when they are cooperative.

Up until approximately 18 months, the toddler explores the world through the mouth so caution needs to be taken when familiarising with the equipment by letting them touch the stethoscope or tongue blade.

Sequence (depends on the purpose of the examination)

- Collect some objective data during the history, which is a less stressful time for the child. While you are focusing on the parent, note the child's gross motor and fine motor skills and gait.
- Start with nonthreatening areas. Save potentially distressing procedures—such as examination of the head, ears, nose or throat—for last.

Early childhood: the preschool child (3–5 or 6 years)

The child at this stage displays developing initiative. The preschooler takes on tasks independently and plans the task and sees it through. A child of this age is often cooperative, helpful and easy to involve. The concept of body image is limited.

Position

- With a 3-year-old child, the parent should be present and may hold the child on their lap.
- A 4- or 5-year-old child usually feels comfortable on the examination table or bed, with the parent present.

Preparation

- A preschooler can talk. Verbal communication becomes helpful now but remember that the child's understanding is still limited. Use short, simple explanations.
- Talk to the child and explain the steps in the examination exactly.
- Do not give the child a choice when there is none. However, as with the toddler, enhance the autonomy of the preschooler by offering choice when possible.
- Allow the child to play with equipment to reduce fears.
- A preschooler likes to help; have the child hold the stethoscope for you.
- Use games. Have the child 'blow out' the light on the penlight as you listen to the breath sounds. Or, pretend to listen to the heart sounds of the child's teddy bear first. One technique that is absorbing to a preschooler is to trace their shape on the examination table paper (Hockenberry & Wilson 2018). You can comment on how big the child is, then fill in the outline with a heart or stomach and listen to this paper doll first. After the examination, the child can take the paper doll home as a souvenir.
- Use a slow, deliberate approach. Do not rush.
- During the examination, give the preschooler needed feedback and reassurance: 'Your tummy feels just fine'.
- Compliment the child on their cooperation.

Sequence (depends on the purpose of the examination)

- Examine the thorax, abdomen and extremities first. Although the preschooler is usually cooperative, continue to assess head, eyes, ears, nose and throat last.

The school-age child (6–12 years)

During the school-age period, the major task of the child is developing industry. The child is developing basic competency in school and in social networks and desires the approval of parents, teachers and friends. When successful, the child has a feeling of accomplishment. During the examination, the child is cooperative and is interested in learning about the body. Language is more sophisticated now, but do not overestimate and treat the school-age child as a small adult. The child's level of understanding does not match that of their speech.

Position

- The school-age child should be sitting on the examination table or bed.

Preparation

- A child in this age group is likely to be shy and modest so you need to be sensitive to their need for privacy and independence. Break the ice with small talk about family, school, friends, music or sports.
- The child should undress themself, leave underpants on and use a gown and drape.
- Demonstrate equipment—a school-age child is curious to know how equipment works.
- Comment on the body and how it works (Figure 9.8). An 8- or 9-year-old child has some understanding of the body and is interested to learn more. It is rewarding to see the child's eyes light up when they hear the heart sounds.

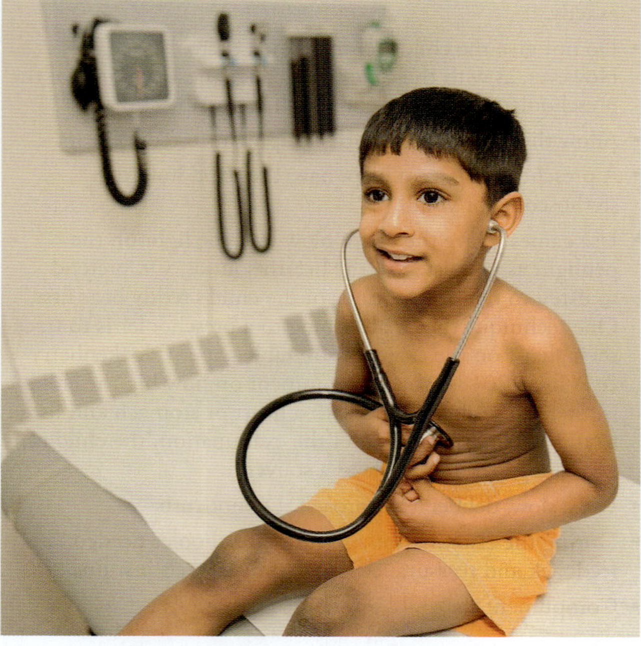

Figure 9.8
Young boy with stethoscope.

Sequence (depends on the purpose of the examination)

- As with the adult, start with examination relevant to the presenting health concern (focused assessment) and continue with a more comprehensive health assessment as needed.

The pre-adolescent/adolescent (10–19 years)

The major task of adolescence is developing a self-identity. This takes shape from various sets of values and different social roles (son or daughter, sibling and student). In the end, each person needs to feel satisfied and comfortable with whom they are. In the process, the adolescent is increasingly self-conscious and introspective. Peer group values and acceptance are important. It is important to gain the adolescent's consent prior to assessment and to ensure confidentiality. While establishing rapport and trust is important, care needs to be taken to maintain professional boundaries (RCH 2019).

Position

- The adolescent should be sitting on the examination table or bed.
- Examine the adolescent alone, without parent or sibling present.

Preparation

- The body is changing rapidly. During the examination, the adolescent needs feedback that their own body is healthy and developing normally.
- The adolescent has keen awareness of body image, often comparing themself to peers. Advise the adolescent of the wide variation among teenagers on the rate of growth and development.
- Communicate with some care. Do not treat the teenager like a child, but do not overestimate and treat them like an adult either.
- The adolescent is usually interested in finding out more about their health. Positive attitudes developed now may last through adult life. Focus your teaching on ways the adolescent can promote wellness.

Sequence (depends on the purpose of the examination)

- As with the adult, start with examination relevant to the presenting health concern (focused assessment) and continue with a more comprehensive health assessment as needed.

The adult

Developmentally, the adult stage spans from young adulthood (20–40 years of age) to older adulthood (85+ years). You will need to adjust your approach depending on the age and state of health of the person you are examining.

Position

- The adult should be sitting on the examination table or bed (Figure 9.9); a frail older adult may need to be supine.

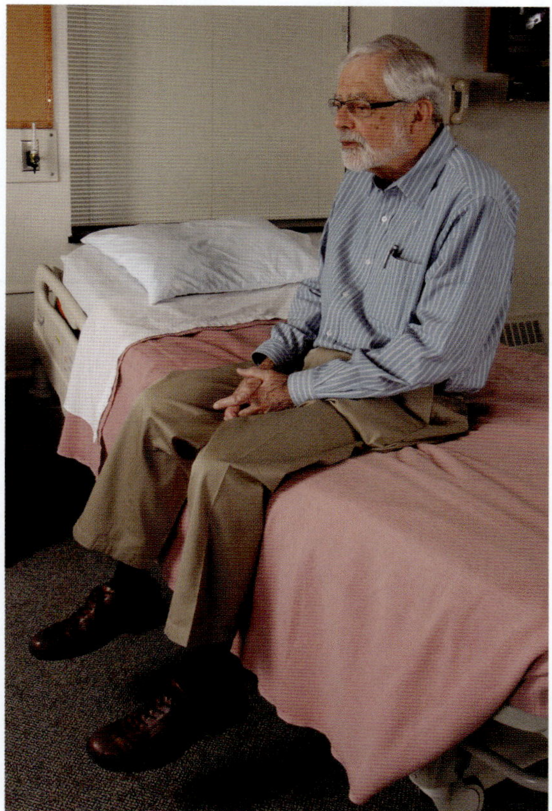

Figure 9.9

- Arrange the sequence to allow as few position changes as possible.

Preparation

- Adjust the pace of the examination to meet the possible slowed pace of the frail older person.
- Allow rest periods when needed if the person is unwell.

Sequence (depends on the purpose of the examination)

- Start with examination relevant to the presenting health concern (focused assessment) and continue with a more comprehensive health assessment as needed. Modify as necessary, particularly if the person is unwell or frail.

BIBLIOGRAPHY

Australian Commission on Safety and Quality in Health Care (ACSQHC). Patient-clinician communication in hospitals – Communicating for safety at transitions of care. 2016. Available at: www.safetyandquality.gov.au/wp-content/uploads/2016/11/Information-sheet-for-healthcare-providers-Improving-patient-clinician-communication.pdf.

Australian Guidelines for the Prevention and Control of Infection in Healthcare. Canberra: National Health and Medical Research Council; 2019. Available at: https://www.safetyandquality.gov.au/our-work/infection-prevention-and-control/guidelines/australian-guidelines-prevention-and-control-infection-healthcare-2019.

Berk LE. Development through the lifespan. 7th ed. Boston: Pearson; 2018.

Duderstadt KG. Pediatric physical examination: an illustrated handbook. 3rd ed. St Louis: Elsevier; 2019.

Erikson E. The life cycle completed (extended version). New York: WW Norton & Company; 1998.

Health, Quality & Safety Commission New Zealand. Hand Hygiene New Zealand. 2019. Available at: www.hqsc.govt.nz/our-programmes/infection-prevention-and-control/projects/hand-hygiene/.

Hockenberry M, Wilson D. Wong's nursing care of infants and children. 11th ed. St Louis: Elsevier/Mosby; 2018.

National Health and Medical Research Council. Australian guidelines for the prevention and control of infection in healthcare. Canberra: 2019. Available at: https://www.nhmrc.gov.au/file/14289/download?token=QNDTcrjY.

Royal Children's Hospital (RCH). Engaging with and assessing the adolescent patient. Clinical Practice Guidelines, Melbourne: Royal Children's Hospital; 2019.

Ryan K, Havers S, Olsen O, et al, editors. 5 moments for hand hygiene: hand hygiene manual. Hand Hygiene Australia; 2018. Available at: www.hha.org.au/component/jdownloads/send/5-implementation/191-hha-manual.

Talley NJ, O'Connor S. Clinical examination: a systematic guide to physical diagnosis. 8th ed. Chatswood, NSW: Elsevier Australia; 2018.

Touhy TA, Jett KF. Ebersole and Hess's gerontological nursing & healthy aging. 5th ed. St Louis: Elsevier/Mosby; 2018.

Website

Hand Hygiene Australia: https://www.hha.org.au

Chapter Ten

General survey and vital signs

Written by Carolyn Jarvis and Ann Eckhardt
Adapted by Helen Forbes

OBJECTIVE DATA

The general survey
Measurement
Vital signs
Additional techniques

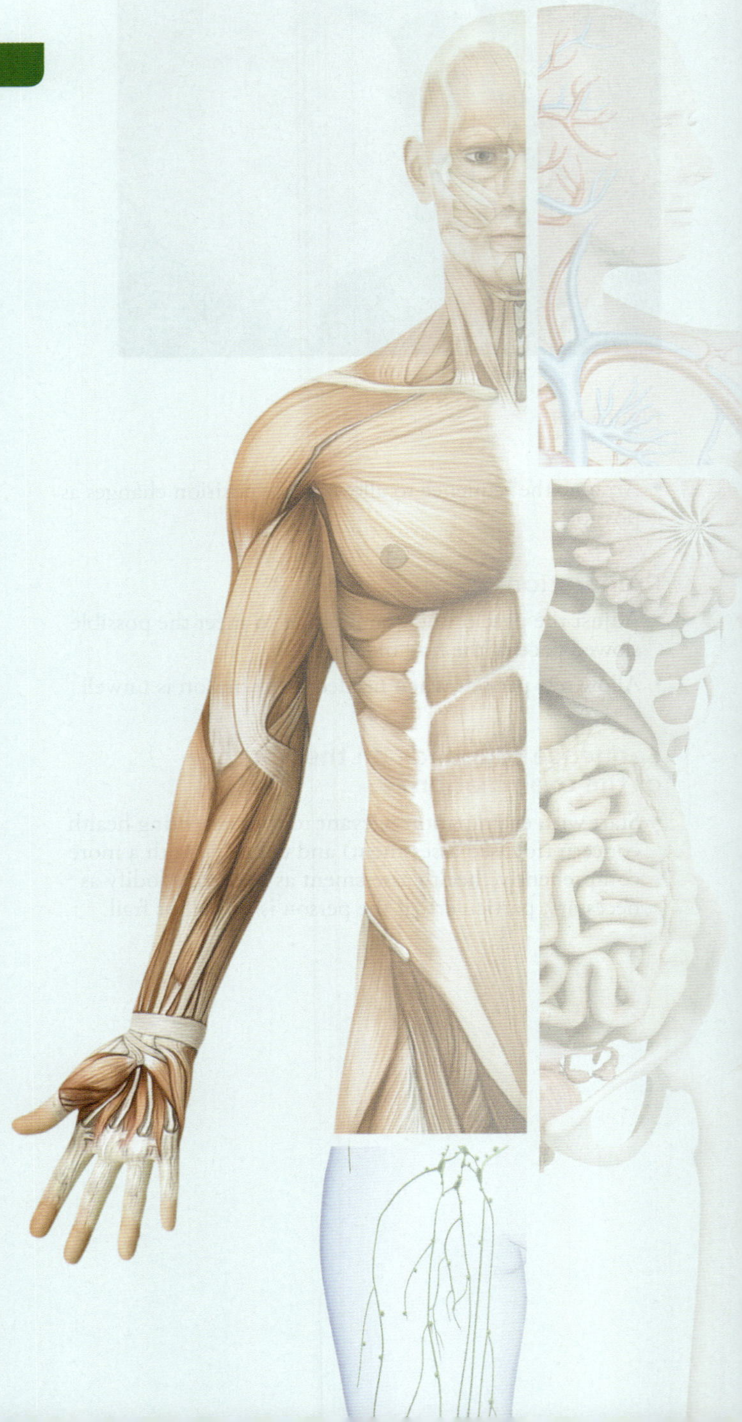

INTRODUCTION

The general survey is a way of ascertaining your impression of the person, includes the general health state and any obvious physical characteristics and usually forms the first part of objective data collection. A general survey begins from the moment you first meet the person (Figure 10.1). What leaves an immediate impression? Does the person look sick, moving slowly or with effort, with shoulders slumped and eyes without lustre or downcast? Is the hospitalised patient conversing with visitors, involved in reading or television or lying perfectly still? Even as you introduce yourself you begin to collect data. Does the person make eye contact or smile? Does the person look relaxed or anxious?

The general survey will give you an overall impression of the person by paying attention to the following characteristics: **physical appearance**, **body structure**, **mobility** and **behaviour**. Following the general survey, you will proceed through the health history, measurements and the vital signs. The sequence of the general survey may vary, depending on the circumstances.

Conducting a general survey each time you encounter the person will alert you to changes that may have taken place that require further assessment. In an emergency situation, the primary survey is used to assess a seriously ill or injured person and is conducted simultaneously with management. Primary survey is used to identify priorities based on the person's condition, injuries, vital signs and/or mechanism of injury (see Chapter 1). Speed and accuracy are essential for patient safety. The primary survey includes assessment of life-threatening conditions such as airway, breathing, circulation, disability (neurological assessment) and exposure (person is undressed and the nurse examines them for injury). A more detailed focused assessment is conducted following the primary survey.

The measurement of vital signs includes measurements of temperature, blood pressure, heart and respiratory rates and oxygen saturation and, as such, are critical indicators of health status, in particular clinical deterioration (see Chapter 30). They reflect interrelationships between body systems, e.g. cardiovascular, respiratory, neurological, endocrine, immune systems and psychological state of the person. Changes in vital signs reflect the body's responses to illness and/or stress. Your approach to measuring vital signs should include informing the person about the procedure, gaining their consent, measuring the vital signs accurately and documenting your findings. Always remember to perform hand hygiene before and after the procedure.

A vital signs chart has been developed by the Australian Commission of Safety and Quality in Health Care for use across Australian hospitals (ACSQHC 2019). This standardised chart enables visualisation of trends in the vital signs and specifies the physiological parameters and other factors that trigger the escalation of care. (See Figure 10.2 for the standardised adult general observation chart 'The Adult Deterioration Detection System (ADDS)'.)

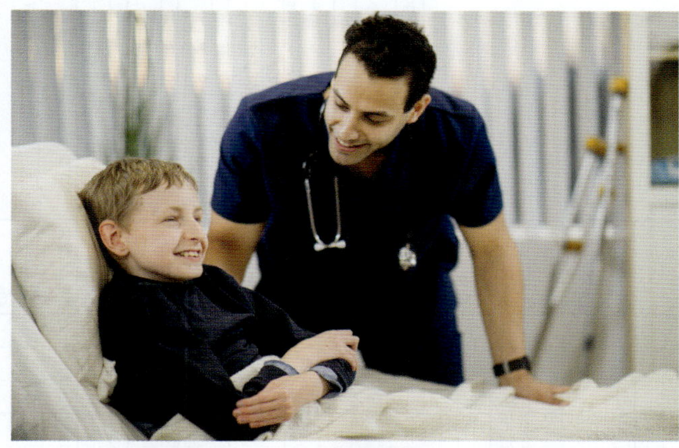

Figure 10.1

DRAFT

DO NOT WRITE IN THIS BINDING MARGIN

Parameter	Row	Date / Time (observations)	Row
Date **Time**			
Respiratory Rate (breaths / min) If respiratory rate ≥ 35 or ≤4, write value in box	Write ≥ 35		Write ≥ 35
	30–34		30–34
	25–29		25–29
	20–24		20–24
	15–19		15–19
	10–14		10–14
	5–9		5–9
	Write ≤ 4		Write ≤ 4
O_2 Saturation (%) If O_2 saturation ≤ 84, write value in box	98–100		98–100
	95–97		95–97
	93–94		93–94
	90–92		90–92
	87–89		87–89
	85–86		85–86
	Write ≤ 84		Write ≤ 84
O_2 Flow Rate (L / min)	≥ 13		≥ 13
	10–12		10–12
	7–9		7–9
	4–6		4–6
	≤ 3		≤ 3
Blood Pressure (mmHg) If systolic BP ≥ 200, write value in box	Write ≥ 200		Write ≥ 200
	190s		190s
	180s		180s
	170s		170s
	160s		160s
	150s		150s
	140s		140s
	130s		130s
	120s		120s
	110s		110s
	100s		100s
	90s		90s
	80s		80s
	70s		70s
	60s		60s
	50s		50s
	40s		40s
Heart Rate (beats / min) If heart rate ≥ 140 or ≤ 30, write value in box	Write ≥ 140		Write ≥ 140
	130s		130s
	120s		120s
	110s		110s
	100s		100s
	90s		90s
	80s		80s
	70s		70s
	60s		60s
	50s		50s
	40s		40s
	Write ≤ 30s		Write ≤ 30s
Temperature (°C) If temperature ≥ 39.1 or ≤ 35.4, write value in box	Write ≥ 39.1		Write ≥ 39.1
	38.5–39.0		38.5–39.0
	38.0–38.4		38.0–38.4
	37.5–37.9		37.5–37.9
	37.0–37.4		37.0–37.4
	36.5–36.9		36.5–36.9
	36.0–36.4		36.0–36.4
	35.5–35.9		35.5–35.9
	Write ≤ 35.4		Write ≤ 35.4
Consciousness If clinically necessary, wake patient to assess and score	Alert		Alert
	To Voice		To Voice
	To Pain		To Pain
	Unresp.		Unresp.
ADDS Scores	Respiratory Rate		**ADDS Scores**
	O_2 Saturation		
	O_2 Flow Rate		
	Systolic BP		
	Heart Rate		
	Temperature		
	Consciousness		
	TOTAL ADDS		
Intervention	E.g. 'a'		E.g. 'a'

UR Number:	
Family name:	
Given names:	
Date of birth: ___/___/___	Sex: ☐M ☐F

(Affix patient identification label here)

Usual/target systolic BP: ___ mmHg Signature: ___

Circle the column showing the patient's usual systolic BP

Score current systolic BP using circled column

Current	190s	180s	170s	160s	150s	140s	130s	120s	110s	100s	90s	80s
Write ≥ 200	0	0	1	1	2	2	2	3	3	4	5	5
190s	0	0	0	1	1	1	2	2	3	3	4	4
180s	0	0	0	0	0	1	1	2	2	3	3	4
170s	1	0	0	0	0	1	1	2	2	3	3	3
160s	1	1	0	0	0	0	0	1	1	2	2	2
150s	1	1	1	0	0	0	0	0	1	1	2	2
140s	2	1	1	1	0	0	0	0	0	1	1	1
130s	2	2	1	1	0	0	0	0	0	0	0	1
120s	2	2	2	1	1	0	0	0	0	0	0	0
110s	3	2	2	2	1	1	0	0	0	0	0	0
100s	3	3	3	2	2	2	1	1	0	0	0	0
90s	4	3	3	3	2	2	2	2	1	1	0	0
80s	Emergency call										1	0
70s–40s	Emergency call											

Adult Deterioration Detection System (ADDS)

If any observation is in a shaded area, add up the Total ADDS Score and take the action required for that score.

- Score 0
- Score 1
- Score 2
- Score 3
- Score 4
- Score 5
- **Emergency call**

Actions Required

Total ADDS Score 1–3

- Increase frequency of observations *[specify frequency]*
- Inform senior nurse and/or Team Leader

Total ADDS Score 4 – 5

- Senior nurse and/or junior medical officer review within 30 minutes

Total ADDS Score 6 – 7

- Senior medical officer review (registrar or above) within 30 minutes
- Request review, and note on the back of this form

Total ADDS Score ≥ 8

- Place Emergency call
- Begin initial life support interventions (support airway, breathing, circulation)
- Advanced life support provider to attend patient immediately

Emergency call if:

- Any observation is in a purple area
- Airway threat
- Respiratory or cardiac arrest
- New drop in O_2 saturation < 90%
- Sudden fall in level of consciousness
- Seizure
- You are seriously worried about the patient but they do not fit the above criteria

ADDS CHART WITH BP TABLE

DRAFT

<INSERT SITE LOGO>

Adult Deterioration Detection System (ADDS) Chart

UR Number: ____________

Family name: ____________

Given names: ____________

Date of birth: ____/____/____ Sex: ☐M ☐F

(Affix patient identification label here)

Other Observation Charts In Use

☐ Alcohol Withdrawal ☐ Insulin Infusion ☐ Pain/Epidural/Patient Controlled Analgesia

☐ Anticoagulant ☐ Neurology

☐ Fluid Balance ☐ Neurovascular

General Instructions

» You must record appropriate observations:
  - On admission
  - At a frequency appropriate for the patient's clinical state.

» You must calculate a Total ADDS Score:
  - If the patient is deteriorating or an observation is in a shaded area
  - Whenever you are concerned about the patient.

» When graphing observations, place a dot (•) in the centre of the box which includes the current observation in its range of values and connect it to the previous dot with a straight line. For blood pressure, use the symbols indicated on the chart.

» Whenever an observation falls within a shaded area, you must enter the ADDS Score for that vital sign in the appropriate row of the ADDS Scores table, unless a modification has been made (see below).

Modifications

- If abnormal observations are to be tolerated for the patient's clinical condition, write the acceptable ranges below (where the ADDS Score will be 0).
- Modifications must be reviewed at least every 72 hours.
- If **any** vital sign needs further modifying, draw two diagonal lines through the entire Modification record in use and write the new acceptable ranges in the next Modification record.

	Modification 1	Modification 2	Modification 3	Modification 4
Respiratory Rate	- breaths / min	- breaths / min	- breaths / min	- breaths / min
O_2 Saturation	- %	- %	- %	- %
O_2 Flow Rate	- L / min	- L / min	- L / min	- L / min
Systolic BP	- mmHg	- mmHg	- mmHg	- mmHg
Heart Rate	- beats / min	- beats / min	- beats / min	- beats / min
Temperature	- °C	- °C	- °C	- °C
Consciousness	-	-	-	-
Doctor's name				
Signature				
Date	/ /	/ /	/ /	/ /
Time	:	:	:	:

DRAFT

UR Number: ____________

Family name: ____________

Given names: ____________

Date of birth: ____/____/____ Sex: ☐M ☐F

(Affix patient identification label here)

Interventions Associated With Abnormal Vital Signs

If you administer an intervention, record here and note letter in Intervention row over page in appropriate time column.

Reference Letter	Intervention (initial if required)
a	
b	
c	
d	
e	
f	
g	
h	

Clinical Review Requests

Review requested Date / / Time : ☐ Ward doctor ☐ ☐ Emergency

Specify reason:

Review requested Date / / Time : ☐ Ward doctor ☐ ☐ Emergency

Specify reason:

Review requested Date / / Time : ☐ Ward doctor ☐ ☐ Emergency

Specify reason:

Additional Observations

Date	
Time	
Blood Glucose Level (mmol / L)	
Weight (kg)	
Bowels	
Urinalysis – Specific gravity	
pH	
Leukocytes	
Blood	
Nitrite	
Ketones	
Bilirubin	
Urobilinogen	
Protein	
Glucose	

DO NOT WRITE IN THIS BINDING MARGIN

Figure 10.2
Adult deterioration detection system (ADDS) chart (vital signs and observations chart).
https://www.safetyandquality.gov.au/sites/default/files/migrated/ADDS-chart-with-blood-pressure-table-2012.pdf

Objective data

Position

General survey—observe as you find the person.
Vital signs—can be performed in bed or in a chair but should be performed at rest. You may require a pillow to support the arm when measuring BP.

Equipment needed

Vital signs chart
Digital vital signs machine (including oral or aural thermometer, oxygen saturation probe and relevant sized blood pressure cuff)
Electronic standing scales (or other type scale)
Height measuring pole
Measuring tape
Hand hygiene solution

PROCEDURES AND NORMAL FINDINGS	ABNORMAL FINDINGS AND CLINICAL ALERTS
The general survey	
The aim is to determine the general state of health and whether the person appears well, chronically unwell or acutely ill.	
Physical appearance	
Observe physical appearance of the person on meeting, then throughout the collection of history information and the physical assessment and throughout the episode of care.	
Age—The person appears their stated age.	Appears older than stated age, as can occur with chronic illness, alcoholism, smoking.
Sex—Sexual development is appropriate for gender and age.	Delayed or precocious puberty. Be aware of assuming that the person identifies as heterosexual, lesbian, gay, bisexual or a particular gender. See Chapters 26 and 27 for more information and guidelines about communicating effectively about sexuality.
Level of consciousness—The person is alert and oriented, attends to your questions and responds appropriately.	Confused, drowsy, lethargic (see Chapter 12) ***Clinical alert:*** Change in conscious state requires immediate further assessment. Consider the need for urgent medical referral.
Skin—Skin is intact. Colour tone is even, pigmentation varying with genetic background, skin is intact with no obvious lesions.	Bleeding or other signs of trauma must be investigated immediately. Pallor: unnaturally pale skin. Jaundice: yellow discolouration. Erythema: redness of the skin. Lesions: (see Chapter 22). Cyanosis: bluish discolouration. ***Clinical alert:*** Presence of cyanosis requires immediate further assessment. Consider the need for urgent medical attention.
Facial features—Facial features are symmetrical with movement, appropriate smiling, frowning.	Immobile, mask-like, asymmetrical, drooping (see Table 12.7, Abnormalities in cranial nerves).

PROCEDURES AND NORMAL FINDINGS	ABNORMAL FINDINGS AND CLINICAL ALERTS
No signs of acute distress are present.	Respiratory signs, e.g. shortness of breath (dyspnoea), wheezing, rapid breathing (tachypnoea), use of accessory muscles, harsh high-pitched wheezing sound made on inspiration or expiration (stridor). Pain, indicated by facial grimace, holding body part, crying, moaning, sweating. Mental state, e.g. acute anxiety, agitation. ***Clinical alert:*** Presence of any of these signs of distress requires immediate attention. Consider the need for urgent medical referral.
Body structure	
Stature—The height appears within normal range for age, genetic heritage (see Measurement below).	Excessively short or tall for age.
Nutrition—The weight appears within normal range for height and body build; body fat distribution is even.	Cachectic, emaciated. Simple obesity, with even fat distribution. Centripetal (truncal) obesity—fat concentrated in face, neck, trunk, with thin extremities, as in Cushing's syndrome. Impressions of cachexia or obesity must be verified by objective measurement.
Symmetry—Body parts look equal bilaterally and are in relative proportion to each other.	Unilateral atrophy: wasting of muscle(s) on one side of the body. Hypertrophy: increased size of a body part. Asymmetrical location of a body part.
Posture—The person stands comfortably erect as appropriate for age. Note the normal 'plumb line' through anterior ear, shoulder, hip, patella, ankle.	Abnormal posture may be associated with neurological, bone or muscle disorders. Rigid spine and neck; moves as one unit (e.g. arthritis). Lordosis: an unusual inward curving of the spine in the lower part of the back. Kyphosis: a permanent curvature of the spine as can be seen in the older person giving a stooped or hunched-over appearance. Scoliosis: an excessive sideways curvature of the spine. Shoulders look slumped.
Position—The person sits comfortably in a chair or on the bed or examination table, arms relaxed at sides, head turned to examiner.	Stiff and tense, ready to spring from chair, fidgety movements. Tripod—leaning forwards with arms braced on chair arms; occurs with chronic pulmonary disease. Sitting straight up and resists lying down (e.g. heart failure). Curled up in fetal position (e.g. acute abdominal pain).
Body build, contour—Proportions are: **1** Arm span (fingertip to fingertip) equals height. **2** Body length from crown to pubis roughly equal to length from pubis to sole of foot.	Elongated arm span, arm span greater than height (e.g. Marfan's syndrome, hypogonadism).
Obvious physical deformities—note any congenital or acquired defects.	Missing extremities or digits; webbed digits; shortened limb.

PROCEDURES AND NORMAL FINDINGS	ABNORMAL FINDINGS AND CLINICAL ALERTS
Mobility	
Observe the person sit, walk and change positions.	
Gait—Normally, the base is as wide as the shoulder width; foot placement is accurate; the walk is smooth, coordinated, even and well balanced; and associated movements, such as symmetrical arm swing, are present.	Exceptionally wide base. Staggering, stumbling. Shuffling, dragging, nonfunctional leg. Limping with injury. Propulsion—difficulty stopping (see Table 12.10).
Range of motion—Note full mobility for each joint and that movement is deliberate, accurate, smooth and coordinated. (See Chapter 20 for information on more detailed testing of joint range of motion.)	Limited joint range of motion. Paralysis—absent movement. Movement jerky, uncoordinated.
No involuntary movement.	Tics, tremors, seizures (see Table 12.9).
Behaviour	
Observation of the facial expression, mood and affect, and quality of speech are performed at the same time as observing behaviour. Clothing and hygiene are evaluated together.	
Facial expression—The person maintains eye contact (unless a cultural taboo exists), expressions are appropriate to the situation, e.g. thoughtful, serious or smiling. (Note expressions both while the face is at rest and while the person is talking.)	Flat, depressed, angry, sad, anxious. However, note that anxiety is common in ill people. Be aware also that some people smile when they are anxious.
Mood and affect—The person is comfortable and cooperative with the examiner and interacts pleasantly.	Agitated, hostile, distrustful, suspicious, crying.
Speech—Articulation (the ability to form words) is clear and understandable.	Alterations in quality of speech such as dysarthria and dysphagia or garbled speech (see Table 12.6, Speech disorders) may occur as a result of neurological disorders (Chapter 12).
The stream of talking is fluent, with an even pace. The person conveys ideas clearly. Word choice is appropriate to context. The person communicates in prevailing language easily or with an interpreter.	Extremes of few words or of constant talking. Inappropriate use of words needs to be further evaluated in a mental status and/or neurological assessment.
Dress—Clothing is appropriate to the climate, looks clean and fits the body and is appropriate to the context and age.	Trousers too large and held up by belt suggest weight loss, as does the addition of new holes in belt. If the belt is moved to a looser fit, it may indicate obesity or ascites. Inappropriate clothing may be related to heat/cold intolerance, mental illness or poverty.
Personal hygiene—The person appears clean and groomed appropriately for their age, occupation and socioeconomic group. (Note that a wide variation of dress and hygiene is 'normal'.)	Abnormal body odours (perspiration, urine, faeces) may be related to inadequate personal hygiene. Abnormal breath odours may be observed such as alcohol, acetone or ammonia.

PROCEDURES AND NORMAL FINDINGS	ABNORMAL FINDINGS AND CLINICAL ALERTS
Hair is groomed, brushed. Women's make-up, if used, is appropriate for age and culture.	In a previously carefully groomed woman, unkempt hair and absent make-up may indicate malaise or illness.
Measurement	
Weight	
Use a standardised *balance* or electronic standing scale. Ask the person to remove their shoes and heavy outer clothing if not in a hospital context before standing on the scale (Figure 10.3). When a sequence of repeated weights is necessary, aim for approximately the same time of day and the same type of clothing worn each time. Record the weight in kilograms. A recent weight loss may be explained by successful dieting and/or exercise program. A weight gain usually reflects overabundant kilojoule intake, unhealthy eating habits and sedentary lifestyle or changes in health status. 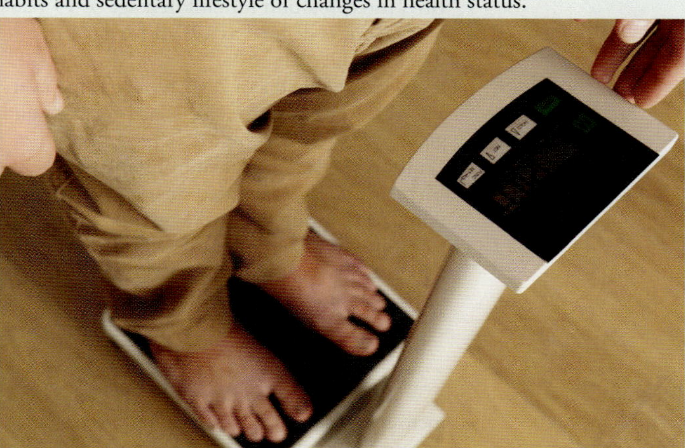 Figure 10.3	An unexplained weight loss may be a sign of a short-term illness (e.g. fever, infection, disease of the mouth or throat) or a chronic illness (endocrine disease, malignancy, mental health dysfunction). Unexplained weight gain may indicate fluid retention, e.g. heart failure.
Height	
Use a wall-mounted device or the measuring pole on the balance scale. Align the extended headpiece with the top of the head. The person should be shoeless, standing straight with gentle traction under the jaw and looking straight ahead. Feet, shoulders and buttocks should be in contact with the hard surface. For bed-bound patients, length can be assessed using a pliable measuring tape to measure the body in sections. Measurements should be taken from the heel to knee, knee to hip, hip to shoulder and shoulder to top of the head. These measurements are then totalled to determine height.	

OBJECTIVE DATA

PROCEDURES AND NORMAL FINDINGS	ABNORMAL FINDINGS AND CLINICAL ALERTS
Body mass index	
Body mass index is a standard measure of weight for height and an indicator of overweight, obesity or protein–calorie malnutrition. BMI formula: $$\text{BMI} = \frac{\text{mass in kg}}{\text{height in m}^2}$$ (See World Health Organization (WHO 2018) BMI classification website: http://apps.who.int/bmi/index.jsp?introPage=intro_3.html) A healthy BMI is a level of 19 or greater to less than 25. Show the person how his or her own weight matches up to the national guidelines for optimal BMI. Compare the person's current weight with that from the previous health visit. Note that BMI overestimates body fat in people who are very muscular and underestimates body fat in older adults who have lost muscle mass.	The cause of weight gain is usually excess kilojoule intake; occasionally it is endocrine disorders, drug therapy (e.g. corticosteroids) or depression. BMI interpretation for adults: <18.5 Underweight 18.5–<25 Normal weight 25.0–<30 Overweight 30.0–<35 Obesity class I 35–<40 Obesity class II 40–45 Obesity class III (AIHW 2018) BMI interpretation for children age 5–19 years; overweight is defined as a BMI for age value over +1 SD. Obesity is defined as a BMI for age value over +2 SD. Refer to percentile charts for boys and girls (WHO 2019). Caution needs to be taken in interpreting BMI since it was validated on a particular population group and it may not be relevant to all groups, e.g. the elite athlete is likely to have a high BMI because of increased muscle mass but would not be considered unhealthy.
Waist circumference	
Waist circumference (WC) alone can be used to predict greater health risk. Excess abdominal fat is an important independent risk factor for disease, over and above that of BMI. If most of the weight is carried around the waist instead of around the hips, the person is at higher risk for heart disease and type 2 diabetes. With the person standing, locate the hip bone—the very top is the iliac crest. Place a measuring tape around the waist, parallel to the floor, at the level of the iliac crest. The tape should be snug but not pinching in the skin. Note the measurement at the end of a normal expiration (Figure 10.4). 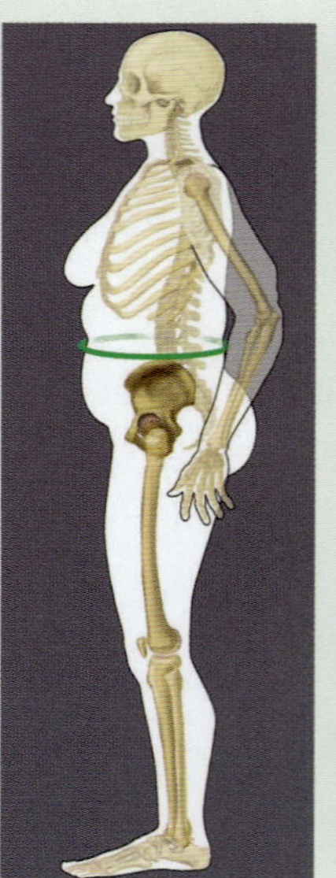 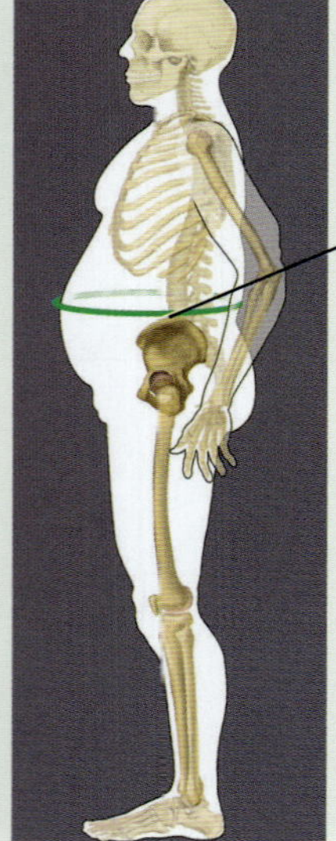 **Figure 10.4** Measuring tape for waist circumference.	A WC >80 cm in women and >94 cm in men increases risk of cardiovascular and metabolic diseases. More than 88 cm for women and > 102 cm for males indicates greatly increased health risk. These measurements can be recorded at each health visit (Talley & O'Connor 2018).

PROCEDURES AND NORMAL FINDINGS	ABNORMAL FINDINGS AND CLINICAL ALERTS
Waist-to-hip ratio	
The waist-to-hip ratio assesses body fat distribution as an indicator of health risk. Obese persons with a greater proportion of fat in the upper body, especially in the abdomen, have android obesity; obese persons with most of their fat in the hips and thighs have gynoid obesity. The equation is: $\text{Waist-to-hip ratio} = \frac{\text{waist circumference}}{\text{hip circumference}}$ For example: If a woman has a 112 cm waist and 101 cm hips, the calculation would be as follows: 112 cm/101 cm = 1.1 waist to hip ratio The desired waist-to-hip ratio for women is 0.8 or less and for men is 1.0 or less.	A waist-to-hip ratio of ≥1.0 in men or ≥0.8 in women is indicative of android (upper body obesity) and increasing risk for obesity-related diseases and early mortality. Increased risk occurs when the measure exceeds 1.0 for men and 0.85 for women (Talley & O'Connor 2018).
Vital signs	
This collection of measurements is used as part of baseline assessment of people, routine monitoring of response to treatments and to detect deterioration. Pulse oximetry, wound or circulation checks and/or pain assessment may also supplement vital signs, according to the person's needs. A consistent, systematic method for measuring vital signs is necessary for accuracy. The order in which the various components of vital signs are taken varies according to need. The frequency of vital sign measurements will also depend on need, and care should be taken so that vital sign measurements are not done unnecessarily. Interpretation of vital sign measurements is always considered in the context of the broader assessment of the person. However, where any one of the vital sign measurements is outside the parameters of normal, further assessment is critical. Document vital signs on the ADDS chart and note the variation of results from previous recordings. If the result falls outside normal parameters, follow instructions on the chart as to further actions (Figure 10.2). As with any procedure, the person requires an explanation and hand hygiene should be undertaken before and after taking vital signs.	It is important that vital signs are correlated with other physical assessment findings. Trends in vital signs are evaluated over time to enable accurate decision making and planning of treatment and/or referral. Vital signs should be taken when the person is at rest and not immediately after ambulating.
Temperature	
Body temperature is the difference between heat produced by metabolism, exercise and activity and heat lost through radiation, evaporation of sweat, convection and conduction. Cellular metabolism requires a stable core temperature ranging between 35.8–37.5°C. Constant core temperature is maintained through homeostasis and is regulated by the hypothalamus.	Body temperature above or below the normal range (35.8–37.5°C) may occur as a consequence of illness, medical treatment or central nervous systems disorders. **Normothermia or afebrile:** Core body temperature is within the normal range (35.8–37.5°C).

PROCEDURES AND NORMAL FINDINGS	ABNORMAL FINDINGS AND CLINICAL ALERTS
Body temperature is influenced by: • **Circadian rhythms.** Body temperature normally fluctuates over the day, with the lowest levels around 4 am and the highest in the late afternoon, between 4 and 6 pm. • **Ovulation.** The menstruation cycle, progesterone secretion occurs with ovulation, creating a 0.15–0.45°C rise in temperature—caused by sharply elevated levels of progesterone—that continues until menses occurs. • **Exercise and stress.** Moderate-to-hard exercise and stress increases body temperature. • **Digestion** causes an elevation in body temperature. • **Extremes of age.** Thermoregulation is less effective in infants, young children and very old people.	**Hypothermia** occurs when the body temperature registers between 25.0°C and 35.0°C. Additional physical changes include skin (cool to touch) and cardiovascular changes (capillary endothelium becomes 'leaky' due to prolonged exposure to cold).
Body temperature can be measured at different body sites using various equipment. Sites include mouth, axilla, external auditory canal, rectum. Temperatures will differ according to selected body site. For example: • Rectal temperatures are usually 0.4°C higher than oral temperatures. • Axillary temperatures are 0.6°C lower than oral temperatures. Site selection depends on conscious state, age and ability to cooperate. Use of the oral route is contraindicated for young children or people who have had facial or nasal surgery.	**Pyrexia** is an elevated temperature due to an increase in the body's temperature set point. Pyrexia is also known as fever or febrile response. **Hyperthermia** or **hyperpyrexia** are terms used to describe a temperature exceeding 39.0°C. Hyperthermia is caused by toxins, e.g. following myocardial infarction, trauma, surgery, malignancy, sepsis and neurological disorders (e.g. stroke, cerebral oedema, brain tumour). Pyrogens cause the thermostat in the hypothalamus to reset to a higher level. ***Clinical alert:*** Sudden increase in temperature usually indicates infection and as such requires further investigation. Report to medical practitioner if temperature exceeds 39.0°C. A febrile person will usually demonstrate pale, cool skin and shiver to generate body heat. This may be followed by vasodilation of the skin and sweating.
Body temperature can be measured in a variety of ways. **A.** The **electronic thermometer** has the advantages of swift and accurate measurement (usually in a few seconds) using safe, unbreakable, disposable probe covers. This type of thermometer can be used in the mouth, axilla or tympanic membrane. The instrument must be fully charged and correctly calibrated. Regardless of the body site used to measure temperature, a disposable probe cover is put on the electronic probe before use on each person. After the measurement has been taken, the probe cover is removed and disposed into suitable waste receptacle. See Figure 10.5.	

PROCEDURES AND NORMAL FINDINGS	ABNORMAL FINDINGS AND CLINICAL ALERTS
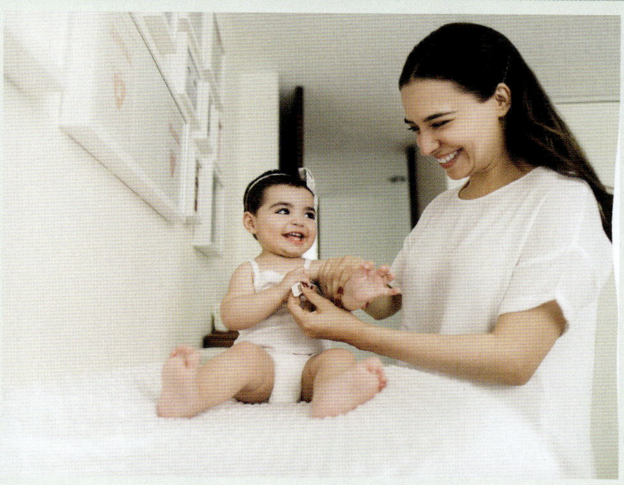 **Figure 10.5** Measuring axillary temperature. https://medical-dictionary.thefreedictionary.com/_/viewer.aspx?path=MosbyMD&name=axillary-temperature-b.jpg&url=https%3A%2F%2Fmedical-dictionary.thefreedictionary.com%2Faxillary%2Btemperature	
B. The **tympanic membrane thermometer** (TMT) is a noninvasive, non-traumatic device that is extremely quick and efficient. The probe tip has the shape of an otoscope (instrument used to inspect the ear). Gently pull the pinna of the ear upwards and backwards and place the covered probe tip in the person's ear canal (see Figure 10.6). Do not force it and do not occlude the canal. Activate the device and you can read the temperature in 2 to 3 seconds. 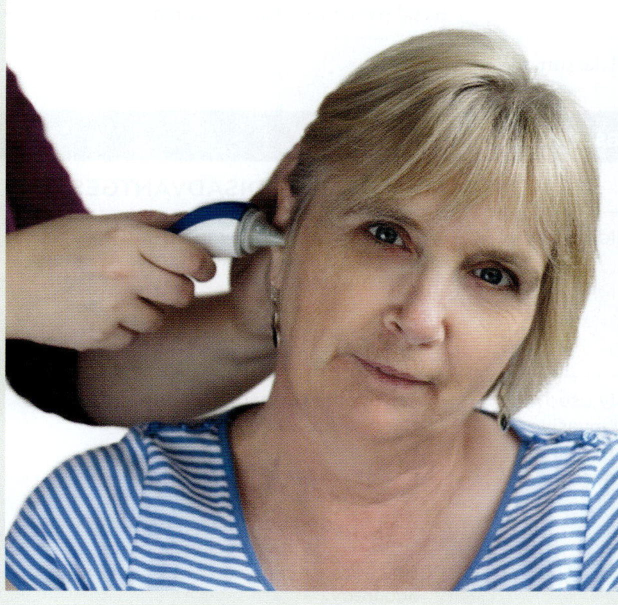 **Figure 10.6** Measuring tympanic temperature. https://opentextbc.ca/vitalsign/chapter/tympanic-temperature/	The tympanic membrane thermometer is not suitable for use in babies under 3 months of age.

PROCEDURES AND NORMAL FINDINGS	ABNORMAL FINDINGS AND CLINICAL ALERTS
C. Strip thermometers are plastic strips, which can be placed on the forehead or in the mouth and change colour to indicate the temperature. The strip is placed on the forehead and read after 1 minute. Read it while the strip is in place. This method is the least accurate of all methods. See Figure 10.7. 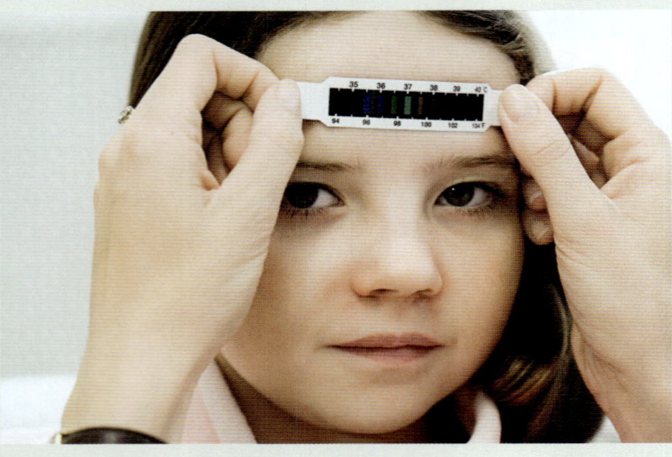 **Figure 10.7** Measuring temperature using a strip thermometer. https://www.dhgate.com/product/forehead-head-strip-thermometer-fever-body/410742771.html	
D. The **infrared thermometer** is a non-invasive temperature measurement method and works on the principle that heat is converted into an electrical signal. The handheld, infrared thermometer is held 3 to 15 cm away from the person's forehead. Activate the device and you can read the temperature in 2 to 3 seconds.	
E. Rectal thermometer is rarely used but, if used, wear gloves, add a lubricated rectal probe cover on an electronic thermometer, insert only 2 to 3 cm into the adult rectum, directed towards the umbilicus.	Extreme care should be taken if temperature is taken via the rectum. Complications such as rectal perforation have occurred.
Document the temperature in degrees Celsius onto the vital signs chart. Make sure to note the route used to obtain the temperature reading.	

TABLE 10.1 Summary of approaches to temperature measurment

SITE	TYPE OF THERMOMETER	USE	ADVANTAGES/DISADVANTGES
Mouth	Digital probe thermometer Strip thermometer	• Older children • Adults	• Reading affected by ingestion of food, fluid, or smoking prior to measurement of temperature • Normal range 35.8–37.5°C • Strip thermometer less accurate than other methods
External auditory canal (tympanic membrane)	Electronic tympanic thermometer	• Commonly used • Minimally invasive • Provides rapid results • Children over 3 months • Adults	• Unsuitable for babies under 3 months • Change probe cover each time temperature taken • Moderate correlation with core temperature • Risk of tympanic membrane perforation • Not reliable in critically ill adults • Presence of cerumen (wax) may affect accuracy

PROCEDURES AND NORMAL FINDINGS	ABNORMAL FINDINGS AND CLINICAL ALERTS

TABLE 10.1 Summary of approaches to temperature measurment—cont'd

SITE	TYPE OF THERMOMETER	USE	ADVANTAGES/DISADVANTGES
Axilla	Digital probe thermometer	Site may be used for people with mouth injuries and/or cannot breathe through their nose	• Less accurate than other methods • Affected by local blood flow, sweat • Moderate concordance with core temperature • Lower than oral temperature • Normal range 34.8–36.3°C • Not recommended for the critically ill person
Forehead	Strip thermometer	Can be used for children, adults	• Less accurate than other methods
Forehead/ temple	Infrared thermometer	• Can be used for any person providing forehead is visible • Portable, handheld, • Non-invasive • Provides rapid results	• Does not reliably reflect core temperature
Rectal	Rectal thermometer	• May be used for people who are critically ill or undergoing complex surgery • Traditionally used to measure core temperature	• Discomfort and risk of rectal perforation • Higher than oral temperature • Found to not be an accurate predictor of core temperature
Invasive temperature measurement	Pulmonary artery, oesophageal, nasopharyngeal, and bladder temperature monitors use thermistors, which are thermally sensitive	• Accurate • Cost effective • Used for critically ill people	• Invasive • Risk of infection/perforation

Pulse

PROCEDURES AND NORMAL FINDINGS	ABNORMAL FINDINGS AND CLINICAL ALERTS
With every beat, the heart pumps an amount of blood—the **stroke volume**—into the aorta. This is about 70 mL in the adult. The force flares the arterial walls and generates a pressure wave, which is felt in the periphery as the **pulse**. Palpating the peripheral pulse gives the rate and rhythm of the heartbeat, as well as local data on the condition of the artery. The *radial* pulse is usually palpated when measuring vital signs.	
Using the pads of your first three fingers, palpate the radial pulse at the flexor aspect of the wrist laterally along the radius bone (Figure 10.8). Push until you feel the strongest pulsation. While it is recommended to count for 60 seconds, if the rhythm is regular, count the number of beats in 30 seconds and multiply by 2. The 30-second interval is the most accurate and efficient when heart rates are normal or rapid and when rhythms are regular. However, if the rhythm is irregular, count for a full minute. Assess the pulse, including (1) rate, (2) rhythm, (3) force (strength) (strong, weak or thready). Document the heart rate on the vital signs chart	Press firmly but not so hard as to obliterate the pulse. Should difficulty be encountered with taking a peripheral pulse, e.g. faint or irregular rhythm, then an apical rate should be taken (see Chapter 17). Pulse force (strength) reflects the volume of blood ejected against the arterial wall with each heart contraction.

OBJECTIVE DATA

PROCEDURES AND NORMAL FINDINGS	ABNORMAL FINDINGS AND CLINICAL ALERTS

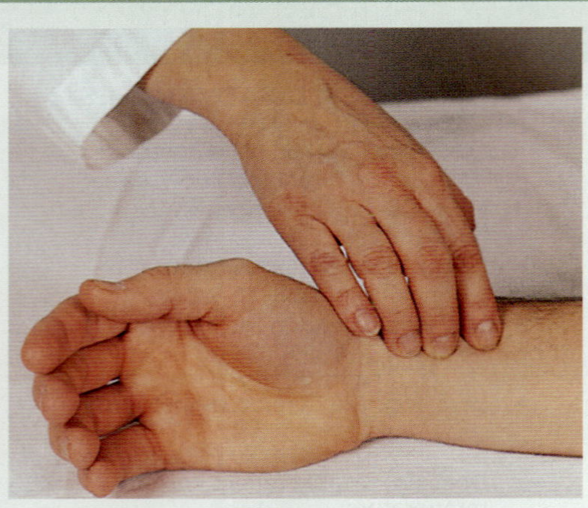

Figure 10.8
Taking a radial pulse.

Rate

In the resting adult, the normal heart rate range is 60 to 100 beats per minute (bpm). The rate normally varies with age, being more rapid in infancy and childhood and more moderate during adult and older years. The rate also varies with gender; after puberty, females have a slightly faster rate than males (Table 10.2).

TABLE 10.2 Normal resting heart rates across age groups

AGE	AVERAGE (BEATS PER MINUTE)	NORMAL LIMITS
Newborn	120	70–190
1 yr	120	80–160
2 yr	110	80–130
4 yr	100	80–120
6 yr	100	75–115
8 yr	90	70–110
10 yr	90	70–110
12 yr		
Female	90	70–110
Male	85	65–105
14 yr		
Female	85	65–105
Male	80	60–100
16 yr		
Female	80	60–100
Male	75	55–95

Many medications affect heart rate, with nearly all people with heart disease taking at least one medication that slows the heart rate.

In the adult, a heart rate less than 60 bpm is **bradycardia**. This occurs normally in the well-trained athlete whose heart muscle develops along with the skeletal muscles. The stronger, more efficient heart muscle pushes out a larger stroke volume with each beat, thus requiring fewer beats per minute to maintain a stable cardiac output.

A more rapid heart rate, over 100 bpm, is **tachycardia**.

Further assessment of abnormal heart rates should be determined by auscultation of the apical pulse (see Chapter 17).

OBJECTIVE DATA

PROCEDURES AND NORMAL FINDINGS	ABNORMAL FINDINGS AND CLINICAL ALERTS

TABLE 10.2 Normal resting heart rates across age groups—cont'd

AGE	AVERAGE (BEATS PER MINUTE)	NORMAL LIMITS
18 yr		
Female	75	55–95
Male	70	50–90
Well-conditioned athlete	May be 50–60	50–100
Adult	74–76	60–100
Over 65 years	74–76	60–100

For descriptions of abnormal rates and rhythms, see Table 16.1.

Rhythm

The rhythm of the heart rate normally has an even tempo.

An irregular rhythm indicates a cardiac arrhythmia.
One irregularity that is commonly found in children and young adults is **sinus arrhythmia**. Here the heart rate varies with the respiratory cycle, speeding up at the peak of inspiration and slowing to normal with expiration. Inspiration momentarily causes a decreased stroke volume from the left side of the heart; to compensate, the heart rate increases. (See Chapter 17 for a full discussion of sinus arrhythmia.) If any other irregularities are felt, auscultate heart sounds for a more complete assessment (Chapter 17).
Tachycardia occurs with fever and also with sepsis, pneumonia, myocardial infarction, pancreatitis.

Force (strength)

The force of the pulse shows the strength of the heart's stroke volume. The pulse force is recorded using a three-point scale:
3+ —Full, bounding
2+ —Normal
1+ —Weak, thready
0—Absent
Make sure your documentation of pulse force (strength) is consistent with that used by your health agency.

A 'weak, thready' pulse reflects a decreased stroke volume (e.g. as occurs with haemorrhagic shock).
A 'full, bounding' pulse denotes an increased stroke volume, as with anxiety, exercise or a number of medical conditions.

Respirations

Normally, a person's breathing is relaxed, regular, automatic and silent. Because most people are unaware of their breathing, do not mention that you will be counting the respirations, because sudden awareness may alter the normal pattern. Instead, maintain your position of counting the radial pulse and unobtrusively count the respirations by placing the person's arm in a relaxed position across the abdomen or lower chest.
Count for 30 seconds or for a full minute if you suspect an abnormality. If you are having difficulty observing the rise and fall of the person's chest wall place your hand on the person's hand.

The optimal method of respiratory rate count involves counting for one full minute, using a stethoscope against the chest when respiratory rate is rapid to ensure all breaths are counted, and counting respiratory rate when the person is at rest.
Clinical alert:
Abnormalities in respiration rates can be a very important early indicator of patient deterioration and must be reported and managed immediately (see Chapter 30 for further discussion of clinical deterioration).

OBJECTIVE DATA

PROCEDURES AND NORMAL FINDINGS	ABNORMAL FINDINGS AND CLINICAL ALERTS

Respiratory rates presented in Table 10.3 show normal respiratory rates across age groups. More detailed assessment on respiratory status is presented in Chapter 19.

TABLE 10.3 Normal respiratory rates

AGE	BREATHS PER MINUTE
Neonate	30–40
1 yr	20–40
2 yr	25–32
8–10 yr	20–26
12–14 yr	18–22
16 yr	12–20
Adult	10–19

Blood pressure

Blood pressure (BP) is the force of the blood pushing against the side of the arterial wall. The strength of the push changes with the stage in the cardiac cycle. The **systolic** pressure is the maximum pressure exerted on the arterial wall during left ventricular contraction or systole. The **diastolic** pressure is the resting pressure exerted by blood on the arterial wall between each contraction or diastole. The **pulse pressure** is the difference between the systolic and diastolic pressures and reflects the stroke volume (Figure 10.9).

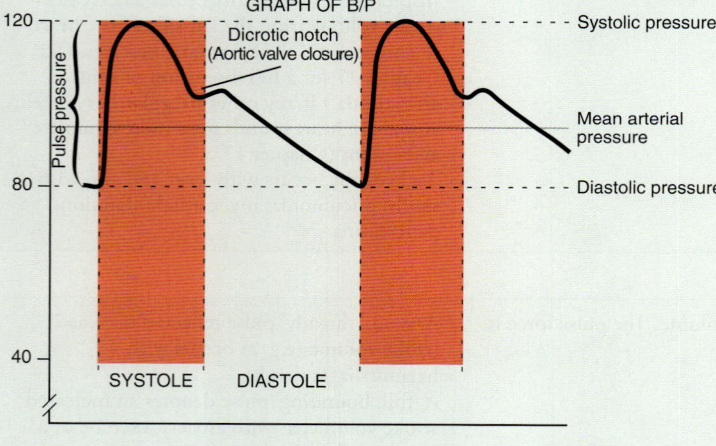

Figure 10.9
Graph of BP.

The average BP in the young adult is 120/80 mmHg, although this varies normally with many factors, such as:

- **Age**. Normally, a gradual rise occurs through childhood and into the adult years (see Figure 10.10).

PROCEDURES AND NORMAL FINDINGS	ABNORMAL FINDINGS AND CLINICAL ALERTS
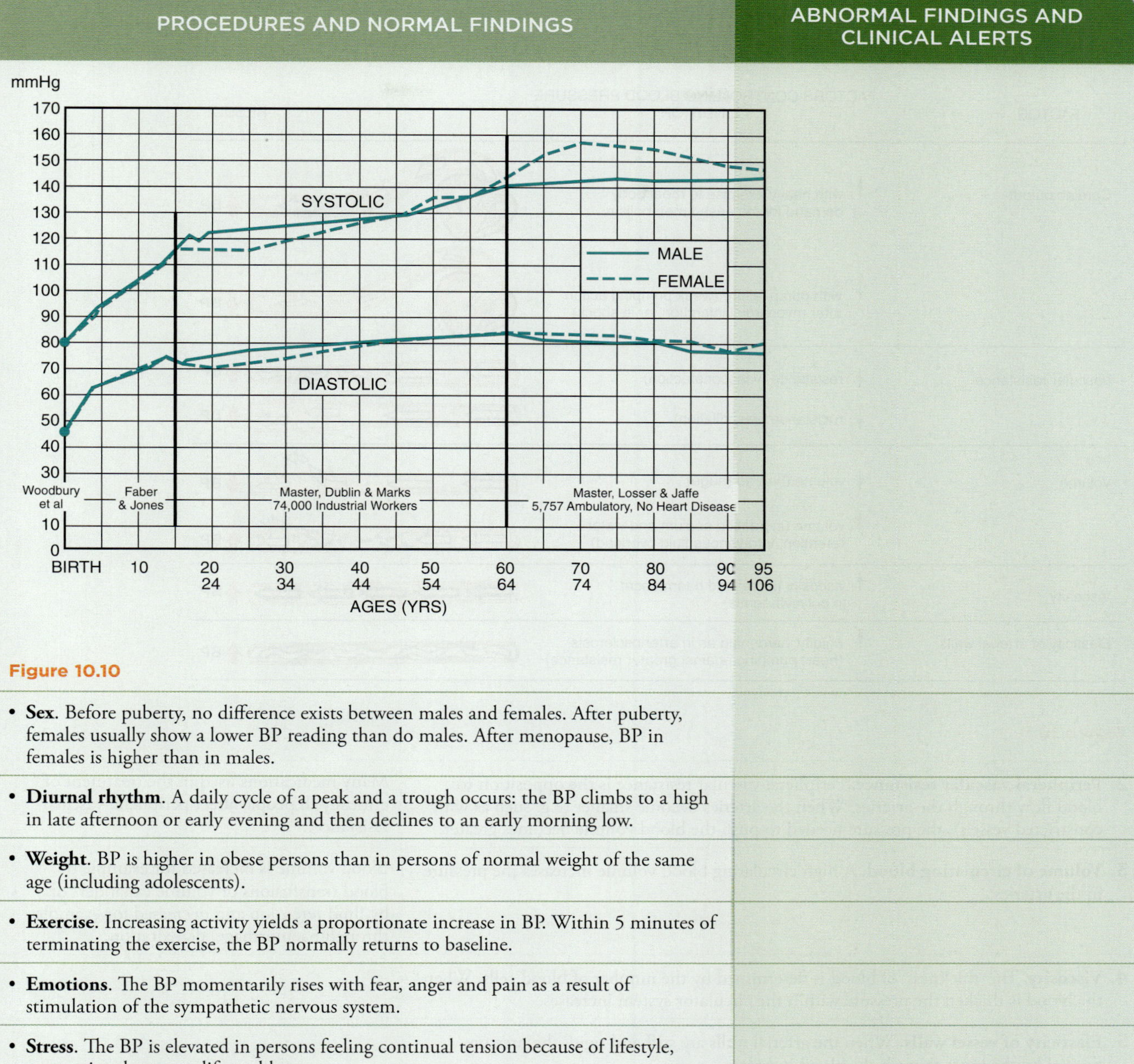 Figure 10.10	
• **Sex.** Before puberty, no difference exists between males and females. After puberty, females usually show a lower BP reading than do males. After menopause, BP in females is higher than in males.	
• **Diurnal rhythm.** A daily cycle of a peak and a trough occurs: the BP climbs to a high in late afternoon or early evening and then declines to an early morning low.	
• **Weight.** BP is higher in obese persons than in persons of normal weight of the same age (including adolescents).	
• **Exercise.** Increasing activity yields a proportionate increase in BP. Within 5 minutes of terminating the exercise, the BP normally returns to baseline.	
• **Emotions.** The BP momentarily rises with fear, anger and pain as a result of stimulation of the sympathetic nervous system.	
• **Stress.** The BP is elevated in persons feeling continual tension because of lifestyle, occupational stress or life problems.	
The level of **BP** is determined by five factors:	
1. **Cardiac output.** The more blood the heart pumps into the blood vessels, the higher the pressure on the arterial walls (Figure 10.11).	

OBJECTIVE DATA

PROCEDURES AND NORMAL FINDINGS	ABNORMAL FINDINGS AND CLINICAL ALERTS

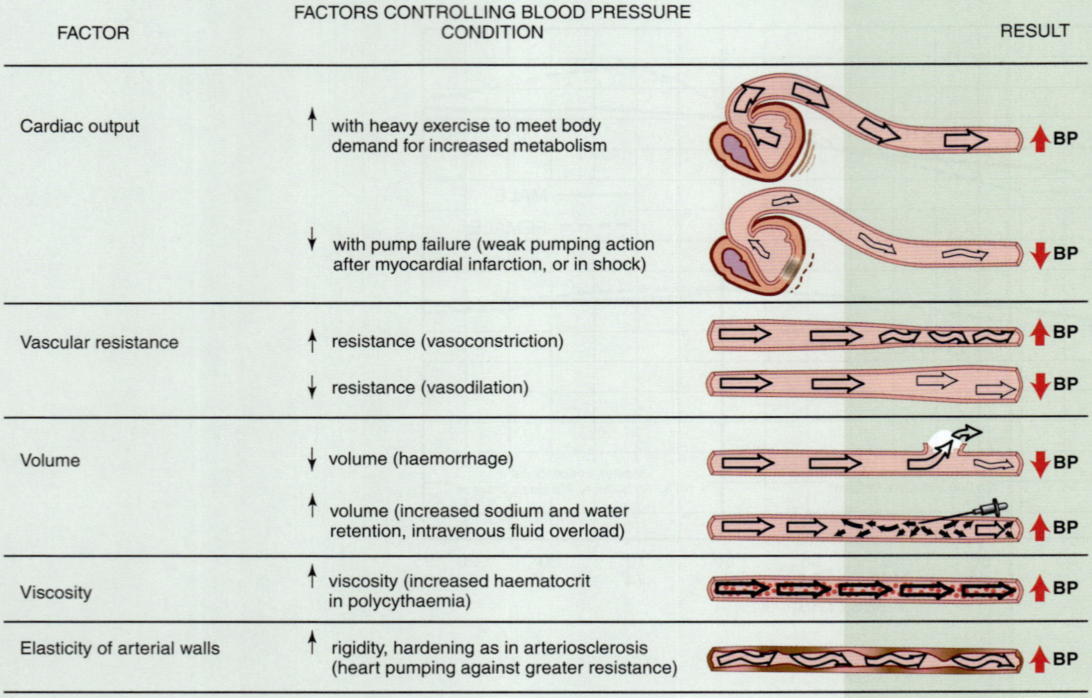

FACTORS CONTROLLING BLOOD PRESSURE

FACTOR	CONDITION	RESULT
Cardiac output	↑ with heavy exercise to meet body demand for increased metabolism	↑ BP
	↓ with pump failure (weak pumping action after myocardial infarction, or in shock)	↓ BP
Vascular resistance	↑ resistance (vasoconstriction)	↑ BP
	↓ resistance (vasodilation)	↓ BP
Volume	↓ volume (haemorrhage)	↓ BP
	↑ volume (increased sodium and water retention, intravenous fluid overload)	↑ BP
Viscosity	↑ viscosity (increased haematocrit in polycythaemia)	↑ BP
Elasticity of arterial walls	↑ rigidity, hardening as in arteriosclerosis (heart pumping against greater resistance)	↑ BP

Figure 10.11

2. Peripheral vascular resistance. Peripheral vascular resistance is the opposition to blood flow through the arteries. When the arteries become smaller (e.g. such as with constricted vessels), the pressure needed to push the blood volume becomes greater.	Many medications used in the treatment of critically ill people affect peripheral vascular resistance.
3. Volume of circulating blood. A high circulating blood volume increases the pressure in the arteries.	Blood volume is increased for example by blood transfusions or volume expanders or by fluid retention and decreased for example through haemorrhage, dehydration.
4. Viscosity. The 'thickness' of blood is determined by the number of blood cells. When the blood is thicker, the pressure within the circulator system increases.	
5. Elasticity of vessel walls. When the arterial walls are stiff and rigid, the pressure needed by the heart to push the blood increases.	
Blood pressure is measured with a stethoscope and an aneroid *sphygmomanometer* or an *electronic blood pressure monitor*.	Regular maintenance and calibration of aneroid manometers or electronic devices is required to ensure accuracy of readings.
Taking a blood pressure manually using an aneroid *sphygmomanometer*. The aneroid gauge must be recalibrated at least once each year and it must rest at zero.	
The cuff consists of an inflatable bladder inside a fabric cover. The width of the cuff should equal 40% of the circumference of the person's arm. The length of the bladder should equal 80% of this circumference.	Ill-fitting or wider cuffs deliver false low readings and narrow cuffs give a false high reading (Talley & O'Connor 2018).
Available cuffs include sizes that fit newborn infants to the extra-large adult. Thigh cuffs are also available and not to the person's age (Figure 10.12). Match the appropriate size cuff to the person's arm size and shape (Figure 8.11).	

PROCEDURES AND NORMAL FINDINGS	ABNORMAL FINDINGS AND CLINICAL ALERTS
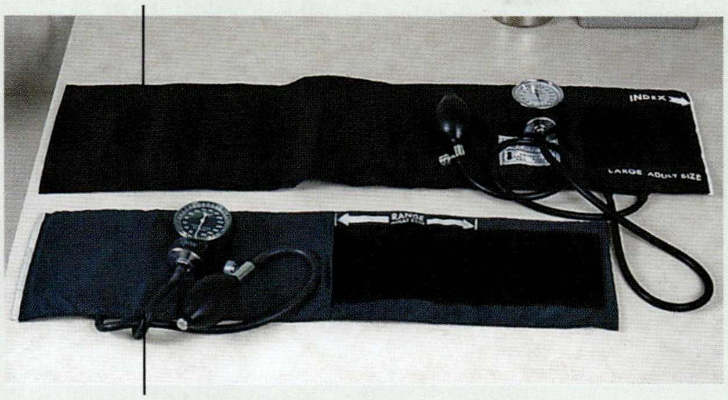 Thigh cuff or large arm cuff Standard adult arm cuff **Figure 10.12**	
A comfortable, relaxed person yields a valid blood pressure. Many people are anxious at the beginning of an examination; allow at least a 5-minutes rest before measuring the BP. Then take two or more BP measurements separated by 2 minutes.	
For each person, verify BP in both arms once, either on admission or for the first complete physical examination. It is not necessary to continue to check both arms for screening or monitoring.	Occasionally, a 5–10 mmHg difference may occur in BP in the two arms (if values are different, use the higher value) (Talley & O'Connor 2018). ***Clinical alert:*** If there is a significant discrepancy in the BP between the two arms, report this finding to a medical practitioner for further assessment as this may be a sign of aortic aneurysm.
The person may be sitting or lying, with the bare arm supported at heart level.	Wait up to 5 min before taking a blood pressure measurement following exertion or position change.
Palpate the brachial artery, which is located just above the antecubital fossa, medial to the biceps tendon. With the cuff deflated, centre it about 2.5 cm above the brachial artery and wrap it evenly and firmly around the arm.	
Now palpate the brachial or the radial artery (Figure 10.13). Inflate the cuff until the artery pulsation is obliterated and then 20–30 mmHg beyond. This will avoid missing an **auscultatory gap**, which is a period when Korotkoff sounds disappear during auscultation (Table 10.3). 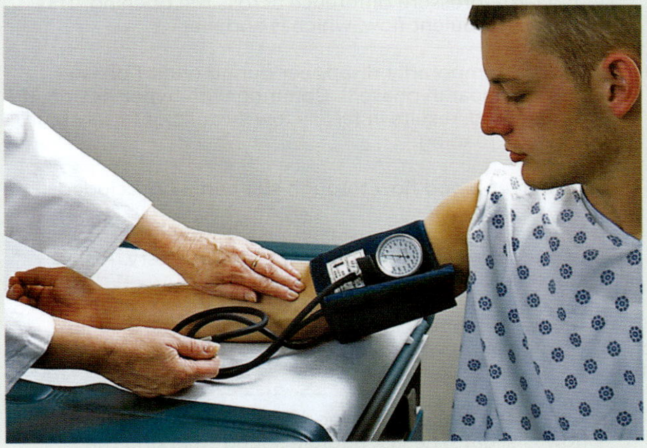 **Figure 10.13**	An auscultatory gap occurs in about 5% of people, most often in hypertension caused by a noncompliant arterial system.

OBJECTIVE DATA

PROCEDURES AND NORMAL FINDINGS	ABNORMAL FINDINGS AND CLINICAL ALERTS
Deflate the cuff quickly and completely; then wait 15 to 30 seconds before reinflating so that the blood trapped in the veins can dissipate. Place the bell of the stethoscope over the site of the brachial artery, making a light but airtight seal (Figure 10.14). The diaphragm endpiece is usually adequate, but the bell is designed to pick up low-pitched sounds such as the sounds of a blood pressure reading. So if you have a bell, use it. 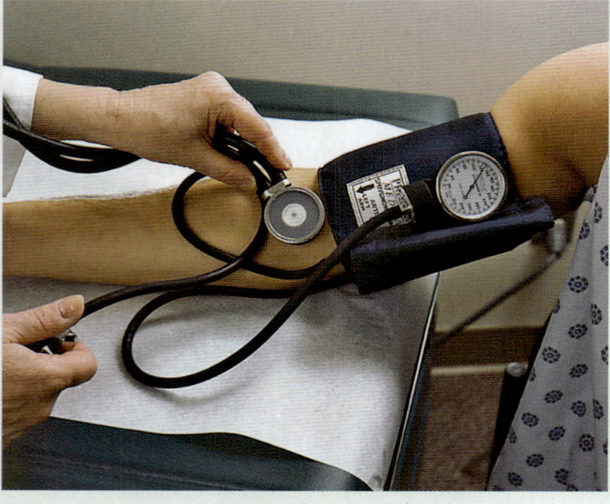 Figure 10.14	Blood pressure measurement is more accurate when using the bell rather than the diaphragm of the stethoscope.
Rapidly inflate the cuff to the maximal inflation level you determined via previous palpation. Then deflate the cuff slowly and evenly, about 2 mmHg per heartbeat. Note the points at which you hear the first appearance of sound, the muffling of sound and the final disappearance of sound. These are phases I, IV and V of **Korotkoff sounds**, which are the components of a BP reading first described by a Russian surgeon in 1905 (see Table 10.4).	

TABLE 10.4 Korotkoff sounds

PHASE	QUALITY	DESCRIPTION	RATIONALE
Cuff correctly inflated	No sound		Cuff inflation compresses brachial artery. Cuff pressure exceeds heart systolic pressure, occluding brachial artery blood flow.
I	Tapping	Soft, clear tapping, increasing in intensity	**Systolic pressure.** As cuff pressure lowers to reach intraluminal systolic pressure, artery opens, and blood first spurts into the brachial artery. Blood is at very high velocity because of the small opening of the artery and large pressure difference across the opening. This creates turbulent flow, which is audible.
Auscultatory gap	No sound	Silence for 30–40 mmHg during deflation; an abnormal finding	Sounds temporarily disappear during end of phase I and reappear in phase II. Common with hypertension. If undetected, results in falsely low systolic or falsely high diastolic reading.
II	Swooshing	Softer murmur follows tapping	Turbulent blood flow through still partially occluded artery.
III	Knocking	Crisp, high-pitched sounds	Longer duration of blood flow through artery. Artery closes just briefly during late diastole.
IV	Abrupt muffling	Sound mutes to a low-pitched, cushioned murmur; blowing quality	Artery no longer closes in any part of cardiac cycle. Change in quality, not intensity.
V	Silence		Decreased velocity of blood flow. Streamlined blood flow is silent. The last audible sound (marking the disappearance of sounds) is **diastolic** pressure. The fifth Korotkoff sound is now used to define diastolic pressure in all age groups.

PROCEDURES AND NORMAL FINDINGS	ABNORMAL FINDINGS AND CLINICAL ALERTS
For all age-groups, the fifth Korotkoff phase is used to define diastolic pressure. However, when a variance greater than 10 to 12 mmHg exists between phases IV and V, record *both* phases along with the systolic reading (e.g. 142/98/80). Clear communication is important because the results significantly affect diagnosis and planning of care. See Table 10.5 for a list of common errors in blood pressure measurement.	**Hypotension**, abnormally low BP; **hypertension**, abnormally high BP (see parameters in Table 10.6 below).

TABLE 10.5 Common errors in blood pressure measurement

COMMON ERROR	RESULT	RATIONALE
Taking blood pressure reading when person is anxious or angry or has just been active	Falsely high	Sympathetic nervous system stimulation
Faulty arm position:		
Above level of heart	Falsely low	Eliminates effect of hydrostatic pressure
Below level of heart	Falsely high	Additional force of gravity added to brachial artery pressure
Person supports own arm	Falsely high diastolic	Sustained isometric muscular contraction
Faulty leg position (e.g. person's legs are crossed)	Falsely high systolic and diastolic	Translocation of blood volume from dependent legs to thoracic area
Inaccurate cuff size (most common error):		
Cuff too narrow for extremity	Falsely high	Needs excessive pressure to occlude brachial artery
Cuff wrap is too loose or uneven, or bladder balloons out of wrap	Falsely high	Needs excessive pressure to occlude brachial artery
Failure to palpate radial artery while inflating:		
Inflating cuff not high enough	Falsely low systolic	Misses initial systolic tapping or may tune in during auscultatory gap (tapping sounds disappear for 10–40 mmHg and then return; common with hypertension)
Inflating cuff too high	Pain	
Pushing stethoscope too hard on brachial artery	Falsely low diastolic	Excessive pressure distorts artery, and sounds continue
Deflating cuff:		
Too quickly	Falsely low systolic or falsely high diastolic	Insufficient time to hear tapping
Too slowly	Falsely high diastolic	Venous congestion in forearm makes sounds less audible
Halting during descent and reinflating cuff to recheck systolic	Falsely high diastolic	Venous congestion in forearm
Failure to wait 1–2 min before repeating entire reading	Falsely high diastolic	Venous congestion in forearm
Any observer error:		
Examiner's 'subconscious bias'; a preconceived idea of what BP reading should be because of person's age, race, gender, weight, history or condition	Error anywhere	Never assume that, because a person appears healthy, their BP will be within normal limits
Examiner's haste		
Faulty technique		
Examiner's digit preference; 'hears' more results that end in zero than would occur by chance alone (e.g. 130/80) Diminished hearing acuity Defective or inaccurately calibrated equipment	Error anywhere	

OBJECTIVE DATA

PROCEDURES AND NORMAL FINDINGS	ABNORMAL FINDINGS AND CLINICAL ALERTS

TABLE 10.6 Abnormalities in blood pressure

HYPOTENSION

In normotensive adults: <95/60
In children: less than expected value for age

Occurs with	Rationale
Acute myocardial infarction	Decreased cardiac output
Shock	Decreased cardiac output
Haemorrhage	Decrease in total blood volume
Vasodilatation	Decrease in peripheral vascular resistance
Addison's disease (hypofunction of adrenal glands)	
As a side effect of treatment for hypertension	

Associated symptoms and signs

In conditions of decreased cardiac output, a low BP is accompanied by an increased pulse, dizziness, diaphoresis, confusion and blurred vision. The skin feels cool and clammy because the superficial blood vessels constrict to shunt blood to the vital organs.
Orthostatic hypotension (postural hypotension) occurs when a normotensive person develops symptoms of low blood pressure when changing from lying or sitting to a standing position. In this case, the blood pressure should be measured in both positions.

HYPERTENSION

Essential or primary hypertension

Essential or primary hypertension accounts for 95% of people with high blood pressure. Obesity, smoking, high salt and alcohol intake and sedentary lifestyle and continued exposure to high levels of stress are known contributing factors.

Secondary hypertension

Secondary hypertension has known causes such as renal disease, endocrine disorders, coarctation of the aorta and others, such use of oral contraceptives, amphetamines, increased intracranial pressure and pre-eclampsia in pregnancy.

CLASSIFICATION OF BLOOD PRESSURE IN ADULTS*

Diagnostic category	*Systolic (mmHg)*		*Diastolic (mmHg)*
Optimal	<120	and	<80
Normal	120–129	and/or	80–84
High normal	130–139	and/or	85–89
Grade 1 (mild) hypertension	140–159	and/or	90–99
Grade 2 (moderate) hypertension	160–179	and/or	100–109
Grade 3 (severe) hypertension	≥180	and/or	≥110
Isolated systolic hypertension	>140	And	<90

*when a person's systolic and diastolic blood pressure falls into different categories the higher diagnostic category applies

OBJECTIVE DATA

PROCEDURES AND NORMAL FINDINGS	ABNORMAL FINDINGS AND CLINICAL ALERTS
Electronic vital signs monitor	
An automated vital signs monitor is commonly used in hospital and clinic settings. The artery pulsations create vibrations that are detected by an electronic sensor. The BP mode is noninvasive and fast and has automatic measurement intervals and a bright numeric display. As with manual BP equipment, accuracy depends on correct cuff selection and placement. A stethoscope is not required when using an electronic blood pressure device. Most electronic BP devices also have probes for thermometry and pulse oximetry (Figure 10.15). 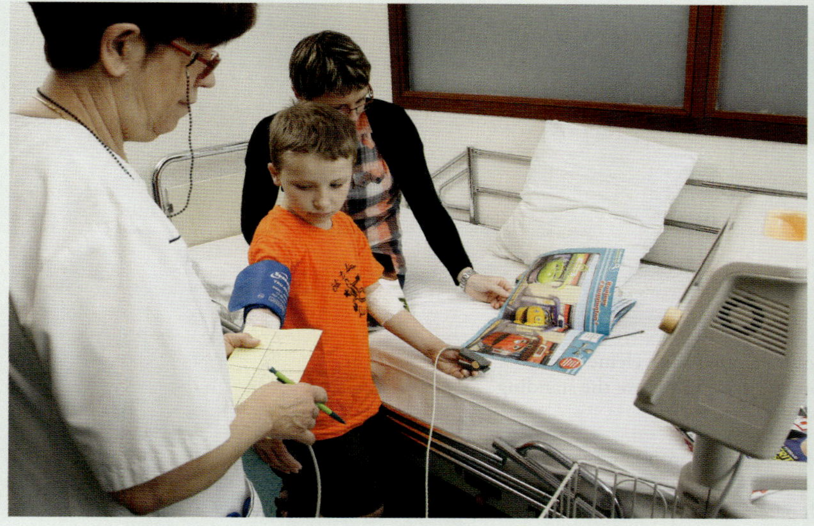 Figure 10.15	Electronic blood pressure devices are not capable of evaluating the quality of the pulse, i.e. force (strength) or rhythm. The device can be programmed to alarm should the blood pressure vary from desired limits. ***Clinical alert:*** The electronic BP monitor cannot sense vibrations of low BP; do not use it with a person who has a systolic BP of <90 mmHg or conditions of an irregular heart rate, shivering, tremors or seizures. If the numeric display does not fit with the person's clinical picture, always validate the measurement with a manual sphygmomanometer and your own stethoscope. Digital and aneroid devices have been found to be similarly accurate (Chong et al 2018).
Orthostatic (or postural) blood pressure measurement	
Take serial measurements of blood pressure: when you suspect • volume depletion; • when the person is known to have hypertension or is taking antihypertensive medications; or • when the person reports fainting (syncope). Have the person rest supine for 2 or 3 min, take baseline readings of BP, then repeat the measurements with the person sitting, then standing. For the person who is too weak or dizzy to stand, assess supine and then sitting with legs dangling. When the position is changed from supine to standing, normally a slight decrease (less than 10 mmHg) in systolic pressure may occur.	**Orthostatic hypotension**, a drop in systolic pressure of more than 20 mmHg. These changes are due to abrupt peripheral vasodilatation without a compensatory increase in cardiac output. Orthostatic changes also occur with prolonged bed rest, older age, hypovolaemia and some medications.
Document the BP on the vital signs chart. Also record the person's position and the arm used.	
Thigh pressure	
Thigh pressures are used when there are no other alternatives. If possible, turn the person into the prone position. (If the person must remain in the supine position, bend the knee slightly.) Wrap a large cuff, 18 to 20 cm, around the lower third of the thigh, centred over the popliteal artery on the back of the knee. Auscultate the popliteal artery for the reading (Figure 10.16). Normally, the systolic value is 10–40 mmHg higher in the thigh than in the arm, and the diastolic pressure ambiguous: 'is the same as normal' or 'is also 10–40 mmHg higher' ?	

OBJECTIVE DATA

PROCEDURES AND NORMAL FINDINGS	ABNORMAL FINDINGS AND CLINICAL ALERTS
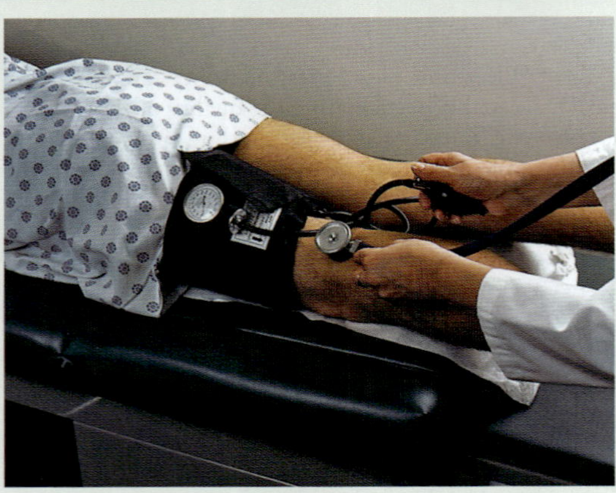 Figure 10.16	
Additional objective data for infants and children	
General survey	
Physical appearance, body structure, mobility—Note the same basic elements as with the adult, with consideration to age and development. Exceptions are the standing toddler who normally has a protuberant abdomen ('toddler lordosis').	
Behaviour—Note the response to stimuli and level of alertness appropriate for age.	
Parental bonding—Note the child's interactions with parents, that parent and child show a mutual response and are warm and affectionate, appropriate to the child's condition. The parent provides appropriate physical care of child and promotes new learning.	Some signs of child abuse are that the child avoids eye contact; the child exhibits no separation anxiety when you would expect it for age; the parent is disgusted by child's odour, sounds, drooling or stools. Deprivation of physical or emotional care (Chapter 5).
Measurement	
Weight. Weigh an infant on an electronic scale. Guard the baby so that they do not fall (Figure 10.17). Weigh to the nearest 10 g for infants and 100 g for toddlers. 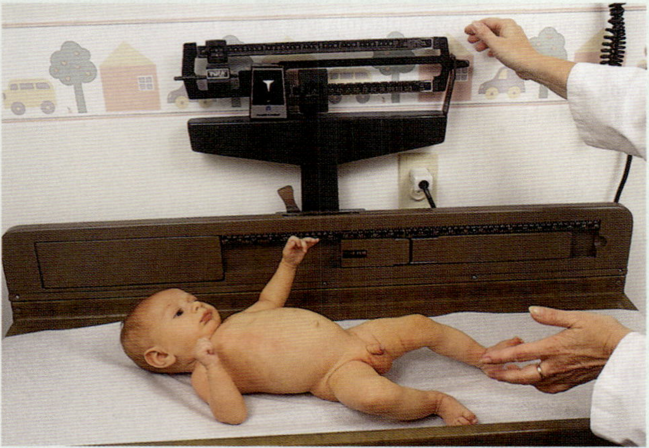 Figure 10.17	

OBJECTIVE DATA

PROCEDURES AND NORMAL FINDINGS	ABNORMAL FINDINGS AND CLINICAL ALERTS
By age 2 or 3 years, use the upright scale. Leave underpants on the child. Use the upright scale with preschoolers and school-age children, maintaining modesty with light clothing (Figure 10.18). 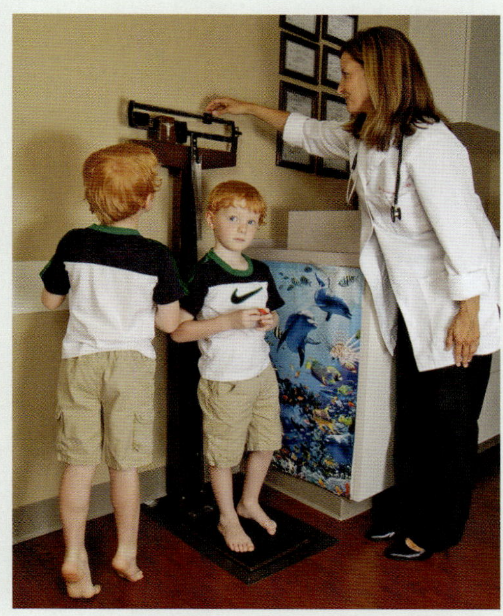 **Figure 10.18**	
Length. Until age 2 years, measure the infant's body length supine by using a horizontal measuring board (Figure 10.19). Hold the head in the midline. Because the infant normally has flexed legs, extend them momentarily by holding the knees together and pushing them down until the legs are flat on the table. Avoid using a tape measure along the infant's length because this is inaccurate. 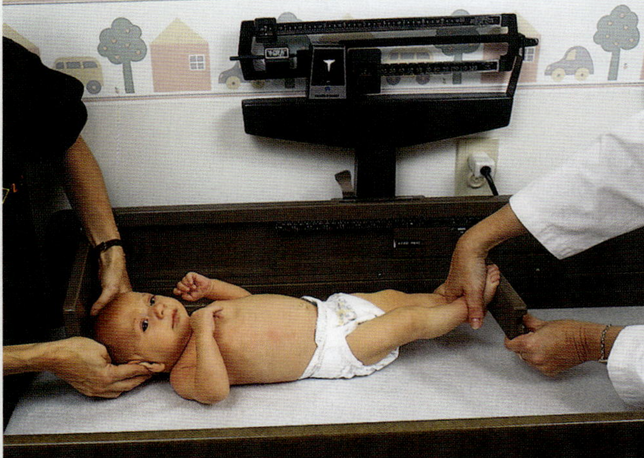 **Figure 10.19**	

PROCEDURES AND NORMAL FINDINGS	ABNORMAL FINDINGS AND CLINICAL ALERTS
For age 2 or 3 years, measure the child's height by standing the child against the pole on the platform scale (Figure 10.20) or back against a flat ruler taped to the wall. (Sometimes a child will stand more erect against the solid wall than against the narrow measuring pole on the scale.) Encourage the child to stand straight and tall and to look straight ahead without tilting the head. The shoulders, buttocks and heels should touch the wall. Hold a book or flat board on the child's head at a right angle to the wall. Mark just under the book, noting the measure to the nearest 1 mm. 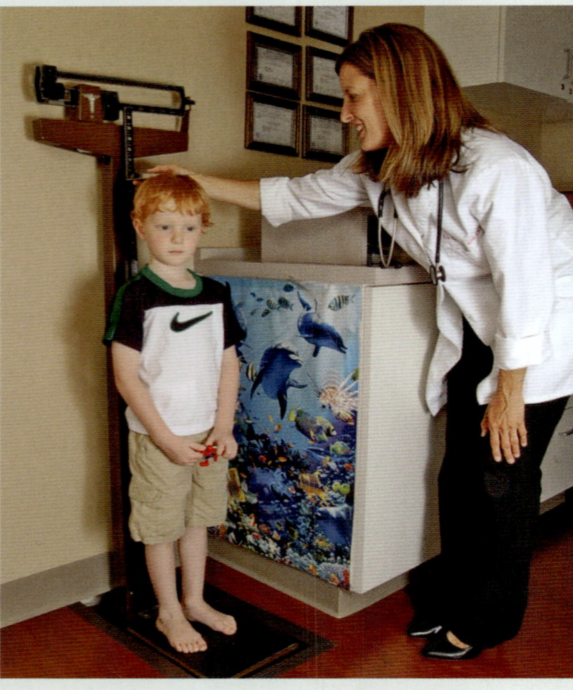 Figure 10.20	
Physical growth is perhaps the best index of a child's general health. The child's height and weight are recorded at every healthcare visit to determine normal growth patterns. The results are plotted on growth charts.	
Healthy childhood growth is continuous but uneven, with rapid growth spurts occurring during infancy and adolescence. Results are more reliable when comparing numerous growth measures over a long time. These charts also compare the individual child's measurements against the general population. Normal limits range from the 5th to the 95th percentile on the standardised charts.	
Use your judgement and consider the ethnic background of the small-for-age child. Explore the growth patterns of the parents and siblings. Be aware that the statistical averages for Australia are based on US charts which are based on norms for Caucasian children and may not necessarily generalise to other ethnic groups.	Further explore any growth measure that: • Falls below the 5th or above the 95th percentile • Shows a wide percentile difference between height and weight—e.g. a 10th percentile height with a 95th percentile weight • Shows that growth has suddenly stopped when it had been steady • Fails to show normal growth spurts during infancy and adolescence.

OBJECTIVE DATA

PROCEDURES AND NORMAL FINDINGS	ABNORMAL FINDINGS AND CLINICAL ALERTS
Head circumference. Measure the infant's head circumference at birth and at each well child visit up to age 2 years and then yearly up to 6 years (Figure 10.21). Circle the tape around the head at the prominent frontal and occipital bones; the widest span is correct. Plot the measurement on standardised growth charts. Compare the infant's head size with that expected for age. A series of measurements is more valuable than a single figure to show the *rate* of head growth. 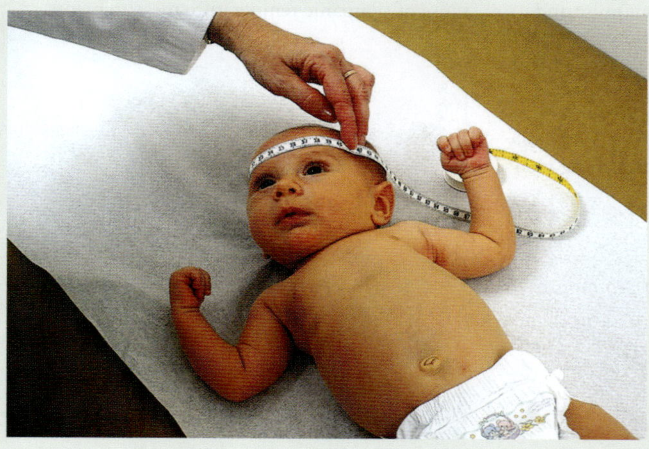 Figure 10.21	
The newborn's head measures about 32–38 cm (average about 34 cm) and is about 2 cm larger than the chest circumference. The chest grows at a faster rate than the cranium; at some time between 6 months and 2 years, both measurements are about the same, and after age 2 years the chest circumference is greater than the head circumference.	Enlarged head circumference occurs with increased intracranial pressure (Chapter 12).
Measurement of the chest circumference is valuable in comparison with the head circumference, but not necessarily by itself. Encircle the tape around the chest at the nipple line. It should be snug, but not so tight that it leaves a mark (Figure 10.22). 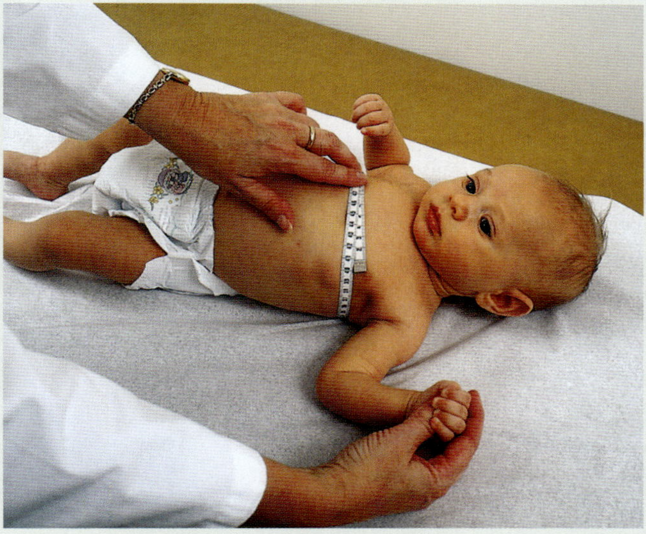 Figure 10.22	

OBJECTIVE DATA

PROCEDURES AND NORMAL FINDINGS	ABNORMAL FINDINGS AND CLINICAL ALERTS
Vital signs	
When taking a child or infant's vital signs, where appropriate ask the parent to assist. The infant or child should be positioned correctly and comfortably prior to and during the procedure.	
Measure vital signs with the same purpose and frequency as you would in an adult. With an *infant*, reverse the order of vital sign measurement to respiration, pulse and temperature. For infants under 3 months of age, take the temperature at the inguinal or axilla sites. For older children take a tympanic, inguinal or axillary temperature. The tympanic temperature measurement is so rapid that it is usually over before the child realises it. Promote the cooperation of the *school-age child* by explaining the procedure completely and encouraging the child to handle the equipment. Your approach to measuring vital signs with the *adolescent* is much the same as with the adult.	Infants must be more than 3 months of age for use of tympanic temperature measurements.
Temperature	
Tympanic. Temperature measurements are commonly used for children >3 months of age (see Figure 10.23). Figure 10.23	Up to ages 6–8 years, children have higher fevers with illness than adults do. Even with minor infections, fevers may elevate to 39.5°C to 40.5°C.
Axillary. The axillary route is safe and accessible and is used for infants <3 months of age. When cold receptors are stimulated, brown fat tissue in the area releases heat through chemical energy, which artificially raises skin temperature. When the axillary route is used, place the tip well into the axilla, and hold the child's arm close to the body.	Oral and rectal routes should not be routinely used to measure the body temperature in children aged from 0 to 5.
Inguinal. The inguinal route is also safe for measuring a child's body temperature. Its results may be closer to core temperature than the axillary site because the inguinal area has a rich supply of blood vessels, it lacks the brown fat tissue that interferes with axillary temperatures and you can form a tight skin-to-skin seal. Abduct the infant's leg and locate the femoral pulse. Place the thermometer probe lateral to the pulse site, and adduct the leg to create a seal.	
Oral. This route may also be used for the child who is old enough to keep the mouth closed. This is usually at age 5 or 6 years, although some 4-year-old children can cooperate.	
Rectal. Use this route with neonates only if a fever is firstly demonstrated by axillary temperature (Royal Children's Hospital 2018). An infant may be supine or side lying, with the examiner's hand flexing the knees up onto the abdomen. An infant also may lie prone across the adult's lap. Separate the buttocks with one hand, and insert the lubricated electronic rectal probe *no further than* 2.5 cm. Any deeper insertion risks rectal perforation because the colon curves posteriorly at 3 cm.	

PROCEDURES AND NORMAL FINDINGS	ABNORMAL FINDINGS AND CLINICAL ALERTS
Normally, rectal temperatures measure higher in infants and young children than in adults, with an average of 37.8°C at 18 months.	
Heart rate	
Palpate or auscultate an apical heart rate with infants and toddlers (see Chapter 17 for location of apex and technique). In children older than 2 years, use the radial site. Count the heart rate for a full minute to take into account normal irregularities, such as sinus arrhythmia. The heart rate normally fluctuates more with infants and children than with adults in response to exercise, emotion and illness.	
Respirations	
Infants and children under 6–7 years are predominantly abdominal breathers. Watch the abdomen for movement, because the respirations are normally more diaphragmatic than thoracic (Figure 10.24). Count a full minute because the pattern varies significantly from rapid breaths to short periods of apnoea. Note the normal rate in Table 10.3. 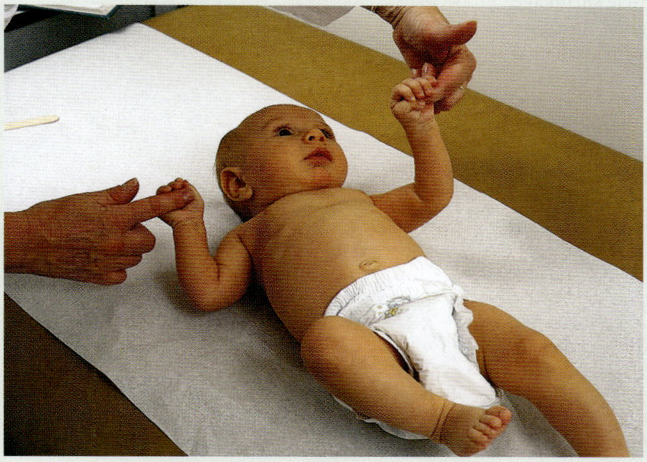 **Figure 10.24**	
Blood pressure	
In children aged 3 years and older and in younger children at risk, measure a routine BP at least annually. For accurate measurement in children, make some adjustment in the choice of equipment and technique. The correct size cuff width must cover two-thirds of the upper arm, and the cuff bladder must completely encircle it.	When it is not possible to use the arm for blood pressure measurement in infants, the lower leg can be used. Crying, eating or sucking can influence blood pressure measurements and should be noted at the time of measurement.
Use a paediatric-sized endpiece on the stethoscope to locate the Koritkoff sounds. If possible, allow a crying infant to become quiet for 5–10 min before measuring the BP; crying may elevate the systolic pressure by 30–50 mmHg. Use the disappearance of sound (phase V Korotkoff) for the diastolic reading in children. Note the guidelines for BP standards based on sex, age and height. These standards give a more precise classification of BP according to body size and avoid misclassifying children who are very tall or very short.	Further explore any blood pressure that is greater than the 95th percentile and refer for diagnostic evaluation.
Children under 3 years of age have such small arm vessels that it is difficult to hear Korotkoff sounds with a stethoscope. Instead, use an electronic BP device which gives a digital readout for systolic and, diastolic blood pressure and heart rate. Or use a *Doppler* ultrasound device to amplify the sounds. This instrument is easy to use and can be used by one examiner. (Note the technique for using the Doppler device; see Figure 10.26 below.)	

PROCEDURES AND NORMAL FINDINGS	ABNORMAL FINDINGS AND CLINICAL ALERTS
Additional objective data for the adult over 65 years	
General survey	
Physical appearance—By the 8th and 9th decades, body contour is sharper, with more angular facial features, and body proportions are redistributed. (See measuring weight and height, above.)	
Posture—A general flexion occurs by the 8th or 9th decade.	
Gait—Older adults often use a wider base to compensate for diminished balance, arms may be held out to help balance and steps may be shorter or uneven.	
Measurement	
Weight. The person over 65 years appears sharper in contour with more prominent bony landmarks than the younger adult. Body weight decreases during the 80s and 90s. This factor is more evident in males, perhaps because of greater muscle shrinkage. The distribution of fat also changes during the 80s and 90s. Even with good nutrition, subcutaneous fat is lost from the face and periphery (especially the forearms), whereas additional fat is deposited on the abdomen and hips.	Obesity can continue into later adult life.
Height. By the 80s and 90s, many people are shorter than they were in their 70s. This results from shortening in the spinal column from thinning of the vertebral discs and shortening of the individual vertebrae and from the postural changes of kyphosis and slight flexion in the knees and hips. Because long bones do not shorten with age, the overall body proportion looks different—a shorter trunk with relatively long extremities.	
Vital signs	
Temperature. Changes in the body's temperature regulatory mechanism leave the person over 65 less likely to have fever but at a greater risk for hypothermia and hyperthermia. Thus the temperature is a less reliable indicator of the older person's true health state. Sweat gland activity is also diminished.	
Heart rate. The normal range of heart rate is 60 to 100 bpm, but the rhythm may be slightly irregular. The radial artery may feel stiff, rigid and tortuous in an older person, although this condition does not necessarily imply vascular disease in the heart or brain. The increasingly rigid arterial wall needs a faster upstroke of blood, so the pulse is actually easier to palpate.	
Respirations. Ageing causes a decrease in vital capacity (the maximum of air the person can expel from the lungs after a maximum inhalation) and a decreased inspiratory reserve volume (the additional amount of air that can be inhaled after a normal inspiration). You may note a shallower inspiratory phase and an increased respiratory rate.	
Blood pressure. The aorta and major arteries tend to harden with age. As the heart pumps against a stiffer aorta, the systolic pressure increases, leading to a widened pulse pressure (see Figure 10.12 for mean BP readings in apparently healthy persons from birth to old age).	
Additional techniques	
Measurement of oxygen saturation	
The **pulse oximeter** is a noninvasive method to assess arterial oxygen saturation (SpO_2). A sensor attached to the person's finger or earlobe has a diode that emits light and a detector that measures the relative amount of light absorbed by oxyhaemoglobin (HbO_2) and deoxygenated (reduced) haemoglobin (Hb). The pulse oximeter compares the ratio of light emitted to light absorbed and converts this ratio into the percentage of oxygen saturation. Because it only measures light absorption of pulsatile flow, the result is arterial oxygen saturation. A healthy person with no lung disease and no anaemia normally has an SpO_2 of 95–100%.	***Clinical alert:*** SpO_2 reading less than 97% requires immediate further investigation. Please note that SpO_2 readings are an approximation of the person's oxygen saturation which can only be accurately measured by arterial blood gas.
Select the appropriate pulse oximeter probe. The finger probe is spring loaded and feels like a clothespin attached to the finger but does not hurt (Figure 10.25)	Nails painted with either brown or black polish or those that have nail extensions may affect results.

OBJECTIVE DATA

PROCEDURES AND NORMAL FINDINGS	ABNORMAL FINDINGS AND CLINICAL ALERTS
Figure 10.25	
An infant has a probe taped to the large toe. Some clinics use single-use probes that stick to the finger or ear instead of the multipatient-use spring-loaded model. If you are using a finger, make sure that the hand is warm to prevent false low readings caused by vasoconstriction. At lower oxygen saturations, the earlobe probe is more accurate. The probe will show both the oxygen saturation and the heart rate. Make sure that the heart rate reading you see on the pulse oximeter matches the palpated heart rate. If it does not correlate with the palpated heart rate, question the accuracy of the result. If this occurs reposition the probe and repeat.	
The Doppler technique	
In many situations, pulse and BP measurement are enhanced by using an electronic device, the *Doppler ultrasonic flowmeter*. Sound varies in pitch in relation to the distance between the sound source and the listener; the pitch is higher when the distance is small, and the pitch lowers as the distance increases. Think of a railway train speeding towards you; its train whistle sounds higher the closer it gets, and the pitch of the whistle lowers as the train fades away.	
In this case, the sound source is the blood pumping through the artery in a rhythmic manner. A handheld transducer picks up changes in sound frequency as the blood flows and ebbs and it amplifies them. The listener hears a whooshing pulsatile beat.	
The Doppler technique is used to locate the peripheral pulse sites (see Chapter 16 for further discussion of this technique). For BP measurement, the Doppler technique will augment Korotkoff sounds (Figure 10.26). Through this technique, you can evaluate sounds that are hard to hear with a stethoscope, such as those in critically ill individuals with a low BP, in infants with small arms and in obese persons in whom the sounds are muffled by layers of fat. Also, proper cuff placement is difficult on the obese person's cone-shaped upper arm. In this situation, you can place the cuff on the more even forearm and hold the Doppler probe over the radial artery. For either location, use the following procedure: Figure 10.26	
• Apply coupling gel to the transducer probe.	
• Turn Doppler flowmeter on.	
• Touch the probe to the skin, holding the probe perpendicular to the artery.	

OBJECTIVE DATA

PROCEDURES AND NORMAL FINDINGS	ABNORMAL FINDINGS AND CLINICAL ALERTS
• A pulsatile whooshing sound indicates location of the artery. You may need to rotate the probe, but maintain contact with the skin. Do not push the probe too hard or you will wipe out the pulse.	
• Inflate the cuff until the sounds disappear; then proceed another 20–30 mmHg beyond that point.	
• Slowly deflate the cuff, noting the point at which the first whooshing sounds appear. This is the systolic pressure.	
• It is difficult to hear the muffling of sounds or a reliable disappearance of sounds indicating the diastolic pressure (phases IV and V of Korotkoff sounds). However, the systolic pressure alone gives valuable data on the level of tissue perfusion and on blood flow through patent vessels.	

BIBLIOGRAPHY

Allan J. Monitoring a pulse in adults. Br J Nurs v 2018;27(21): 1237–39.

Australian Bureau of Statistics (ABS). Hypertension and measured high blood pressure. 2019. Available at: https://www.abs.gov.au/ausstats/abs@.nsf/Lookup/by%20Subject/4364.0.55.001~2017-18~Main%20Features~Hypertension%20and%20measured%20high%20blood%20pressure~60.

Australian Commission on Safety and Quality in Health Care (ACSQHC). Observation and response charts. 2019. Available at: https://www.safetyandquality.gov.au/our-work/recognising-and-responding-to-clinical-deterioration/observation-and-response-charts/.

Australian Government Department of Health. Healthy weight guide. 2019. Available at: http://healthyweight.health.gov.au/wps/portal/Home/home/!ut/p/a1/04_Sj9CPykssy0xPLMnMz0vMAfGjzOI9jFxdDY1MDD3dzbycDTzNLfwsfP2AAsbGQAWRQAUGOICjASH94fpRYCXO7o4eJuYQD0mFkYGni5OHi7mlr4GBp5mUAV4rCjIjTDIdFRUBADr1DFv/dl5/d5/L2dBISEvZ0FBIS9nQSEh/.

Cardona-Morrell M, Prgomet M, Lake R, et al. Vital signs monitoring and nurse–patient interaction: a qualitative observational study of hospital practice. Int J Nurs Stud 2016;56:9–16.

Chong JY, Quek ZL, Thanapalan D, et al. Comparison between mercury manometer, digital device and aneroid device in blood pressure measurements. Public Health Prevent Med 2018;4(2):35–43.

Esler D. Hypertension: high prevalence and a positive association with obesity among Aboriginal and Torres Strait Islander youth in far north Queensland. Aust N Z J Public Health 2016;40(S1):S65–9.

Flenady T, Dwyer T, Applegarth J. Accurate respiratory rates count: So should you! Australas Emerg Nurs J 2017;20:45–7.

Heart Foundation. Is my blood pressure normal? 2019. Available at: https://www.heartfoundation.org.au/your-heart/know-your-risks/blood-pressure/is-my-blood-pressure-normal.

Hockenberry MJ, Wilson D (eds). Wong's nursing care of infants and children. 11th ed. Edinburgh: Elsevier; 2018.

Kallioinen N, Hill A, Horswill MS, et al. Sources of inaccuracy in the measurement of adult patients' resting blood pressure in clinical settings: a systematic review. J Hypertens 2017;35(3):421–41.

Kellett J, Sebat F. Make vital signs great again – a call for action. Eur J Intern Med 2017;45:13–19.

Knecht K, Seller J, Alpert B. Korotkoff sounds in neonates, infants, and toddlers. Am J Cardiol 2009;103(8):1165–7.

Lambe K, Currey J, Considine J. Frequency of vital sign assessment and clinical deterioration in an Australian Emergency Department. Australas Emerg Nurs J 2016;19: 217–22.

Milutinovic D, Repic G, Arandelovic B. Clinical nurses' knowledge level on pulse oximetry: a descriptive multi-centre study. Intensive Crit Care Nurs 2016;37:19–26.

Minzola DJ, Keele R. Relationship of tympanic and temporal temperature modalities to core temperature in pediatric surgical patient. AANA Journal 2018;86(1):19–26.

Ministry of Health New Zealand. Annual update of key findings 2017/18: New Zealand health survey. Wellington: Ministry of Health; 2019. Available at: https://www.health.govt.nz/publication/annual-update-key-results-2016-17-new-zealand-health-survey.

Ministry of Health New Zealand. Tier 1 statistics 2017/18: New Zealand health survey. Available at: https://www.health.govt.nz/publication/tier-1-statistics-2017-18-new-zealand-health-survey.

Ministry of Health New Zealand. High blood pressure, nd. Available at: www.moh.govt.nz/notebook/nbbooks.nsf/0/b5deda9a12dace3b4c25677d00720599/$FILE/ttp_c4.pdf, https://www.cdc.gov/growthcharts/.

Muntner P, Shimbo D, Carey RM, et al. Measurement of blood pressure in humans: a scientific statement from the American Heart Association. Hypertension 2019;73(5):e35–66.

National Health and Medical Research Council/Ministry of Health New Zealand. Nutrient reference values for Australia and New Zealand. 2014. Available at: www.nrv.gov.au.

National Heart Foundation of Australia. Guideline for the diagnosis and management of hypertension in adults – 2016. Melbourne: National Heart Foundation of Australia; 2016. Available at: https://www.heartfoundation.org.au/images/uploads/publications/PRO-167_Hypertension-guideline-2016_WEB.pdf.

Oguz F, Yildiz I, Varkal MA, et al. Axillary and tympanic temperature measurement in children and normal values for ages. Pediatr Emerg Care 2018;34(3):169–73.

Osborne S, Douglas C, Reid C, et al.; RBWH Patient Assessment Research Council. The primacy of vital signs – acute care nurses'

OBJECTIVE DATA

and midwives' use of physical assessment skills: a cross sectional study. Int J Nurs Stud 2015;52(5):951–62.

Royal Children's Hospital. Clinical practice guideline on the febrile child. Melbourne, Australia: RCH; 2018. Available at: https://www.rch.org.au/clinicalguide/guideline_index/Febrile_child/.

Stergiou G. Accuracy of automated blood pressure measurement in children. Hypertension 2017;69(6):1000–6.

Talley NJ, O'Connor S. Clinical examination. 8th ed. Chatswood, NSW: Elsevier; 2018.

Tanner RM. White-coat effect among older adults: data from the Jackson heart study. J Clin Hypertens 2016;18(2):139-45.

Türe E, Yazar A. How should we measure body temperature in the pediatric emergency department? Which one is the most accurate? Pediatr Infect Dis J 2019;14(03):121–6.

Wang Z, Knight S, Wilson A, et al. Blood pressure and hypertension for Australian Aboriginal and Torres Strait Islander people. Eur J Cardiovasc Prev Rehabil 2006;13(3):438–43.

Weheida S, Mohammed E, Aly M. Blood pressure measurements: factors affecting readings accuracy. Nurs Health Sci 2017;6(5): 71–86.

World Health Organization (WHO). BMI classification.2018. Available at: http://apps.who.int/bmi/index.jsp?introPage=intro_3.html.

World Health Organization (WHO). Growth reference 5–19 years. 2019. Available at: http://www.who.int/growthref/who2007_bmi_for_age/en/.

Unit 3

Assessing mental health, neurological and sensory function

Chapter Eleven
Mental health assessment

Adapted by Rebecca Corbett

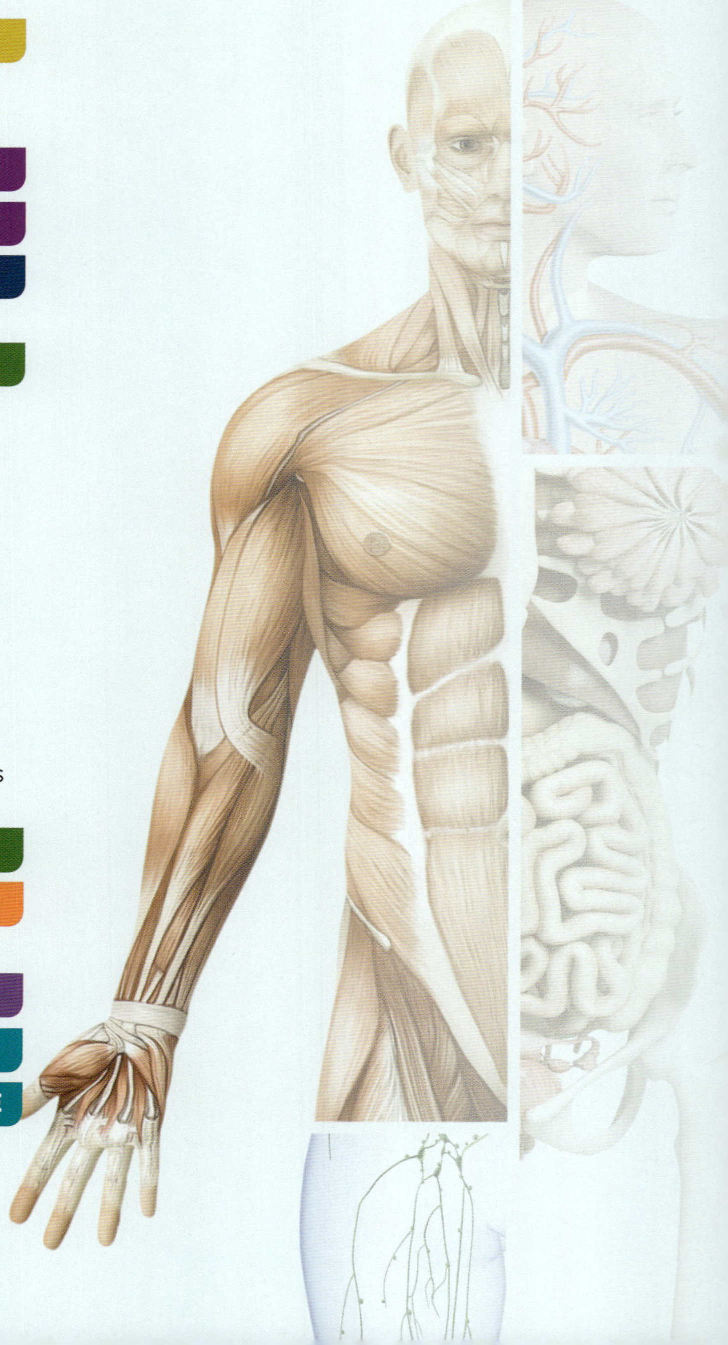

INTRODUCTION

When considering the background issues related to mental health assessment you may need to review the anatomy and physiology related to neurological assessment which is detailed in Chapter 12. In this chapter (Chapter 11), the relevant terms related to mental status assessment are defined. Mental illness presents one of the five greatest burdens of disease worldwide, with some authors more recently arguing mental illness may even be the greatest global burden of disease in terms of years lived with disability (Vigo et al 2016). One in five (20%) of Australians aged 16–85 years meet the diagnostic criteria for a high prevalence (common) mental disorder such as anxiety disorder, depression and substance use disorder in any given year (Australian Institute of Health and Welfare (AIHW) 2020). Approximately 3% of the population meet the criteria for a less common but high impact mental disorder with such as schizophrenia, schizo-affective disorder, severe depression and bipolar disorder (AIHW 2020). Age of onset for mental illness is usually between 15 and 25 years, and 1 in 7 (14%) of children aged 4–17 years meet the diagnostic criteria for a mental health disorder (Lawrence et al 2015). This has significant developmental and functional implications for study, work, relationships and the emerging sense of self. People with mental illnesses are over-represented in the healthcare system, as co-occurring physical and mental health disorders are common (Harris et al 2018).

Mental illness increases the likelihood of physical illness, which in turn can contribute to poor mental health (AIHW 2019, Harris et al 2018). Mental illness will often also present with physical symptoms such as tiredness, palpitations, gastrointestinal upset or lack of appetite—this is because the mind and body are interrelated and function in unison. People with serious mental illness are also more likely to smoke tobacco, have a poor diet, live a sedentary lifestyle and live in poverty, but are less likely to seek out health services than the general population (AIHW 2018a). This lack of help seeking is often due to stigma experienced from healthcare providers; whereby those with a mental illness are treated differently, thereby experiencing shame and embarrassment when seeking help. Diagnostic overshadowing also frequently occurs in emergency departments and primary health settings where the person with a diagnosed mental illness will be assessed and treated for their mental health issues, not the physical health issues they have presented with (Australian Commission on Safety and Quality in Health Care (ACSQHC) 2018). Those with serious mental illness therefore have up to 30% shorter life expectancy than the general population. This is largely due to untreated or poorly managed health conditions such as diabetes and cardiovascular disease, complicated by long-term treatment with psychotropic medications (AIHW 2018b).

There has been significant social change in the way people experiencing a mental illness are viewed and treated in the Australian healthcare setting in recent years (Commonwealth of Australia 2017). The consumer movement, which is a social and political movement representing the rights and views of those with mental illness, has demanded that treatment approaches change to reflect inclusive, respectful, person-centred care (ACSQHC 2018). Contemporary mental healthcare across the world now promotes the consumer as expert in their own recovery journey, and does not assume that symptom control is the primary treatment goal (Australian Government, National Mental Health Commission 2017). The aim of mental health assessment is to identify cognitive, behavioural, mental and physical conditions, issues and risks of harm to the person as well as the identification of circumstances that may impact these risks.

Structure and function

DEFINING MENTAL STATUS

Mental status is a measure of a person's emotional, psychological and behavioural functioning. Mental health and wellbeing are more than just the absence of illness. Mental health can mean life satisfaction through the achievement of one's potential in work, in caring relationships, in society and within the self. Mental health is relative and ongoing. This means it impacts and is impacted by internal and external stressors. Everyone has 'good' and 'bad' days. Mentally well people display resilience in the face of adversity, having the capacity to attribute meaning to difficult life events and restore a sense of balance. Coping strategies, connectedness to others, help seeking and meaningful engagement in work/study and community all contribute to psychological resilience (Graber et al 2015).

The stress surrounding a traumatic life event such as the death of a loved one or serious illness may disrupt the balance, causing transient dysfunction. Mental status assessment during a traumatic life event can identify remaining strengths and help the individual mobilise resources and use coping skills. It would be normal to identify disruption to mental status during and after a traumatic life event. Most people will begin to recover their previously experienced levels of functioning from trauma within approximately 4 weeks (American Psychiatric Association (APA) 2013) and grief within a period of 12 months (6 months for children) (APA 2013). Poverty, exposure to violence, sexual abuse, problematic substance use, lack of social support, parental mental illness, chronic health issues and lack of education all impact on mental health and recovery including trauma and grief.

A **mental disorder** is apparent when a person's response is much greater than the expected reaction to a traumatic life event such as being diagnosed with a serious illness, or when the person does not begin to show signs of recovery/return to functioning. A mental disorder is defined as a significant behavioural or psychological *pattern* that is associated with distress such as a painful symptom or disability affecting function, and which has a significant risk of pain, disability or death or a loss of freedom (APA 2013). Mental disorders include:

- **organic disorders** due to brain disease of *known* specific organic cause (delirium, dementia, intoxication and withdrawal) and;
- **psychiatric mental illness** in which organic aetiology has not yet been established (anxiety disorder or schizophrenia).

THE LANGUAGE OF MENTAL HEALTH ASSESSMENT

Most aspects of mental status cannot be scrutinised directly like the characteristics of skin or heart sounds. Its functioning is inferred through assessment of an individual's responses and behaviours.

Consciousness: being aware of one's own existence, feelings and thoughts and aware of the environment. It also describes the level of wakefulness in the individual. This is the most elementary of mental status functions which can be objectively assessed using the Glasgow Coma Scale (see Chapter 12).

Language: using the voice to communicate one's thoughts and feelings. This is a basic tool of humans and its loss has a heavy social impact on the individual. Language is the direct medium through which thoughts are expressed and thereby assessed. Language formation is also a highly complex cognitive function and its impairment is a key early indicator of many neurological as well as psychiatric conditions. The absence or delay of language development in children is a strong indicator of an underlying condition or may be due to trauma in the child's environment.

Mood and affect: both of these elements deal with the prevailing emotions; **affect** is a temporary expression of feelings—it is visible to the assessor in the form of facial expressions and expressed emotions—and **mood** is pervasive over time (weeks rather than days)—how the person feels internally—and is not always visible to the assessor.

Orientation: the awareness of the objective world in relation to the self, specifically time, place and person.

Attention: the power of concentration, the ability to focus on one specific thing without being distracted by many environmental or internal stimuli.

Memory: the ability to lay down and store experiences and perceptions for later recall. *Recent* memory evokes day-to-day events; *remote* memory brings up years' worth of experiences.

Abstract reasoning: pondering a deeper meaning beyond the concrete and literal. Abstract reasoning ability will give some cues to level of intelligence.

Thought process: the *way* a person thinks; the formation, sequence, relatedness, speed, availability and logic of thoughts.

Thought content: *what* the person thinks—specific ideas, beliefs, fears, preoccupations and the use of words.

Perceptions: what the person perceives in the environment through the senses and through their body as a whole.

DEVELOPMENTAL CONSIDERATIONS

Infants and children

The maturation of emotional and cognitive functioning is described in detail in Chapter 3. It is difficult to separate and trace the development of just one aspect of mental status. All aspects are interdependent. For example, consciousness is rudimentary at birth because the cerebral cortex is not yet developed; the infant cannot distinguish the self from the mother's body. Consciousness gradually develops along with language, so that by 18 to 24 months the child learns that it is separate from objects in the environment and has words to express this. We can also trace language development: from the differentiated crying at 4 weeks, the cooing at 6 weeks, through one-word sentences at 1 year to multi-word sentences at 2 years. Yet the concept of language as a social tool of communication occurs at around 4 to 5 years of age, coinciding with the child's readiness to play cooperatively with other children.

Attention gradually increases in span through preschool years so that, by school age, most children are able to sit and concentrate on their work for a period of time. Some children are late in developing concentration. School readiness coincides with the development of the thought process; around age 7, thinking becomes more logical and systematic, and the child is able to reason and understand. Abstract thinking, the ability to consider a hypothetical situation, usually develops between ages 12 and 15, although a few adolescents never achieve it. Healthy physical, psychological, emotional and social development is all dependent on the formation of trusting attachments with parents or caregivers (Goldberg et al 2009). Where there has been trauma, physical or sexual abuse or neglect in the child's environment there will be a disruption to development. Prolonged physical illness can also affect a child's mental health. This may present itself in many ways in the healthcare setting; possibly in regressed, sexualised or angry behaviour, developmental delay, excessive fear, passivity or clinginess. Should you observe any unusual behaviour while assessing children and young people, a further enquiry is warranted. Childhood trauma is a strong precursor to the development of mental disorders. Perinatal issues such as physical illness, mental illness, birth trauma and stress can also affect the mental health and psychological development of a child. It is pertinent to ask some basic screening questions of parents about pregnancy, childbirth and maternal and paternal mental health after birth when assessing a child. This information can be documented in the clinical history and will be very helpful should further psychiatric assessment be required.

Family history of mental illness and the nature and disposition of the child are important factors to assess for and document. Shy, sensitive, easily distressed children are more likely to develop depression and anxiety. Most childhood mental illness will first manifest as anxiety. Mood and anxiety disorders also commonly occur with other health and medical conditions, including asthma, insulin resistance and other chronic medical conditions and might affect treatment adherence for these conditions (Sztein & Lane 2016).

Late adulthood (65+ years)

The ageing process leaves the parameters of mental status mostly intact. There is no decrease in general knowledge and little or no loss in vocabulary. Response time is slower than in youth; it takes a bit longer for the brain to process information and react to it. Thus performance on timed intelligence tests may be lower for the ageing person—not because intelligence has declined, but because it takes longer to respond to the questions. The slower response time affects new learning; if a new presentation is rapidly paced, the older person does not have time to respond to it later.

Recent memory, which requires some processing (e.g. medication instructions, 24-hr diet recall, names of new acquaintances), is somewhat decreased with ageing. Remote memory is not affected (see Chapter 12).

Age-related changes in sensory perception can affect mental status. For example, vision loss may result in apathy, social isolation and depression (see Chapter 14). Hearing changes are common in older adults (see the discussion of presbycusis in Chapter 15). Age-related hearing loss involves high frequencies of sound. Consonants are high-frequency sounds, so older people who have difficulty hearing them have problems with normal conversation. This problem produces frustration, suspicion and social isolation and also makes the person look confused.

Older adults, if physically well, are generally happy and satisfied with their lives compared to the general population. It should not be assumed that it is normal for older adults to be depressed. Mental health concerns in older people should be assessed and treated. The era of older adulthood contains more potential for loss than do earlier eras, such as loss of loved ones, loss of job status and prestige, loss of income and the loss of an energetic and resilient body. The grief and despair surrounding these losses can affect mental health. These losses can result in disorientation, disability or depression. Depression is highly treatable in all ages, and if detected in the older person, the nurse may need to take a strong advocacy position in order for them to be correctly treated. Adults over the age of 85 years have a higher suicide rate than the general population; this is particularly so for males. While the prevalence of depression occurring in older adults is decreasing, aetiology can be attributed to many complex reasons, including loneliness, social isolation and physical health issues (AIHW 2018a). It is therefore very important that the nurse screens for mental illness in older adults, as there will often not be a previous history.

CULTURAL AND SOCIAL CONSIDERATIONS

There is a significant correlation with the development of mental health issues with specific cultural groups and social circumstances within the Australian and New Zealand communities. Refer to Chapter 4 for in-depth discussion of these issues. Different cultural groups have their own explanatory models of health and illness, and their own accepted cultural practices with regards to interacting with health professionals. Mental illness can be poorly understood and stigmatised in many cultural groups; which in turn may negatively impact the help-seeking behaviours of those suffering distressing symptoms. In particular, Aboriginal and Torres Strait Islander Australians are in a very high risk group for suicide (twice the rate for general population), and are often over-represented in the health system in general due to multiple overlapping vulnerabilities. Careful consideration of cultural issues must be incorporated into assessment of Aboriginal and Torres Strait Islander people. It is relevant for all healthcare providers to train in cultural sensitivity and competence, as this skill set applies across healthcare settings and can help guide the nurse in how to ask sensitive and difficult questions.

People who have arrived in Australia or New Zealand as either asylum seekers awaiting refugee status or refugees (confirmed status) will have endured significant hardship and suffering throughout the various stages of their journey. This may include exposure to torture, violence (at a personal, family or community level), sexual assault, persecution, extreme deprivation and loss of loved ones in the pre-migration period. The migration period also involves great hardship and uncertainty with people waiting many years in camps or detention centres before finding refuge. Families are often separated during the migration phase and it is quite normal for mental health and wellbeing of refugees/asylum seekers to be profoundly affected. Depression, anxiety, substance use disorder and post-traumatic stress disorder are commonly associated with prolonged migration experiences (AIHW 2018a). Each person is unique in their resilience and capacity to manage change, and it is therefore important to always use a strengths-based approach in mental health assessment, whereby a person's courage and survival is acknowledged and respected and existing skills are built upon.

The main risks for people from culturally and linguistically diverse (CALD) backgrounds relate to social exclusion due to language and cultural barriers, and lack of understanding of the health care system (Victorian Government 2016). The most significant strategy a nurse can employ when assessing people from CALD backgrounds is to use a properly trained interpreter whenever possible. Using family members to interpret may seem convenient; however, issues of privacy may mean the person is not honest about stressors, suicide and other risks in the presence of family. Additionally, when using untrained/personally involved family/friends, incorrect explanation of medical information and filtering or misunderstanding of assessment data may occur. Mental health concerns are fraught with fear, lack of understanding and high levels of emotion for most people. In many cultures, there is great stigma and shame associated with mental illness, and healthcare workers may be viewed as authority figures that are not trustworthy. In order to properly understand the cultural impact/sensitivities around mental illness for each person, and to decrease exclusion and fear, correct communication needs to occur via an interpreter (see Chapter 7 for information on working effectively with interpreters).

WHEN TO PERFORM A MENTAL STATUS ASSESSMENT

Mental status assessment documents a dysfunction and determines how that dysfunction affects self-care and engagement in everyday life. As with any assessment, it is always important to determine the previous level of functioning and the length of time the disruption has been experienced. All diagnostic parameters for mental disorders require a length of time during which the cluster of symptoms has been experienced (APA 2013). (see Chapter 7 for information on working effectively with interpreters; see also Figure 11.1 for suicide first aid guidelines for people from immigrant and refugee backgrounds.)

It is necessary to perform a full mental status examination when you discover any abnormality in affect or behaviour, and in the following situations:

- Family members are concerned about a person's recent behavioural changes, such as memory loss, strange or unusual/out of character behaviour, disturbance to sleep and appetite or social withdrawal.
- Brain lesions (trauma, tumour and cerebrovascular accident/stroke). A mental status assessment documents any emotional or cognitive change associated with the lesion. Not recognising these changes hinders care planning and creates problems with social readjustment. It can be very helpful in planning interventions to have a snapshot of a person's mental status.
- Aphasia (the impairment of language ability secondary to brain damage, substance intoxication or withdrawal or other psychiatric presentations). A mental status examination assesses language dysfunction as well as any emotional problems associated with it, such as depression or agitation.
- Symptoms of psychiatric illness, such as responding to stimuli not visible to the assessor, expressions of hopelessness, self-neglect or disruption to usual functioning (care of children, attendance at work).
- Onset of mental illness usually develops over time (days or weeks/months); whereas organic causes such as delirium or drug-induced psychosis have a more sudden onset (hours to days).

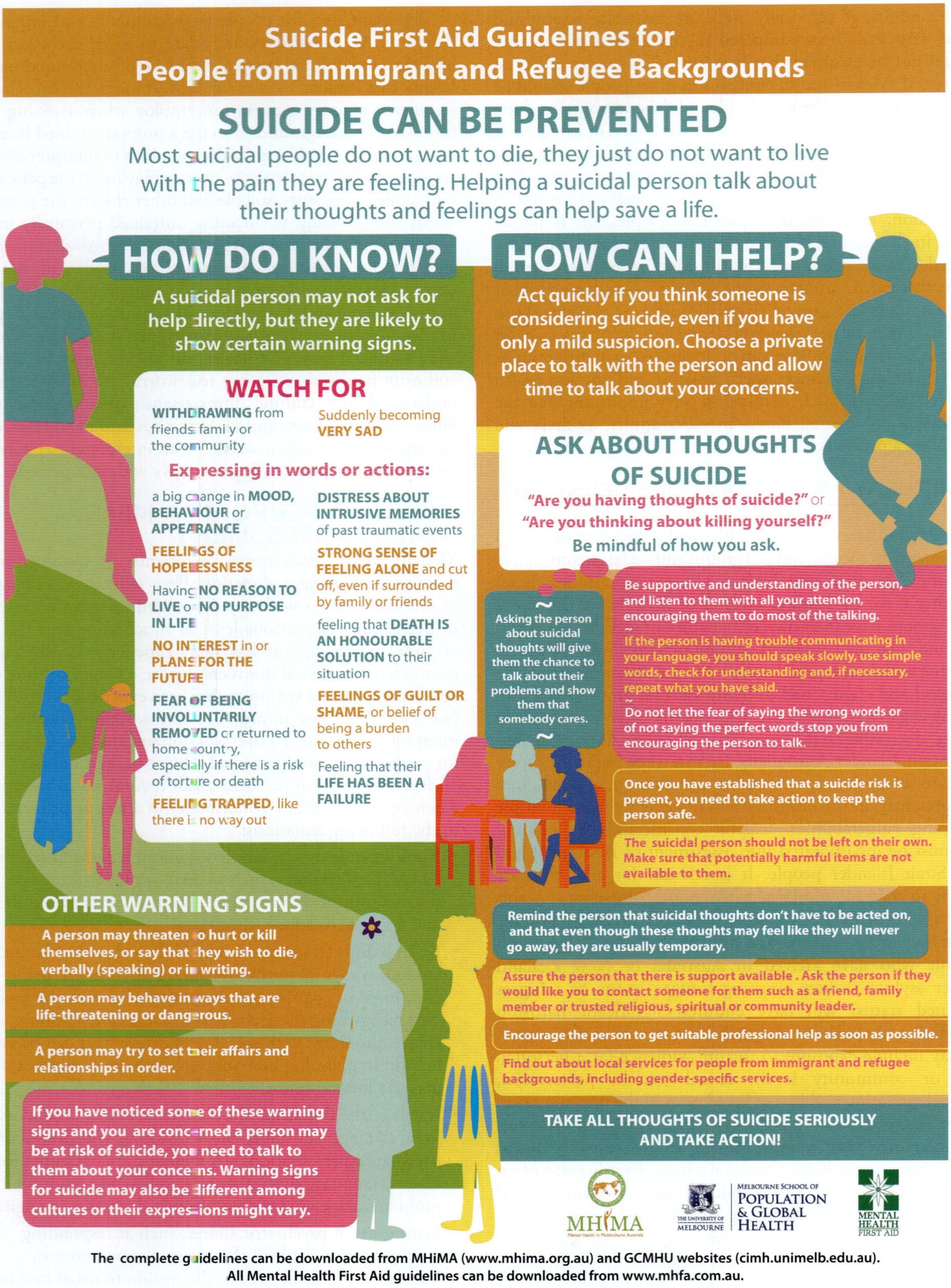

Suicide First Aid Guidelines for People from Immigrant and Refugee Backgrounds

SUICIDE CAN BE PREVENTED

Most suicidal people do not want to die, they just do not want to live with the pain they are feeling. Helping a suicidal person talk about their thoughts and feelings can help save a life.

HOW DO I KNOW?

A suicidal person may not ask for help directly, but they are likely to show certain warning signs.

WATCH FOR

WITHDRAWING from friends, family or the community

Suddenly becoming **VERY SAD**

Expressing in words or actions:

a big change in **MOOD, BEHAVIOUR** or **APPEARANCE**

FEELINGS OF HOPELESSNESS

Having **NO REASON TO LIVE** or **NO PURPOSE IN LIFE**

NO INTEREST in or **PLANS FOR THE FUTURE**

FEAR OF BEING INVOLUNTARILY REMOVED or returned to home country, especially if there is a risk of torture or death

FEELING TRAPPED, like there is no way out

DISTRESS ABOUT INTRUSIVE MEMORIES of past traumatic events

STRONG SENSE OF FEELING ALONE and cut off, even if surrounded by family or friends

feeling that **DEATH IS AN HONOURABLE SOLUTION** to their situation

FEELINGS OF GUILT OR SHAME, or belief of being a burden to others

Feeling that their **LIFE HAS BEEN A FAILURE**

OTHER WARNING SIGNS

A person may threaten to hurt or kill themselves, or say that they wish to die, verbally (speaking) or in writing.

A person may behave in ways that are life-threatening or dangerous.

A person may try to set their affairs and relationships in order.

If you have noticed some of these warning signs and you are concerned a person may be at risk of suicide, you need to talk to them about your concerns. Warning signs for suicide may also be different among cultures or their expressions might vary.

HOW CAN I HELP?

Act quickly if you think someone is considering suicide, even if you have only a mild suspicion. Choose a private place to talk with the person and allow time to talk about your concerns.

ASK ABOUT THOUGHTS OF SUICIDE

"Are you having thoughts of suicide?" or "Are you thinking about killing yourself?"

Be mindful of how you ask.

~ Asking the person about suicidal thoughts will give them the chance to talk about their problems and show them that somebody cares. ~

Be supportive and understanding of the person, and listen to them with all your attention, encouraging them to do most of the talking.

~ If the person is having trouble communicating in your language, you should speak slowly, use simple words, check for understanding and, if necessary, repeat what you have said.

~ Do not let the fear of saying the wrong words or of not saying the perfect words stop you from encouraging the person to talk.

Once you have established that a suicide risk is present, you need to take action to keep the person safe.

The suicidal person should not be left on their own. Make sure that potentially harmful items are not available to them.

Remind the person that suicidal thoughts don't have to be acted on, and that even though these thoughts may feel like they will never go away, they are usually temporary.

Assure the person that there is support available. Ask the person if they would like you to contact someone for them such as a friend, family member or trusted religious, spiritual or community leader.

Encourage the person to get suitable professional help as soon as possible.

Find out about local services for people from immigrant and refugee backgrounds, including gender-specific services.

TAKE ALL THOUGHTS OF SUICIDE SERIOUSLY AND TAKE ACTION!

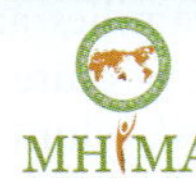

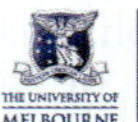

MELBOURNE SCHOOL OF POPULATION & GLOBAL HEALTH

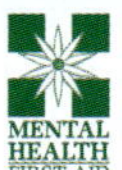

The complete guidelines can be downloaded from MHiMA (www.mhima.org.au) and GCMHU websites (cimh.unimelb.edu.au). All Mental Health First Aid guidelines can be downloaded from www.mhfa.com.au.

Figure 11.1
Suicide First Aid Guidelines for People from Immigrant and Refugee Backgrounds
Source: Colucci E. et al., (2018). Suicide first aid guidelines for assisting persons from immigrant or refugee background: a Delphi study. Advances in Mental Health, 16(2), 105-116 https://doi.org/10.1080/18387357.2018.1469383

Subjective data

Nurses are in a key position to screen for mental illness, offer holistic assessment and support and referrals to specialist services for treatment. The nurse's role as advocate is very important for those experiencing mental distress, because mental illness can invoke feelings of fear, helplessness and powerlessness. Empathic, caring support at the point of entry to any health setting can play a significant role in positive mental health outcomes.

Nurses routinely conduct mental status assessments across a variety of clinical settings including accident and emergency departments, surgical and medical wards, general practitioner clinics, community health settings, aged person's services, midwifery settings or post-hospitalisation in the person's home. When assessing mental status in a person's own environment, take note of whether they are attending to their home, family, hygiene and commitments as observed in their environment. This will give you an indicator of how the person is managing life's demands each day.

When collecting subjective information, keep in mind the main domains of the Mental Status Examination (MSE). The language and categories described in the MSE can help you to formulate your observations and give you a common language for your documentation, as well as communicate to other health professionals should you be concerned about clinical deterioration of mental state. They can also help you to think about the types of questions you may ask the person. It is essential that you employ a caring, respectful, nonjudgemental approach so that a therapeutic relationship can be formed (Sommers-Flanagan & Sommers-Flanagan 2017). It is also important that you honour each person as an expert in their own health experience, so that you work collaboratively and respectfully alongside the person. This approach will allow you to enquire about the very personal domains of mental health assessment with warmth and respect (Sommers-Flanagan & Sommers-Flanagan 2017).

1. Presenting concern
2. History of present illness
3. Mental health history
4. Current and past health history
5. Family history
6. Interpersonal relationships/resources
7. Values, beliefs or spiritual resources
8. Coping and stress management
9. Sleep and rest
10. Health and lifestyle management
11. Risk of harm to self or others

Setting

Choose a quiet, private and respectful space and ensure the person is comfortable. Give them your full attention, sit at the same level, use a warm and confident approach and open body language (Sommers-Flanagan & Sommers-Flanagan 2017).

Practice note: Before you commence the assessment, introduce yourself to the person, confirm the person's identity, discuss the purpose and scope of the assessment, clarify any questions the person may have and obtain verbal consent from the person to perform the assessment.

SUBJECTIVE DATA

ASSESSMENT GUIDELINES	CLINICAL SIGNIFICANCE AND CLINICAL ALERTS
1. Presenting concern	
A suggested approach: • 'I would like to ask you some questions about why you are here today. Some of the questions may appear personal and intrusive but will assist me to help work out what might be happening and how we can help you. Is that OK? Everything we discuss will remain confidential and will only be shared to help you and keep you safe.' From the presenting concern, the person may be able to provide you with some insight into their symptoms and other healthcare issues. Responses to these questions will guide the sequence to the rest of the subjective data collection. Take cues from the person and what they say.	The person may present for treatment following a traumatic event or with new symptoms/behaviours or an exacerbation of a current diagnosis. The nurse is uniquely placed to offer compassionate, person-centred assessment and may be the only clinician who detects a mental health concern. Often people feel extremely vulnerable and have told their very personal story many times. It can be very exposing and thus is important that the nurse assures discretion. Establishing rapport with the person is the first step in developing a therapeutic relationship. It is important to note that mental illness and medical problems may be interlinked. How the person responds to questions is just as important as what the person says. Taking note of both will help you to develop insight into the person's problems and their perception of the problems.

SUBJECTIVE DATA

ASSESSMENT GUIDELINES	CLINICAL SIGNIFICANCE AND CLINICAL ALERTS
2. History of present illness (if relevant)	
• Can you tell me how you have been feeling? • What symptoms have you been experiencing? • Have you been feeling down/depressed/hopeless? • When did they start? Have you been feeling like this for weeks? Months? • How frequent are the symptoms? Are these feelings there first thing in the morning? Do they last all day? Have they changed over time? • What level of distress have you been feeling? (Scale of 1–10) • What factors make them worse? Is there anything that helps? What have you tried? • What factors make them better? Are there situations that make you feel worse? • Are you experiencing any other associated symptoms? (e.g. insomnia, reduced or increased appetite) Should there be any hesitancy to answer questions, you could use statements such as 'You were talking about … Can you tell me more about that?'	Use of open-ended questions enables the person to tell their story and explain their experiences. Social determinants of health such as poverty, exposure to violence and lack of education or rurality all contribute to how a person will experience and manage life challenges such as illness (World Health Organization 2018). ***Clinical alert:*** If the person answers yes, then depression should be explored in detail. See Tables 11.2 and 11.7. The person should be referred to a mental health nurse or medical practitioner. Hearing the person's perception of their illness/symptoms and challenges helps the nurse to understand the person's situation but it is important to note that the person experiencing a mental health crisis may not believe a mental health problem exists. In situations like this it is important to get further information from relevant people such as parents, children, spouse, best friend, teacher, police officers and/or other healthcare providers.
3. Mental health history (if relevant)	
• Have you ever seen someone for mental or emotional concerns? Do you know if you were given a diagnosis? • What treatment/s did you receive? This may include counselling or talking therapy with a psychologist, medications or other types of treatment such as electroconvulsive therapy. • How effective was the treatment?	***Clinical alert:*** Many people will not receive a formal diagnosis and if they do they may not be made aware of what that is. Many clinicians not trained to diagnose will assign a label that is incorrect, unhelpful and misinformed. Only psychiatrists and psychologists are formally trained in diagnostics. All other labels are diagnostic impressions.
4. Current and past health history	
• Have you had any accidents/injuries? • Have you had any serious or chronic medical illnesses or surgery? • If relevant, ask about pregnancy, health during and after.	Known illnesses, such as substance use disorder, hyperthyroidism, chronic renal disease or head injury could affect your interpretation of the findings.
5. Family history	
• Any family history of mental illness?	Family history of mental illness is clinically relevant, especially with low prevalence disorders.

ASSESSMENT GUIDELINES	CLINICAL SIGNIFICANCE AND CLINICAL ALERTS
6. Interpersonal relationships/resources	
• Do you have a home at the moment? Where do you live? Who do you live with? Are you renting or are you buying your own home? • What is your educational level? • What is your current employment or social welfare payment? • How would you describe your role in the family? • Can you please describe your relationships with family, friends and co-workers? • Who can you go to for support if you have a problem with work, your health or personal problems? • How do you fill in your time? If any of this information has already been obtained through an admission assessment or collected by another health professional there is no need to ask for this information again; instead confirm the details with the person.	***Clinical alert:*** These questions are sensitive and should be asked compassionately and kindly. As mental health deteriorates, so too do relationships and this will often be the tipping point for presentation. It would be normal for the person to become emotional when describing their situation and appropriate for the nurse to offer comfort, validation and reassurance. People often feel a lot of shame that they aren't coping as they normally would. Homelessness, including temporary accommodation and couch surfing, can have a significant impact on mental health and wellbeing. If you suspect that the person is experiencing family violence, refer to Chapter 5 for specific questions and approach to assessment.
7. Values, beliefs or spiritual resources	
• Does your religious faith or spirituality play an important part in your life? • Do you identify with any specific cultural group? • Are there some cultural health practices that are important to you?	
8. Coping and stress management	
• What do you consider to be the most significant stressors in your life, especially in the last year? • How has that affected you? • What is it about your present situation that is most worrying for you? • What methods have you tried to relieve stress and were these helpful?	If this information has already been revealed then use clinical judgement to leave out questions and avoid repetition of painful information.
9. Sleep and rest	
• What time do you usually go to sleep? • Do you have difficulty getting to sleep? If so how do you manage it? Do you have difficulty staying asleep? • What time do you usually get up? • Do you feel refreshed in the morning after sleep?	Often insomnia will either be initial (difficulty getting to sleep) or early morning waking (3 or 4 am and ruminating).
10. Health and lifestyle management	
• What treatment have you received for your physical and mental health problem? • What are your current medications? Have you had any side effects? • Do you smoke cigarettes? At what age did you start? How many packs do you smoke per day? How many years have you smoked? Have you ever tried to quit? • How much and how often do you drink alcohol? When was your last drink? How much did you drink at that time? What do you drink? In the last week how many days would you say you drank alcohol? • Do you use illicit drugs? How often? What type of drug? Refer to Chapter 6 for screening tools for substance abuse. • Activity and exercise—refer to Chapters 17, 19 and 20 for specific questions. • Nutrition—refer to Chapter 21 for specific questions.	Side effects of current prescribed medications such as contraceptives or corticosteroids may cause confusion or depression. See Table 11.1 for definitions and typical symptoms of substance use disorders.
11. Risk of harm to self or others	
This information is elicited in the thought content component of the mental status examination in the objective data section	

SUBJECTIVE DATA

Objective data

In the following assessment, you are asked to examine all aspects of the person in comparison to what would be in the normal range for their age, gender, education, social position, cultural norms and the current environment. You should not expect the person to perform at a higher level on the mental status examination than their usual educational and behavioural level. You are looking for congruence: does what you see concur with what the person says and what you know? Use the categories below to assess the person's mental state at that moment in time, and then enquire whether this is different from their usual way of being.

The full Mental Status Examination (MSE) is a systematic assessment of psychological, emotional and behavioural functioning. It is part of a suite of assessments conducted in the clinical setting in order to form a holistic picture of the person in the context of their psychosocial history. While the history provides context and backdrop to the person's story, the MSE provides a snapshot of what is happening right here, right now. The MSE also provides a benchmark at this point in time against which future assessments can be measured, and changes can be noted. The quality and accuracy of your documentation is very important for the next clinician to ascertain what has changed in the mental status.

An MSE can be done through routine observation, conversation and interaction with the person. When a person is hospitalised for a mental health problem it is not necessary to formally ask all the questions in the MSE each shift. However, the nurse will be interacting with the person and observing their behaviour which should be documented. When a person is mentally unwell, their mental state may change frequently, often due to the effects of the person's environment and current stressors. If you observe unusual or significant change in the person's behaviour, you would complete the full MSE.

Domains of the MSE:

- Appearance and behaviour
- Mood and affect
- Speech
- Thought process and thought content
- Perception
- Cognition
- Judgement and insight.

Equipment needed

Pencil, paper, reading material
An MSE prompter card is very helpful

PROCEDURES AND NORMAL FINDINGS	ABNORMAL FINDINGS AND CLINICAL ALERTS
Appearance and behaviour	
The assessment of appearance and behaviour begins at the moment the nurse observes the person. Be careful to use clear, nonjudgemental descriptors which consider the person's culture.	
Level of consciousness. The person is awake, alert and attentive.	Drowsy, sedated, lethargic, yawning, hypervigilant, hyper-aroused, distracted, easily startled.
Physical characteristics. Gender, age, appears stated age, race, physical build, distinguishing features, injuries, physical disabilities, sounds or odours emanating from the person.	When a person appears older or younger than stated age this has clinical significance with regards to past history of the person.
Posture and engagement. Posture is erect and position is relaxed, sitting, lying in bed or standing. The person is facing towards you and is engaged in the process.	Sitting on edge of chair or curled in bed, tense muscles, folded arms, turned away, restless pacing occurs with anxiety, paranoia, agitated depression and hyperthyroidism. Sitting slumped in chair, psychomotor retardation occurs with depression and some organic brain diseases. Unusual posturing or gesturing (catatonia, schizophrenia), unusual gait or rigidity of movement (autism, antipsychotic side effects).

PROCEDURES AND NORMAL FINDINGS	ABNORMAL FINDINGS AND CLINICAL ALERTS
Body movements. Body movements are voluntary, deliberate, coordinated and smooth and even.	Restless, fidgety movements or hyperkinetic appearance occur with anxiety. Apathy and psychomotor slowing occur with depression and organic brain disease. Tics and stereotypical movements occur with psychotic disorders, autism and severe depression. Abnormal posturing and bizarre gestures occur with schizophrenia.
Dress. Dress is appropriate for setting, season, age, gender and social group. Clothing is clean, fits and is put on appropriately.	Inappropriate dress can occur with organic brain syndrome. Dress which appears suited to the opposite sex may indicate gender role confusion/gender identity issues. Eccentric dress combination and bizarre make-up occurs with schizophrenia or manic phase of bipolar affective disorder. Soiled, torn clothing and lack of footwear may indicate disorganisation, homelessness or self-neglect due to depression.
Grooming and hygiene. The person is clean and well groomed; hair is neat and clean; women have moderate or no make-up; men are shaved or beard or moustache is well groomed. Nails are clean (though some jobs leave nails chronically dirty).	Unilateral neglect (total inattention to one side of body) occurs following some strokes. Inappropriate dress, poor hygiene and lack of concern with appearance may occur with depression, schizophrenia and severe Alzheimer's disease. Meticulously dressed and groomed appearance and fastidious manner may occur with obsessive-compulsive disorders. ***Clinical alert:*** A dishevelled appearance in a previously well-groomed person is significant. Use care in interpreting clothing that is dishevelled, bizarre or in poor repair, piercings and tattoos, because these sometimes reflect the person's economic status or a deliberate fashion trend (especially among adolescents).
Facial expression. The expression is appropriate to the situation and responds to the topic. There is comfortable eye contact unless precluded by cultural norm.	Flat, mask-like expression can occur with parkinsonism, depression, psychosis (thought disorder), hyperthyroidism and myasthenia gravis. Grimacing, frowning and grinning that are incongruent may occur with psychosis. Perplexed, confused expression may occur with dementia and psychosis; suspicious, fearful expression and darting eyes with paranoia. Response to hallucinations can affect facial expression (e.g. preoccupation, smiling).
Mood and affect	
Mood is the internal feeling state. It usually persists over time: hours, days, weeks. It is the subjective way the person feels. Affect is the external expressed emotion and can be observed by others in facial expression, tone and expressed emotion.	See Table 11.2 Abnormalities of mood and affect.
Mood. Euthymic (normal mood) may fluctuate mildly throughout the day or over time, with good and bad days, but generally is manageable, consistent with life events, able to be improved through enjoyable activities/social supports/meaningful activities.	Mood is the subjective and pervasive emotional state, impacting on functioning and relationships. If depressed, one feels down and sad all the time, nothing is enjoyable, nothing is easy. Depression can range from mild to severe, and can also manifest in anger. Rating the mood from 1–10 can be useful. Deterioration in mood can be very gradual and the person may not realise their mood has become depressed. If mood is elevated, the person feels elated, speedy, irritable, powerful, energetic and often does not feel they need to sleep. Elevated mood ranges from hypomanic to hypermanic. A person who has an anxiety disorder may describe feeling worried, tense, frightened and nervous most of the time.

OBJECTIVE DATA

PROCEDURES AND NORMAL FINDINGS	ABNORMAL FINDINGS AND CLINICAL ALERTS
Affect. A normal affect is emotional expression that can be observed that is congruent with the situation, responsive and reactive. It has a range from happy to sad and is observable.	Affect can range from flat, blunted, expressionless to exaggerated and dramatic. It may not be congruent with the topic and stated mood (grinning when talking about mother's death) or inappropriate to topic. The range may be restricted, mask-like without reactivity. Congruence of mood and affect are very important clinical indicators of psychosis, in particular.
Other measures affected by mood. Normal mood fluctuations will generally not affect sleep, appetite, enjoyment, libido and memory for long periods of time. One may have one or two nights of poor sleep, but balance is quickly recovered. Asking about these factors are excellent objective measures of mood overall.	Sleep will often be disturbed (hypo- or hypersomnia) with a pattern of difficulty falling asleep, staying asleep or early morning waking. Appetite will be reduced or increased, with marked weight loss. Anhedonia (lack of pleasure in previously enjoyable activities) is common. Decreased libido or increased with mania.
Speech	
Speech reveals the content, order, speed of thought as well as possible organic concerns or intoxication.	Disruptions to the normal structure, flow and formations of speech reveal a great deal about cognitive function, education and mental state.
In people without disability, speech will be spontaneous, audible, clear, expressive, at the correct volume, pitch, rate and rhythm and be age appropriate.	Abnormal speech may reveal physical or cognitive difficulties with speaking (such as after a stroke or oral surgery or slurring with intoxication) or with the formation of language due to mood or thought disorder. Depression may cause mutism, slow or quiet speech. Psychosis may cause nonsensical, jumbled speech of a strange pace or pitch. Elevated mood may cause rapid, pressured speech or grandiose tones. Paranoia may cause hushed, secretive speech.
The pace of the conversation is moderate, in keeping with the other person and stream of talking is fluent.	Slow, monotonous speech with parkinsonism, depression. Rapid-fire, pressured and loud talking occurs with manic or hypomanic episodes.
Articulation (ability to form words) is clear and understandable.	Dysarthria is distorted speech; see Table 12.6. Misuse of words; omits letters, syllables or words; transposes words: occurs with aphasia. Circumlocution or repetitious abnormal patterns: neologism, echolalia. See Table 11.3.
Word choice is effortless and appropriate to educational level. The person completes sentences, occasionally pausing to think.	Unduly long word-finding or failure in word search occurs with aphasia. Thought blocking occurs with depression and psychosis.
Thought processes and content	
Thought processes cannot be objectively observed, as they are internal and personal, but can be inferred through language and observation of behaviour. Thought processes have a usual, logical and coordinated profile; when thought processes are disrupted, this can be observed in a number of ways.	
Ask yourself, 'Does this person make sense? Can I follow what the person is saying?' The *way* a person thinks should be logical, goal directed, coherent and relevant. The person should complete a thought.	Illogical, unrealistic thought processes. Digression from initial thought. Ideas run together. Evidence of blocking (person stops in middle of thought). See Tables 11.3 and 11.4.
Thought content. What is the person thinking about? You may need to enquire quite specifically here and follow a line of enquiry to reveal the content of thoughts. This is a very important part of the assessment.	Delusions, obsessions, compulsions. See Table 11.4. Suicidal thoughts, homicidal thoughts (violent ideation), preoccupation with guilt or hopelessness, paranoia, phobias. Is the person aware that their thoughts are unusual?

OBJECTIVE DATA

PROCEDURES AND NORMAL FINDINGS	ABNORMAL FINDINGS AND CLINICAL ALERTS
Screen for suicidal thoughts. When the person expresses feelings of sadness, hopelessness, despair or grief, it is important to assess any possible risk of physical harm to themselves. Begin with more general questions. If you hear affirmative answers, continue with more specific questions: • Have you ever felt so down you thought of suicide? • Are you thinking about suicide now, or have you been thinking about it today? • Do you have a plan of how you might kill yourself? • What would happen if you were dead? • How would other people react if you were dead? It is very difficult to question people about possible suicidal ideas, especially for beginning nurses. Examiners fear invading privacy and may have their own normal denial of death and suicide. However, the risk is far greater if you skip these questions when you have the slightest idea that they are appropriate. You may be the only health professional to pick up clues of suicide risk. You are responsible for encouraging the person to talk about suicidal thoughts. While not all suicide deaths can be prevented, the very effort of asking kindly and confidently has a profound protective impact. For the people who are ambivalent about dying, and they are the majority, you can buy time so the person can be helped to find an alternative route through the situation. Most people who think about suicide do not go on to attempt suicide. Share any concerns you have about a person's suicidal ideation with a mental health professional. The questions need to be specific and direct; 'hurt yourself' is too ambiguous, as it could mean self-injury only. A person who has suicidal thoughts will often feel very relieved to be able to tell someone. Make a determination about the level of risk based on your screening. If the answer is 'yes' to many of the risk alerts, the risk is higher. If you feel the risk is moderate or above, do not leave the person alone and seek specialist mental health support.	A precise suicide plan (which includes a specific method with materials already collected, such as a rope for hanging) to take place in the next 24–48 hours using a lethal method constitutes a very high risk. ***Clinical alert:*** **Important clues and warning signs of suicide:** • Prior suicide attempts • Family member or close friend who has suicided • Feelings of pain and desperation (physical and mental) • Depression, hopelessness • Social withdrawal, running away • Self-injury • Hypersomnia or insomnia • Slowed psychomotor activity • Anorexia • A mental disorder • Increased risk taking • Minimal supports/alone • Verbal suicide messages (defeat, failure, worthlessness, loss, giving up, desire to kill self) • Death themes in art, jokes, writing, behaviours • Saying goodbye (giving away prized possessions) Additional content on mental disorders is listed in Tables 11.5, 11.6, 11.7 and 11.8. See also Figure 11.1 for suicide first aid guidelines for people from immigrant and refugee backgrounds.
Perception	
Disturbances of perception can take the form of hallucinations, illusions, derealisation (things not seeming real), déjà vu or depersonalisation (one's person, body or self does not feel real).	Auditory, tactile, visual, gustatory, olfactory hallucinations occur in the absence of external stimuli. Illusions, hallucinations. See Table 11.9. Auditory and visual hallucinations occur with psychiatric and organic brain disease and with psychedelic drugs. Tactile hallucinations occur with alcohol withdrawal. Gustatory and olfactory hallucinations are more common with organic brain issues or severe psychotic depression (smelling and tasting foul things like faeces).
Cognitive functions	
Cognition is the ability to think, reason, know, understand and remember. It is dependent on brain function and should be formally tested if there is a suspected deficit, so that later testing can compare to previous scores/results. If you think there is something unusual in a person's cognition, it is worth exploring with the family/carer as well as the person. A family will often adjust to changes without noticing, as cognitive decline can be gradual. By making enquiries as to whether anything has changed in the person's behaviour, you prompt the family to reflect. Again, you may be the first person to screen for these changes.	Abnormal findings are more likely to occur with organic disorders and less likely to occur with mental illness such as psychosis. Where a person has a pre-existing mental illness, cognitive decline may be less obvious. Medication interactions and side effects can cause significant cognitive disturbances; e.g. serotonergic syndrome (from selective serotonin reuptake inhibitors (SSRIs)) may cause sudden racing, suicidal thoughts.

PROCEDURES AND NORMAL FINDINGS	ABNORMAL FINDINGS AND CLINICAL ALERTS
Orientation	
You can discern orientation through the course of the interview, or ask for it directly, using tact. 'Some people have trouble keeping up with the dates while in the hospital. Do you know today's date?' • Time: day of week, date, year, season • Place: where person lives, present location, type of building, name of city and state • Person: own name, age, who examiner is, type of worker Many hospitalised people normally have trouble with the exact date but are fully oriented on the remaining items.	Disorientation occurs with organic brain disorders, such as delirium and dementia. Orientation is usually lost in this order—first to time, then to place and rarely to person. It is unusual for a person with psychosis to be disoriented, other than to perhaps the date; however, a severely depressed person may be disoriented to time/date due to withdrawal from functioning and psychomotor slowing. Anorexia nervosa causing an electrolyte imbalance may cause disruption to cognition (thinking, decision making) but this will not usually affect orientation.
Attention and concentration are related, with attention being the ability to focus on someone or something (such as the assessment) and concentration being the ability to sustain that attention over time. Check the person's ability to concentrate by noting whether they complete a thought without wandering. Note any distractibility or difficulty attending to you. Or, give a series of directions to follow and note the correct sequence of behaviours, such as 'Please take this glass of water with your left hand, drink from it, shift it to your right hand, and place it on the table'. Note that attention span commonly is impaired in people who are anxious, fatigued or drug intoxicated.	Digression from initial thought. Irrelevant replies to questions. Easily distracted, 'stimulus bound', i.e. any new stimulus quickly draws attention. Confusion, negativism. It would be common to see disturbance in attention with most acute psychiatric presentations such as psychosis, moderate-to-severe depression, mania, severe anxiety. This occurs as a result of disruption to thought processes and preoccupations with thought content. Confusion, rather than distractibility, is more evident with dementia or delirium (such as trying to urinate in a cupboard, thinking it is a toilet, or putting clothes on incorrectly).
Recent memory. Assess recent memory in the context of the interview by the 24-hr diet recall or by asking the time the person arrived at the agency. Ask questions you can corroborate. This screens for the occasional person who confabulates or makes up answers to fill in the gaps of memory loss. For people who appear depressed or anxious, ask if they are forgetting things like appointments, where they left their keys and so on. Ask if they have a favourite television program and, if so, can they still watch from beginning to end?	Recent memory deficit occurs with organic disorders, e.g. delirium, dementia, amnestic syndrome or Korsakoff's syndrome in chronic alcoholism. Short-term memory issues are very common in depression and anxiety; this occurs as a result of internal distraction rather than organic issues. The person will often be aware of their difficulty and may feel quite distressed by it. If there is reduced capacity to concentrate on previously enjoyed activities, this can help you ascertain a timeline of deterioration.
Remote memory. In the context of the interview, ask the person verifiable past events, e.g. ask to describe past health, the first job, birthday and anniversary dates, and historical events that are relevant for that person.	Remote memory is lost when cortical storage area for that memory is damaged, such as in Alzheimer's dementia or any disease that damages the cerebral cortex. There should be no effect on remote memory with psychiatric illness; however, episodes of hospitalisation or traumatic events may be partially remembered due to medications and trauma responses (fight or flight mechanism interfering with the laying down of long-term memories).
New learning—the Four Unrelated Words Test. This tests the person's ability to lay down new memories. It is a highly sensitive and valid memory test. It requires more effort than does the recall of personal or historic events. It also avoids the danger of unverifiable material. To the person, say, 'I am going to say four words. I want you to remember them. In a few minutes I will ask you to recall them'. To be sure the person has understood, have the words repeated. Pick four words with semantic and phonetic diversity: **1.** brown **1.** fun **2.** honesty **2.** carrot **3.** tulip **3.** ankle **4.** eyedropper **4.** loyalty	People with Alzheimer's dementia score a zero- or one-word recall. Impaired new learning ability also occurs with anxiety (due to inattention and distractibility) and depression (due to lack of effort mobilised to remember). See also Mini-Mental State Examination below.
After 5 min, ask for the recall of the four words. To test the duration of memory, ask for a recall at 10 min and at 30 min. The normal response for persons under 60 years is an accurate three- or four-word recall after a 5-, 10- and 30-min delay.	

OBJECTIVE DATA

PROCEDURES AND NORMAL FINDINGS	ABNORMAL FINDINGS AND CLINICAL ALERTS
Additional testing for persons with aphasia	
Word comprehension. Point to articles in the room, parts of the body and articles from pockets, and ask the person to name them.	Aphasia is the loss of the ability to speak or write coherently, or to understand speech or writing, due to a stroke. See Table 12.6. Confabulation (making up words/stories to cover for deficits) is more common in early dementia; neologisms (made-up words) may be exhibited in psychotic presentations.
Reading. Ask the person to read available print. Be aware that reading is related to educational level. Use caution that you are not just testing literacy.	Reading and writing are important in planning health teaching and rehabilitation.
Writing. Ask the person to make up and write a sentence. Note coherence, spelling and parts of speech (the sentence should have a subject and verb).	
Higher intellectual function	
These tests measure problem-solving and reasoning abilities. Results are closely related to the person's general intelligence and must be assessed considering educational and cultural background. Tests of higher intellectual functioning have been used to discriminate between organic brain disease and psychiatric disorders; errors on the tests indicate organic dysfunction. Although they have been widely used, there is little evidence that most of these tests are valid in detecting organic brain disease. Furthermore, most of these tests have little relevance for daily clinical care. Thus, many time-honoured standard tests of higher intellectual function are not discussed here, such as fund of general knowledge, digit span repetition, calculation, proverb interpretation and similarities to test abstract reasoning or hypothetical situations to test judgement.	Should you assess that a person has some cognitive deficits that warrant formal testing, e.g. you suspect a person may have impaired cognition due to long-term alcohol use, they can be referred to a neuropsychologist for specialist testing. This may be relevant when trying to arrange consent for surgery, or when considering care of children, for example.
Insight and judgement	
Insight is a person's ability to reflect on their current situation, inclusive of illness, with a level of self-awareness and self-understanding. Insight affects a person's judgement, which in turn affects the decisions that they make. A person with well-developed insight and judgement will generally make decisions about their health, work, family and recreation that consider risks and benefits. This does not mean people will not take risks, as dignity of risk is afforded to all people in life. This is part of free will and learning by mistakes. Judgement can be considered to be impaired when a person takes excessive, ill-thought-out and out-of-character risks.	A person with limited insight may not agree that they have an illness or that they have any problems. They therefore may make risky or impulsive decisions (e.g. driving after having no sleep, not taking medications that keep them alive, leaving children unattended to go out or frequent unprotected sexual encounters). Impaired judgement can be a helpful indicator of overall coping and is often seen in depression (doesn't care, self-neglect, taking risks), anxiety (can't decide, paralysed by fear), elevated mood (promiscuity, spending), pain (impulsivity), psychosis (acting on paranoia, impulsive risk taking). Sometimes people who have very high risk factors and poor insight and judgement will be treated against their will under the Mental Health Act (MHA) in their state. This will only occur if they meet strict legal criteria and there are many oversight and checking mechanisms built into each MHA to ensure treatment is appropriate and cannot be delivered in a less restrictive manner.
A person exercises judgement when they can compare and evaluate the alternatives in a situation and reach an appropriate course of action. Rather than testing the person's response to a hypothetical situation (e.g. 'What would you do if you found a stamped, addressed envelope lying on the footpath?'), you should be more interested in the person's judgement about daily or long-term life goals, the likelihood of acting in response to delusions or hallucinations and the capacity for violent or suicidal behaviour.	Impaired judgement (unrealistic or impulsive decisions, wish fulfilment) occurs with intellectual disability, emotional dysfunction, schizophrenia, mood disorders, substance use disorders, anxiety disorders, personality disorders and organic brain disease. ***Clinical alert:*** When you are assessing a person's judgement, you are also trying to estimate or predict how risky the person's actions may be based on how they are thinking now. This is complex and difficult to do. If you are worried about the person's safety now or in the near future, it is important to seek senior/specialist assessment. A person who presents a high level of risk will often be rapidly changing and unpredictable in their behaviour.

PROCEDURES AND NORMAL FINDINGS	ABNORMAL FINDINGS AND CLINICAL ALERTS
To assess judgement in the context of the interview, note what the person says about job plans, social or family obligations and plans for the future. Job and future plans should be realistic, considering the person's health situation. Also, ask the person to describe the rationale for personal healthcare, and how they decided about whether or not to comply with prescribed health regimens. The person's actions and decisions should be realistic.	

Mini-Mental State Examination

The Mini-Mental State Examination tool is a simplified scored form of the cognitive functions of the mental status examination (Folstein et al 1975) (see Table 11.10 for several sample questions) It is quick and easy, includes a standard set of only 11 questions and requires only 5–10 minutes to administer. It is useful for both initial and serial measurement, so you can demonstrate worsening or improvement of cognition over time and with treatment. It concentrates only on cognitive functioning, not on mood or thought processes. It is a valid detector of organic disease, thus it is a good screening tool to detect dementia and delirium and to differentiate these from psychiatric mental illness. The maximum score on the test is 30; people with normal mental status average 27. Scores between 24 and 30 indicate no cognitive impairment.	Scores that occur with dementia and delirium are classified as follows: 18–23 = mild cognitive impairment; 0–17 = severe cognitive impairment.

TABLE 11.10 Mini-Mental State Examination (MMSE)

MMSE Sample Items

Orientation to time
'What is the date?'

Registration
'Listen carefully. I am going to say three words. You say them back after I stop.
Ready? Here they are ...
APPLE (pause), PENNY (pause), TABLE (pause). Now repeat those words back to me.' (Repeat up to 5 times, but score only the first trial.)

Naming
'What is this?' (Point to a pencil or pen.)

Reading
'Please read this and do what it says.' (Show examinee the words on the stimulus form.)
CLOSE YOUR EYES

Additional objective data for infants and children

The mental status assessment of infants and children covers behavioural, cognitive and psychosocial development, and examines how the child is coping with their environment. Essentially, you will follow the same guidelines as for the adult, with special consideration for developmental milestones. Your best examination 'technique' arises from thorough knowledge of developmental milestones as described in Chapter 3. Abnormalities are often problems of *omission*; the child does not achieve a milestone you would expect. The parent's health history, especially the sections on the developmental history and personal history, yields most of the mental status data.	Most mental illness in children will manifest as anxiety, depression, withdrawal and social (conduct) problems initially. Anxiety can manifest in repetitive and stereotypical behaviours such as tics, rocking and rituals. Persistent toileting problems may occur as a sign of mental illness in children. Children who are experiencing abuse or neglect will often come to the attention of school teachers and healthcare services. They may exhibit developmental delay, emotional dysregulation (anger, distress, and withdrawal), aggression, sexualised behaviours or regression. Children who have suffered abuse may also disassociate (have periods when they seem absent/blank) as a means of self-protection (Sadock et al 2017).

OBJECTIVE DATA

PROCEDURES AND NORMAL FINDINGS	ABNORMAL FINDINGS AND CLINICAL ALERTS
In addition, the Denver II screening test (see Chapter 3) gives you a chance to interact directly with the young child to assess mental status. For the child from birth to 6 years of age, the Denver II helps identify those who may be slow in development in behavioural, language, cognitive and psychosocial areas. An additional language test is the Denver Articulation Screening Exam. For primary school-age children, ages 7 to 11, who have grown beyond the age when developmental milestones are very useful, the 'Behavioural checklist' (Table 11.11) is an additional tool that can be given to the parent along with the history. It covers five major areas: mood, play, school, friends and family relations. It is easy to administer and takes about 5 min.	Aggressive, abusive, destructive or isolative behaviours warrant assessment. Extreme clinginess, fear, distress, crying or bizarre behaviour should all be assessed. Self-injury is a very clear indicator of emotional distress. Self-injury can take the form of cutting, scratching, hair tearing, self-punching, head banging, burning, swallowing objects or inserting objects.

TABLE 11.11 Behavioural checklist

1 Prefers to play alone	15 Seems afraid of someone or something
2 Gets hurt in major accidents	16 Is nervous and jumpy
3 Does he/she ever play with fire?	17 Has a nervous habit
4 Has difficulties with teachers	18 Does not show feelings
5 Gets poor grades in school	19 Fights with other children
6 Is absent from school	20 Is understanding of other people's feelings
7 Becomes angry easily	21 Refuses to share
8 Daydreams	22 Shows jealousy
9 Feels unhappy	23 Takes things that are not theirs
10 Acts younger than other children their age	24 Blames others for their troubles
11 Does not listen to parents	25 Prefers to play with children not their age
12 Does not tell the truth	26 Gets along well with grownups
13 Unsure of themself	27 Teases others
14 Has trouble sleeping	

Scoring is a point system: 0—never; 1—sometimes; 2—often. Scoring is reversed for items 20 and 26. Scores between 15 and 22 indicate closer following; scores above 22 warrant psychiatric evaluation.

From Jellinek M, Evans N, Knight R: Use of a behavior checklist on a pediatric inpatient unit, *Journal of Pediatrics* 94:156-158, 1979.

Additional objective data for the adolescent

For the adolescent, follow the same guidelines as described for the adult. It is important to assess the adolescent away from, as well as with parents, to allow for confidential material to be discussed. This will allow you to screen for health risks such as sexual risk taking or substance use.	Excessive risk-taking behaviour, excessive substance use, school refusal, promiscuity, self-injury, eating disorders.

Additional objective data for the adult over 65 years

While for most people older age may present a time of significant life changes and some sense of loss, the previously resilient person will cope and adjust to these life changes with appropriate support. The majority of older Australians are happy and resilient. Social inclusion, meaningful engagement in life, physical activity and effective treatment of health issues will assist the older person to maintain good mental health. Health screening, early detection and health education are crucial nursing roles which can prevent mental illness developing or worsening in older people. People in this age group experiencing mental illness often get missed by health professionals because no one asks the question 'Is this the best health this person can obtain?' Older people are often left to suffer with mental health issues unnecessarily for longer than younger people because as a society we assume mental decline and depression are normal in older age. Nurses need to advocate for the highest level of attainable health for all of their patients, regardless of age (Wand et al 2019).	

OBJECTIVE DATA

PROCEDURES AND NORMAL FINDINGS	ABNORMAL FINDINGS AND CLINICAL ALERTS
It is important to conduct even a brief examination of all older people admitted to the hospital. Confusion is common in ageing people and is easily misdiagnosed. Between a third and a half of older adults admitted to acute care medical and surgical services show varying degrees of confusion already present. In the community, about 5% of adults over 65 and almost 20% of those over 75 have some degree of clinically detectable impaired cognitive function (Draper 2014). Check sensory status before assessing any aspect of mental status. Vision and hearing changes due to ageing may alter alertness and leave the person looking confused. When older people cannot hear your questions, the results of the test may be inaccurate. Follow the same guidelines as described for the younger adult with these *additional* considerations:	Depression and anxiety in older adults is not normal and should not be expected or tolerated by health professionals. Older adults will become depressed when there is a co-occurring physical issue that is not being managed, they are in pain or they have a medical condition that affects independence and mobility. Depression can be easily treated when correctly assessed for, and this will, in turn, greatly improve adherence to other medical regimens and overall functioning. The nurse is very well placed to screen for depression and anxiety and refer for further assessment and treatment.
Behaviour	
Level of consciousness. In a hospital or extended care setting, the Glasgow Coma Scale (see Chapter 12) is a quantitative tool that is useful in testing consciousness in ageing persons in whom confusion is common. It gives a numerical value to the person's eye-opening responses: best verbal and best motor. This system avoids ambiguity when numerous examiners care for the same person.	
Cognitive functions	
Orientation. Many ageing persons experience social isolation, loss of structure without a job, a change in residence or some short-term memory loss. These factors affect orientation, and this person may not provide the precise date or complete name of agency. You may consider ageing persons oriented if they know *generally* where they are and the present period. That is, consider them oriented to time if the year and month are correctly stated. Orientation to place is accepted with the correct identification of the type of setting (e.g. the hospital) and the name of the town.	People with Alzheimer's disease and other dementias do not improve their performance on subsequent trials.
New learning. In people of normal cognitive function, an age-related decline occurs in performance in the Four Unrelated Words Test described above. Persons in the eighth decade average two of four words recalled over 5 min. They will improve their performance at 10 and 30 min after being reminded by verbal cues (e.g. 'one word was a colour; a common flower in Holland is ____________').	
Supplemental mental status examination	
There are two predominant supplemental mental status examination scales used in the Australian context. Firstly, the Geriatric Depression Scale (Shives 2012) indicates the level of depression a person may be experiencing but is not used to determine cognitive impairment, whereas the Psychogeriatric Assessment Scale (PAS) is administered to assess for clinical changes in dementia, depression and cognitive impairment (Jorm & Mackinnon 2016).	

Summary Checklist

MENTAL HEALTH ASSESSMENT

Subjective data

1. Presenting concern
2. History of present illness
3. Mental health history
4. Current and past health history
5. Family history
6. Interpersonal relationships/resources
7. Values, beliefs or spiritual resources
8. Coping and stress management
9. Sleep and rest
10. Health and lifestyle management
11. Risk of harm to self or others

Objective data (Mental status examination)

1. Appearance
   - Posture
   - Body movements
   - Dress
   - Grooming and hygiene
2. Behaviour
   - Level of consciousness
   - Facial expression
3. Mood and affect
   - Speech (quality, pace, articulation, word choice)
4. Cognitive functions
   - Orientation
   - Attention span
   - Recent and remote memory
   - New learning—the Four Unrelated Words Test
5. Judgement and insight
6. Perform the Mini-Mental State Examination

PROMOTING A HEALTHY LIFESTYLE

HEALTH PROMOTION—ARE YOU OK? (R U OK?)

R U OK? day was founded as a national day of action to prevent suicide. The mission of the R U OK? Foundation is to encourage people to connect meaningfully and support each other in particular those who are undergoing significant life problems.

The goals of the R U OK? Foundation are to:

a. Boost our confidence to meaningfully connect and ask about life's ups and downs
b. Nurture our sense of responsibility to regularly connect and support others
c. Strengthen our sense of belonging because we know people are there for us
d. Be relevant, strong and dynamic

The R U OK? Foundation has developed four simple steps to encourage connection when someone you know or care about is not behaving as they normally would.

1. **Ask**—are you OK?
2. **Listen**—without judgement
3. **Encourage Action**

For example, you could ask:

a. What have you done to manage a similar situation in the past?
b. How would you like me to support you?
c. What is something you could do for yourself right now?

4. **Check in**—put a reminder in your diary to follow up in a couple of days/weeks. If they are really struggling, follow up sooner. Stay in touch and be there for the person.

R U OK? has a website with many resources to help people ask questions and support a person who is having difficulties. See https://www.ruok.org.au/about-us

Documentation and critical thinking

FOCUSED ASSESSMENT: CLINICAL CASE STUDY

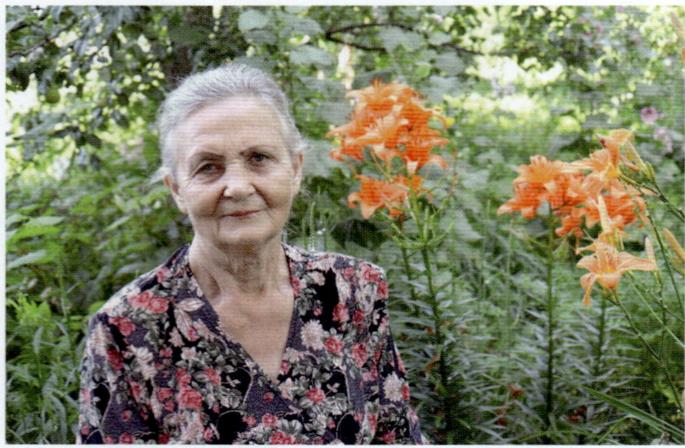

Context

Lola Peters is a 79-year-old married woman, with a recent hospitalisation for evaluation of increasing memory loss, confusion and socially inappropriate behaviour. During this hospitalisation, Mrs Peters has undergone a series of medical tests, including a negative lumbar puncture test, normal electroencephalogram (EEG) and a benign head computed tomography (CT) scan. Her physician now suggests a diagnosis of senile dementia of the Alzheimer's type (SDAT).

Subjective

She has been irritable with friends and has left a supermarket with items she did not pay for. Her family reports that Mrs Peters' hygiene and grooming standards have decreased; she eats very little and has lost weight, does not sleep through the night, has angry emotional outbursts that are unlike her former demeanour and does not recognise her younger grandchildren. Her husband reports that she has drifted away from the stove while cooking, allowing food to burn on the stovetop. He has found her wandering through the house in the middle of the night, unsure of where she was. She used to 'talk on the phone for hours' but now he has to push her into conversations. Mood described by family as angry and irritable, with some social withdrawal.

Objective

Appearance: Sitting quietly, somewhat slumped, picking on loose threads on her dress. Hooded, zippered windcheater top worn over dress. Hair is gathered in loose ponytail with stray wisps. No make-up.

Behaviour: Awake and gazing at hands and lap. Expression is flat and vacant. Will make eye contact when called by name, although gaze quickly shifts back to lap. Speech is a bit slow but articulate; some trouble with word choice.

Mood and affect: Appears distracted and sad during interview.

Thought processes and content: Experiences blocking in train of thought, needs prompting to answer questions. Thought content is logical. Acts with hostility and suspicion towards family members. No suicidal ideation, no delusions evident.

Cognitive functions: Oriented to person and place. Can state the season, but not the day of the week or the year. Is not able to repeat the correct sequence of complex directions involving lifting and shifting glass of water to the other hand. Scores a one-word recall on the Four Unrelated Words Test. Cannot tell examiner how she would plan a grocery shopping trip.

Mini-Mental State Examination score is 17, and shows poor recall ability and marked difficulty with serial 7s.

Collaborative problem

Probable Alzheimer type dementia

Problem statements/nursing diagnoses

Chronic confusion related to probable dementia

Impaired social interaction related to probable dementia

Impaired memory related to probable dementia

Risk for injury as related to wandering and poor concentration

Self-care deficit related to confusion and memory loss

Increased family stressors related to change in health status

Abnormal findings

TABLE 11.1 Substance use disorders

The American Psychiatric Association *Diagnostic and Statistical Manual of Mental Disorders*, 5th edition refers to **substances** as agents taken non-medically to alter mood or behaviour. Substance use disorders may be diagnosed as mild, moderate or severe, depending on the number of symptoms present. See also Chapter 29 for more information about substance abuse.

Intoxication: ingestion of substance produces behavioural or psychological changes due to effects on the central nervous system and may include disturbances of perception, wakefulness, thinking, attention, judgement, psychomotor activity and social behaviour.

Problematic use will involve two or more of the following over a 12-month period: daily use needed to function, craving for the substance, inability to stop despite desire to or effort, impaired social and occupational functioning, recurrent use when it is physically hazardous, substance-related legal problems, significant time spent seeking, using or recovering from the substance use.

Dependence: physiological dependence on substance.

Tolerance: requires increased amount of substance to produce same effect.

Withdrawal: cessation of substance produces a syndrome of physiological and psychological symptoms.

Alcohol intoxication and withdrawal

Alcohol intoxication is characterised by the recent consumption of alcohol with the presence of at least one of the following:

- Uncoordinated body movements
- Slurred or incoherent speech
- Reduced attention or memory abilities
- Involuntary eye movement and stupor or coma.

Changes in behaviour or psychological functions are clearly noticeable and generally problematic. These changes include: aggression, changes in mood, compromised judgement and inappropriate sexual decisions.

Alcohol withdrawal can develop within several hours to several days after a reduction or complete termination of alcohol consumption, provided such consumption has been heavy and prolonged. Symptoms will usually present as:

- Nausea and vomiting
- Increase in sweating or pulse rate
- Anxiety, insomnia, visual and auditory disturbances
- Illusions, hallucinations, agitation and generalised tonic-clonic seizures.

These symptoms will severely impact the individual and their daily functioning in social and occupational areas.

Sedatives/hypnotics

Sedative intoxication is characterised by the recent consumption of a sedative, hypnotic or anxiolytic, with the presence of at least one of the following:

- Uncoordinated body movements
- Slurred or incoherent speech, reduced attention or memory abilities
- Involuntary eye movement and stupor or coma.

Maladaptive behaviour and psychological variations are clearly noticeable immediately after use and are generally problematic. They include aggression, changes in mood, compromised judgement and inappropriate sexual decisions.

Sedative withdrawal can develop within several hours to several days after a reduction or complete termination of sedative, hypnotic or anxiolytic consumption, provided such consumption has been heavy and prolonged. Symptoms will usually present as:

- Nausea and vomiting
- Increase in sweating or pulse rate
- Anxiety, tonic-clonic seizures, insomnia
- Visual and auditory illusions and hallucinations
- Hand tremors and agitation.

These symptoms will severely impact the individual and their daily functioning in social and occupational areas.

Cannabis (marijuana)

Cannabis intoxication is characterised by the recent use of the substance, with the presence of at least two of the following within 24 h:

- Increased appetite
- Dry mouth
- Conjunctival injection (redness)
- Tachycardia.

Significant changes in behaviour and psychological functions will develop during or shortly after cannabis use and these include euphoria, reduced motor coordination, anxiety, diminished judgement, a sense of slowed time and social withdrawal.

Cannabis withdrawal will present as:

- An increase in nervousness or anxiety, an upsurge in irritability, feelings of heightened anger
- Aggression and difficulty in sleeping, which may include nightmares or unsettling dreams.

(Continued)

TABLE 11.1 Substance use disorders—cont'd

Individuals will be restless and show signs of a depressed mood, with a lack of appetite and resulting weight loss.

Pain in the abdominal area, shaking and tremors, fever, chills, headache and sweating may be present in isolation or in accompaniment with each other and will cause distress and physical discomfort.

Stimulants including cocaine or amphetamines

Stimulant intoxication is characterised by recent use of an amphetamine, stimulant or other substance such as cocaine. At least two signs or symptoms will present themselves shortly after the stimulant has been ingested. These include:

- Dilation of the pupils
- Elevated or reduced blood pressure
- Perspiration, chills, nausea or vomiting
- Confusion, involuntary muscle movement, seizures
- Muscle weakness, weight loss, psychomotor agitation
- Chest pain, respiratory depression, tachycardia or bradycardia.

Behavioural and psychological changes such as euphoria and changes to anxiety, anger, sociability and judgement will develop during stimulant use or shortly after and will be problematic for the individual.

Stimulant withdrawal occurs after a reduction or termination of prolonged use of an amphetamine, cocaine or other stimulant. Changes to physiological function, accompanied by a sense of unease or depression, will usually develop within a few hours to several days and will include:

- Insomnia and vivid or unpleasant dreams
- Fatigue
- Increased appetite and retardation or agitation of movement and coordination.

These changes will cause distress and impairment to the individual in important areas of daily functioning.

Opioids

Opioid intoxication is characterised by the recent use of an opioid substance, with one or more of the following symptoms presenting during use or immediately after ingestion:

- Slurred speech
- Constriction of the pupils
- Drowsiness, reduced levels of attention and/or memory and, in severe cases, coma.

Opioid use will initially create feelings of euphoria in the individual, followed by apathy and other problematic behavioural and psychological changes such as agitated movements, impaired judgement and dysphoria.

Opioid withdrawal occurs after a reduction or termination of prolonged use, over several weeks or more, of opioids. Withdrawal symptoms will present within minutes to several days after a reduction or cessation of use, or after the use of an opioid antagonist:

- Nausea or vomiting
- Pupil dilation
- Sweating, muscle aches
- Piloerection and a change in mood (dysphoria) are common.

Rhinorrhoea and lacrimation may also be present, with most withdrawal cases showing three or more of the above.

TABLE 11.2 Abnormalities of mood and affect

TYPE OF MOOD OR AFFECT	DEFINITION	CLINICAL EXAMPLE
Flat affect (blunted affect)	Lack of emotional response; no expression of feelings; voice monotonous and face immobile	No emotional response when telling a sad story about the death of their dog, face and voice remain expressionless
Depression	Sad, gloomy, dejected; symptoms have a physical dimension of tiredness, no energy, no appetite	'I feel so empty, I just don't want to see anyone. I just don't enjoy anything anymore ...'
Elation	Joy and optimism, overconfidence, increased motor activity, not necessarily pathological	'Wow, this is so exciting, I'm so happy. I just can't sit still ...'
Euphoria	Excessive wellbeing, unusually cheerful or elated, which is inappropriate considering physical and mental condition, implies a pathological mood	'I am high.' 'I feel like I'm flying.' 'I feel on top of the world.'
Anxiety	Worried, uneasy, apprehensive from the anticipation of a danger whose source is unknown. Physical symptoms such as butterflies, dizziness, jelly legs and palpitations are very common	'I just know that something bad is going to happen, please don't leave me alone ...'

TABLE 11.2 Abnormalities of mood and affect—cont'd

TYPE OF MOOD OR AFFECT	DEFINITION	CLINICAL EXAMPLE
Fear	Worried, uneasy, apprehensive; external danger is known and identified	Scared about coming into hospital, shaking and pale
Irritability	Annoyed, easily provoked, impatient, often presents as sarcastic and hostile	Person internalises a feeling of tension, and a seemingly mild stimulus 'sets them off'. 'I told you I hate carrots ... you are so stupid, you never listen!'
Rage	Furious, loss of control	Person has expressed violent behaviour towards self or others
Ambivalence	The existence of opposing emotions towards an idea, object, person, common with depression and anxiety which causes indecision and emotional distress/paralysis.	'I just can't decide whether to go to work or call in sick ... I can't decide about anything...'
Lability	Rapid shift of emotions	Person expresses euphoric, tearful, angry feelings in rapid succession
Incongruent affect	Affect clearly discordant with the content of the person's speech	Laughs while discussing admission for liver biopsy

Abnormal findings for advanced practice

TABLE 11.3 Abnormalities of thought process (formal thought disorder)

TYPE OF PROCESS	DEFINITION	CLINICAL EXAMPLE
Blocking	Sudden interruption in train of thought, unable to complete sentence, usually occurs with psychosis	The person will stop mid-sentence and when they resume talking are not aware what happened or of the previous topic
Confabulation	Fabricates events to fill in memory gaps, frequently occurs with dementia	Gives detailed description of his long walk around the hospital although you know Mr J remained in his room all afternoon
Neologism	Coining a new word; invented word has no real meaning except for the person; may condense several words	'I'll have to turn on my thinkilator'
Circumlocution	Round-about expression, substituting a phrase when cannot think of name of object	Says 'the thing you open the door with' instead of 'key'.
Circumstantiality	Talks with excessive and unnecessary detail, talks around a topic, but eventually reaches the point	'When was my surgery? Well, I was 27, I was living with my aunt, she's the one with psoriasis, she had it bad that year because of the heat, the heat was worse then than it was in the summer of 2009 ...'
Tangentiality	The topic of conversation repeatedly goes off on a tangent and does not return to the original topic without frequent redirection	When asked about a family member's health, the person diverts on to describing their choice of clothing and does not mention their health
Loosening associations	Shifting from one topic to an unrelated topic; person seems unaware that topics are unconnected. There may be some connection between topics but there is no logic to their connection	'My boss is angry with me and it wasn't even my fault. (pause) I saw that movie too, Lord of the Rings. I felt really bad about it. But she kept trying to land the aeroplane and she never knew what was going on.'
Flight of ideas	Abrupt change, rapid skipping from topic to topic, practically continuous flow of accelerated speech; topics usually have recognisable associations or are plays on words	'Take this pill? The pill is blue. I feel blue. (sings) She wore blue velvet.'

(Continued)

TABLE 11.3 Abnormalities of thought process (formal thought disorder)—cont'd

TYPE OF PROCESS	DEFINITION	CLINICAL EXAMPLE
Word salad	Incoherent mixture of words, phrases and sentences; illogical, disconnected, includes neologisms	'Beauty, red based five, pigeon, the street corner, sort-of.'
Perseveration	Persistent repeating of verbal or motor response, even with varied stimuli. The person seems stuck on a topic	'I'm going to lock the door, lock the door. I walk every day and I lock the door. I usually take the dog and I lock the door.'
Echolalia	Imitation, repeats others' words or phrases, often with a mumbling, mocking or mechanical tone	Nurse: 'I would like you to take your pill.' Patient (mocking): 'Take your pill. Take your pill.'
Clanging	Word choice based on sound, not meaning, includes nonsense rhymes and puns	'My feet are cold. Cold, bold, told. The bell tolled for me.'

TABLE 11.4 Abnormalities of thought content

TYPE OF CONTENT	DEFINITION	CLINICAL EXAMPLE
Phobia	Strong, persistent, irrational fear of an object or situation; feels driven to avoid it	Birds, spiders, snakes, heights, enclosed spaces, flying
Preoccupations such as hypochondriasis	Morbid worrying about their own health, feels sick with no actual basis for that assumption	Preoccupied with the fear of having cancer; any symptom or physical sign means cancer
Obsession	Unwanted, persistent thoughts or impulses; logic will not purge them from consciousness; experienced as intrusive and senseless	Violence (parent having repeated impulse to kill a loved child); contamination (becoming infected by water from the shower)
Compulsion	Unwanted repetitive, purposeful act; driven to do it; the ritualistic behaviour reduces anxiety and discomfort or prevents some dreaded event	Handwashing, counting, checking and rechecking, touching. 'If I clean my hands with bleach every time I touch a door handle my mother won't die in an accident...'
Delusions	Firm, fixed, false beliefs; irrational; the delusional belief does not alter despite objective evidence to the contrary	Grandiose—person believes they are God, famous or that they have a special mission to complete to save the human race. Paranoid/persecutory: the person feels they are being followed, harassed, poisoned or people are trying to harm them
Violent ideation (suicidal and homicidal)	Intrusive preoccupation with ideas of one's own death, plans to suicide, thoughts of harming others, thoughts of revenge	'I just don't feel like my life is worth living anymore. I wish I was dead, I'm in so much pain'

TABLE 11.5 Delirium and major neurocognitive disorder (dementias)

DELIRIUM

The American Psychiatric Association *Diagnostic and Statistical Manual of Mental Disorders,* 5th edition describes delirium as a direct result of a medical condition, exposure to toxin or a substance withdrawal or intoxication issue. It can also be due to multiple aetiologies and is diagnosed in the absence of any pre-existing or evolving neurocognitive disorders or a diminished level of alertness, e.g. coma. The disturbance can develop rapidly, generally within hours to a few days and is punctuated by:

- Fluctuating level of attention, with a reduced ability to focus and sustain thoughts and awareness
- Orientation, perception, visuospatial ability and language may also be affected
- Delirium can often be confused with psychosis.

MAJOR NEUROCOGNITIVE DISORDER

Major neurocognitive disorders can be due to a number of diseases and medical conditions such as HIV infection, Parkinson's disease, Alzheimer's disease, traumatic brain injury, Lewy body disease, vascular disease, prion disease, Huntington's disease, frontotemporal lobar degeneration and substance or medication use and abuse. The American Psychiatric Association *Diagnostic and Statistical Manual of Mental Disorders,* 5th edition describes major neurocognitive disorder as a significant decline from the previously observed level of cognitive function within complex attention, learning and memory, perceptual-motor skills, executive function and social cognition. The cognitive deficit will interfere with daily function and severely impact on independence, with the individual relying on assistance with activities that require complex thought processes, such as paying bills and medication doses. The impairment should be documented by clinical assessment and standardised neuropsychological testing. It does not occur exclusively in the context of delirium and any deficits should also be assessed to ensure they are not associated with another mental disorder such as schizophrenia or major depressive disorder.

TABLE 11.6 Schizophrenia

The American Psychiatric Association *Diagnostic and Statistical Manual of Mental Disorders,* 5th edition describes the characteristics of schizophrenia as:

- Hallucinations
- Delusions
- Disorganised thinking and speech (formal thought disorder).

These symptoms will be present for a considerable amount of time over a period of 1 month. Other symptoms that may also be present include disorganised or catatonic behaviour and a lack of emotional expression and motivation (negative symptoms). The disturbance will persist for 6 months or more; however, this may include periods of residual or prodromal symptoms during which only negative symptoms are present or reduced levels of hallucinations, delusions and formal thought disorder are evident. Schizophrenia will have a significant impact on functioning in personal areas such as self-care and relationships and occupational functioning. If no major depressive episodes, manic episodes or mood episodes have occurred concurrently with the active symptoms or have been minimally present, then schizoaffective disorder and depressive or bipolar disorder with psychotic features can be eliminated. If the individual has a history of a communication disorder or autism spectrum disorder that presented in childhood, schizophrenia can only be diagnosed if prominent hallucinations and delusions are present for at least 1 month, in addition to the other primary symptoms of schizophrenia.

TABLE 11.7 Depressive disorder and bipolar disorder

MAJOR DEPRESSIVE EPISODE

A major depressive episode is defined by the American Psychiatric Association *Diagnostic and Statistical Manual of Mental Disorders,* 5th edition as an individual showing a loss of interest or pleasure in daily life and activities and/or a depressed mood with at least three of the following symptoms consistently over a 2-week period:

- Fatigue
- Psychomotor retardation or agitation
- Excessive sleepiness or insomnia almost every day
- Noticeable weight loss or weight gain with the accompanying decrease or increase in appetite or, in children, a failure to meet expected weight gains
- Recurring suicidal thoughts or an obsession with death without a specific plan for how to commit suicide
- Indecisiveness, lack of concentration, interrupted thought processes and feelings of worthlessness.

Important areas of functioning such as occupational, social and interpersonal relationships will be significantly affected by these symptoms.

MANIC EPISODE

A manic episode is described by the American Psychiatric Association *Diagnostic and Statistical Manual of Mental Disorders,* 5th edition as a defined change in mood, activity or energy lasting at least 1 week, with continually elevated or irritable moods or amplified purpose-driven activity present for most of the day. Noticeable changes in behaviour will be obvious with three or more of the following symptoms present, four if the mood is only irritable:

- Decreased need for sleep, grandiosity or inflated self-esteem
- Excessive talking or a feeling that the individual must keep talking
- Racing thoughts, flight of ideas, easily distracted
- Excessive risk taking in pleasurable activities that could lead to negative consequences such as unwise business decisions, unsafe sexual encounters and unrestrained shopping binges.

Manic episodes can severely impact occupational functioning and social and interpersonal interaction and may necessitate hospitalisation if there are psychotic features or the risk of harm to the individual and those around them.

TABLE 11.8 Anxiety disorders

PANIC ATTACK

A panic attack is a set of symptoms, not a mental disorder, and can occur in the presence of other disorders such as major depressive disorder or medical conditions such as vestibular disorders.

The American Psychiatric Association *Diagnostic and Statistical Manual of Mental Disorders,* 5th edition defines a panic attack as an abrupt surge of intense fear or intense discomfort that will reach a peak within minutes. As a result, the individual will change their behaviour related to the attacks and will avoid situations that may trigger panic attacks. Individuals will also show persistent concern about future panic attacks and the consequences. Four or more of the following symptoms will occur during a panic attack:

- Sweating, palpitations or an accelerated heart rate
- The sensation of shortness of breath, shaking or trembling
- Chest pain, nausea, sensation of choking
- Abdominal discomfort, lightheadedness or feeling dizzy
- Feeling detached from oneself or from reality
- Fear of losing control or a fear of dying
- Numbness or tingling and a feeling of heat or chills.

Other culture-specific symptoms such as a sore neck, tinnitus, out-of-control screaming or crying and headache may also be present.

(Continued)

TABLE 11.8 Anxiety disorders—cont'd

AGORAPHOBIA
Agoraphobia is defined by the American Psychiatric Association *Diagnostic and Statistical Manual of Mental Disorders,* 5th edition as an increased anxiety or fear of two or more of the following situations: • Open spaces such as parks, bridges or markets • Enclosed spaces such as cinemas or elevators • Using public transport • Being alone outside of the home and being in a crowd or standing in line. These situations almost always create anxiety or fear in the individual and, as a result, they will either avoid them entirely or require the assistance of a companion to help them endure the intense emotions. These emotions are consistent and typically last 6 months or more and impact upon daily functioning. Individuals with agoraphobia believe escape from the above situations will be difficult or that help will not be available to them in the event of an incapacitating or embarrassing event within those situations. This anxiety or fear is, however, out of proportion to the actual danger and sociocultural context. The fear, anxiety and avoidance will be exacerbated if another medical condition is present such as Parkinson's disease or inflammatory bowel disease. Agoraphobia should not be diagnosed if the symptoms can be attributed to another mental disorder such as obsessive-compulsive disorder, social anxiety disorder, body dysmorphic disorder, separation anxiety disorder or post-traumatic stress disorder. Agoraphobia should be diagnosed in conjunction with panic disorder if the individual meets the criteria for both disorders.
PANIC DISORDER
An individual who has persistent panic attacks and is constantly worried about future panic attacks is diagnosed as having panic disorder. Changes in behaviour, e.g. avoidance of unfamiliar locations, are common and individuals suffering panic disorder will often predict a catastrophic outcome from a minor physical symptom or medication side effect. They may believe a headache signals a deadly brain tumour or that an ache in a limb signifies bone cancer. Panic disorder represents the highest number of medical visits amongst anxiety disorders and this disorder is heightened further when combined with agoraphobia. Individuals with panic disorder are often absent from work or school, which leads to both economic costs and disruption to social and interpersonal functioning. Persistent full-symptom panic attacks as part of panic disorder lead to an increased risk of disability and a poorer quality of life.
SOCIAL ANXIETY DISORDER (SOCIAL PHOBIA)
The American Psychiatric Association *Diagnostic and Statistical Manual of Mental Disorders,* 5th edition describes social anxiety disorder as an anxiety or marked fear about one or more social situations in which the individual will be exposed to scrutiny from others. This can include: • Social interactions such as meeting new people or holding a conversation with an individual or group • Eating or drinking in public • Performing in front of others such as public speaking. These situations will always incite anxiety or fear and the individual believes that they will act in a way or show symptoms that will lead to negative responses from others: responses such as rejection, offence or a feeling of embarrassment. The fear or anxiety of these situations is persistent, lasting 6 months or more. Children will present differently by crying, throwing tantrums, being clingy, freezing or failing to speak in social situations, and these symptoms must be present during interactions with their peers, not just when they are among adults. Individuals who suffer from social anxiety disorder will avoid situations that bring on their anxiety or fear or, if they are forced to endure them, it will be with intense fear or anxiety. These emotions, however, are out of proportion to the actual danger posed by the situation or its context. Social anxiety disorder should not be diagnosed if the symptoms can be attributed to another mental disorder such as autism spectrum disorder, panic disorder or body dysmorphic disorder, or to the effects of substance abuse or another medical condition.
GENERALISED ANXIETY DISORDER
An individual with generalised anxiety disorder will find it difficult to control their excessive anxiety and worry about occasions, activities or performance (such as related to work) over a period of 6 months or more. The apprehensive expectation will be associated with three or more of the following symptoms, with some of the symptoms presenting consistently: • Difficulty concentrating and directing thought • Feeling on edge and restless, interrupted sleep, issues falling asleep • Fatigue, muscle aches and pains and irritability. Generalised anxiety disorder will severely impact social and interpersonal relationships and occupational functioning. The disorder should not be diagnosed if it is attributable to the effects of another medical condition such as hyperthyroidism or the effects of drug abuse or medication. It can also be confused with symptoms from other mental disorders such as anxiety in panic attacks and panic disorder, obsessions in obsessive-compulsive disorder, negative assessment in social anxiety disorder, gaining weight in anorexia nervosa, perceived flaws in body dysmorphic disorder, separation in separation anxiety disorder, reliving traumatic events in post-traumatic stress disorder, delusional beliefs in schizophrenia or delusional disorder, physical complaints in somatic symptom disorder and serious illness in illness anxiety disorder.

TABLE 11.8 Anxiety disorders—cont'd

TRAUMA AND STRESS-RELATED DISORDERS
Post-traumatic stress disorder
The American Psychiatric Association *Diagnostic and Statistical Manual of Mental Disorders,* 5th edition defines post-traumatic stress disorder as exposure to serious injury, sexual violence or threatened or actual death. The individual will have directly experienced the traumatic event, witnessed in person the event as it happened to another person or learnt of the traumatic event as it occurred to a close family member or friend. In the case of death, threatened or actual, the event must have been either accidental or violent. Repeated exposure to traumatic events, such as police officers repeatedly dealing with details of child abuse and paramedics responding to injured and deceased patients, also applies; however, this criterion does not apply to individuals who view these events through media such as television, photographs or movies unless this relates directly to their work. The defining criteria apply to adults, adolescents and children over the age of 6 years.
Post-traumatic stress disorder will present with involuntary and recurrent upsetting memories of the traumatic event with dissociative reactions such as flashbacks, during which the individual may feel that the event is reoccurring. In children over 6 years this can show through repetitive play in which the theme of the trauma is expressed. Distressing dreams in adults will include events and content that relate to the traumatic event; however, in children, the dreams will most likely include no recognisable content. Psychological distress and physiological reactions to cues that symbolise an aspect of the event will be intense and prolonged and sufferers will show persistent avoidance of those cues, stimuli or anything and anyone that triggers memories, thoughts and feelings of the event.
Negative changes in mood and cognitions will be present with two or more of the following symptoms over a period of 1 month or more: • Consistent distorted thoughts about the cause of the traumatic event leading to the individual blaming themselves or others • A persistent negative emotional state including negativity relating to the world at large or the individual's self-worth • An inability to remember a key part of the traumatic event, usually due to dissociative amnesia • Noticeably diminished interest and participation in everyday activities • Lack of positive emotions such as an inability to feel happy and feelings of detachment from others.
Changes in arousal and reactions associated with the traumatic event will last for longer than 1 month and will present with two or more of the following: • Reckless or self-destructive behaviour • Verbal or physical aggression towards other people or inanimate objects • Hyper-vigilance, lack of concentration • Interrupted sleep or trouble falling asleep and an amplified startle response. These symptoms and disturbances will severely impact on occupational, social and interpersonal functioning. When diagnosing post-traumatic stress disorder, clinicians should specify whether the dissociative symptoms meet the above criteria and if the individual experiences consistent symptoms of either of the following: persistent feelings of depersonalisation, feeling detached from oneself, of no connection to one's body or mental thought processes while there is a sense of time moving slowly, or a recurrent feeling of derealisation in which the individual feels as though stuck in a dream-like world distorted from reality. This subtype can only be applied if the dissociative symptoms are not attributable to the effects of substance abuse, such as blackouts during alcohol intoxication or a different medical condition such as complex partial seizures.

TABLE 11.9 Abnormalities of perception

TYPE OF PERCEPTION	DEFINITION	CLINICAL EXAMPLE
Hallucination	Sensory perceptions for which there are no external stimuli; may strike any sense: visual, auditory, tactile, olfactory, gustatory, somatic	Visual: seeing an image (ghost) of a person who is not there; auditory: hearing voices (one or many, even hundreds) or music/sounds
Illusion	Misperception of an actual stimulus, by any sense	Folds of bedsheets appear to be animated, jumper on end of bed appears to be a cat
Depersonalisation (lack of ego boundaries)	Loss of identity, feels estranged, perplexed about own identity and meaning of existence	'I don't feel real.' 'I feel like I'm not really here.'

BIBLIOGRAPHY

American Psychiatric Association. Diagnostic and statistical manual of mental disorders. 5th ed. Washington DC: American Psychiatric Association; 2013.

Australian Commission on Safety and Quality in Health Care. National Safety and Quality Health Service standards user guide for health services providing care for people with mental health issues. Sydney: ACSQHC; 2018.

Australian Commission on Safety and Quality in Health Care. National Consensus Statement: essential elements for recognising and responding to deterioration in a person's mental state. Sydney: ACSQHC; 2017.

Australian Government, National Mental Health Commission. The Fifth National Mental Health and Suicide Prevention Plan. Barton, ACT: 2017. Available at: https://www.mentalhealthcommission.gov.au/monitoring-and-reporting/fifth-plan/5th-national-mental-health-and-suicide-prevention.

Australian Institute of Health and Welfare. Australia's health 2018. Canberra: AIHW; 2018a. Available at: https://www.aihw.gov.au/reports/australias-health/australias-health-2018/contents/table-of-contents.

Australian Institute of Health and Welfare. Mental health services—in brief 2018. Cat. no. HSE 211. Canberra: AIHW; 2018b. Available at: https://www.aihw.gov.au/reports/mental-health-services/mental-health-services-in-australia-in-brief-2018/contents/table-of-contents.

Australian Institute of Health and Welfare. Mental health services—in brief 2019. Cat. no. HSE 228. Canberra: AIHW; 2019. Available at: https://www.aihw.gov.au/getmedia/f7395726-55e6-4e0a-9c1c-01f3ab67c193/aihw-hse-228-in-brief.pdf.aspx?inline=true.

Australian Institute of Health and Welfare. Mental health services in Australia. 2020. Available at: https://www.aihw.gov.au/reports/mental-health-services/mental-health-services-in-australia.

Department of Health and Ageing (DOHA). Mental health in multicultural Australia (MHiMA): strategic plan 2012–2014. Building capacity and supporting inclusion. Canberra: DOHA; 2012.

Draper BM. Suicidal behaviour and suicide prevention in later life. Maturitas 2014;79(2):179–183.

Evans K, Nizette D, O'Brien A. Psychiatric and mental health nursing. 4rd ed. Chatswood, NSW: Elsevier; 2016.

Folstein M, Folstein S, McHugh P. 'Mini-mental state': a practical method for grading the cognitive state of patients for the clinician. J Psychiatr Res 1975;12:189–198.

Garlick R, Koch S. The older adult and mental illness. In: Edward K, Munro I, Welch I, et al, editors. Mental health nursing: dimensions of praxis. 3rd ed. Melbourne: Oxford University Press; 2018.

Goldberg S, Muir R, Kerr J. Attachment theory: social, developmental, and clinical perspectives. New York: Routledge; 2009.

Graber R, Pichon F, Carabine E. Psychological resilience: state of knowledge and future research agendas. Working paper 425. London: Overseas Development Institute (ODI); 2015. Available at: https://www.alnap.org/system/files/content/resource/files/main/9872.pdf.

Harris B, Duggan M, Batterham P, et al. Australia's Mental and Physical Health Tracker: Background Paper, Australian Health Policy Collaboration issues paper no. 2018-02. Melbourne: AHPC; 2018. Available at: https://www.vu.edu.au/sites/default/files/australias-mental-and-physical-health-tracker-background-paper.pdf.

Jellinek MS, Murphy JM, Little M, et al. Use of the Pediatric Symptom Checklist to screen for psychosocial problems in pediatric primary care: a national feasibility study. Arch Pediatr Adolesc Med 1999;153:254–260.

Jorm A, Mackinnon, A. Psychogeriatric assessment scales user's guide. 4th ed. Canberra: Commonwealth Department of Health; 2016

Lawrence D, Johnson S, Hafekost J, et al. The mental health of children and adolescents. Report on the second Australian Child and Adolescent Survey of Mental Health and Wellbeing. Canberra: Department of Health; 2015. Available at: https://www1.health.gov.au/internet/main/publishing.nsf/Content/9DA8CA21306FE6EDCA257E2700016945/$File/child2.pdf.

Rosen A, Rosen T, McGorry P. The human rights of people with severe and persistent mental illness: can conflicts between dominant and non-dominant paradigms be reconciled? In: Dudley M, Silove D, Gale F, editors. Mental health and human rights: vision, praxis, and courage. Oxford: Oxford University Press; 2012.

Sadock B, Sadock V, Ruiz P. Kaplan and Sadock's comprehensive textbook of psychiatry. 10th ed. Philadelphia: Lippincott, Williams & Wilkins; 2017.

Santhanam-Martin R, Fraser N, Jenkins A, et al. Evaluation of cultural responsiveness using a transcultural secondary consultation model. Transcult Psychiatry 2017;54(4):488–501. doi:10.1177/1363461517724984.

Shives R. Basic concepts of psychiatric-mental health nursing. Philadelphia: Lippincott, Williams & Wilkins; 2012.

Sommers-Flanagan J, Sommers-Flanagan R. Clinical interviewing. 6th ed. New Jersey: John Wiley & Sons; 2017.

Sztein D, Lane W. Examination of the comorbidity of mental illness and somatic conditions in hospitalized children in the United States using the Kids' Inpatient Database, 2009. Hosp Pediatr 2016;6(3):126–34.

Victorian Government, Department of Health and Human Services. Delivering for diversity – Cultural diversity plan 2016–2019. Melbourne: Victorian Government, Department of Health and Human Services; 2016.

Vigo D, Thornicroft G, Atun R. Estimating the true global burden of mental illness. Lancet Psychiatry 2016;3(2):171–178.

Wand APF, Peisah C, Draper B, et al. Carer insights into self-harm in the very old: a qualitative study. Int J Geriatr Psychiatry 2019;34(4):594–600.

World Health Organization (WHO). Mental health: strengthening our response. WHO; 2018. Available at: https://www.who.int/news-room/fact-sheets/detail/mental-health-strengthening-our-response.

Chapter Twelve
Neurological assessment

Written by Carolyn Jarvis
Adapted by Bronwyn Coulton

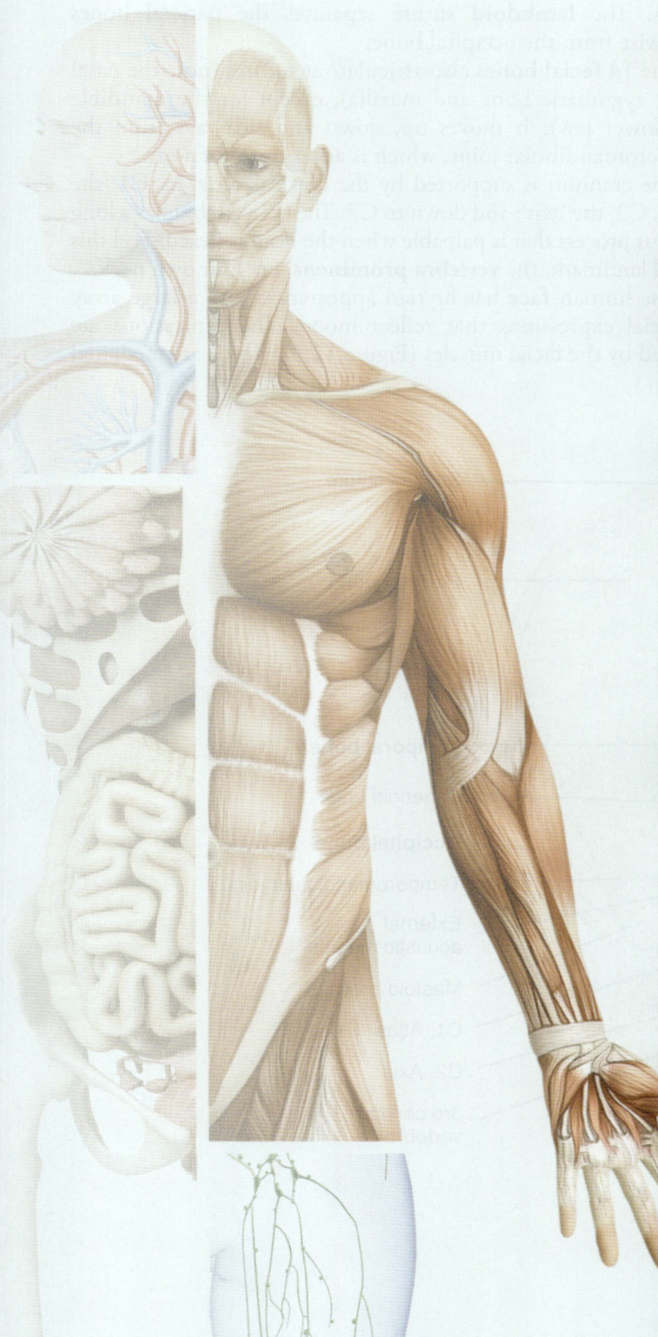

INTRODUCTION

The head and neck are important structures to consider when assessing neurological function. These structures support and protect parts of the nervous system.

The nervous system can be divided into two parts—central and peripheral. The **central nervous system** (CNS) includes the brain and spinal cord. The **peripheral nervous system** (PNS) includes the 12 pairs of cranial nerves, the 31 pairs of spinal nerves and all their branches. The peripheral nervous system carries sensory (afferent) messages *to* the CNS from sensory receptors, motor (efferent) messages *from* the CNS out to muscles and glands, as well as autonomic messages that govern the internal organs and blood vessels. You may also need to review the structure and function related to the peripheral vascular system (Chapter 16) as often neurological and vascular assessment is conducted concurrently. You will also need to review the structure and function of the visual pathways and visual fields, and visual light reflexes which are described in Chapter 14.

Structure and function

THE HEAD

The **skull** is a rigid bony box that protects the brain and special sense organs, and it includes the bones of the cranium and the face (Figure 12.1). Note the location of these **cranial bones**: frontal, parietal, occipital and temporal. Use these names to describe any of your findings in the corresponding areas.

The adjacent cranial bones unite at meshed immovable joints called the **sutures**. The bones are not firmly joined at birth; this allows for the mobility and change in shape needed for the birth process. The sutures gradually ossify during early childhood. The **coronal** suture *crowns* the head from ear to ear at the union of the frontal and parietal bones. The **sagittal** suture *separates* the head lengthwise between the two parietal bones. The **lambdoid** suture separates the parietal bones crosswise from the occipital bone.

The 14 **facial bones** also articulate at sutures (note the nasal bone, zygomatic bone and maxilla), except for the mandible (the lower jaw). It moves up, down and sideways from the temporomandibular joint, which is anterior to each ear.

The cranium is supported by the cervical vertebra: C1, the 'atlas'; C2, the 'axis'; and down to C7. The C7 vertebra has a long spinous process that is palpable when the head is flexed. Feel this useful landmark, the **vertebra prominens**, on your own neck.

The human **face** has myriad appearances and a large array of facial expressions that reflect mood. The expressions are formed by the facial muscles (Figure 12.2), which are mediated

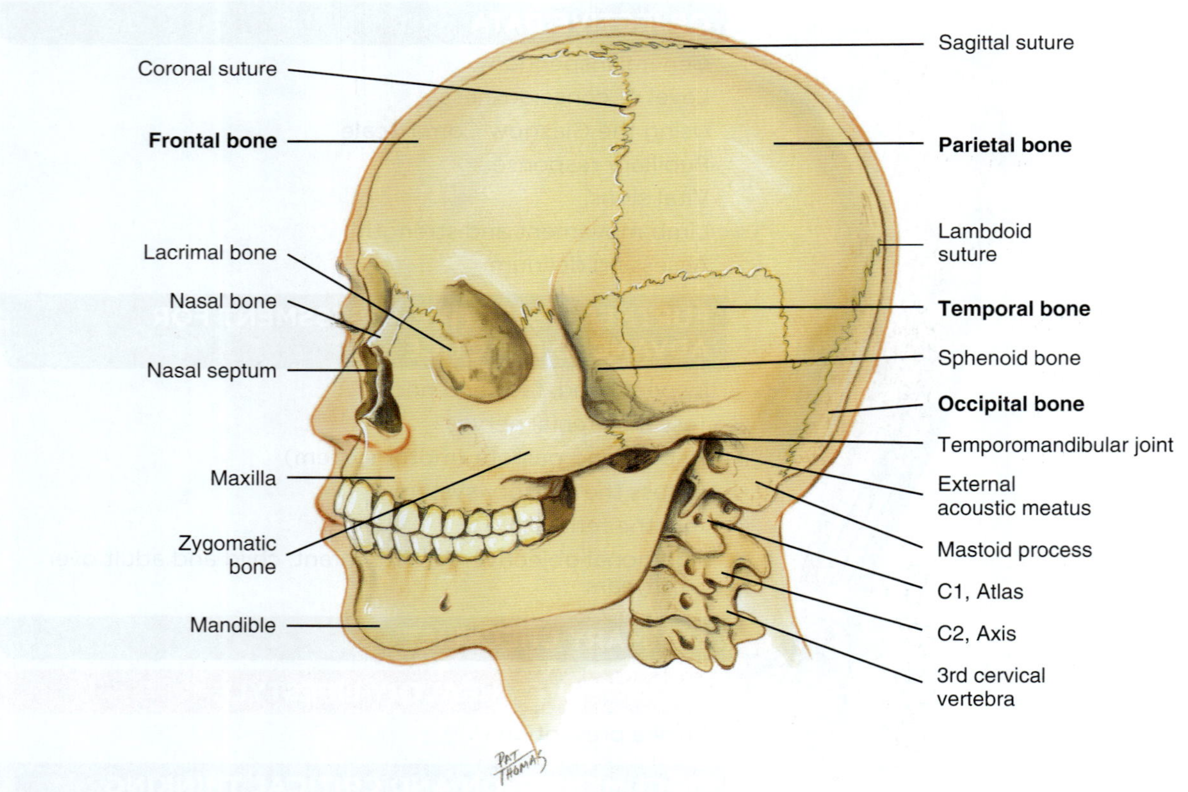

Figure 12.1

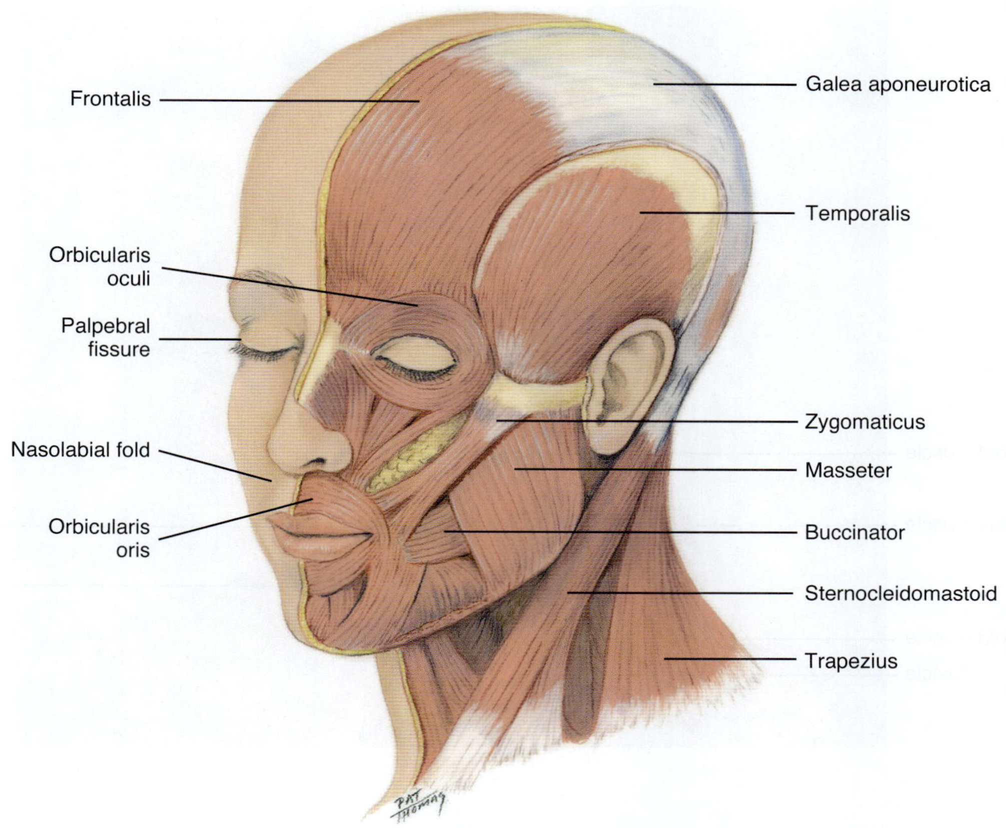

Figure 12.2

by cranial nerve VII, the facial nerve. Facial muscle function is symmetrical bilaterally, except for an occasional quirk or wry expression.

Facial structures also are symmetrical; the eyebrows, eyes, ears, nose and mouth appear about the same on both sides. The palpebral fissures—the openings between the eyelids—are equal bilaterally. Also, the nasolabial folds, the creases extending from the nose to each corner of the mouth, should look symmetrical. Facial sensations of pain or touch are mediated by the three sensory branches of cranial nerve V, the trigeminal nerve.

THE NECK

The **neck** is delimited by the base of the skull and inferior border of the mandible above, and by the manubrium sterni, the clavicle, the first rib and the first thoracic vertebra below. Think of the neck as a *conduit* for the passage of many structures, which are lying in close proximity: vessels, muscles, nerves, lymphatics and viscera of the respiratory and digestive systems. Blood vessels include the common and internal carotid arteries and their associated veins. The internal carotid branches off the common carotid and runs inwards and upwards to supply the brain; the external carotid supplies the face, salivary glands and superficial temporal area. The carotid artery and internal jugular vein lie beneath the sternocleidomastoid muscle. The external jugular vein runs diagonally across the sternomastoid muscle.

The major **neck muscles** are the **sternocleidomastoid** and the **trapezius** (Figure 12.3); they are innervated by cranial nerve XI, the spinal accessory. The sternocleidomastoid muscle arises from the sternum and the medial part of the clavicle and extends diagonally across the neck to the mastoid process behind the ear. It accomplishes head rotation and head flexion. The two trapezius muscles form a trapezoid shape on the upper back. Each arises from the occipital bone and the vertebrae and extends, fanning out to the scapula and clavicle. The trapezius muscles move the shoulders and extend and turn the head.

The sternocleidomastoid muscle divides each side of the neck into two triangles. The **anterior triangle** lies in front, between the sternocleidomastoid and the midline of the body, with its base up along the lower border of the mandible and its apex down at the suprasternal notch. The **posterior triangle** is behind the sternocleidomastoid muscle, with the trapezius muscle on the other side and with its base along the clavicle below. It contains the posterior belly of the omohyoid muscle. These triangles are helpful guidelines when describing findings in the neck.

THE CENTRAL NERVOUS SYSTEM

The brain is made up of three main parts; Prosencephalon (or forebrain), consisting of the cerebrum, thalamus, hypothalamus and limbic system; Mesencephalon (or midbrain), consisting

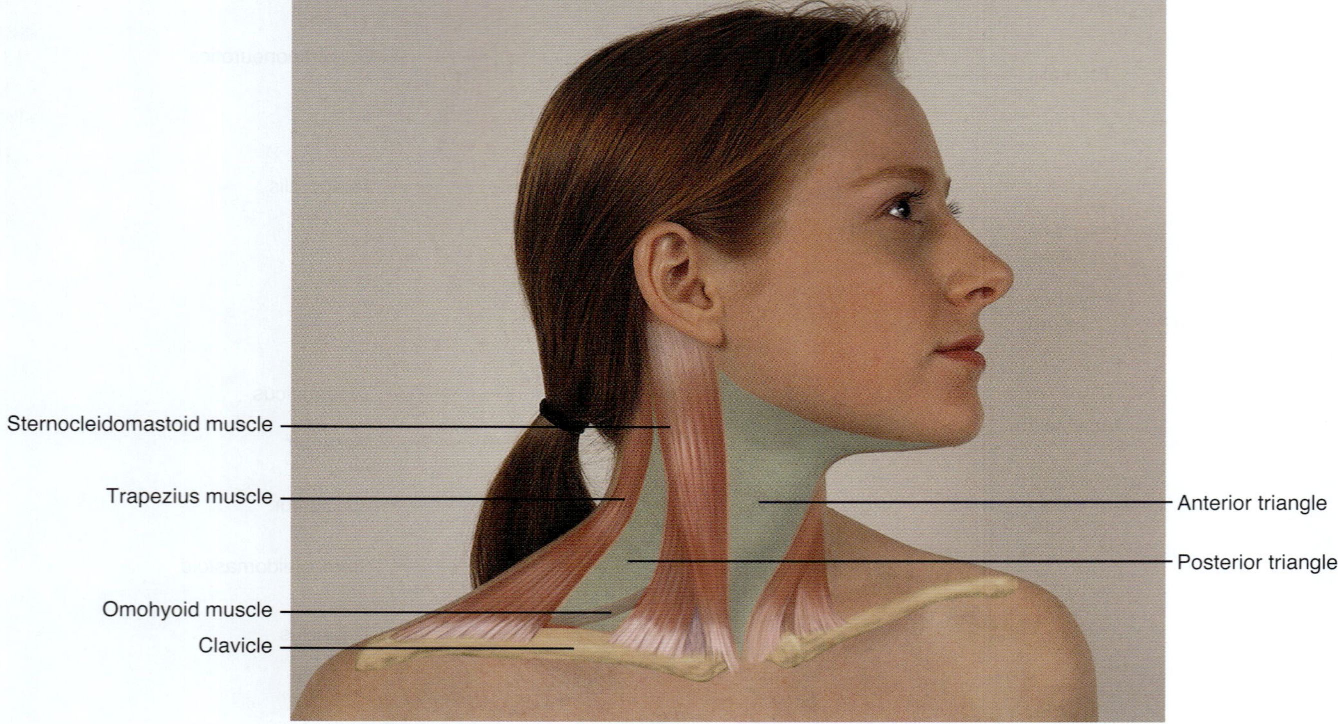

Figure 12.3

of the tectum and tegmentum; and Rhombencephalon (or hindbrain), consisting of the cerebellum, pons and medulla.

Cerebral cortex. The cerebral cortex is the cerebrum's outer layer of nerve cell bodies, which looks like 'grey matter' because it lacks myelin. Myelin is the white insulation on the axon that increases the conduction velocity of nerve impulses.

The cerebral cortex is the centre for humans' highest functions, governing thought, memory, reasoning, sensation, language and voluntary movement (Figure 12.4). Each half of the cerebrum is a **hemisphere**; the left hemisphere is dominant in most people (95%), including those who are left-handed.

Each hemisphere is divided into four main **lobes**: frontal, parietal, temporal and occipital. The lobes have certain areas that mediate specific functions.

- The **frontal** lobe has areas concerned with reasoning, concentration, personality, behaviour, emotions and intellectual function. The frontal lobe also contains the frontal eye fields, responsible for vision.
- The precentral gyrus of the frontal lobe is the primary centre involved in voluntary contralateral movement.
- The **parietal** lobe's postcentral gyrus is the primary centre for the interpretation of contralateral sensation. Additionally, in the non-dominant hemisphere it is important in visual/proprioception, and in the dominant hemisphere it is important in calculation.
- The **occipital** lobe is the primary visual receptor centre, some visual reflexes and involuntary smooth eye movements.
- The **temporal** lobe behind the ear has the primary auditory reception centre, language function, learning and memory.
- **Wernicke's area** in the temporal lobe is associated with language comprehension. When damaged in the person's dominant hemisphere, *receptive* or *Wernicke's aphasia* results. The person hears sound, but it has no meaning, like hearing a foreign language.
- **Broca's area** (inferior part of the dominant frontal lobe) in the frontal lobe mediates motor speech. When injured in the dominant hemisphere the person may experience *expressive aphasia* (cannot talk at all) or *expressive dysphasia* (difficulty in communicating). The person can understand language and knows what they want to say, but cannot express what they want to say.

Damage to any of these specific cortical areas produces a corresponding loss of (usually contralateral) function: motor weakness, paralysis, loss of sensation or impaired ability to understand and process language. Damage occurs when the highly specialised neurological cells are affected by trauma or deprived of their blood supply, such as when a cerebral artery becomes occluded, or when vascular bleeding or vasospasm occurs.

Basal ganglia. The basal ganglia are large bands of grey matter buried deep within the two cerebral hemispheres that form the subcortical associated motor system (the extrapyramidal system) (Figure 12.5). They help to initiate and coordinate movement and control; for example, the arm-swing alternating with the legs during walking.

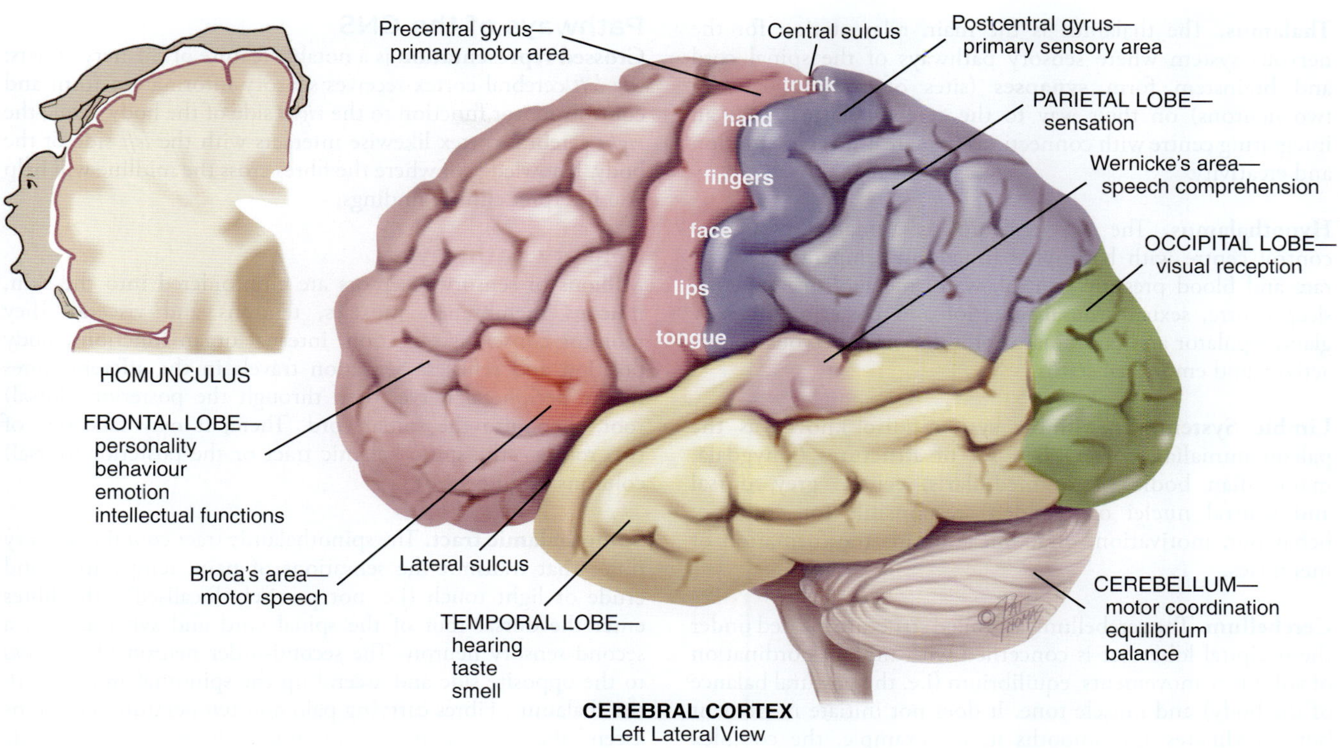

Figure 12.4
Cerebral cortex left lateral view

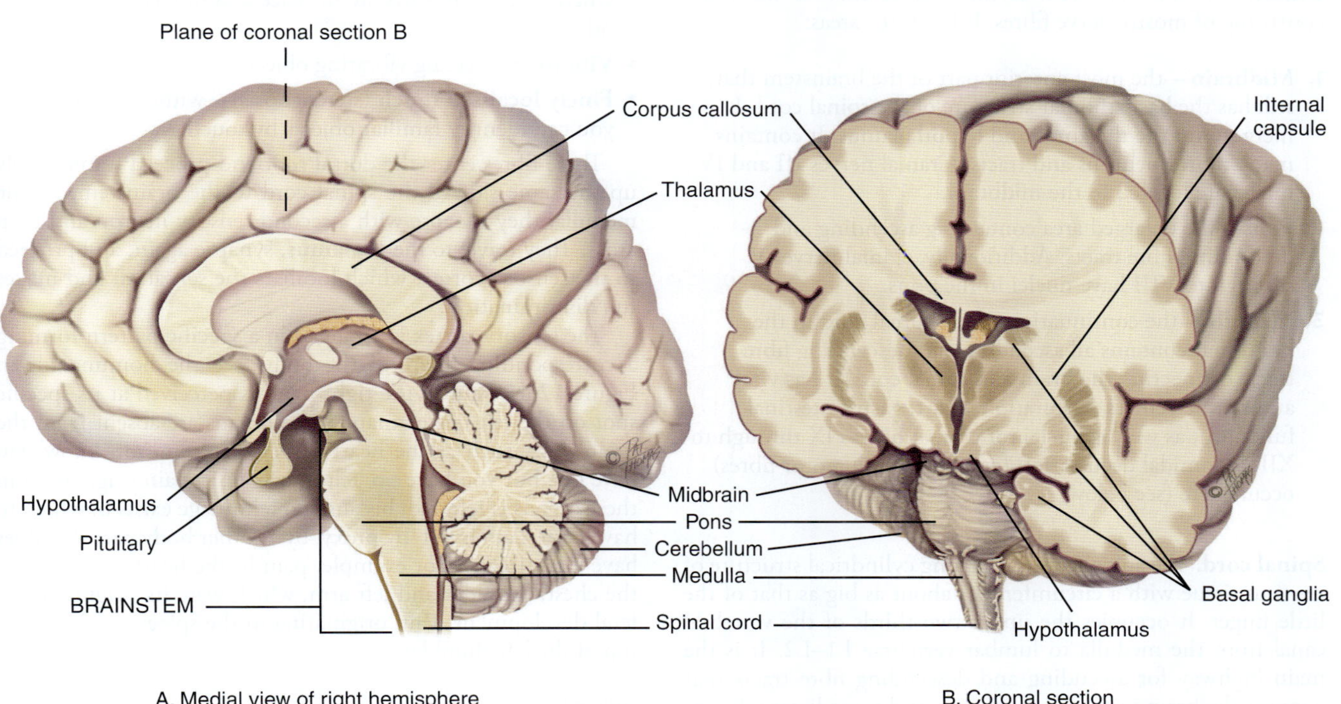

Figure 12.5
Components of the central nervous system

Thalamus. The thalamus is the main relay station for the nervous system where sensory pathways of the spinal cord and brainstem form **synapses** (sites of contact between two neurons) on their way to the cerebral cortex. It is an integrating centre with connections that are crucial to emotion and creativity.

Hypothalamus. The hypothalamus is a major respiratory control centre with basic vital functions: temperature, heart rate and blood pressure control, water metabolism, appetite, sleep centre, sexual arousal, anterior and posterior pituitary gland regulator and coordinator of autonomic nervous system activity and emotional status.

Limbic System. The limbic system (also known as the paleomammalian cortex) is a set of structures (amygdala, mammalian bodies, stria medullaris, central grey, dorsal and ventral nuclei of Gudden) responsible for emotion, behaviour, motivation, olfaction and aids the formation of memories.

Cerebellum. The cerebellum is a coiled structure located under the occipital lobe that is concerned with motor coordination of voluntary movements, equilibrium (i.e. the postural balance of the body) and muscle tone. It does not initiate movement but coordinates and smooths it; for example, the complex and quick coordination of many different muscles needed in playing the piano, swimming or juggling. It is like the 'automatic pilot' on an aeroplane in that it adjusts and corrects the voluntary movements, but operates entirely below the conscious level.

Brainstem. The brainstem is the central core of the brain consisting of mostly nerve fibres. It has three areas:

1. **Midbrain**—the most anterior part of the brainstem that still has the basic tubular structure of the spinal cord. It merges into the thalamus and hypothalamus. It contains many motor neurons and tracts. Cranial nerves III and IV nuclei are located in the midbrain.
2. **Pons**—the enlarged area containing ascending and descending fibre tracts. Additionally, cranial nerves V through to VIII have nuclei in the pons.
3. **Medulla**—the continuation of the spinal cord in the brain that contains all ascending and descending fibre tracts connecting the brain and spinal cord. It has vital autonomic centres (respiration, heart, gastrointestinal function), as well as nuclei for cranial nerves IX through to XII. Pyramidal decussation (crossing of the motor fibres) occurs here (see below).

Spinal cord. The spinal cord is the long cylindrical structure of nervous tissue with a circumference about as big as that of the little finger. It occupies the upper two-thirds of the vertebral canal from the medulla to lumbar vertebrae L1–L2. It is the main highway for ascending and descending fibre tracts that connect the brain to the spinal nerves, and it mediates reflexes. Its nerve cell bodies, or grey matter, are arranged in a butterfly shape with anterior and posterior 'horns'.

Pathways of the CNS

Crossed representation is a notable feature of the nerve tracts: the *left* cerebral cortex receives sensory information from and controls motor function to the *right* side of the body, while the *right* cerebral cortex likewise interacts with the *left* side of the body. Knowledge of where the fibres cross the midline will help you interpret clinical findings.

Sensory pathways

Millions of sensory receptors are embroidered into the skin, mucous membranes, muscles, tendons and viscera. They monitor conscious sensation, internal organ functions, body position and reflexes. Sensation travels in the afferent fibres in the peripheral nerve, then through the posterior (dorsal) root, then into the spinal cord. There, it may take one of two routes—the spinothalamic tract or the posterior (dorsal) columns (Figure 12.6).

Spinothalamic tract. The spinothalamic tract contains sensory fibres that transmit the sensations of pain, temperature and crude or light touch (i.e. not precisely localised). The fibres enter the dorsal root of the spinal cord and synapse with a second sensory neuron. The second-order neuron fibres cross to the opposite side and ascend up the spinothalamic tract to the thalamus. Fibres carrying pain and temperature sensations ascend the *lateral* spinothalamic tract, whereas those of crude touch form the *anterior* spinothalamic tract. At the thalamus, the fibres synapse with a third sensory neuron, which carries the message to the sensory cortex for full interpretation.

Posterior (dorsal) columns. These fibres conduct the sensations of position, vibration and finely localised touch.

- **Position** (proprioception)—without looking, you know where your body parts are in space and in relation to each other
- **Vibration**—feeling vibrating objects
- **Finely localised touch** (stereognosis)—without looking, you can identify familiar objects by touch.

These fibres enter the dorsal root and proceed immediately up the same side of the spinal cord to the brainstem. At the medulla, they synapse with a second sensory neuron and then cross. They travel to the **thalamus**, synapse again, and proceed to the sensory cortex, which localises the sensation and makes full discrimination.

The sensory cortex is arranged in a specific pattern forming a corresponding 'map' of the body (see the homunculus in Figure 12.4). Pain in the right hand is perceived at its specific spot on the left cortex map. Some organs are absent from the brain map, such as the heart, liver or spleen. You know you have one but you have no 'felt image' of it. Pain originating in these organs is referred, because no felt image exists in which to have pain. Pain is felt 'by proxy' by another body part that does have a felt image. For example, pain in the heart is referred to the chest, shoulder and left arm, which were its neighbours in fetal development. Pain originating in the spleen is felt on the top of the left shoulder.

Motor pathways

Corticospinal or pyramidal tract. (Figure 12.7) The area has been named 'pyramidal' because it originates in pyramid-shaped

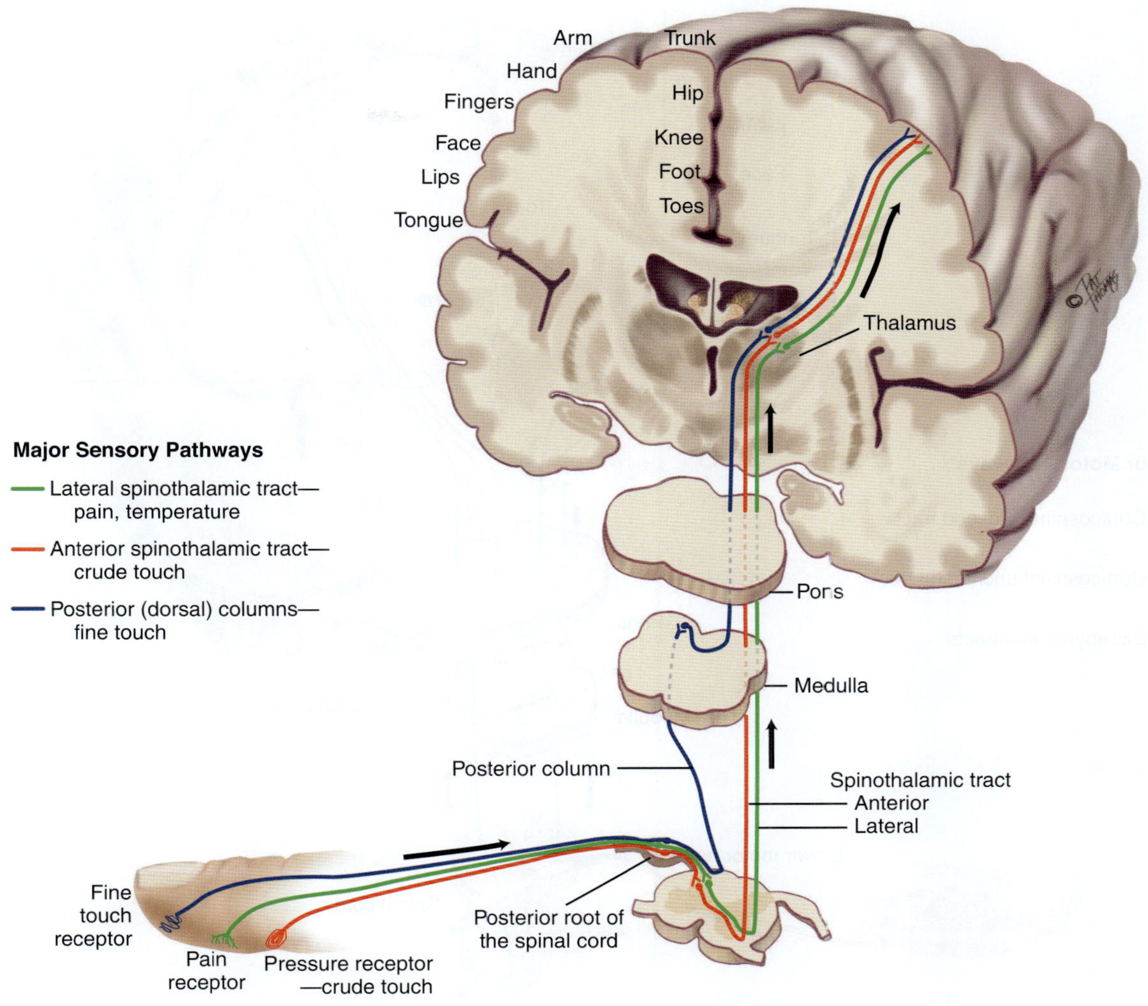

Figure 12.6
Major sensory pathways

cells in the motor cortex. Motor nerve fibres originate in the motor cortex and travel to the brainstem, where they cross to the opposite or contralateral side (*pyramidal decussation*) and then pass down in the lateral column of the spinal cord. At each cord level, they synapse with a lower motor neuron contained in the anterior horn of the spinal cord. Ten per cent of corticospinal fibres do *not* cross, and these descend in the anterior column of the spinal cord. Corticospinal fibres mediate voluntary movement, particularly very skilled, discrete, purposeful movements, such as writing.

The corticospinal tract is a newer, 'higher' motor system which humans have that permits very skilled and purposeful movements. The tract's origin in the motor cortex is arranged in a specific pattern called *somatotopic organisation*. It is another body map, this one of a person, or *homunculus*, hanging 'upside down' (see Figure 12.4). Body parts are not equally represented on the map, and the homunculus looks distorted. To use political terms, it is more like an electoral map than a geographic map. That is, body parts whose movements are relatively more important to humans (e.g. the hand) occupy proportionally more space on the brain map.

Extrapyramidal tracts. The extrapyramidal tracts include all the motor nerve fibres originating in the motor cortex, basal ganglia, brainstem and spinal cord that are *outside* the pyramidal tract. This is a phylogenetically older, 'lower', more primitive motor system. These subcortical motor fibres maintain muscle tone and control body movements, especially gross automatic movements, such as walking.

Cerebellar system. This complex motor system coordinates movement, maintains equilibrium and helps maintain posture. The cerebellum receives information about the position of muscles and joints, the body's equilibrium and what kind of motor messages are being sent from the cortex to the muscles. The information is integrated, and the cerebellum uses feedback pathways to exert its control back on the cortex or down to

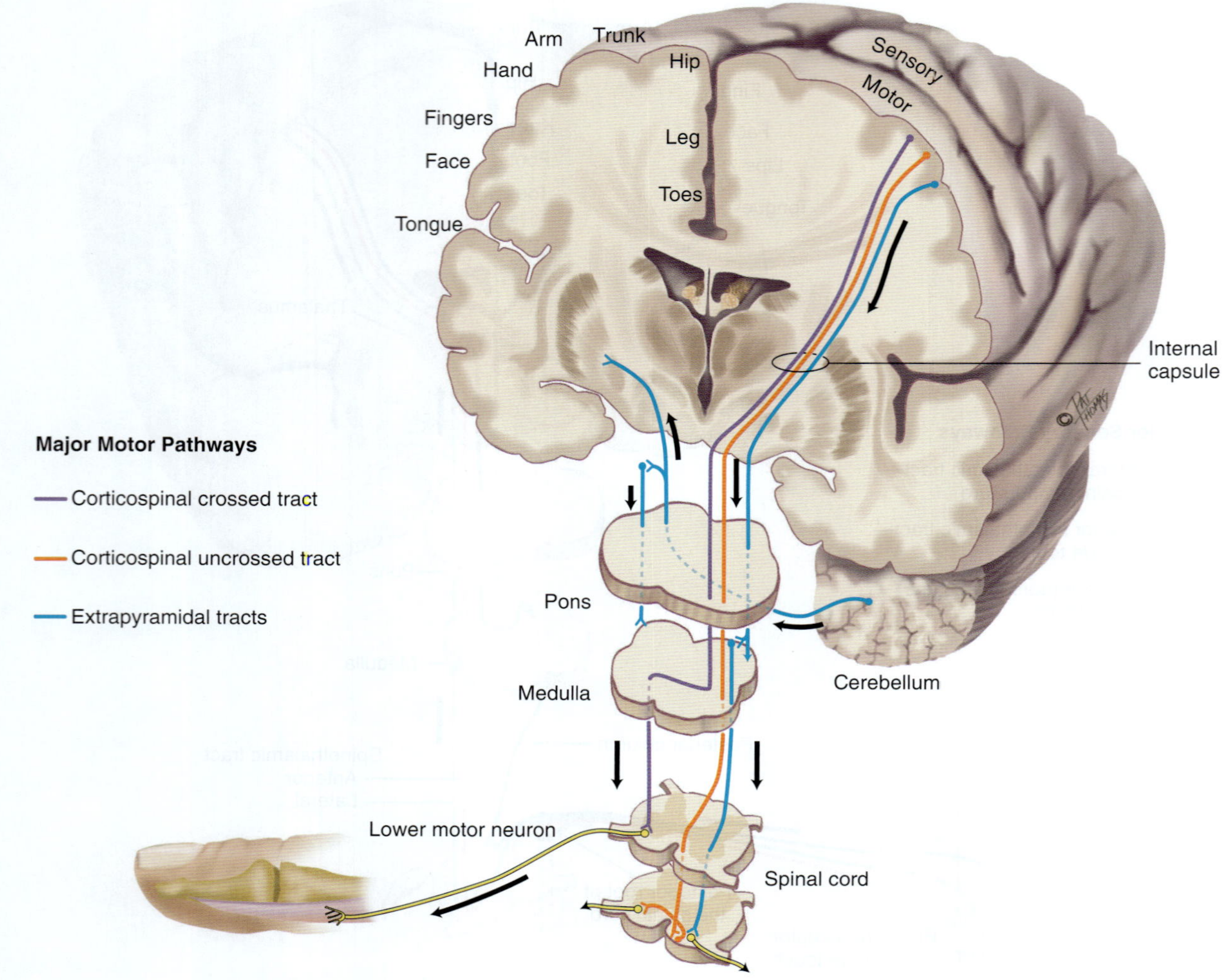

Figure 12.7
Major motor pathways

lower motor neurons in the spinal cord. This entire process occurs on a subconscious level.

Upper and lower motor neurons

Upper motor neurons are a complex of all the descending motor fibres that can influence or modify the lower motor neurons. Upper motor neurons are located completely within the CNS. The neurons convey impulses from motor areas of the cerebral cortex to the lower motor neurons in the anterior horn cells of the spinal cord. Examples of upper motor neurons are corticospinal, corticobulbar and extrapyramidal tracts. Examples of upper motor neuron diseases are stroke, cerebral palsy and multiple sclerosis. See Figure 12.8.

Lower motor neurons are located mostly in the peripheral nervous system. The cell body of the lower motor neuron is located in the anterior grey column of the spinal cord, but the nerve fibres extend from here to the muscle. The lower motor neuron is the 'final common pathway', because it funnels many neural signals here and it provides the final direct contact with the muscles. Any movement must be translated into action by lower motor neuron fibres. Examples of lower motor neurons are cranial nerves and spinal nerves of the peripheral nervous system. Examples of lower motor neuron diseases are Bell's palsy in cranial nerve lesions and in spinal cord lesions, poliomyelitis and motor neuron disease.

THE PERIPHERAL NERVOUS SYSTEM

A **nerve** is a bundle of fibres *outside* the CNS. The peripheral nerves carry input to the CNS via their sensory afferent fibres and deliver output from the CNS via the efferent fibres.

Reflex arc

Reflexes are basic defence mechanisms of the nervous system. They are involuntary, operating below the level of conscious control and permitting a quick reaction to potentially painful or damaging situations. Reflexes also help the body maintain balance and appropriate muscle tone. There are four types of reflexes: (1) **deep tendon reflexes** (myotatic), for example,

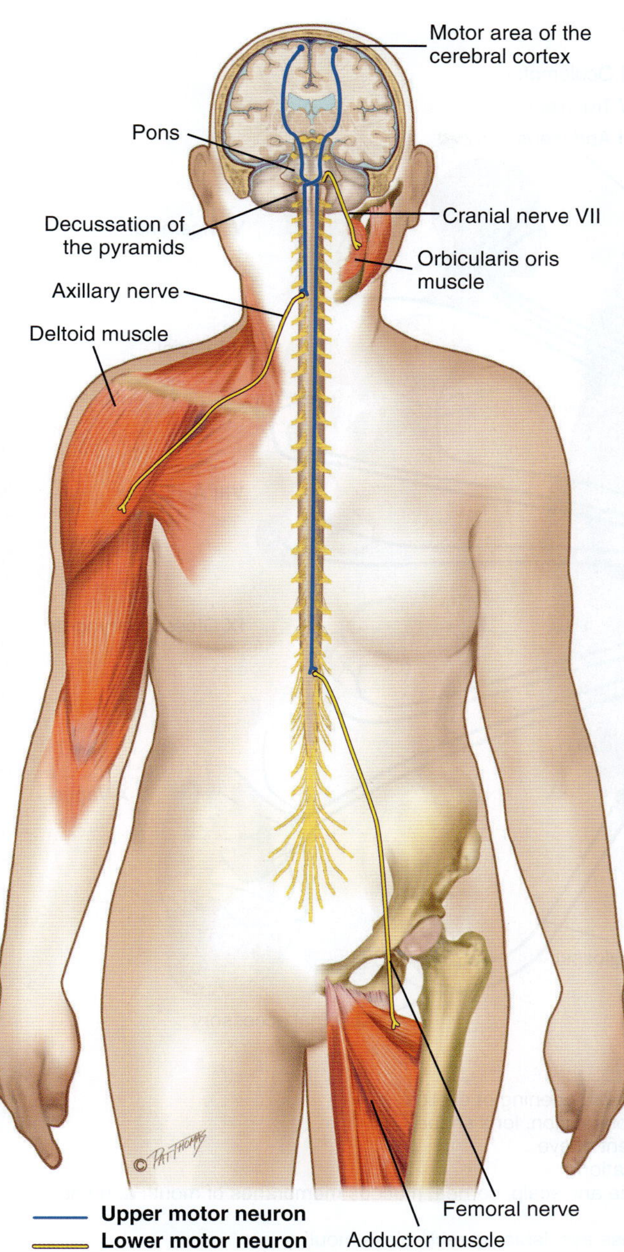

Figure 12.8

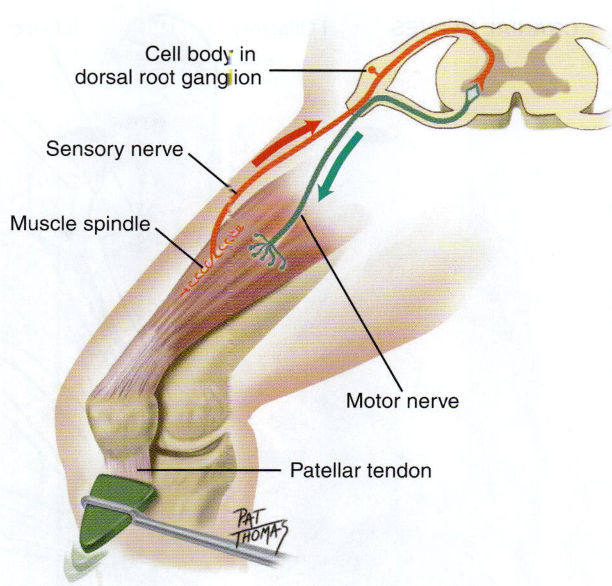

Figure 12.9
Reflex arc

patellar or knee jerk; (2) **superficial**, for example, corneal reflex, abdominal reflex; (3) **visceral** (organic), for example, pupillary response to light and accommodation; and (4) **pathological** (abnormal), for example, Babinski's or extensor plantar reflex.

The fibres that mediate the reflex are carried by a specific spinal nerve. In the simplest reflex, tapping the tendon stretches the muscle spindles in the muscle, which activates the sensory afferent nerve. The sensory afferent fibres carry the message from the receptor and travel through the dorsal root into the spinal cord (Figure 12.9). They synapse directly in the cord with the motor neuron in the anterior horn. Motor efferent fibres leave via the ventral root and travel to the muscle, stimulating a sudden contraction.

The deep tendon (myotatic or stretch) reflex has five components: (1) an intact sensory nerve (afferent); (2) a functional synapse in the cord; (3) an intact motor nerve fibre (efferent); (4) the neuromuscular junction; and (5) a competent muscle.

Cranial nerves

Cranial nerves are lower motor neurons that enter and exit the brain rather than the spinal cord (Figure 12.10). Cranial nerves I and II extend from the cerebrum; cranial nerves III–XII extend from the lower diencephalon and brainstem. The 12 pairs of cranial nerves supply primarily the head and neck, except the vagus nerve (Lat. *vagus*, or wanderer, as in 'vagabond') which, apart from supplying some sensory (tympanic membrane, external auditory canal, external ear and pharynx) and motor function (muscles of the palate, pharynx and larynx), also travels to the heart, respiratory muscles, stomach and gallbladder.

Spinal nerves

The 31 pairs of **spinal nerves** arise from the length of the spinal cord and supply the rest of the body. They are named for the region of the spine from which they exit: eight cervical, twelve thoracic, five lumbar, five sacral and one coccygeal. They are 'mixed' nerves because they contain both sensory and motor fibres. The nerves enter and exit the cord through roots—sensory afferent fibres through the posterior or dorsal roots, and motor efferent fibres through the anterior or ventral roots.

The nerves exit the spinal cord in an orderly ladder. Each nerve innervates a particular segment of the body. **Dermal segmentation** is the cutaneous distribution of the various spinal nerves.

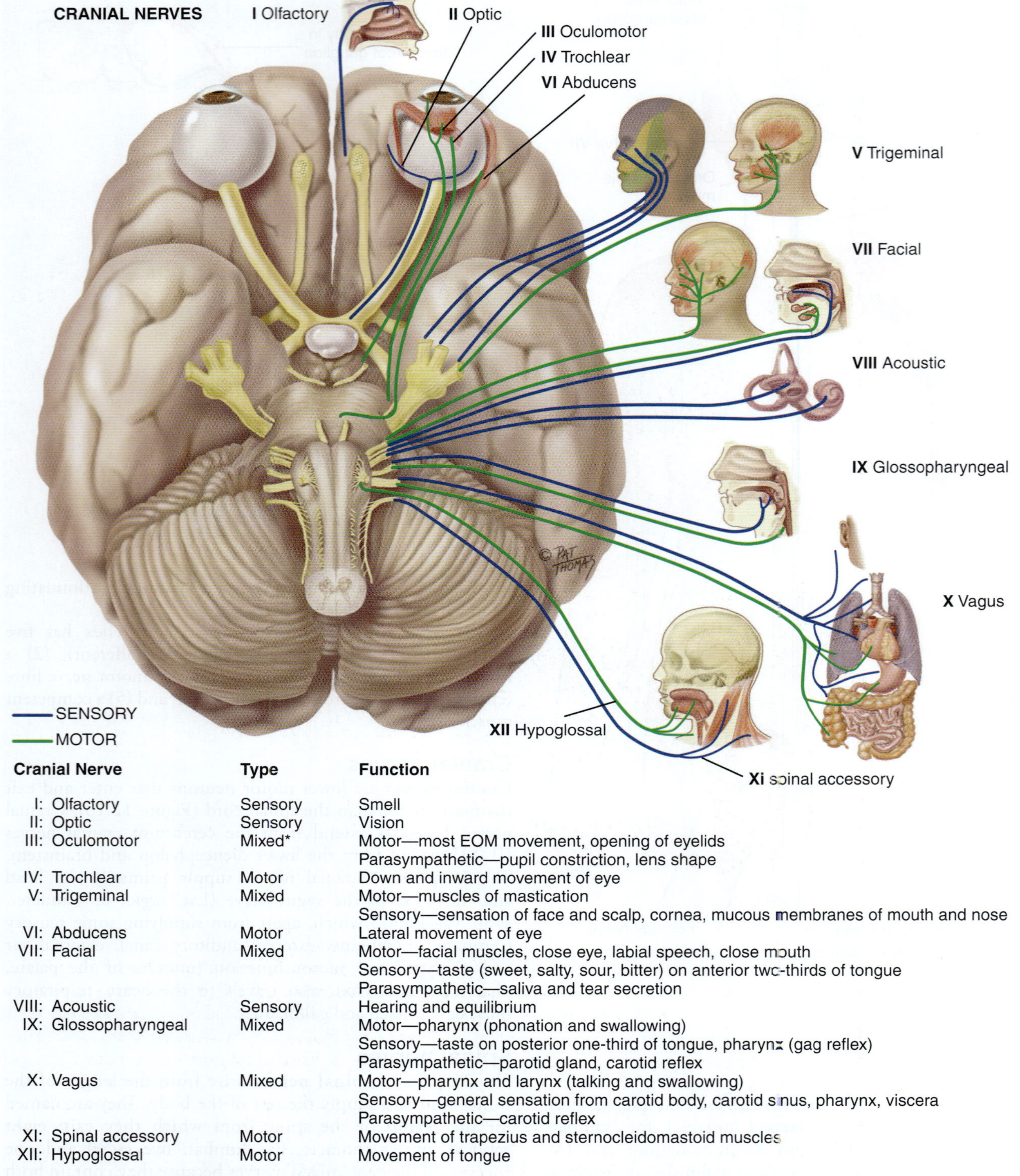

Cranial Nerve	Type	Function
I: Olfactory	Sensory	Smell
II: Optic	Sensory	Vision
III: Oculomotor	Mixed*	Motor—most EOM movement, opening of eyelids
		Parasympathetic—pupil constriction, lens shape
IV: Trochlear	Motor	Down and inward movement of eye
V: Trigeminal	Mixed	Motor—muscles of mastication
		Sensory—sensation of face and scalp, cornea, mucous membranes of mouth and nose
VI: Abducens	Motor	Lateral movement of eye
VII: Facial	Mixed	Motor—facial muscles, close eye, labial speech, close mouth
		Sensory—taste (sweet, salty, sour, bitter) on anterior two-thirds of tongue
		Parasympathetic—saliva and tear secretion
VIII: Acoustic	Sensory	Hearing and equilibrium
IX: Glossopharyngeal	Mixed	Motor—pharynx (phonation and swallowing)
		Sensory—taste on posterior one-third of tongue, pharynx (gag reflex)
		Parasympathetic—parotid gland, carotid reflex
X: Vagus	Mixed	Motor—pharynx and larynx (talking and swallowing)
		Sensory—general sensation from carotid body, carotid sinus, pharynx, viscera
		Parasympathetic—carotid reflex
XI: Spinal accessory	Motor	Movement of trapezius and sternocleidomastoid muscles
XII: Hypoglossal	Motor	Movement of tongue

**Mixed* refers to a nerve carrying a combination of fibres: motor + sensory; motor + parasympathetic; or motor + sensory + parasympathetic.

Figure 12.10
Cranial nerves

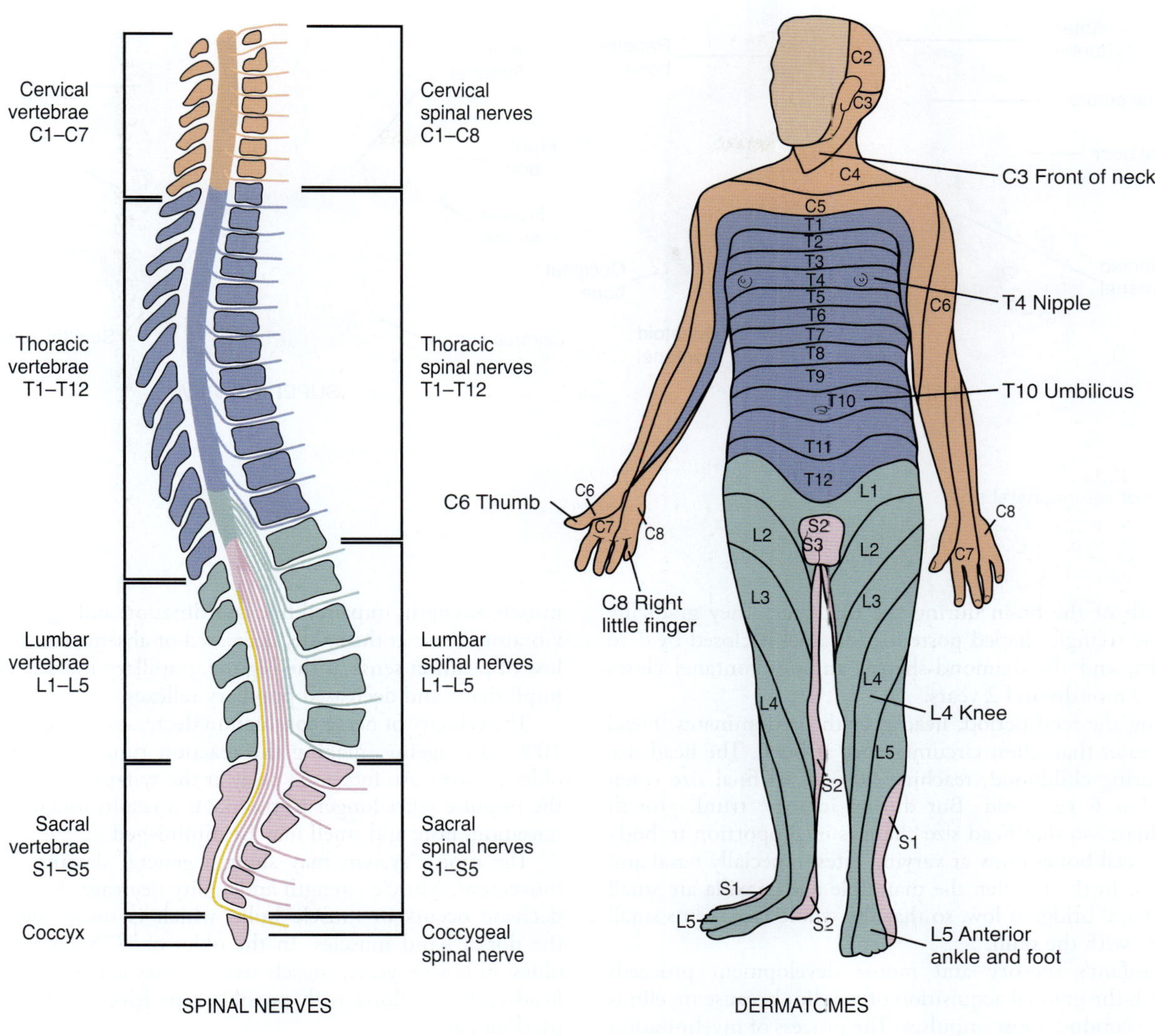

Figure 12.11
Spinal nerves dermatomes

A **dermatome** is a circumscribed skin area that is supplied mainly from one spinal cord segment through a particular spinal nerve (Figure 12.11). The dermatomes overlap, which is a form of biological insurance. That is, if one nerve is severed, most of the sensations can be transmitted by the one above and the one below. Do not attempt to memorise all dermatome segments; just focus on the following as useful landmarks:

- The **thumb**, **middle finger**, and **fifth finger** are each in the dermatomes of **C6**, **C7** and **C8**.
- The **axilla** is at the level of **T1**.
- The **nipple** is at the level of **T4**.
- The **umbilicus** is at the level of **T10**.
- The **groin** is in the region of **L1**.
- The **knee** is at the level of **L4**.

Somatic and autonomic nervous system

The peripheral nervous system is composed of cranial nerves and spinal nerves. These nerves carry fibres that can be divided functionally into two parts—somatic and autonomic. The somatic fibres innervate the skeletal (voluntary) muscles; the autonomic fibres innervate smooth (involuntary) muscles, cardiac muscle and glands. The autonomic system mediates unconscious activity. Although a description of the autonomic system is beyond the scope of this book, its overall function is to maintain homeostasis of the body.

DEVELOPMENTAL CONSIDERATIONS

Infants and children

The bones of the neonatal skull are separated by sutures and by **fontanels**, the spaces where the sutures intersect (Figure 12.12). These membrane-covered 'soft spots' allow

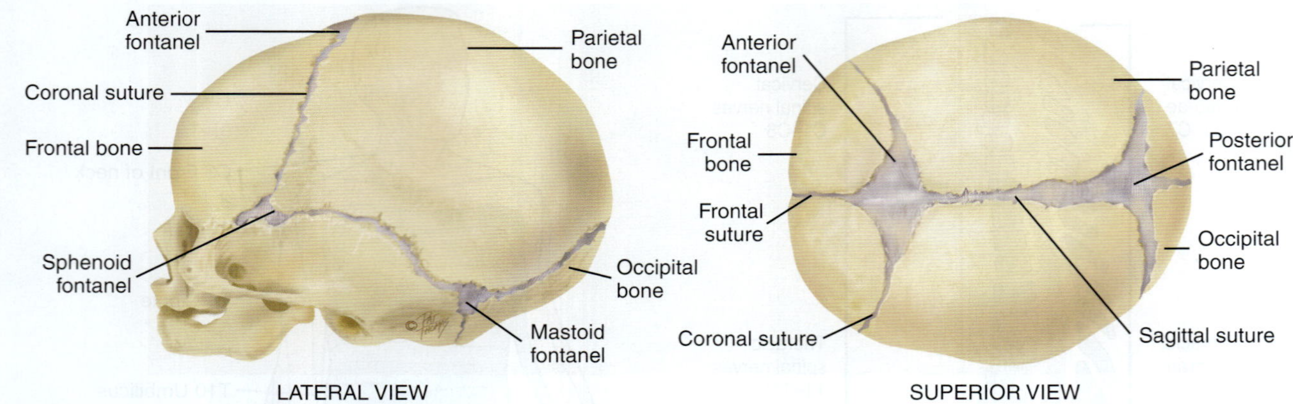

Figure 12.12
Bones of the neonatal skull

for growth of the brain during the first year. They gradually ossify; the triangle-shaped posterior fontanel is closed by 1 to 2 months, and the diamond-shaped anterior fontanel closes between 9 months and 2 years.

During the fetal period, head growth predominates. Head size is greater than chest circumference at birth. The head size grows during childhood, reaching 90% of its final size when the child is 6 years old. But during infancy, trunk growth predominates so that head size changes in proportion to body height. Facial bones grow at varying rates, especially nasal and jaw bones. In the toddler, the mandible and maxilla are small and the nasal bridge is low, so that the whole face seems small compared with the skull.

The infant's sensory and motor development proceeds along with the gradual acquisition of myelin, because myelin is needed to conduct most impulses. The process of myelinisation follows a cephalocaudal and proximodistal order (head, neck, trunk and extremities). This is just the order we observe the infant gaining motor control (lifts head, lifts head and shoulders, rolls over, moves whole arm, uses hands, walks). As the milestones are achieved, each is more complex and coordinated. Milestones occur in an orderly sequence, although the exact age of occurrence may vary.

The ability to localise sensation is also rudimentary at birth. The newborn needs a strong stimulus and then responds by crying and with whole body movements. As myelinisation develops, the infant is able to localise the stimulus more precisely and to make a more accurate motor response.

Late adulthood (65+ years)

As a person ages, the facial bones and orbits may appear more prominent, and the facial skin sags as a result of decreased elasticity, decreased subcutaneous fat and decreased moisture in the skin. The normal ageing process causes a general atrophy with a steady loss of neurons in the brain and spinal cord (Muller et al 2011). The loss of neurons causes a decrease in weight and volume of the brain. Neuron loss leads many older people to show signs that, in the younger adult, would be considered abnormal, such as general loss of muscle bulk, loss of muscle tone in the face, in the neck and around the spine, decreased muscle strength, impaired fine coordination and agility, loss of vibratory sense at the ankle, decreased or absent Achilles reflex, loss of position sense at the big toe, pupillary miosis, irregular pupil shape and decreased pupillary reflexes.

The velocity of nerve conduction decreases between 5% and 10% with ageing, making the reaction time slower in some older persons. An increased delay at the synapse also occurs, so the impulse takes longer to travel. As a result, touch and pain sensation, taste and smell may be diminished.

The motor system may show a general slowing down of movement. Muscle strength and agility decrease. A generalised decrease occurs in muscle bulk, which is most apparent in the dorsal hand muscles. In the older-old (75–84 years) and oldest old (85+ years) muscle tremors may occur in the hands, head and jaw, along with possible repetitive facial grimacing (dyskinesias).

Ageing is accompanied by a progressive decrease in cerebral blood flow and oxygen consumption. In some people this causes dizziness and a loss of balance with position change, which needs to be taken into account, for example when standing from a sitting position. When they are in good health, older people walk about as well as they did during their middle and younger years, but they tend to have slower and more deliberate movements.

Alzheimer's Disease and other dementias

Dementia is the term used to describe the symptoms of a large group of illnesses which cause a progressive decline in a person's functioning. It is a broad term used to describe a loss of memory, intellect, rationality, social skills and physical functioning. There are many types of dementia, including Alzheimer's Disease, vascular dementia and Lewy Body Disease. Dementia is the second leading cause of death of Australians (and the leading cause of death amongst Australian females). It is also the leading cause of disability for older Australians (over age 65) and the third leading cause of disability burden overall. In 2019, there are approximately 447,115 Australians living with dementia and more 1.5 million Australians involved in the care of someone with dementia. Currently, there is no cure for the disease. See Table 12.1.

Delirium in hospitalised older adults

Delirium is an acute confusional state that occurs very commonly in hospitalised older adults and is largely preventable. One third of general medical patients over the age of 70 years will experience delirium and there are several predisposing (baseline) or precipitating (contributing) factors which increase the risk of a patient developing delirium. Delirium is associated with poor short-term and long-term outcomes and has been independently associated with risk of death, and so early diagnosis and appropriate management of delirium is essential (including addressing any reversible causes and providing interventions to reduce the incidence, severity and duration of delirium). However, studies show that only 12–35% of delirium cases are recognised. This is perhaps partly because historically the condition has been variably described and there was not a well-defined criterion for diagnosis, but also because delirium is associated with many complex underlying medical conditions and can be hard to recognise (Inouye et al 2014, Marcantonio 2017).

In recent years there have been significant advances in the recognition and management of delirium in Australia. The Diagnostic and Statistical Manual of Mental Disorders, 5th edition (DSM-5 2013) describes diagnostic criteria for delirium and the Confusion Assessment Method (CAM) algorithm, demonstrated to be an effective bedside tool for the identification of delirium, has been widely implemented into Australian acute healthcare settings.

The presence of delirium requires all of the following criteria to be met (DSM-5 2013):

- Disturbance in attention and awareness
- Disturbance develops acutely and tends to fluctuate in severity
- At least one additional disturbance in cognition
- Disturbances are not better explained by a pre-existing dementia
- Disturbances do not occur in the context of a severely reduced level of arousal or coma
- Evidence of an underlying organic cause or causes.

CULTURAL AND SOCIAL CONSIDERATIONS

Many neurological health issues have profound impact on the person and their family. Some will be progressive and chronic, for example Parkinson's disease and multiple sclerosis; others have acute onset such as head or spinal cord injury or stroke. Many people will have ongoing cognitive and functional difficulties which will affect their ability to live a full and active life.

Stroke is a serious health problem in the Australian and New Zealand community. Stroke occurs when an artery supplying blood to the brain either suddenly becomes blocked or begins to bleed (Stroke Foundation Australia 2017).

Stroke has a high prevalence and incidence and is a leading cause of death and disability worldwide. The prevalence of stroke is similar in Australian males and females (1.7%). Australians living in regional areas are up to 19% more likely to suffer a stroke than those living in metropolitan areas (Stroke Foundation 2020). The incidence of new stroke in Australia equates to one stroke every 9 minutes (Stroke Foundation 2017).

Stroke is more common in older age groups; 67% of people who had a stroke were aged 65 years and over (AIHW 2017). However, stroke is not just a disease of older people; young people are also at risk. While the median age for stroke in Australia is around 75 years, one in every four strokes occurs in a person aged less than 65 years. Compared to older people, young people with stroke tend to take longer to seek medical attention, are less likely to receive rehabilitation and have more unmet needs in relation to psychosocial functioning and return to work. Though there is a lack of solid local trend evidence, rates of stroke in young people are increasing worldwide due to an increase in modifiable risk factors such as obesity, hypertension and diabetes (Brain Injury Australia 2016).

Aboriginal and Torres Strait Islander people are 1.5 times as likely to die from stroke as non-Indigenous Australians. They are younger too: their median age is 58 compared to 75 for non-Indigenous Australians. They also have poorer access to in-patient rehabilitation, secondary prevention to reduce risk of further stroke and community support to aid long-term recovery (Stroke Foundation 2017).

Stroke is largely a preventable health problem with modifiable risk factors such as high blood pressure, atrial fibrillation, hyperlipidaemia and smoking (Talley & O'Connor 2018). It is the high prevalence of these risk factors in Aboriginal and Torres Strait Islander people and Māori and Pacific Islander people that accounts for the high incidence of stroke in these groups (AIHW 2017, Stroke Foundation of New Zealand 2019). For further discussion of stroke risk factors, symptoms and prevention see the section titled 'Promoting a healthy lifestyle—stroke prevention' later in this chapter. See Table 12.2 Ischaemic and Haemorrhagic Stroke.

Subjective data

Assessment of neurological function is an important assessment area for nurses in a variety of healthcare settings and is part of a primary survey which is undertaken when first meeting a person, particularly in an emergency situation. The extent of the questioning and examination will depend on the person's main health concern.

Subjective assessment of neurological function investigates a variety of symptoms such as headache, dizziness, seizures, tremors, weakness, un-coordination, numbness or tingling, dysphagia and dysphasia. Symptoms such as these can impact the individual's safety and capacity to perform their activities of daily living. There may also be effects on the nutritional state of the person, their relationships and capacity to work. In addition, significant past history and environmental/occupational hazards are also explored. Neurological subjective assessment is performed in conjunction with assessment of the individual's mental state, vision, hearing, ability to smell, taste and touch and their position sense. The focused health assessment interview aims to clarify any presenting symptoms in the person's own words, after which you will need to carefully question the person to obtain further detail.

1. Presenting concern
2. Headache
3. Neck pain, limitation of motion
4. Pain
5. Head injury
6. Dizziness/vertigo
7. Seizures
8. Tremors and involuntary movements
9. Weakness
10. Un-coordination
11. Numbness or tingling
12. Visual disturbances and deafness
13. Difficulty swallowing
14. Difficulty speaking
15. Relevant health and family history
16. Health and lifestyle management
17. Environmental/occupational hazards

Practice note: Before you commence the assessment, introduce yourself to the person, confirm the person's identity, discuss the purpose and scope of the assessment, clarify any questions the person may have and obtain verbal consent from the person to perform the assessment.

ASSESSMENT GUIDELINES	CLINICAL SIGNIFICANCE AND CLINICAL ALERTS
1. Presenting concern	
• Do you feel that you have any problems concerning your ability to think, your memory, hearing, vision, sensation or with movement and coordination? It is important to ascertain the person's perception of their presenting health concern. • If they do perceive a problem—how does this impact on their quality of life?	
2. Headache	
Have you experienced any unusually frequent or severe headaches? • When did this start? How often does this occur? Gradual, over hours, or a day? Or, suddenly, over minutes, or less than 1 hour? • Ever had *this kind* of headache before? • Where in your head do you feel the headaches? In the front, side, over the temple area, behind your eyes, like a band around the head, in the sinus area or in the back of the head? Do the headaches seem to be associated with anything?	***Clinical alert:*** If a person reports any sudden onset of headache of increasing severity they should be referred to a medical practitioner for urgent further assessment. For location, character, duration, timing triggers of headaches, see Table 12.3.
• Is pain localised on one side, or all over?	Unilateral or bilateral (e.g. with cluster headaches pain is always unilateral and always on the same side of the head).
• Character. Throbbing (pounding, shooting) or aching (vice-like, constant pressure, dull)?	Character is typically vice-like with tension headache, throbbing with migraine or temporal arteritis.
• Is it mild, moderate or severe?	Quality—often severe with migraine, or excruciating with cluster headache.
• Course and duration. What time of day do the headaches occur: morning, evening, awaken you from sleep? • How long do they last? Hours, days? • Have you noted any daily headaches, or several within a time period?	Migraines occur about two per month, each lasting 1 to 3 days; one to two cluster headaches occur per day, each lasting 30 min to 2 hours for 1 or 2 months; then complete remission may last for months or years.

ASSESSMENT GUIDELINES	CLINICAL SIGNIFICANCE AND CLINICAL ALERTS
• Precipitating factors. What brings it on: activity or exercise, work environment, emotional upset, anxiety, alcohol?	Alcohol ingestion and daytime napping typically precipitate cluster headaches, whereas alcohol, letdown after stress, menstruation and eating chocolate or cheese precipitate migraines.
• Associated factors. Any relation to other symptoms: any nausea and vomiting? (Note which came first, headache or nausea.) Any vision changes, pain with bright lights, neck pain or stiffness, fever, weakness, moodiness, stomach problems?	Nausea, vomiting and visual disturbances are associated with migraines; eye reddening and tearing, eyelid drooping, rhinorrhoea and nasal congestion are associated with cluster headaches; anxiety and stress are associated with tension headaches; neck rigidity and fever are associated with meningitis or encephalitis.
• Do you have any other illness?	Hypertension, fever, hypothyroidism and vasculitis produce headaches.
• What makes it worse: movement, coughing, straining, exercise?	
• Pattern. Any family history of headache? • What is the frequency of your headaches: once a week? Are your headaches occurring more frequently? • Are they getting worse? Or are they getting better? • (For females) When do they occur in relation to your menstrual periods?	Migraines are associated with family history of migraine.
• Effort to treat. What seems to help: going to sleep, medications, positions, rubbing the area?	With migraines, people lie down to feel better, whereas with cluster headaches they need to move—even to pace the floor—to feel better.
• Coping strategies. How have these headaches affected your self-care, or your ability to function at work, home and socially?	
3. Neck pain	
Have you experienced any neck pain?	
• Onset. How did the pain start: injury, car accident, after lifting, from a fall? Or with a fever? Or did it have a gradual onset?	Acute onset of stiffness with headache and fever occurs with meningeal inflammation.
• Location. Does the pain radiate? To the shoulders, arms?	
• Associated symptoms. Any limitations to range of motion, numbness or tingling in shoulders, arms or hands?	
• Precipitating factors. What movements cause pain? Do you need to lift or bend at work or home?	
• Does stress seem to bring it on?	
• Coping strategies. Able to do your work, to sleep?	Pain creates a vicious circle. Tension increases pain and disability, which produces more anxiety.

SUBJECTIVE DATA

ASSESSMENT GUIDELINES	CLINICAL SIGNIFICANCE AND CLINICAL ALERTS
4. Other pain	
Do you have any pain in any other part of the body? • Intensity (using a numerical rating scale)—how would you rate your pain at the moment? At its worst, it is ... what? At its best, it is ... what? • Quality: Is it dull, sharp pressure, burning? • Onset/duration: When does it occur and for how long? • Relief of pain: Do you use medication or other strategies for relief of pain? • Effect of pain: How does the pain affect your work, any functional limitations, emotional status, concentration, appetite and relationship with others?	Refer to Chapter 13 for further discussion of pain assessment.
5. Head injury	
Have you ever had any **head injury**? Or have you sought healthcare because of a head injury? Please describe. • How did this occur? (Describe the mechanism.) Can you show me where on your head the injury occurred? • Did you have a loss of consciousness? For how long? • Were there any other effects such as nausea, vomiting, drowsiness, amnesia or confusion?	In some circumstances you might be obtaining this information from another person if the person is unable to respond or remember. While non-specific, any report of the following symptoms should prompt consideration of the diagnosis of concussion and warrants further investigation and follow up. **a.** Somatic (e.g. headache), cognitive (e.g. feeling like in a fog) and/or emotional symptoms (e.g. lability) **b.** Physical signs (e.g. loss of consciousness, amnesia, neurological deficit) **c.** Balance impairment (e.g. gait unsteadiness) **d.** Behavioural changes (e.g. irritability) **e.** Cognitive impairment (e.g. slowed reaction times) **f.** Sleep/wake disturbance (e.g. somnolence, drowsiness). ***Clinical alert:*** any change in conscious state should be referred to the responsible medical or nurse practitioner. The presence of nausea, vomiting, drowsiness or confusion can indicate rising intracranial pressure and the person should be urgently referred to the responsible medical or nurse practitioner for further assessment.
6. Dizziness/vertigo	
Do you ever feel lightheaded, experience a swimming sensation or feel faint? • When have you noticed this? How often does it occur? Does it occur with activity, change in position?	People often find it difficult to discriminate between dizziness and vertigo. Dizziness is often described as a period of light-headedness and maybe associated with a drop in BP. Syncope is a sudden loss of strength, a temporary loss of consciousness (a faint) due to lack of cerebral blood flow, e.g. low BP.
• Do you ever feel a sensation called **vertigo**, a rotational spinning sensation? Do you feel as if the room is spinning or that your head is spinning? Did this come on suddenly or gradually?	Vertigo is a sense of rotational spinning caused by neurological disease in the vestibular apparatus in the ear or in the vestibular nuclei in the brainstem.

ASSESSMENT GUIDELINES	CLINICAL SIGNIFICANCE AND CLINICAL ALERTS
7. Seizures	
Have you ever had any seizures (sometimes referred to as convulsions or fits)? When did they start? How often do they occur? • Course and duration: When a seizure starts, do you have any warning sign? What type of sign? • Motor activity: Where in your body do the seizures begin? Do the seizures travel through your body? On one side or both? Does your muscle tone seem tense or limp? • Any associated signs: colour change in face or lips, loss of consciousness (for how long?), automatisms (eyelid fluttering, eye rolling, lip smacking, vocalisation), incontinence? • Postictal (phase—after the seizure): Are you told you spend time sleeping? Do you have any confusion, weakness, headache or muscle ache? • Precipitating factors: Does anything seem to bring on the seizures: activity, discontinuing medication, flashing lights, fatigue and stress? • Are you on any medication? If so, what is the medication? • Coping strategies: How have the seizures affected daily life, occupation?	**Seizures** occur with epilepsy, a paroxysmal disease characterised by altered or loss of consciousness, involuntary muscle movements and sensory disturbances. However, an isolated seizure does not mean the person has epilepsy. **Aura** is a subjective sensation that precedes a seizure; it could be auditory, visual or motor.
8. Tremors and involuntary movements	
Do you ever experience shakes or **tremors** in the hands or face? When did these start? • Do they seem to grow worse with anxiety, intention or rest? • Are they relieved with rest, activity, alcohol? Do they affect daily activities? • Are you on any medication? If so, what is the medication?	Tremor is an involuntary shaking, vibrating or trembling. Often people will not report shakes or tremors without being directly asked about them. However, these may be signs that you observe during an assessment. You can use these questions to explore this observation. See Table 12.7 for further information.
9. Weakness	
• Do you experience any **weakness** or problem moving any part of the body? • Is this generalised or local? • Does weakness occur with any particular movement? (e.g. with proximal or large muscle weakness, it may be hard to get up out of a chair or reach for an object; with distal or small muscle weakness, it is hard to open a jar, write, use scissors or walk without tripping.) • Is there a fatiguable element (i.e. does the weakness get worse with repeated actions, or is it worst at the end of the day?)	**Paresis** is a partial or incomplete paralysis. **Paralysis** is a loss of motor function due to a lesion in the neurological or muscular system or loss of sensory innervation.
10. Lack of coordination	
• Do you experience any problem with **coordination**? • Any problem with balance when walking? • Do you lean to one side? • Any falling? • Which way? • Do your legs seem to give way? • Any clumsy movement?	**Dysmetria** is the inability to control range of motion of muscles.

SUBJECTIVE DATA

ASSESSMENT GUIDELINES	CLINICAL SIGNIFICANCE AND CLINICAL ALERTS
11. Numbness or tingling	
• Do you have any **numbness or tingling** in any part of the body? • Does it feel like pins and needles? • When did this start? • Where do you feel it? • Does it occur with activity?	**Paraesthesia** is an abnormal sensation, e.g. burning, tingling. ***Clinical alert:*** If the person is experiencing dizziness, tremor, paralysis, lack of coordination or paraesthesia there will be an impact of these symptoms on the person's ability to manage activities of daily living.
12. Visual disturbances and deafness	
• Have you experienced any periods of visual disturbances (such as double vision (diplopia), blurred vision (amblyopia), light intolerance (photophobia)) or visual loss? If so, when did this occur? One eye or both eyes? Sudden or gradual onset? How long did it last? What did you do about it? • Have you experienced any periods of deafness or changes in your hearing (such as ringing sound)? If so, when did this occur? Was it on one side or both? Sudden or gradual onset? How long did it last? Have you been exposed to loud noise in your workplace or recreationally? What did you do about it? See also Chapter 15 for further assessment of hearing.	***Clinical alert:*** visual disturbances can be signs of a problem within the eye or symptoms of other neurological health issues. A person with a sudden change in vision should be referred for urgent medical assessment. Unilateral deafness is likely to be the result of a nerve lesion (e.g. acoustic neuroma or trauma) and the person should be referred for an assessment by a medical practitioner (Talley & O'Connor 2018). For further information on causes of hearing loss refer to Chapter 15.
13. Difficulty swallowing (dysphagia)	
• Have you experienced a problem with swallowing? Does this occur with solids or liquids? Have you experienced excessive saliva, drooling?	**Dysphagia** is difficulty with swallowing. See Chapter 21 for further discussion of swallow assessment. ***Clinical alert:*** difficulty with swallowing can pose serious risk to a person's airway and requires further detailed assessment.
14. Difficulty speaking	
• Do you experience any problem **speaking**: for example, with forming words or with saying what you intended to say? When did you first notice this? How long did it last?	**Dysarthria** is difficulty forming words. **Dysphasia** is difficulty with language comprehension or expression (see Table 12.4).
15. Relevant health and family history	
• Stroke, head injury, spinal cord injury, hypertension, meningitis or encephalitis, mental health problems, family history of neurological health issues, degenerative neurological disease?	Many common medications can cause neurological symptoms. For example, major tranquillisers can have the side effect of sedation, parkinsonian tremor and ataxia; antihypertensive drugs can cause postural dizziness and fainting (Talley & O'Connor 2018).
16. Health and lifestyle management	
• Review of current medications. • Ask about smoking history (predisposition to cerebrovascular disease), alcohol use and illicit drug use.	

ASSESSMENT GUIDELINES	CLINICAL SIGNIFICANCE AND CLINICAL ALERTS
17. Environmental/occupational hazards	
• Are you exposed to any environmental/occupational hazards: for example, insecticides, organic solvents, lead?	
Additional history for infants and children	
1. Did you (the mother) have any health problems during the pregnancy: for example, any infections or illnesses, medications taken, preeclampsia, hypertension, alcohol or drug use, type 1 and type 2 diabetes? • You should also ask the parent whether the infant or child has undergone regular assessment with a Maternal & Child Health Nurse.	Prenatal history may affect infant's neurological development.
2. Please tell me about this baby's birth. Was the baby at term or premature? Birth weight? • Any birth trauma? Did the baby breathe immediately? • Were you told the baby's Apgar scores? • Any congenital defects?	
3. Reflexes: What have you noticed about the baby's behaviour? Do the baby's sucking and swallowing seem coordinated? When you touch the cheek, does the baby turn their head towards the touch? Does the baby startle with a loud noise or shake of crib? Does the baby grasp your finger?	
4. Does the child seem to have any problem with balance? Have you noted any unexplained falling, clumsy or unsteady gait, progressive muscular weakness, problem with going up or down stairs, problem with getting up from lying position?	If occurs, may not be noticed until starts to walk in late infancy. Screen for muscular dystrophy.
5. Has this child had any seizures? Please describe. Did the seizure occur with a high fever? Did any loss of consciousness occur—how long? How many seizures occurred with this same illness (if occurred with high fever)?	Seizures may occur with high fever in infants and toddlers. Or seizures may be a sign of neurological disease.
6. Did this child's motor or developmental milestones seem to come at about the right age? Does this child seem to be growing and maturing normally to you? How does this child's development compare to siblings or to age mates?	
7. Do you know if your child has had any environmental exposure to lead?	Chronically elevated lead levels may cause a developmental delay, a loss of a newly acquired skill or no clinical signs may be present.
8. Have you been told about any learning problems in school: problems with attention span, cannot concentrate, hyperactive?	
9. Any family history of: seizure disorder, cerebral palsy, muscular dystrophy?	
Additional history for the adult over 65 years	
1. Do you experience any problem with dizziness? Does this occur when you first sit or stand up, when you move your head, when you get up and walk just after eating? Does this occur with any of your medications?	Diminished cerebral blood flow and diminished vestibular response may produce staggering with position change, which increases risk of falls.
• (For men) Do you ever get up at night and then feel faint while standing to urinate? • How does dizziness affect your daily activities? Are you able to drive safely and to manoeuvre within your house safely? • What safety modifications have you applied at home?	Micturition syncope is a temporary loss of consciousness while urinating and is thought to be caused by a sudden positional drop in blood pressure.

SUBJECTIVE DATA

ASSESSMENT GUIDELINES	CLINICAL SIGNIFICANCE AND CLINICAL ALERTS
2. Have you noticed any decrease in memory, change in mental function? Have you felt any sense of confusion? Did this seem to come on suddenly or gradually? Has a family member expressed concern about your memory or ability to make decisions?	
3. Have you ever noticed any tremor? Is this in your hands or face? Is this worse with: anxiety, activity, rest? Does the tremor seem to be relieved with: alcohol, activity, rest? Does the tremor interfere with daily or social activities?	Tremor is relieved by alcohol, although this is not a recommended treatment. Assess if the person is abusing alcohol in an effort to relieve tremor.
4. Have you ever had any sudden vision change, fleeting blindness? Did this occur along with weakness? Did you have any loss of consciousness?	***Clinical alert:*** these symptoms can be characteristic of decreased blood flow to the brain and require more detailed medical investigation.

Objective data

There are three main types of objective neurological examinations—ongoing neurological observations, a screening examination and a complete examination.

The most common objective neurological assessment performed by nurses is **ongoing neurological observations ('neuro obs')**. This type of assessment is conducted on persons with demonstrated neurological deficits who require periodic or ongoing assessments. Most hospitals have specific charts to guide you in this assessment and for ease in recording the data. The assessment data is presented in graphic form and usually includes the Glasgow Coma Scale (see Figure 12.13 below), pupillary response and vital signs.

You would perform a **routine neurological screening assessment** (items identified in following sections) on seemingly well persons who have no significant subjective findings from the history.

You would perform a **complete neurological assessment** on persons who have neurological symptoms (e.g. change in conscious state, headache, weakness, loss of coordination) or who have shown signs of neurological dysfunction. The complete neurological assessment sequence are described in the advanced practice section below.

Preparation

People who have recent head trauma, neurological surgery, stroke or a neurological deficit due to a systemic disease process must be monitored closely for any improvement or deterioration in neurological status and for any indication of increasing intracranial pressure. Signs of increasing intracranial pressure signal impending cerebral disaster and potential death and require early and prompt intervention.

Equipment needed

Neurological observations chart
Penlight torch
Hand hygiene solution

PROCEDURES AND NORMAL FINDINGS	ABNORMAL FINDINGS AND CLINICAL ALERTS
General inspection (ongoing neurological observations and routine neurological screening assessment)	
Neurological assessment begins as soon as you see the person. This enables the clinician to quickly determine the the extent of the neurological assessment that is required. As you undertake the subjective data collection you will also be making observations of the following.	
Alertness • Do they appear to be aware of their surroundings? • Conscious • Unconscious • Drowsy/stupor	This will enable the clinician to determine how to proceed with the neurological assessment. ***Clinical alert:*** If any suspicion of change to conscious state the Glasgow Coma Scale should be conducted (Figure 12.13).

PROCEDURES AND NORMAL FINDINGS	ABNORMAL FINDINGS AND CLINICAL ALERTS
Posture • Straight • Listing to one side	This may indicate a previous or current neurological condition.
Dysmorphic features • Facial expressions (facies) • Skull shape and size • Skeleton, spine, hands and feet • Skin	Dysmorphic features may indicate underlying congenital neurological conditions and may require a complete neurological examination by a specialist practitioner.
Hygiene and grooming • Cleanliness • Body odours • Appropriate dress for age and environment	The ability to care for oneself is often demonstrated in how we present ourselves. Although this may indicate underlying mental health concerns it may also indicate neurological disorder of the brain, in particular the frontal lobe.

Affect, attitude, mood
• Behaviour: Are they acting appropriately to their current situation?
• Note speech
  – Volume (see Table 12.6 for common speech disorders)
  – Appropriateness
  – Incomprehensible
• Facial expressions
  – Grimacing
  – Contorting their face
  – Smiling
• Does what they convey relate to their facial expression?
• Do they appear relaxed?
• Can they make and maintain eye contact?
	The ability to interact with others may be inhibited by either neurological or mental health conditions.

Supports • Glasses • Hearing aids • Walking stick • Communication board • Tracheostomy	Supports may determine to what extent the neurological examination can be performed.
Movement • Coordinated • Guarded • Un-coordinated	
Muscles • Bulk • Atrophy • Fasciculations	May indicate underlying medical conditions which may affect the neurological assessment.

OBJECTIVE DATA

PROCEDURES AND NORMAL FINDINGS	ABNORMAL FINDINGS AND CLINICAL ALERTS
Level of consciousness (ongoing neurological observations and routine neurological screening assessment)	
A *change* in the level of consciousness is the single most important factor in this assessment. A change can be subtle. Note the ease of arousal and state of awareness and orientation. A person is fully alert when: • their eyes are open or open spontaneously at your approach; • they are oriented to person, place and time; and • they are able to follow verbal commands appropriately.	Note any decreasing level of consciousness, disorientation, memory loss, uncooperative behaviour or even complacency in a previously combative person. ***Clinical alert:*** If the person is not fully alert, increase the amount of stimulus used in this order: • Light touch on person's arm • Vigorous shake of shoulder • Pain applied (pressure to nailbed, pinch trapezius muscle. Be careful not to inflict trauma/bruising on the person. If the person is not responding there is no point in repeatedly continuing to inflict pain. Note your findings and report any changes to a medical practitioner.
Assess orientation by asking questions about: • Person—own name, occupation, • Place—where person is, nature of building, city, state • Time—day of week, month, year	***Clinical alert:*** If any sudden change in the person's orientation to person, place or time, complete a Glasgow Coma Scale score and then report the findings to the medical practitioner immediately.
Vary the questions during repeat assessments so that the person is not merely memorising answers. Note the quality and the content of the verbal response; articulation, fluency, manner of thinking; and any deficit in language comprehension or production (see Chapter 7).	***Clinical alert:*** If the person cannot speak fluent English or if English is not their first language, you may need to get the assistance of a qualified interpreter to ensure accuracy in the assessment.
If the person cannot speak, you will have to ask questions that require a nod or shake of the head, 'Are we in a hospital?' 'Are you at home?' 'Are we in (location/place)?'	
Using the Glasgow Coma Scale (ongoing neurological observations)	
The Glasgow Coma Scale (GCS) was developed as an accurate and reliable **quantitative** tool that assesses the functional state of the brain as a whole (Figure 12.13). The GCS is a standardised, objective assessment that defines the level of consciousness by giving it a numeric value. This universal scale has good interrater reliability (Teasdale et al 2014) and enhances interprofessional communication by providing a common language.	Where possible, have one nurse conduct the assessments over a shift time frame. This will increase the reliability of the data over time. Before handing over to the next shift nurse, take the time to conduct the test together to increase the reliability of the data between the two nurses.
The scale is divided into three areas: **eye opening, verbal response** and **motor response**. Each area is rated separately, and a number is given for the person's best response. The three numbers are added: • the total score reflects the brain's functional level. • a fully alert, normal person has a score of 15, whereas a score of 7 or less reflects coma. • serial assessments are plotted on a graph to illustrate visually whether the person is stable, improving or deteriorating.	A score of 15 indicates normal consciousness A score of 7 indicates coma A score of 3 indicates a deep coma ***Clinical alert:*** any downward trend (a change in score of 2 or more) in the GCS score should be urgently reported for medical review.

PROCEDURES AND NORMAL FINDINGS | ABNORMAL FINDINGS AND CLINICAL ALERTS

GLASGOW COMA SCALE (GCS)			
(E) Eye opening - indicates the person's level of arousal	Open spontaneously	4	If the eyes are closed by swelling record as - C
	Open to sound or speech	3	
	Open to pressure or painful stimuli	2	
	None/no eye opening	1	
(V) Best verbal response - appropriateness of the person's speech	Orientated to time, place, person	5	If the person has a tracheostomy record as - T
	Confused	4	
	Inappropriate words	3	
	Incomprehensible sounds	2	
	Silent/no verbal response	1	
(M) Best motor response - awareness/ability to respond by movement	Obeys commands	6	Usually record the best arm response
	Localises to painful stimuli	5	
	Withdraws from painful stimuli	4	
	Abnormal flexion to painful stimuli (decorticate)	3	
	Abnormal extension to painful stimuli (decerebrate)	2	
	No motor response	1	
	Total GCS score/15 =		

Figure 12.13
Glasgow Coma Scale
Adapted from Institute of Neurological Sciences. (2015). *Glasgow Coma Scale: Do it this way.* NHS Greater Glasgow and Clyde. https://www.glasgowcomascale.org/downloads/GCS-Assessment-Aid-English.pdf?v=3; Mehta, R., & Chinthapalli, K. (2019). Glasgow coma scale explained. *BMJ,* 365, l1296.

Eye opening

Best eye opening response:

- Note the person's ability to open their eyes spontaneously.
- If the person does not open their eyes spontaneously, note whether they open their eyes to your request asking them to open their eyes (record if they open their eyes to speech).
- If they do not open their eyes to speech, apply painful stimuli as described above (start with light touch and increase as necessary).
- If they do not open their eyes to painful stimuli, record no response.

Verbal response

Best verbal response:

- Check the person's orientation to person, place, time (follow the instructions detailed above).
- Assess clarity and appropriateness of words/speech or note if there is no verbal response.
- If the person is unable to speak due to an endotracheal tube or tracheostomy tube, record this on the chart.

OBJECTIVE DATA

PROCEDURES AND NORMAL FINDINGS	ABNORMAL FINDINGS AND CLINICAL ALERTS

Motor Response

Best motor response:

Ask the person, 'Can you wriggle your fingers (or toes)?'

- If the person can wriggle their fingers even faintly they are scored as obeying commands.
- This procedure also tests level of consciousness by noting the person's ability to follow commands.
- If the person cannot obey your commands, you would then assess the person's best motor response to a painful stimuli.
- For the person with decreased level of consciousness, movement may occur spontaneously and as a result of noxious stimuli such as airway suctioning.

In response to painful stimulus, if the person:

- moves their hand above the nipple line, record **'localising to pain'**
- moves their body away from the pain but does not localise, record **withdraws from pain**
- bends their arm at the elbow, record '**flexion**'.
- extends their elbows and internally rotates their wrists, record '**extension to painful stimuli**'
- If there is no physical response to painful stimulus, record '**no response**'

Pupillary response (ongoing neurological observations and routine neurological screening assessment)

- To test the pupillary light reflex, darken the room and ask the person to gaze into the distance. (This dilates the pupils.)
- Shine a fine light beam (from a penlight torch) in from the side and note the response. Normally you will see (1) constriction of the same-sided pupil (a direct light reflex) and (2) simultaneous constriction of the other pupil (a consensual light reflex).
- Note the size, shape and symmetry of both pupils.
- Both pupils should constrict briskly. (Allow for the effects of any medication that could affect pupil size and reactivity.)

Increasing intracranial pressure causes a sudden, unilateral, dilated and nonreactive pupil. Cranial nerve III runs parallel to the brainstem. When increasing intracranial pressure pushes the brainstem down (brain herniation or 'coning'), it puts pressure on cranial nerve III, causing pupil dilatation.

Unequal, slowed response.

Clinical alert: Report changes in the pupil size immediately for urgent medical review. You should continue to perform ongoing neurological observations.

In the acute care setting, gauge the pupil size in millimetres, both before and after the light reflex. Normally, the resting size is 3, 4 or 5 mm and decreases equally in response to light (Figure 12.14). This indicates that both pupils measure 3 mm in the resting state and that both constrict to 1 mm in response to light. A graduated scale printed on a handheld vision screener or taped onto a tongue blade facilitates your measurement (Figure 12.15).

Clinical documentation: Record the normal response to all these manoeuvres as PERRLA, or **P**upils **E**qual, **R**ound, **R**eact to **L**ight and **A**ccommodation.

Pupil sizes in millimetres	
1 mm	●
2 mm	●
3 mm	●
4 mm	●
5 mm	●
6 mm	●
7 mm	●
8 mm	●

Figure 12.14

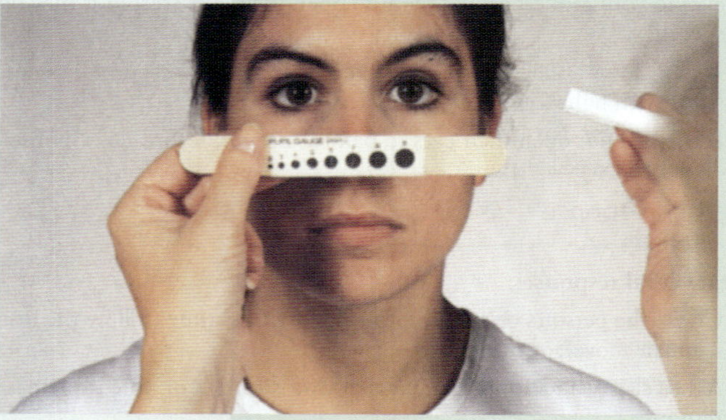

Figure 12.15

PROCEDURES AND NORMAL FINDINGS	ABNORMAL FINDINGS AND CLINICAL ALERTS
Vital signs (ongoing neurological observations)	
Measure the temperature, pulse, respiration and blood pressure as often as the person's condition warrants. Vital signs should always be performed after neurological assessment as the act of performing these activities may elicit painful response to eye opening rather than to name.	Although they are vital to the overall assessment of the critically ill person, pulse and blood pressure are notoriously unreliable parameters of CNS deficit. Any changes are late consequences of rising intracranial pressure. ***Clinical alert:*** **The Cushing reflex** shows signs of increasing intracranial pressure: blood pressure—sudden elevation with widening pulse pressure; pulse—decreased rate, slow and bounding. This requires urgent medical referral.
Limb movement and strength (ongoing neurological observations and routine neurological screening assessment)	
Upper extremities • You can check upper arm strength by checking hand grasps. • Ask the person to squeeze your fingers. Offer your two fingers, one on top of the other, so that a strong hand grasp does not hurt your knuckles (Figure 12.16). • Do not place fingers in the palm of the person's hand as some people with diffuse brain damage, especially frontal lobe injury, have a grasp that is a reflex only. 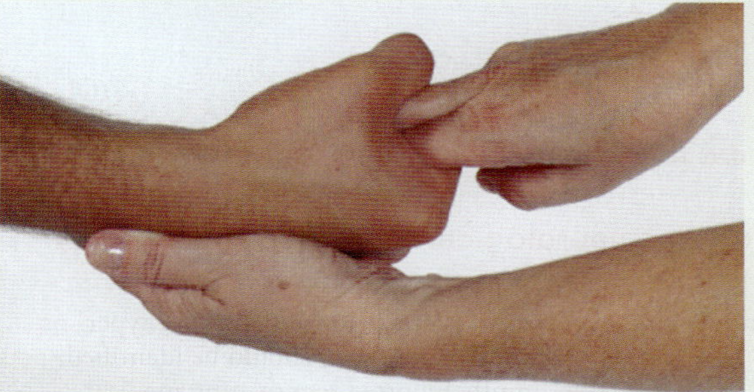 Figure 12.16	Unequal grasp. ***Clinical alert:*** Changes to limb movement, strength and/or balance can put the person at risk of falling and or being unable to perform activities of daily living. In such a situation a detailed assessment is required to be performed by a nurse or medical practitioner.
• Alternatively, ask the person to lift each hand or to hold up one finger. • You can also check upper extremity strength by palmar drift. Ask the person to extend both arms forwards or halfway up, palms up, eyes closed and hold for 10 to 20 seconds (Figures 12.17A and 12.17B). • Normally, the arms stay steady with no downward drift. 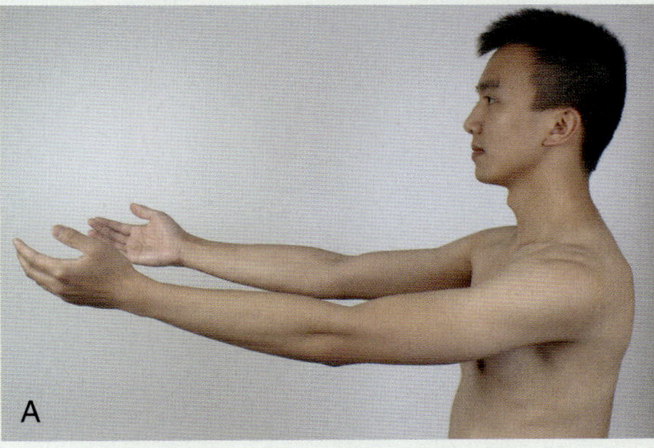 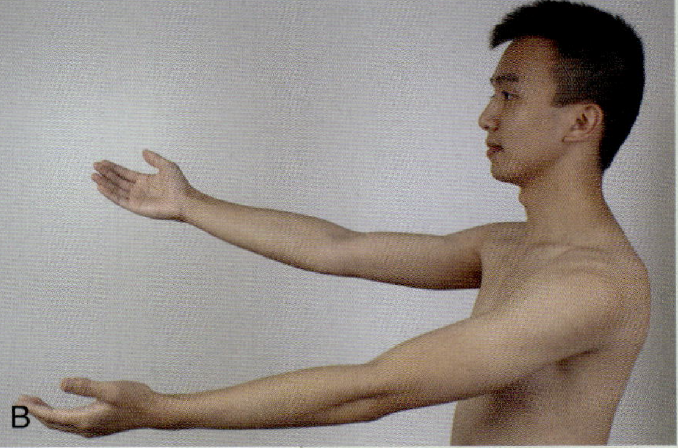 Figure 12.17	

PROCEDURES AND NORMAL FINDINGS	ABNORMAL FINDINGS AND CLINICAL ALERTS
Lower extremities • Check lower extremities by asking the person to do straight leg raises. • Ask the person to lift one leg at a time straight up off the bed (Figure 12.18). • Full strength allows the leg to be lifted 90 degrees. If multiple trauma, pain or equipment exclude this motion, ask the person to push one foot at a time against your hand's resistance, 'like putting your foot on the accelerator pedal of your car' (Figure 12.19).	Unequal resistance. Changes in motor function may indicate pathological conditions of the spinal cord or cerebral cortex. Disorders of the neurological system may affect muscle tone and strength.

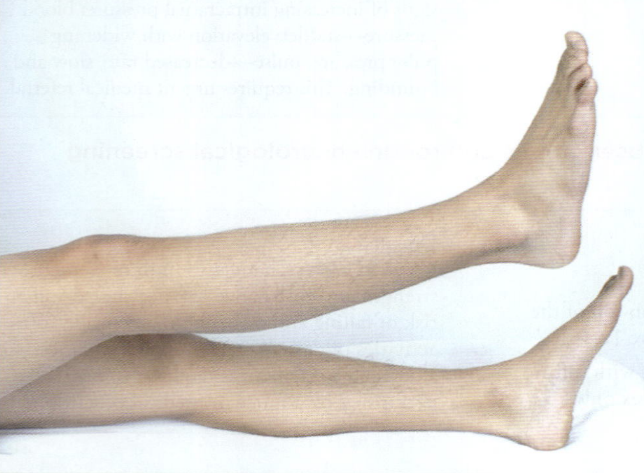

Figure 12.18

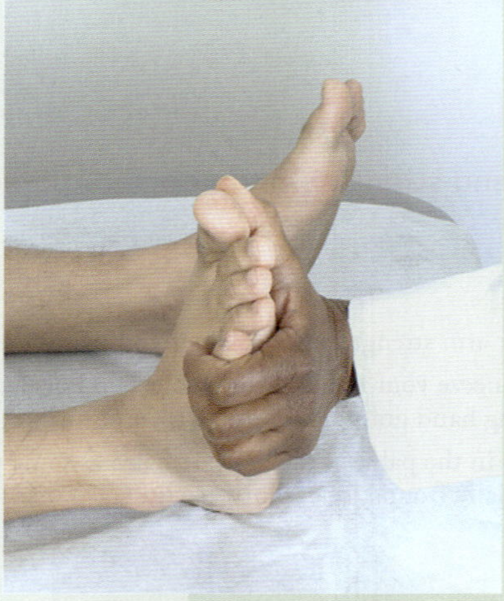

Figure 12.19

Assessing delirium (ongoing neurological observations and routine neurological screening assessment)

For recognising delirium in hospitalised patients use the Confusion Assessment Method (CAM) (Marcantonio 2017). The presence of delirium requires the presence of features 1 and 2 and either 3 or 4: **1.** Acute change in mental status with fluctuating course **AND** **2.** Inattention **AND EITHER** **3.** Disorganised thinking **OR** **4.** Altered level of consciousness	***Clinical alert:*** Signs of delirium (hyper- or hypoactive delirium) should be identified, promptly reported to a treating medical clinician, carefully documented (i.e. using a validated tool, such as the Confusion Assessment Method) and closely monitored. Measures should be taken to identify and, whenever possible, predict or eliminate potential contributing factors. Escalating or fluctuating conscious state in delirium may be an indicator of increased risk of morbidity and mortality. See also Chapter 30.

OBJECTIVE DATA

Further objective assessment for advanced practice

The assessments described in the following sections require advanced skill and scope of practice. Nurses working in specialist settings need to develop these skills.

Preparation

In addition to the assessment strategies described above, use the following sequence for a complete neurological examination.

1. Mental health (see Chapter 11)
2. Head, face and neck
3. Cranial nerves
4. Motor system
5. Sensory system
6. Reflexes

Equipment needed

Neurological observations chart
Hand hygiene solution
Penlight torch
Tongue blade
Cotton swab
Cotton ball
Tuning fork (128 Hz or 256 Hz)
Percussion hammer
(Possibly) familiar aromatic substances, e.g. peppermint, coffee, vanilla

PROCEDURES AND NORMAL FINDINGS	ABNORMAL FINDINGS AND CLINICAL ALERTS
Inspect head, face and neck	
Inspect and palpate the skull	
Note the general size and shape. **Normocephalic** is the term that denotes a round symmetrical skull that is appropriately related to body size. Be aware that 'normal' includes a wide range of sizes.	Abnormalities: microcephaly (abnormally small head); macrocephaly (abnormally large head)—as occurs in hydrocephaly, acromegaly, Paget's disease.
To assess shape, place your fingers in the person's hair and palpate the scalp. The skull normally feels symmetrical and smooth. The cranial bones that have normal protrusions are the forehead, the lateral edge of each parietal bone, the occipital bone and the mastoid process behind each ear. There is no tenderness to palpation.	Note lumps, depressions or abnormal protrusions.
Temporal area Palpate the temporal artery above the zygomatic (cheek) bone between the eye and top of the ear.	The artery looks more tortuous and feels hardened and tender with temporal arteritis.
The temporomandibular joint is just below the temporal artery and anterior to the tragus. Palpate the joint as the person opens the mouth and note normally smooth movement with no limitation or tenderness.	Crepitation, limited range of motion or tenderness.
Inspect the face	
Facial expression Appropriateness to behaviour or reported mood. Anxiety is common in the hospitalised or ill person.	Hostility or embarrassment. Tense, rigid muscles may indicate anxiety or pain; a flat affect may indicate depression; excessive smiling may be inappropriate.
Shape and symmetry of facial structures May vary somewhat among people, they should always be largely symmetrical. Note symmetry of eyebrows, palpebral fissures, nasolabial folds and sides of the mouth. Note any abnormal facial structures (coarse facial features, exophthalmos, changes in skin colour or pigmentation) or any abnormal swelling. Also note any involuntary movements (tics) in the facial muscles. Normally none occur.	Marked asymmetry with central brain lesion (e.g. stroke) or with peripheral cranial nerve VII damage (Bell's palsy). See Table 12.15. Oedema in the face occurs first around the eyes (periorbital) and the cheeks where the subcutaneous tissue is relatively loose. Note rhythmic movement of jaw, tics, fasciculations or excessive blinking.

OBJECTIVE DATA

PROCEDURES AND NORMAL FINDINGS	ABNORMAL FINDINGS AND CLINICAL ALERTS
Inspect and palpate the neck	
Symmetry Head position is centred in the midline, and the accessory neck muscles should be symmetrical. The head should be held erect and still.	Head tilt occurs with muscle spasm. Rigid head and neck occur with arthritis.
Range of motion (ROM) Note any limitation of movement during active motion. Ask the person to touch the chin to the chest, turn the head to the right and left, try to touch each ear to the shoulder (without elevating shoulders) and to extend the head backwards. When the neck is supple, motion is smooth and controlled.	Note pain at any particular movement. Note ratchety or limited movement from cervical arthritis or inflammation of neck muscles. The arthritic neck is rigid; the person turns at the shoulders rather than at the neck.
Muscle strength Test muscle strength and the status of cranial nerve XI by trying to resist the person's movements with your hands as the person shrugs the shoulders and turns the head to each side.	
Palpate for swelling, masses, pulsations As the person moves the head, note enlargement of the salivary glands and lymph glands. Normally no enlargement is present. Note a swollen parotid gland when the head is extended; look for swelling below the angle of the jaw. Also, note thyroid gland enlargement. Normally none is present.	Thyroid enlargement may be a unilateral lump, or it may be diffuse and look like a doughnut lying across the lower neck (see Table 12.8).
Also note any obvious pulsations. The carotid artery runs medial to the sternocleidomastoid muscle, and it creates a brisk localised pulsation just below the angle of the jaw. Normally, there are no other pulsations while the person is in the sitting position (see Chapter 17).	
Test the cranial nerves	
Cranial nerve I—olfactory nerve	
Do not test routinely. Test the sense of smell in those who report loss of smell, those with head trauma and those with altered mental status, and when the presence of an intracranial lesion is suspected. First, assess patency by occluding one nostril at a time and asking the person to sniff. Then, with the person's eyes closed, occlude one nostril and present an aromatic substance. Use familiar, conveniently obtainable and non-noxious smells, such as coffee, toothpaste, orange, vanilla, soap or peppermint.	You cannot test smell when air passages are occluded with upper respiratory infection or with sinusitis. **Anosmia**—decrease or loss of smell occurs bilaterally with tobacco smoking, allergic rhinitis and cocaine use.
Normally, a person can identify an odour on each side of the nose. Smell is normally decreased bilaterally with ageing. Any asymmetry in the sense of smell is important.	Unilateral loss of smell in the absence of nasal disease is **neurogenic anosmia** (see Table 12.5).
Cranial nerve II—optic nerve	
Test visual acuity and test visual fields by confrontation (see Chapter 14).	Visual field loss (see Table 14.5).
Using the ophthalmoscope, examine the ocular fundus to determine the colour, size and shape of the optic disc (see Chapter 14).	Papillo-oedema with increased intracranial pressure; optic atrophy (see Table 14.9).
Cranial nerves III, IV and VI—oculomotor, trochlear and abducens nerves	
Palpebral fissures are usually equal in width or nearly so (see Figure 14.1).	Ptosis (drooping) occurs with myasthenia gravis, dysfunction of cranial nerve III or Horner's syndrome (see Table 14.2).

PROCEDURES AND NORMAL FINDINGS	ABNORMAL FINDINGS AND CLINICAL ALERTS
Check pupils for size, regularity, equality, direct and consensual light reaction and accommodation (see above and Chapter 14).	Increasing intracranial pressure causes a sudden, unilateral, dilated and nonreactive pupil. ***Clinical alert:*** report this finding immediately to medical practitioner. You should continue to perform ongoing neurological observations.
Assess extraocular movements by the cardinal positions of gaze (see Chapter 14). Nystagmus is a back-and-forth oscillation of the eyes. End-point nystagmus, a few beats of horizontal nystagmus at extreme lateral gaze, occurs normally. Assess any other nystagmus carefully, noting: • Presence of abnormal movement in one or both eyes. • *Pendular* movement (oscillations move equally left to right) or *jerk* (a quick phase in one direction, then a slow phase in the other). Classify the jerk nystagmus in the direction of the quick phase. • Amplitude. Judge whether the degree of movement is fine, medium or coarse. • Frequency. Is it constant, or does it fade after a few beats? • Plane of movement. Horizontal, vertical, rotary or a combination?	**Strabismus** (deviated gaze) or limited movement **Nystagmus** occurs with disease of the vestibular system, cerebellum or brainstem. Nystagmus leads to low vision: symptoms include: blurred vision and a reduction in depth perception which may put the person at risk of injury, falls or an inability to manage their activities of daily living.
Cranial nerve V—trigeminal nerve	
Motor function. Assess the muscles of mastication by palpating the temporal and masseter muscles as the person clenches the teeth (Figure 12.20). Muscles should feel equally strong on both sides. Next, try to separate the jaws by pushing down on the chin; normally you cannot. 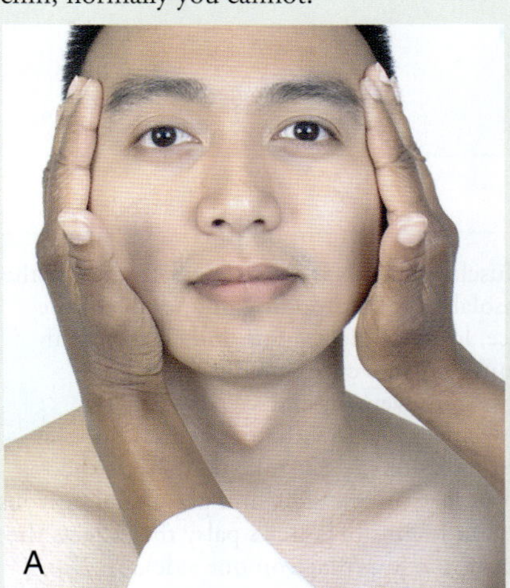 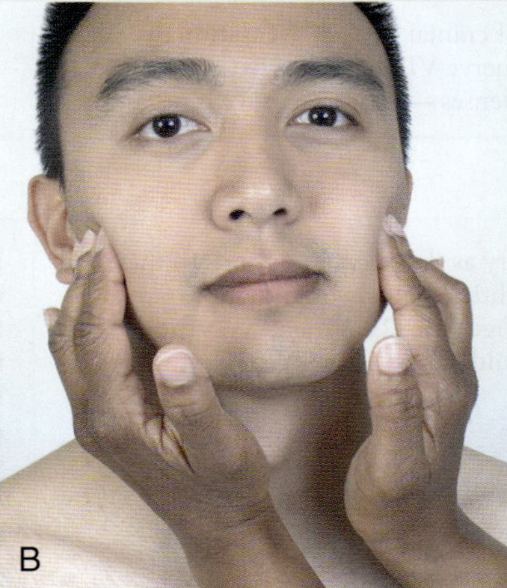 **Figure 12.20**	Decreased strength on one or both sides. Asymmetry in jaw movement. Pain with clenching of teeth. ***Clinical alert:*** abnormalities in ability to chew may result in nutritional issues.
Sensory function. With the person's eyes closed, test light touch sensation by touching a cotton wisp to these designated areas on person's face: forehead, cheeks and chin (Figure 12.21). Ask the person to say 'Now', whenever the touch is felt. This tests all three divisions of the nerve: (1) ophthalmic, (2) maxillary and (3) mandibular.	Decreased or unequal sensation.

PROCEDURES AND NORMAL FINDINGS	ABNORMAL FINDINGS AND CLINICAL ALERTS
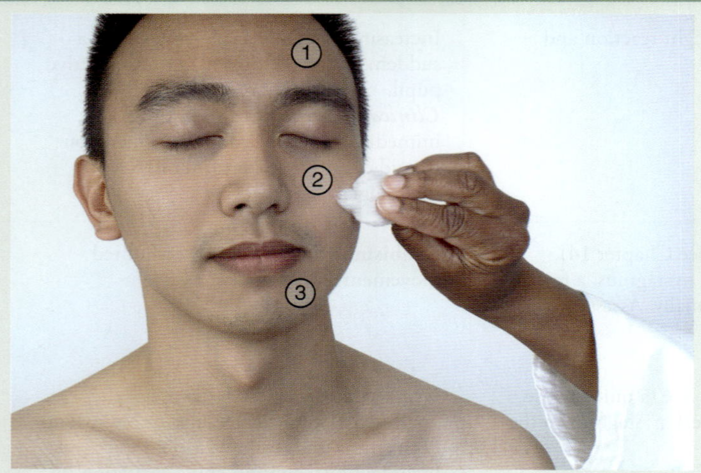 Figure 12.21	
Corneal reflex. This test is done if there is a current or induced altered conscious state occurring as a result of a general anaesthetic. This test may also be done for people who have abnormal facial sensation or abnormalities of facial movement, for example Bell's palsy. Normally, a person will blink bilaterally and frequently. If the person is not able to blink, then a wisp of clean cotton wool can be used to elicit the corneal reflex. This is done with the person looking forwards. Bring the wisp of cotton wool in laterally and lightly touch the cornea of the eye. This procedure tests the sensory afferent pathway of cranial nerve V (sensation of cornea) and the motor efferent pathway of cranial nerve VII (muscles that close the eye). Check to see if the person is wearing contact lenses—assist to remove if necessary.	No blink occurs with a lesion of cranial nerve V or cranial nerve VII paralysis. ***Clinical alert:*** lack of blink reflex can result in corneal abrasions, infection and dryness.
Cranial nerve VII—facial nerve	
Motor function. Note mobility and facial symmetry as the person responds to these requests: smile (Figure 12.22), frown, close eyes tightly (against your attempt to open them), lift eyebrows, show teeth and puff cheeks (Figure 12.23). Then, press the person's puffed cheeks in, and note that the air should escape equally from both sides. 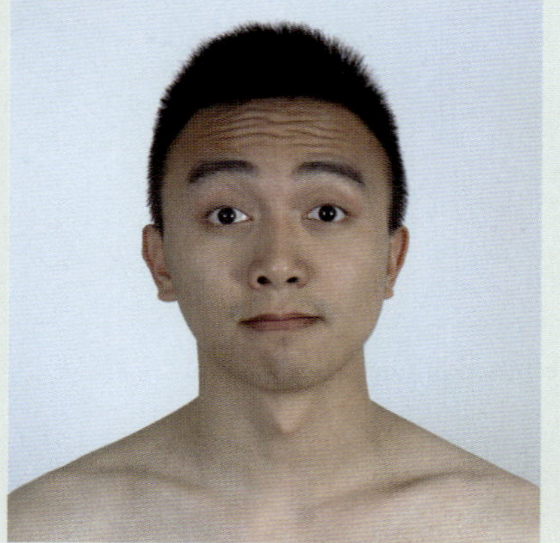 Figure 12.22 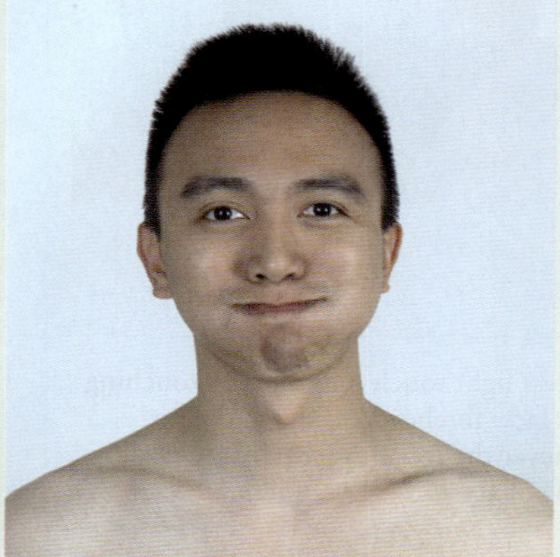 Figure 12.23	Muscle weakness is shown by flattening of the nasolabial fold, drooping of one side of the face, lower eyelid sagging and escape of air from only one cheek that is pressed in. Loss of movement and asymmetry of movement occur with both central nervous system lesions (e.g. stroke that affects the lower face on one side) and peripheral nervous system lesions (e.g. Bell's palsy that affects the upper *and* lower face on one side). ***Clinical alert:*** facial nerve weakness can result in difficulty in chewing food and control of saliva in the mouth.

OBJECTIVE DATA

PROCEDURES AND NORMAL FINDINGS	ABNORMAL FINDINGS AND CLINICAL ALERTS
Sensory function. Do not test routinely. Test only when you suspect facial nerve injury. When indicated, test sense of taste by applying to the tongue a cotton applicator covered with a solution of sugar, salt or lemon juice (sour). Ask the person to identify the taste.	
Cranial nerve VIII—acoustic (vestibulocochlear) nerve	
Test hearing acuity by assessing the person's ability to hear normal conversation: by the whispered voice test (see Chapter 15).	
Cranial nerves IX and X—glossopharyngeal and vagus nerves	
Motor function. Depress the tongue with a tongue blade, and note pharyngeal movement as the person says 'ahhh' or yawns; the uvula and soft palate should rise in the midline, and the tonsillar pillars should move medially.	Absence or asymmetry of soft palate movement. Uvula deviates to side. Asymmetry of tonsillar pillar movement.
If motor function abnormalities are detected or the person reports swallowing difficulties, touch the posterior pharyngeal wall with a tongue blade and note the gag reflex. Also note that the voice sounds smooth and not strained.	Hoarse or brassy voice occurs with vocal cord dysfunction; nasal twang occurs with weakness of soft palate.
Sensory function. Cranial nerve IX does mediate taste on the posterior one-third of the tongue, but technically this sensation is too difficult to test.	***Clinical alert:*** abnormalities in the function of the glossopharyngeal and vagus nerves are likely to compromise the person's airway.
Cranial nerve XI—spinal accessory nerve	
Examine the sternocleidomastoid and trapezius muscles for equal size. Check equal strength by asking the person to rotate the head forcibly against resistance applied to the side of the chin (Figure 12.24). Then ask the person to shrug the shoulders against resistance (Figure 12.25). These movements should feel equally strong on both sides. 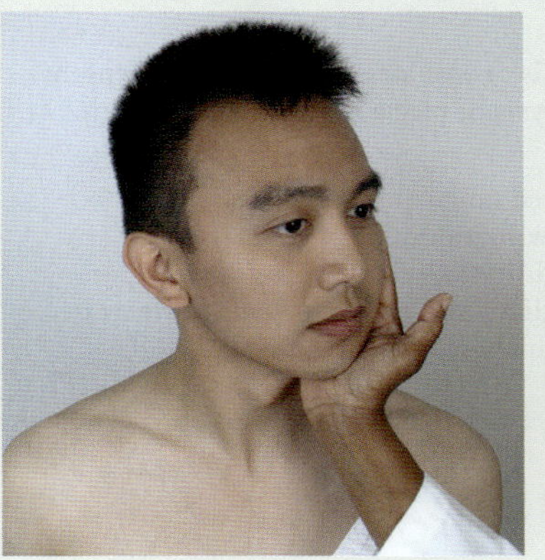 Figure 12.24 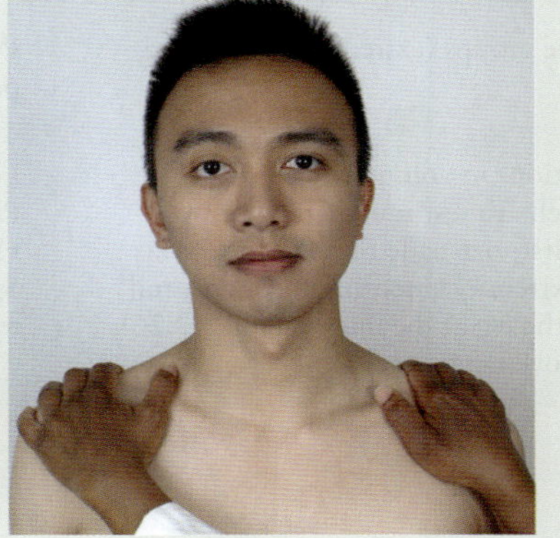 Figure 12.25	Atrophy. Muscle weakness or paralysis.
Cranial nerve XII—hypoglossal nerve	
Inspect the tongue. No wasting or tremors should be present. Note the forward thrust in the midline as the person protrudes the tongue. Also ask the person to say 'light, tight, dynamite', and note that lingual speech (sounds of letters l, t, d, n) is clear and distinct.	Atrophy. Fasciculations. Tongue deviates to side with lesions of the hypoglossal nerve (when this occurs, deviation is towards the paralysed side). ***Clinical alert:*** abnormalities in the function of the hypoglossal nerve are likely to compromise the person's airway.

PROCEDURES AND NORMAL FINDINGS	ABNORMAL FINDINGS AND CLINICAL ALERTS

TABLE 12.4 Summary—testing cranial nerve function of adults

CRANIAL NERVE	RESPONSE
I	Not tested routinely—should have sense of smell in both nostrils. Sense of smell does decrease with age.
II, III, IV, VI	Optical blink reflex—shine light in open eyes, note rapid closure Size, shape, equality of pupils Eyes follow movement
V	Chewing Sensation Ophthalmic Maxillary Mandibular
VII	Facial movements symmetrical when smiling
VIII	Facial muscles
IX, X	Swallowing, gag reflex Coordinated swallowing
XII	Movement of the tongue

Inspect and palpate motor system

Muscles

PROCEDURES AND NORMAL FINDINGS	ABNORMAL FINDINGS AND CLINICAL ALERTS
Size. As you proceed through the examination, inspect all muscle groups for size. Compare the right side with the left. Muscle groups should be within the normal size limits for age and should be symmetrical bilaterally. When muscles in the extremities look asymmetrical, measure each in centimetres and record the difference. A difference of 1 cm or less is not significant. Note that it is difficult to assess muscle mass in very obese people.	**Atrophy**—abnormally small muscle with a wasted appearance; occurs with disuse, injury, lower motor neuron disease such as polio, diabetic neuropathy. **Hypertrophy**—increased size and strength; occurs with isometric exercise.
Strength. (See Chapter 20.) Test the power of muscle groups (extremities, neck and trunk) simultaneously.	**Paresis** or weakness is diminished strength; **paralysis** or plegia is absence of strength.
Tone. Tone is the normal degree of tension (contraction) in voluntarily relaxed muscles. It shows as a mild resistance to passive stretch. To test muscle tone, move the extremities through a passive range of motion. First, persuade the person to relax completely, to 'go loose like a rag doll'. Move each extremity smoothly through a full range of motion. Support the arm at the elbow and the leg at the knee (Figure 12.26). Normally, you will note a mild, even resistance to movement.	Limited range of motion. Pain with motion. **Flaccidity**—decreased resistance, hypotonic. **Spasticity and rigidity**—types of increased resistance (see Table 12.8).

PROCEDURES AND NORMAL FINDINGS	ABNORMAL FINDINGS AND CLINICAL ALERTS
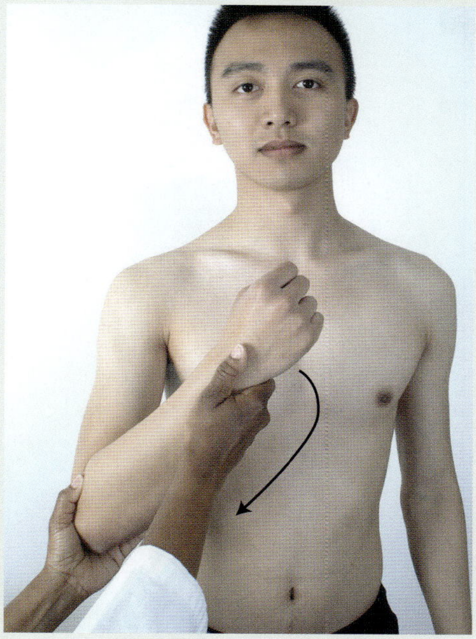 Figure 12.26	
Involuntary movements. Normally, no involuntary movements occur. If they are present, note their location, frequency, rate and amplitude. Note if the movements can be controlled at will.	Tic, tremor, fasciculation, myoclonus, chorea and athetosis (see Table 12.7).
Cerebellar function	
Balance tests	
Gait. Observe as the person walks 5 to 10 m, turns and returns to the starting point. Normally, the person moves with a sense of freedom. The gait is smooth, rhythmic and effortless; the opposing arm swing is coordinated; the turns are smooth. The step length is about 40 cm from heel to heel.	Stiff, immobile posture. Staggering or reeling. Wide base of support. Lack of arm swing or rigid arms. Unequal rhythm of steps. Slapping of foot. Scraping of toe of shoe. Ataxia—un-coordinated or unsteady gait (see Table 12.8).
Tandem walking. Ask the person to walk a straight line in a heel-to-toe fashion (tandem walking) (Figure 12.27). This decreases the base of support and will accentuate any problem with coordination. Normally, the person can walk straight and stay balanced.	

PROCEDURES AND NORMAL FINDINGS	ABNORMAL FINDINGS AND CLINICAL ALERTS
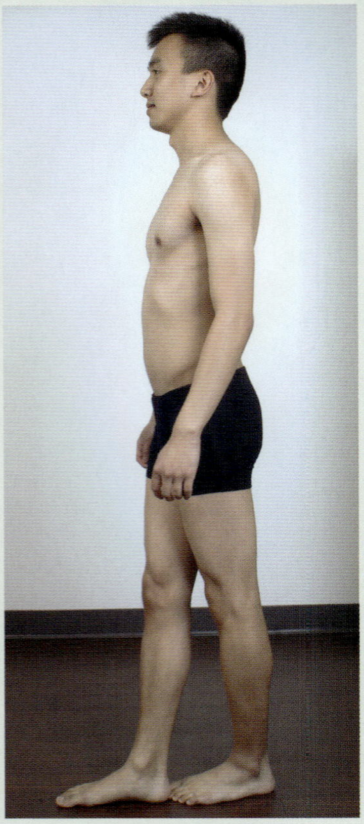 **Figure 12.27** Tandem walking	
You may also test for balance by asking the person to walk on their toes, then on their heels for a few steps.	Muscle weakness in the legs prevents this.
The Romberg test. Ask the person to stand up with feet together and arms at the sides. Once in a stable position, ask the person to close the eyes and to hold the position (Figure 12.28). Wait about 20 seconds. Normally, a person can maintain posture and balance even with the visual orienting information blocked, although slight swaying may occur. Stand close to catch the person in case they fall.	Sways, falls, widens base of feet to avoid falling. Positive Romberg sign is loss of balance that occurs when closing the eyes. You eliminate the advantage of orientation with the eyes, which had compensated for sensory loss. A positive Romberg sign occurs with cerebellar ataxia (multiple sclerosis, alcohol intoxication), loss of proprioception and loss of vestibular function.

PROCEDURES AND NORMAL FINDINGS	ABNORMAL FINDINGS AND CLINICAL ALERTS
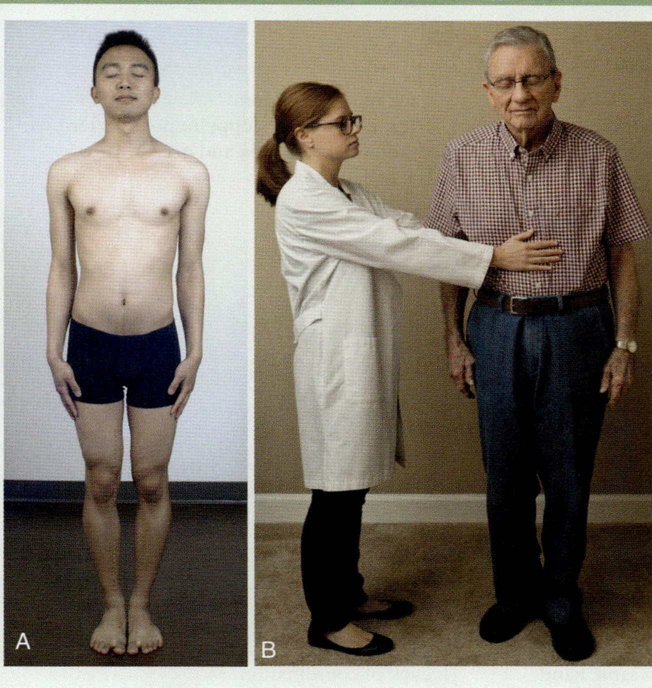 **Figure 12.28** Romberg test	
Ask the person to perform a shallow knee bend first on one leg, then the other either standing alone or lightly supporting themselves by holding on to a bench or stable chair (Figure 12.29A and 12.29B). Alternatively the person can be asked to rise from a chair without using the arm rests for support. This demonstrates normal position sense, muscle strength and cerebellar function. 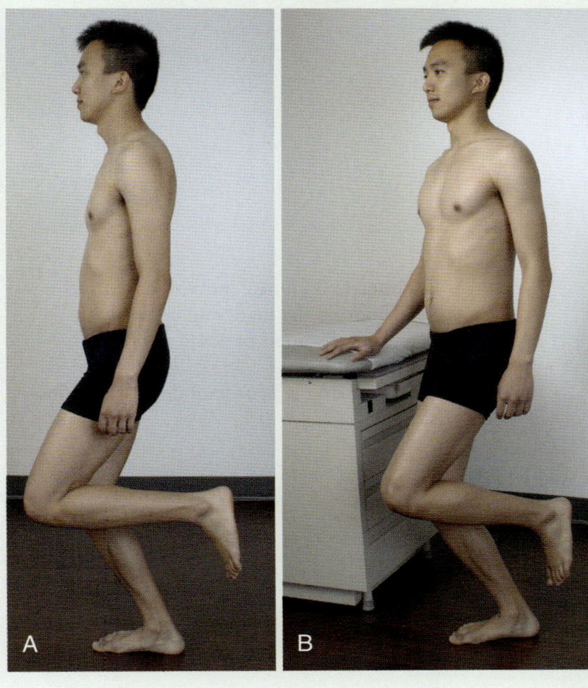 **Figure 12.29**	Unable to perform knee bend because of weakness in quadriceps muscle or hip extensors.

PROCEDURES AND NORMAL FINDINGS	ABNORMAL FINDINGS AND CLINICAL ALERTS
Coordination and skilled movements	
Rapid alternating movements (RAM). Ask the person to pat the knees with both hands, lift up, turn hands over and pat the knees with the backs of the hands (Figure 12.30A and 12.30B). Then ask the person to do this faster. Normally, this is done with equal turning and a quick rhythmic pace. 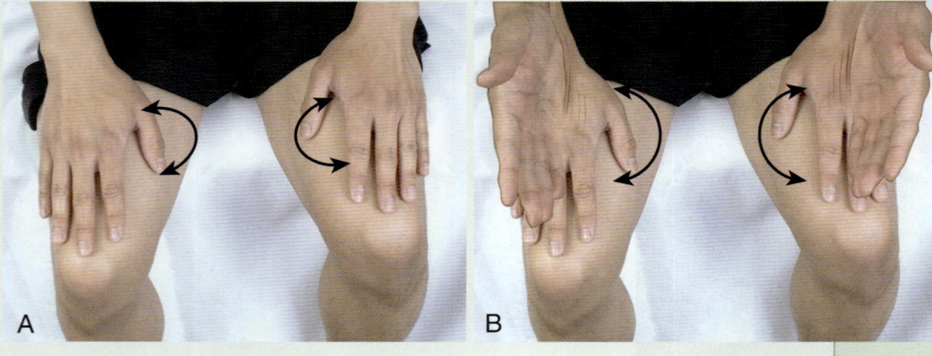 Figure 12.30	Lack of coordination. Slow, clumsy and sloppy response is termed **dysdiadochokinesia** and occurs with cerebellar disease.
Alternatively, ask the person to touch the thumb to each finger on the same hand, starting with the index finger, then reverse direction (Figure 12.31). Normally, this can be done quickly and accurately. 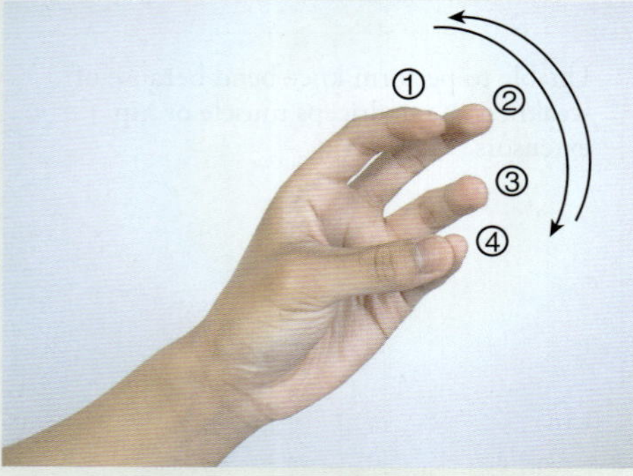 Figure 12.31	Lack of coordination.
	Dysmetria is clumsy movement with overshooting the mark and occurs with cerebellar disorders or acute alcohol intoxication. **Past-pointing** is a constant deviation to one side.
Finger-to-finger test. With the person's eyes open, ask them to use the index finger to touch your finger, then their own nose (Figure 12.32). After a few times move your finger to a different spot. The person's movement should be smooth and accurate.	

PROCEDURES AND NORMAL FINDINGS	ABNORMAL FINDINGS AND CLINICAL ALERTS
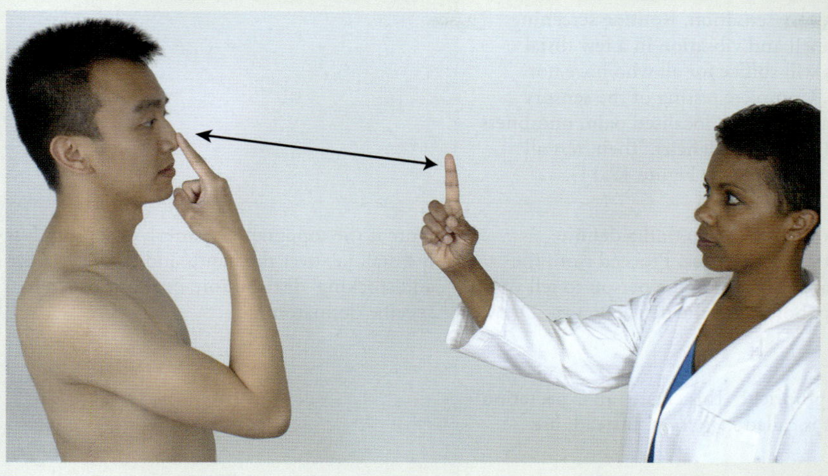 Figure 12.32	
Finger-to-nose test. Ask the person to close the eyes and to stretch out the arms. Ask the person to touch the tip of their nose with each index finger, alternating hands and increasing speed. Normally this is done with accurate and smooth movement.	Misses nose. Worsening of coordination when the eyes are closed occurs with cerebellar disease or alcohol intoxication.
Heel-to-shin test. Test lower extremity coordination by asking the person, who is in a supine position, to place the heel on the opposite knee, and run it down the shin from the knee to the ankle (Figure 12.33). Normally, the person moves the heel in a straight line down the shin. 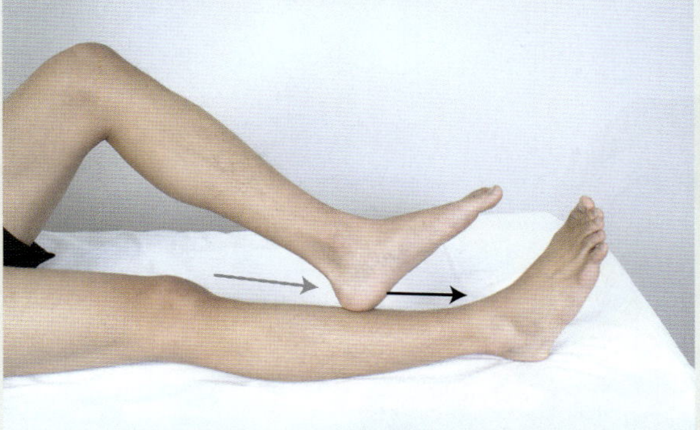 Figure 12.33	Lack of coordination, heel falls off shin; occurs with cerebellar disease.
Assess the sensory system	
Ask the person to identify various sensory stimuli in order to test the intactness of the peripheral nerve fibres, the sensory tracts and higher cortical discrimination.	***Clinical alert:*** abnormalities in sensory perception can pose an injury risk such as burns and pressure injury.
Ensure validity of sensory system testing by making sure the person is alert, cooperative and comfortable and has an adequate attention span. Otherwise, you may get misleading and invalid results. Testing of the sensory system can be fatiguing. If the person is tired you may need to repeat the examination later or to break it into parts.	

OBJECTIVE DATA

PROCEDURES AND NORMAL FINDINGS	ABNORMAL FINDINGS AND CLINICAL ALERTS
You do not need to test the entire skin surface for every sensation. Routine screening procedures include testing superficial pain, light touch and vibration in a few distal locations and testing stereognosis (see below). This will suffice for all who have not demonstrated any neurological symptoms or signs. Complete testing of the sensory system is warranted in those with neurological symptoms (e.g. localised pain, numbness and tingling) or when you discover abnormalities (e.g. motor deficit). Then, test all sensory modalities and cover most dermatomes of the body (see Figure 12.11).	
Compare sensations on symmetrical parts of the body. When you find a definite decrease in sensation, map it out by systematic testing in that area. Proceed from the point of decreased sensation towards the sensitive area. By asking the person to tell you where the sensation changes, you can map the exact borders of the deficient area. Draw your results on a diagram.	Note if the topographic pattern of sensory loss is distal, i.e. over the hands and feet in a 'glove and stocking' distribution, or if it is over a specific dermatome.
Avoid asking leading questions, 'Can you feel this pinprick?' This creates an expectation of how the person should feel the sensation, which is called *suggestion*. Instead, use unbiased directions such as, 'What can you feel?'	
The person's eyes should be closed during each of the tests. Take time to explain what will be happening and exactly how you expect the person to respond.	
Spinothalamic tract	
Pain. Pain is tested by the person's ability to perceive a pinprick. Break a tongue blade lengthwise, forming a sharp point at the fractured end and a dull spot at the rounded end. Lightly apply the sharp point or the dull end to the person's body in a random, unpredictable order (Figure 12.34). Ask the person to say 'sharp' or 'dull', depending on the sensation felt. (Note that the sharp edge is used to test for pain; the dull edge is used as a general test of the person's responses.) Discard tongue blade. 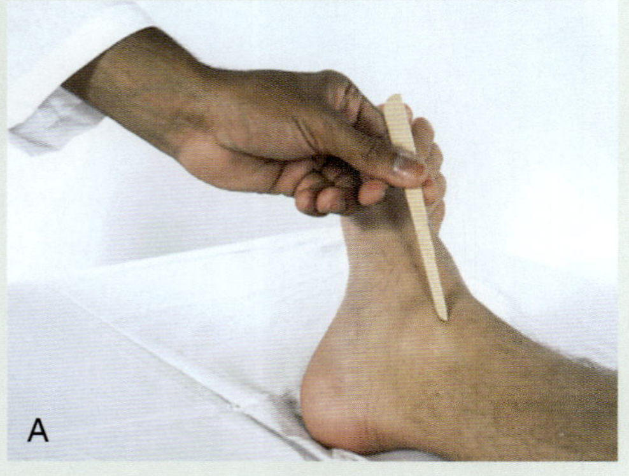 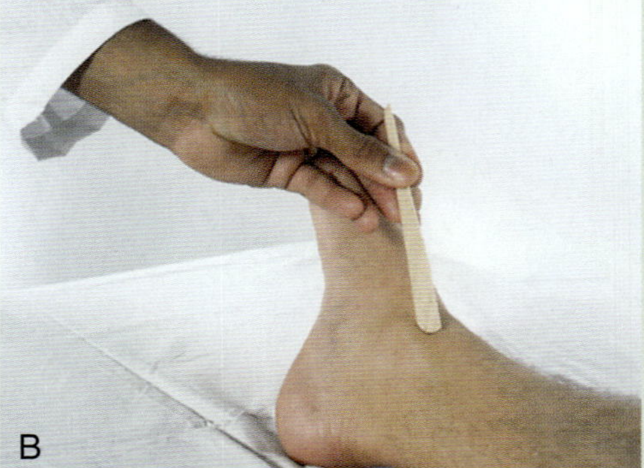 **Figure 12.34**	**Hypoalgesia**—decreased pain sensation. **Analgesia**—absent pain sensation. **Hyperalgesia**—increased pain sensation.
Temperature. Test temperature sensation only when pain sensation is abnormal; otherwise, you may omit it because the fibres' tracts are much the same. Place a metal object (for example the flat side of a tuning fork) on the skin; the metal is almost always cold. Ask the person to describe the sensation.	
Light touch. Apply a wisp of cotton to the skin. Stretch a cotton ball to make a long end and brush it over the skin in a random order of sites and at irregular intervals (Figure 12.35). This prevents the person from responding just from repetition. Include the arms, forearms, hands, chest, thighs and legs. Ask the person to say 'now' or 'yes' when touch is felt. Compare symmetrical points.	**Hypoaesthesia**—decreased touch sensation. **Anaesthesia**—absent touch sensation. **Hyperaesthesia**—increased touch sensation.

PROCEDURES AND NORMAL FINDINGS	ABNORMAL FINDINGS AND CLINICAL ALERTS
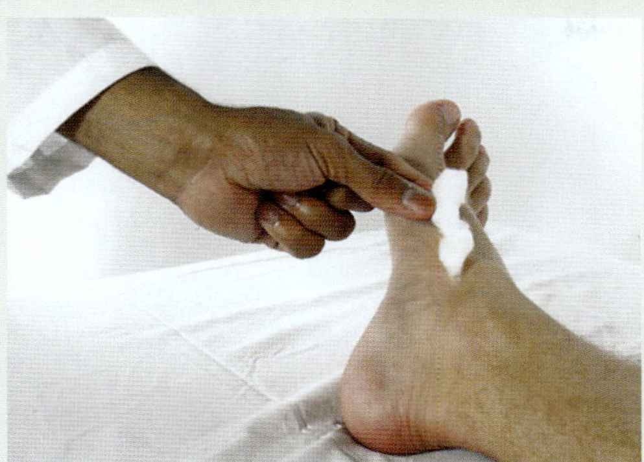 Figure 12.35	
Posterior column tract	
Vibration. Test the person's ability to feel vibrations of a tuning fork over bony prominences. Use a low-pitch tuning fork (128 Hz or 256 Hz) because its vibration has a slower decay. Strike the tuning fork on the heel of your hand, and hold the base on a bony surface of the fingers and great toe (Figure 12.36). Ask the person to indicate when the vibration starts and stops. If the person feels the normal vibration or buzzing sensation on these distal areas, you may assume proximal spots are normal and proceed no further. If no vibrations are felt, move proximally and test ulnar processes and ankles, patellae and iliac crests. Compare the right side with the left side. If you find a deficit, note whether it is gradual or abrupt. 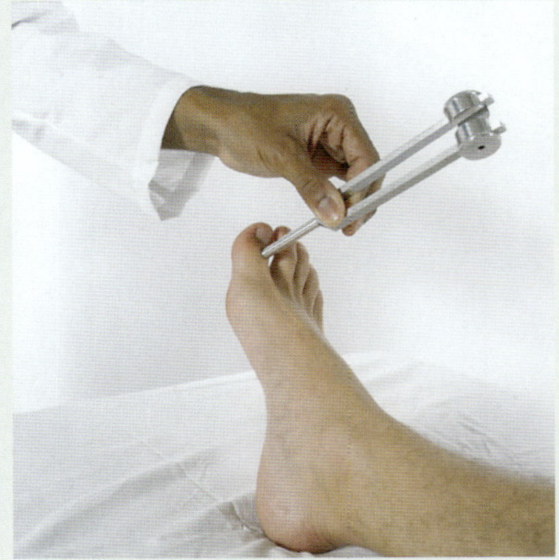 Figure 12.36	Unable to feel vibration. Loss of vibration sense occurs with peripheral neuropathy, e.g. type 1 and type 2 diabetes and alcoholism. Often, this is the first sensation lost. Peripheral neuropathy is worse at the feet and gradually improves as you move up the leg, as opposed to a specific nerve lesion, which has a clear zone of deficit for its dermatome.
Position (kinaesthesia). Test the person's ability to perceive passive movements of the extremities. Move a finger or the big toe up and down, and ask the person to tell you which way it is moved (Figure 12.37). The test is done with the eyes closed, but to be sure it is understood, have the person watch a few trials first. Vary the order of movement up or down. Hold the digit by the sides, since upwards or downwards pressure on the skin may provide a clue as to how it has been moved. Normally, a person can detect movement of a few millimetres.	Loss of position sense.

OBJECTIVE DATA

PROCEDURES AND NORMAL FINDINGS	ABNORMAL FINDINGS AND CLINICAL ALERTS
Figure 12.37	
Tactile discrimination (fine touch). The following tests also measure the discrimination ability of the sensory cortex. As a prerequisite, the person needs a normal or near-normal sense of touch and position sense.	Problems with tactile discrimination occur with lesions of the sensory cortex or posterior column.
Stereognosis. Test the person's ability to recognise objects by feeling their forms, sizes and weights. With the eyes closed, place a familiar object (paper clip, key, coin, cotton ball or pencil) in the person's hand and ask the person to identify it (Figure 12.38). Normally, a person will explore it with the fingers and correctly name it. Test a different object in each hand; testing the left hand assesses right parietal lobe functioning. Figure 12.38 Stereognosis	**Astereognosis**—inability to identify object correctly. Occurs in sensory cortex lesions, e.g. stroke.
Graphaesthesia. Graphaesthesia is the ability to 'read' a number by having it traced on the skin. With the person's eyes closed, use a blunt instrument to trace a single digit number or a letter on the palm (Figure 12.39). Ask the person to tell you what it is. Graphaesthesia is a good measure of sensory loss if the person cannot make the hand movements needed for stereognosis, as occurs in arthritis.	Inability to distinguish number occurs with lesions of the sensory cortex.

OBJECTIVE DATA

PROCEDURES AND NORMAL FINDINGS	ABNORMAL FINDINGS AND CLINICAL ALERTS
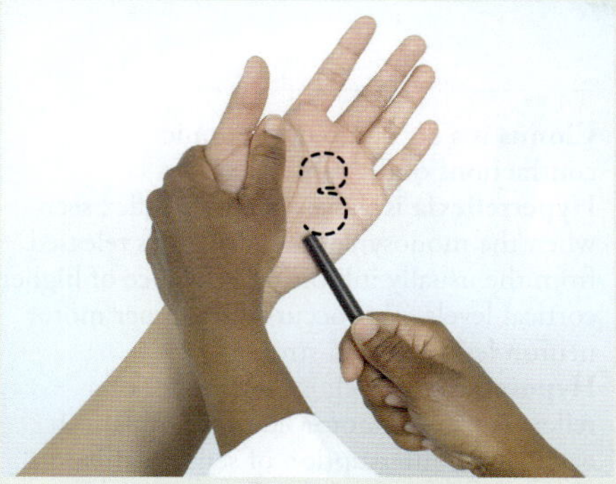 **Figure 12.39** Graphaesthesia	
Two-point discrimination. Test the person's ability to distinguish the separation of two simultaneous pin points on the skin. Apply the two points of an opened paper clip lightly to the skin in ever-closing distances. Note the distance at which the person no longer perceives two separate points. The level of perception varies considerably with the region tested; it is most sensitive in the fingertips (2 to 8 mm) and least sensitive on the upper arms, thighs and back (40 to 75 mm).	An increase in the distance it normally takes to identify two separate points occurs with sensory cortex lesions.
Extinction. Simultaneously touch both sides of the body at the same point. Ask the person to state how many sensations are felt and where they are. Normally, both sensations are felt.	The ability to recognise only one of the stimuli occurs with sensory cortex lesion; the stimulus is extinguished on the side *opposite* the cortex lesion.
Point location. Touch the skin, and withdraw the stimulus promptly. Tell the person, 'Put your finger where I touched you'. You can perform this test simultaneously with light touch sensation.	With a sensory cortex lesion, the person cannot localise the sensation accurately, even though light touch sensation may be retained.
Test the reflexes	
Stretch, or deep tendon reflexes (DTRs)	
Measurement of the stretch reflexes reveals the intactness of the reflex arc at specific spinal levels as well as the normal override on the reflex of the higher cortical levels.	
For an adequate response, the limb should be relaxed and the muscle partially stretched. Stimulate the reflex by directing a short, snappy blow of the reflex hammer onto the muscle's insertion tendon. Use a relaxed hold on the hammer.	
As with the percussion technique, the action takes place at the wrist. Strike a brief, well-aimed blow, and bounce up promptly; do not let the hammer rest on the tendon. Use the pointed end of the reflex hammer when aiming at a smaller target such as your thumb on the tendon site; use the flat end when the target is wider or to diffuse the impact and prevent pain.	

PROCEDURES AND NORMAL FINDINGS	ABNORMAL FINDINGS AND CLINICAL ALERTS
Use just enough force to get a response. Compare right and left sides—the responses should be equal.	
The reflex response is graded on a 4-point scale: 4+ Very brisk, hyperactive with clonus, indicative of disease 3+ Brisker than average, may indicate disease 2+ Average, normal 1+ Diminished, low normal 0 No response. This is a subjective scale and requires some clinical practice. Even then, the scale is not completely reliable because no standard exists to say *how* brisk a reflex should be to warrant a grade of 3+. Also, a wide range of normal exists in reflex responses. Healthy people may have diminished reflexes or they may have brisk ones. Your best plan is to interpret the deep tendon reflexes *only* within the context of the rest of the neurological assessment, and findings over time.	**Clonus** is a set of rapid, rhythmic contractions of the same muscle. **Hyperreflexia** is the exaggerated reflex seen when the monosynaptic reflex arc is released from the usually inhibiting influence of higher cortical levels. This occurs with upper motor neuron lesions, e.g. a stroke. **Hyporeflexia**, which is the absence of a reflex, is a lower motor neuron problem. It occurs with interruption of sensory afferents or destruction of motor efferents and anterior horn cells, e.g. spinal cord injury.
Sometimes the reflex response fails to appear. Try further encouragement of relaxation, varying the person's position or increasing the strength of the blow. **Reinforcement** is another technique to relax the muscles and enhance the response (Figure 12.40). Ask the person to perform an isometric exercise in a muscle group somewhat away from the one being tested. For example, to enhance a patellar reflex, ask the person to lock the fingers together and 'pull'. Then strike the tendon. To enhance a biceps response, ask the person to clench the teeth or to grasp the thigh with the opposite hand. 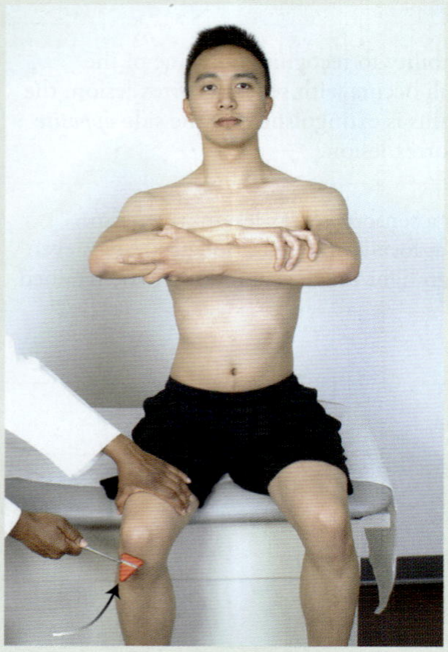 **Figure 12.40** Reinforcement	
Biceps reflex (C5 to C6). Support the person's forearm on yours; this position relaxes, as well as partially flexes, the person's arm. Place your thumb on the biceps tendon and strike a blow on your thumb. You can feel as well as see the normal response, which is contraction of the biceps muscle and flexion of the forearm (Figure 12.41).	

PROCEDURES AND NORMAL FINDINGS	ABNORMAL FINDINGS AND CLINICAL ALERTS
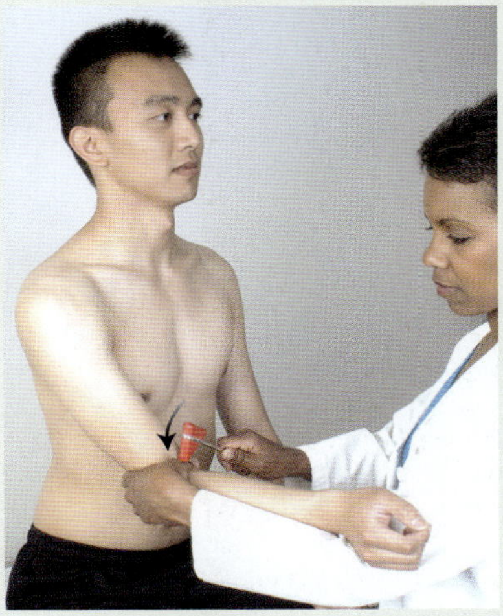 **Figure 12.41** Biceps reflex	
Triceps reflex (C7 to C8). Tell the person to let the arm 'just go dead' as you suspend it by holding the upper arm. Strike the triceps tendon directly just above the elbow (Figure 12.42). The normal response is extension of the forearm. Alternatively, hold the person's wrist across the chest to flex the arm at the elbow, and tap the tendon. 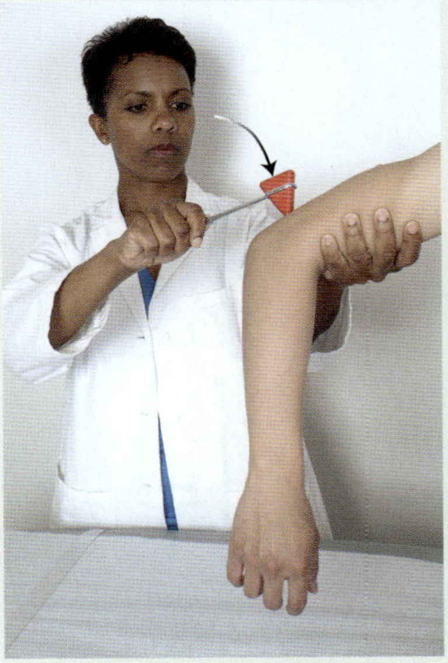 **Figure 12.42** Triceps reflex	
Brachioradialis reflex (C5 to C6). Hold the person's thumbs to suspend the forearms in relaxation. Strike the forearm directly, about 2 to 3 cm above the radial styloid process (Figure 12.43). The normal response is flexion and supination of the forearm.	

OBJECTIVE DATA

PROCEDURES AND NORMAL FINDINGS	ABNORMAL FINDINGS AND CLINICAL ALERTS
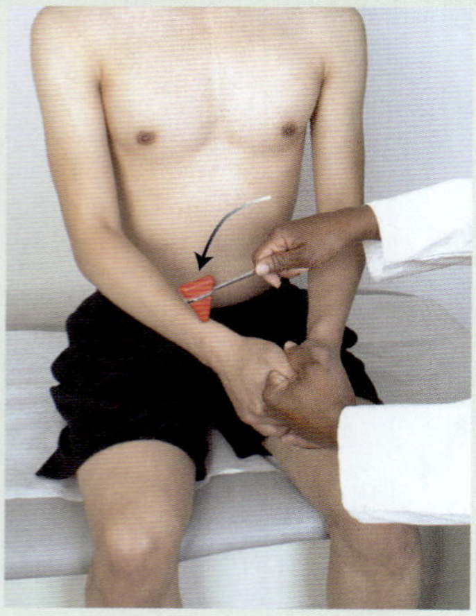 **Figure 12.43** Brachioradialis reflex	
Quadriceps reflex ('knee jerk') (L2 to L4). Let the lower legs dangle freely to flex the knee and stretch the tendons. Strike the tendon directly just below the patella (Figure 12.44). Extension of the lower leg is the expected response. You will also palpate contraction of the quadriceps. 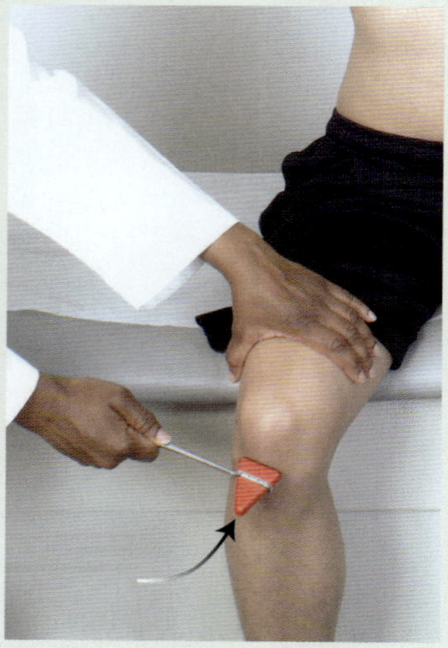 **Figure 12.44** Quadriceps reflex	
For the person in the supine position, use your own arm as a lever to support the weight of one leg against the other leg. This manoeuvre also flexes the knee (Figure 12.45).	

OBJECTIVE DATA

PROCEDURES AND NORMAL FINDINGS	ABNORMAL FINDINGS AND CLINICAL ALERTS
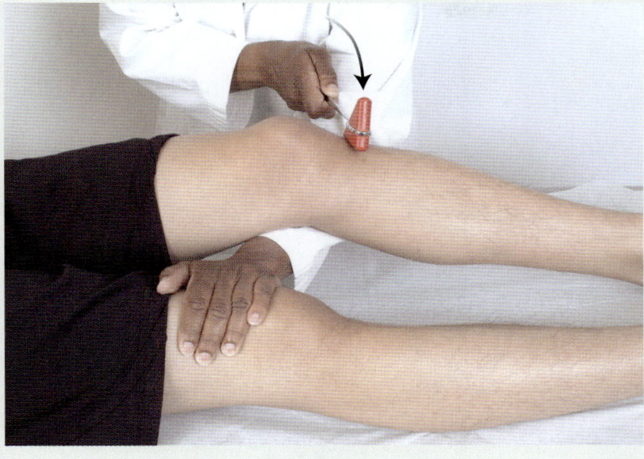 **Figure 12.45** Supine quadriceps reflex	
Achilles reflex ('ankle jerk') (L5 to S2). Position the person with the knee flexed and the hip externally rotated. Hold the foot in dorsiflexion, and strike the Achilles tendon directly (Figure 12.46). Feel the normal response as the foot plantar flexes against your hand. 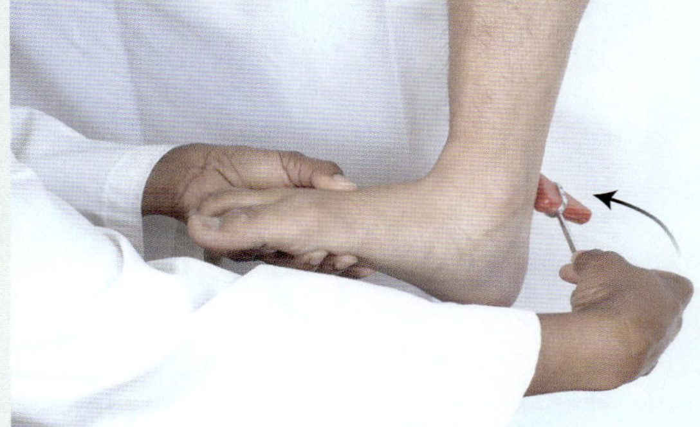 **Figure 12.46** Achilles reflex	
For the person in the supine position, flex one knee and support that lower leg against the other leg so that it falls 'open'. Dorsiflex the foot and tap the tendon (Figure 12.47).	

OBJECTIVE DATA

PROCEDURES AND NORMAL FINDINGS	ABNORMAL FINDINGS AND CLINICAL ALERTS
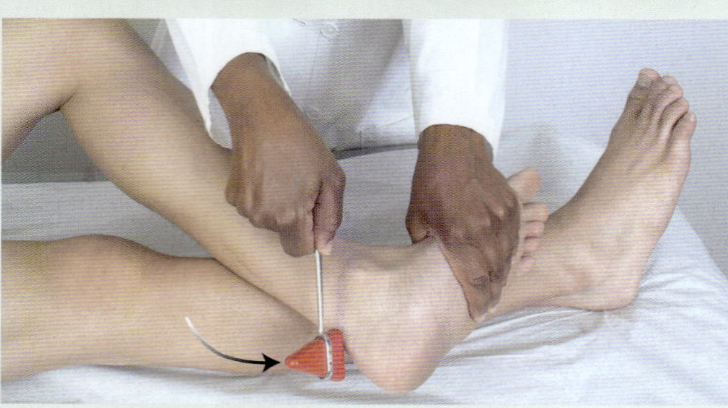 **Figure 12.47** Supine achilles reflex	
Clonus. Test for clonus, particularly when the reflexes are hyperactive. Support the lower leg in one hand. With your other hand, move the foot up and down a few times to relax the muscle. Then stretch the muscle by briskly dorsiflexing the foot. Hold the stretch (Figure 12.48). With a normal response, you feel no further movement. When clonus is present, you will feel and see rapid rhythmic contractions of the calf muscle and movement of the foot. 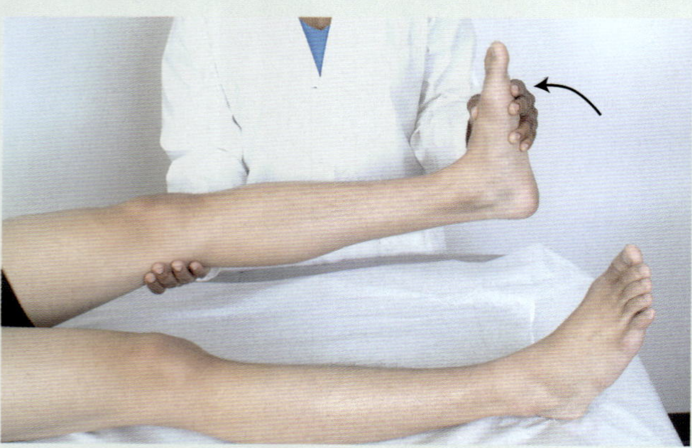 **Figure 12.48**	**Clonus** is repeated reflex muscular movements. A hyperactive reflex with sustained clonus (lasting as long as the stretch is held) occurs with upper motor neuron disease.
Superficial (cutaneous) reflexes	
Here, the sensory receptors are in the skin rather than in the muscles. The motor response is a localised muscle contraction.	
Abdominal reflexes—upper (T8 to T10), lower (T10 to T12). Have the person assume a supine position, with the knees slightly bent. Use the handle end of the reflex hammer, a wood applicator tip or the end of a split tongue blade to stroke the skin. Move from the side of the abdomen towards the midline at both the upper and the lower abdominal levels (Figure 12.49). The normal response is ipsilateral contraction of the abdominal muscle with an observed deviation of the umbilicus towards the stroke. When the abdominal wall is very obese, pull the skin to the opposite side and feel it contract towards the stimulus.	Superficial reflexes are absent with diseases of the pyramidal tract, e.g. they are absent on the contralateral side with stroke.

PROCEDURES AND NORMAL FINDINGS	ABNORMAL FINDINGS AND CLINICAL ALERTS
Abdominal reflex Cremasteric reflex **Figure 12.49**	
Cremasteric reflex (L1 to L2). This is not routinely done. On the male, lightly stroke the inner aspect of the thigh with the reflex hammer or tongue blade (see Figure 12.49). Note elevation of the ipsilateral testicle.	Absent in both upper motor neuron and lower motor neuron lesions.
Plantar reflex (L4 to S2). Position the thigh in slight external rotation. With the reflex hammer, draw a light stroke up the lateral side of the sole of the foot and inwards across the ball of the foot, like an upside-down J (Figure 12.50A). The normal response is plantar flexion of the toes and inversion and flexion of the forefoot.	Except in infancy, the abnormal response is dorsiflexion of the big toe and fanning of all toes, which is a positive **Babinski sign**, also called 'upgoing toes' (Figure 12.50B). This occurs with upper motor neuron disease of the corticospinal (or pyramidal) tract.

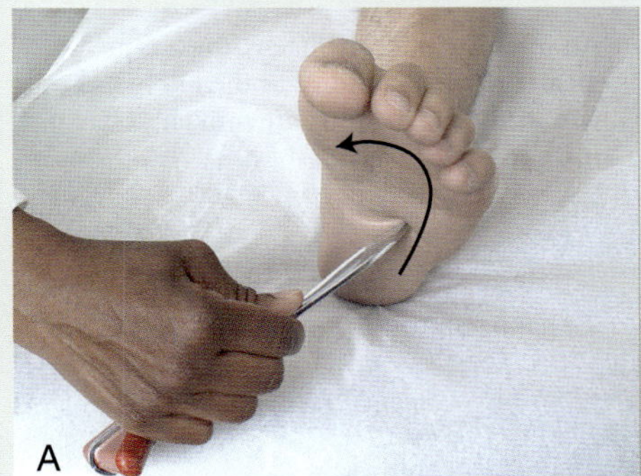

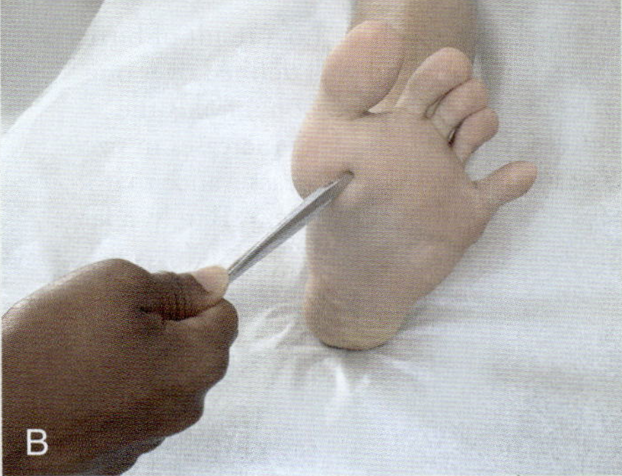

Figure 12.50
Plantar reflex

Additional objective assessment for infants and toddlers

Skull

Measure an infant's **head size** with measuring tape at periodic health checks up to age 2 years, then yearly up to age 6 years. (Measurement of head circumference is presented in detail in Chapter 3.)	Note an abnormal increase in head size or failure to grow.

OBJECTIVE DATA

PROCEDURES AND NORMAL FINDINGS	ABNORMAL FINDINGS AND CLINICAL ALERTS
The newborn's head measures about 32 to 38 cm (average around 34 cm), and is 2 cm larger than chest circumference. At age 2 years, both measurements are the same. During childhood the chest circumference grows to exceed head circumference by 5 to 7 cm.	**Microcephalic**—head size below norms for age. **Macrocephalic**—an enlarged head for age, or rapidly increasing in size (e.g. hydrocephalus (increased cerebrospinal fluid)).
Observe the infant's head from all angles, not just the front. The contour should be symmetrical. Some variation occurs in normal head shapes.	Frontal bulges, or 'bossing', occur with prematurity or rickets.
Two common variations in the newborn cause the shape of the skull to look markedly asymmetrical: A **caput succedaneum** is oedematous swelling and ecchymosis of the presenting part of the head caused by birth trauma (Figure 12.51). It feels soft, and it may extend across suture lines. It gradually resolves during the first few days of life and needs no treatment. 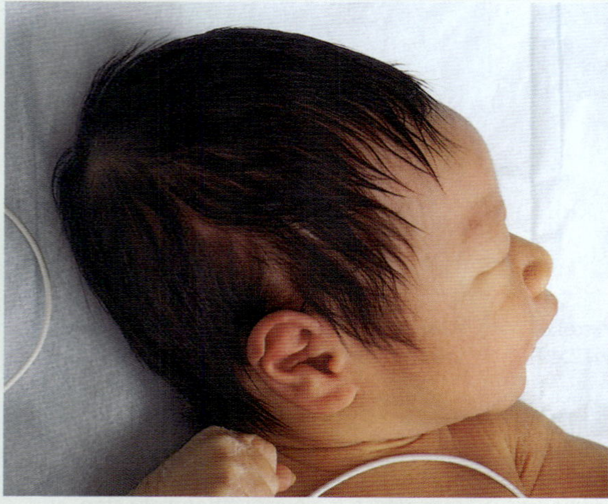 **Figure 12.51** Caput succedaneum	
A **cephalhaematoma** is a subperiosteal haemorrhage, which is also a result of birth trauma (Figure 12.52A and 12.52B). It is soft, fluctuant and well defined over one cranial bone because the periosteum (i.e. the covering over each bone) holds the bleeding in place. It appears several hours after birth and gradually increases in size. No discolouration is present but it looks bizarre, so parents need reassurance that it will be reabsorbed during the first few weeks of life without treatment. Rarely, a large haematoma may persist to 3 months. 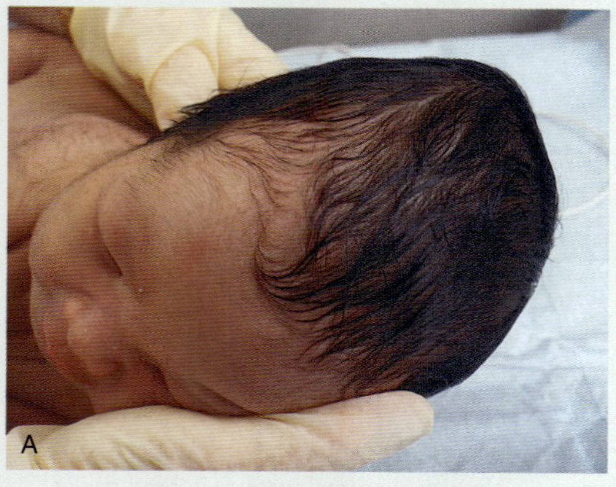 **Figure 12.52** Cephalhaematoma	An infant with cephalhaematoma is at greater risk for jaundice as the red blood cells within the haematoma are broken down and reabsorbed.

PROCEDURES AND NORMAL FINDINGS	ABNORMAL FINDINGS AND CLINICAL ALERTS
As you palpate the newborn's head, the suture lines feel like ridges. By 5 to 6 months, they are smooth and not palpable.	Sutures palpable when the child is older than 6 months.
A newborn's head may feel asymmetrical and the involved ridges more prominent due to **moulding** of the cranial bones during engagement and passage through the birth canal. Moulding is overriding of the cranial bones; usually, the parietal bone overrides the frontal or occipital bone. Reassure parents that this lasts only a few days or a week. Babies delivered by caesarean section are noted for their evenly round heads. Also, some asymmetry may occur if an infant continually sleeps in one position; this is a flattening of the dependent cranial bone, usually the occiput.	Marked asymmetry, as in **craniosynostosis**, a severe deformity caused by premature closure of the sutures. Premature closing of the sutures results in a long, narrow head. Flattening also occurs with rickets or developmental delay.
Gently palpate the skull and **fontanels** while the infant is calm and somewhat in a sitting position (crying, lying down or vomiting may cause the anterior fontanel to look full and bulging). The skull should feel smooth and fused except at the fontanels. The fontanels feel firm, slightly concave and well-defined against the edges of the cranial bones. You may see slight arterial pulsations in the anterior fontanel.	A true tense or bulging fontanel occurs with acute increased intracranial pressure. Depressed and sunken fontanels occur with dehydration or malnutrition. Marked pulsations occur with increased intracranial pressure.
The posterior fontanel may not be palpable at birth. If it is, it measures 1 cm and closes by 1 to 2 months. The anterior fontanel may be small at birth and enlarge to 2.5 by 2.5 cm. A large diameter of 4 to 5 cm occasionally may be normal under 6 months. A small fontanel is usually normal. The anterior fontanel closes between 9 months and 2 years. Early closure may be insignificant if head growth proceeds normally.	Delayed closure or larger-than-normal fontanel size occurs with hydrocephalus, Trisomy 21, hypothyroidism or rickets. A small fontanel is a sign of microcephaly, as is early closure.
Note the infant's **head posture** and **head control**. The infant can turn the head side to side by 2 weeks and shows the **tonic neck reflex** when supine and the head is turned to one side (extension of same arm and leg, flexion of opposite arm and leg). The tonic neck reflex disappears between 3 and 4 months, then the head is maintained in the midline. Head control is achieved by 4 months, when the baby can hold the head erect and steady when pulled to a vertical position.	Tonic neck reflex beyond 5 months may indicate brain damage. In children, head tilt occurs with habit spasm, poor vision and brain tumour. Head lag after 4 months may indicate developmental delay.
Face	
Check **facial features** for symmetry, appearance and presence of swelling. Note symmetry of wrinkling when the infant cries or smiles (e.g. both sides of the lips rise and both sides of forehead wrinkle). Parotid gland enlargement is seen best when the infant/toddler sits and looks up at the ceiling; the swelling appears below the angle of the jaw.	Unilateral immobility indicates nerve damage (central or peripheral) (e.g. note angle of mouth droop on paralysed side). Some facies are characteristic of congenital abnormalities or chronic allergy. See Table 12.9.
Neck	
An infant's neck looks short; it lengthens during the first 3 to 4 years. You can see the neck better by supporting the infant's shoulders and tilting the head back a little. This positioning also enhances palpation of the trachea, which is buried deep in the neck. Feel for the row of cartilaginous rings in the midline or just slightly to the right of midline.	A short neck or webbing (loose fan-like folds) may indicate congenital abnormality (e.g. Trisomy 21 or Turner's syndrome) or it may occur alone.
Assess muscle development with gentle passive ROM. Cradle the infant's head with your hands and turn it side to side and test forward flexion, extension and rotation. Note any resistance to movement, especially flexion.	Head tilt and limited ROM occur with **torticollis** (wryneck), or from sternocleidomastoid muscle injury during birth or a congenital defect. Resistance to flexion (nuchal rigidity) and pain on flexion indicate meningeal irritation or meningitis.
The neurological system shows dramatic growth and development during the first year of life. Assessment includes noting that milestones you normally would expect for each month have indeed been achieved, and that the early, more primitive reflexes cease at the appropriate developmental stage.	Failure to attain a skill by expected time. Persistence of reflex behaviour beyond the normal time.

PROCEDURES AND NORMAL FINDINGS	ABNORMAL FINDINGS AND CLINICAL ALERTS
At birth, the newborn is very alert, with the eyes open and demonstrates strong, urgent sucking. The normal cry is loud, lusty and even angry. The next 2 or 3 days may be spent mostly sleeping as the baby recovers from the birth process. After that, the pattern of sleep and waking activity is highly variable; it depends on the baby's individual body rhythm as well as external stimuli.	A high-pitched, shrill cry or cat-sounding screech occurs with CNS damage. A weak, groaning cry or expiratory grunt occurs with respiratory distress.
The behavioural assessment should include your observations of the infant's spontaneous waking activity, responses to environmental stimuli and social interaction with the parents and others.	***Clinical alert:*** Lethargy, hyporeactivity, hyperirritability and parent's report of significant change in behaviour all warrant referral.
By 2 months of age, the baby smiles responsively and recognises the parent's face. Babbling occurs at 4 months, and one or two words (mama, dada) are used nonspecifically after 9 months.	

TABLE 12.5 Summary—testing cranial nerve function of infants

CRANIAL NERVE	RESPONSE
II, III, IV, VI	Optical blink reflex—shine light in open eyes, note rapid closure Size, shape, equality of pupils Regards face or close object Eyes follow movement
V	Rooting reflex, sucking reflex
VII	Facial movements (e.g. wrinkling forehead and nasolabial folds) symmetrical when crying or smiling
VIII	Loud noise yields Moro reflex (until 4 months) Acoustic blink reflex—infant blinks in response to a loud hand clap 30 cm from head (avoid making air current) Eyes follow direction of sound
IX, X	Swallowing, gag reflex Coordinated sucking and swallowing
XII	Pinch nose, infant's mouth will open and tongue rise in midline

The motor system

Observe spontaneous motor activity for smoothness and symmetry. Smoothness of movement suggests proper cerebellar function, as does the coordination involved in sucking and swallowing. To screen gross and fine motor coordination, use the Denver II test with its age-specific developmental milestones. You also can assess movement by testing the reflexes listed in the following section. Note their smoothness of response and symmetry. Also, note whether their presence or absence is appropriate for the infant's age.	Delay in motor activity occurs with brain damage, cognitive delay, peripheral neuromuscular damage, prolonged illness and parental neglect.

OBJECTIVE DATA

PROCEDURES AND NORMAL FINDINGS	ABNORMAL FINDINGS AND CLINICAL ALERTS
Assess muscle tone by first observing resting posture. The newborn favours a flexed position; extremities are symmetrically folded inwards, the hips are slightly abducted and the fists are tightly flexed (Figure 12.53). Infants born by breech delivery, however, do not have flexion in the lower extremities. 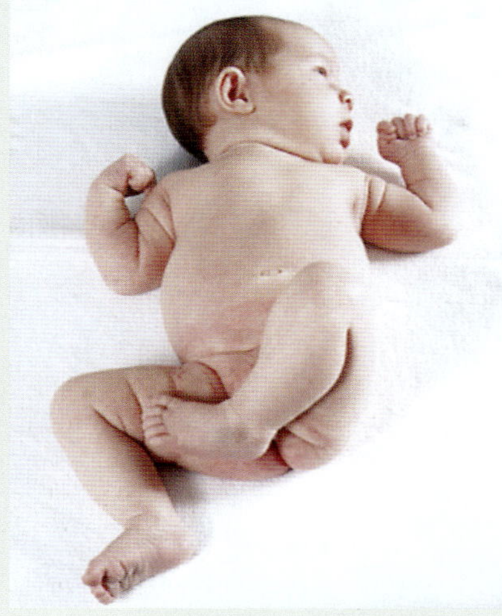 **Figure 12.53**	Abnormal postures: **Frog position**—hips abducted and almost flat against the table, externally rotated (only normal after breech delivery). **Opisthotonos**—head arched back, stiffness of neck and extension of arms and legs; occurs with meningeal or brainstem irritation and kernicterus (see Table 12.12). Extension of limbs may occur with intracranial haemorrhage. Any type of continual asymmetry, e.g. asymmetry of upper limbs occurs with **brachial plexus palsy**.
After 2 months of age, flexion gives way to gradual extension, beginning with the head and continuing in a cephalocaudal direction. Now is the time to check for spasticity; none should be present. Test for spasticity by flexing the infant's knees onto the abdomen and then quickly releasing them. They will unfold but not too quickly. Also, gently push the head forward—the baby should comply.	**Spasticity** is an early sign of cerebral palsy. After releasing flexed knees, legs will quickly extend and adduct, even to a 'scissoring' motion when spasticity is present. Also, the baby often resists head flexion and extends back against your hand when spasticity is present.
The fists are normally held in tight flexion for the first 3 months. Then the fists open for part of the time. A purposeful reach for an object with both hands occurs around 4 months of age, a transfer of an object from hand to hand at 7 months of age, a grasp using fingers and opposing thumb at 9 months of age and a purposeful release at 10 months of age. Babies are normally ambidextrous for the first 18 months.	Note persistent one-hand preference in baby younger than 18 months of age, which may indicate a motor deficit on the opposite side.
Head control is an important milestone in motor development. You can incorporate the following two movements into every infant assessment to check the muscle tone necessary for head control.	
First, with the baby supine, pull to a sit holding the wrists and note head control (Figure 12.54). The newborn will hold the head almost in the same plane as the body, and it will balance briefly when the baby reaches a sitting position, then flop forward. (Even a premature infant shows some head flexion.) At 4 months of age, the head stays in line with the body and does not flop.	Because development progresses in a cephalocaudal direction, head lag is an early sign of brain damage. ***Clinical alert:*** After 6 months of age, refer any baby with failure to hold head in midline when sitting.

PROCEDURES AND NORMAL FINDINGS	ABNORMAL FINDINGS AND CLINICAL ALERTS
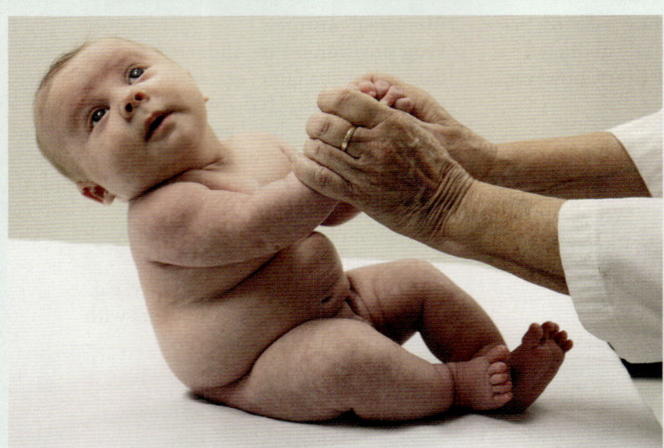 **Figure 12.54**	
Second, lift up the baby in a prone position, with one hand supporting the chest (Figure 12.55). The term newborn holds the head at an angle of 45 degrees or less from horizontal, the back is straight or slightly arched and the elbows and knees are partly flexed. 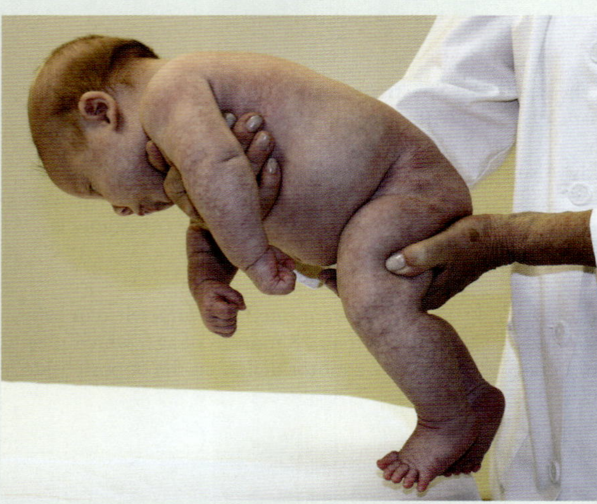 **Figure 12.55**	
At 3 months of age, the baby raises the head and arches the back, as in a swan dive. This is the **Landau reflex**, which persists until 18 months of age.	Head lag, a limp, floppy trunk and dangling arms and legs. Absence of the reflex indicates motor weakness, upper motor neuron disease or cognitive delay.

PROCEDURES AND NORMAL FINDINGS	ABNORMAL FINDINGS AND CLINICAL ALERTS
Assess muscle strength by noting the strength of sucking and of spontaneous motor activity. Normally, no tremors are present, and no continual over shooting of the mark occurs when reaching (Figure 12.56). 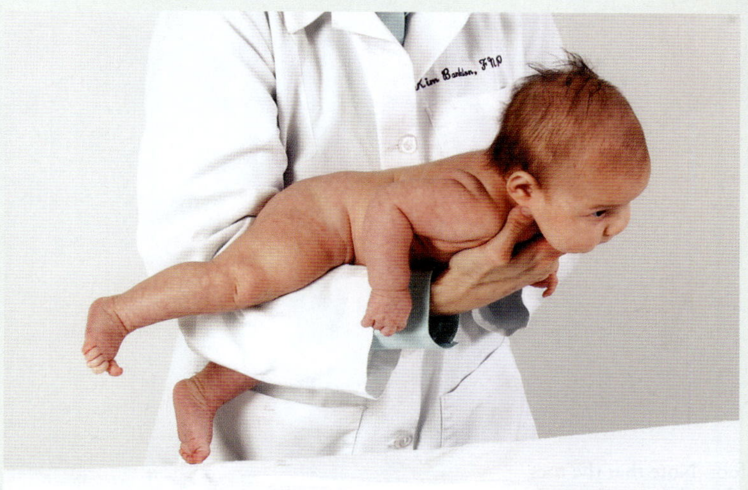 **Figure 12.56**	
The sensory system	
You will perform very little sensory testing with infants and toddlers. The newborn normally has hypoaesthesia and requires a strong stimulus to elicit a response. The baby responds to pain by crying and a general reflex withdrawal of all limbs. By 7 to 9 months of age, the infant can localise the stimulus and shows more specific signs of withdrawal. Other sensory modalities are not tested.	Unusually rapid withdrawal is **hyperaesthesia**, which occurs with spinal cord lesions, CNS infections, increased intracranial pressure, peritonitis. No withdrawal is decreased sensation, which occurs with decreased consciousness, cognitive delay, spinal cord or peripheral nerve lesions.
The motor system—reflexes	
Infantile automatisms are reflexes that have a predictable timetable of appearance and departure. The reflexes most commonly tested are listed in the following section. For the screening examination, you can just check the rooting, grasp, tonic neck and Moro reflexes.	
Rooting reflex. Brush the infant's cheek near the mouth. Note whether the infant turns the head towards that side and opens the mouth. Appears at birth and disappears at 3 to 4 months.	
Sucking reflex. Touch the lips and offer your gloved little finger to suck. Note strong sucking reflex. The reflex is present at birth and disappears at 10 to 12 months.	
Palmar grasp. Place the baby's head midline to ensure symmetrical response. Offer your finger from the baby's ulnar side, away from the thumb. Note tight grasp of all the baby's fingers (Figure 12.57). Sucking enhances grasp. Often you can pull baby to a sit from grasp. The reflex is present at birth, is strongest at 1 to 2 months and disappears at 3 to 4 months.	The palmar grasp reflex is absent with brain damage and with local muscle or nerve injury. Persistence of palmar grasp reflex after 4 months of age occurs with frontal lobe lesion.

PROCEDURES AND NORMAL FINDINGS	ABNORMAL FINDINGS AND CLINICAL ALERTS
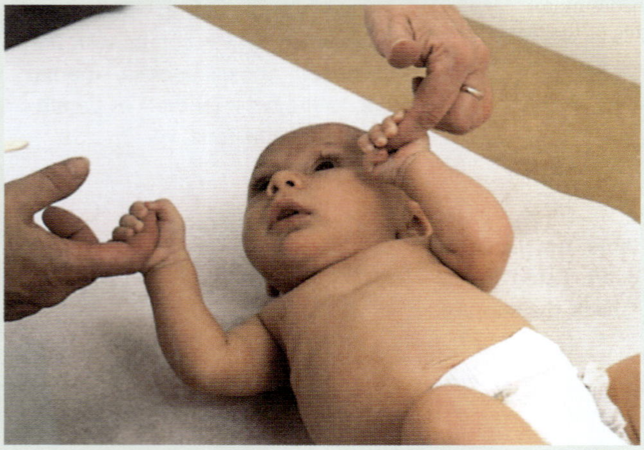 Figure 12.57	
Plantar grasp. Touch your thumb at the ball of the baby's foot. Note that the toes curl down tightly (Figure 12.58). The reflex is present at birth and disappears at 8 to 10 months. 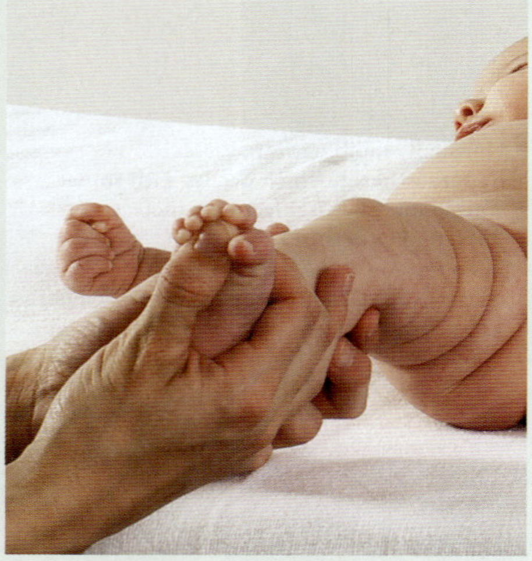 Figure 12.58	
Babinski's reflex. Stroke your finger up the lateral edge and across the ball of the infant's foot. Note fanning of toes (positive Babinski's reflex) (Figure 12.59). The reflex is present at birth and disappears (changes to the adult response) by 24 months of age (variable).	Positive Babinski's reflex after 2 or 2½ years of age occurs with pyramidal tract disease.

OBJECTIVE DATA

PROCEDURES AND NORMAL FINDINGS	ABNORMAL FINDINGS AND CLINICAL ALERTS
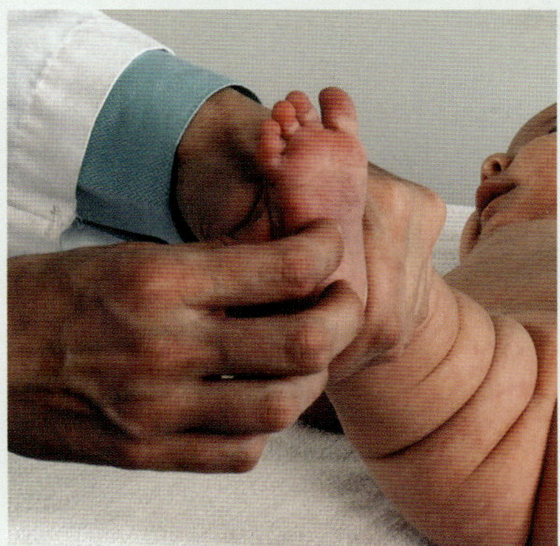 Figure 12.59	
Tonic neck reflex. With the baby supine, relaxed or sleeping, turn the head to one side with the chin over shoulder. Note ipsilateral extension of the arm and leg and flexion of the opposite arm and leg; this is the 'fencing' position. If you turn the infant's head to the opposite side, positions will reverse (Figure 12.60). The reflex appears by 2 to 3 months, decreases at 3 to 4 months and disappears by 4 to 6 months. 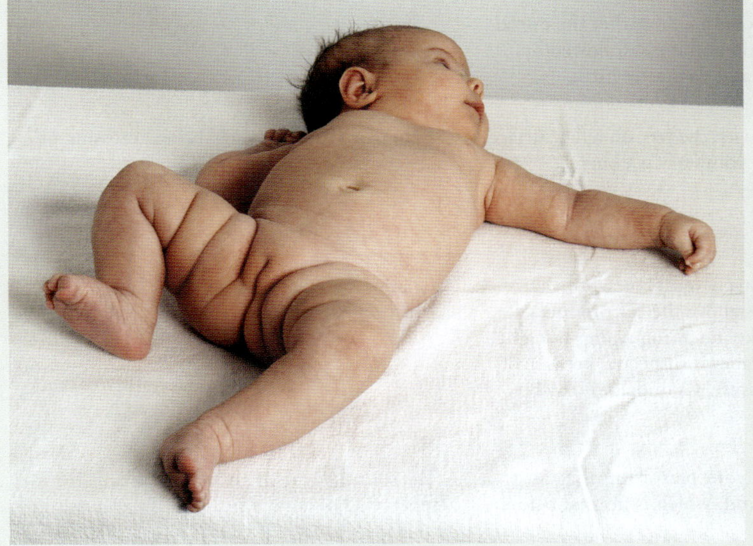 Figure 12.60	Persistence later in infancy occurs with brain damage.
Moro reflex. Startle the infant by jarring the crib, making a loud noise or supporting the head and back in a semi-sitting position and quickly lowering the infant to 30 degrees. The baby looks as if they are hugging a tree. That is, symmetrical abduction and extension of the arms and legs, fanning fingers and curling of the index finger and thumb to C position occur. The infant then brings in both arms and legs (Figure 12.61). The reflex is present at birth, and disappears at 1 to 4 months.	Absence of the Moro reflex in the newborn or persistence after 5 months of age indicates severe CNS injury. Absence of movement in just one arm occurs with fracture of the humerus or clavicle and with brachial nerve palsy. Absence in one leg occurs with a lower spinal cord problem or a dislocated hip. A hyperactive Moro reflex occurs with tetany or CNS infection.

OBJECTIVE DATA

PROCEDURES AND NORMAL FINDINGS	ABNORMAL FINDINGS AND CLINICAL ALERTS
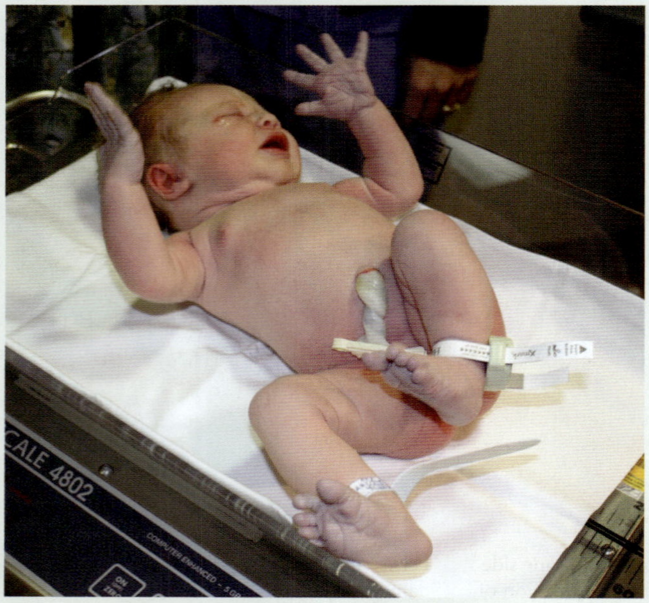 **Figure 12.61** Moro reflex	
Placing reflex. Hold the infant upright under the arms, close to a table. Let the dorsal 'top' of foot touch the underside of table. Note flexing of hip and knee, followed by extension at the hip, to place foot on table. Reflex appears at 4 days after birth.	
Stepping reflex. Hold the infant upright under the arms, with the feet on a flat surface. Note regular alternating steps. The reflex disappears before voluntary walking.	**Extensor thrust**, or 'scissoring'; crossing of lower extremities.
Special procedures	
Palpation. Craniotabes is a softening of the skull's outer layer. With a newborn, pressure along the suture of the parietal and occipital bones above the ear produces a snapping sensation because of the pliable skull bone. It is like indenting a ping-pong ball and feeling it snap back. Do not attempt this unless craniotabes is suspected because of other abnormal findings, and even then avoid excessive pressure. Craniotabes may be normal, especially with premature infants.	Craniotabes may occur with rickets, hydrocephaly or congenital syphilis.
Percussion. With an infant, you may directly percuss with your plexor finger against the head surface. This yields a resonant or 'cracked pot' sound, which is normal before closure of the fontanels.	The sound occurs with hydrocephalus from separation of cranial sutures (Macewen's sign).
Auscultation. Bruits are common in the skull in children under 4 or 5 years of age or in children with anaemia. They are systolic or continuous and are heard over the temporal area.	After 5 years of age, bruits indicate increased intracranial pressure, aneurysm or arteriovenous shunt.
	If you suspect an abnormal head size or an intracranial lesion refer to medical practitioner for further assessment.
Additional objective assessment for children	
Use the same sequence of neurological assessment as with the adult, with the omissions or modifications mentioned in the following section.	

OBJECTIVE DATA

PROCEDURES AND NORMAL FINDINGS	ABNORMAL FINDINGS AND CLINICAL ALERTS
Behaviour	
Assess the child's general behaviour during play activities, reaction to parent and cooperation with parent and with you. Complete details are described in Chapter 11.	
Cranial nerves	
Smell and taste are almost never tested, but if you need to test the child's sense of smell (cranial nerve I), use a scent familiar to the child such as peanut butter or orange peel. When testing visual fields (cranial nerve II) and cardinal positions of gaze (cranial nerves III, IV, VI), you often need to gently immobilise the head, or the child will track with the whole head. Make a game out of asking the child to imitate your funny 'faces' (cranial nerve VII); thus, the child has fun and you win a friend.	
Motor system	
Much of the motor assessment can be derived from watching the child undress and dress and manipulate buttons. This indicates muscle strength, symmetry, joint range of motion and fine motor skills. Use the Denver II test to screen gross and fine motor skills that are appropriate for the child's specific age. Be familiar with developmental milestones described in Chapter 3 for each age. Note the child's gait during both walking and running. Allow for the normal wide-based gait of the toddler and the normal knock-kneed walk of the preschooler. Normally, the child can balance on one foot for about 5 seconds by 4 years of age, can balance for 8 to 10 seconds at 5 years of age and can hop at 4 years. Children enjoy performing these tests (Figure 12.62). 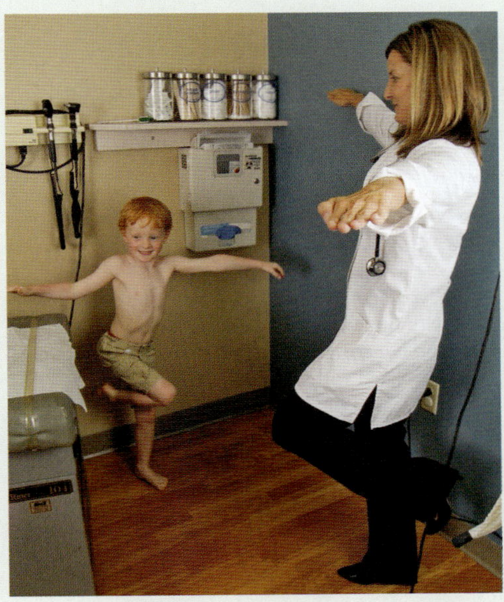 **Figure 12.62**	**Muscle hypertrophy** or **atrophy** occurs with muscular dystrophy. Muscle weakness. Lack of coordination. Causes of motor delay are listed earlier in the infant section. Staggering, falling. Weakness climbing up or down stairs occurs with muscular dystrophy. Broad-based gait beyond toddlerhood, scissor gait (see Table 12.8). Failure to hop after 5 years of age indicates un-coordination of gross motor skill.
Observe the child as they rise from a supine position on the floor to a sitting position, and then to a stand. Note the muscles of the neck, abdomen, arms and legs. Normally, the child curls up in the midline to sit up, then pushes off with both hands against the floor to stand (Figure 12.63).	Weak pelvic muscles are a sign of muscular dystrophy; from the supine position, the child will roll to one side, bend forward to all four extremities, plant hands on legs and literally 'climb' up themself. This is **Gower's sign**.

PROCEDURES AND NORMAL FINDINGS	ABNORMAL FINDINGS AND CLINICAL ALERTS
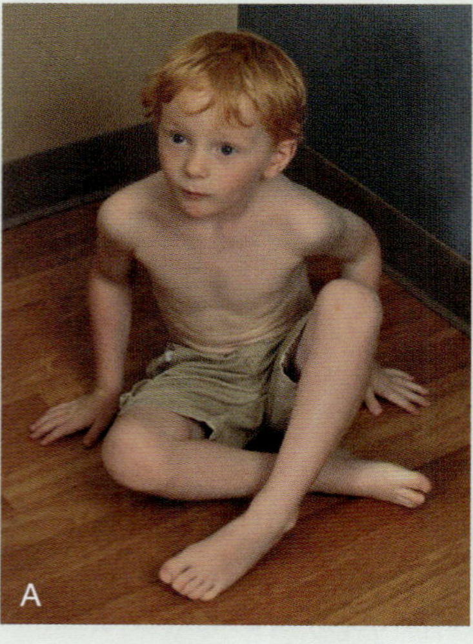 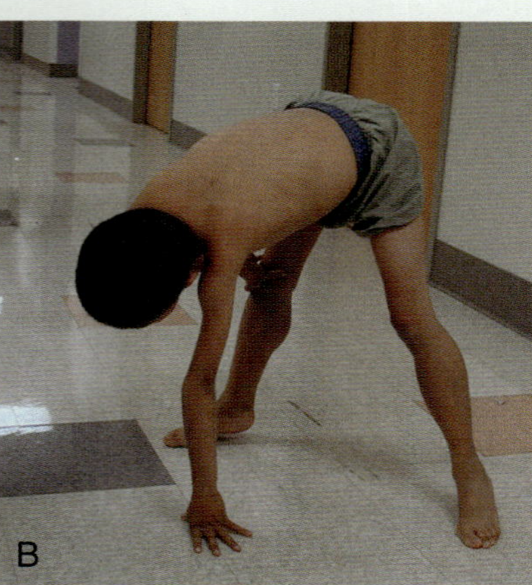 **Figure 12.63**	
Assess fine coordination by using the finger-to-nose test if you can be sure the young child understands your directions. Demonstrate the procedure first, then ask the child to do the test with the eyes open, then with the eyes closed. Fine coordination is not fully developed until the child has reached 4 to 6 years of age. Consider it normal if a younger child can bring the finger to within 2 to 5 cm of the nose.	Failure of the finger-to-nose test with the eyes open indicates gross un-coordination; failure of the test with the eyes closed indicates minor un-coordination or lack of position sense.
Sensation	
Testing sensation is very unreliable in toddlers and preschoolers. You may test light touch by asking the child to close the eyes and then to point to the spot where you touch or tickle. Testing of vibration, position, stereognosis, graphaesthesia or two-point discrimination usually is not done on a child younger than 6 years of age. Also, do not test for perception of superficial pain. In children older than 6 years of age, you may perform sensory testing as with adults. Use a fractured tongue blade if you need to test superficial pain.	Sensory loss occurs with decreased consciousness, mental deficiency or spinal cord or peripheral nerve dysfunction.
Reflexes	
The deep tendon reflexes are usually not tested in children younger than 5 years of age due to lack of cooperation in relaxation. When you need to test deep tendon reflexes in a young child, use your finger to percuss the tendon. Use a reflex hammer only with an older child. Coax the child to relax, or distract and percuss discreetly when the child is not paying attention. The knee jerk is present at birth, then the ankle jerk and brachial reflex appear and the triceps reflex is present at 6 months.	Hyperactivity of deep tendon reflexes occurs with upper motor neuron lesion, hypocalcaemia and hyperthyroidism and with muscle spasm associated with early poliomyelitis. Decreased or absent reflexes occur with a lower motor neuron lesion, muscular dystrophy and flaccidity or flaccid paralysis. Clonus may occur with fatigue, but it usually indicates hyperreflexia.
Additional objective assessment for the adult over 65 years	
Use the same examination as used with the younger adult. The findings discussed in the following sections are normal variants due to ageing.	
Cranial nerves	
Although the cranial nerves mediating taste and smell are not usually tested, they may show some decline in function.	
Motor system	
Any decrease in muscle bulk is most apparent in the hand, as seen by guttering between the metacarpals. These dorsal hand muscles often look wasted, even with no apparent arthropathy. The grip strength remains relatively good.	Hand muscle atrophy is worsened with disuse and degenerative arthropathy.

PROCEDURES AND NORMAL FINDINGS	ABNORMAL FINDINGS AND CLINICAL ALERTS
Tremors occasionally occur. These benign tremors include an intention tremor of the hands, head nodding (as if saying yes or no) and tongue protrusion. **Dyskinesias** are the repetitive stereotyped movements in the jaw, lips or tongue that may accompany senile tremors. No associated rigidity is present.	Tfremors associated with Parkinson's disease are accompanied by rigidity and slowness and weakness of voluntary movement.
The gait may be slower and more deliberate than that in the younger person, and it may deviate slightly from a midline path.	Absence of a rhythmic reciprocal gait pattern is seen in Parkinson's disease and hemiparesis (see Table 12.8).
The rapid alternating movements, e.g. pronating and supinating the hands on the thigh, may be more difficult to perform by the ageing adult.	
Sensory	
After 65 years of age, loss of the sensation of vibration at the ankle malleolus is common and is usually accompanied by loss of the ankle jerk. Position sense in the big toe may be lost, although this is less common than vibration loss. Tactile sensation may be impaired. The ageing person may need stronger stimuli for light touch and especially for pain.	Note any difference in sensation between right and left sides, which may indicate a neurological deficit.
Reflexes	
The deep tendon reflexes are less brisk. Those in the upper extremities are usually present, but the ankle jerks are commonly lost. Knee jerks may be lost, but this occurs less often.	
The plantar reflex may be absent or difficult to interpret. Often, you will not see a definite normal flexor response. However, you still should consider a definite extensor response to be abnormal.	
The superficial abdominal reflexes may be absent, probably because of stretching of the musculature through pregnancy or obesity.	

Summary Checklist

NEUROLOGICAL ASSESSMENT

Subjective data

1. Presenting concern
2. Headache
3. Neck pain
4. Pain
5. Head injury
6. Dizziness/vertigo
7. Seizures
8. Tremors and involuntary movements
9. Weakness
10. Lack of coordination
11. Numbness or tingling
12. Disturbances or deafness
13. Dysphagia
14. Difficulty speaking
15. Relevant health and family history
16. Health and lifestyle management
17. Environmental/occupational hazards

Objective data

1. General inspection
2. Level of consciousness
3. Using the Glasgow Coma Scale
4. Pupillary response
5. Vital signs
6. Limb movement and strength
7. Assessing delirium

PROMOTING A HEALTHY LIFESTYLE

STROKE PREVENTION

Symptoms, non-modifiable and well-documented modifiable risk factors for stroke

According to the Stroke Foundation Australia (2020) stroke is a leading cause of long-term disability and death. A stroke occurs when the blood flow is interrupted to a part of the brain. The most common type is an ischaemic stroke, occurring when a blood clot blocks a blood vessel in the brain. Less common is a haemorrhagic stroke, which occurs when a blood vessel in the brain ruptures and causes bleeding. The symptoms and after-effects of a stroke depend on which area of the brain is affected and to what extent. This can make a stroke difficult to diagnose. However, early recognition of symptoms and prompt treatment are essential.

The **most common** symptoms of stroke include:

1. Sudden weakness or numbness in the face, arms or legs, especially when it is on one side of the body
2. Sudden confusion, trouble speaking or understanding speech
3. Sudden changes in vision, such as blurry vision or partial or complete loss of vision in one or both eyes
4. Sudden trouble walking, dizziness and/or loss of balance or coordination
5. Sudden severe headache with no reason or explanation.

Less common symptoms of stroke include:

1. Sudden nausea and/or vomiting
2. Brief loss of consciousness, including fainting.

Stroke symptoms usually do not cause pain, which is why many people ignore them or delay seeking medical attention. Sometimes, people can have a 'mini-stroke' or transient ischaemic attack (TIA). In these cases, the stroke symptoms last only temporarily and then disappear, often within an hour. Because the symptoms 'go away', people too often do not report them or seek medical attention. However, a TIA is a warning sign that should not be ignored. When people experience chest pain, they seek medical attention, to rule out a heart attack. Having a TIA should also prompt people to seek medical attention to rule out the possibility of a future stroke.

The Stroke Foundation Australia (2020) has devised an easy-to-remember acronym to assist the general public in recognising the signs and symptoms of stroke quickly and calling for an ambulance. The acronym is F.A.S.T.

- **F**ace Check the person's face—has their mouth drooped?
- **A**rm Can they lift both arms?
- **S**peech Is their speech slurred? Do they understand you?
- **T**ime Time is critical—if you see any of these signs call the emergency number (000 in Australia; 111 in New Zealand).

Stroke can strike anyone without warning. People need to be aware of their stroke risk and take steps to change the risk factors they can control.

Well-documented modifiable risk factors for stroke include:

1. History of cardiovascular disease including hypertension, atrial fibrillation, dyslipidaemia and asymptomatic carotid stenosis
2. Cigarette smoking
3. Type 1 and type 2 diabetes
4. Sickle cell disease
5. Postmenopausal hormone therapy
6. Diet and nutrition
7. Physical inactivity
8. Obesity

Non-modifiable risk factors for stroke include:

1. Age
2. Gender—strokes are generally more prevalent in men than in women. However, exceptions are in 35- to 44-year-olds and ≥85 years of age—groups in which women have slightly greater age-specific stroke incidence than do men
3. Low birth weight
4. Ethnicity—Aboriginal and Torres Strait Islander people have higher stroke incidence and mortality rates than other Australians
5. Genetic factor disorders (e.g. Marfan's syndrome, Fabry's disease, cerebral autosomal dominant arteriopathy with sub-cortical infarcts and leucoencephalopathy (CADASIL)

Non-modifiable risk factors for stroke may help to identify those who, in conjunction with well-documented modifiable risks, are at highest risk of stroke and who may benefit from more rigorous treatment of modifiable risk factors.

Stroke Foundation Australia:
https://strokefoundation.org.au

Stroke Foundation of New Zealand:
http://www.stroke.org.nz

Documentation and critical thinking

FOCUSED ASSESSMENT: CLINICAL CASE STUDY

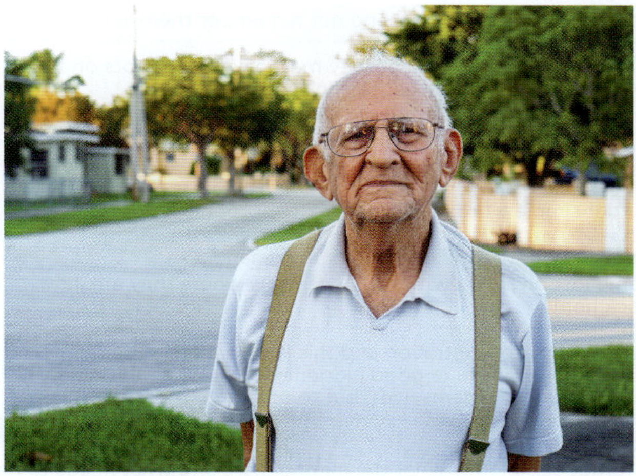

Context

It is bedside handover at change of shift. The registered nurse is undertaking a baseline assessment of Mr Bob Williams' neurological status at the start of the shift in conjunction with the RN that has been caring for him on the morning shift.

Mr Williams is a aged 80 years retired builder who lives with his son in a single-storey house that he owns, with an unknown number of stairs at front and back doors. He was previously living independently performing his activities of daily living without assistance of others. He was initially referred to neurosurgery department after a two-month history of increasing confusion and generalised malaise, which led his general practitioner to order a computed tomography (CT) scan, which showed a left-sided cerebral lesion. Four hours ago, Mr Williams returned to the ward from the operating room following a craniotomy and biopsy of a left temporal parietal lesion.

Subjective

Mr Williams is currently stating that he is 'on the way to the bus stop'. This is despite being reoriented to time, place and person.

Objective

Mental status: Dressed in hospital gown, lying in bed he appears alert with appropriate eye contact, listening intently to history. Speech is slow, requires great effort, and voice tone is very soft. Verbal content confused to place and time.

Eye opening in response to speech.

Motor: Obeying commands. Right hand grip weak, right arm drifts, right leg weak. Spasticity in right arm and leg muscles, limited range of motion on passive motion.

Pupillary response: Size 3 mm, equal, and responding briskly to light.

Glasgow Coma Scale score: 13/15. No change from previous assessment.

Collaborative problem

Deteriorating cognitive and neurological function related to brain tumour

Impaired physical mobility related to neuromuscular impairment

Problem statements/nursing diagnoses

Impaired verbal communication related to effects of neurological condition

Impaired physical mobility related to neuromuscular impairment

Self-care deficits: feeding, bathing, toileting, dressing/grooming related to muscular weakness

Risk for injury related to neuromuscular impairment

Abnormal findings

TABLE 12.1 Warning signs of dementia	
Recent memory loss that affects job skills	• It is normal to forget meetings, colleagues' names or a business associate's telephone number occasionally, but then remember them later. • A person with dementia may forget things more often, and not remember them later.
Difficulty performing familiar tasks	• Busy people can be so distracted from time to time that they may leave the carrots on the stove and only remember to serve them when the meal has finished. • A person with dementia might prepare a meal and not only forget to serve it, but also forget they made it.
Problems with language	• Everyone has trouble finding the right word sometimes. • A person with dementia may forget simple words or substitute inappropriate words.
Disorientation of time and place	• It is normal to forget the day of the week or your destination for a moment. • People with dementia can become lost on their own street, not know where they are, how they got there or how to get back home.
Poor or decreased judgement	• Dementia affects a person's memory and concentration and this in turn affects their judgement. Many activities, such as driving, require good judgement and when this ability is affected, the person will be a risk, not only to themselves, but to others on the road.
Problems with abstract thinking	• Managing finances can be difficult for anyone. • Someone with dementia could forget completely what the numbers are and what needs to be done with them.
Misplacing things	• Anyone can temporarily misplace a wallet or keys. • A person with dementia may repeatedly put things in inappropriate places.
Changes in mood or behaviour	• Everyone becomes sad or moody from time to time. • Someone with dementia can have rapid mood swings from calm to tears to anger, for no apparent reason.
Changes in personality	• People's personalities can change a little with age. • A person with dementia can become suspicious or fearful, or just apathetic and uncommunicative. They may also become dis-inhibited, over-familiar or more outgoing than previously.
Loss of initiative	• It is normal to tire of housework, business activities or social obligations. • The person with dementia may become very passive and require cues prompting them to become involved.

Adapted from the Dementia Australia website: https://www.dementia.org.au/information/diagnosing-dementia

TABLE 12.2 Ischaemic and haemorrhagic stroke

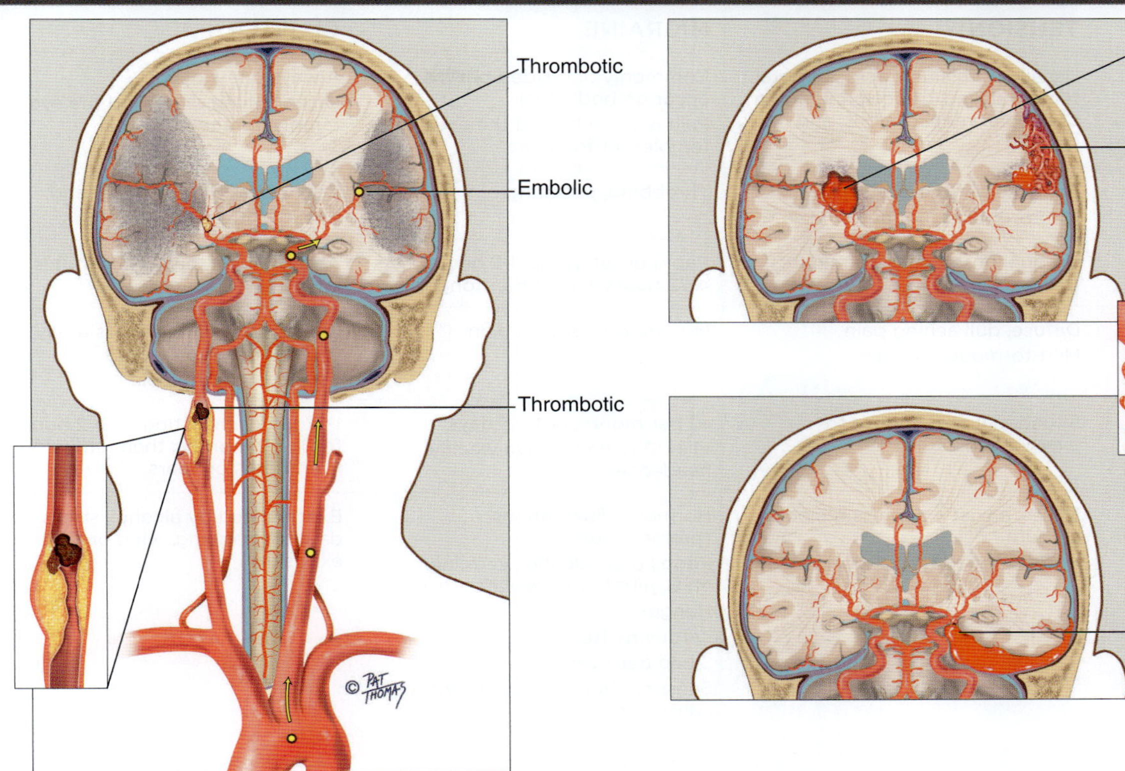

Ischaemic stroke is a sudden interruption of blood flow to the brain and accounts for 87% of all strokes. These are of two types. **Thrombotic** strokes result from atherosclerotic plaque formation. A vulnerable plaque ruptures, and a local thrombus forms that deprives the brain tissue in the region of crucial oxygen and glucose. **Embolic** strokes result from a travelling clot caused by atrial fibrillation or flutter, recent heart attack, growth around prosthetic heart valves, and endocarditis. Acute ischaemic stroke symptoms include unilateral facial droop, arm drift, weakness or paralysis on one half of the body, difficulty speaking or understanding speech, confusion, sudden onset of dizziness, loss of balance, clouding of vision.

Haemorrhagic stroke results from acute rupture and bleeding from a weakened artery in the brain and accounts for only 13% of all strokes. Most are intracerebral haemorrhages caused by ruptured aneurysm, arteriovenous malformation, disturbed coagulation cascade, tumour or cocaine abuse. Arteriovenous malformations are congenital networks of arteries and veins that do not have capillaries in between and are at risk for rupture. Think of a snarl of tendrils. A subarachnoid haemorrhage is less common and is due to an aneurysm between the base of the cerebral cortex and the arachnoid layer of the meninges. Symptoms include sudden severe headache, nausea and vomiting, sudden loss of consciousness and focal seizures.

TABLE 12.3 Primary headaches

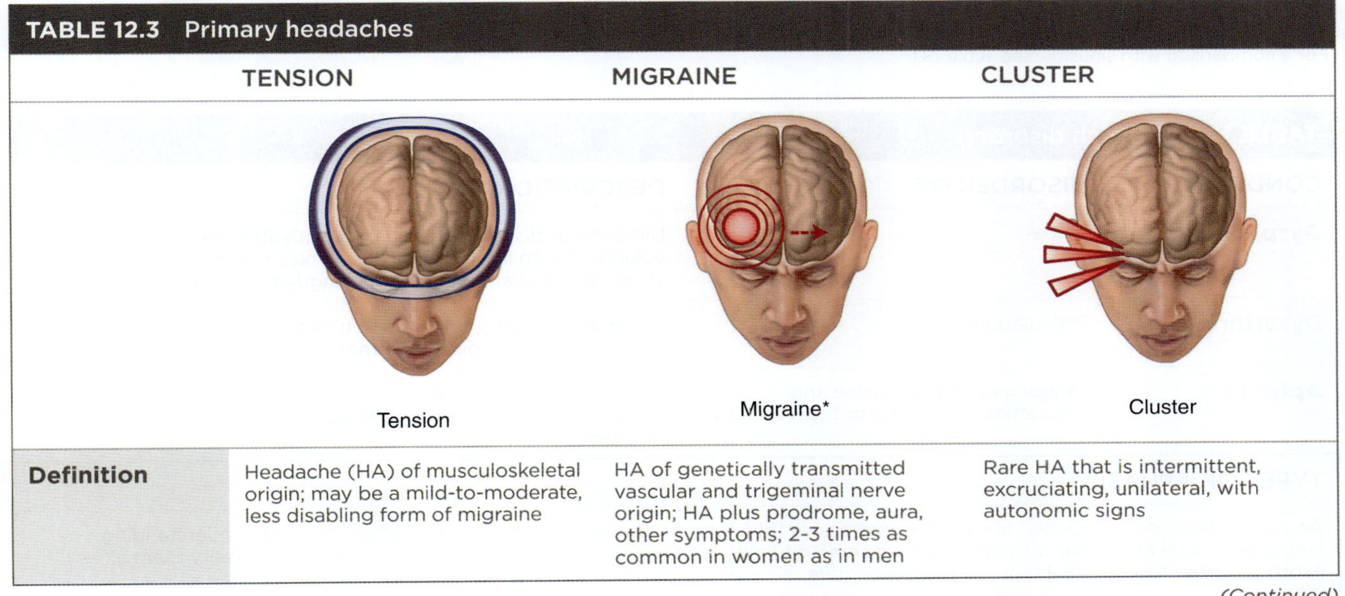

	TENSION	MIGRAINE	CLUSTER
Definition	Headache (HA) of musculoskeletal origin; may be a mild-to-moderate, less disabling form of migraine	HA of genetically transmitted vascular and trigeminal nerve origin; HA plus prodrome, aura, other symptoms; 2-3 times as common in women as in men	Rare HA that is intermittent, excruciating, unilateral, with autonomic signs

(Continued)

TABLE 12.3 Primary headaches—cont'd

	TENSION	MIGRAINE	CLUSTER
Location	Usually both sides, across frontal, temporal, and/or occipital region of head: forehead, sides, and back of head	Commonly one-sided but may occur on both sides Pain is often behind the eyes, the temples, or forehead	Always one-sided Often behind or around the eye, temple, forehead, cheek
Character	Bandlike tightness, vicelike Nonthrobbing, nonpulsatile	Throbbing, pulsating	Continuous, burning, piercing, excruciating
Duration	Gradual onset, lasts 30 minutes to days	Rapid onset, peaks 1-2 hours, lasts 4-72 hours, sometimes longer	Abrupt onset, peaks in minutes, lasts 45-90 min
Quantity and severity	Diffuse, dull aching pain Mild-to-moderate pain	Moderate-to-severe pain	Can occur multiple times a day, in "clusters," lasting weeks Severe, stabbing pain
Timing	Situational, in response to overwork, posture	≈2 per month, last 1-3 days ≈1 in 10 patients have weekly headaches	1-2/day, each lasting ½ to 2 hours for 1 to 2 months; then remission for months or years
Aggravating symptoms or triggers	Stress, anxiety, depression, poor posture Not worsened by physical activity	Hormonal fluctuations (premenstrual) Foods (e.g., alcohol, caffeine, MSG, nitrates, chocolate, cheese) Hunger Letdown after stress Sleep deprivation Sensory stimuli (e.g., flashing lights or perfumes) Changes in weather Physical activity	Exacerbated by alcohol, stress, daytime napping, wind or heat exposure
Associated symptoms	Fatigue, anxiety, stress Sensation of a band tightening around head, of being gripped like a vice Sometimes photophobia or phonophobia	Aura (visual changes such as blind spots or flashes of light, tingling in an arm or leg, vertigo) Prodrome (change in mood, behavior, hunger, cravings, yawning) Nausea, vomiting, photophobia, phonophobia, abdominal pain Person looks sick Family history of migraine	Ipsilateral autonomic signs: Nasal congestion or runny nose, watery or reddened eye, eyelid drooping, miosis Feelings of agitation
Relieving factors, efforts to treat	Rest, massaging muscles in area, NSAID medication	Lie down, darken room, use eyeshade, sleep, take NSAID early, try to avoid opioid	Need to move, pace floor

*For a comparison with sinusitis, see Table 18.1.

TABLE 12.6 Speech disorders

CONDITION	DISORDER OF	DESCRIPTION
Dysphonia	Voice	Difficulty or discomfort in talking, with abnormal pitch or volume, due to laryngeal disease. Voice sounds hoarse or whispered, but articulation and language are intact.
Dysarthria	Articulation	Distorted speech sounds; speech may sound unintelligible; basic language (word choice, grammar, comprehension) intact.
Aphasia	Language comprehension and production secondary to brain damage	True language disturbance, defect in word choice and grammar or defect in comprehension; defect is in higher integrative language processing.
TYPES OF APHASIA		
An earlier dichotomy classified aphasias as expressive (difficulty producing language) or receptive (difficulty understanding language). Since all people with aphasia have some difficulty with expression, beginning examiners tend to classify them all as expressive. The following system is more descriptive.		

TABLE 12.6 Speech disorders—cont'd

Condition	Description
Global aphasia	The most common and severe form. Spontaneous speech is absent or reduced to a few stereotyped words or sounds. Comprehension is absent or reduced to only the person's own name and a few select words. Repetition, reading and writing are severely impaired. Prognosis for language recovery is poor. Caused by a large lesion that damages most of the combined anterior and posterior language areas.
Broca's aphasia	Expressive aphasia. The person can understand language but cannot express themself using language. This is characterised by nonfluent, dysarthric and effortful speech. The speech is mostly nouns and verbs (high-content words) with few grammatic fillers, termed 'agrammatic' or 'telegraphic' speech. Repetition and reading aloud are severely impaired. Auditory and reading comprehensions are surprisingly intact. Lesion is in anterior language area called the motor speech cortex or Broca's area.
Wernicke's aphasia	Receptive aphasia. The linguistic opposite of Broca's aphasia. The person can hear sounds and words but cannot relate them to previous experiences. Speech is fluent, effortless and well-articulated but has many paraphasias (word substitutions that are malformed or wrong) and neologisms (made-up words) and often lacks substantive words. Speech can be totally incomprehensible. Often, there is a great urge to speak. Repetition, reading and writing also are impaired. Lesion is in posterior language area called the association auditory cortex or Wernicke's area.

(For a discussion of other types of aphasia (e.g. conduction, anomic, transcortical), please consult a neurology text.)

TABLE 12.7 Abnormalities in cranial nerves

NERVE	TEST	ABNORMAL FINDINGS	POSSIBLE CAUSES
I: Olfactory	Identify familiar odours	Anosmia	Upper respiratory infection (temporary); tobacco or cocaine use; fracture of cribriform plate or ethmoid area; frontal lobe lesion; tumour in olfactory bulb or tract
II: Optic	Visual acuity	Defect or absent central vision	Congenital blindness, refractive error, acquired vision loss from numerous diseases (e.g. stroke, type 1 and type 2 diabetes), trauma to globe or orbit (see discussion of cranial nerve III)
	Visual fields	Defect in peripheral vision, hemianopsia	
	Shine light in eye	Absent light reflex	
	Direct inspection	Papillo-oedema Optic atrophy Retinal lesions	Increased intracranial pressure Glaucoma Type 1 and type 2 diabetes
III: Oculomotor	Inspection	Dilated pupil, ptosis, eye turns out and slightly down	Paralysis in cranial nerve III from internal carotid aneurysm, tumour, inflammatory lesions, uncal herniation with increased intracranial pressure
	Extraocular muscle movement	Failure to move eye up, in, down	Ptosis from myasthenia gravis, oculomotor nerve palsy, Horner's syndrome
	Shine light in eye	Absent light reflex	Blindness, drug influence, increased intracranial pressure, CNS injury, circulatory arrest, CNS syphilis
IV: Trochlear	Extraocular muscle movement	Failure to turn eye down or out	Fracture of orbit, brainstem tumour
V: Trigeminal	Superficial touch—three divisions Corneal reflex	Absent touch and pain, paraesthesias No blink	Trauma, tumour, pressure from aneurysm, inflammation, sequelae of alcohol injection for trigeminal neuralgia
	Clench teeth	Weakness of masseter or temporalis muscles	Unilateral weakness with cranial nerve V lesion; bilateral weakness with upper or lower motor neuron disorder
VI: Abducens	Extraocular muscle movement to right and left sides	Failure to move laterally, diplopia on lateral gaze	Brainstem tumour or trauma, fracture of orbit

(Continued)

TABLE 12.7 Abnormalities in cranial nerves—cont'd

NERVE	TEST	ABNORMAL FINDINGS	POSSIBLE CAUSES
VII: Facial	Wrinkle forehead, close eyes tightly	Absent or asymmetric facial movement	Bell's palsy (lower motor neuron lesion) causes paralysis of entire half of face
	Smile, puff cheeks Identify tastes	Loss of taste	Upper motor neuron lesions (stroke, tumour, inflammatory) cause paralysis of lower half of face, leaving forehead intact Other lower motor neuron causes of paralysis: swelling from ear or meningeal infections
VIII: Acoustic	Hearing acuity	Decrease or loss of hearing	Inflammation, occluded ear canal, otosclerosis, presbycusis, drug toxicity, tumour
IX: Glossopharyngeal	Gag reflex	See cranial nerve X	
X: Vagus	Phonates 'ahh'	Uvula deviates to side	Brainstem tumour, neck injury, cranial nerve X lesion
	Gag reflex	No gag reflex	Vocal cord weakness
	Note voice quality	Hoarse or brassy Nasal twang Husky	Soft palate weakness Unilateral cranial nerve X lesion
	Note swallowing	Dysphagia, fluids regurgitate through nose	Bilateral cranial nerve X lesion
XI: Spinal accessory	Turn head, shrug shoulders against resistance	Absent movement of sternocleidomastoid or trapezius muscles	Neck injury, torticollis
XII: Hypoglossal	Protrude tongue Wiggle tongue from side to side	Deviates to side Slowed rate of movement	Lower motor neuron lesion Bilateral upper motor neuron lesion

TABLE 12.8 Abnormalities in muscle tone

CONDITION	DESCRIPTION	ASSOCIATED WITH
Flaccidity	Decreased muscle tone or *hypotonia*; muscle feels limp, soft and flabby; muscle is weak and easily fatigued	Lower motor neuron injury anywhere from the anterior horn cell in the spinal cord to the peripheral nerve (peripheral neuritis, poliomyelitis, Guillain-Barré syndrome). Early stroke and spinal cord injury are flaccid at first.
Spasticity	Increased tone or *hypertonia*; increased resistance to passive lengthening; then may suddenly give way (clasp-knife phenomenon)	Upper motor neuron injury to corticospinal motor tract, e.g. paralysis with stroke (chronic stage)
Rigidity	Constant state of resistance (lead-pipe rigidity); resists passive movement in any direction; dystonia	Injury to extrapyramidal motor tracts, e.g. basal ganglia with Parkinsonism
Cogwheel rigidity	Type of rigidity in which the increased tone is released by degrees during passive range of motion so it feels like small regular jerks	Parkinsonism

TABLE 12.9 Abnormalities in muscle movement

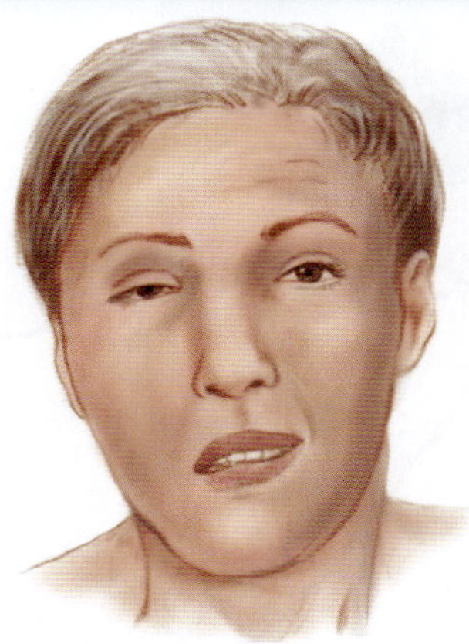

Paralysis

Decreased or loss of motor power due to problem with motor nerve or muscle fibres. Causes: acute—trauma, spinal cord injury, stroke, poliomyelitis, polyneuritis, Bell's palsy; chronic—muscular dystrophy, diabetic neuropathy, multiple sclerosis; episodic—myasthenia gravis.

Patterns of paralysis: *hemiplegia*—spastic or flaccid paralysis of one side (right or left) of body and extremities; *paraplegia*—symmetrical paralysis of both lower extremities; *quadriplegia*—paralysis in all four extremities; *paresis*—weakness of muscles rather than paralysis.

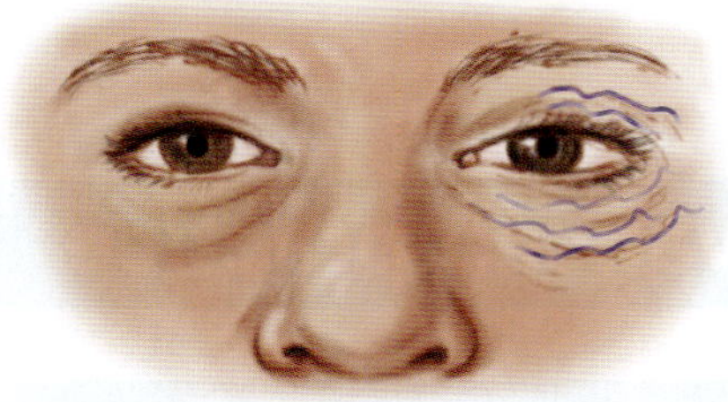

Fasciculation

Rapid, continuous twitching of resting muscle or part of muscle, without movement of limb, which can be seen or palpated. Types: fine—occurs with lower motor neuron disease, associated with atrophy and weakness; coarse—occurs with cold exposure or fatigue and is not significant.

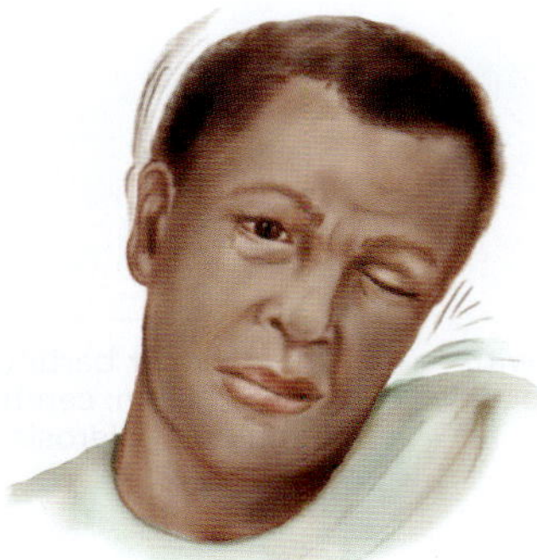

Tic

Involuntary, compulsive, repetitive twitching of a muscle group, e.g. wink, grimace, head movement, shoulder shrug; due to a neurological cause, e.g. tardive dyskinesias, Tourette's syndrome or psychogenic cause (habit tic).

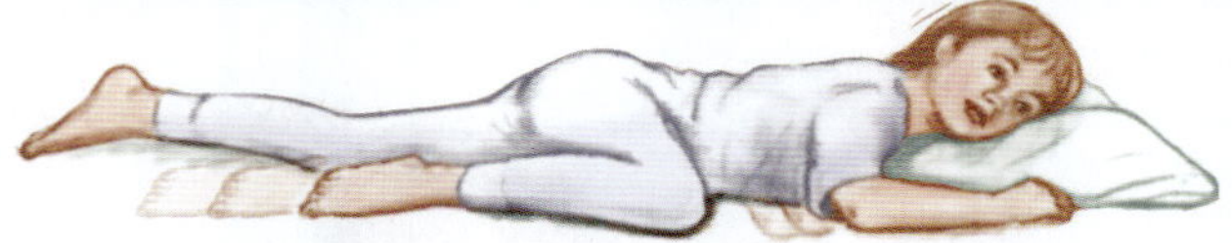

Myoclonus

Rapid, sudden jerk or a short series of jerks at fairly regular intervals. A hiccup is a myoclonus of diaphragm. Single myoclonic arm or leg jerk is normal when the person is falling asleep; myoclonic jerks are severe with tonic-clonic seizures.

Tremor

Involuntary contraction of opposing muscle groups. Results in rhythmic, back-and-forth movement of one or more joints. May occur at rest or with voluntary movement. All tremors disappear while sleeping. Tremors may be slow (3 to 6 per second) or rapid (10 to 20 per second).

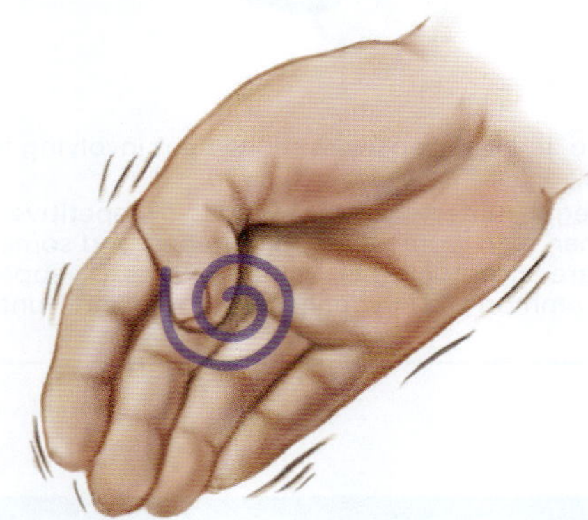

Rest tremor

Coarse and slow (3 to 6 per second); partly or completely disappears with voluntary movement, e.g. 'pill rolling' tremor of Parkinsonism, with thumb and opposing fingers.

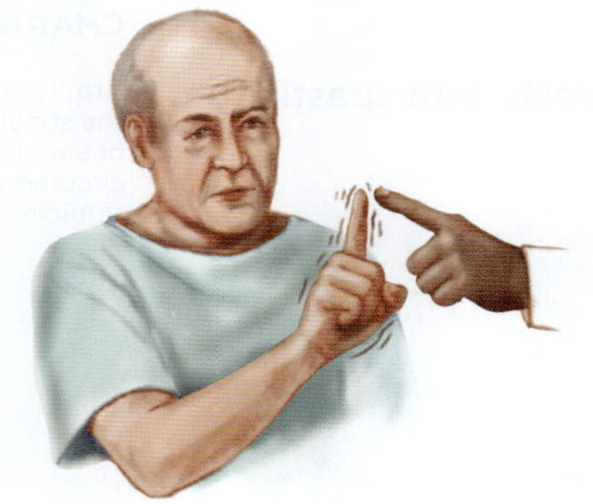

Intention tremor

Rate varies; worse with voluntary movement. Occurs with cerebellar disease and multiple sclerosis.

Essential tremor (familial)—a type of intention tremor; most common tremor with older people. Benign (no associated disease) but causes emotional stress in business or social situations. Improves with the administration of sedatives, propranolol, alcohol, but use of alcohol is discouraged because of the risk of addiction.

(Continued)

TABLE 12.9 Abnormalities in muscle movement—cont'd

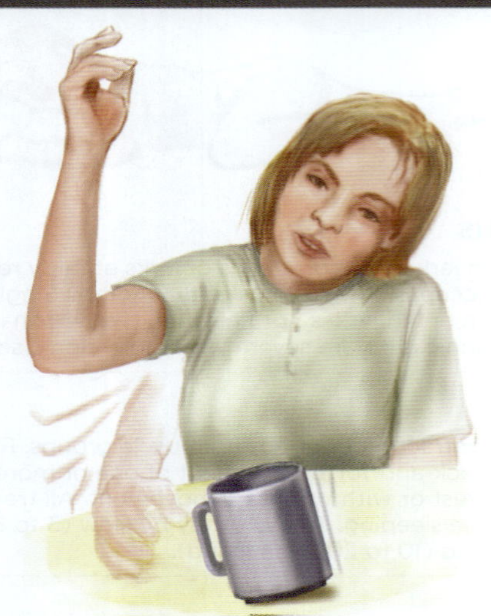	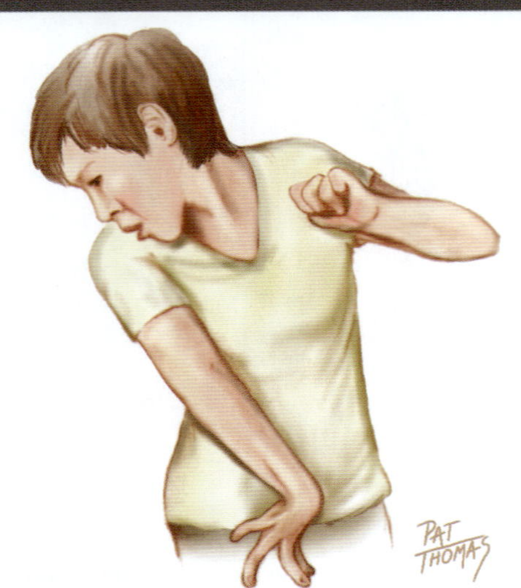
Chorea Sudden, rapid, jerky, purposeless movement involving limbs, trunk or face. Occurs at irregular intervals, not rhythmic or repetitive, more convulsive than a tic. Some are spontaneous, and some are initiated; all are accentuated by voluntary acts. Disappears with sleep. Common with Sydenham's chorea and Huntington's disease.	**Athetosis** Slow, twisting, writhing, continuous movement, resembling a snake or worm. Involves distal part of limb more than the proximal part. Occurs with cerebral palsy. Disappears with sleep. 'Athetoid' hand—some fingers are flexed and some are extended.

Abnormal findings for advanced practice

TABLE 12.10 Abnormal gaits

TYPE	CHARACTERISTIC APPEARANCE	POSSIBLE CAUSES
Hemiparesis with spasticity	Arm is immobile against the body, with flexion of the shoulder, elbow, wrist, fingers and adduction of shoulder. The leg is stiff and extended and circumducts with each step (drags toe in a semicircle)	Upper motor neuron lesion of the corticospinal tract, e.g. stroke, trauma
Cerebellar ataxia	Staggering, wide-based gait; difficulty with turns; un-coordinated movement with positive Romberg sign	Alcohol or barbiturate effect on cerebellum; cerebellar tumour; multiple sclerosis

TABLE 12.10 Abnormal gaits—cont'd

TYPE	CHARACTERISTIC APPEARANCE	POSSIBLE CAUSES
Parkinsonian (festinating)	Posture is stooped; trunk is pitched forwards; elbows, hips and knees are flexed. Steps are short and shuffling. Hesitation to begin walking, and difficult to stop suddenly. The person holds the body rigid. Walks and turns body as one fixed unit. Difficulty with any change in direction	Parkinsonism
Scissors	Knees cross or are in contact, like holding an orange between the thighs. The person uses short steps, and walking requires effort	Paraparesis of legs, multiple sclerosis
Steppage or footdrop	Slapping quality—looks as if walking up stairs and finds no stair there. Lifts knee and foot high and slaps it down hard and flat to compensate for footdrop	Weakness of peroneal and anterior tibial muscles; due to lower motor neuron lesion at the spinal cord, e.g. poliomyelitis, Charcot-Marie-Tooth disease (an inherited peripheral neuropathy)
Waddling	Weak hip muscles—when the person takes a step, the opposite hip drops, which allows compensatory lateral movement of pelvis. Often, the person also has marked lumbar lordosis and a protruding abdomen	Hip girdle muscle weakness due to muscular dystrophy, dislocation of hips
Short leg	Leg length discrepancy >2.5 cm. Vertical telescoping of affected side, which dips as the person walks. Appearance of gait varies depending on amount of accompanying muscle dysfunction	Congenital dislocated hip; acquired shortening due to disease, trauma

TABLE 12.11 Characteristics of upper and lower motor neuron lesions

	UPPER MOTOR NEURON LESION	LOWER MOTOR NEURON LESION
Weakness/paralysis	In muscles corresponding to distribution of damage in pyramidal tract lesion; usually in hand grip, arm extensors, leg flexors	In specific muscles served by damaged spinal segment, ventral root or peripheral nerve
Location	Descending motor pathways that originate in the motor areas of cerebral cortex and carry impulses to the anterior horn cells of the spinal cord	Nerve cells that originate in the anterior horn of spinal cord or in brainstem, and carry impulses by the spinal nerves or cranial nerves to the muscles, the 'final common pathway'
Example	Stroke	Poliomyelitis, herniated intervertebral disc
Muscle tone	Increased tone; spasticity	Loss of tone, flaccidity
Bulk	May have some atrophy from disuse; otherwise normal	Atrophy (wasting), may be marked
Abnormal movements	None	Fasciculations
Reflexes	Hyperreflexia, ankle clonus; diminished or absent superficial abdominal reflexes; positive Babinski's sign	Hyporeflexia or areflexia; no Babinski's sign, no pathological reflexes
Possible nursing diagnoses	Risk for contractures; impaired physical mobility	Impaired physical mobility

TABLE 12.12 Common patterns of motor system dysfunction

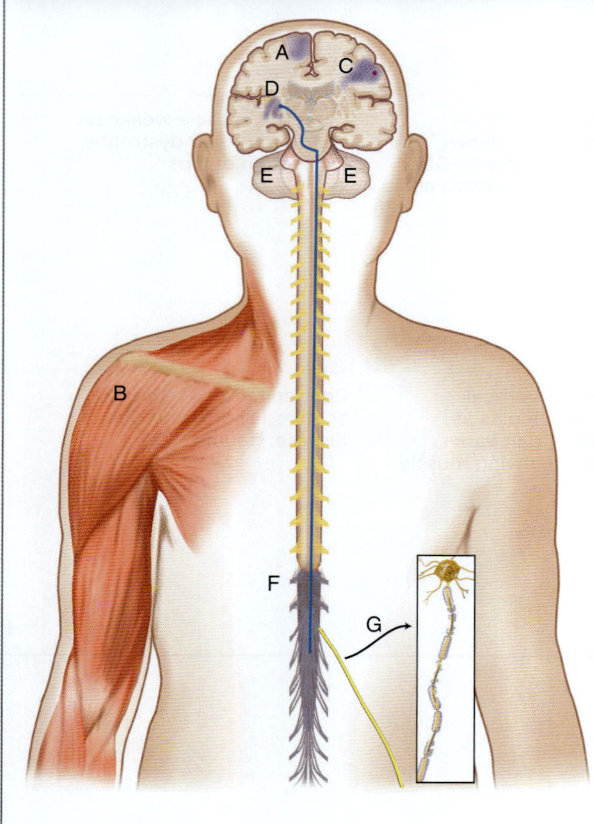

A—Cerebral palsy. Mixed group of paralytic neuromotor disorders of infancy and childhood; due to damage to cerebral cortex caused by a developmental defect, intrauterine meningitis or encephalitis, birth trauma, anoxia or kernicterus.

B—Muscular dystrophy. Chronic, progressive wasting of skeletal musculature, which produces weakness, contractures and, in severe cases, respiratory dysfunction and death. Onset of symptoms occurs in childhood. Many types exist; the most severe is Duchenne's dystrophy, characterised by the waddling gait described in Table 12.10.

C—Hemiplegia. Damage to corticospinal tract, e.g. stroke. Upper motor neuron damage occurs above the pyramidal decussation crossover, so motor impairment is on contralateral (opposite) side. Initially flaccid when the lesion is acute; later, the muscles become spastic and abnormal reflexes appear. Characteristic posture: arm—shoulder adducted, elbow flexed, wrist pronated, leg extended; face—weakness only in lower muscles. Hyperreflexia and possible clonus occur on the involved side; loss of corneal, abdominal and cremasteric reflexes; positive Babinski's and Hoffman's reflexes.

D—Parkinsonism. Defect of extrapyramidal tracts, in the region of the basal ganglia, with loss of the neurotransmitter dopamine. Classic triad of symptoms: tremor, rigidity, akinesia. Also slower monotonous speech and diminutive writing. Body tends to stay immobile; facial expression is flat, staring, expressionless; excessive salivation occurs; reduced eye blinking (see Table 12.17). Posture is stooped; equilibrium is impaired; loses balance easily; gait is described in Table 12.10. Parkinsonian tremor; cogwheel rigidity on passive range of motion.

E—Cerebellar. A lesion in one hemisphere produces motor abnormalities on the ipsilateral side. Characterised by ataxia, lurching forward of affected side while walking, rapid alternating movements are slow and arrhythmic, finger-to-nose test reveals ataxia and tremor with overshoot or undershoot, and eyes display coarse nystagmus.

F—Paraplegia. Lower motor neuron damage caused by spinal cord injury. A severe injury or complete transection initially produces 'spinal shock', which is defined as no movement or reflex activity below the level of the lesion. Gradually, deep tendon reflexes reappear and become increased, flexor spasms of legs occur; and finally, extensor spasms of legs occur; these spasms lead to prevailing extensor tone.

TABLE 12.13 Common patterns of sensory loss

TYPE	CHARACTERISTICS	POSSIBLE CAUSES
Peripheral neuropathy 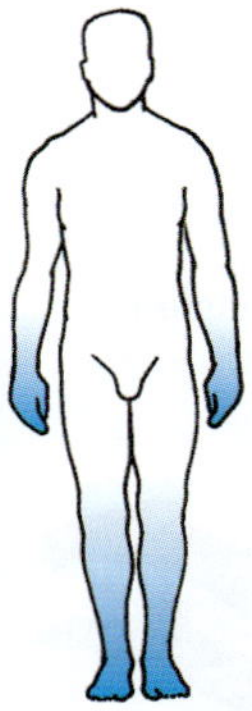	Loss of sensation involves all modalities. Loss is most severe distally (feet and hands); response improves as stimulus is moved proximally (glove-and-stocking anaesthesia). Anaesthesia zone gradually merges into a hypoaesthesia zone, then gradually becomes normal.	Type 1 and type 2 diabetes, chronic alcoholism, nutritional deficiency
Individual nerves or roots 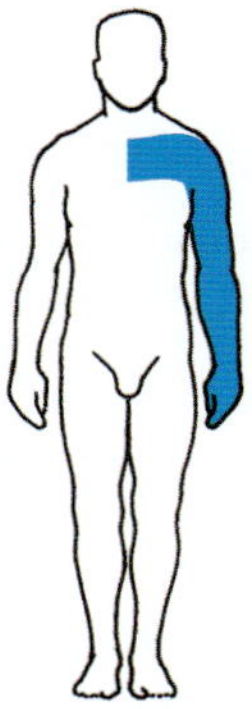	Decrease or loss of all sensory modalities. Area of sensory loss corresponds to distribution of the involved nerve.	Trauma, vascular occlusion
Spinal cord hemisection (Brown-Séquard syndrome) 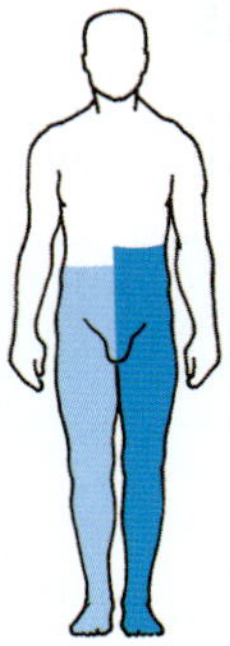	Loss of pain and temperature, contralateral side, starting one to two segments below the level of the lesion. Loss of vibration and position discrimination on the ipsilateral side, below the level of the lesion.	Meningioma, neurofibroma, cervical spondylosis, multiple sclerosis
Complete transection of the spinal cord 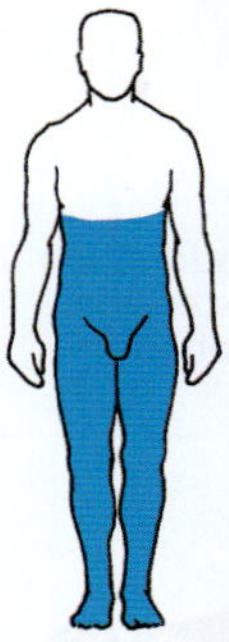	Complete loss of all sensory modalities below the level of the lesion. Condition is associated with motor paralysis and loss of sphincter control.	Spinal cord trauma, demyelinating disorders, tumour
Thalamus 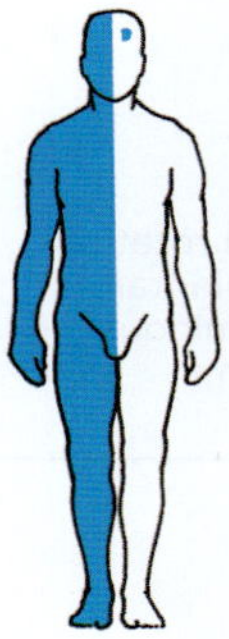	Loss of all sensory modalities on the face, arm and leg on the side contralateral to the lesion.	Vascular occlusion
Cortex 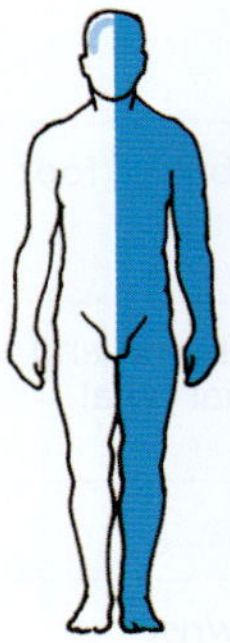	Since pain, vibration and crude touch are mediated by thalamus, little loss of these sensory functions occurs with a cortex lesion. Loss of discrimination occurs on the contralateral side. Loss of graphaesthesia, stereognosis, recognition of shapes and weights, finger finding.	Cerebral cortex, parietal lobe lesion, e.g. stroke

TABLE 12.14 Abnormal postures

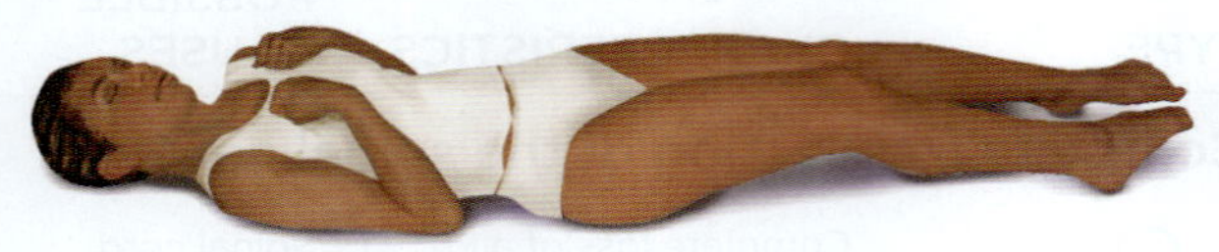

Decorticate rigidity

Upper extremities—flexion of arm, wrist and fingers; adduction of arm, i.e. tight against thorax. Lower extremities—extension, internal rotation, plantar flexion. This indicates hemispheric lesion of cerebral cortex.

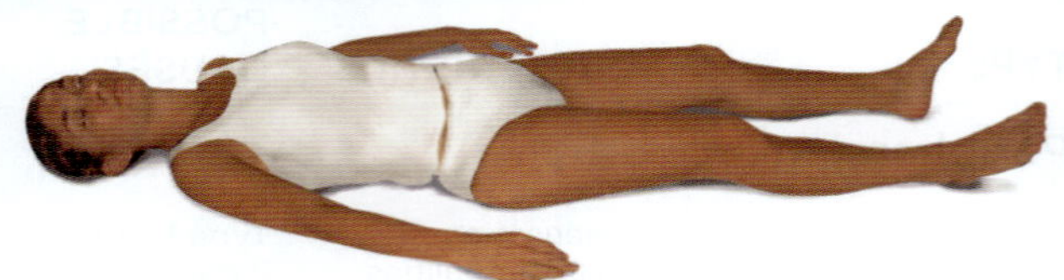

Flaccid quadriplegia

Complete loss of muscle tone and paralysis of all four extremities, indicating completely nonfunctional brainstem.

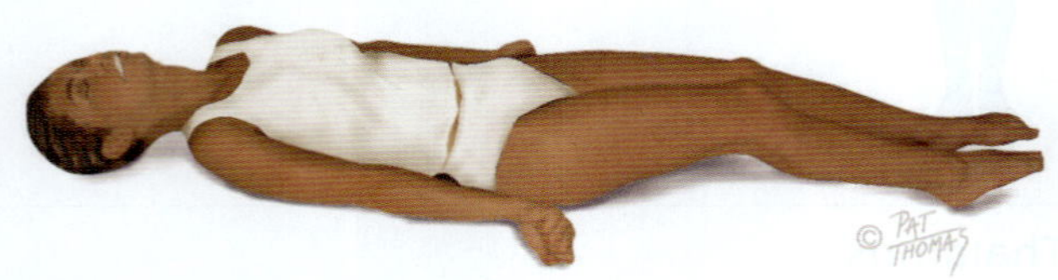

Decerebrate rigidity

Upper extremities stiffly extended, adducted, internal rotation, palms pronated. Lower extremities stiffly extended, plantar flexion; teeth clenched; hyperextended back. More ominous than decorticate rigidity; indicates lesion in brainstem at midbrain or upper pons.

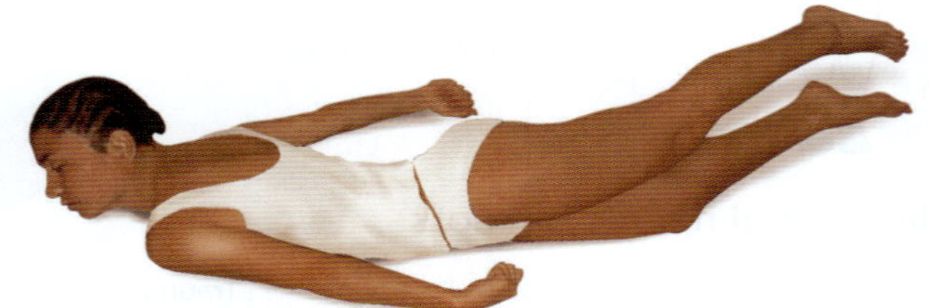

Opisthotonos

Prolonged arching of the back, with head and heels bent backwards. This indicates meningeal irritation.

TABLE 12.15 Pathological reflexes

REFLEX	METHOD OF TESTING	ABNORMAL RESPONSE (REFLEX IS PRESENT)	INDICATIONS
Babinski	Stroke lateral aspect and across ball of foot	Extension of great toe, fanning of toes	Corticospinal (pyramidal) tract disease, e.g. stroke, trauma
Oppenheim	Using heavy pressure with your thumb and index finger, stroke anterior medial tibial muscle	Same as above	Same
Gordon	Firmly squeeze calf muscles	Same as above	Same
Hoffman	With the person's hand relaxed, wrist dorsiflexed, fingers slightly flexed, sharply flick nail of distal phalanx of middle or index finger	Clawing of fingers and thumb	Same
Kernig	In flat-lying supine position, raise leg straight or flex thigh on abdomen, then extend knee	Resistance to straightening (because of hamstring spasm), pain down posterior thigh	Meningeal irritation, e.g. meningitis, infections
Brudzinski	With one hand under the neck and other hand on person's chest, sharply flex chin on chest, watch hips and knees	Resistance and pain in neck, with flexion of hips and knees	Meningeal irritation, e.g. meningitis, infections

TABLE 12.16 Frontal release signs

REFLEX	
Snout 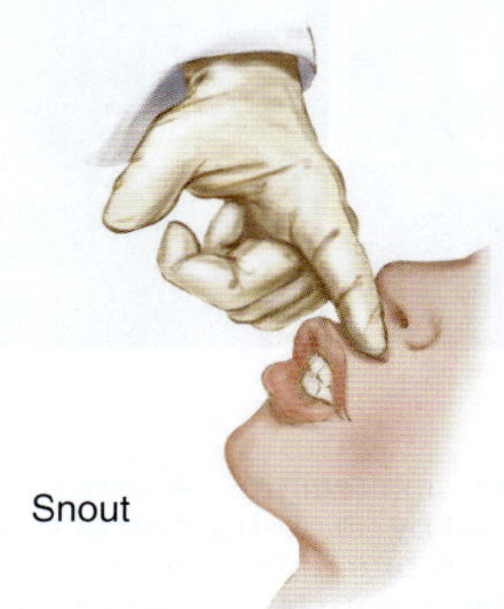 Snout	*Method of testing* Gently percuss oral region Abnormal response (reflex is present) Puckers lips *Indications* Frontal lobe disease, cerebral degenerative disease (Alzheimer's), motor neuron disease, corticobulbar lesions
Sucking 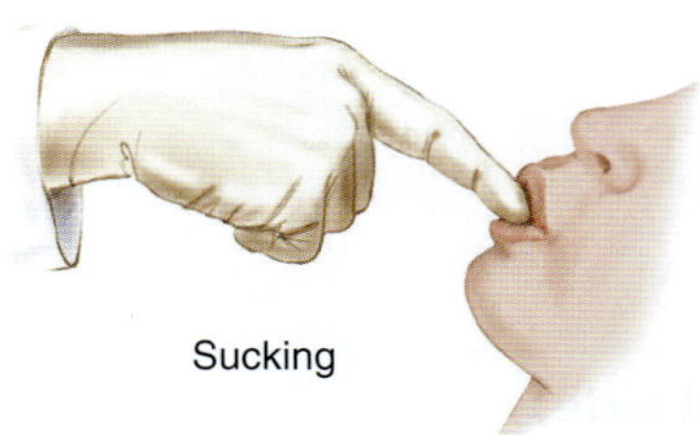 Sucking	*Method of testing* Touch oral region Abnormal response (reflex is present) Sucking movement of lips, tongue, jaw, swallowing *Indications* Same as for snout reflex
Grasp 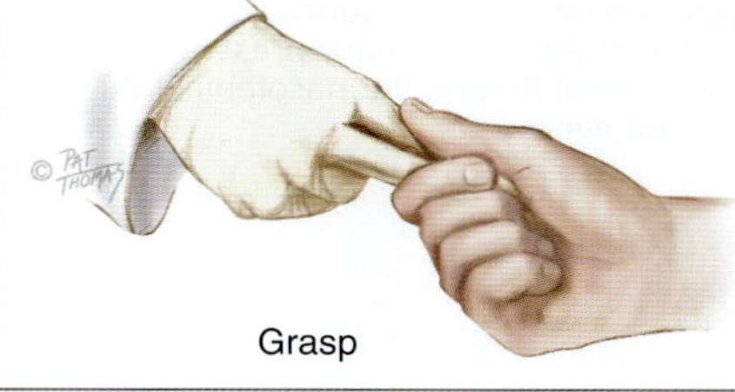 Grasp	*Method of testing* Touch palm with your finger Abnormal response (reflex is present) Uncontrolled, forced grasping (grasp is usually last of these signs to appear, so its presence indicates severe disease) *Indications* When unilateral, frontal lobe lesion on contralateral side; when bilateral, diffuse bifrontal lobe disease

TABLE 12.17 Abnormal facial appearances with neurological disorders

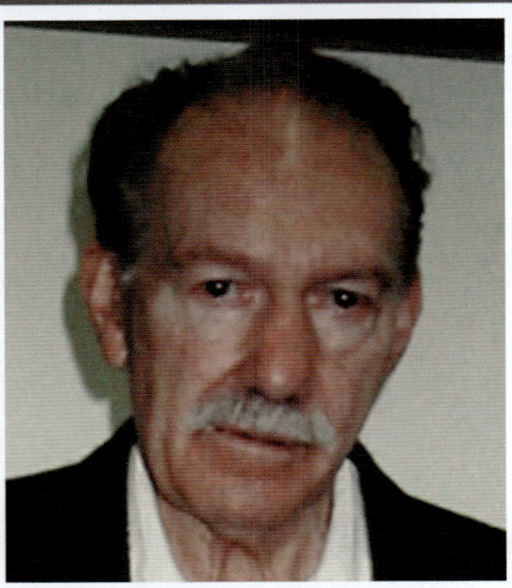

Parkinson's syndrome

A deficiency of the neurotransmitter dopamine and degeneration of the basal ganglia in the brain. The immobility of features produces a face that is flat and expressionless, 'mask-like', with elevated eyebrows, staring gaze, oily skin and drooling.

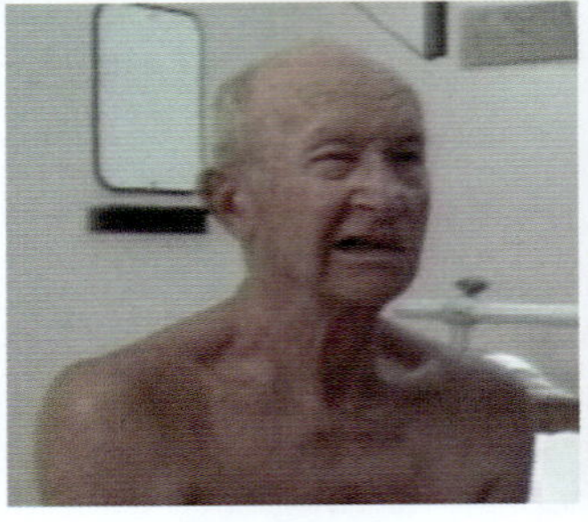

Stroke

An **upper motor neuron** lesion (**central**). A stroke is an acute neurological deficit caused by an obstruction of a cerebral vessel, as in atherosclerosis, or a rupture in a cerebral vessel. Note paralysis of lower facial muscles, but also note that the upper half of the face is not affected because of the intact nerve from the unaffected hemisphere. The person is still able to wrinkle the forehead and close the eyes.

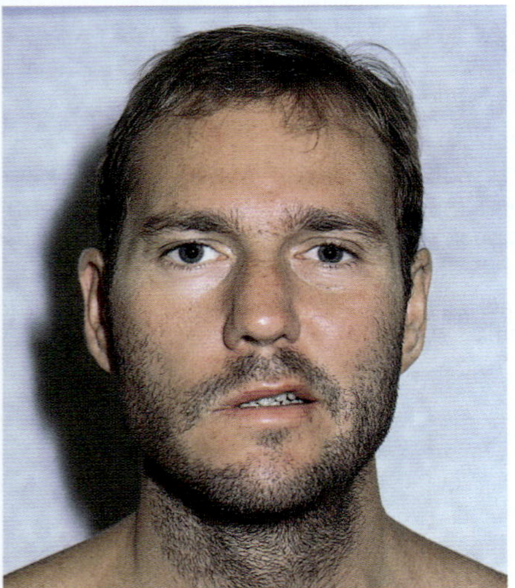

Bell's palsy (right side)

A **lower motor neuron** lesion (**peripheral**), producing cranial nerve VII paralysis, which is almost always unilateral. It has a rapid onset and its cause is currently thought to be the herpes simplex virus (HSV). Note complete paralysis of half of the face; the person cannot wrinkle forehead, raise eyebrows, close eye, whistle or show teeth on the right side. Usually presents with smooth forehead, wide palpebral fissure, flat nasolabial fold, drooling and pain behind the ear.

BIBLIOGRAPHY

American Psychiatric Association. Diagnostic and statistical manual of mental disorders. 5th ed. Arlington, VA: American Psychiatric Association; 2013.

Australian Institute of Health and Welfare (AIHW). Australia's Health 2018 Report. Canberra: AIHW; 2017. Available at: https://www.aihw.gov.au/reports/australias-health/australias-health-2018/contents/table-of-contents.

Brain Injury Australia. Position paper: young stroke. August 2016. Available at: https://www.braininjuryaustralia.org.au/brain-injury-australia-3/.

Feigin VL, Roth GA, Naghavi M, et al for the Global Burden of Diseases, Injuries, and Risk Factors Study 2013 and Stroke Experts Writing Group*: Global burden of stroke and risk factors in 188 countries, during 1990–2013: a systematic analysis for the Global Burden of Disease Study 2013. Lancet. 2016;15:913–24.

Greenshields S. Neurological assessment in children and young people. British Journal of Nursing. 2019;28(16):1056–9.

Harrison-Dening K. Recognition and assessment of dementia in primary care. Practice Nursing. 2019;30(9):438-43.

Hickey J, Strayer AL. The clinical practice of neurological & neurosurgical nursing. 8th ed., Philadelphia: Wolters Kluwer Health.

Kirschen MP, Lourie K, Snyder M, et al. Routine neurological assessments by nurses in the pediatric intensive care unit. Critical Care Nurse. 2019;39(3):20–32.

Marcantonio ER. Delirium in hospitalized older adults. N Engl J Med. 2017;377:1456–66.

McCrory P, Meeuwisse W, Dvorak J, et al. Consensus statement on concussion in sport—the 5th international conference on concussion in sport held in Berlin, October 2016. Br J Sports Med. 2018;51:838–47.

Muller M, Appelman AP, van der Graaf Y, et al. Brain atrophy and cognition: interaction with cerebrovascular pathology? Neurobiol Aging. 2011;32(5):885–93.

Stroke Foundation Australia. National stroke audit of acute services. 2017. Available at: https://informme.org.au/en/stroke-data/Acute-audits.

Stroke Foundation Australia. Stroke in Australia: no postcode untouched. 2017. Available at: https://strokefoundation.org.au/What-we-do/Research/Research-resources/No-postcode-untouched.

Stroke Foundation of New Zealand. Facts and FAQs. 2020. Available at: https://www.stroke.org.nz/facts-and-faqs.

Stroke Foundation Australia. About stroke. 2020. Available at: https://strokefoundation.org.au/About-Stroke.

Talley NJ, O'Connor S. Clinical examination: a systematic guide to physical diagnosis. 8th ed. Chatswood: Elsevier; 2018.

Teasdale G, Maas A, Lecky F, et al. The Glasgow Coma Scale at 40 years: standing the test of time. Lancet Neurol. 2014;13(8):844–54.

Websites

Dementia Australia: https://www.dementia.org.au/information/diagnosing-dementia

Glasgow Coma Scale: https://www.glasgowcomascale.org

Chapter Thirteen

Pain assessment

Written by Carolyn Jarvis and Sarah Jarvis
Adapted by Mari Botti

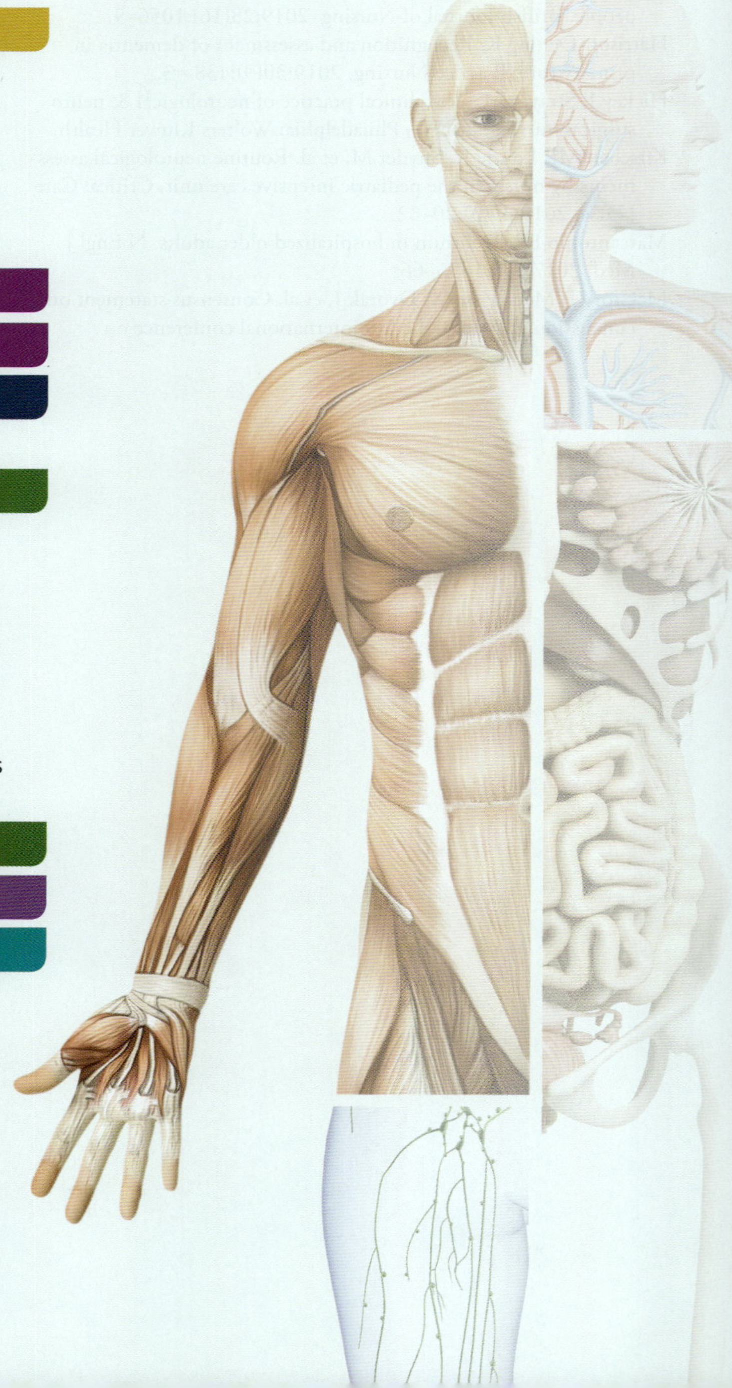

INTRODUCTION

The International Association for the Study of Pain (IASP) endorses the definition of pain as 'an unpleasant sensory and emotional experience associated with actual or potential tissue damage, or described in terms of such damage' (Merskey & Bogduk 1994). Almost 50 years ago, McCaffery introduced the often quoted definition of '… pain is what the person says it is and exists whenever he or she says it does' (McCaffery 1968). The recognition that pain is more than a physiological manifestation and that the person experiencing pain is the most reliable source (or 'gold-standard') for understanding their pain experience has shaped the way pain is assessed clinically.

The purpose of pain assessment is to, where possible, establish the person's perception of their experience of pain, identify how pain interferes with physical and psychosocial wellbeing and provide a baseline for decisions about pharmacological and non-pharmacological treatment, self-management and response to treatment.

Structure and function

Pathological pain develops by two main processes: **nociceptive** (Figure 13.1) and/or **neuropathic** processing. It is important to understand how these two types of pain develop because people present with distinguishing sensations and respond differently to analgesics. An accurate pain assessment enables clinicians to more accurately select effective strategies to interrupt pain processing along multiple points within the pain messaging system and ultimately provide improved pain relief.

NEUROANATOMICAL PATHWAY

Pain is a highly complex and subjective experience that originates from the central (CNS) or peripheral nervous system (PNS) or both. Specialised peripheral sensory nerve endings called **nociceptors** are designed to detect painful sensations from the periphery and transmit them to the central nervous system. Nociceptors are located within the skin, joints, connective tissue, muscle, and the thoracic, abdominal and pelvic viscera. These nociceptors can be stimulated directly by trauma or injury or secondarily by chemical mediators that are released from the site of tissue damage.

Nociceptors carry the pain signal to the central nervous system by two primary sensory (or afferent) fibres: **A-delta** and **C-fibres** (Figure 13.1). A-delta fibres are myelinated and large in diameter, thus they transmit the pain signal rapidly to the CNS. Very localised, short-term and sharp sensations result from A-delta fibre stimulation. In contrast, C-fibres are unmyelinated and smaller, and they transmit the signal more *slowly*. These secondary sensations are diffuse and aching and they persist after the initial injury.

Peripheral sensory A-delta and C-fibres enter the spinal cord by posterior nerve roots within the dorsal horn by the tract of Lissauer. The fibres synapse with **interneurons** located within a specified area of the cord called the **substantia gelatinosa**. A cross section shows that the grey matter of the spinal cord is divided into a series of consecutively numbered laminae (layers of nerve cells) (see Figure 13.1). The substantia gelatinosa is lamina II, which receives sensory input from various areas of the body. The pain signals then cross over to the other side of the spinal cord and ascend to the brain via the **anterolateral spinothalamic tract**. When pain is poorly controlled over an extended period of time, structural plasticity and reorganisation of pain pathways occurs. Cells within the dorsal horn become altered in size and function, and this damage is associated with nociceptive hypersensitivity (Kuner & Flor 2017).

NOCICEPTIVE PAIN

Nociception is the term used to describe how noxious stimuli are typically perceived as pain. Nociceptive pain develops when *functioning and intact* nerve fibres in the periphery and the CNS are stimulated. It is triggered by events outside the nervous system from actual or potential tissue damage. Nociception can be divided into four phases: (1) transduction, (2) transmission, (3) perception and (4) modulation (Figure 13.2).

Initially, the first phase of **transduction** occurs when a noxious stimulus in the form of traumatic or chemical injury, burn, incision or tumour takes place in the periphery. The periphery includes the skin, as well as somatic and visceral structures. These injured tissues then release a variety of chemicals, including substance P, histamine, prostaglandins, serotonin and bradykinin. These chemicals are neurotransmitters that transmit a pain message, or action potential, along sensory afferent nerve fibres to the spinal cord. These nerve fibres terminate in the dorsal horn of the spinal cord. Because the initial afferent fibres stop in the dorsal horn, a second set of neurotransmitters carry the pain impulse across the synaptic cleft to the dorsal horn neurons. These neurotransmitters include substance P, glutamate and adenosine triphosphate (ATP).

In the second phase, known as **transmission**, the pain impulse moves from the level of the spinal cord to the brain. Within the spinal cord, at the site of the synaptic cleft are opioid receptors that can block this pain signalling with endogenous opioids or with exogenous opioids if they are administered. However, if left uninterrupted, the pain impulse moves to the brain via various ascending fibres within the spinothalamic tract to the thalamus. Once the pain impulse moves through the thalamus, the message is dispersed to higher cortical areas via mechanisms that are not clearly understood at this time.

The third phase, **perception**, indicates the conscious awareness of a painful sensation. Cortical structures such as the limbic system account for the emotional response to pain, and somatosensory areas can characterise the sensation. Only when the noxious stimuli are interpreted in these higher cortical structures can this sensation be identified as 'pain'.

Lastly, the pain message is inhibited through the phase of **modulation**. Fortunately, our bodies have a built-in mechanism that will eventually slow down and stop the processing of a painful stimulus. If not for pain modulation, the experience of pain would continue from childhood injuries to adulthood. To inhibit and block the pain impulse, descending pathways from the brainstem to the spinal cord produce a third set of

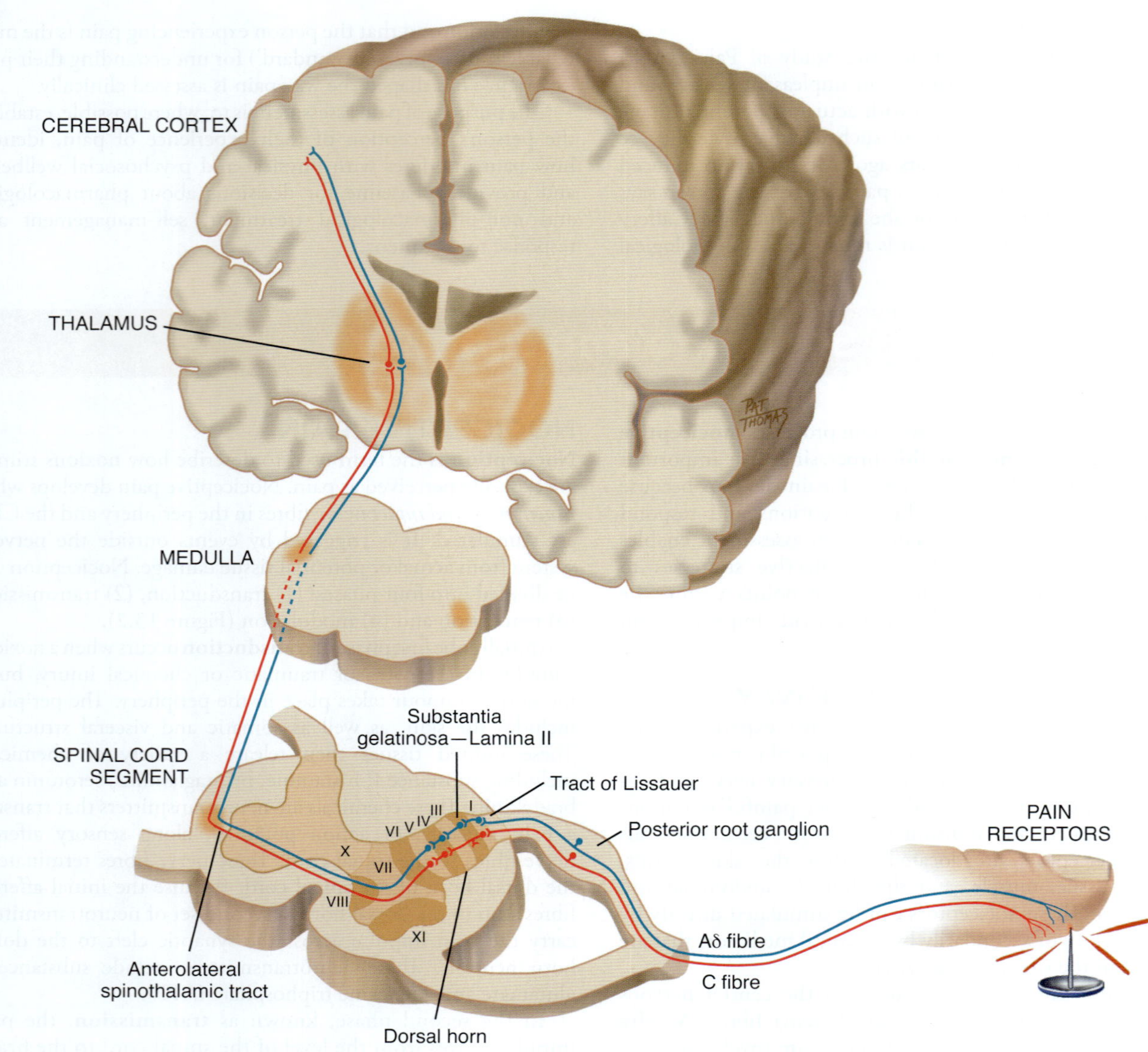

Figure 13.1

neurotransmitters that slow down or impede the pain impulse, producing an analgesic effect. These neurotransmitters include: serotonin; noradrenaline; neurotensin; gamma-aminobutyric acid (GABA); and our own endogenous opioids, β-endorphins, enkephalins and dynorphins.

Normal nociceptive processing is protective and can be a warning signal that injury is about to take or has taken place (Schug et al 2015). We quickly learn to move our hand away from a hot stove. Other examples of nociceptive pain include a skinned knee, kidney stones, menstrual cramps, muscle strain, venipuncture or arthritic joint pain. Nociceptive pain is typically predictable and time limited based on the extent of the injury.

NEUROPATHIC PAIN

Neuropathic pain is pain that does not adhere to the typical and rather predictable phases in nociceptive pain. It is pain due to a lesion or disease in the somatosensory nervous system (IASP 2019a). Neuropathic pain implies abnormal processing of the pain message from an injury to the nerve fibres. This type of pain is the most difficult to assess and treat. Pain is often perceived long after the site of the injury heals, and it evolves into a chronic condition.

Nociceptive pain can change into a neuropathic pain pattern over time when pain has been poorly controlled. This is because of the constant irritation and inflammation caused by a pain stimulus, which alters nerve cells, making them more sensitive to any future stimulus.

Conditions and treatments that may cause neuropathic pain include diabetes mellitus, herpes zoster (shingles), HIV/AIDS, sciatica, trigeminal neuralgia, phantom limb pain and chemotherapy. Further examples include CNS lesions such as stroke, multiple sclerosis, and tumour. Pain sustained on a neurochemical level cannot be identified by X-ray imaging,

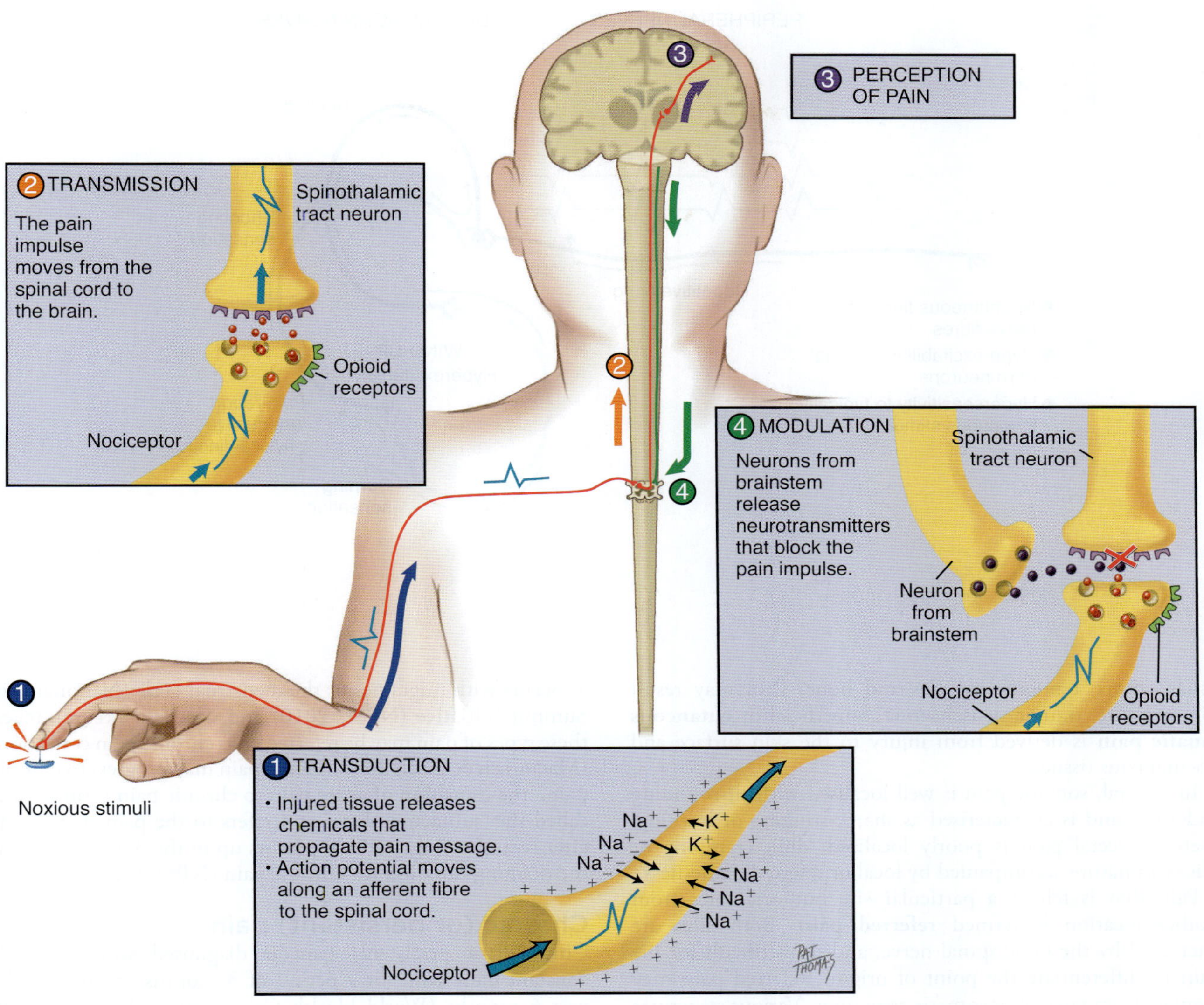

Figure 13.2

computerised axial tomography (CAT) scan or traditional magnetic resonance imaging (MRI). Recent advances in noninvasive neuroimaging techniques allow us to study the structural, functional and neurochemical changes in the brain caused by nociception (Morton et al 2016). Pain researchers are using functional MRI (fMRI) to visualise changes in brain activity while people experience pain. When these images are shown to a person in real time, they can learn to use neurofeedback to help control pain. Researchers are able to better understand how pain is processed and how cognitive influences (e.g. fear and anxiety) impact the experience of pain.

The abnormal processing of the neuropathic pain impulse can be continued by the PNS or CNS. An injury to peripheral neurons can result in spontaneous and repetitive firing of nerve fibres, almost seizure-like activity (Figure 13.3). Neuropathic pain may be sustained centrally in a phenomenon known as neuronal 'wind-up'. Central neuron hyper-excitability leads to maintenance of neuropathic pain. In neuropathic pain, even minor stimuli cause significant pain (Banasik & Copstead 2019).

SOURCES OF PAIN

Physical pain sources are based on their origin. **Visceral** pain originates from the larger interior organs (i.e. kidneys, stomach, intestines, gallbladder and pancreas). It is often described as dull, deep, squeezing or cramping. The pain can stem from direct injury to the organ, or from stretching of the organ from tumour, ischaemia, distension or severe contraction. Examples of visceral pain include ureteric colic, acute appendicitis, ulcer pain and cholecystitis. The pain impulse is transmitted by ascending nerve fibres and nerve fibres of the autonomic nervous system (ANS). That is why visceral pain often presents in association with autonomic responses such as vomiting, nausea, pallor and diaphoresis.

Somatic pain originates from musculoskeletal tissues or the body surface and can be classified as deep or superficial. **Deep somatic pain** comes from sources such as the blood

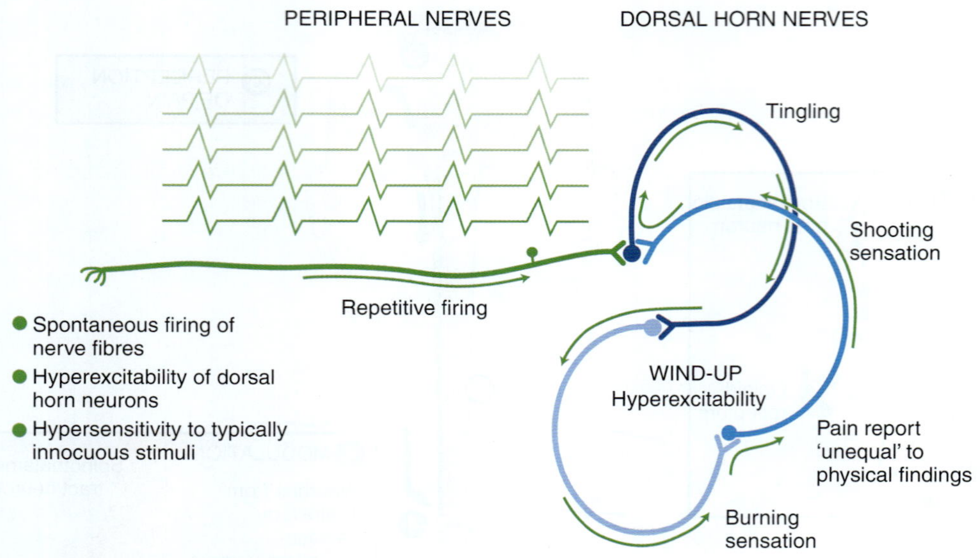

Figure 13.3
Neuropathic mechanisms.

vessels, joints, tendons, muscles and bone. Pain may result from pressure, trauma or ischaemia. Superficial or **cutaneous somatic pain** is derived from injury to the skin surface and subcutaneous tissues.

In general, somatic pain is well localised with surrounding tenderness and is characterised as sharp, stinging or burning, whereas visceral pain is poorly localised, dull, cramping or colicky in nature accompanied by local or referred tenderness.

Pain that is felt at a particular site but originates from another location is termed **referred pain**. Both sites are innervated by the same spinal nerve, and it is difficult for the brain to differentiate the point of origin. Referred pain may originate from visceral or somatic structures. Various structures maintain their same embryonic innervations. For example, an inflamed appendix in the right lower quadrant of the abdomen may have referred pain in the periumbilical area, or the pain from acute coronary syndrome may be felt in the left arm or neck. It is useful to have knowledge of areas of referred pain for diagnostic purposes (see Table 23.3: Common Sites of Referred Abdominal Pain).

TYPES OF PAIN

Pain can be classified by its duration into acute or chronic (also referred to as *persistent*) categories. The duration can provide information on possible underlying mechanisms and thus inform treatment decisions.

Acute pain

Acute pain is short term and self-limiting, often following a predictable trajectory and dissipates after an injury heals. Acute pain serves a self-protective purpose, warning the individual of actual or potential tissue damage. Examples of acute pain include surgery, trauma and kidney stones. Incident pain is a type of pain that occurs predictably with certain movements. Examples include pain in the lower back on standing or turning from side to side. Acute pain may also present as recurrent pain, as occurs with migraines or the menstrual cycle (National Pain Summit Initiative (NPSI) 2010) and, in these circumstances, these types of pain may be referred to as chronic pain conditions (Macintosh & Elson 2008). Acute pain may progress to chronic pain. The transition of acute pain to chronic pain is sometimes called the 'sub-acute phase' and refers to the pain that occurs after tissue healing and that persists up to the 3 months that is the defining duration for chronic pain (NPSI 2010).

Chronic (or persistent) pain

Chronic (or persistent) pain is diagnosed when there is constant daily pain for a period of 3 months or more in the past 6 months (World Health Organization (WHO) 2019). Chronic pain originates from abnormal processing of pain fibres in peripheral or central sites (Banasik & Copstead 2019) and often the source of pain is unknown.

Chronic pain can be further divided into:

- *Chronic primary pain.* This is chronic pain in one or more anatomical regions characterised by significant emotional distress or functional disability.
- *Chronic cancer-related pain.* This pain type often parallels the pathology created by the tumour cells. The pain is induced by tissue necrosis or stretching of an organ by the growing tumour. The pain fluctuates within the course of the disease.
- *Chronic post surgical or post traumatic pain* is pain developing or increasing in intensity after a surgical procedure or a tissue injury and persisting beyond the healing process (greater than 3 months).
- *Chronic secondary musculoskeletal pain* is associated with conditions such as arthritis, low back conditions or fibromyalgia.
- *Chronic secondary visceral pain* is persistent or recurrent pain originating from internal organs of the head/neck regions and of the thoracic, abdominal and pelvic cavities.

- *Chronic neuropathic pain* is pain caused by a lesion or disease of the somatosensory nervous system. See Table 13.3.
- *Chronic secondary headache or orofacial pain* comprises all headache and orofacial pain disorders that have an underlying cause and occur on at least 50% of the days in the last 3 months. The duration of the pain is at least 4 hours (untreated) (WHO 2019).

Chronic pain does not stop when the injury heals. It persists after the predicted trajectory associated with injury. Chronic pain outlasts its protective purpose, and the level of pain intensity does not correspond with the physical findings. Chronic pain may not respond readily to therapy and, unfortunately, many people with chronic pain are not believed and are often labelled as malingerers, attention seekers, drug seekers and so forth (Henschke et al 2009, Shaw & Lee 2010). There are many misconceptions held by clinicians and carers about chronic pain that can influence how pain is assessed and treated. These misconceptions include overemphasis on the contributing role of psychological factors on pain experience and misunderstandings about the meanings of pain tolerance (Shaw & Lee 2010). In Australia, it is estimated that 3.24 million people are living with chronic pain and as such it is a significant problem that has an estimated annual cost of $73.2 billion in terms of health service costs, financial costs and loss of healthy life (Deloitte Access Economics 2019).

Breakthrough pain

Breakthrough pain is a transient spike in pain level, moderate to severe in intensity, in an otherwise controlled pain syndrome. It can result from end-of-dose medication failure. This occurs when a person taking a long-acting opioid has a recurrence of pain before the next scheduled dose. Treatment of end-of-dose failure includes shortening the interval between doses or increasing the dose of medication. Breakthrough pain can also be the result of incident or episodic pain. This is a predictable breakthrough pain that may be triggered by a physical stimulus such as a return to activity after surgery or from a psychological event.

The experience of pain is a complex biopsychosocial phenomenon. We are only now developing an understanding of pain at the cellular level, but more research is needed to fully understand the complexities of the pain experience. We still rely on the person's report as the best indicator of pain, but researchers continue to explore whether pain and certain objective measures (e.g. biomarkers) are associated with one another. When treating people with acute or chronic pain, it is important to frequently assess pain scores to evaluate the effectiveness of the treatment used. It is also important to talk to people about what pain score they consider tolerable.

Complex Regional Pain Syndrome (CRPS)

Complex regional pain syndrome (CRPS), also known as Reflexive Sympathetic Dystrophy or Sudeck's Atrophy, is a chronic progressive nerve condition, characterised by burning pain, swelling, stiffness and discolouration of the affected extremity. It affects both men and women (although the prevalence is higher in women), usually around the age of 40 to 60 years and occurs weeks to months after a nerve injury (e.g. carpal tunnel syndrome, leg fracture, stroke or surgery). The prevalence of CRPS in Australia is not known but is estimated to account for 2–5% of adult and 20% of children seen in pain clinics (Palmer 2015).

The pathophysiology involves a complex interaction of sensory, motor and autonomic nerves and the immune system (Figure 13.4). The nerve injury may modify the usual pain pathway, causing a neuropathic 'wind-up' or 'short circuit' mechanism.

A key feature is that a typically innocuous stimulus (e.g. a light brush of a cotton ball or clothing) can create a severe, intense painful response. Subjective data include burning pain often disproportionate to the degree of injury and joint pain during movement. Objective data include swelling, disappearance of skin wrinkles, cool skin temperature, discolouration, brittle nails and atrophic changes (pale, dry, shiny skin and muscle atrophy). Treatment includes high doses of a combination of medications (e.g. prednisolone, amitriptyline, pregabalin and clonidine) to reduce symptoms and physical therapy to regain limb function. There is limited evidence for prevention strategies, but providing effective analgesia after surgery or trauma is recommended (Palmer 2015).

EFFECTS AND USE OF OPIOIDS

Opioid medications must connect with **mu-opioid receptors** to achieve pain-relieving effects. Mu-opioid receptors are located throughout the body. There are high concentrations of mu-opioid receptors in the brain, including in the periaqueductal grey region, the thalamus, the cingulate cortex and the insula; these receptors regulate pain perception (Volkow & McLellan 2016). Further, mu receptors in the amygdala mediate the emotional response to pain, and mu receptors in the ventral tegmental area and nucleus accumbens mediate the perception of wellbeing and pleasure. Thus, opioid medications produce pain relief and euphoria. As to the side-effects of opioid medications, mu receptors in the brainstem can lead to respiratory depression, and mu receptors in the small intestine produce troublesome constipation (Figure 13.5). Mu receptors in the dorsal horn of the spinal cord and peripheral nerves modulate the perception of pain.

Mu receptors are also responsible for the physical dependence associated with continued use of opioid pain medications (Burcham & Rosenthal 2016, Volkow & McLellan 2016). Physical dependence means only that repeated dosing will lead to a predictable physical reaction when the drug is withdrawn abruptly after prolonged use; this is **not** the same as addiction. Certainly the stimulation of mu receptors in the reward system of the brain can lead to addiction, especially when opioids are delivered rapidly, as happens when opioids are used for pleasure and reward, or as can happen to persons in pain after months of opioid medication exposure (Volkow & McLellan 2016). Refer to Chapters 6 and 11 for information relevant to substance abuse, withdrawal from opioids and mental health.

While opioid medications are effective in the management of severe pain, they also cause a variety of side-effects based on the mechanism of action. Opioid medications are indispensable in treating certain types of pain (e.g. cancer pain, end-of-life pain, trauma and postoperative pain) and remain the mainstay of systemic analgesia for the treatment of moderate to severe acute pain (Schug et al 2015) but care should be taken in the long-term use of opioids.

In 2017, the US Department of Health and Human Services declared the opioid crisis a public health emergency

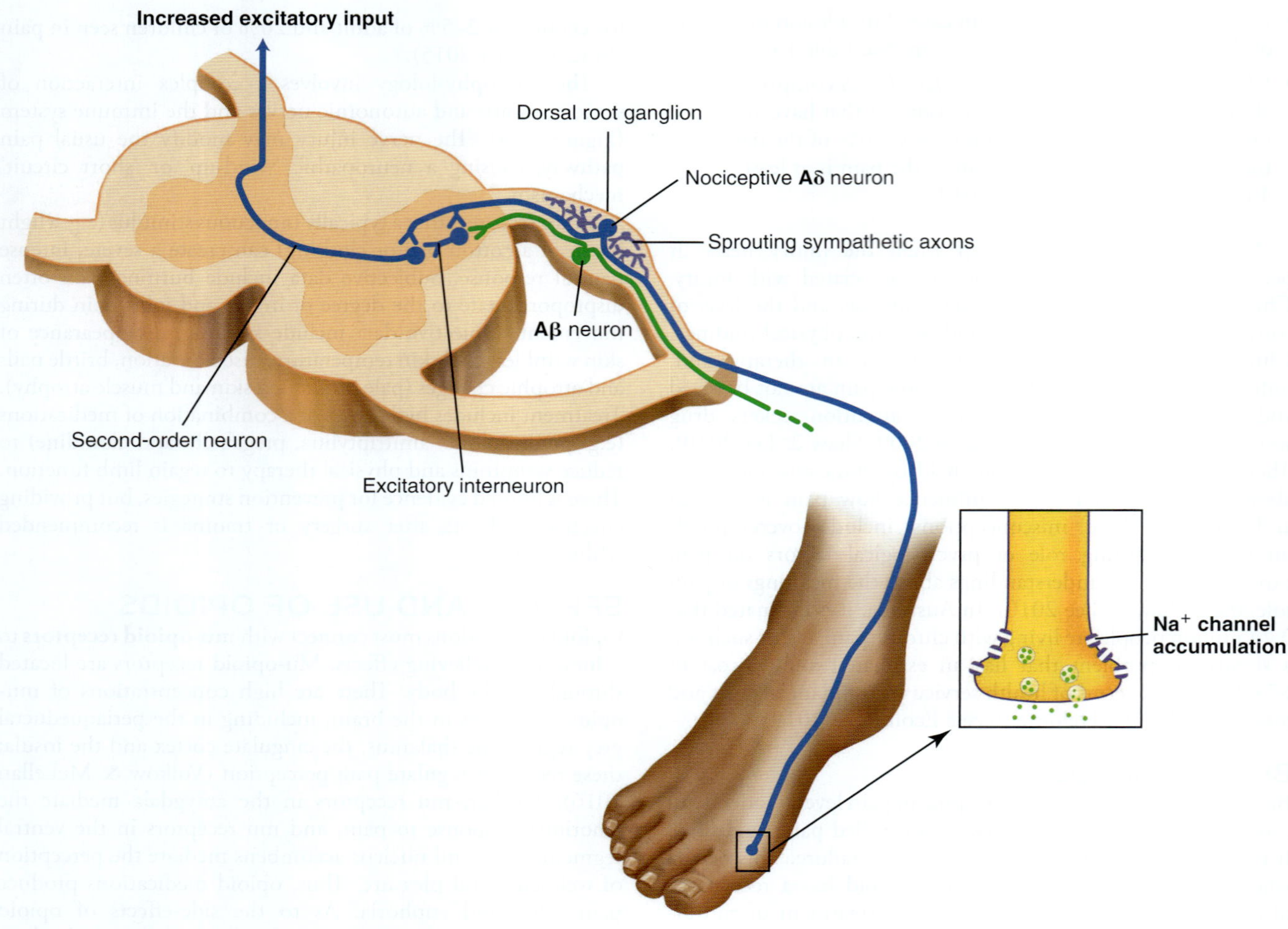

Figure 13.4
Complex regional pain syndrome.

and announced a strategy to combat the epidemic. The 'opioid epidemic' has been linked to the increase in prescriptions and misuse of opioid medications. In the US, although research indicates that the amount of pain experienced is stable, the prescription of opioids has quadrupled. It is estimated that more than 130 people die every day in the US due to opioid overdose, and 115 million Americans misuse prescription opioids (Centers for Disease Control and Prevention 2018, NIH National Institute on Drug Abuse 2019, Volkow & McLellan 2016).

According to an Australian government report (Brown & Morgan 2019), there is little evidence that Australia has experienced the same trajectory of the problem as seen in the US. However, there is evidence of an increase in harm associated with pharmaceutical opioids and heroin. As such, there is a recognised need to introduce measures in Australia to reduce the harm associated with pharmaceutical opioids (Campbell et al 2019, Larance et al 2018). See Chapter 6 for further discussion of substance abuse.

While caution is needed in the use of opioids, we must also recognise that people in pain need adequate pain management. Addressing adequate pain management capability and appropriate education on opioid prescribing is necessary for all healthcare providers to ensure the safe use of pharmaceutical opioids while ensuring that people receive appropriate treatment.

DEVELOPMENTAL CONSIDERATIONS

Infants and children

Infants have the same capacity for pain as adults. During fetal development, ascending sensory fibres, neurotransmitters and connections to the thalamus are developed by 20 weeks gestation. However, immaturity of the cortex and lack of conscious awareness may prevent the fetus from experiencing emotional 'pain' until 30 weeks gestation. Conscious or not, pain-producing invasive fetal procedures elicit a stress response, and pain during gestation should be avoided until more is known about fetal pain. If invasive procedures must be performed on a developing fetus, adequate analgesia is necessary (Sekulic et al 2016). During the postnatal period, there is functional and structural immaturity in the nociceptive pathways that affects the pattern of activity in the infant's central nervous system (Fitzgerald & Walker 2009). This immaturity means that there is less discrimination between noxious and non-noxious stimuli. In addition, inhibitory networks and neurotransmitters are in

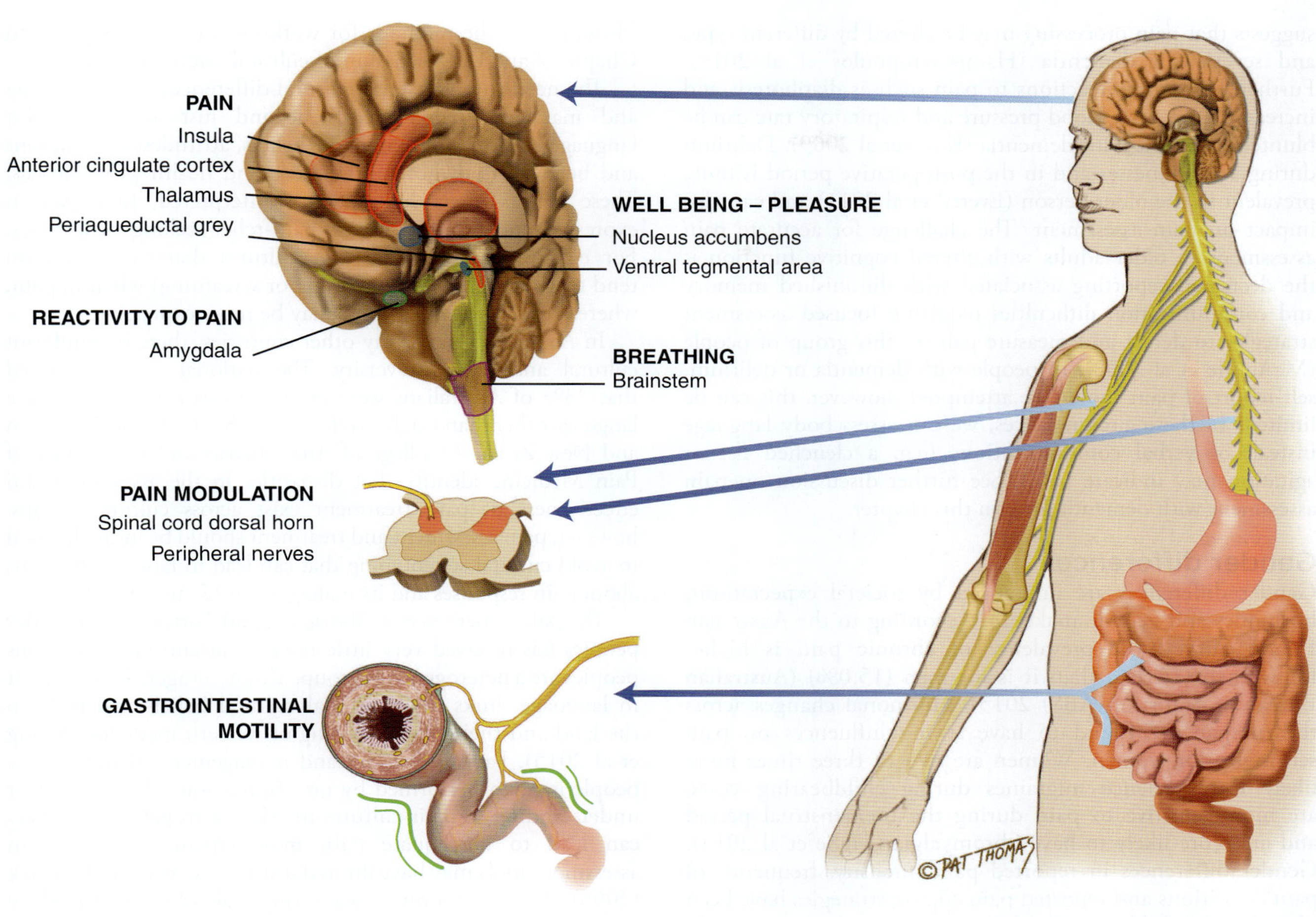

Figure 13.5
Response of mu receptor activation.

insufficient supply in early development (Fitzgerald 1987). Therefore, the neonate, contrary to popular belief, is rendered more sensitive to painful stimuli than the older child.

Preverbal infants are at high risk for under-treatment of pain because of persistent myths and beliefs that infants have lower sensitivity to pain or do not remember pain (Schultz et al 2009, Shrestha-Ranjit & Manias 2010). Repetitive and poorly controlled pain in infants (daily heel sticks, venipunctures) can result in long-term adverse consequences such as neurodevelopmental problems, poor weight gain and learning disabilities (Walker et al 2009, Walker 2013). Regardless of age, adequate use of analgesics during painful procedures is necessary (Banasik & Copstead 2019).

Late Adulthood (65+ years)

The ageing population and advances in anaesthetic and surgical techniques have resulted in an increase in the age of people undergoing major surgery (Australian Institute of Health and Welfare 2017). In addition, older people are more likely to have chronic pain conditions. The most common pain-producing conditions for ageing adults include pathologies such as arthritis, osteoarthritis, osteoporosis, peripheral vascular disease, cancer, peripheral neuropathies, ischaemic heart disease and chronic constipation. According to the Australian and New Zealand College of Anaesthetists and Faculty of Pain Acute Pain Management Guidelines (Schug et al 2015), there are many factors that combine to make effective pain management difficult in older adults. These include the higher incidence of comorbid conditions and concurrent medications, age-related changes in physiology, pharmacodynamics and pharmacokinetics and altered responses to pain.

Although pain is a common experience among individuals 65 years of age and older, it is *not* a normal process of ageing. People over the age of 65 report more chronic pain and demonstrate a reduced tolerance to experimental pain than do people under the age of 65 (Cole et al 2010). Pain indicates pathology or injury. Pain should never be considered something to tolerate or accept in one's later years. Unfortunately, many clinicians and older adults wrongfully assume that pain should be expected in ageing, which leads to fewer investigations and less aggressive treatment. Older adults have additional fears about becoming dependent on others, undergoing invasive procedures, taking pain medications and having a financial burden.

Altered cognitive function may present a challenge for pain assessment within this group, and the available evidence suggests that pain processing may be altered by different types and severity of dementia (Hadjistavropoulos et al 2014). Further, autonomic reactions to pain such as diaphoresis and increased heart rate, blood pressure and respiratory rate can be blunted in people with dementia (Kunz et al 2009). Delirium during acute illnesses and in the postoperative period is more prevalent in the older person (Evered et al 2011) and can also impact on pain assessment. The challenge for accurate pain assessment in older adults with altered cognitive function is the decreased reporting associated with diminished memory and communication difficulties requiring focused assessment strategies to detect and measure pain in this group of people (McAuliffe et al 2008). In people with dementia or delirium, self-report of pain should be attempted; however, this can be limited. In these circumstances, we can assess body language instead of verbal communications (e.g. a clenched fist or agitation may indicate pain). See further discussion on pain assessment with dementia later in this chapter.

Gender differences

Gender differences are influenced by societal expectations, hormones and genetic make-up. According to the Australian Health Survey, the prevalence of chronic pain is higher for women (16.9%) than it is for men (15.0%) (Australian Bureau of Statistics (ABS) 2015). Hormonal changes across the lifespan are found to have strong influences on pain sensitivity for women. Women are two to three times more likely to experience migraines during childbearing years, are more sensitive to pain during the premenstrual period and are more likely to have fibromyalgia (Tighe et al 2014). Gender differences in reported pain intensity, frequency of pain conditions and reported pain coping strategies have been identified in children and adolescents from the age of eight onwards (Boerner et al 2014).

Findings from the Human Genome Project indicate that a pain gene exists, which helps to explain why some people feel more/less pain even with the same stimulus. Efforts are being made to tailor pharmacological agents to improve pain treatment based upon genetic sequencing (Packiasabapathy & Sadhasivam 2018).

CULTURAL AND SOCIAL CONSIDERATIONS

When clinicians speak a language or belong to a culture different from the person experiencing pain, the risk increases for misunderstanding, under-reporting and undertreating. Please review the methods for working with an interpreter in Chapter 7 and the discussion of cultural safety in Chapter 4.

The need to understand cultural differences when assessing and managing pain extends beyond just accounting for language. Culture influences the beliefs, attitudes, expectations and behaviours of both individuals and health professionals. These factors affect how pain is interpreted, how pain is expressed and the individual's pain-relief-seeking behaviours. For example, individuals from cultures that value stoicism tend to avoid vocalising (moaning or screaming) when in pain, whereas other cultural groups may be more expressive.

In Australia, as in many other countries, there is significant cultural and ethnic diversity. The national census revealed that 33% of Australians were born overseas and 21% spoke a language other than English at home (ABS 2017). The Australian and New Zealand College of Anaesthetists and the Faculty of Pain Medicine identify that disparities in the assessment and effectiveness of pain treatment exist across cultural groups; however, pain assessment and treatment should be individualised to avoid cultural stereotyping that can lead to false assumptions about pain responses and its management (Schug et al 2015).

The pain experience of Aboriginal and Torres Strait Islander peoples has received very little research attention. Indigenous peoples are a heterogeneous group. This heterogeneity is evident in language, links to traditional cultural beliefs and links to the land and their understanding of western medicine (Schug et al 2015). Pain assessment and management of Indigenous people is often performed by non-Indigenous clinicians. Poor understanding of their cultures in relation to pain experiences can lead to inadequate pain management. Current pain assessment tools may have limited utility. According to Fenwick (2006), the use of a numerical rating scale of 0 to 10 is likely to produce inaccurate pain assessment as some Indigenous languages do not have a conceptual recognition of certain numbers. Pain behaviours and language that may be unique to Indigenous people such as averting their eyes or turning their head away or feigning sleep can be misinterpreted and pain may be undertreated. The use of verbal description of pain and involving Aboriginal health workers to assist in communication should be encouraged (Taylor & Guerin 2014).

The experience of pain is more layered than just physical suffering. Pain and the expression of pain are influenced by social, cultural, emotional and spiritual concerns. It is imperative that pain assessment is thorough for all people, recognising that a lack of outward signs of pain does not indicate an absence of pain.

Subjective data

Pain is a highly subjective and personal experience, hence the subjective report is the most reliable indicator of pain. The assessment of pain includes a thorough history, physical examination and an evaluation of associated functional impairment (Macintyre et al 2015). Some people may be reluctant to discuss having pain for fear of dependency on others, the fear of further testing or invasive procedures, the cost and fear of taking pain killers or becoming drug addicted. During the interview you must establish an empathetic and caring rapport with any person, child or adult to gain trust.

Practice note: Before you commence the assessment, introduce yourself to the person, confirm the person's identity, discuss the purpose and scope of the assessment, clarify any questions the person may have and obtain verbal consent from the person to perform the assessment.

ASSESSMENT GUIDELINES	CLINICAL SIGNIFICANCE AND CLINICAL ALERTS
Initial pain assessment	
1. Do you have pain? Discomfort or soreness? Tell me in your own words.	Some people report pain only when it is severe. Try a variety of words.
2. Where is your pain? Tell me about all the places you have pain.	Pain may be localised or occur in multiple sites.
3. When did your pain start? What were you doing when the pain started? Is it constant or does it come and go?	Identifies onset and duration. Chronic pain persists after injury heals; it is pain that occurs for 3 months or longer.
4. What does your pain feel like? • Burning, stabbing, aching • Throbbing, firelike, squeezing • Cramping, sharp, itching, tingling • Shooting, crushing, sharp, dull	Identifies quality of pain and helps differentiate between nociceptive and neuropathic pain mechanisms. Neuropathic pain is described as burning, shooting and tingling. Nociceptive pain originating from visceral sites is described as aching if localised and cramping if poorly localised. Somatic site pain is described as throbbing/aching.
5. How much pain do you have now? Refer to various intensity scales, for example the 0–10 numerical rating scale. Refer to Pain Assessment Tools below.	Identifies current intensity and represents pain at rest.
6. How much pain do you have when you move? Refer to various intensity scales, for example the 0–10 numerical rating scale.	Identifies intensity of pain with activity. This pain is referred to as dynamic pain.
7. What makes your pain better or worse? (e.g. behavioural, pharmacological and nonpharmacological interventions) Which medicines control your pain? Are doses adequate? How often do you take pain medicines?	Identifies alleviating and aggravating factors. Evaluates effectiveness of current treatment. ***Clinical alert:*** If a person has unrelieved or increasing pain which is not relieved by current treatment plan, report to medical to practitioner.
8. How much does your pain interfere with your ability to: Do activities in bed such as turning, repositioning or sitting up? Do activities out of bed such as walking, sitting in a chair or standing? What does the pain prevent you from doing?	Identifies the dynamic nature of pain and the degree of impairment or effect on quality of life.
9. How does pain affect your sleep and mood?	Identifies degree of impairment and quality of life. Mood (feeling anxious or depressed) and sleep (falling asleep and staying asleep) may be particularly relevant for chronic pain.
10. Do you experience any other symptoms along with the pain (nausea, vomiting, dizziness, heart racing, difficulty sleeping or fatigue)?	Will aid in detection, assessment and treatment. Unfortunately, clinical staff may inadvertently interpret an altered sleeping pattern, particularly day sleeping, as 'comfort' and fail to properly assess the person's pain and also may fail to provide appropriate pharmacological intervention.
11. What does this pain mean to you? Why do you think you are having pain?	Can identify myths, misconception, beliefs, such as 'I'm getting old'. Can reveal feelings of fear, depression or helplessness.

ASSESSMENT GUIDELINES	CLINICAL SIGNIFICANCE AND CLINICAL ALERTS
12. What are your expectations of, and preferences for, pain treatment?	Assists in planning pain relief interventions that reflects patient preferences and satisfaction with pain relief outcomes.
As an alternative to the questions above you can collect a complete pain health history using the PQRST mnemonic described in Table 13.1.	

SUBJECTIVE DATA

TABLE 13.1 PQRST Method of pain assessment

P = Provocation/Palliation What were you doing when the pain started? What caused it? What makes it better? Worse? What seems to trigger it? Stress? Position? Certain activities? What relieves it? Medications, massage, heat/cold, changing position, being active, resting? What aggravates it? Movement, bending, lying down, walking, standing?
Q = Quality/Quantity What does it feel like? Use words to describe the pain, such as sharp, full, stabbing, burning, crushing, throbbing, nauseating, shooting, twisting or stretching.
R = Region/Radiation Where is the pain located? Does it radiate? Where? Does it feel as if it travels/moves around? Did it start elsewhere and is now localised to one spot?
S = Severity Scale How severe is the pain on a scale of 0 to 10, with zero being no pain and 10 being the worst pain ever? Does it interfere with activities? How bad is it at its worst? Does it force you to sit down, lie down or slow down? How long does an episode last?
T = Timing When/at what time did the pain start? How long did it last? How often does it occur: Hourly? Daily? Weekly? Monthly? Is it sudden or gradual? What were you doing when you first experienced it? When do you usually experience it: Daytime? Night? Early morning? Are you ever awakened by it? Does it lead to anything else? Is it accompanied by other signs and symptoms? Does it ever occur before, during or after meals? Does it occur seasonally?

From Crozer Keystone Center for Nursing Excellence: PQRST method facilitates accurate pain assessment. Available at www.crozerkeystone.org/healthcare-professionals/nursing.

PAIN ASSESSMENT TOOLS

Pain is multidimensional in scope, encompassing physical, affective and functional domains. Assessment of pain varies in complexity depending on the context of pain and the ability of people to communicate their pain. Various tools have been developed to capture unidimensional aspects such as intensity or multidimensional components.

The choice of tool depends on its purpose, time involved in its administration and the person's ability to comprehend and complete the tool. Self-assessment pain scales can be used reliably for most people with mild-to-moderate cognitive impairment (Pautex et al 2005), although dementia and delirium can limit a person's ability to report pain.

In situations of acute pain and pain as a symptom of trauma or disease, assessment of the presence, intensity (at rest and with movement) and location of pain enables characterisation of pain and evaluation of the effectiveness of treatment. The following practice points will help you get the most useful information from the pain tool.

- The assessment tool should be used consistently before and after treatment to see whether the treatment has been effective.
- When first using a tool, familiarise the person with the format and purpose of the tool.
- It may be useful to enlarge the print for individuals with impaired vision.
- Where possible, involve an interpreter when the person's first language is other than English.
- For people with low literacy you will need to read out the statements/questions on the pain tool.
- Ask the person to rate and evaluate all their pain sites.
- Some pain tools allow for only one pain rating score, therefore if the person has pain at more than one site, you will need to document the pain score for each site.

Multidimensional pain assessment tools are more useful for chronic pain conditions or particularly problematic acute pain problems. These tools provide more information about the characteristics of pain and its impact on the individual. A few examples include the Initial Pain Assessment, the Brief Pain Inventory and the McGill Pain Questionnaire.

In the **Initial Pain Assessment** (McCaffery & Pasero 1999), the clinician asks the person to answer eight questions concerning location, intensity, quality, duration and aggravating/relieving factors. Further, the clinician adds questions about manner of expressing pain and the effects of pain that impairs quality of life (Figure 13.6).

Initial Pain Assessment Tool

Date ____________
Patient's Name ______________________ Age ____________ Room ____________
Diagnosis ______________________ Physician ____________
Nurse ____________

1. LOCATION: Patient or nurse mark drawing.

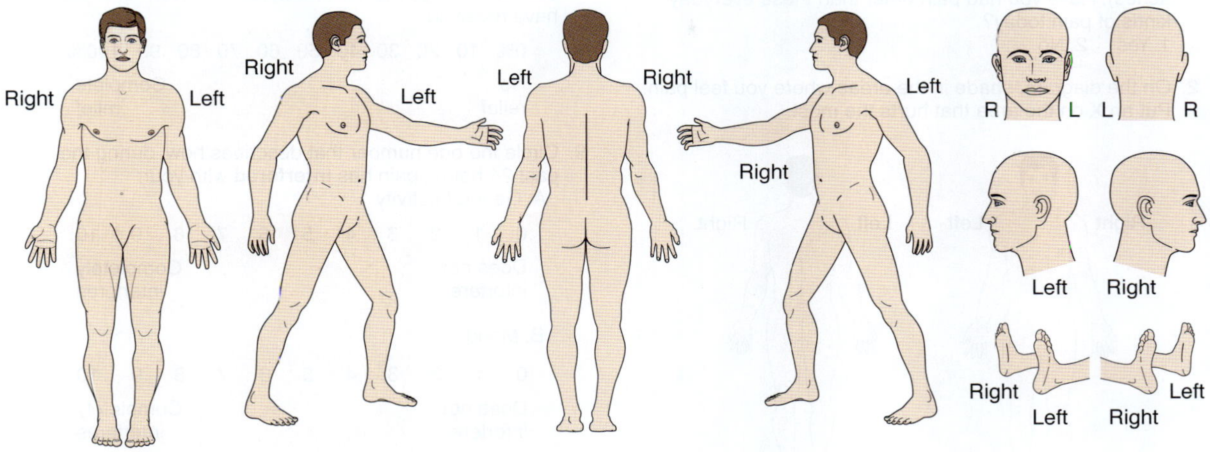

Right Left Right Left Left Right Left Right
R L L R
Left Right
Right Left Left Right

2. INTENSITY: Patient rates the pain. Scale used ____________
 Present: ____________
 Worst pain gets: ____________
 Best pain gets: ____________
 Acceptable level of pain: ____________
3. QUALITY: (Use patient's own words, e.g. prick, ache, burn, throb, pull, sharp.) ____________
4. ONSET, DURATION, VARIATION, RHYTHMS: ____________
5. MANNER OF EXPRESSING PAIN: ____________
6. WHAT RELIEVES THE PAIN? ____________
7. WHAT CAUSES OR INCREASES THE PAIN? ____________
8. EFFECTS OF PAIN: (Note decreased function, decreased quality of life.)
 Accompanying symptoms (e.g. nausea) ____________
 Sleep ____________
 Appetite ____________
 Physical activity ____________
 Relationship with others (e.g. irritability) ____________
 Emotions (e.g. anger, suicidal, crying) ____________
 Concentration ____________
 Other ____________
9. OTHER COMMENTS: ____________
10. PLAN: ____________

Figure 13.6
Initial Pain Assessment Tool.

Brief Pain Inventory

Date:___/___/___ Time:________

Name:____________________

Last First Middle initial

1. Throughout our lives, most of us have had pain from time to time (such as minor headaches, sprains and toothaches). Have you had pain other than these everyday kinds of pain today?
   1. Yes 2. No
2. On the diagram, shade in the areas where you feel pain. Put an X on the area that hurts the most.

Right Left Left Right

3. Please rate your pain by circling the one number that best describes your pain at its **worst** in the past 24 hours.

0	1	2	3	4	5	6	7	8	9	10
No pain										Pain as bad as you can imagine

4. Please rate your pain by circling the one number that best describes your pain at its **least** in the past 24 hours.

0	1	2	3	4	5	6	7	8	9	10
No pain										Pain as bad as you can imagine

5. Please rate your pain by circling the one number that best describes your pain on the **average**.

0	1	2	3	4	5	6	7	8	9	10
No pain										Pain as bad as you can imagine

6. Please rate your pain by circling the one number that tells how much pain you have **right now**.

0	1	2	3	4	5	6	7	8	9	10
No pain										Pain as bad as you can imagine

7. What treatments or medications are you receiving for your pain?

____

____

8. In the past 24 hours, how much **relief** have pain treatments or medications provided? Please circle the one percentage that most shows how much relief you have received.

0%	10	20	30	40	50	60	70	80	90	100%
No relief										Complete relief

9. Circle the one number that describes how, during the past 24 hours, pain has **interfered** with your:

A: General activity

0	1	2	3	4	5	6	7	8	9	10
Does not interfere										Completely interferes

B: Mood

0	1	2	3	4	5	6	7	8	9	10
Does not interfere										Completely interferes

C: Walking ability

0	1	2	3	4	5	6	7	8	9	10
Does not interfere										Completely interferes

D: Normal work (includes both work outside the home and housework)

0	1	2	3	4	5	6	7	8	9	10
Does not interfere										Completely interferes

E: Relations with other people

0	1	2	3	4	5	6	7	8	9	10
Does not interfere										Completely interferes

F: Sleep

0	1	2	3	4	5	6	7	8	9	10
Does not interfere										Completely interferes

G: Enjoyment of life

0	1	2	3	4	5	6	7	8	9	10
Does not interfere										Completely interferes

Figure 13.7
Brief pain inventory.

The **Brief Pain Inventory** (Cleeland & Ryan 1994, Poquet & Lin 2010) asks the person to rate the pain within the past 24 hours using graduated scales (0–10) with respect to its impact on areas such as mood, walking ability and sleep. It is available in multiple languages (Figure 13.7). The **Short-Form McGill Pain Questionnaire** (Melzack 1987) asks the person to rank a list of descriptors in terms of their intensity and to give an overall intensity rating to their pain. The short form only takes 2 to 3 minutes to complete.

Pain rating scales are **unidimensional** and are intended to reflect pain intensity. They come in various forms. Pain rating scales can indicate baseline intensity, track changes due

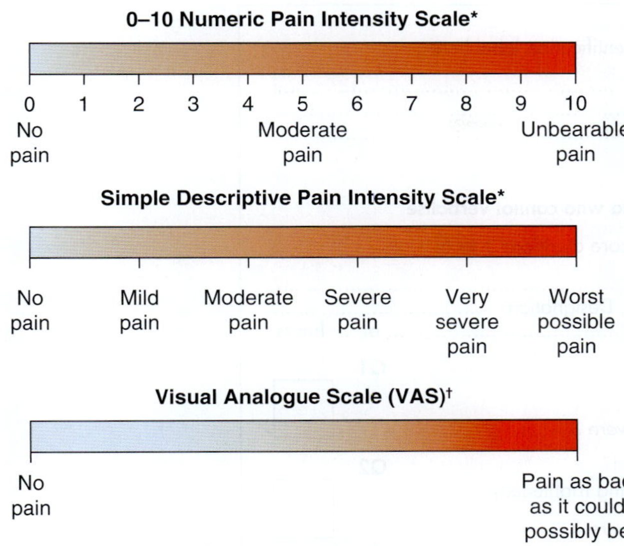

Figure 13.8
Numerical rating scale.

to changing disease state or recovery and give some degree of evaluation of treatment.

Numerical rating scales (NRS) can be administered verbally or visually along a vertical or horizontal line (Figure 13.8). Typically patients are asked to choose a number that rates the level of pain, with 0 being no pain and the highest anchor, 10, indicating the worst pain possible. The use of a numerical rating scale makes recording pain intensity among various clinicians easier and more consistent. The **Visual Analogue Scale** is a numerical scale that allows patients to place a mark along a 10-cm line from no pain to the worst pain possible. There are minor variations in the anchors used for these scales.

An alternative to numerical scales is the use of **categorical scales** such as the simple **Verbal Descriptor Scale (VDS)** where words are used to describe the magnitude of pain. The words describe different levels of pain intensity, such as *no pain*, *mild pain*, *moderate pain* and *severe pain*. The words can be converted to *numeric scores* (e.g. 0, 1, 2, 3, 4, 5).

Frail older adults may find the **numerical rating scales** abstract and have difficulty responding, especially with a fluctuating chronic pain experience and will therefore often respond to scales such as the **Verbal Descriptor Scale**, in which words are selected rather than numbers. Again, it is essential to teach the person how to use the scale to enhance accuracy. There also needs to be awareness that personal, linguistic and cultural differences may affect interpretation of the descriptor words (Scott & McDonald 2008). In situations where the person cannot communicate their pain because of altered conscious state, impaired cognition, language or developmental constraints, pain assessment needs to be modified to encompass behavioural and physiological manifestations of pain.

TOOLS FOR ASSESSING PAIN IN PEOPLE WITH DEMENTIA

A number of observational pain assessment scales have been developed and used in people with varying degrees of dementia. A commonly used scale in Australia is the Abbey Pain Scale (Abbey et al 2004) (Figure 13.9). This scale is a one-page assessment tool where the presence and severity of six observable cues (vocalisation, facial expression, change in body language, behavioural change, physiological change and physical changes) are scored to provide a total pain score.

The PAINAD scale is a simple, reliable and validated five-item observational tool that evaluates common behaviours: breathing; vocalisation; facial expression; body language and consolability (Warden et al 2002) (Figure 13.10). Specific behaviours in these categories are quantified from 0 to 2, with a total score of 0–10. This is consistent with the commonly used 0–10 score on other pain assessment tools. For the PAINAD, a score of 4 or more indicates the need for pain management.

TOOLS FOR INFANTS AND CHILDREN

Most pain research on infants has focused on acute, procedural pain. We have a limited understanding of how to assess chronic pain in the infant. At this time, there is no one assessment tool that adequately identifies pain in the infant. Using a multidimensional approach for the whole infant is encouraged. Assessment of pain in infants and children requires the use of age- and context-appropriate assessment tools. It is recommended that behavioural and physiological signs are evaluated in conjunction with a child's self-report of pain (Schug et al 2015).

Because infants are preverbal and incapable of self-report, pain assessment is dependent exclusively upon behavioural and physiological cues. Refer to the Objective Data section below. It is important to emphasise the understanding that infants *do* feel pain but are vulnerable to having their pain not recognised or underestimated.

Children 2 years of age can report pain and point to its location. They cannot rate pain intensity at this developmental level. It is helpful to ask the parent or caregiver what words their child uses to report pain (e.g. ouch, sore). Be aware that some children will try to be 'grown up and brave' and often deny having pain in the presence of a stranger or if they are fearful of receiving a 'needle'.

Rating scales can be introduced at 3–4 years of age (Schug et al 2015). **The Faces Pain Scale – Revised (FPS-R)** has six drawings of faces that show pain intensity. The child is given an explanation that each face is a person with 'no pain' on the left (score of 0) to 'very much pain' on the right (score of 10) (Figure 13.11). The FPS-R has realistic facial expressions, with a furrowed brow and horizontal mouth. The advantage of the FPS-R is that it avoids smiles or tears so that children will not confuse pain intensity with happiness or sadness (IASP 2019b).

One tool that has been developed for postoperative pain in preterm and term neonates is the **CRIES** developed by Krechel and Bildner (1995). It measures physiological and behavioural indicators on a 3-point scale (Figure 13.12).

The **FLACC scale** (Merkel et al 1997) was developed to assess pain in young children and has been shown to have good

Place identification label here

Name: ....
DOB: ....
Room No: ....

ABBEY PAIN SCALE

For measurement of pain in people with dementia who cannot verbalise

How to use scale: While observing the resident, score questions 1 to 6.

Name of person completing the scale: ....
Date: .... Time: .... Designation: ....
Latest pain relief given was .... at .... hours.

Q1 Vocalisation — Q1 ☐
(e.g. whimpering, groaning, crying)
Absent 0 *Mild 1* *Moderate 2* *Severe 3*

Q2 Facial expression — Q2 ☐
(e.g. looking tense, frowning, grimacing, looking frightened)
Absent 0 *Mild 1* *Moderate 2* *Severe 3*

Q3 Change in body language — Q3 ☐
(e.g. fidgeting, rocking, guarding part of body, withdrawn)
Absent 0 *Mild 1* *Moderate 2* *Severe 3*

Q4 Behavioural change — Q4 ☐
(e.g. increased confusion, refusing to eat, alteration in usual patterns)
Absent 0 *Mild 1* *Moderate 2* *Severe 3*

Q5 Physiological change — Q5 ☐
(e.g. temperature, pulse or blood pressure outside normal limits, perspiring, flushing or pallor)
Absent 0 *Mild 1* *Moderate 2* *Severe 3*

Q6 Physical changes — Q6 ☐
(e.g. skin tears, pressure areas, arthritis, contractures, previous injuries)
Absent 0 *Mild 1* *Moderate 2* *Severe 3*

Add scores for 1–6 and record here — **Total Pain Score** ☐

Now tick the box that matches the Total Pain Score

0–2 No pain	3–7 Mild	8–13 Moderate	14+ Severe

Finally, tick the box which matches the type of pain

Chronic	Acute	Acute on Chronic

Figure 13.9
The Abbey Pain Scale. Abbey J, et al (2004)

interrater reliability and validity in children aged 2–7 years (Willis et al 2002). The FLACC scale is a simple framework that enables pain behaviours to be assessed objectively and quantified. The scale is comprised of five categories of pain behaviours: F = face, L = legs, A = activity, C = cry, C = consolability. Each category receives a score of 0–2 to provide a total pain score range of 0–10 (Figure 13.13). The FLACC is recommended by the Australian Department of Health for use in emergency triage. Note that these tools assess acute pain. No biological markers have been identified for long-term chronic pain in infants or children. Therefore, evaluate the whole individual.

Pain Assessment In Advanced Dementia (PAINAD) Scale

	0	1	2	Score
Breathing Independent of Vocalisation	Normal	Occasional laboured breathing, short period of hyperventilation	Noisy laboured breathing, long period of hyperventilation, Cheyne-Stokes respirations	
Negative Vocalisation	None	Occasional moan or groan, low level of speech with a negative or disapproving quality	Repeated troubled calling out, loud moaning or groaning, crying	
Facial Expression	Smiling or inexpressive	Sad, frightened, frown	Facial grimacing	
Body Language	Relaxed	Tense, distressed pacing, fidgeting	Rigid, fists clenched, knees pulled up, pulling or pushing away, striking out	
Consolability	No need to console	Distracted or reassured by voice or touch	Unable to console, distract or reassure	
			TOTAL	

Figure 13.10
Pain Assessment in Advanced Dementia (PAINAD) Scale.

Faces Pain Scale — Revised (FPS-R)

In the following instructions, say 'hurt' or 'pain', whichever seems right for a particular child.

'These faces show how much something can hurt. This face [point to left-most face] **shows no pain. The faces show more and more pain** [point to each from left to right] **up to this one** [point to right-most face] **— it shows very much pain. Point to the face that shows how much you hurt** [right now].'

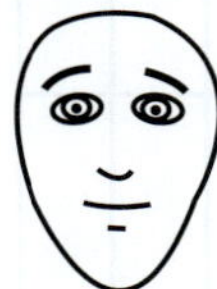
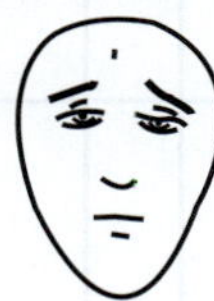
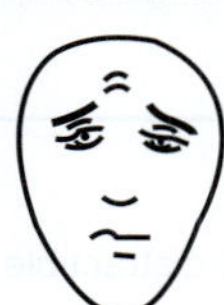
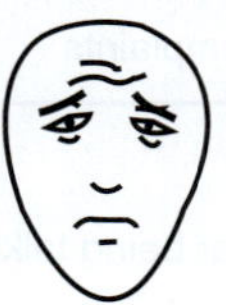
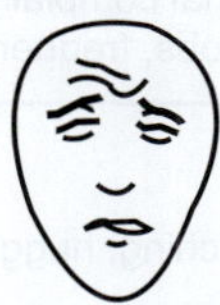
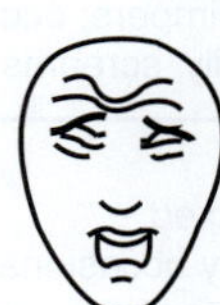

Score the chosen face 0, 2, 4, 6, 8 or 10, counting left to right, so '0' = 'no pain' and '10' = 'very much pain'. Do not use words like 'happy' and 'sad'. This scale is intended to measure how children feel inside, not how their face looks.

Sources. Hicks CL, von Baeyer CL, Spafford P, et al. The Faces Pain Scale—Revised: toward a common metric in pediatric pain measurement. *Pain, 93*, 173–83. Bieri D, Reeve R, Champion GD, et al. The Faces Pain Scale for the self-assessment of the severity of pain experienced by children: development, initial validation and preliminary investigation for ratio scale properties. *Pain, 41*, 139–50.

Figure 13.11
Wong-Baker FACES Pain Rating Scale.
(From Hockenberry MJ et al. Wong's essentials of pediatric nursing, 7th edn. St. Louis, 2005, p. 1259. Used with permission. Copyright, Mosby.)

CRIES Neonatal Postoperative Pain Measurement Score

	0	1	2
Crying	No	High-pitched	Inconsolable
Requires O_2 for sat >95%	No	<30% from baseline	>30% from baseline
Increased vital signs	HR and BP = or < preop	HR or BP ↑ <20% of preop	HR or BP ↑ >20% of preop
Expression	None	Grimace	Grimace/grunt
Sleepless	No, continuously asleep	Wakes at frequent intervals	Constantly awake

Figure 13.12
CRIES Neonatal Postoperative Pain Measurement Score. Krechel & Bildner (1995)

FLACC Behavioral Pain Scale (Infants and Toddlers)

DATE/TIME						
Face 0 - No particular expression or smile 1 - Occasional grimace or frown, withdrawn, disinterested 2 - Frequent to constant quivering chin, clenched jaw						
Legs 0 - Normal position or relaxed 1 - Uneasy, restless, tense 2 - Kicking, or legs drawn up						
Activity 0 - Lying quietly, normal position, moves easily 1 - Squirming, shifting back and forth, tense 2 - Arched, rigid, or jerking						
Cry 0 - No cry (awake or asleep) 1 - Moans or whimpers; occasional complaint 2 - Crying steadily, screams or sobs, frequent complaints						
Consolability 0 - Content, relaxed 1 - Reassured by occasional touching, hugging or being talked to, distractible 2 - Difficult to console or comfort						
TOTAL SCORE						

Figure 13.13
FLACC Behavioral Pain Scale (Infants and Toddlers).

OBJECTIVE DATA

Objective data

Preparation

Objective assessment of pain is sometimes necessary in circumstances when verbalisation of pain is not possible. The objective data collection process including the use of pain assessment tools can help you further understand the person's experience and the nature of the pain. Consider whether this is an acute or chronic condition. Recall that physical findings may not always support the person's pain complaints, particularly for chronic pain syndromes. Pain should not be discounted when objective physical evidence is not found. Based on the person's pain report, make every effort to reduce or eliminate the pain with appropriate analgesic and nonpharmacological intervention.

Equipment needed

Hand hygiene solution
Tape measure to measure circumference of swollen joints or extremities
Tongue depressor
Penlight

PROCEDURES AND NORMAL FINDINGS	ABNORMAL FINDINGS AND CLINICAL ALERTS
General inspection	
Identify pain-related features through observation of alteration in mobility or guarding. Observe for changes in facial expression, posture, gait or mood.	For example, abdominal pain may result in a hunched posture; appearance of tiredness or grimacing; uneven gait such as limping, which may indicate site of injury.
When the individual cannot verbally communicate their pain, you can (to a limited extent) identify pain using behavioural cues.	People react to painful stimuli with a wide variety of behaviours. Behaviours are influenced by many factors, including the nature of the pain (acute versus chronic), age, and cultural and gender expectations.
Acute pain behaviours	
Acute pain involves autonomic responses and has a protective purpose. Individuals experiencing moderate to intense levels of pain *may* exhibit the following behaviours. Observe the person for guarding, grimacing, vocalisations such as moaning, agitation, restlessness, stillness, diaphoresis or change in vital signs.	This list of behaviours is not exhaustive because they should not be used exclusively to deny or confirm the presence of pain. For example, in a postoperative patient, pulse and blood pressure can be altered by fluid volume, medications and blood loss.
Chronic (persistent) pain behaviours	
Observe for chronic pain behaviours such as bracing, rubbing, diminished activity, sighing and change in appetite. Sleeping is one way people behave in response to chronic pain in order to self-distract.	
Limbs and joints	
If the pain is located in a limb or joint, note the size and contour of the joint/limb. Measure circumference of the involved joint/limb for comparison with baseline. Check active or passive range of motion (see complete technique, Chapter 20). Joint motion normally causes no tenderness, pain or crepitation.	Swelling, inflammation, injury, deformity, diminished range of motion, increased pain on palpation and crepitation (an audible and palpable crunching that accompanies movement).
Muscles and skin	
Inspect the skin and tissue for colour, swelling, temperature and any masses or deformity.	Bruising, lesions, open wounds, tissue damage, atrophy, bulging, change in hair distribution, heat or cold and pallor or redness.
To assess for changes in sensation, ask the person to close their eyes. Test the person's ability to perceive sensation by breaking a tongue depressor in two lengthwise. Lightly press the sharp and blunted ends on the skin in a random fashion and ask the person to identify it as sharp or dull (see Figure 12.34A and 12.34B). This test will help you identify location and extent of altered sensation.	Absent pain sensation (**analgesia**); increased pain sensation (**hyperalgesia**); or if a severe pain sensation is evoked with a stimulus that does not normally induce pain (e.g. the blunt end of the tongue blade, cotton ball, clothing) (**allodynia**).
Abdomen	
If the pain is located in the abdomen, observe for contour and symmetry. Palpate superficially for muscle guarding and organ size (for discussion of complete technique see Chapter 23). Note any areas of referred pain (see Table 23.22).	Swelling, bulging, herniation, inflammation and muscle guarding. Leave any reported area of tenderness until last so as not to cause guarding or unnecessary discomfort. Observe person's face and nonverbal responses, such as drawing up of legs, guarding, groaning while palpating. ***Clinical alert:*** If the person experiences any significant abdominal tenderness on palpation stop the examination and refer the person to a medical practitioner for further assessment.
Other pain sites	
For example, chest, mouth, face, nose, ear, lips, tongue, throat or symptoms such as dysuria, constipation, pain on breathing refer to relevant chapters within the text for assessment guidelines.	

OBJECTIVE DATA

OBJECTIVE DATA

PROCEDURES AND NORMAL FINDINGS	ABNORMAL FINDINGS AND CLINICAL ALERTS
Vital signs	
A check of vital signs is recommended to determine any physiological change.	Vital sign changes may include tachycardia, high or low blood pressure, raised respiratory rate, pallor and perspiration. ***Clinical alert:*** A lack of change in vital signs is not a reliable indicator of the person's pain state. Be aware that tachycardia and tachypnoea also occur with anxiety and fear and are not specific to pain. However, poorly controlled pain can result in systemic physiological change. See Table 13.2.
Functional impact of pain	
Measure pain intensity scores on movement and with deep breathing and coughing. Assess ability to sit upright by self, move and self-care. Can use the **Functional Activity Scale (FAS)**, the purpose of which is to assess whether a patient can undertake a certain activity (Scott & McDonald 2008).	The FAS has a simple three-level ranked categorical score: A—No limitation (the person is able to undertake the activity without limitation due to pain) (pain intensity score typically 0–3 on a 0–10 scale), B—Mild limitation (the person is able to undertake the activity but experiences moderate to severe pain) (pain intensity score is typically 4–10), C—Significant limitation (the person is unable to complete the activity due to pain or pain treatment-related side effects independent of pain intensity scores).
Additional objective data for the adult over 65 years	
Pain should not be considered a 'normal' part of ageing. When the older adult reports a history of conditions such as osteoarthritis, peripheral vascular disease, cancer, osteoporosis, angina or chronic constipation, be alert and anticipate a pain problem. Observe behavioural cues, such as changes in functional status. For example, changes in dressing, walking, toileting, eating or involvement in daily activities. Slowness and rigidity may be apparent. Look for a sudden onset of acute confusion, which may indicate poorly controlled pain.	***Clinical alert:*** Sudden onset of acute confusion may indicate poorly controlled pain. However, you will need to rule out other competing explanations such as infection, adverse reaction to medications or delirium.
Adults with cognitive impairment and disability The person with cognitive impairment may report pain, but may not be able to describe the pain, discern variations in pain, recall severity of pain or alert others about their pain. When this is the case, then observation of pain behaviours is an important component of pain assessment. Observe for restlessness, frowning and grimacing or sounds such as grunting or groaning. It is strongly suggested that the Abbey Pain Scale or similar is used.	These behaviours can be used to assess pain but may not always be valid indicators of pain in non-verbal adults.
Additional objective data for infants and children	
General inspection Look for changes in temperament, expression and activity. For example, observe facial activity and body movements. Crying can be described in terms of its presence or absence, duration and amplitude or pitch. Observe for facial expressions (e.g. taut tongue, bulging brow, eye squeeze, nasolabial furrow). If a procedure or disease process is known to induce pain in adults (e.g. surgery, injury, cancer), it *will* induce pain in the infant or child.	Because the sympathetic nervous system is engaged particularly in acute episodes of pain, physiological changes take place that may indicate the presence of pain. These include sweating, increases in blood pressure and heart rate, vomiting, nausea and changes in oxygen saturation. However, like the adult, these physiological changes cannot be used exclusively to confirm or deny pain because of other factors such as stress, medications and fluid changes.

Summary Checklist

Subjective data

1. Initial pain assessment
2. Pain assessment tools

Objective data

1. General inspection (acute pain behaviours and chronic pain behaviours)
2. Limbs and joints
3. Muscles and skin
4. Abdomen
5. Other pain sites
6. Vital signs
7. Functional impact of pain

Documentation and critical thinking

FOCUSED ASSESSMENT: CLINICAL CASE STUDY 1

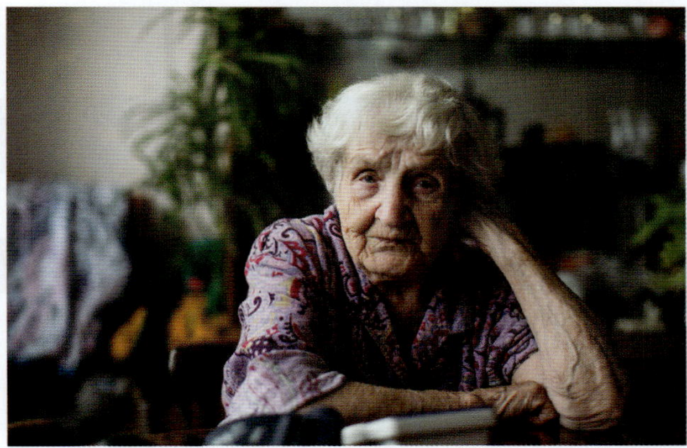

Context

Mrs Maria Alberici is an 85-year-old Italian-Australian female with a 20-year history of osteoarthritis.

Subjective

Mrs Alberici reports increased pain and stiffness in her hips and knees for the past month. No radiation of pain, tingling or numbness in lower extremities. Having difficulty getting in and out of the bath and dressing herself. Describes pain as aching, with 'good and bad days'. Becomes frustrated when asked to rate her pain intensity. Replies 'I don't know what number to give; it hurts a lot, on and off'. Takes Panadol Osteo, two tablets, when the pain 'really gets bad', with some degree of relief. Restricts her activities, such as walking to the local shops, because she 'hurts too much'.

Objective

Localised tenderness noted upon palpation of knees; unable to fully flex knees. Crepitus noted in both knee joints. Swelling noted. Rubs lower knee area frequently. Gait slow and unsteady. Facial expression tense, clenching teeth.

Collaborative problem

Chronic pain related to osteoarthritis of hips and knees

Problem statements/nursing diagnoses

Chronic pain related to osteoarthritis of hips and knees

Partial self-care deficit: hygiene and dressing related to pain in knees

Impaired mobility related to painful knees

FOCUSED ASSESSMENT: CLINICAL CASE STUDY 2

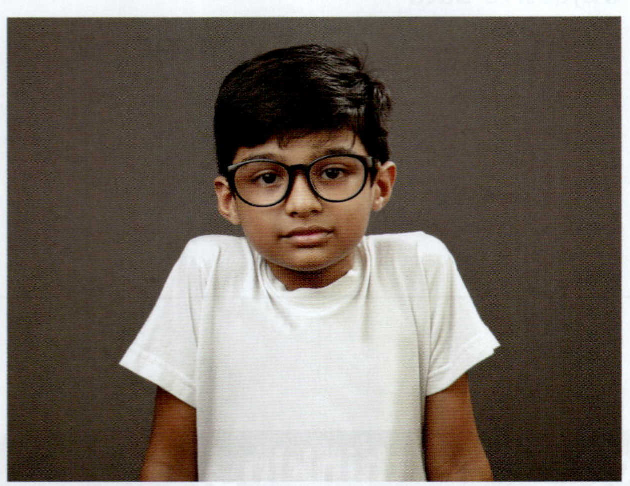

Context

Vivaan Patel is a 7-year-old boy who has just undergone a laparoscopic appendectomy. He is awake, but his eyes are closed and he is lying flat on the bed without movement.

Subjective

When asked if he is in pain, Vivaan states 'a little', however, he rates pain as +8 using the Faces Pain Scale.

Objective

Requiring assistance to move in the bed. Speaks only when spoken to.

Diaphoretic, flushed, grimaces with slight touch.

Vital Signs: Temp 37°C oral, BP 122/72 mmHg, HR 126 bpm, RR 22/min.

Lungs: Clear on auscultation. Pulse oximetry 98% on room air.

Abdomen: Hypoactive bowel sounds, tenderness on light palpation, dressings dry and intact at surgical sites.

Collaborative problem

Acute postoperative pain

Problem statements/nursing diagnoses

Acute postoperative pain related to surgical wound

Abnormal Findings

TABLE 13.3 Peripheral neuropathy
Peripheral neuropathy (PN) is symmetrical damage to peripheral nerves (feet or hands), resulting in pain without stimulation of the nerves. This is a common neuropathic pain characterised by numbness and tingling, with interspersed shooting or lancinating pain that is not attributed to a specific nociceptive source. Diabetic neuropathy is a common complication of diabetes and may relate to demyelination of the larger peripheral nerves, with an increase in smaller myelinated nerves. Other aetiologies may include ischaemic damage to nerves or hyperglycaemia, causing changes in nerve microenvironment. Patients experience burning pain in feet bilaterally, which is often worse at night.
Chemotherapy Induced PN occurs during or after chemotherapy treatment for cancer. The risk increases with the number or agents used in the course of treatment, higher cumulative doses of neurotoxic agents, pre-existing neuropathy from diabetes or other causes and older age. The symptoms depend on the nerves affected and include: tingling ('pins and needles'); burning pain that can be severe and constant or may come and go; decreased sensation; increased sensitivity to touch, temperature or pressure and muscle weakness (Brown et al 2019). NOTE: With any cancer survivor, you must address any new onset of pain promptly to rule out pathological recurrence of cancer.

TABLE 13.2 Physiological changes from poorly controlled pain

Pain is not a benign symptom. Poorly controlled acute pain and chronic pain have negative impacts on physiological systems.

PHYSIOLOGICAL SYSTEM	ACUTE PAIN RESPONSES
Cardiac	Tachycardia Elevated blood pressure Increased myocardial oxygen demand Increased cardiac output
Pulmonary	Hypoventilation Hypoxia Decreased cough Atelectasis
Gastrointestinal	Nausea Vomiting Ileus
Renal	Oliguria Urinary retention
Musculoskeletal	Spasm Joint stiffness
Endocrine	Increased adrenergic activity
Central nervous system	Fear Anxiety Fatigue
Immune	Impaired cellular immunity Impaired wound healing
Poorly controlled chronic pain	Depression Isolation Limited mobility and function Confusion Family distress Diminished quality of life

BIBLIOGRAPHY

Abbey J, Piller N, De Bellis A et al. The Abbey pain scale: A 1-minute numerical indicator for people with end-stage dementia. International J Palliat Med 2004;10(1):6–13.

American Pain Society (APS). Principles of analgesic use. 7th ed. Chicago: APS; 2016.

Australian Bureau of Statistics (ABS). National Health Survey: First Results. Australia. 2014–15. Cat. No. 4364.0.55.001; 2015.

Australian Bureau of Statistics (ABS). Cultural Diversity in Australia. Census of Population and Housing: Reflecting Australia – Stories from the census 2016. 2017. Available at: https://www.abs.gov.au/ausstats/abs@.nsf/Lookup/by%20Subject/2071.0~2016~Main%20Features~Cultural%20Diversity%20Data%20Summary~30.

Australian Institute of Health and Welfare. Admitted patient care 2015–16: Australian hospital statistics. Canberra: AIHW, Health services series no.75. Cat. no. HSE 185; 2017.

Banasik JL, Copstead LE. Pathophysiology. 6th ed. St Louis: Elsevier; 2019.

Boerner KE, Birnie KA, Caes L, et al. Sex differences in experimental pain among healthy children: a systematic review and meta-analysis. Pain 2014;155(5):983–93.

Brown R, Morgan A. The opioid epidemic in North America: Implications for Australia. Trends & issues in crime and criminal justice no. 578. Canberra: Australian Institute of Criminology; 2019. Available at: https://aic.gov.au/publications/tandi/tandi578.

Brown TJ, Sedhom R, Gupta A. Chemotherapy induced peripheral neuropathy. JAMA Oncology Patient Page February 28. 2019. doi:10.1001/jamaoncol.2018.6771.

Burchum JR, Rosenthal LD. Lehne's pharmacology for nursing care. 9th ed. St Louis: Elsevier; 2016.

Campbell G, Lintzeris N, Gisev N, et al. Regulatory and other responses to the pharmaceutical opioid problem. Med J Aust 2019;210(1):6–8.e1. doi:10.5694/mja2.12047

Centers for Disease Control and Prevention. Opioid overdose. 2018. Available at: https://www.cdc.gov/drugoverdose/data/index.html.

Cole LJ, Farrell MJ, Gibson SJ, Egan GF. Age-related differences in pain sensitivity and regional brain activity evoked by noxious pressure. Neurobiol Aging 2010;31:494–503.

Cleeland CS, Ryan KM. Pain assessment: global use of the brief pain inventory. Ann Acad Med Singap 1994;23(2):129–38.

ABNORMAL FINDINGS

Deloitte Access Economics. The cost of pain in Australia. 2019. Available at: https://www.painaustralia.org.au/static/uploads/files/the-cost-of-pain-in-australia-final-report-12mar-wfxbrfyboams.pdf.

DeVon HA, Piano MR, Hoppensteadt DA. The association of pain with protein inflammatory biomarkers: A review of the literature. Nurs Res 2014;63(1):51–62.

Evered L, Scott DA, Silbert B, et al. Postoperative cognitive dysfunction is independent of type of surgery and anesthetic. Anesth Analg 2011;112(5):1179–85.

Fenwick C. Assessing pain across the cultural gap: central Australian Indigenous people's pain assessment. Contemp Nurse 2006;22(2): 218–27.

Fitzgerald M. Pain and analgesia in neonates. Trends Neurosci 1987;19(9):344–6.

Fitzgerald M, Walker SM. Infant pain management: a developmental neurobiological approach. Nat Clin Pract Neurol 2009;5(1): 35–50.

Hadjistavropoulos T, Herr K, Prkachin KM, et al. Pain assessment in elderly adults with dementia. Lancet Neurol 2014;13:1216–27.

Henschke N, Maher CG, Refshauge KM, et al. Characteristics of patients with acute low back pain presenting to primary care in Australia. Clin J Pain 2009;25(1):5–11.

International Association for the Study of Pain (IASP). Neuropathic pain. 2019a. Available at: https://www.iasp-pain.org/Advocacy/GYAP.aspx?ItemNumber=5054.

International Association for the Study of Pain (IASP). Faces pain scale—revised. 2019b. Available at: https://www.iasp-pain.org/Education/Content.aspx?ItemNumber=1519.

Kuner R, Flor H. Structural plasticity and reorganisation in chronic pain. Nat Rev Neurosci 2017;18:20–30.

Kunz M, Mylius V, Schepelmann K, Lautenbacher S. Effects of age and mild cognitive impairment on the pain response system. Gerontology 2009;55:674–82.

Krechel SW, Bildner J. CRIES: a new neonatal postoperative pain measurement score. Initial testing of validity and reliability. Paediatr Anaesth 1995;5(1):53–61.

Larance B, Degenhardt L, Peacock A, et al. Pharmaceutical opioid use and harm in Australia: The need for proactive and preventative responses. Drug Alcohol Rev 2018;37:S203–5.

Macintosh C, Elson S. Chronic pain: clinical features, assessment and treatment. Nurs Stand 2008;23(5):48–56.

Macintyre PE, Schug SA. Acute pain management: a practical guide. 4th ed. Florida: CRC Press; 2015.

McAuliffe L, Nay R, O'Donnell M, et al. Pain assessment in older people with dementia: literature review. J Adv Nurs 2008;65(1):2–10.

McCaffery M. Nursing practice theories related to cognition, bodily pain, and main-environment interactions. Los Angeles: University of Los Angeles; 1968.

McCaffery M, Pasero C. Pain: clinical manual. 2nd ed. St Louis: Mosby; 1999.

Melzack R. The short-form McGill pain questionnaire. Pain 1987;30:191–7.

Merkel SI, Voepel-Lewis T, Shayevitz JR, et al. The FLACC: A behavioral scale for scoring postoperative pain in young children. Pediatr Nurs 1997;23(3):293–7.

Merskey H, Bogduk N. Classification of chronic pain, IASP taskforce on taxonomy. Seattle: IASP Press, Updated 22 May, 2012; 1994.

Morton DL, Sandhu JS, Jones AK. Brain imaging of pain: State of the art. J Pain Res 2016;9:613–24.

National Pain Summit Initiative. National pain strategy. Pain management for all Australians. 2010. Available at: www.painsummit.org.au.

NIH National Institute on Drug Abuse. Opioid overdose crisis. 2019. Available at: https://www.drugabuse.gov/drugs-abuse/opioids/opioid-overdose-crisis#one.

Packiasabapathy S, Sadhasivam S. Gender, genetics, and analgesia: understanding the differences in response to pain relief. J Pain Res 2018;11:2729–39.

Palmer G. Complex regional pain syndrome. Aust Prescr 2015;38(3):82.

Pautex S, Herrmann F, Le Louis P. Feasibility and reliability of four pain self-assessment scales and correlation with an observational rating scale in hospitalised elderly demented patients. J Gerontol A Biol Sci Med Sci 2005;60(4):524–9.

Poquet N, Lin C. The Brief Pain Inventory (BPI). J Physiother 2010;62:52.

Schug SA, Palmer GM, Scott DA, et al. APM:SE working group of the Australian and New Zealand College of Anaesthetists and Faculty of Pain Medicine (2015), Acute Pain Management: Scientific evidence. 4th ed. Melbourne: ANZCA & FPM; 2015.

Schultz M, Loughran-Fowlds A, Spence K. Neonatal pain: a comparison of the beliefs and practices of junior doctors and current best evidence. J Paediatr Child Health 2009;46:23–8.

Sekulic S, Gebauer-Bukurov K, Cvijanovic M, et al. Appearance of fetal pain could be associated with maturation of the mesodiencephalic structures. J Pain Res 2016;9:1031–8.

Scott DA, McDonald WM. Assessment, measurement and history. In Macintyre PE, Rowbotham D, Walker S, editors. Textbook of clinical pain management; acute pain. 2nd ed. London: Hodder Arnold; 2008.

Shaw S, Lee A. Student nurses' misconceptions of adults with chronic nonmalignant pain. Pain Manag Nurs 2010;11(1): 2–14.

Shrestha-Ranjit JM, Manias E. Pain assessment and management practice in children following surgery of the lower limb. J Clin Nurs 2010;19:118–28.

Taylor K, Guerin P. Health care and indigenous Australians. South Yarra, Vic: Palgrave Macmillan; 2014.

Tighe PJ, Riley JL, Fillingim RB. Sex differences in the incidence of severe pain events following surgery: A review of 333,000 pain scores. Pain Med 2014;15(8):1390–404.

Volkow ND, McLellan AT. Opioid abuse in chronic pain—Misconceptions and mitigation strategies. N Eng J Med 2016;374(13):1253–63.

Walker SM, Franck LS, Fitzgerald M, et al. Longterm impact of neonatal intensive care and surgery on somatosensory perception in children born extremely preterm. Pain 2009;141(1–2):79–87.

Walker SM. Biological and neurodevelopmental implications of neonatal pain. Clin Perinatol 2013;40(3):471–91.

Warden V, Hurley AC, Volicer L. Development and psychometric evaluation of the Pain Assessment in Advanced Dementia (PAINAD) scale. J Am Med Dir Assoc 2002;4(1):9–15.

Willis MH, Merkel SI, Voepel-Lewis T, et al. FLACC Behavioral Pain Assessment Scale: a comparison with the child's self-report. Pediatr Nurs 2002;29(3):195–8.

World Health Organization (WHO). International Classification of Diseases: ICD-11 for Mortality and Morbidity Statistics (Version 04/2019) – Chronic pain. 2019. Available at: https://icd.who.int/browse11/l-m/en#/http%3a%2f%2fid.who.int%2ficd%2fentity%2f1581976053.

Chapter Fourteen

Eye assessment

Written by Carolyn Jarvis
Adapted by Amanda Wylie

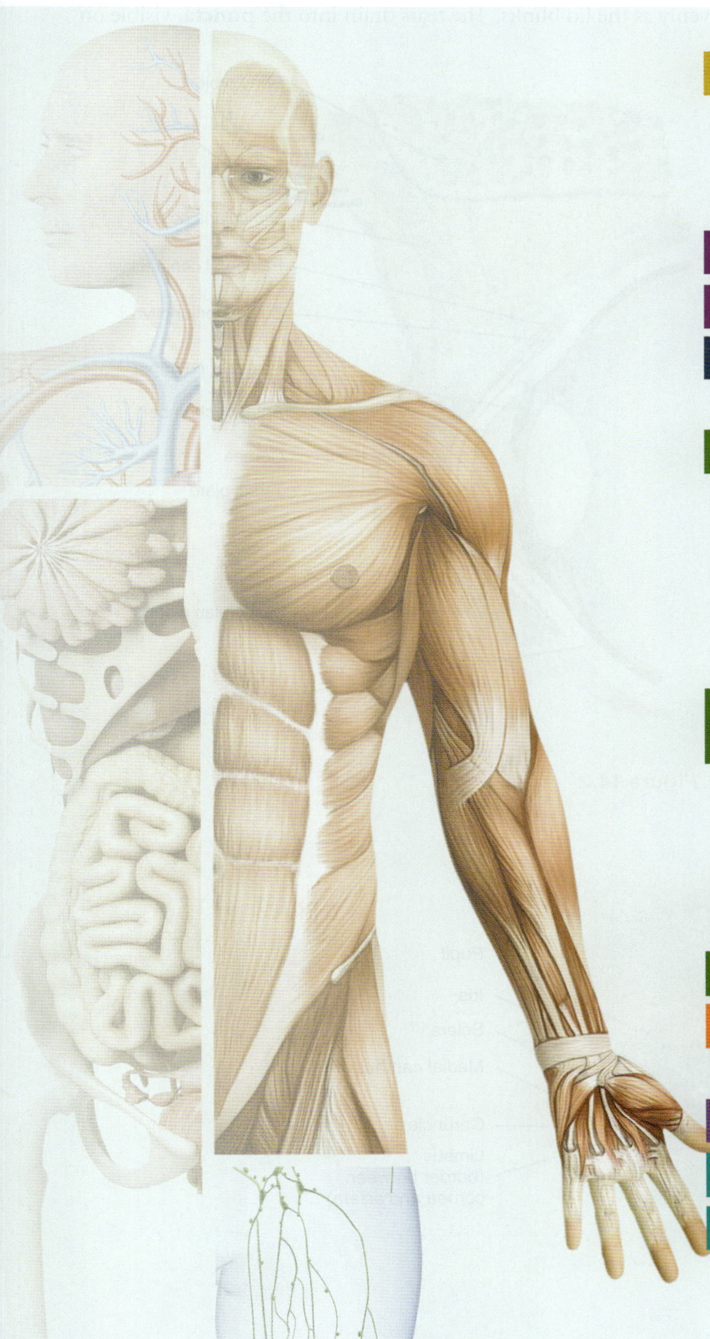

INTRODUCTION

As the eye is the major source of sensory information, the brain is heavily involved in the function of vision. Any alteration in vision has an impact on function and safety that needs to be considered in planning care. Processing visual information takes place in the cerebral cortex and the visual association area occupies most of the occipital lobe. It is the largest of all the cortical sensory areas in the occipital lobe (Marieb & Keller 2018). In this chapter we review the external and internal anatomy of the eye and accessory muscles, visual pathways, visual fields and visual light reflexes. This information is also relevant to neurological system assessment (see Chapter 12).

Structure and function

EXTERNAL ANATOMY

Because this sense is so important to humans, the eye is well protected by the bony orbital cavity, which is surrounded with a cushion of orbital fat. The **eyelids** are like two movable shades that further protect the eye from injury, strong light and dust. The upper eyelid is the larger and more mobile one. The eyelashes are short hairs in double or triple rows that curve outwards from the lid margins, filtering out dust and dirt.

When closed, the lid margins approximate completely. When open, the upper lid covers the upper part of the iris and the lower lid sits just at the **limbus**, the border between the cornea and sclera. The elliptical open space between the eyelids is called the **palpebral fissure** (Figure 14.1). The **canthus** is the corner of the eye, the angle where the lids meet. At the inner canthus, the **caruncle** is a small fleshy mass containing sebaceous glands.

Within the upper lid, **tarsal plates** are strips of connective tissue that give it shape (Figure 14.2). The tarsal plates contain the **meibomian glands**, modified sebaceous glands that secrete an oily lubricating material onto the lids. This stops the tears from overflowing and evaporating, and helps to form an airtight seal when the lids are closed.

The exposed white part of the eye (sclera) has a transparent protective covering, the **conjunctiva**. The conjunctiva is a thin mucous membrane folded like an envelope between the eyelids and the eyeball. The *palpebral* conjunctiva lines the lids and is clear, with many small blood vessels. It forms a deep recess or pocket and then folds back over the eye. The *bulbar* conjunctiva overlays the eyeball, with the white sclera showing through. At the limbus the conjunctiva merges with the cornea. The cornea covers and protects the iris and pupil.

The **lacrimal apparatus** provides constant irrigation to keep the conjunctiva and cornea moist and lubricated (Figure 14.3). The **lacrimal gland**, in the upper outer corner over the eye, secretes aqueous tears. The tears wash across the eye and are drawn up evenly as the lid blinks. The tears drain into the **puncta**, visible on

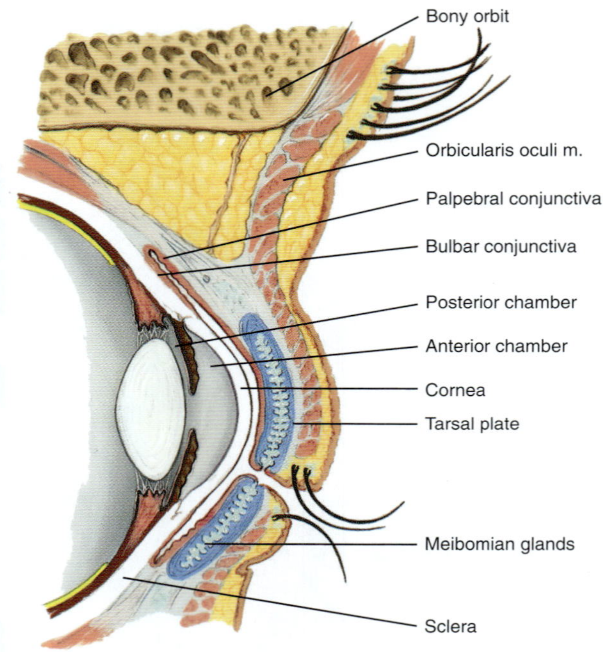

Figure 14.2

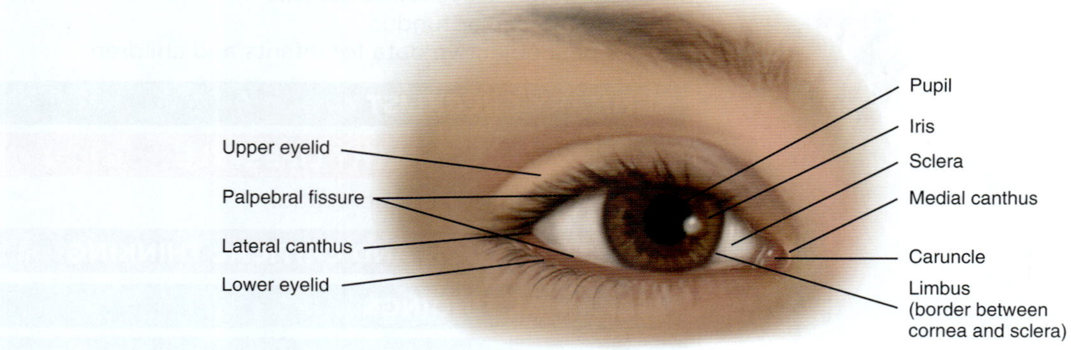

Figure 14.1

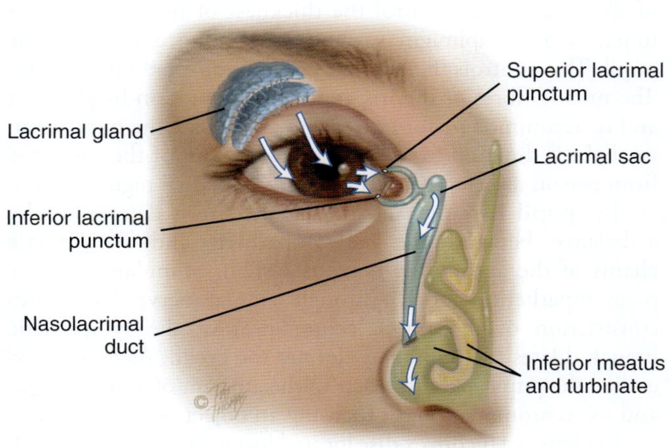

Figure 14.3

the upper and lower lid rims at the inner canthus. The tears then drain into the nasolacrimal sac, through the 7.5 cm **nasolacrimal duct** and empty into the inferior meatus inside the nose. A tiny fold of mucous membrane prevents air from being forced up the nasolacrimal duct when the nose is blown.

Extraocular muscles. Six muscles attach the eyeball to its orbit (Figure 14.4A and 14.4B) and serve to direct the eye to points of the person's interest. These extraocular muscles give the eye both straight and rotary movement. The four straight, or *rectus*, muscles are the superior, inferior, lateral and medial rectus muscles. The two slanting, or *oblique*, muscles are the superior and inferior oblique muscles.

Each muscle is coordinated, or yoked, with one in the other eye. This ensures that when the two eyes move, their axes always remain parallel (called *conjugate movement*). Parallel axes are important because the human brain can tolerate seeing only one image. Although some animals can perceive two different pictures through each eye, human beings have a binocular, single-image visual system. This occurs because our eyes move as a pair. For example, the two yoked muscles that

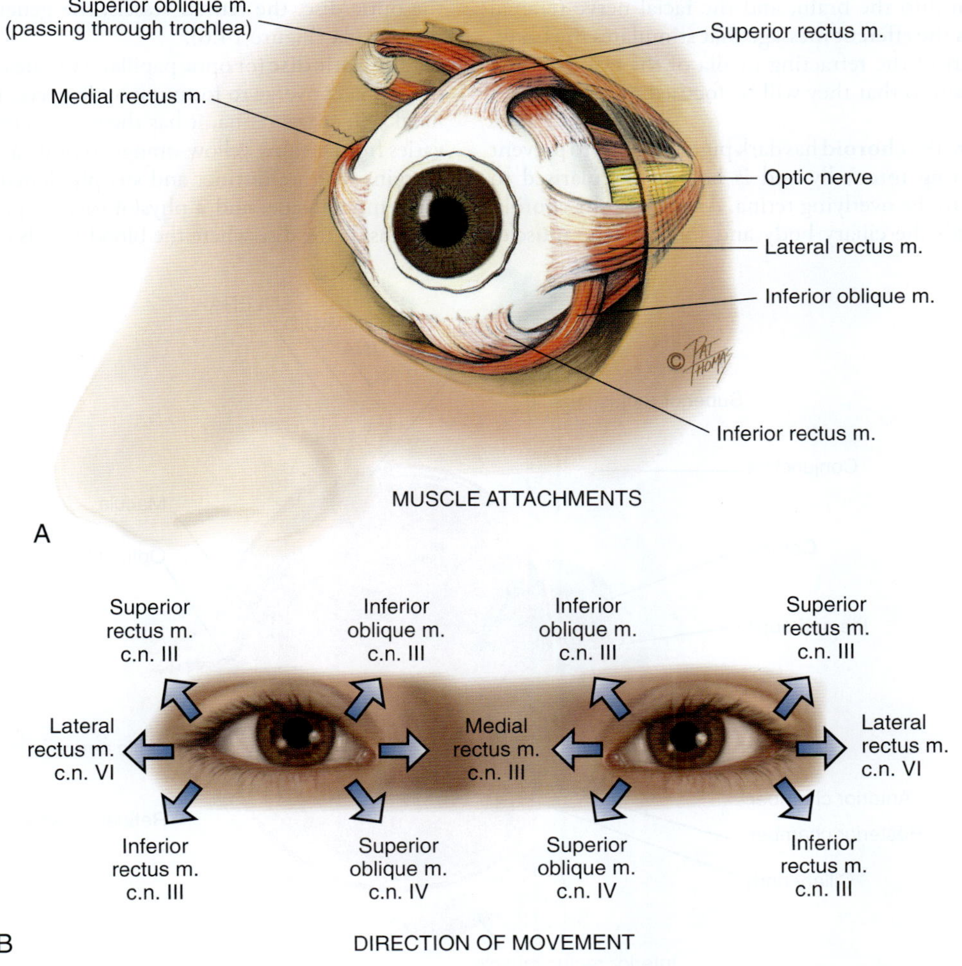

Figure 14.4

allow looking to the far right are the right lateral rectus and the left medial rectus.

Movement of the **extraocular muscles** (below) is stimulated by three **cranial nerves**. Cranial nerve VI, the abducens nerve, innervates the lateral rectus muscle (which abducts the eye); cranial nerve IV, the trochlear nerve, innervates the superior oblique muscle; and cranial nerve III, the oculomotor nerve, innervates all the rest—the superior, inferior and medial rectus and the inferior oblique muscles. Note that the superior oblique muscle is located on the superior aspect of the eyeball, but when it contracts, it enables the person to look downwards and inwards.

INTERNAL ANATOMY

The eye is a sphere composed of three concentric coats: (1) the outer fibrous **sclera and cornea**, (2) the middle vascular **choroid, ciliary body and iris** and (3) the inner nervous **retina** (Figure 14.5).

The outer layer. The **sclera** is a tough, protective, white covering. It is continuous anteriorly with the smooth, transparent cornea, which covers the iris and pupil.

The **cornea** is very sensitive to touch; contact with a wisp of cotton stimulates a blink in both eyes, called the *corneal reflex*. The trigeminal nerve (cranial nerve V) carries the afferent sensation into the brain, and the facial nerve (cranial nerve VII) carries the efferent message that stimulates the blink. The cornea is part of the refracting media of the eye, bending incoming light rays so that they will be focused on the retina.

The middle layer. The **choroid** has dark pigmentation to prevent light from reflecting internally and is heavily vascularised to deliver nutrients to the overlying retina. Anteriorly, the choroid is continuous with the ciliary body and the iris. The muscles of the ciliary body control the thickness of the lens. The iris functions as a diaphragm, varying the opening at its centre, the pupil. This controls the amount of light admitted into the eye. The muscle fibres of the iris contract the pupil in bright light and to accommodate for near vision, and dilate the pupil when the light is dim and for far vision. The colour of the iris varies from person to person, dependent on individual pigmentation.

The **pupil** is round and regular. Its size is determined by a balance between the parasympathetic and sympathetic chains of the autonomic nervous system. Stimulation of the parasympathetic branch, through cranial nerve III, causes constriction of the pupil. Stimulation of the sympathetic branch dilates the pupil and elevates the eyelid. As mentioned earlier, the pupil size also reacts to the amount of ambient light and to accommodation, or focusing an object on the retina.

The **lens** is a biconvex disc located just posterior to the pupil. The transparent lens serves as a refracting medium, keeping a viewed object in continual focus on the retina. Its thickness is controlled by the ciliary body; the lens bulges for focusing on near objects and flattens for far objects.

The inner layer. The **retina** is the visual receptive layer of the eye in which light waves are changed into nerve impulses. The retinal structures viewed through the ophthalmoscope are the optic disc, the retinal vessels, the general background and the macula (Figure 14.6).

The **optic disc** (or optic papilla) is the area in which fibres from the retina converge to form the optic nerve. Located towards the nasal side of the retina, it has these characteristics: a colour that varies from creamy yellow-orange to pink; a round or oval shape; margins that are distinct and sharply demarcated, especially on the temporal side; and a physiological cup, the smaller circular area inside the disc where the blood vessels exit and enter.

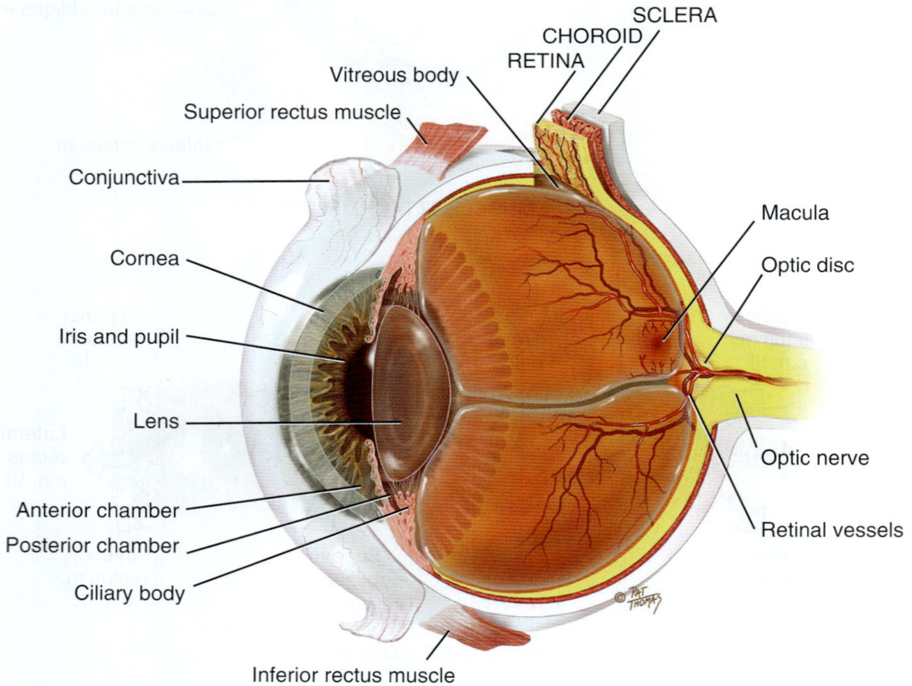

Figure 14.5

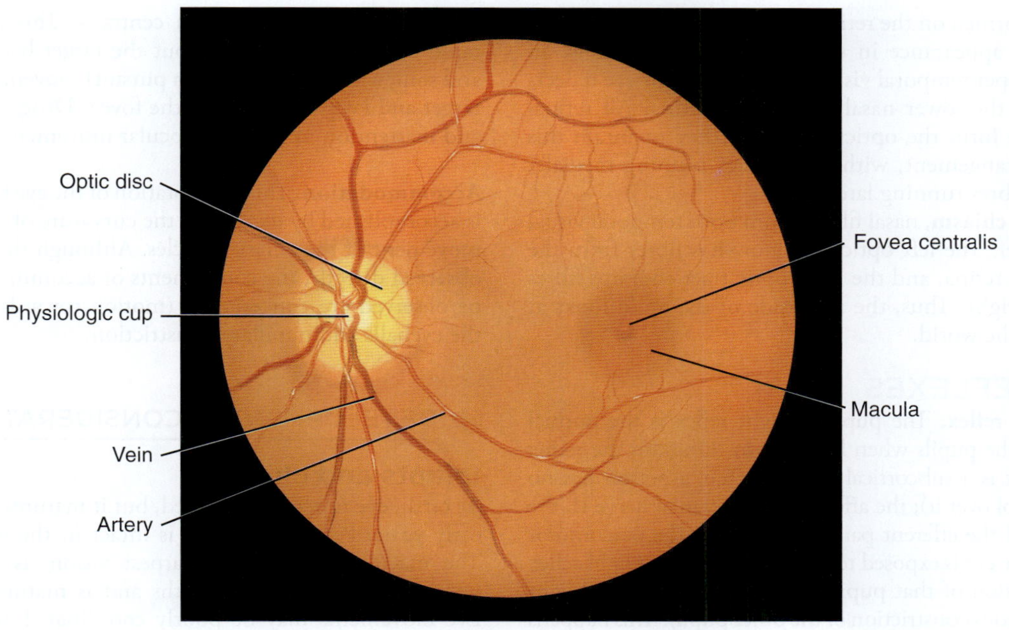

Figure 14.6

The **retinal vessels** normally include a paired artery and vein extending to each quadrant, growing progressively smaller in calibre as they reach the periphery. The arteries appear brighter red and narrower than the veins, and the arteries have a thin sliver of light on them (the arterial light reflex). The general background of the fundus varies in colour, depending on the person's skin colour. The **macula** is located on the temporal side of the fundus. It is a slightly darker pigmented region surrounding the **fovea centralis**; these areas are responsible for the most detailed and colour vision. The macula receives and transduces light from the centre of the visual field.

The eye is divided into **anterior** and **posterior segments**. The **anterior segment** is from the clear cornea to the posterior part of the lens. The anterior segment is divided into two chambers. The **anterior chamber** is from the clear cornea to the front of the iris. The **posterior chamber** lies behind the iris to the posterior lens. Both chambers of the anterior segment contain the clear, watery **aqueous humour** that is produced continually by the ciliary body. The continuous flow of fluid serves to deliver nutrients to the surrounding tissues and to drain metabolic wastes. Intraocular pressure is determined by a balance between the amount of aqueous humour produced and resistance to its outflow through the trabecular meshwork in the anterior chamber. The **posterior segment** of the eye is from the posterior lens to the retina. It is filled with a gelatinous, transparent substance called **vitreous humour**.

VISUAL PATHWAYS AND VISUAL FIELDS

Objects reflect light. The light rays are refracted through the transparent media (cornea, aqueous humour, lens and vitreous body) and strike the retina. The retina transforms the light stimulus into nerve impulses that are conducted through the optic nerve and the optic tract to the visual cortex of the occipital lobe (Figure 14.7).

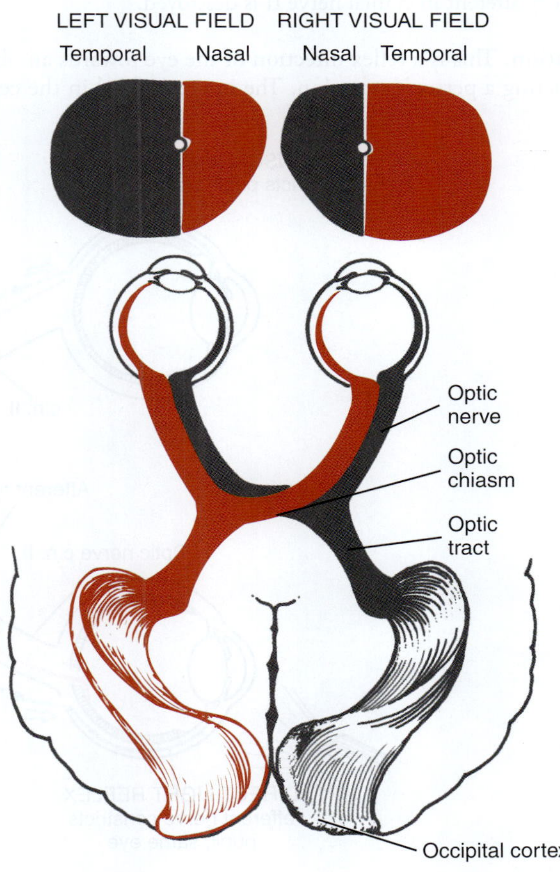

Figure 14.7
Visual pathways (viewed from above).

The image formed on the retina is upside down and reversed from its actual appearance in the outside world. That is, an object in the upper temporal visual field of the right eye reflects its image onto the lower nasal area of the retina. All retinal fibres collect to form the optic nerve, but they maintain this same spatial arrangement, with nasal fibres running medially and temporal fibres running laterally.

At the **optic chiasm**, nasal fibres (from both temporal visual fields) cross over. The left optic tract now has fibres from the left half of each retina, and the right optic tract contains fibres only from the right. Thus, the right side of the brain looks at the left side of the world.

VISUAL REFLEXES

Pupillary light reflex. The pupillary light reflex is the normal constriction of the pupils when bright light shines on the retina (Figure 14.8). It is a subcortical reflex arc (i.e. a person has no conscious control over it); the afferent link is cranial nerve II, the optic nerve, and the efferent path is cranial III, the oculomotor nerve. When one eye is exposed to bright light, a direct light reflex occurs (constriction of that pupil), as well as a consensual light reflex (simultaneous constriction of the other pupil). This happens because the optic nerve carries the sensory afferent message in and then synapses with both sides of the brain. For example, consider the light reflex in a person who is blind in one eye. Stimulation of the normal eye produces both a direct and a consensual light reflex. Stimulation of the blind eye causes no response because the sensory afferent in cranial nerve II is destroyed.

Fixation. This is a reflex direction of the eye towards an object attracting a person's attention. The image is fixed in the centre of the visual field, the fovea centralis. This consists of very rapid ocular movements to put the target back on the fovea, and somewhat slower (smooth pursuit) movements to track the target and keep its image on the fovea. Drugs, alcohol, fatigue and inattention impair these ocular movements.

Accommodation. This is adaptation of the eye for near vision. It is accomplished by increasing the curvature of the lens through movement of the ciliary muscles. Although the lens cannot be observed directly, the components of accommodation that can be observed are convergence (motion towards) of the axes of the eyeballs and pupillary constriction.

DEVELOPMENTAL CONSIDERATIONS

Infants and children

At birth, eye function is limited, but it matures fully during the early years. Peripheral vision is intact in the newborn infant. The macula, the area of sharpest vision, is absent at birth but is developing by 4 months and is mature by 8 months. Eye movements may be poorly coordinated at birth. By 3–4 months of age, the infant establishes binocularity and can fixate on a single image with both eyes simultaneously. Most neonates (80%) are born farsighted; this gradually decreases after 7–8 years of age.

In structure, the eyeball reaches adult size by 8 years. At birth, the iris shows little pigment, and the pupils are small. The lens is nearly spherical at birth, growing flatter throughout life. Its consistency changes from that of soft plastic at birth to rigid glass in old age.

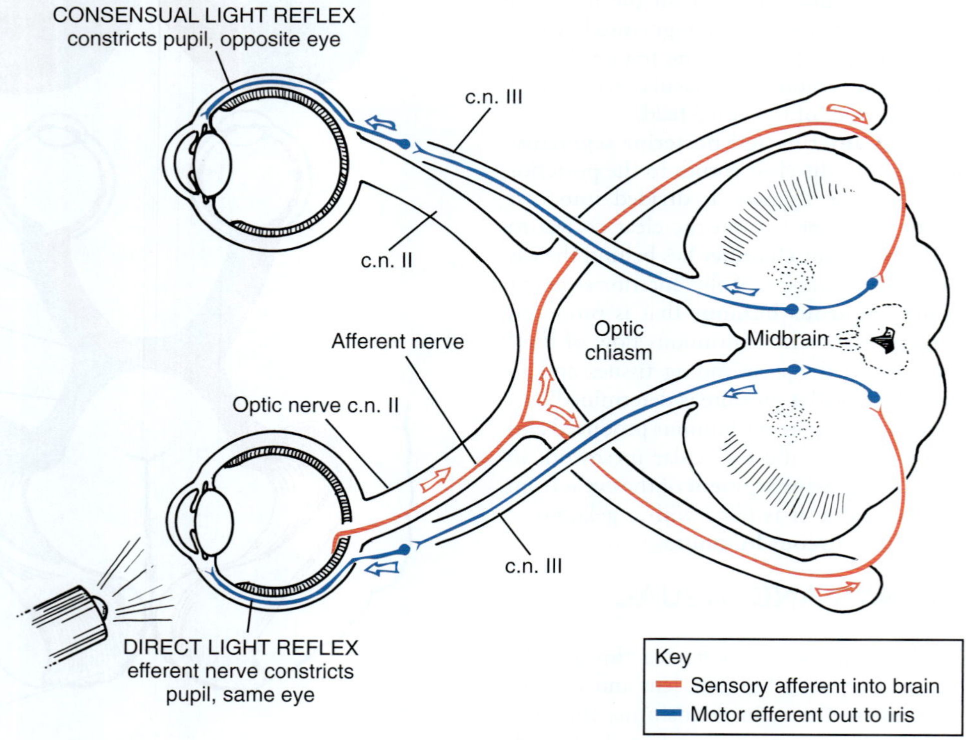

Figure 14.8

Late adulthood (65+ years)

Internationally, over 285 million people are visually impaired, though 80% of visual impairment can be avoided or cured. In Australia, vision disorders are common and are often related to ageing. In 2016, more than 453,000 Australians were living with vision impairment or blindness. This included up to 432,800 non-Indigenous Australians aged 50 years or older and up to 18,300 Indigenous Australians aged 40 years or older (Foreman et al 2016). Approximately 90% of vision impairment in both Indigenous and non-Indigenous Australians is preventable or treatable (Foreman et al 2016). Similarly, in New Zealand, 11% of adults over 65 years experience vision impairment, compared with 2% for adults aged 15–44 (Statistics New Zealand 2014).

Changes in eye structure contribute greatly to the distinct facial changes of the ageing person. The skin loses its elasticity, causing wrinkling and drooping; fat tissues and muscles atrophy; and the external eye structures appear sunken (see Figure 14.15 later in this chapter).

Visual acuity may diminish gradually after 50 years of age, and even more so after 70 years. The leading cause of vision impairment in Australia is *uncorrected refractive error* and *cataract*. Other notable causes are *age-related macular degeneration*, *diabetic retinopathy* and *glaucoma* (Foreman et al 2016). These are explained as:

1. **Uncorrected refractive error:** this is a condition where the light that passes through the front of the eye fails to focus precisely on the retina. This causes long or short sightedness and difficulties changing focus. Approximately 63.39% of Indigenous Australians and 61.69% of non-Indigenous Australians are affected by this condition (Foreman et al 2016).
2. **Cataract**, or lens opacity, results from a degeneration of proteins in the natural lens as the adult ages. Between the ages of 65 and 74, 50% of people will have cataract formation, and in those over 75 years of age, the prevalence increases to 70% (Harper 2010). In 2016, cataracts were the leading cause of visual impairment in Indigenous Australians (40%), affecting 20.22% of the population compared to 13.93% of non-Indigenous Australians (Foreman et al 2016). In New Zealand, the prevalence of cataract varies from approximately 0.1% in 60–69 year olds to 15% in the population aged over 90 (Taylor & Mapp 2010).
3. **Age-related macular degeneration (AMD)** is the breakdown of cells in the macula of the retina. There are two types of AMD: *non-neovascular or atrophic* (dry), the most common form; and *neovascular* (wet) the most severe form. It is a progressive, late-onset degenerative disease that affects central vision. Peripheral vision is not affected, so the person can usually manage self-care and will not become completely disabled. Over the past decade, understanding of the risk factors of the disease, along with advances in treatment options have seen a reduction in the progression of the disease leading to a decrease in vision impairment and blindness due to AMD (Mitchell et al 2018). It is still the most common form of visual impairment in non-Indigenous Australians (71%) over the age of 50 and has a prevalence of 1.09% in Indigenous Australians (Foreman et al 2016).
4. **Glaucoma** is the term used for a large group of disorders. The common factors in all glaucomas are damage to the optic nerve (optic neuropathy), loss of visual field and irreversible loss of vision. This is often associated with elevation of intraocular pressure (Harper 2010). The prevalence of glaucoma is estimated to be 5.46% in Indigenous Australians and 0.55% in non-Indigenous Australians (Foreman et al 2016). Chronic or primary open-angle glaucoma is the most common type and involves a gradual loss of peripheral vision that is usually unnoticed. As damage becomes extensive, symptoms such as reduced field of vision are noticeable. It is worth noting that while high intraocular pressure has been associated with glaucoma, this is now considered a risk factor as opposed to a criterion for diagnosis (Jonas et al 2017).
5. **Retinopathy** refers to microvascular damage of the retina, which may develop slowly or rapidly, leading to blurred vision and progressive vision loss. Retinopathy is most often associated with chronic hypertension and type 1 or type 2 diabetes (Smith et al 2012). Diabetic retinopathy is caused by complex neuronal, glial and microvascular abnormalities that disrupt retinal function. Diabetic macular oedema and proliferative diabetic retinopathy are the major sight-threatening end points of diabetes (Lechner et al 2017). Occurrence of diabetic retinopathy is most often associated with duration of disease, poor glycaemic control, chronic hypertension, pregnancy, smoking and diabetic nephropathy. Almost everyone with type 1 diabetes and more than 60% of those with type 2 diabetes will develop some form of diabetic eye disease (Dirani 2013, Lechner et al 2017). There are two types of diabetic retinopathy: *non-proliferative retinopathy*, the most common form, and *proliferative retinopathy*, the most severe form which leads to irreversible blindness. In its early forms, diabetic eye disease may be asymptomatic, which is why regular eye examinations for persons with diabetes is vital. It is the leading cause of irreversible blindness in Australian adults (Dirani 2013). See Table 14.10.

Aside from these leading causes of eye disease, other conditions are seen. With ageing **lacrimal glands** involute, causing decreased tear production and a feeling of dryness and burning (known as *dry eye disease*). This is more common in women and with age (Findlay & Reid 2018). The **cornea** may show an infiltration of degenerative lipid material around the limbus. This is known as *arcus senilis* (see Figure 14.16 later in this chapter.) As the person grows older, pupil size decreases and the lens progressively hardens and loses its ability to change shape (accommodate); this leads to a decreased ability to focus on close objects with no coinciding changes to distance vision. This is known as **presbyopia**. As these changes occur progressively with age, symptoms will usually manifest in the early to mid-40s and necessitate the use of reading glasses (Smith et al 2012). Inside the posterior segment of the eye, **floaters** (vitreous opacities) may appear as a result of vitreous degeneration. People commonly describe these as blobs, spots or cobwebs in their vision.

CULTURAL AND SOCIAL CONSIDERATIONS

Australia and New Zealand are culturally diverse societies and the health practitioner will need to be familiar with specific variations and disease incidences that affect different cultural groups. Structural differences are evident in the palpebral fissures and epicanthic fold in individuals' eyes. Examples of this include narrowed palpebral fissures in persons of Asian origin, which in non-Asian individuals may be diagnostic of a serious congenital anomaly like Trisomy 21 (Down syndrome) (see Table 14.2).

Variability exists in the colour of the iris and in retinal pigmentation, with darker irides having darker retinas behind them. Individuals with light retinas generally have better night vision but can have pain in an environment that has too much light.

Specific populations within Australia and New Zealand are at higher risk for certain diseases that affect the eye. These groups include: Aboriginal and Torres Strait Islanders, Māori, the older adult, people with diabetes, those with a family history of eye disease and those who are considered marginalised and disadvantaged (Department of Health and Ageing 2015).

Prevalence of eye disease is three times higher in the Aboriginal and Torres Strait Islander community compared with the non-Indigenous community, and 90% of vision loss in Aboriginal and Torres Strait Islanders is preventable or treatable (Foreman et al 2016, AIHW 2017). Cataract, diabetic retinopathy, under-corrected refractive error and trachoma are the leading causes of blindness and vision impairment in Aboriginal and Torres Strait Islander communities (Foreman et al 2017).

Retinopathy is the third highest occurring eye disease. Diabetic retinopathy is more prevalent in Aboriginal and Torres Strait Islander populations in Australia and the Māori and Pacific Islander population in New Zealand than in non-Indigenous populations (Foreman et al 2017, Harvey 2010). This is due to higher rates of diabetes in these populations (New Zealand Ministry of Health 2018).

Trachoma is an infectious disease of the eye caused by *Chlamydia trachomatis* and is a significant factor in ocular morbidity within the Aboriginal community (Taylor et al 2014). Significant reductions in the incidence of trachoma in these populations have been made in recent years (Dirani et al 2017).

The higher rate of vision loss in these populations can be attributed to barriers to access and delays in diagnosis. Barriers to accessing eye healthcare include: health service barriers (infrastructure and systems, cost, transport and distance, interpreters, escorts, consent, trust of specialists); community (family influence, community influence, culture and beliefs); individual (ignorance, stoicism, fear, beliefs, demographics, other illnesses) (Foreman et al 2017, Boudville et al 2013). With cataract-related blindness being higher in Aboriginal and Torres Strait Islander populations and the surgery rate less than other Australians, there appears to be a marked under-provision of resources to these populations (Razavi et al 2018). Similarly, Māori and Pacific Islander populations have a higher prevalence of cataract after the age of 50 than other New Zealanders (Taylor & Mapp 2010).

Subjective data

Vision enables people to perform daily tasks and to learn about the world that surrounds them. The eye is the sensory organ of vision, which is the major source of sensory information. Disorders of the eye can affect so many parts of an individual's functional life. Accurate, systematic assessment can identify issues and provide focus for early treatment that may lead to sight preservation.

Subjective data can lead the nurse to focus more specifically on aspects of the eye examination, particularly in identifying symptoms that will not necessarily be evident in objective assessment. Other body systems that can affect the eye that you might consider when focusing your specific assessment questions include the cardiovascular, vascular and neurological systems. Eye assessment can also detect abnormalities that impact on other body systems such as the musculoskeletal system; such abnormalities might cause a risk of falling or the inability to complete activities of daily living independently. Subjective data assessment focuses on the following:

1. Presenting concern
2. Vision difficulty (decreased acuity, blurring, blind spots)
3. Pain
4. Strabismus (turned eye), diplopia (double vision)
5. Redness, swelling
6. Watering, discharge
7. History of ocular problems
8. Glaucoma
9. Use of glasses or contact lenses
10. Health and lifestyle management
11. Adjustment to vision loss (if relevant).

Practice note: Before you commence the assessment, introduce yourself to the person, confirm the person's identity, discuss the purpose and scope of the assessment, clarify any questions the person may have and obtain verbal consent from the person to perform the assessment.

ASSESSMENT GUIDELINES	CLINICAL SIGNIFICANCE AND CLINICAL ALERTS
1. Presenting concern	
Do you feel you have any problem with your vision or your eyes? It is important to ascertain the person's perception of their vision and eye health. If a problem is perceived ask, 'How does this impact on your quality of life?'	

ASSESSMENT GUIDELINES	CLINICAL SIGNIFICANCE AND CLINICAL ALERTS
2. Vision difficulty (decreased acuity, blurring, blind spots)	
• Any **difficulty seeing** or any blurring? Did this begin suddenly, or progress slowly?	Any decrease in vision has an impact on function and safety, which needs to be considered in planning care. ***Clinical alert:*** Any sudden change or new change in vision requires immediate referral to a medical practitioner.
• Is it in one eye or both eyes?	Loss or change in visual field in both eyes indicates the problem is after the *optic chiasm in the visual pathway*. Thus, the person may have suffered a stroke, brain injury or a tumour may be present.
• Is it constant, or does it come and go (intermittent)? How long does it last?	
• What part of the vision is affected? Is there a blind spot? Does it move as you shift your gaze? Any loss of peripheral vision?	If the central vision or colour vision is affected this suggests a problem with the *macula or optic nerve*. If only one part of the visual field is affected then *brain or visual pathway disease* may be present.
	Scotoma, a blind spot in the visual field surrounded by an area of normal or decreased vision, occurs with glaucoma and with optic nerve and visual pathway disorders.
• Is the vision distorted?	When straight lines look wavy (metamorphopsia), this may indicate *macular disease*, for example macular degeneration.
• Do spots move in front of your eyes (floaters)? Is there one or are there many? In one or both eyes? Are there also 'flashes' of light seen?	Floaters are common with myopia or after middle age as a result of condensed vitreous fibres. ***Clinical alert:*** Usually not significant, but acute onset of floaters ('shade' or 'cobwebs'), especially with associated 'flashes', may occur with retinal detachment. These people require immediate referral to a medical practitioner.
• Are there any halos/rainbows around objects? Or rings around lights?	Halos around lights occur with acute angle-closure glaucoma. ***Clinical alert:*** Halos with associated pain require immediate referral to a medical practitioner.
• Is there any trouble seeing in dim light (night blindness)?	Night blindness occurs with optic atrophy, glaucoma or vitamin A deficiency.
3. Pain	
• Is there any **eye pain**? Please describe. • Does it come on suddenly?	***Clinical alert:*** *Sudden onset* of eye symptoms (pain, floaters, blind spot, loss of peripheral vision) may be an emergency (such as acute glaucoma or foreign body). Refer immediately.

SUBJECTIVE DATA

SUBJECTIVE DATA

ASSESSMENT GUIDELINES	CLINICAL SIGNIFICANCE AND CLINICAL ALERTS
• Quality of pain. • Is it sharp, stabbing pain or pain with bright light (photophobia)? • Is burning or itching present? • Is there a foreign body sensation or grittiness? • Or deep aching? Or headache in the brow area, or behind the eye? • Is there scalp tenderness, pain in jaw when chewing?	**Photophobia** is inability to tolerate light. It is often associated with ocular inflammation. Itchy eyes are often due to allergic conjunctivitis. Grittiness is often due to dry eyes or blepharitis (inflammation of the eyelid), especially in the older adult. See Table 14.3 for further details. Note: some common eye problems cause no pain (e.g. refractive errors, cataract, open-angle glaucoma, detached retina). ***Clinical alert:*** In older people, headache with scalp tenderness and pain on chewing may indicate temporal arteritis, which is vision and life threatening. Refer to a medical practitioner immediately.
4. Strabismus (turned eye), diplopia (double vision)	
• Any history of crossed eyes? Now or in the past? Does this occur with eye fatigue? • Do you ever see double? Is this constant, or does it come and go? In one eye or both?	**Strabismus** is a deviation in the anteroposterior axis of the eye. **Diplopia** is the perception of two images of a single object. This type of visual change can significantly impact on a person's daily life.
5. Redness, swelling	
• Any redness or swelling in the eyes or eyelids? • Is one or both eyes affected?	
• Is there a history of: – Trauma or injury to the eye? – Eye disease or operations? – Any infections presently or in the past? When do/did these occur? Was this in a particular time of year? – Recent viral upper respiratory tract infection? – Contact lens wear?	Eye infections may be a result of bacterial, viral or fungal sources. Foreign-body-introduced infections are common from contact lens use, injuries, seasonal variations (pollens) and environmental factors (e.g. swimming in contaminated water). Recent viral upper respiratory tract infection can be associated with viral conjunctivitis. Advice should be given to the person regarding infection control measures to protect the unaffected eye and household members. ***Clinical alert:*** Eye infections can be very contagious and require immediate treatment by a medical practitioner.
6. Watering, discharge	
• Have you noticed **watering** or excessive tearing?	**Lacrimation** (tearing) and **epiphora** (excessive tearing) are due to increased reflex tearing (due to dry eye, soreness or irritants) or obstruction in drainage of tears.
• Do you have any **discharge**? Does it feel like there is anything in the eye that should not be there? Is it hard to open your eyes in the morning? What colour is the discharge? • How do you remove this from the eyes?	Purulent discharge is thick and yellow. Crusts often form at night. This is commonly associated with bacterial conjunctivitis. Assess hygiene practices and knowledge of cross-contamination. More common in children. ***Clinical alert:*** A person with discharge and associated pain, photophobia and decreased vision requires urgent referral.

ASSESSMENT GUIDELINES	CLINICAL SIGNIFICANCE AND CLINICAL ALERTS
7. History of ocular problems	
• Any family history of ocular problems? • Any history of injury or surgery to the eye? • Is there any history of allergies? • Is there any history of diseases with ocular manifestations such as type 1 or type 2 diabetes, hypertension, thyroid disease, cardiac disease, high cholesterol, migraine?	Some eye diseases have a genetic component; a family history of eye disease or blindness may be significant. Allergens may cause irritation of conjunctiva or cornea (e.g. make-up, contact lens solution, pollens).
8. Glaucoma	
• Have you ever been tested for **glaucoma**? What were the results? When were you tested for glaucoma? • Is there any family history of glaucoma?	Glaucoma is associated with increased intraocular pressure. Where there is a family history of glaucoma or if the person is more than 40 years of age, they should be advised to have regular eye examinations.
• If you have glaucoma, how do you manage your eye drops?	Adherence to the treatment regimen is often a problem, as treatment manages the disease but does not cure it. Assess ability to administer eye drops.
9. Use of glasses or contact lenses.	
• Do you wear **glasses** or **contact lenses**? How do they work for you? How long have you needed these?	
• Has your prescription been stable? When was the last time your prescription was checked? Was it changed?	
• If you wear contact lenses, are there any problems such as pain, photophobia, watering or swelling?	
• What type of contact lens do you wear? • How do you care for contacts? How long do you wear them? How do you clean them? • Do you remove them/wear them for certain activities?	Assess self-care behaviours as below. Some of these questions will only need to be asked once.
10. Health and lifestyle management.	
• When was your last vision test? Who tested it? • Have you ever had a colour vision test?	The current recommendation is that individuals should have their eyes tested every 2 years, or more often if recommended by a health professional or if there is a change in the vision. In Australia, optometrists provide most eye examinations free of charge under Medicare. In New Zealand, the Ministry of Health provides funding for children and low income families.
• Are there any environmental conditions at home or at work that may affect your eyes? For example, flying sparks, metal shards, smoke, dust, chemical fumes? If so, do you wear goggles to protect your eyes?	Provide education to prevent work-related eye injury (e.g. an auto mechanic with a foreign body from metal working or radiation damage from welding).
• What medications are you taking? Are they systemic or topical? • Do you take any medication specifically for the eyes?	Some medications have ocular side effects, e.g. prednisone may cause cataracts or increased intraocular pressure. Others can dilate or constrict the pupil, thus making it difficult to accommodate changes in light.

SUBJECTIVE DATA

ASSESSMENT GUIDELINES	CLINICAL SIGNIFICANCE AND CLINICAL ALERTS
11. Adjustment to vision loss (if relevant).	
• How has your life changed (roles and relationships, employment, nutrition, activity and exercise, history of recent falls)? • What are some of the strategies you use to manage (for example a change in layout within the home, reduced social activity)? • Do you need additional lighting or magnification? • Have you been referred to/are a current client of support services (e.g. Vision Australia)? • Do you use books with large print, audio books, Braille?	Be alert to people in a hospital setting or new to residential care who are vision impaired. They may require additional supports until they find their way around in new surroundings. They are at significant risk of injury. A constant spatial layout eases navigation through the home. If a person is an existing client of support services, collaboration with the service will assist in planning care.
Additional subjective data for infants and children (Questions for parents or guardian)	
• Did the mother have any vaginal infections at time of delivery?	Genital herpes and gonorrhoea vaginitis may have ocular sequelae for the newborn.
• Have you noticed any visual difficulties in your child? • Have you noticed a 'turned' or 'crossed' eye? • Does the child have routine vision testing at school? • Does your child have reading problems or complain of difficulty seeing the screens, whiteboard or TV? • Have you noticed a white or pale pupil in a photograph? (Usually the pupil should appear black or red.) • Which safety measures do you use to protect your child's eyes from trauma? Do you inspect toys? • Have you taught the child safe care with sharp objects and how to carry and how to use them? (Can include specifics such as not looking directly at the sun.)	The parent is most often the one to detect vision problems. While eye examinations are available under Medicare, vision testing in schools varies between States in Australia. Free testing for children is available in New Zealand through the Ministry of Health. An interruption in the pupillary red reflex indicates opacity in the cornea, lens or ocular media. This is often detected in family photographs. ***Clinical alert:*** An absent red reflex occurs with congenital cataracts or retinal disorders. A white reflex or 'pupil' may indicate a serious intraocular tumour (retinoblastoma). The child should be referred urgently.
Additional subjective data for adults over 65 years	
• Have you had to decrease any of your usual activities, such as reading, driving or sewing? Had difficulty using equipment, for example the telephone or computer?	Age-related macular degeneration causes a loss in central vision acuity that can impact on activities of daily living.
• Have you experienced a loss of independence, such as problems climbing stairs, crossing the road or driving?	Age-related macular degeneration can result in loss of depth perception or decreased central vision. The person should be referred to a medical practitioner.
• Is there a history of cataracts? Any loss or progressive blurring of vision? Have you had cataract surgery? • Do you suffer from glare sensitivity, e.g. from lights when driving at night?	**Cataract** is opacity of the crystalline lens and commonly occurs in persons over the age of 60. It is usually a bilateral condition, although degree of progression may vary between eyes. Cataract can cause glare sensitivity due to the opacities in the lens scattering light, rather than focusing it.
• Do your eyes ever feel dry, burn or water excessively? What do you do for this?	Decreased tear production may occur with ageing. Use of artificial lubricants can improve comfort for these persons.

Objective data

Objective data assists the nurse to complete the eye assessment by collecting verifiable data, which is information gained by physical examination and any investigations. Generalist nurses do not usually perform the majority of physical assessment techniques related to eye examination. However, nurses working in specialist centres, emergency departments, primary care and community settings may develop advanced skill in using more complex assessment techniques such as use of eye assessment equipment (e.g. tonometers, Snellen charts, etc). Documentation of this data also takes a specific form and needs to follow a logical sequence (e.g. visual acuity documented as 6/6 means the person can read to line 6 on the Snellen chart at 6 m distance from the chart). Visual acuity is often the focal point of the objective data collected.

Preparation

Have the person sitting comfortably in an upright position where possible. The examiner should sit or stand opposite the person so that they can maintain a straight back. Ensure the examination takes place in a well-lit environment.

Equipment needed

Opaque card or occluder
Penlight
Hand hygiene solution

PROCEDURES AND NORMAL FINDINGS	ABNORMAL FINDINGS AND CLINICAL ALERTS
General inspection	
Already you will have noted the person's ability to move around the room, with vision functioning well enough to avoid obstacles and respond to your directions. Also note the facial expression, looking specifically for squinting, grimacing and so on. Note also the person's head posture and facial symmetry.	Note groping with hands while walking and squinting or craning forwards. Abnormal head posture may indicate a problem with a particular area of the visual field. Asymmetrical facial appearance may indicate nerve involvement.
Inspect external ocular structures	
Begin with the most external points, and logically work your way inwards.	
Eyebrows	
Normally the eyebrows are present bilaterally, move symmetrically as the facial expression changes and have no scaling or lesions.	Hypothyroidism often causes the lateral third of brow to be absent. Unequal or absent movement of brows may be present with nerve damage. Scaling occurs with seborrhoea.
Eyelids and lashes	
The upper lids normally overlap the superior part of the iris, and approximate completely with the lower lids when closed. The skin is intact without redness, swelling, discharge or lesions.	Hyperthyroidism causes lid lag. Incomplete closure of lids creates risk for corneal damage. ***Ectropion*** occurs when lower lid turns outwards, ***entropion*** is when the lower lid turns inwards. Both of these findings are abnormal and can predispose the person to corneal damage and eye infection (see Table 14.2). **Ptosis** is drooping of upper lid. For examples of eyelid abnormalities and lesions see Tables 14.2 and 14.3.
The **palpebral fissures** are horizontal in non-Asian people, whereas Asian people normally have an upward slant to the eye.	**Blepharospasm** is increased blink rate that occurs in spasms. It can be an inability to open eyelid. This is usually due to inflammation or malfunction of cranial nerves V and VII. It can occur in exposure to bright lights.

PROCEDURES AND NORMAL FINDINGS	ABNORMAL FINDINGS AND CLINICAL ALERTS
Note that the eyelashes are evenly distributed along the lid margins and curve outwards. Observe that the eyelid area is free of redness, swelling or rash.	**Xanthelasma** is raised yellowish plaques on the nasal portion of the eyelid; these are often associated with lipid disorders but can be a normal finding (see Figure 14.17). Periorbital oedema, when the lids are swollen, may indicate local infection or systemic conditions (see Table 14.2). ***Clinical alert:*** **Orbital cellulitis** is an acute purulent inflammation of the cellular tissue of the orbit. It is an ophthalmic emergency. The person should be referred urgently (see Table 14.2).
Eyeballs	
The eyeballs are aligned normally in their sockets with no protrusion or sunken appearance.	**Exophthalmos** (protruding eyes) and **enophthalmos** (sunken eyes) (see Table 14.2). Exophthalmos can be associated with thyroid eye disease and may result in exposure (drying) of the cornea.
Conjunctiva and sclera	
Ask the person to look up. Using your thumbs, slide the lower lids down along the bony orbital rim. Take care not to push against the eyeball. Inspect the exposed area (Figure 14.9). The eyeball looks moist and glossy. Numerous small blood vessels normally show through the transparent conjunctiva. Otherwise, the conjunctivae are clear and show the normal colour of the structure below—pink over the lower lids and white over the sclera. Note any colour change, swelling or lesions. 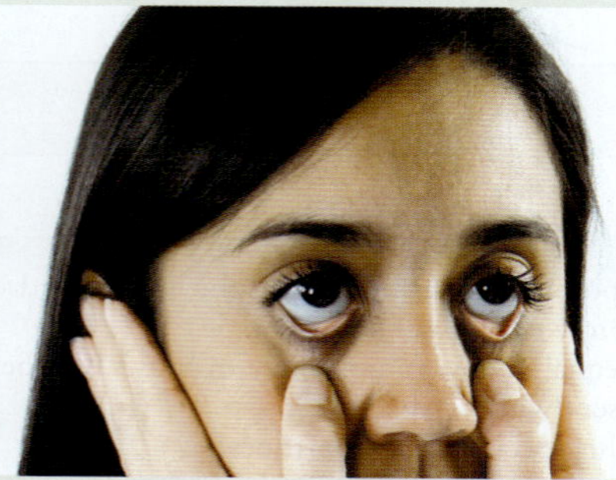 **Figure 14.9** Sclera.	Note abnormal findings such as general reddening (see Table 14.6). Pallor near the outer canthus of the lower lid may indicate anaemia (the inner canthus normally contains less pigment).
The sclera is china white, although those with dark pigmented skin occasionally have a grey-blue or 'muddy' colour to the sclera. You may see small brown macules (like freckles) on the sclera, which are normal and should not be confused with foreign bodies or petechiae. 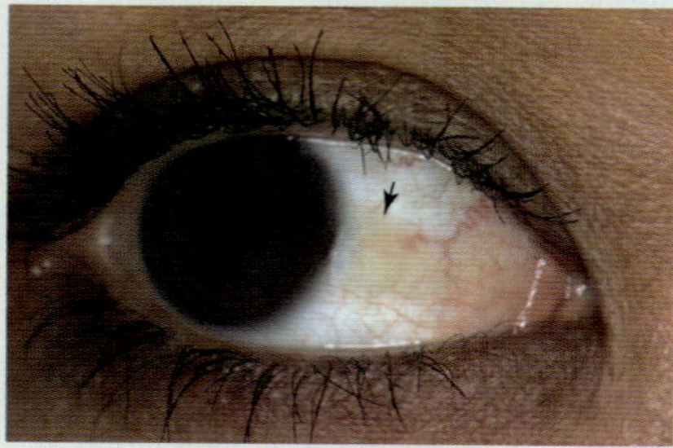 **Figure 14.10** Pinguecula.	**Scleral icterus** is an even yellowing of the sclera extending up to the cornea, indicating jaundice. Note any tenderness, foreign body, discharge or lesions. **Pinguecula** growth on conjunctiva due to chronic ultraviolet light or other environmental exposure—see Figure 14.10.

PROCEDURES AND NORMAL FINDINGS	ABNORMAL FINDINGS AND CLINICAL ALERTS
Inspect anterior eyeball structures	
Cornea and lens	
Shine a light from the side across the cornea, and check for smoothness and clarity. This oblique view highlights any abnormal irregularities in the corneal surface. There should be no opacities (cloudiness) in or on the cornea, the anterior chamber or the lens behind the pupil. Do not confuse an **arcus senilis** with an opacity.	A **corneal abrasion** causes irregular ridges in reflected light, producing a shattered look to light rays (see Table 14.7). This is associated with foreign body sensation or pain. **Arcus senilis** is a grey-white arc or circle around the limbus due to deposition of lipid material. It is a normal finding in ageing persons (see Figure 14.16). **Pterygium** is an abnormal triangular growth over the cornea and sclera (Table 14.7).
Iris and pupil	
The iris normally appears flat, with a round regular shape and even colouration. Note the size, shape and equality of the pupils. Normally the pupils appear round, regular and of equal size in both eyes. In the adult, resting size is from 3 to 5 mm. A small number of people (5%) normally have pupils of two different sizes, which is termed **anisocoria** (Table 14.4).	***Clinical alert***: Look for irregular pupil shape. Ask if this is old or new. Irregularly shaped pupils may indicate intraocular inflammation or infection, previous eye surgery or injury. Although they may be normal, all unequally sized pupils should be investigated to rule out central nervous system injury, tumour or local trauma.
To test the **pupillary light reflex**, darken the room and ask the person to gaze into the distance (this dilates the pupils). Ensure you have a strong, bright light. Advance a light in from the side and note the response. Normally you will see (1) constriction of the same-sided pupil (a *direct light reflex*) and (2) simultaneous constriction of the other pupil (a *consensual light reflex*). See Chapter 12 for further detail. Always advance the light in from the *side* to test the light reflex. If you advance from the front, the pupils will constrict to accommodate for near vision and confuse the test results.	Abnormal findings include: Dilated pupils. Dilated and fixed pupils. Constricted pupils. Unequal or no response to light (see Table 14.4). Some systemic medications (such as opioids) or eye drops can effect the size of the pupil.
Visual acuity—test vision	
A simple but effective method for most nurses includes asking the person to read a magazine or brochure (to test near vision) and a sign or clock on the wall (for distance vision), making the necessary adjustments for people who read a language other than English or who are unable to read. The information gained will assist you to adjust health information to meet the person's individual needs and to make referrals to other health professionals as necessary. Advanced practice nurses may use a range of techniques to test visual acuity (see section titled 'Further objective assessment for advanced practice').	Visual acuity only assesses the person's macular function. Even if a person has good visual acuity, they can be visually impaired due to other eye problems.
Visual field—confrontation test	
This is a gross measure of peripheral vision. It compares the person's peripheral vision with your own, assuming yours is normal (Figure 14.11). Position yourself at eye level with the person, about 60 cm away. Direct the person to cover one eye with an opaque card, and with the other eye to look straight at you. Cover your own eye opposite to the person's covered one. You are testing the uncovered eye. Hold a pencil or your flicking finger as a target midline between you and the other person, and slowly advance it in from the periphery in several directions.	

PROCEDURES AND NORMAL FINDINGS	ABNORMAL FINDINGS AND CLINICAL ALERTS
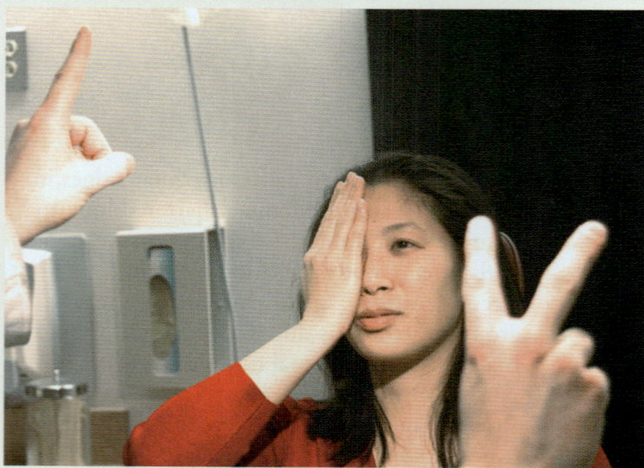 **Figure 14.11**	
Ask the person to say 'now' as the target is first seen; this should be just as you see the object also. (This works with all but the temporal visual field, with which you would need a 1.8 m arm to avoid being seen initially! With the temporal direction, start the object somewhat behind the person.) Estimate the angle between the anteroposterior axis of the eye and the peripheral axis where the object is first seen. Normal results are about 50 degrees upwards, 90 degrees temporal, 70 degrees down and 60 degrees nasal (Figure 14.12). 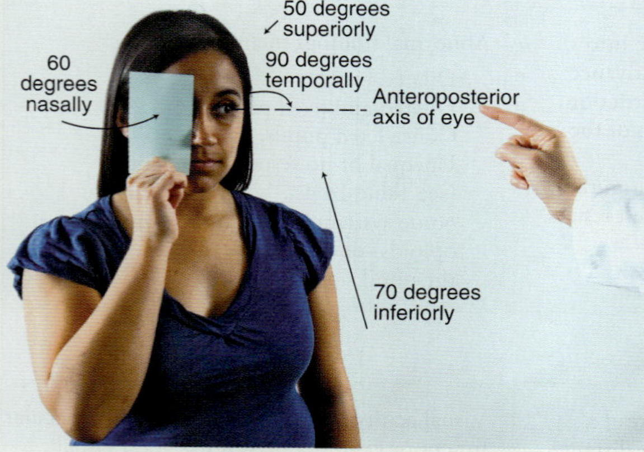 **Figure 14.12** Range of peripheral vision.	Abnormalities in peripheral vision can occur following stroke or head injury or with abnormalities of the eye or visual pathway. (See Table 14.5.) Visual field loss can lead to risk of injury due to bumping into objects or falling and has implications for driving.
Additional objective data for infants and children (birth to 12 years)	
The eye examination is often deferred at birth because of transient oedema of the lids from birth trauma. The eyes should be examined within a few days and at every well-child visit thereafter. Currently, in Australia, there is limited consistency in how and when visual screening is performed in children. This includes inconsistencies in number of vision checks recommended, when age screening is undertaken, the tools and procedures used, the personnel conducting screening and referral and follow-up of the screening (White et al 2017).	***Clinical alert:*** prevalence data of common visual conditions in Australian children is inconsistent. In 2008, there were more than 411,000 cases of long-term eye disorders among children, with most of these being long- and short-sightedness (AIHW 2008). **Amblyopia** (poor or indistinct vision in an eye that is otherwise physically normal) affects approximately 1.9% of children (Pai et al 2012). Strabismus (turned eye) affects 0.3–7.3% (Morcos & Wright 2009).

PROCEDURES AND NORMAL FINDINGS	ABNORMAL FINDINGS AND CLINICAL ALERTS
Test **light perception** using the blink reflex; the neonate blinks in response to bright light (Figure 14.13). Also, the pupillary light reflex shows that the pupils constrict in response to light. These reflexes indicate that the lower portion of the visual apparatus is intact. But you cannot infer that the infant can *see*; that requires later observation to show that the brain has received images and can interpret them. 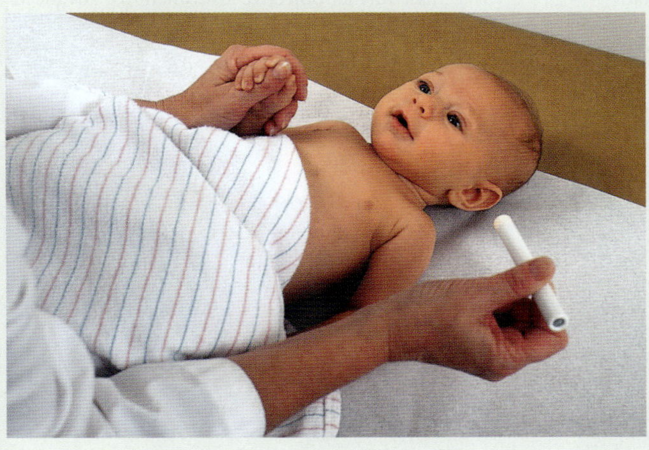 Figure 14.13	***Clinical alert:*** Look for absence of blinking, and pupillary light reflex, especially after 3 weeks, as this may indicate blindness.
As you introduce an object to the infant's line of vision, note these attending behaviours: **Birth to 2 weeks**—Refusal to reopen eyes after exposure to bright light; increasing alertness to object; infant may fixate on an object. **By 2 to 4 weeks**—Infant can fixate on an object. **By 1 month**—Infant can fixate and follow a light or bright toy. **By 3 to 4 months**—Infant can fixate, follow and reach for the toy. **By 6 to 10 months**—Infant can fixate and follow the toy in all directions.	Centre for Community Child Health (2009) advises that available evidence suggests screening for vision should be undertaken from 18 months of age and no later than 5 years of age, in addition to the standard neonatal check. Exceptions are made for newborns with existing congenital vision conditions.
External eye structures. Inspect the ocular structures as described in the earlier section. A neonate usually holds the eyes tightly shut. Do not attempt to pry them open; that just increases contraction of the orbicularis oculi muscle. Hold the newborn supine and gently lower the head; the eyes will open. Also, the eyes will open when you hold the infant at arm's length and slowly turn the infant in one direction. In addition to inspecting the ocular structures, this also tests the vestibular function reflex. That is, the baby's eyes will look in the same direction as the body is being turned. When the turning stops, the eyes will shift to the opposite direction after a few quick beats of nystagmus. Also termed 'doll's eyes', this reflex disappears by 2 months of age.	
Eyelids and lashes. Normally, the upper lids overlie the superior part of the iris. In newborns the *setting-sun sign* is common. The eyes appear to deviate down, and you see a white rim of sclera over the iris. It may show as you rapidly change the neonate from a sitting to a supine position.	The setting-sun sign also occurs with hydrocephalus as the globes protrude. Blank sunken eyes accompany malnutrition, dehydration and a severe illness.

OBJECTIVE DATA

PROCEDURES AND NORMAL FINDINGS	ABNORMAL FINDINGS AND CLINICAL ALERTS
Many infants have an *epicanthal fold*, an excess skinfold extending over the inner corner of the eye, partly or totally overlapping the inner canthus. It occurs frequently in children of Asian descent and in 20% of other children. In children of non-Asian descent, it disappears as the child grows, usually by 10 years of age. While they are present, epicanthal folds give a false appearance of malalignment, termed **pseudostrabismus** (Figure 14.14). Yet the corneal light reflex is normal. **Figure 14.14** Pseudostrabismus.	The **corneal light reflex** is assessed by shining a bright torch towards both eyes from in front of the child. When the eyes are correctly aligned the light reflection from the torch will appear in the same location on each cornea. (See further objective assessment for advanced practice.)
Infants of Asian descent normally have an upward slant of the palpebral fissures. Entropion, a turning inward of the eyelid, is found normally in some children of Asian descent. If the lashes do not abrade the corneas, it is not significant.	An upward lateral slope together with epicanthal folds and hypertelorism (large spacing between eyes) occurs with people with trisomy 21 (Down syndrome) (see Table 14.2).
Conjunctiva and sclera. The conjunctiva should be clear and show the normal colour of the structure below—pink over the lower lids and white over the sclera. Note any colour change or discharge. The sclera should be white and clear, although it may have a blue tint as a result of thinness at birth. The lacrimal glands are not functional at birth.	Conjunctivitis infections account for most general practice encounters involving children with eye conditions ***Clinical alert:*** Ophthalmia neonatorum (conjunctivitis of the newborn) is a purulent discharge caused by a bacterial or viral agent from the birth canal. Refer to medical practitioner.
Iris and pupils. The iris normally is blue or slate grey in light-skinned newborns and brown in dark-skinned infants. By 6–9 months, the permanent colour is differentiated. Brushfield's spots, or white specks around the edge of the iris, occasionally may be normal.	Absence of iris colour occurs with albinism. This results in poor vision due to excess light entering the eye. Brushfield's spots usually suggest Trisomy 21 (Down syndrome).
The **crystalline lens** of a newborn is colourless, clear and spherical.	**Cataract,** opacity of the crystalline lens, can occur congenitally. When a torch is shone in the eye, a white reflex in the pupil may be seen.
A searching nystagmus is common just after birth. The pupils are small but constrict to light.	***Clinical alert:*** Abnormality: Constant nystagmus, prolonged setting-sun sign, marked strabismus and slow lateral movements suggest vision loss. Refer to a medical practitioner.
Additional objective data for the adult over 65 years	
Ocular structures. The eyebrows may show a loss of the outer one-third to one-half of hair because of a decrease in hair follicles. The remaining brow hair is coarse (Figure 14.15). As a result of atrophy of elastic tissues, the skin around the eyes may show wrinkles or crow's feet. The upper lid may be so elongated as to rest on the lashes, resulting in a **pseudoptosis**.	

OBJECTIVE DATA

PROCEDURES AND NORMAL FINDINGS	ABNORMAL FINDINGS AND CLINICAL ALERTS
Figure 14.15 Pseudoptosis.	
The eyes may appear sunken from atrophy of the orbital fat. Also, the orbital fat may herniate, causing bulging at the lower lids and inner third of the upper lids.	Look for ectropion (lower lid dropping away) and entropion (lower lid turning in) (see Table 14.2).
The lacrimal apparatus may decrease tear production, causing the eyes to look dry and lustreless. The person may report a burning sensation or grittiness. **Pingueculae** commonly show on the sclera (see Figure 14.10). These yellowish elevated nodules are due to a thickening of the bulbar conjunctiva from prolonged exposure to sun, wind and dust. Pingueculae appear at the 3 and 9 o'clock positions—first on the nasal side, then on the temporal side.	Distinguish pinguecula from the abnormal **pterygium**, also an opacity on the bulbar conjunctiva, but one that grows over the cornea (see Table 14.7). This subsequently disrupts the normal tear film, often causing a foreign body sensation.
The cornea may look cloudy with age. An **arcus senilis** is commonly seen around the cornea (Figure 14.16). This is a grey-white arc or circle around the limbus; it is due to deposition of lipid material. As more lipid accumulates, the cornea may look thickened and raised, but the arcus has no effect on vision. **Figure 14.16** Arcus senilis.	
Xanthelasma are soft, raised yellow plaques occurring on the lids at the inner canthus (Figure 14.17). They commonly occur around the fifth decade of life and more frequently in women. They occur with both high and normal blood levels of cholesterol and have no pathological significance.	

OBJECTIVE DATA

PROCEDURES AND NORMAL FINDINGS	ABNORMAL FINDINGS AND CLINICAL ALERTS
Figure 14.17 Xanthelasma.	
Pupils are small in old age, and the pupillary light reflex may be slowed. The lens loses transparency and looks opaque.	**Cataract** is opacity of the crystalline lens and commonly occurs in persons over the age of 60. It is usually a bilateral condition, although degree of progression may vary between eyes. Cataract can also occur due to metabolic disease, certain medications or trauma.

Further objective assessment for advanced practice

The assessments described in the following sections require advanced skill and scope of practice. Nurses working in specialist eye hospitals and clinics and some community and emergency nurses need to develop these skills.

Preparation

The person should be positioned at the distance specified from the eye chart (e.g. 3 m or 6 m). The examination environment should be well lit.

Equipment needed

In addition to the equipment listed previously you will require:

- Snellen eye chart and pinhole occluder
- Handheld visual screener (near vision card)
- Applicator stick
- Ophthalmoscope
- Amsler grid
- Hand hygiene solution

PROCEDURES AND NORMAL FINDINGS	ABNORMAL FINDINGS AND CLINICAL ALERTS
Inspect extraocular muscle function	
Corneal light reflex (the Hirschberg test)	
Assess the parallel alignment of the eye axes by shining a light towards the person's eyes. Direct the person to stare straight ahead as you hold the light about 30 cm away. Note the reflection of the light on the corneas; it should be in exactly the same spot on each eye. See the bright white dots in asymmetrical corneal light reflex in Figure 14.18 for symmetry of the corneal light reflex. Some asymmetry (where one light falls off centre) under 6 months is normal. 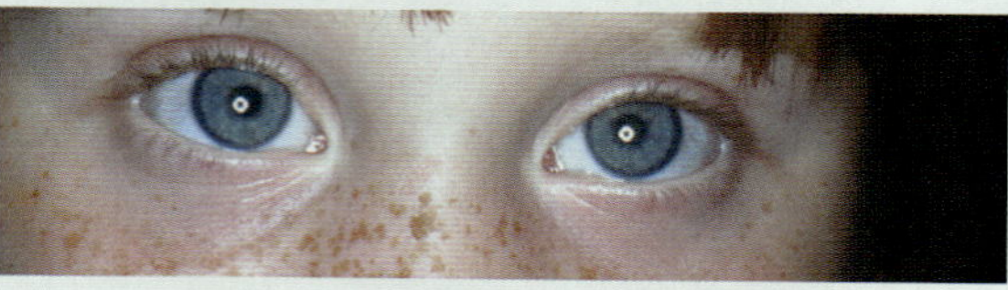 **Figure 14.18** Corneal light reflex	Asymmetry of the light reflex indicates deviation in alignment from eye muscle weakness or paralysis. If you see this, perform the cover test.

PROCEDURES AND NORMAL FINDINGS	ABNORMAL FINDINGS AND CLINICAL ALERTS
Cover test	
This test detects small degrees of deviated alignment by interrupting the fusion reflex that normally keeps the two eyes parallel. Ask the person to stare straight ahead at your nose even though the gaze may be interrupted. With an opaque card, cover one eye. As it is covered, note the uncovered eye. A normal response is a steady fixed gaze (Figure 14.19A).	If the eye 'jumps' to fixate on the designated point, it was out of alignment before. Meanwhile, the macular image has been suppressed on the covered eye. If muscle weakness exists, the covered eye will drift into a relaxed position.
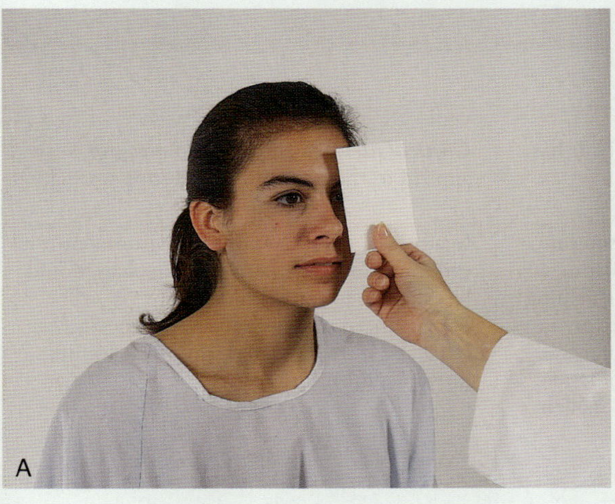 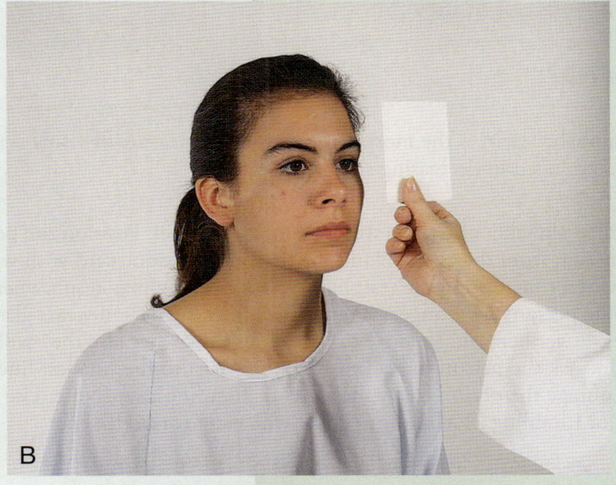 **Figure 14.19** Cover test	
Now uncover the eye and observe it for movement. It should stare straight ahead (Figure 14.19B). If it jumps to re-establish fixation, eye muscle weakness exists. Repeat with the other eye.	A **phoria** is a mild weakness noted only during the cover test. **A tropia** is a constant malalignment of the eyes (see Table 14.1c).
Diagnostic positions test	
Leading the eyes through the six cardinal positions of gaze will elicit any muscle weakness during movement (Figure 14.20). Ask the person to hold the head steady and to follow the movement of your finger, pen or penlight only with the eyes. Hold the target back about 30 cm so the person can focus on it comfortably, and move it to each of the six positions, hold it momentarily, then back to centre. Progress clockwise. A normal response is parallel tracking of the object with both eyes.	When eye movement is not parallel there is an abnormality. Failure to follow in a certain direction indicates weakness of an extraocular muscle (EOM) or dysfunction of the cranial nerve innervating it (see cranial nerves for each direction in Table 14.1).
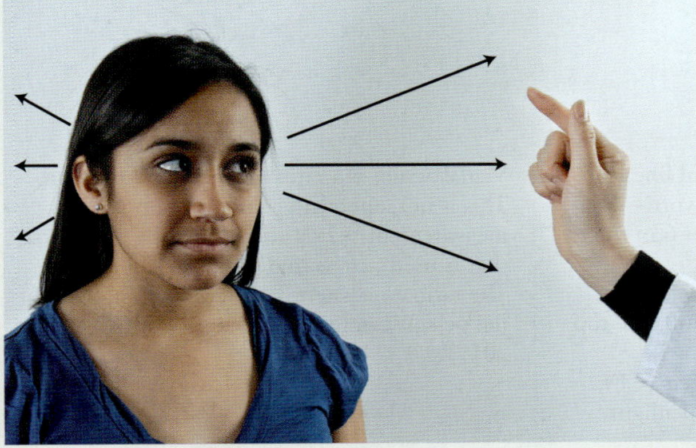 **Figure 14.20** Diagnostic positions test.	

PROCEDURES AND NORMAL FINDINGS	ABNORMAL FINDINGS AND CLINICAL ALERTS
In addition to parallel movement, note any **nystagmus**, a fine oscillating movement best seen around the iris. Mild nystagmus at extreme lateral gaze is normal; nystagmus at any other position is not.	**Nystagmus** is caused by disease of the semicircular canals in the ears, a paretic eye muscle, multiple sclerosis or brain lesions.
Finally, note that the upper eyelid continues to overlap the superior part of the iris, even during downward movement. You should not see a white rim of sclera between the lid and the iris. If noted, this is termed 'lid lag'.	Lid lag occurs with hyperthyroidism.
Test central—visual acuity	
Snellen eye chart	
The Snellen alphabet chart is the most commonly used measure of visual acuity. It has lines of letters arranged in decreasing size.	***Clinical alert:*** Ensure that no pressure is applied to the ocular surface during testing.
Place the Snellen alphabet chart in a well-lit spot at eye level. Position the person on a mark exactly 6 m from the chart. Hand the person an opaque card with which to shield one eye at a time during the test; inadvertent peeking may result when shielding the eye with the person's own fingers (Figure 14.21). If the person wears glasses or contact lenses, leave them on. Remove only reading glasses because they will blur distance vision. Ask the person to read through the chart to the smallest line of letters possible. Encourage the person to try the next smallest line also. (Note: Use a Snellen picture chart or tumbling 'E' chart for people who cannot read letters.) 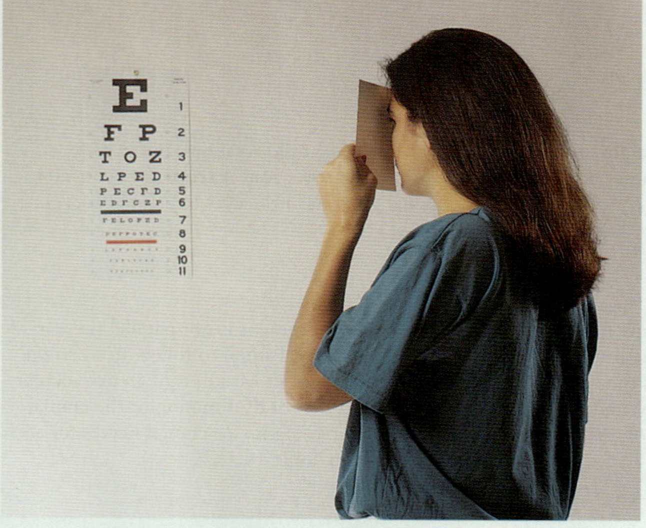 **Figure 14.21**	In a typical medical/surgical environment it is extremely unlikely that a Snellen chart would be available to test vision acuity. For advanced practice nurses, use the Snellen chart and note hesitancy, squinting, leaning forwards, misreading letters.
Record the result using the numeric fraction at the end of the last successful line read. Indicate whether the person missed any letters or if corrective lenses were worn—for example, 'right 6/12, with glasses' (with the right eye, at the test distance of 6 m the person read to line 12 with their glasses on). If the person is unable to see even the largest letters, shorten the distance to the chart until the top letter is seen and record that distance (e.g. '4/60' at 4 m, line 60 (the top letter) was read). If visual acuity is even lower, assess whether the person can count your fingers (CF), see hand movement (HM) or distinguish light perception (PL) from your penlight. The standard distance for these tests is 30 cm. If the person is unable to perceive light vision is recorded as 'no perception of light' (NPL).	Visual acuity is a ratio recorded as a fraction. This is not a percentage of vision, but a measurement that is affected by the eye chart that is used (e.g. 6 m or 3 m Snellen chart). The ratio equals test distance/smallest line that the person can read the majority of (Marsden 2017).

PROCEDURES AND NORMAL FINDINGS	ABNORMAL FINDINGS AND CLINICAL ALERTS
Normal visual acuity is 6/6 using a 6 m chart and means, 'You can read at 6 m what the normal eye could have read at 6 m'.	Impaired vision may be due to refractive error, opacity in the media (cornea, lens, vitreous) or disorder in the retina or optic pathway. In Australia, a visual acuity of 6/12 or better with both eyes is the legal driving limit. Visual acuity of 6/18 or worse is termed moderate vision Impairment (World Health Organization 2019). A person with visual acuity of 6/60 or worse in the better eye is considered legally blind and may be eligible for various entitlements and assistance (AIHW 2016).
Pinhole test	
A pinhole test is used when visual acuity is diminished. A pinhole occluder (solid occluder with multiple 19 gauge needle holes) is held over the eye in place of the standard occluder and the test is performed as described above. Results are recorded noting that the pinholes were used to look through, e.g. right eye 6/6 with pinhole.	A test using the pinhole mask can identify those people with poor vision due to refractive error, and in some cases of cataract or corneal scarring. The mask has very small holes in the area in front of the pupil. People who have visual acuity improved with the pinhole should be referred for examination and treatment by an eye care practitioner as their visual acuity is likely to be due to refractive error rather than a disease process.
Near vision	
For people over 40 years of age or for those who report increasing difficulty reading, a test of near vision is performed. A handheld vision screener with various sizes of print, with each size attributed a number (e.g. a Jaeger card) is used (Figure 14.22). Hold the card in good light at a comfortable reading distance (about 35 cm from the eye). Test each eye separately, with glasses on. Near visual acuity is recorded in point notation (the same as for computer font), which relates to the smallest line of print the person reads comfortably. A person with normal near vision can read 4-point type at 35 cm. The person should be able to read without hesitancy and without moving the card closer or further away. 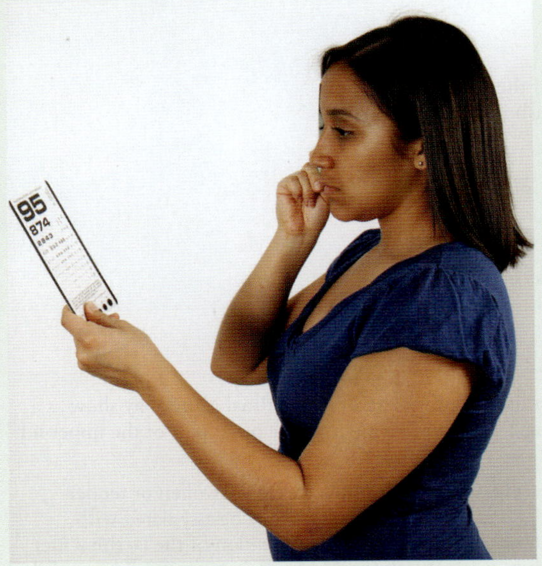 Figure 14.22 Near vision test	**Presbyopia**, the decrease in the lens' ability to accommodate with ageing, is suspected when the person moves the card further away. In case you do not have a Jaeger card, normal newspaper print is 8-point type (N8).

OBJECTIVE DATA

PROCEDURES AND NORMAL FINDINGS	ABNORMAL FINDINGS AND CLINICAL ALERTS
Inspect external ocular structures	
Eversion of the upper lid	
This manoeuvre is not part of the normal examination, but it is useful when you must inspect the conjunctiva of the upper lid, as with eye pain or suspicion of a foreign body. Most people are apprehensive of any eye manipulation. Enhance their cooperation by using a calm and gentle, yet deliberate, approach.	***Clinical alert:*** Eyelid eversion should not be attempted if a penetrating eye injury is suspected.
1. Ask the person to keep both eyes open and look down. This relaxes the eyelid, whereas closing it would tense the orbicularis muscle. 2. Slide the upper lid up along the bony orbit to lift up the eyelashes. 3. Grasp the lashes between your thumb and forefinger and gently pull down and outwards. 4. With your other hand, place the tip of an applicator stick on the upper lid above the level of the internal tarsal plates (Figs 14.23A).	Eyelid eversion is a skill that should be practised. It is most easily performed on older people due to the normal atrophy of eyelid tissues associated with age.
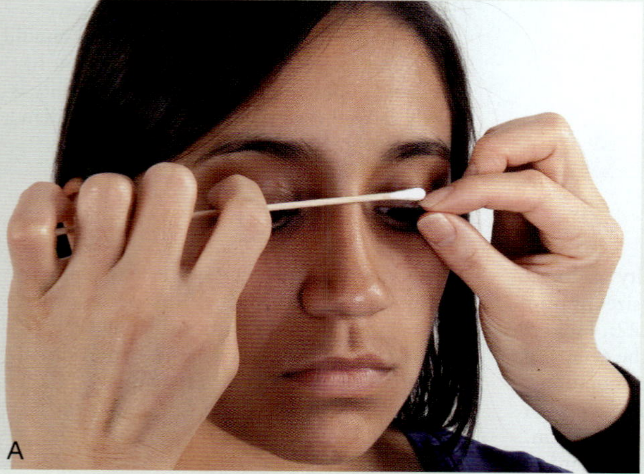 A 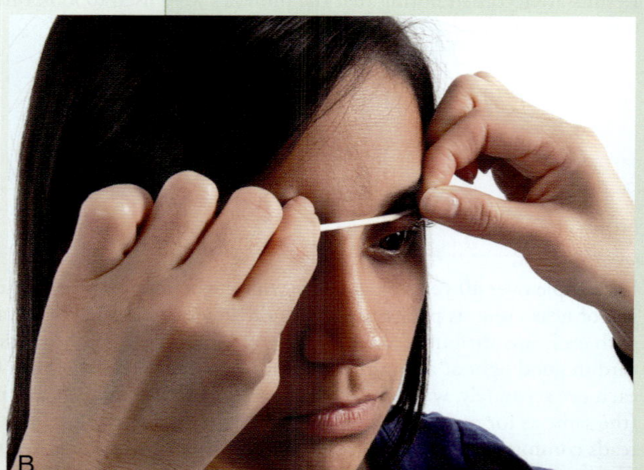 B **Figure 14.23** Eyelid eversion	
5. Gently push down with the stick as you lift the lashes up. This uses the edge of the tarsal plate as a fulcrum and flips the lid inside out. Take special care not to push in on the eyeball. 6. Secure the everted position by holding the lashes against the bony orbital rim (Figure 14.23B). 7. Inspect for any colour change, swelling, lesion or foreign body. 8. To return to normal position, gently pull the lashes outwards as the person looks up.	
Lacrimal apparatus	
Ask the person to look down. With your thumbs, slide the outer part of the upper lid up along the bony orbit to expose under the lid. Inspect for any redness or swelling.	Swelling of the lacrimal gland may show as a visible bulge in the outer part of the upper lid.
Normally, the puncta drain the tears into the lacrimal sac. Presence of excessive tearing may indicate blockage of the nasolacrimal duct. Check this by pressing the index finger against the sac, just inside the lower orbital rim, not against the side of the nose (Figure 14.24). Pressure will slightly evert the lower lid, but there should be no other response to pressure.	Note if puncta are red, swollen or tender to pressure. This may be associated with **dacryocystitis** (infection of the lacrimal sac). Watch for any regurgitation of fluid out of the puncta, which confirms duct blockage.

OBJECTIVE DATA

PROCEDURES AND NORMAL FINDINGS	ABNORMAL FINDINGS AND CLINICAL ALERTS
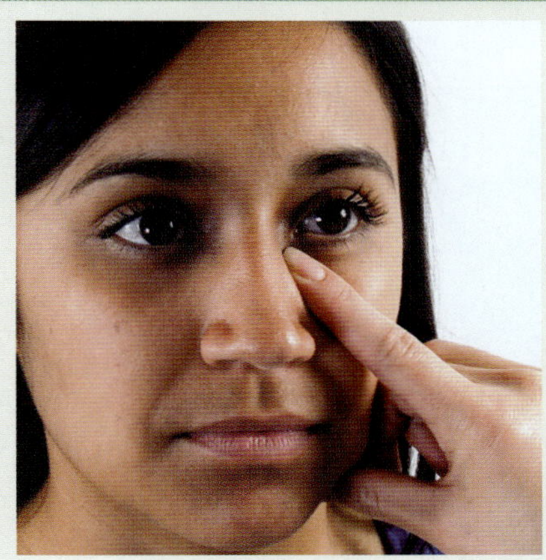 **Figure 14.24** Punctal inspection	
Inspect anterior eyeball structures	
Test pupillary response to **accommodation** by asking the person to focus on a distant object (Figure 14.25). This process dilates the pupils. Then have the person shift the gaze to a near object, such as your finger held about 7–8 cm from the nose. A normal response includes (1) pupillary constriction and (2) convergence of the axes of the eyes.	Note any absence of constriction or convergence or an asymmetric response.
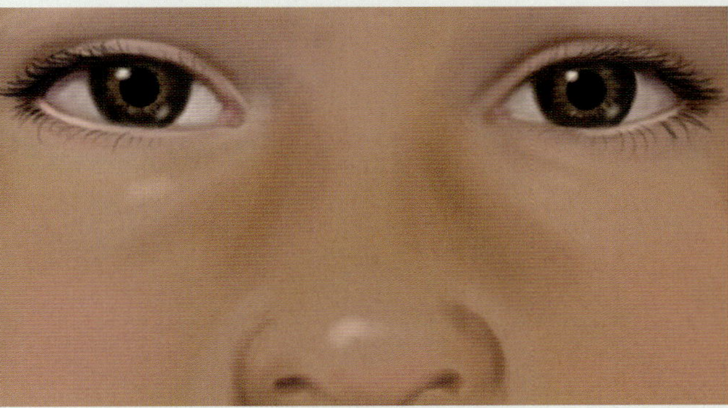 Far vision—pupils dilate 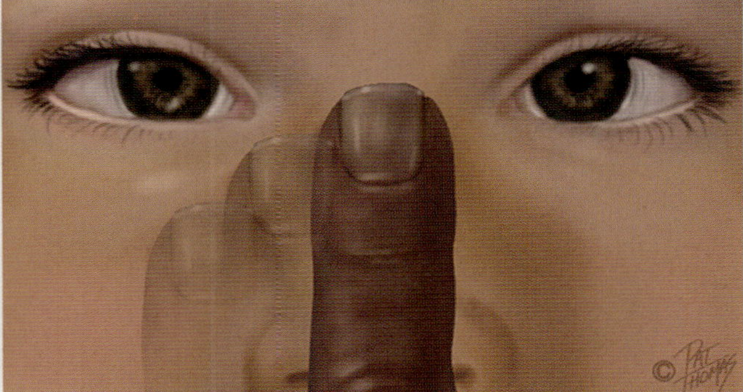 Near vision—pupils constrict **Figure 14.25** Pupillary response to accommodation	
Test for relative afferent papillary defect (RAPD) by performing the 'swinging torch test'. Dim or turn off room lights and use the brightest light available. Ask the person to focus in the distance. First observe the **pupillary light reflex** (as described earlier), noting *direct* and *consensual* constriction of the pupil in response to the light. Next, move the light briskly from one eye to the other. A normal response is for each pupil to **constrict** when the torch is shone on it. A relative pupillary defect (abnormal response) is when the torch is swung from one eye to the other and the pupil of the illuminated eye **dilates** (becomes larger) instead of constricting as is normal (Talley & O'Connor 2018).	The presence of a relative afferent pupil defect alerts you that the person has seriously reduced visual acuity (Talley & O'Connor 2018).

OBJECTIVE DATA

PROCEDURES AND NORMAL FINDINGS	ABNORMAL FINDINGS AND CLINICAL ALERTS
Inspect the ocular fundus	
The ophthalmoscope enlarges your view of the eye so that you can inspect the *media* (anterior chamber, lens, vitreous) and the *ocular fundus* (the internal surface of the retina). It accomplishes this by directing a beam of light through the pupil to illuminate the inner structures. The ophthalmoscope should function as an appendage of your own eye. This takes some practice. Practise holding the instrument and focusing at objects around the room before you approach the person. Hold the ophthalmoscope right up to your eye, braced firmly against the cheek and brow. Extend your index finger onto the lens selector dial so that you can refocus as needed during the procedure without taking your head away from the ophthalmoscope to look. Now look about the room, moving your head and the instrument together as one unit. Keep both your eyes open; just view the field through the ophthalmoscope.	
The ophthalmoscope contains a set of lenses that control the focus (Figure 14.26). The unit of strength of each lens is the *diopter*. The black numbers indicate a positive diopter; they focus on objects nearer in space to the ophthalmoscope. The red numbers show a negative diopter and are for focusing on objects further away. **Figure 14.26** Ophthalmoscope	
To examine a person, darken the room to help dilate the pupils. Remove eyeglasses from yourself or the other person; they obstruct close movement and you can compensate for their correction by using the diopter setting. Contact lenses may be left in; they pose no problem as long as they are clean. Dilating eye drops are not needed during a screening examination. When indicated, they dilate the pupils for a wider look at the fundus background and macular area. Eye drops are used only when history of angle closure glaucoma can be completely ruled out, because dilating the pupils in the presence of glaucoma can precipitate an acute episode. Care should also be taken when dilating the pupils of persons with high degrees of long-sightedness, as they are also predisposed to angle closure.	
Select the large round aperture with the white light for the routine examination. If the pupils are small, use the smaller white light. The light must have maximum brightness; replace old or dim batteries.	Although the instrument has other shape and coloured apertures, these are rarely used in a screening examination.

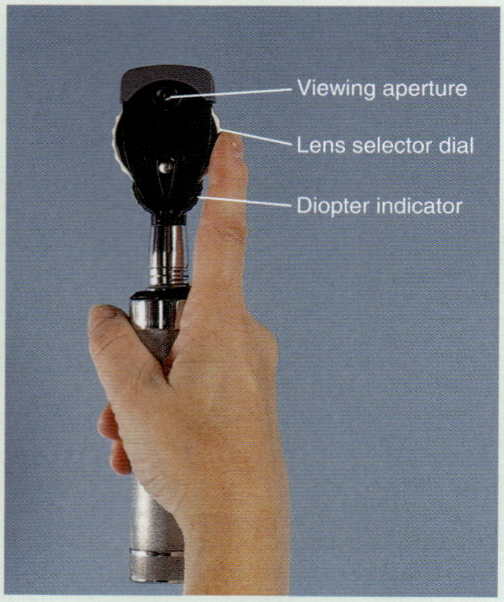

PROCEDURES AND NORMAL FINDINGS	ABNORMAL FINDINGS AND CLINICAL ALERTS
Tell the person, 'Please keep looking at that light switch (or mark) on the wall across the room, even though my head will get in the way'.	Staring at a distant fixed object helps to dilate the pupils and to hold the retinal structures still.
Match sides with the person. That is, hold the ophthalmoscope in your *right* hand up to your *right* eye to view the person's *right* eye. You must do this to avoid bumping noses during the procedure. Place your free hand on the person's shoulder or forehead (Figure 14.27A). This helps orient you in space, because once you have the ophthalmoscope in position, you have only a very narrow range of vision. Also, your thumb can anchor the upper lid and help prevent blinking. **Figure 14.27A** Examination using an ophthalmoscope	
Begin about 25 cm away from the person at an angle about 15 degrees lateral to the person's line of vision. Note the red glow filling the person's pupil. This is the *red reflex*, caused by the reflection of your ophthalmoscope light off the inner retina. Keep sight of the red reflex, and steadily move closer to the eye. If you lose the red reflex, the light has wandered off the pupil and onto the iris or sclera. Adjust your angle to find it again.	
As you advance, adjust the lens to +6 and note any opacity in the media. These appear as dark shadows or black dots interrupting the red reflex. Normally, none are present.	Cataracts appear as opaque black areas against the red reflex (see Table 14.8).
Progress towards the person until your foreheads almost touch (Figure 14.27B). Adjust the diopter setting to bring the ocular fundus into sharp focus. If you and the person have normal vision, this should be at 0. Moving the diopters compensates for nearsightedness or farsightedness. Use the red lenses for nearsighted eyes and the black for farsighted eyes (Figure 14.28). **Figure 14.27B** Examination using an ophthalmoscope	

PROCEDURES AND NORMAL FINDINGS	ABNORMAL FINDINGS AND CLINICAL ALERTS

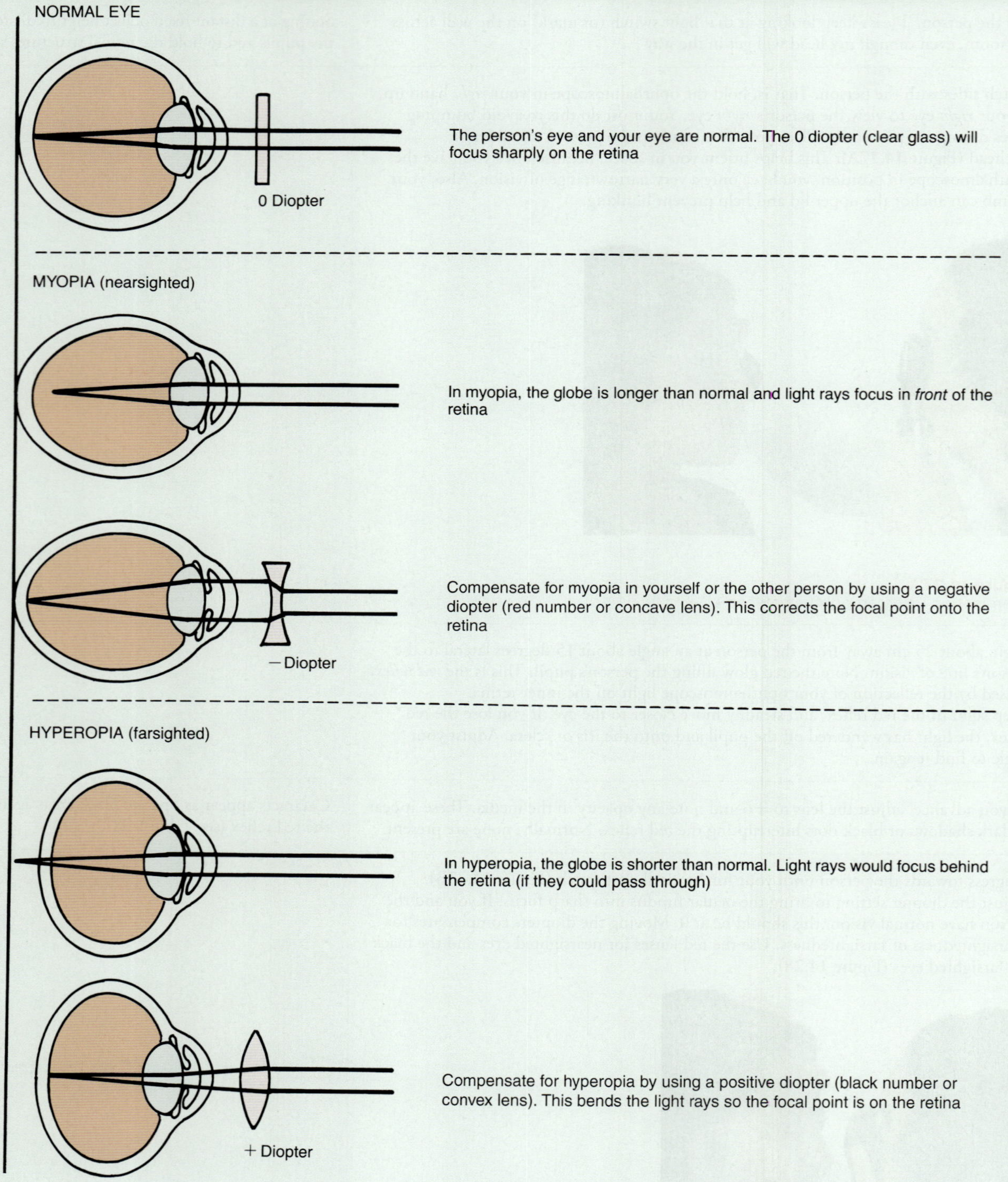

Figure 14.28
Using lenses in the ophthalmoscope

PROCEDURES AND NORMAL FINDINGS	ABNORMAL FINDINGS AND CLINICAL ALERTS
Moving in on the 15-degree lateral line should bring your view just to the optic disc. If the disc is not in sight, track a blood vessel as it grows larger and it will lead you to the disc. Systematically inspect the structures in the ocular fundus: (1) optic disc, (2) retinal vessels, (3) general background and (4) macula (Figure 14.29).	Note the illustration here shows a large area of the fundus. Your actual view through the ophthalmoscope is much smaller—slightly larger than 1 disc diameter.

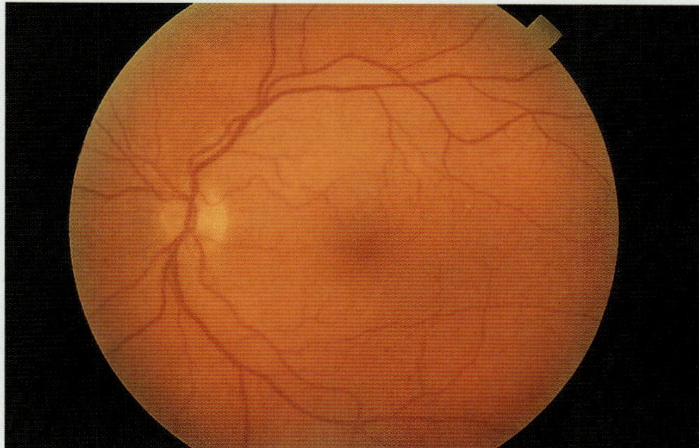

Figure 14.29
Normal ocular fundus.

Optic disc

The most prominent landmark is the optic disc, located on the nasal side of the retina. Explore these characteristics:

PROCEDURES AND NORMAL FINDINGS	ABNORMAL FINDINGS AND CLINICAL ALERTS
1. Colour The outer 'rim' is usually pink with a paler central excavated 'cup'.	Note pallor, hyperaemia (excess of blood flow to the area).
2. Shape Round or oval and flat.	Note irregular shape.
3. Margins Distinct and sharply demarcated, although the nasal edge may be slightly fuzzy.	Look for blurred margins and disc swelling (papillo-oedema). Swollen optic discs may indicate high intracranial pressure.
4. Cup–disc ratio Distinctness varies. When visible, physiological cup is a brighter yellow-white than rest of the disc. Its width is not more than half the disc diameter (Figure 14.30).	Discs are abnormally 'cupped' in glaucoma (have an enlarged and deepened central cup or high cup–disc ratio). The cup can extend to the disc border (see Table 14.9).

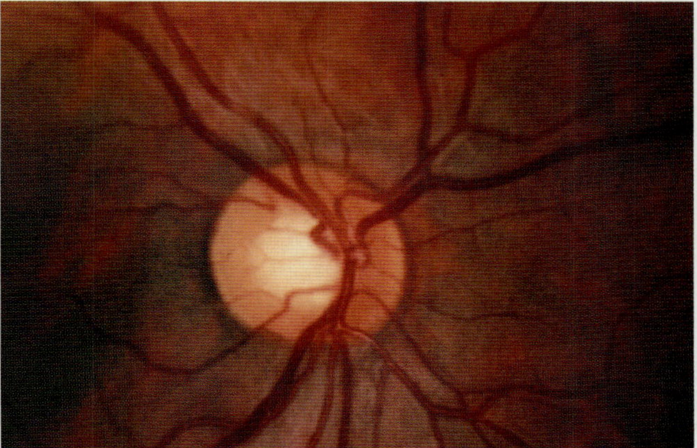

Figure 14.30
Normal optic disc.

PROCEDURES AND NORMAL FINDINGS	ABNORMAL FINDINGS AND CLINICAL ALERTS
Two normal variations may occur around the disc margins. A **scleral crescent** is a grey-white new moon shape (Figure 12.31). It occurs when pigment is absent in the choroid layer and you are looking directly at the sclera. A **pigment crescent** is black; it is due to accumulation of pigment in the choroid.	
Figure 14.31 Scleral crescent.	
The diameter of the disc, or DD, is a standard of measure for other fundus structures. To describe a finding, note its clock-face position as well as its relationship to the disc in size and distance (e.g. '… at 5:00, 3 DD from the disc').	
General background of the fundus	
The colour normally varies from light red to dark brown-red, generally corresponding with the person's skin colour. Your view of the fundus should be clear; no lesions should obstruct the retinal structures.	Abnormal lesions: haemorrhages, exudates, microaneurysms. These are often associated with diabetic retinopathy. See Table 14.10.
Macula	
The macula is 1 DD in size and located 2 DD temporal to the disc. Inspect this area last in the fundoscopic examination. A bright light on this area of central vision causes some watering and discomfort and pupillary constriction. Note that the normal colour of the area is somewhat darker than the rest of the fundus but is even and homogeneous. Clumped pigment may occur with ageing.	Clumped pigment occurs with trauma or retinal detachment.
Within the macula, you may note the foveal light reflex. This is a tiny white glistening dot reflecting your ophthalmoscope light.	Haemorrhage or exudate in the macula occurs with senile macular degeneration.
Additional objective data for infants and children (birth to 12 years)	
Visual fields	
Assess peripheral vision with the confrontation test in children older than 3 years when the preschooler is able to stay in position. As with the adult, the child should see the moving target at the same time as your normal eyes do. Often a young child forgets to say 'now' or 'stop' as the moving object is seen. Rather, note the instant the child's eyes deviate or head shifts position to gaze at the moving object. Match this nearly automatic response with your own sighting.	Usually only performed by advanced practice nurses.
External muscle function	
Testing for **strabismus** (squint or turned eye) is an important screening measure during early childhood. Strabismus causes disconjugate vision because one eye deviates off the fixation point. To avoid diplopia or unclear images, the brain begins to suppress data from the weak eye (a suppression scotoma). Then visual acuity in this otherwise normal eye begins to deteriorate from disuse. Early recognition and treatment are essential to restore binocular vision. Diagnosis after 6 years of age has a poor prognosis. Test malalignment by the corneal light reflex and the cover test.	Untreated strabismus can lead to permanent visual damage and can impact on a child's general development and learning. The resulting loss of vision from disuse is termed **amblyopia** and is commonly referred to as 'lazy eye'.

PROCEDURES AND NORMAL FINDINGS	ABNORMAL FINDINGS AND CLINICAL ALERTS
Corneal light reflex	
Check the **corneal light reflex** by shining a light towards the child's eyes. The light should be reflected at exactly the same spot in the two corneas (see Figure 14.18). Some asymmetry (where one light falls off centre) under 6 months of age is normal.	***Clinical alert:*** Asymmetry in the corneal light reflex after 6 months is abnormal and must be referred.
Cover test	
Perform the **cover test** on all children as described above. Some examiners omit the opaque card and place a hand on the child's head. The examiner's thumb extends down and blocks vision over the eye without actually touching the eye. You can use a familiar character puppet to attract the child's attention. The normal results are the same as those listed in the adult section.	
A brightly coloured toy can be used as a target to assess function of the extraocular muscles during the early weeks. An older infant can sit on the parent's lap as you move the toy in all directions. After 2 years of age, direct the child's gaze through the six cardinal positions of gaze. You may stabilise the child's chin with your hand to prevent them from moving the entire head.	
Visual acuity	
The child's age determines the screening measures used. With a newborn, test visual reflexes and attending behaviours. Until children reach school age, naming letters on visual acuity charts such as the Snellen chart is usually not possible (see Figure 14.21). By the age of 4, most children can complete a recognition acuity task, which involves either naming or matching letters or pictures of standard sizes. Testing may include: • Picture charts • Letter charts • Nonsense symbol recognitions.	At-risk groups for further eye problems include those born prematurely, those with multiple disabilities and children in remote Aboriginal and Torres Strait Islander communities. For children in remote communities, education and health assessment needs to be tailored towards detection of uncorrected refractive error and prevention of trachoma (Centre for Community Child Health 2009).
In Australia and New Zealand, the Sheridan-Gardiner test is widely used for testing visual acuity in children who cannot yet read or those who are illiterate (Anstice & Thomson 2014). This test is conducted by providing the child with a seven-letter card and the examiner with a set of single-letter cards corresponding in size to Snellen letters. The child is then asked to point on their card to the letter shown to them by the examiner. For children above 3 years of age, the examiner may use cards containing lines of letters.	
Colour vision	
Colour blindness (red–green) is an inherited recessive X-linked trait affecting about 8% of males and 0.4% of females. Only 5% of people who are colour blind have blue colour blindness—for these people this is not inherited but a change in the chromosome during development. In assessment, this may be identified when children are not able to recognise different colours and separate items by colour.	'Colour deficient' is a more accurate term, because the condition is relative and not disabling. Often, it is just a social inconvenience, although it may affect the person's ability to discern traffic lights, or it may affect school performance when colour is a learning tool. Abnormal colour vision may also affect employment later in life.
The ocular fundus	
The amount of data gathered during the fundoscopic examination depends on the child's ability to hold the eyes still and on your ability to glean as much data as possible in a brief period of time.	
A complete fundoscopic examination is difficult to perform on an infant, but the **red reflex** could be checked when the infant fixates at the bright light for a few seconds. Note any interruption in the light reflex. Position the infant (up to 18 months) lying on the table. The fundus appears pale, and the vessels are not fully developed. There may be no foveal light reflection because the macula area will not be mature until 1 year. Inspect the fundus of the young child and school age child as described in the preceding section on the adult. Allow the child to handle the equipment. Explain why you are darkening the room and that you will leave a small light on. Assure the child that the procedure will not hurt. Direct the young child to look at an appealing picture, perhaps a toy or an animal, during the examination.	An interruption in the red reflex indicates opacity in the cornea, lens or ocular media. This may be due to congenital cataract, retinal disorder or a serious intraocular tumour (retinoblastoma). Papillo-oedema is rare in the infant because the fontanels and open sutures will absorb any increased intracranial pressure if it occurs. ***Clinical alert:*** Any child with an abnormal red reflex should be referred urgently.

PROCEDURES AND NORMAL FINDINGS	ABNORMAL FINDINGS AND CLINICAL ALERTS
Additional objective data for the adult over 65 years	
Visual acuity	
Perform the same examination as described in the adult section. Central acuity may decrease, particularly after 70 years of age. Peripheral vision may be diminished.	
Central visual field	
To assess the central visual field an **Amsler grid** test is used. This is a small sheet of paper with a grid of black lines on it (see Figure 14.32). To use the grid, ask the person to cover one eye at a time, with glasses on if usually worn. Holding the grid about 30 cm away, ask them to focus on the central dot and ask if the lines look clear and straight (Macular Disease Foundation Australia n.d.).  **Figure 14.32** Amsler grid	Amsler grid testing is used to assess the central visual field. People with macular disease, for example age-related macular degeneration, will often report the lines on the grid look distorted, curved or missing. These people may also report that straight lines, such as the edges of doors or windows, look wavy (metamorphopsia).
The ocular fundus	
Retinal structures generally have less shine. The blood vessels look paler, narrower and attenuated. Arterioles appear paler and straighter, with a narrower light reflex. More arteriovenous crossing defects occur.	
A normal development on the retinal surface is *drusen*, or benign degenerative hyaline deposits (Figure 14.33). They are small, round, yellow dots that are scattered haphazardly on the retina. Although they do not occur in a pattern, they are usually symmetrically placed in the two eyes. They have no effect on vision. 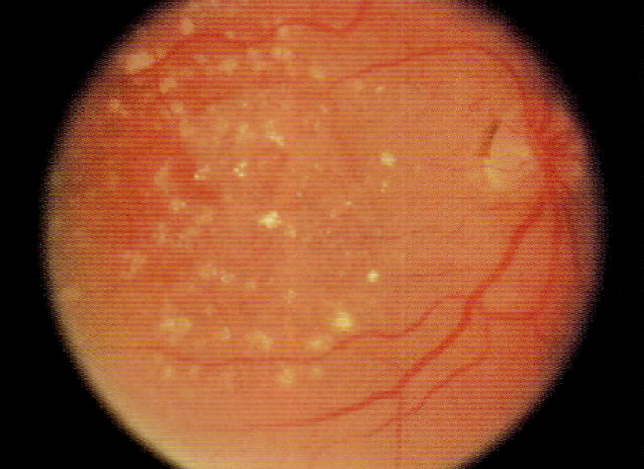 **Figure 14.33** Drusen.	**Drusen** are easily confused with the abnormal finding *hard exudates*, which occur with a more circular or linear pattern. Drusen in the macular area occur with age-related macular degeneration.

OBJECTIVE DATA

Summary Checklist

EYE ASSESSMENT

Subjective data

1. Presenting concern
2. Vision difficulty
3. Pain
4. Strabismus
5. Redness, swelling
6. Watering, discharge
7. History of ocular problems
8. Glaucoma
9. Use of glasses or contact lenses
10. Health and lifestyle management
11. Adjustment to vision loss

Objective data

1. General inspection
2. Inspect external ocular structures
3. Inspect anterior eyeball structures
4. Visual acuity—test vision

PROMOTING A HEALTHY LIFESTYLE

AGE-RELATED MACULAR DEGENERATION

Age related macular degeneration (AMD) is the most common cause of visual impairment in people over the age of 50 years in the developed world, and contributes 71% of blindness in non-Indigenous Australians (Deloitte Access Economics 2011, Foreman et al 2017). AMD impairs central vision by progressive destruction of the macula, and impacts significantly on a person's quality of life and independence. This includes affecting their ability to read, recognise faces, drive a car and watch TV. As this is often a bilateral condition, people with AMD often fear complete blindness. They require reassurance that peripheral vision is unaffected, meaning that 'navigational' vision is preserved.

The disease can be classified into early (not visually impairing) and late (visually impairing) stages. Late AMD can be further divided into 'wet' (neovascular changes) and 'dry' (atrophic changes) forms. Non-modifiable risk factors that increase the speed of progression of the disease include age, genetic factors and ethnicity (e.g. Caucasian). Cigarette smoking is the major lifestyle risk factor predicting the presence and development of AMD. Dietary antioxidants also play a role in the occurrence, prevention and treatment of the disease.

Recent developments in the treatment of wet AMD have resulted in some success in slowing the progression of vision loss, and in some cases achieving an improvement in vision. There is currently no effective treatment for dry AMD (Mitchell et al 2018, Deloitte Access Economics 2011). Prevention is the first approach to reducing vision loss in persons affected by AMD. These measures focus on modifiable risk factors. By controlling such risk factors as smoking, alcohol, high body mass index (BMI) and inadequate diet, the onset of AMD may be delayed (Mitchell et al 2018).

The advanced practice nurse plays an important role in assessment of risk and screening for AMD. This forms part of any comprehensive eye evaluation.

The person at risk of AMD or with signs of early AMD needs information and advice to slow or delay the onset or progression of the disease. This should include:

1. Information on how to quit smoking, including referral to support services if appropriate
2. Advice on controlling weight and exercising regularly
3. Advice on eating a well-balanced diet, including:
   - Eat fish two to three times a week, dark green leafy vegetables and fresh fruit daily, and a handful of nuts a week. Limit fats and oils.
   - Choose low glycaemic index (GI) carbohydrates instead of high GI whenever possible.
4. Considering a suitable dietary supplement in consultation with an eye health professional (several supplements are currently available, formulated specifically for persons who are at risk of AMD or who have been diagnosed with the disease)
5. Using the Amsler grid daily to check for symptoms of AMD, e.g. distortion of lines or missing areas
6. Providing adequate protection for eyes from sunlight exposure, including for those who are very young
7. Encouragement to have regular eye examinations and referral to an eye health professional for further assessment and treatment as required.

Websites

Macular Degeneration Foundation Australia: https://www.mdfoundation.com.au

Macular Degeneration New Zealand: http://mdnz.org.nz

(Macular Disease Foundation Australia and Macular Degeneration New Zealand)

OBJECTIVE DATA

Documentation and critical thinking

FOCUSED ASSESSMENT: CLINICAL CASE STUDY

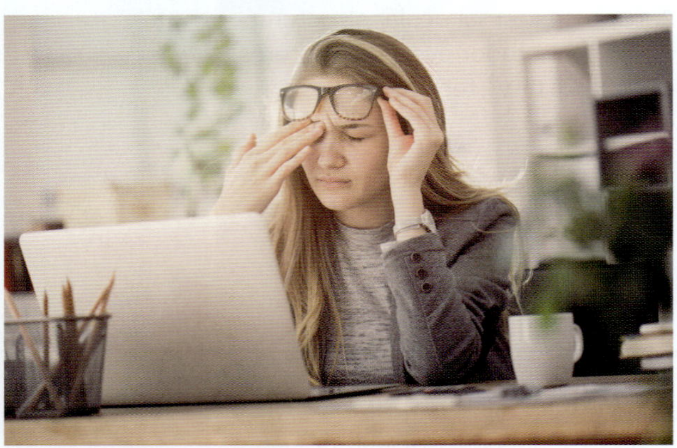

Context

Jane Jensen is an 18-year-old female who has attended the primary care clinic complaining of red, gritty eyes.

Subjective

States her right eyelid was 'stuck together', red and gritty when she woke up that morning. The left eye has become progressively red and gritty during the course of the day, with both eyes now affected equally. She says her vision is 'the same as it usually is'. She doesn't complain of pain, but finds very bright lights uncomfortable (mild photophobia). She has a gritty, foreign body sensation in both eyes. She states there has been some thick, yellow discharge from her eyes during the day. There is no history of trauma or eye injury. Jane does not wear contact lenses. Apart from the problem with her eyes, Jane has been otherwise well.

Objective

Eyelids are slightly red and oedematous, and the conjunctivae are quite red. When the lower lid is pulled away from the eyeball, the forniceal conjunctiva are noted to be very red and mucopurulent discharge is seen in the lower fornix.

On inspection with a pen torch, there is no obvious injury to the conjunctiva, although Jane finds the bright light uncomfortable. The pupils are equal, round and briskly reactive to light.

Collaborative problem

Probable eye infection—refer to medical practitioner for further assessment and swabs for micro and culture.

Problem statements/nursing diagnoses

Discomfort related to photophobia, mucopurulent discharge and foreign body sensation

Potential for spread of infection related to knowledge deficit of hygiene and infection control practices

Abnormal findings

TABLE 14.1 Extraocular muscle dysfunction

Asymmetrical corneal light reflex	
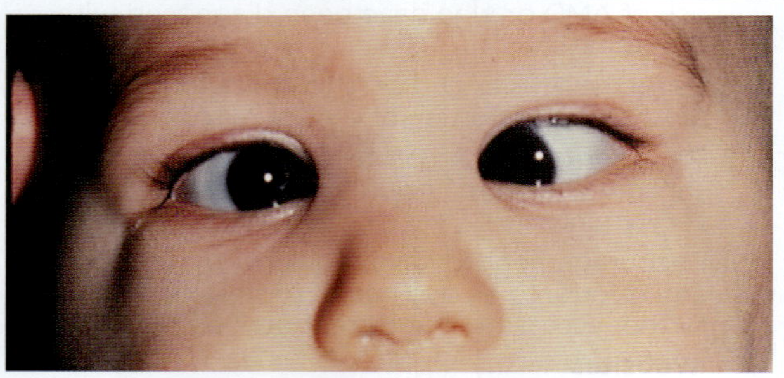 A Eso*tropia*—inward turn of the eye. **Strabismus** is true disparity of the eye axes. This constant malalignment is also termed *tropia* and is likely to cause amblyopia.	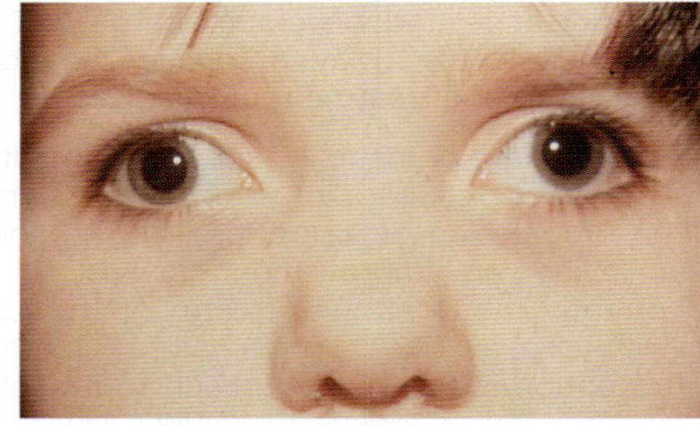 B Exo*tropia*—outward turning of the eyes.

ABNORMAL FINDINGS

TABLE 14.1 Extraocular muscle dysfunction—cont'd

Cover test

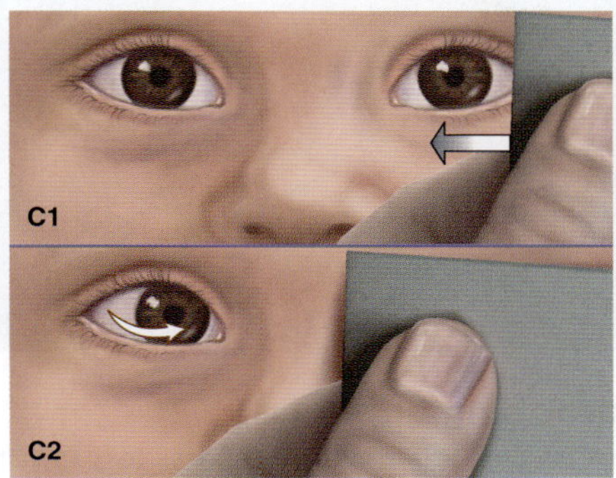

C Right, or uncovered eye, is weaker

Uncovered eye—if it jumps to fixate on designated point, it was out of alignment before (i.e. when you cover the stronger eye (C1), the weaker eye now tries to fixate (C2)).

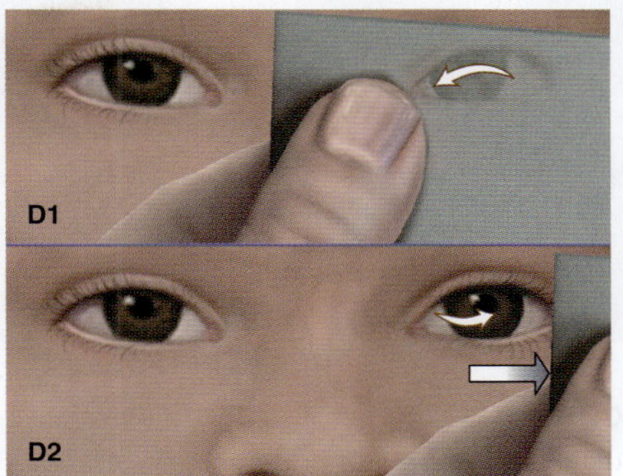

D Left, or uncovered eye, is weaker

Covered eye—if this is the weaker eye, once macular image is suppressed it will drift to relaxed position (D1).

As eye is uncovered—if it jumps to reestablish fixation (D2), weakness exists.

Phoria—mild weakness, apparent only with the cover test and less likely to cause amblyopia than a tropia but still possible.

Esophoria—nasal (inward) drift.

Exophoria—temporal (outward) drift.

Diagnostic positions test

Paralysis apparent during movement through six cardinal positions of gaze.

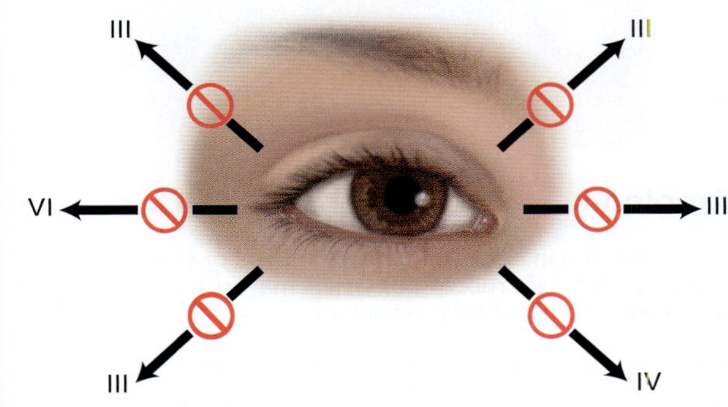

If eye will not turn:	Indicates paralysis in:	or cranial nerve
Straight nasal	Medial rectus	III
Up and nasal	Inferior oblique	III
Up and temporal	Superior rectus	III
Straight temporal	Lateral rectus	VI
Down and temporal	Inferior rectus	III
Down and nasal	Superior oblique	IV

From Zitelli BJ, Davis HW: *Atlas of pediatric physical diagnosis*, 5th ed. St Louis, 2007, Mosby.

TABLE 14.2 Abnormalities in the eyelids

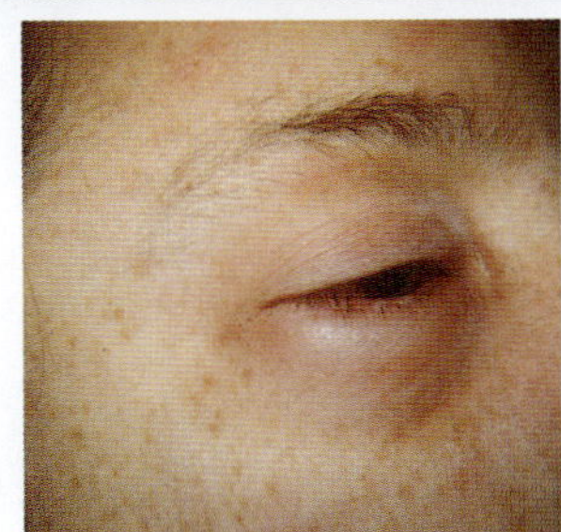

Periorbital oedema

Lids are swollen and puffy. Lid tissues are loosely connected so excess fluid is easily apparent. This occurs with local infections; crying; and systemic conditions such as congestive heart failure, renal failure, allergy, hypothyroidism (myxoedema).

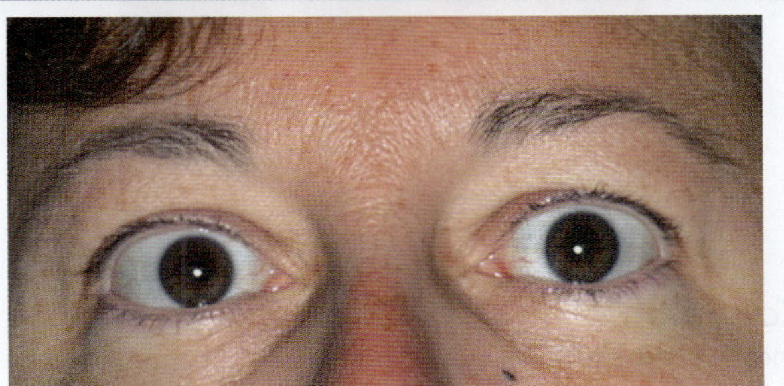

Exophthalmos (protruding eyes)

Exophthalmos is a forward displacement of the eyeballs and widened palpebral fissures. Note 'lid lag': the upper lid rests well above the limbus and white sclera is visible. Acquired bilateral exophthalmos is associated with thyrotoxicosis.

(Continued)

TABLE 14.2 Abnormalities in the eyelids—cont'd

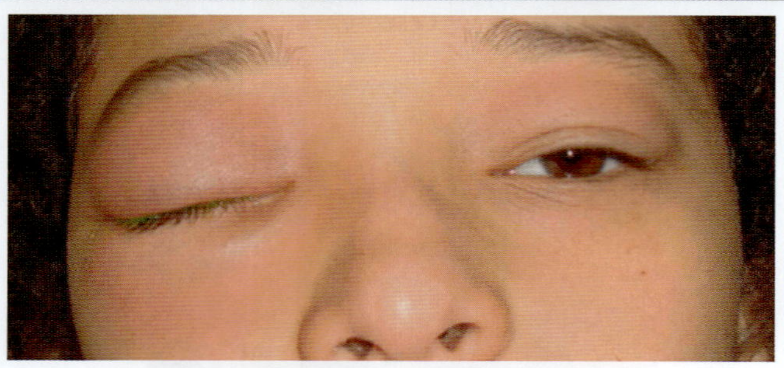

Orbital cellulitis

Orbital cellulitis is a severe and potentially life-threatening infection of the orbit soft tissues. Symptoms may include severe pain, blurred vision, diplopia (double vision), fever and malaise. Severe swelling and redness of the eyelid, with proptosis and decreased movement, is seen. The eyeball itself is also red. These people require urgent referral.

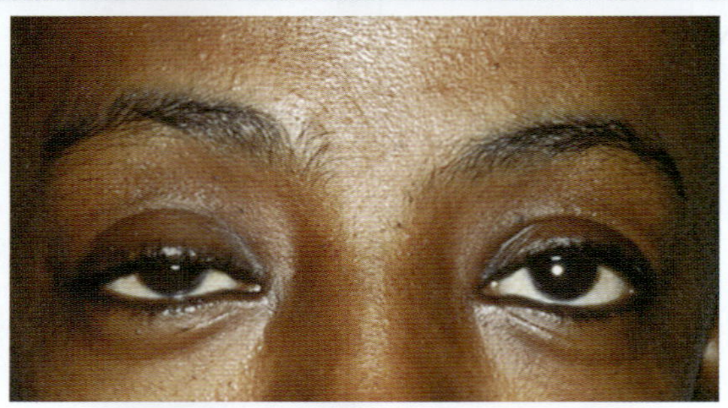

Ptosis (drooping upper lid)

Ptosis occurs from neuromuscular weakness (e.g. myasthenia gravis with bilateral fatigue as the day progresses), oculomotor cranial nerve III damage or sympathetic nerve damage (e.g. Horner's syndrome). It is a positional defect that gives the person a sleepy appearance and impairs vision.

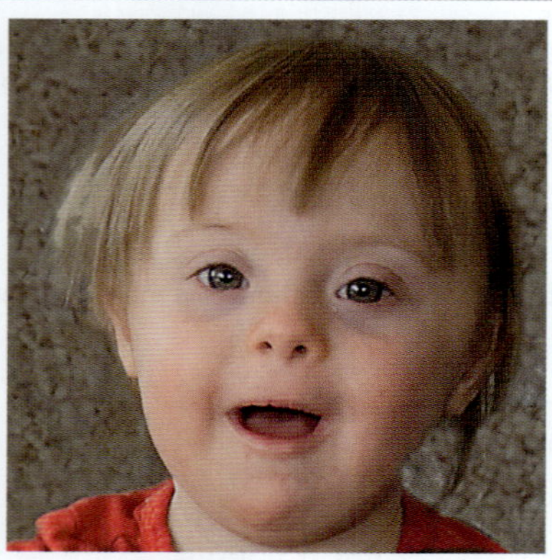

Upward palpebral slant

Although normal in many children, when combined with epicanthal folds, hypertelorism (large spacing between the eyes) and Brushfield spots (light-coloured areas in outer iris), indicates Trisomy 21 (Down syndrome).

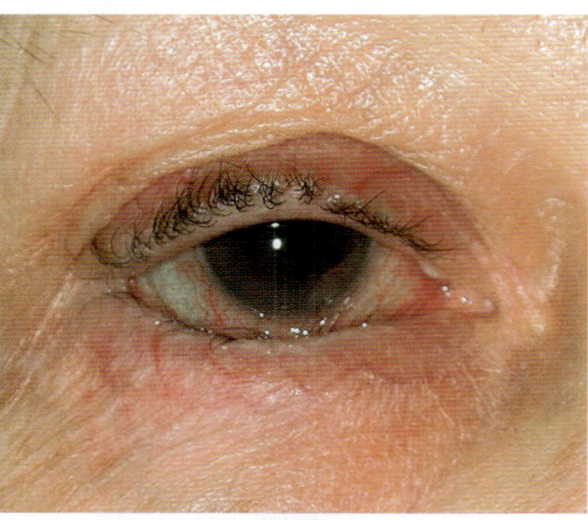

Entropion

The lower lid rolls in because of spasm of lids or scar tissue contracting. Constant rubbing of lashes may irritate cornea. The person feels a 'foreign body' sensation.

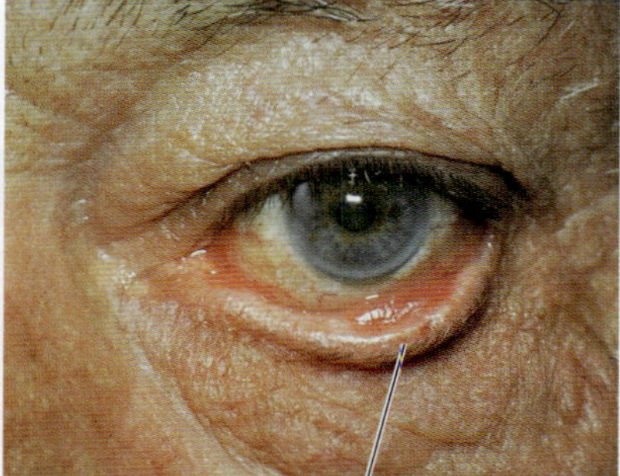

Ectropion

The lower lid is loose and rolling out, does not approximate to eyeball. Puncta cannot siphon tears effectively, so excess tearing results. The eyes feel dry and itchy because the tears do not drain correctly over the corner and towards the medial canthus. Exposed palpebral conjunctiva increases risk for inflammation. Occurs in ageing as a result of atrophy of elastic and fibrous tissues but may result from trauma.

TABLE 14.3 Lesions on the eyelids

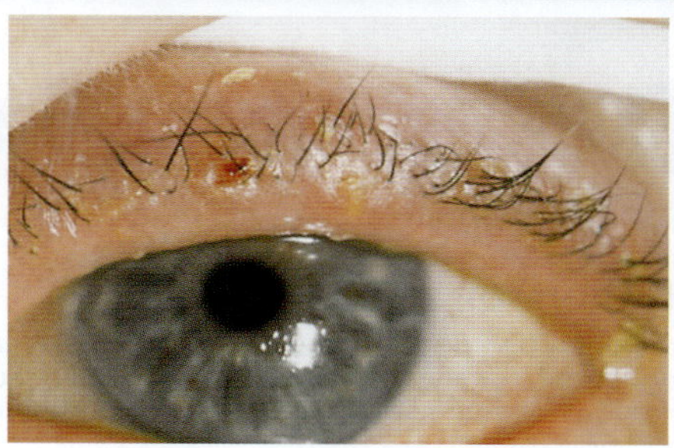

Blepharitis (inflammation of the eyelids)

Red, scaly, greasy flakes and thickened, crusted lid margins occur with staphylococcal infection or seborrhoeic dermatitis of the lid edge. Symptoms include burning, itching, tearing, foreign body sensation and some pain.

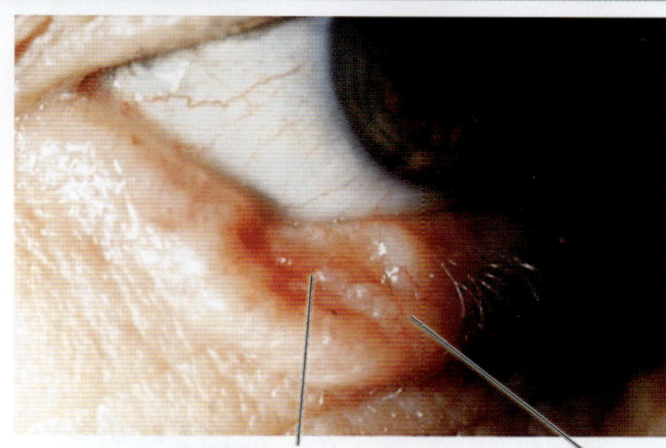

Basal cell carcinoma

Basal cell carcinoma occurs most often on the lower lid and presents as a small, painless nodule with central ulceration and sharp, rolled-out pearly edges. It occurs in older adults, associated with ultraviolet exposure and light skin tones. It is locally invasive, but metastases are rare (Rosner & Fabian 2014).

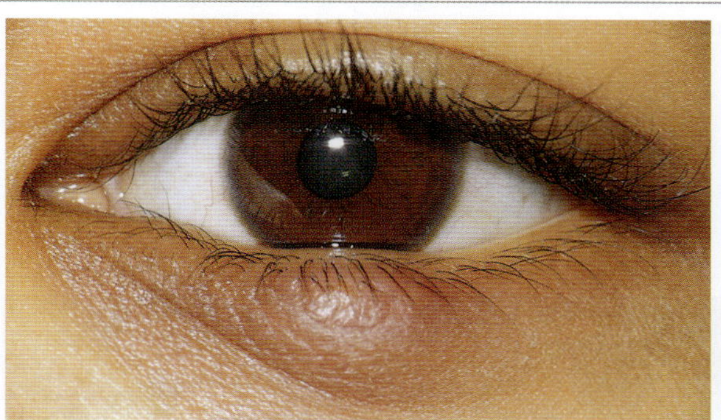

Chalazion

A beady nodule protruding on the lid, chalazion is an infection or retention cyst of a meibomian gland. It is a nontender, firm, discrete swelling with freely movable skin overlying the nodule. If it becomes inflamed, it points inside and not on lid margin (in contrast with stye).

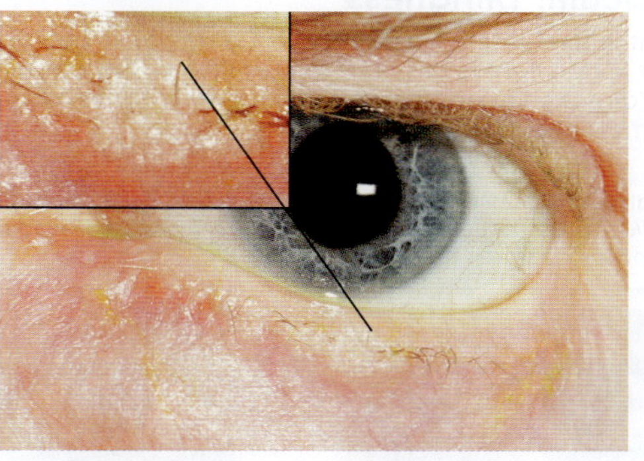

Squamous cell carcinoma

Squamous cell carcinoma is a rarer form of eyelid tumour, but can be life threatening if it extends into the orbit. The lesion can be plaque-like, nodular or ulcerating. It does not usually have vascularisation (Kanski & Bowling 2011). Immediate referral is required.

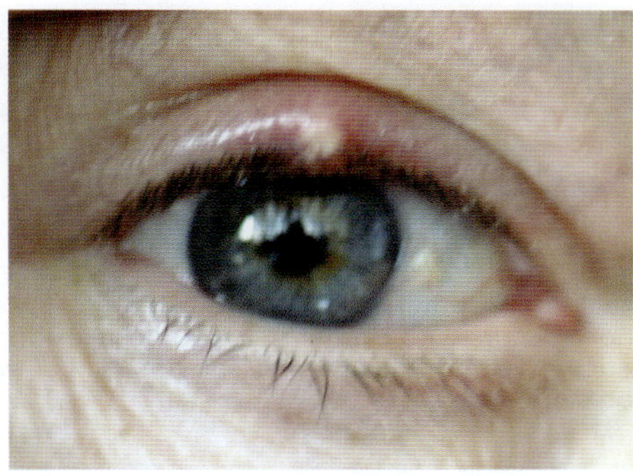

Hordeolum (stye)

Hordeolum is a localised staphylococcal infection of the hair follicles at the lid margin. It is painful, red and swollen—a pustule at the lid margin. Rubbing the eyes can cause cross-contamination and development of another stye.

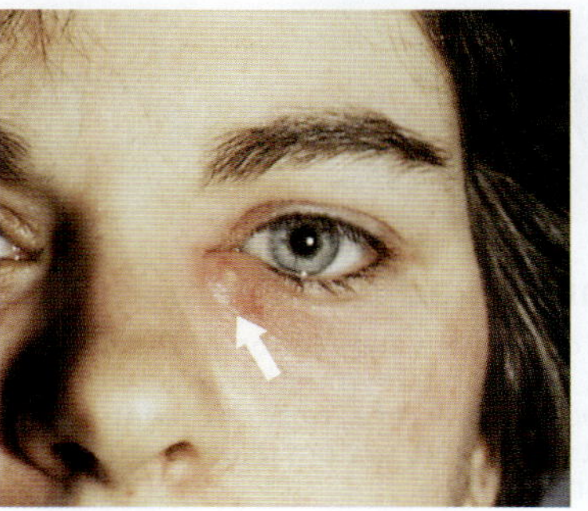

Dacryocystitis (Inflammation of the Lacrimal Sac)

Dacryocystitis is infection and blockage of sac and duct. Pain warmth, redness and swelling occur below the inner canthus towards the nose. Tearing is present. Pressure on sac yields purulent discharge from puncta.

Dacryoadenitis is an infection of the lacrimal gland (not illustrated). Pain, swelling and redness occur in the outer third of the upper lid. It occurs with mumps, measles and infectious mononucleosis or from trauma.

TABLE 14.4 Abnormalities in the pupil

A Unequal pupil size—anisocoria

Although this exists normally in 5% of the population, consider central nervous system disease.

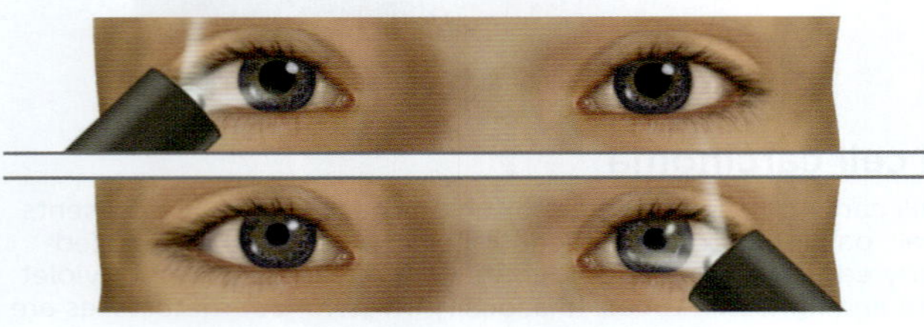

B Monocular blindness

When light is directed to the blind eye, no response occurs in either eye. When light is directed to normal eye, both pupils constrict (direct and consensual response to light) as long as the oculomotor nerve is intact.

From Friedman NJ, Kaiser PK, Pineda A: *Massachusetts ear & eye infirmary illustrated manual of ophthalmology*, 3rd edn. Philadelphia, 2009, Saunders.

C Constricted and fixed pupils—miosis

Miosis occurs with the use of pilocarpine drops for glaucoma treatment, the use of narcotics, with iritis and with brain damage of pons.

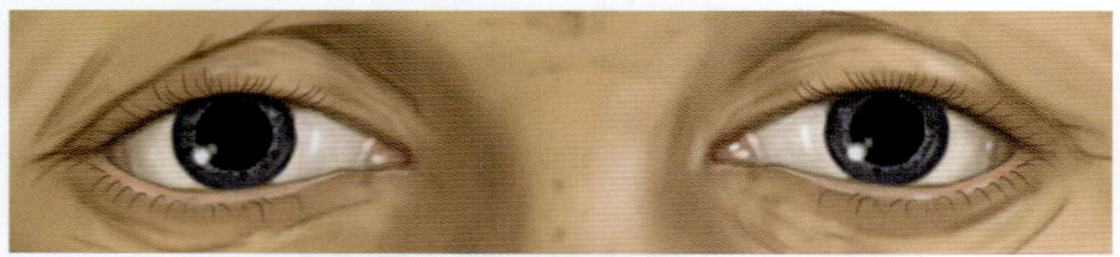

D Dilated and fixed pupils—mydriasis

Enlarged pupils occur with stimulation of the sympathetic nervous system, reaction to sympathomimetic drugs, use of dilating drops, acute glaucoma, past or recent trauma. Also, they herald central nervous system injury, cardiorespiratory arrest or deep anaesthesia.

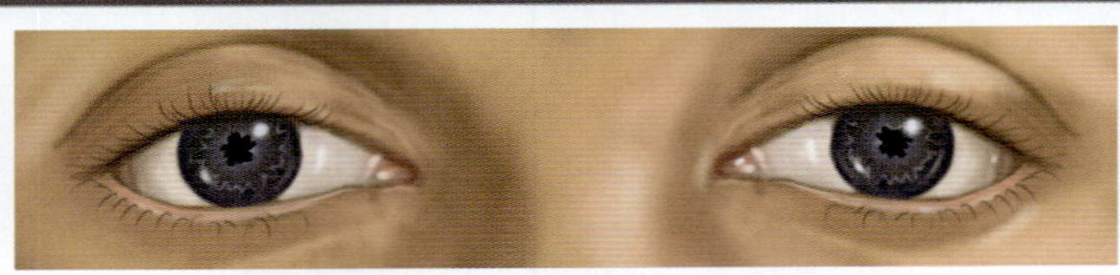

E Argyll Robertson pupil

No reaction to light, pupil does constrict with accommodation. Small and irregular bilaterally. Argyll Robertson pupil occurs with central nervous system syphilis, brain tumour, meningitis and chronic alcoholism.

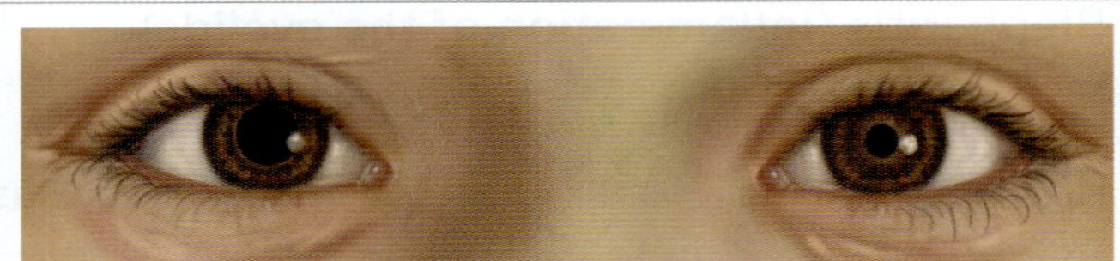

F Tonic pupil (Adie's pupil)

Sluggish reaction to light and accommodation. Tonic pupil is usually unilateral, a large regular pupil that does react, but sluggishly after long latent time. No pathological significance.

G Cranial nerve III damage

Unilateral dilated pupil with no reaction to light or accommodation, occurs with oculomotor nerve damage. May also have ptosis with eye deviating down and laterally.

H Horner's syndrome

Unilateral, small, regular pupil does react to light and accommodation. Occurs with Horner's syndrome, a lesion of the sympathetic nerve. Also, note ptosis and absence of sweat (anhidrosis) on same side.

Abnormal findings for advanced practice

TABLE 14.5 Visual field loss

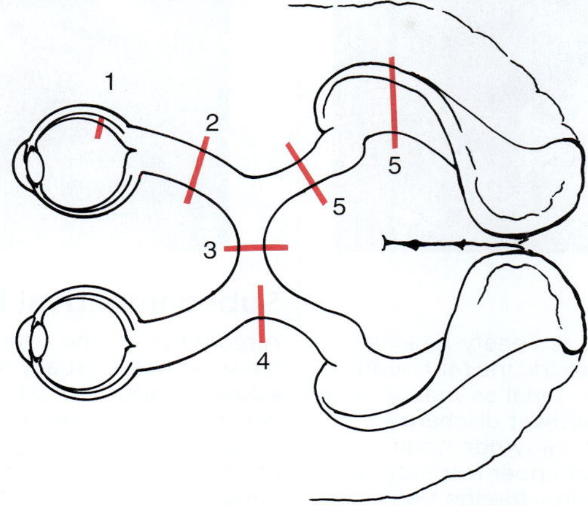

1. Retinal damage.
   - Macula—central blind area (e.g. diabetes):

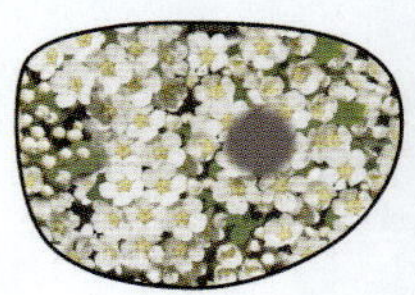 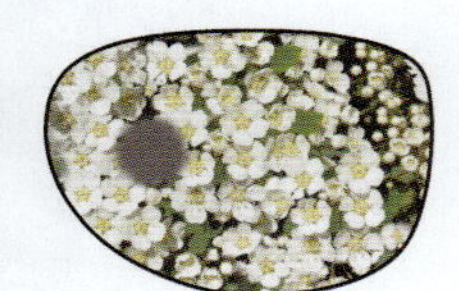

2. **Lesion in globe or optic nerve.**
Injury here yields one blind eye, or unilateral blindness:

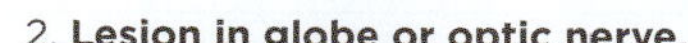

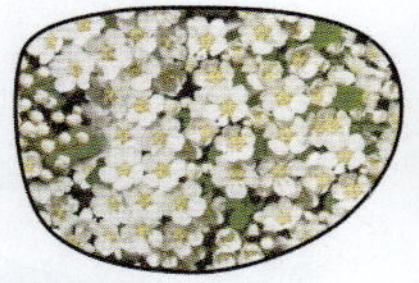 

- Localised damage—blind spot (scotoma) corresponding to particular area:

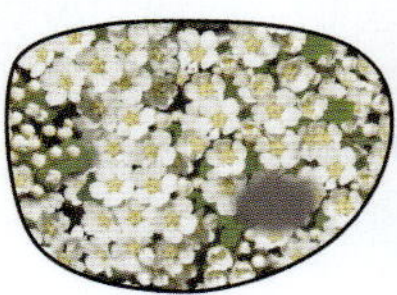 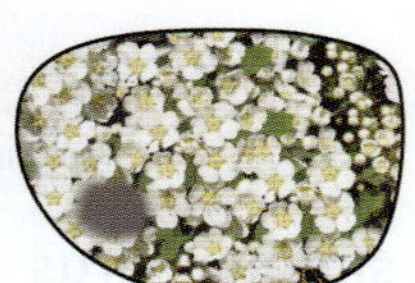

3. **Lesion at optic chiasm** (e.g. pituitary tumour)—injury to crossing fibres only yields a loss of nasal part of each retina and a loss of both temporal visual fields. Bitemporal (heteronymous) hemianopsia:

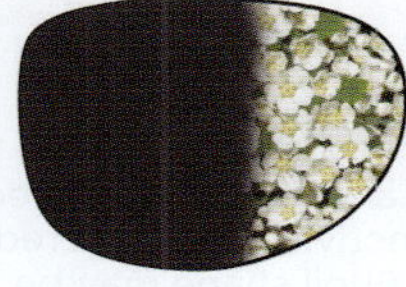 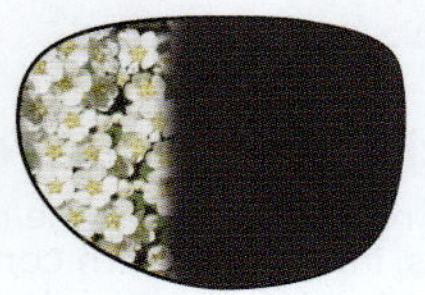

- Increasing intraocular pressure—decrease in peripheral vision (e.g. glaucoma). Starts with paracentral scotoma in early stage:

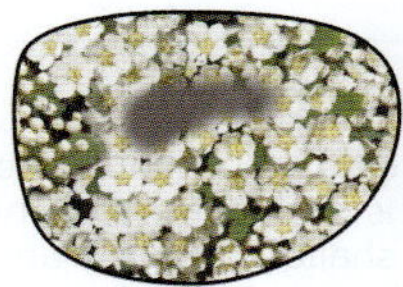 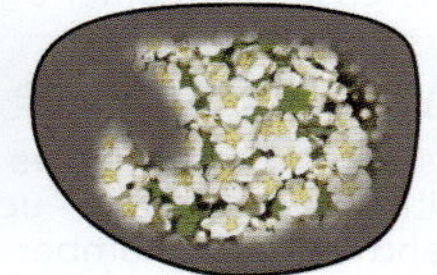

4. **Lesion of outer uncrossed fibres at optic chiasm** (e.g. aneurysm of left internal carotid artery exerts pressure on uncrossed fibres). Injury yields left nasal hemianopsia:

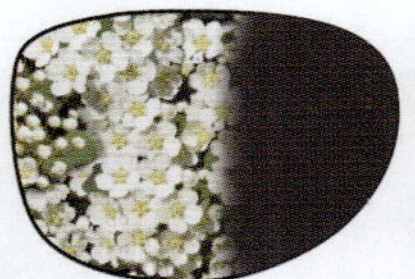 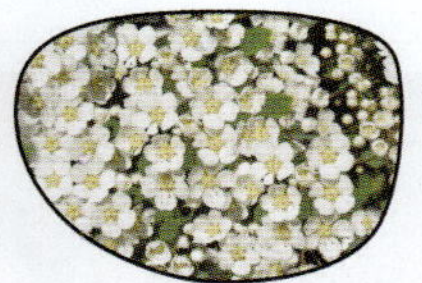

- **Retinal detachment.** Person has shadow or diminished vision in one quadrant or half of visual field:

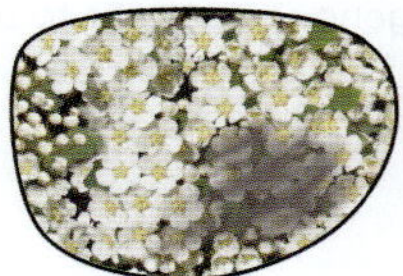 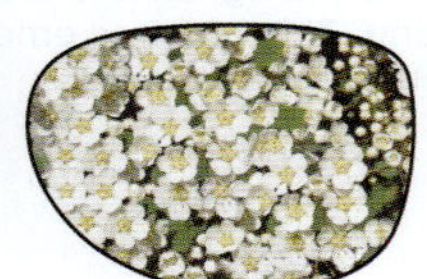

5. **Lesion R optic tract or R optic radiation.**
Visual field loss in R nasal and L temporal fields.
Loss of same half visual field in both eyes is homonymous hemianopsia:

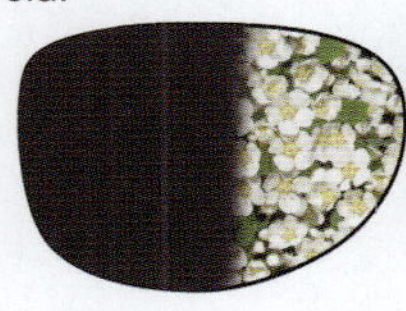 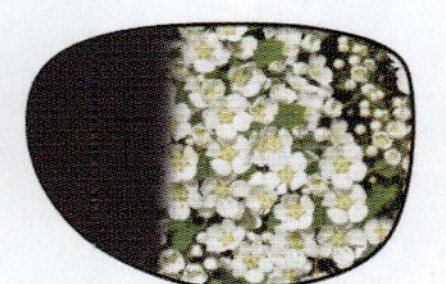

TABLE 14.6 Red eye—vascular disorders

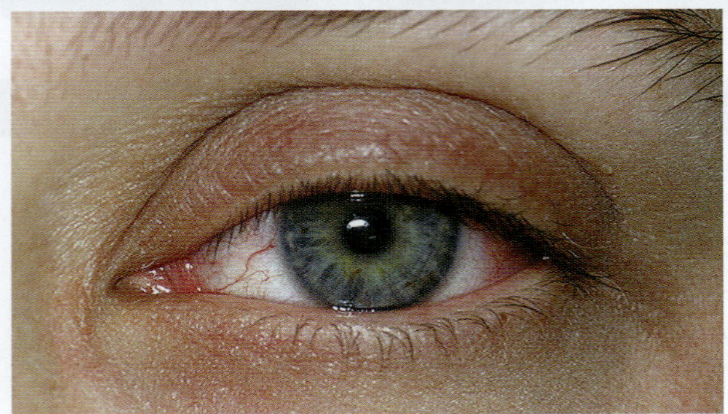

Conjunctivitis

Infection of the conjunctiva, 'red eye', has red beefy-looking vessels at periphery but usually clearer around iris (although here it is severe). This is common from bacterial or viral infection, allergy or chemical irritation. Purulent discharge accompanies bacterial infection. Preauricular lymph node is often swollen and painful, with a history of upper respiratory infection. Symptoms include itching, burning, foreign body sensation and eyelids stuck together on awakening.

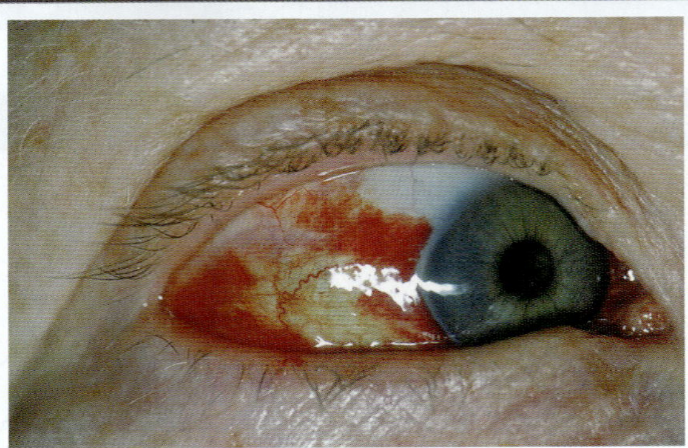

Subconjunctival haemorrhage

A red patch on the sclera, subconjunctival haemorrhage looks alarming but is usually not serious. The red patch has sharp edges like a spot of paint, although here it is extensive. It occurs from increased intraocular pressure from coughing, sneezing, weight lifting, labour during childbirth, straining at stool or trauma. Seen more commonly in persons taking anticoagulation medications.

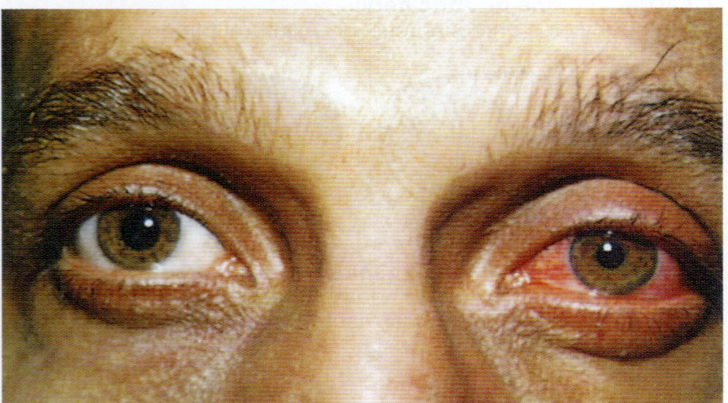

Iritis (circumcorneal redness)

Deep dull red halo around the iris and cornea. Note red is around iris, in contrast with conjunctivitis, in which redness is more prominent at the periphery. Pupil shape may be irregular from swelling of iris. Person also has marked photophobia, constricted pupil, blurred vision and throbbing pain. Requires immediate medical intervention.

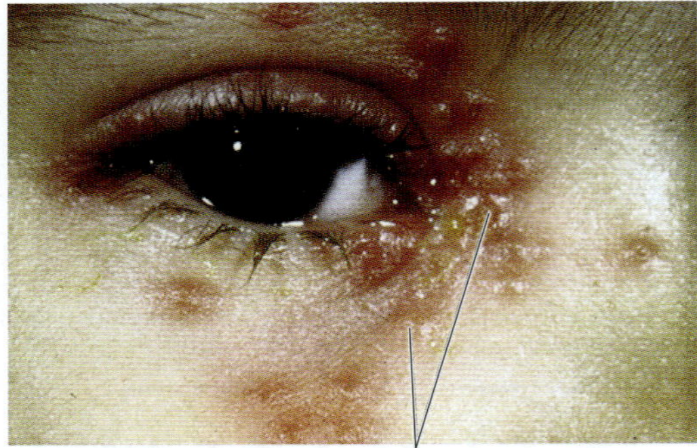

Herpes simplex virus

Lid vesicles from primary HSV, associated with fever, preauricular lymphadenopathy. **Herpes zoster ophthalmicus** is a serious presentation of shingles involving the ophthalmic nerve. May have prodrome: numbness and tingling or burning along nerve route, fever, headache, malaise. Signs are acute, painful reddened conjunctivae; unilateral maculopapular rash with vesicles and ulcers; and ocular signs that threaten vision. Severity increases with older age.

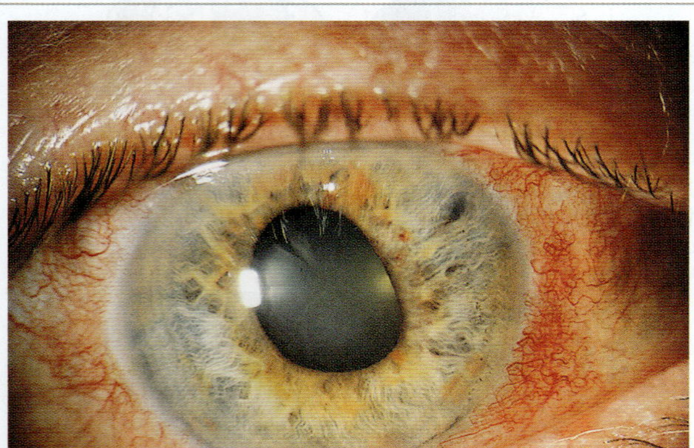

Primary angle-closure glaucoma

Angle-closure glaucoma shows a circumcorneal redness around the iris, with a dilated pupil. Pupil is oval, dilated; cornea looks 'steamy'; and anterior chamber is shallow. Primary angle-closure glaucoma occurs with sudden increase in intraocular pressure from blocked anterior chamber outflow. The person experiences a sudden decrease in vision, sudden eye pain and halos around lights. It is often accompanied by nausea and vomiting. This requires emergency treatment to avoid permanent vision loss.

TABLE 14.6 Red eye—vascular disorders—cont'd

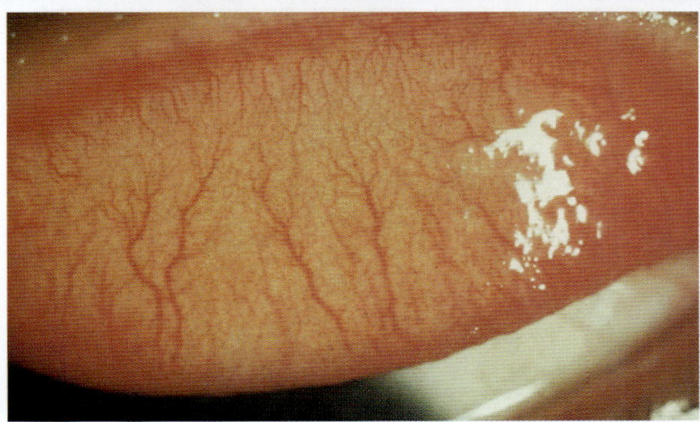

Allergic Conjunctivitis

Note the upper lid, conjunctiva, and cornea are inflamed from seasonal allergen (e.g., pollen, spores) or persistent allergen (e.g., house dust mite, animal dander). Symptoms include eye itching (not present in nonallergic conditions), redness, watering, discomfort. It does not obscure vision. Signs are diffuse redness of conjunctivae, lid swelling, upper tarsal surface that shows velvety thickening, redness, small papillae (shown above).

TABLE 14.7 Abnormalities on the cornea, iris and anterior chamber

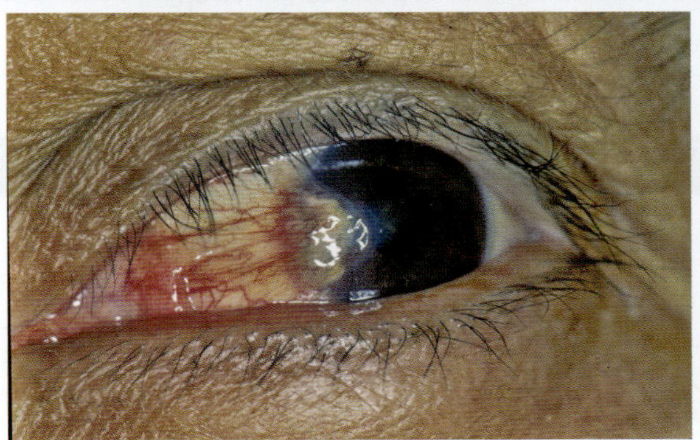

Pterygium

A triangular opaque wing of bulbar conjunctiva overgrows towards the centre of the cornea. It looks membranous, translucent and yellow to white, usually invades from nasal side and it may obstruct vision as it covers pupil. Occurs usually from chronic exposure to UV light. People who live in hot, dry, sunny regions are more likely to develop pterygia.

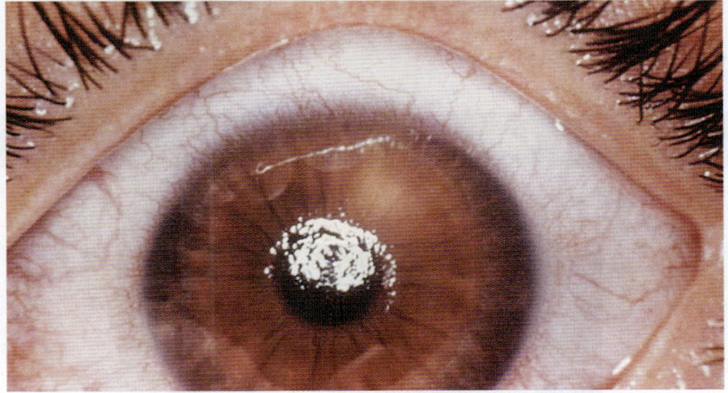

Corneal abrasion

This is the most common result of a blunt eye injury, but irregular ridges usually visible only when fluorescein stain reveals yellow-green abraded area. Top layer of corneal epithelium is damaged, from scratches or poorly fitting or overworn contact lenses. Because the area is rich in nerve endings, the person feels intense pain, a foreign body sensation and lacrimation, redness and photophobia.

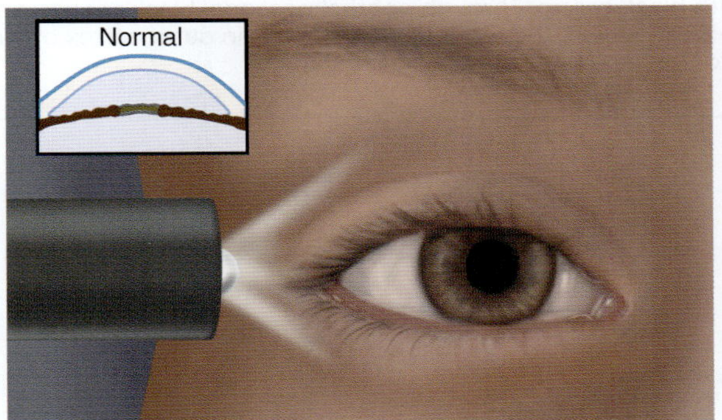

Normal anterior chamber (for contrast)

A light directed across the eye from the temporal side illuminates the entire iris evenly because the normal iris is flat and creates no shadow.

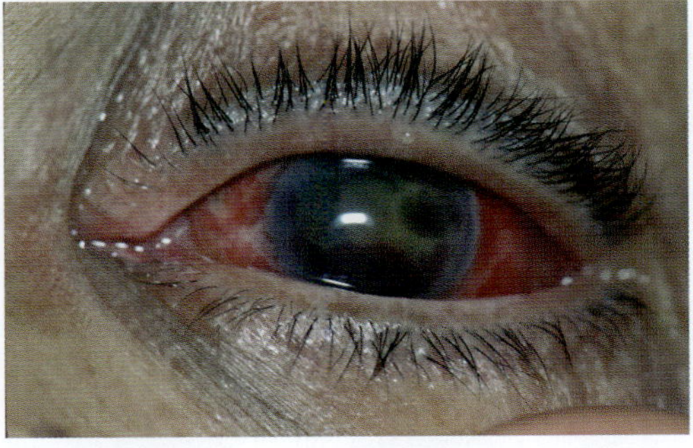

Hyphaema

Blood in anterior chamber is a serious result of blunt trauma (a fist or a tennis ball) or spontaneous haemorrhage. Suspect scleral rupture or major intraocular trauma. Note that gravity settles blood.

(Continued)

TABLE 14.7 Abnormalities on the cornea, iris and anterior chamber—cont'd

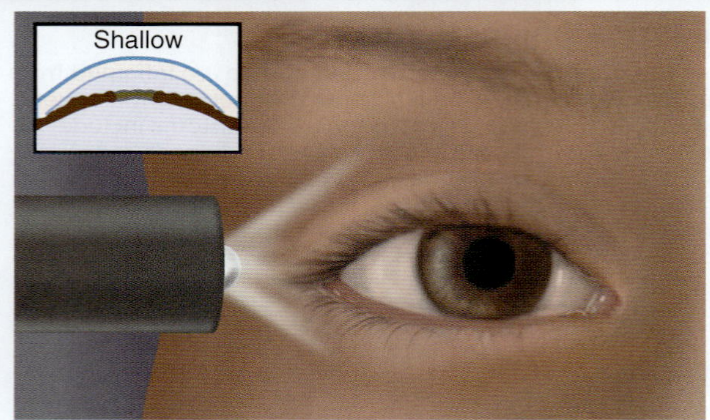

Shallow anterior chamber

The iris is pushed anteriorly because of increased intraocular pressure. Because direct light is received from the temporal side, only the temporal part of the iris is illuminated; the nasal side is shadowed, the 'shadow sign'. This may be a sign of acute angle-closure glaucoma; the iris looks bulging because aqueous humour cannot circulate.

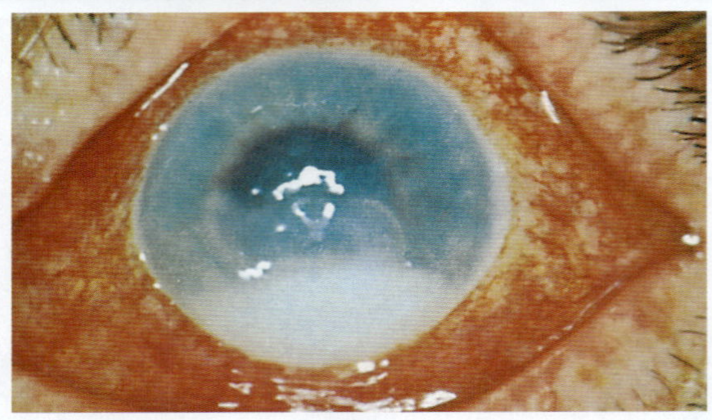

Hypopyon

Purulent matter in anterior chamber occurs with intraocular inflammation, such as iritis, or intraocular infection.

TABLE 14.8 Lens opacities

Senile cataracts

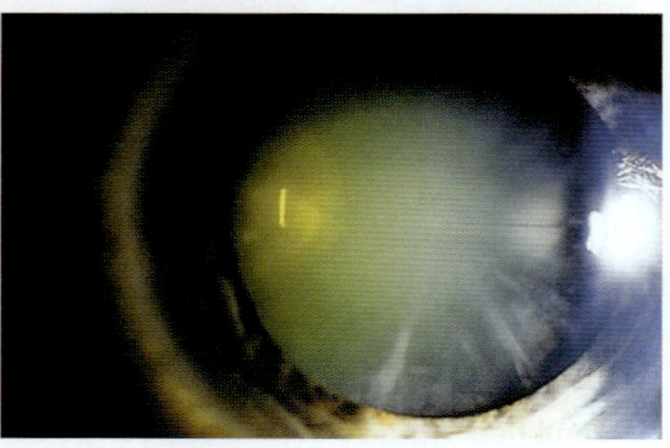

Central grey opacity—nuclear cataract

Nuclear cataract shows as an opaque grey surrounded by black background as it forms in the centre of lens nucleus. Through the ophthalmoscope, it looks like a black centre against the red reflex. It begins after age 40 years and develops slowly, gradually obstructing vision.

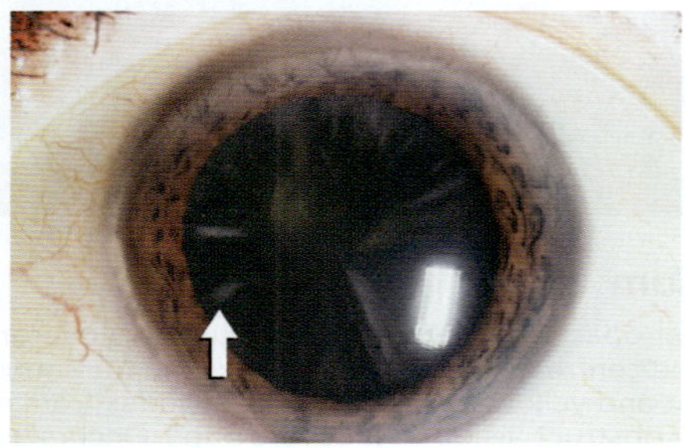

Star-shaped opacity—cortical cataract

Cortical cataract shows as asymmetrical, radial, white spokes with black centre. Through ophthalmoscope, black spokes are evident against the red reflex. This forms in outer cortex of lens, progressing faster than nuclear cataract.

TABLE 14.9 Optic disc abnormalities

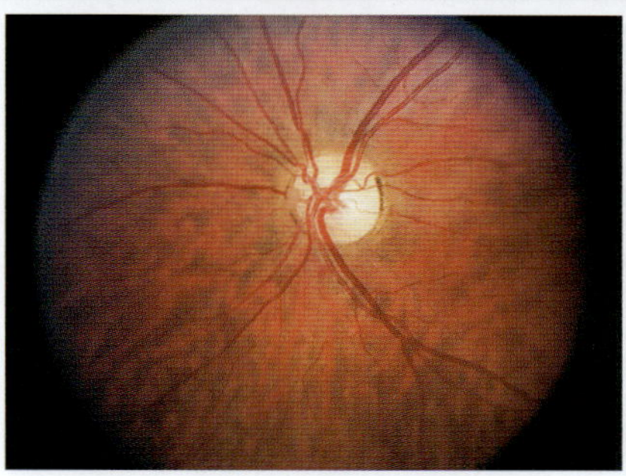

Optic atrophy (disc pallor)

Optic atrophy is a white or grey colour of the disc as a result of partial or complete death of the optic nerve. This results in decreased visual acuity, decreased colour vision and decreased contrast sensitivity.

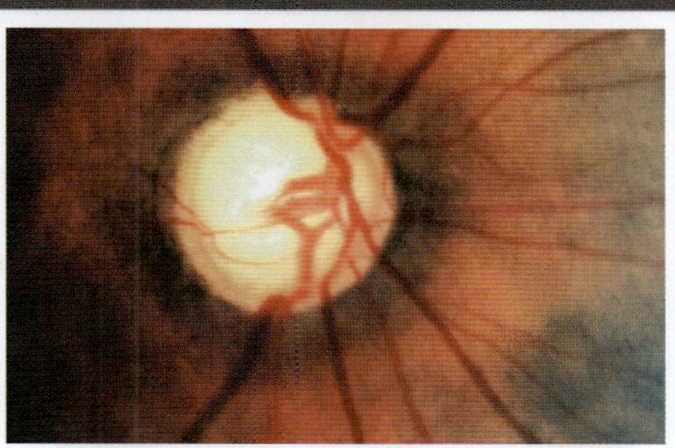

Excessive cup–disc ratio

With primary, open-angle glaucoma, the increased intraocular pressure decreases blood supply to retinal structures. The physiological cup enlarges to more than half of the disc diameter, vessels appear to plunge over edge of cup and the vessels are displaced nasally. This is asymptomatic, although the person may have decreased vision or visual field defects in the late stages of glaucoma.

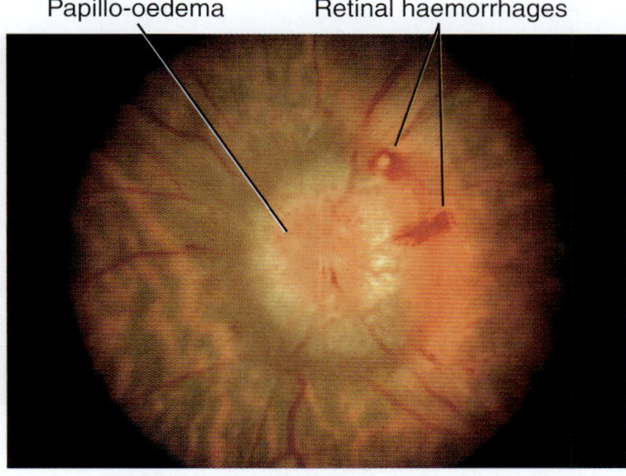

Papillo-oedema

Increased intracranial pressure causes venous stasis in the globe, showing redness, congestion and elevation of the disc; blurred margins; haemorrhages; and absent venous pulsations. This is a serious sign of intracranial pressure, usually caused by a space-occupying mass (e.g. a brain tumour or haematoma). Visual acuity is not affected.

TABLE 14.10 Retinal vessel and background abnormalities

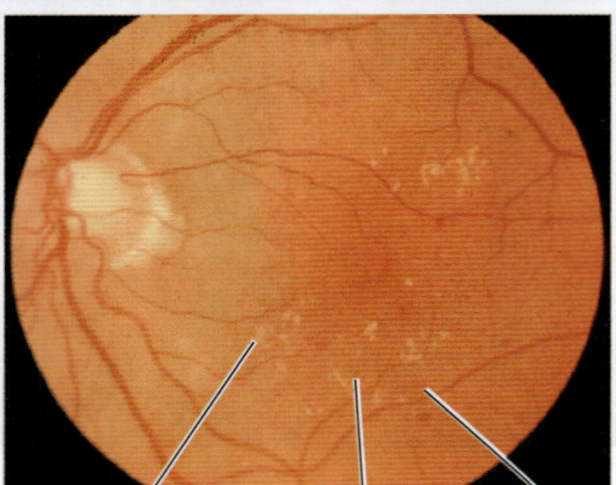

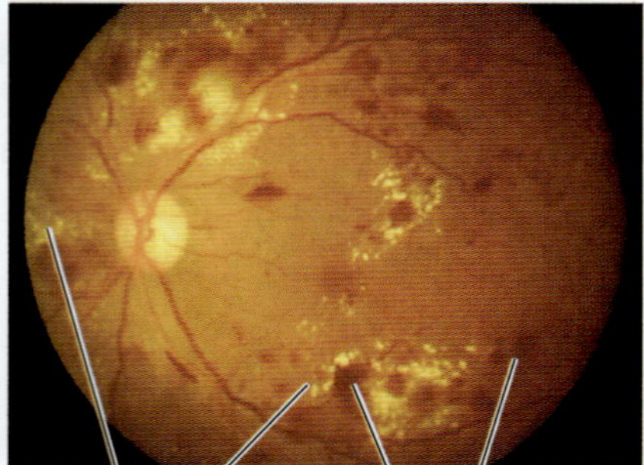

Diabetic retinopathy

Microaneurysms

Microaneurysms (top image) are round punctate red dots that are localised dilations of a small vessel. Their edges are smooth and discrete. The vessel itself is too small to view with the ophthalmoscope; only the isolated red dots are seen. This occurs with diabetes.

Intraretinal haemorrhages

Dot-shaped haemorrhages

Dot-shaped haemorrhages are deep intraretinal haemorrhages that look splattered on (lower image). They may be distinguished from microaneurysms by the blurred irregular edges. Flame-shaped haemorrhages are superficial retinal haemorrhages that look linear and spindle-shaped. They occur with hypertension.

Exudates

Soft exudates or 'cotton wool-like' areas (both images). They are arteriolar microinfarctions that envelop and obscure the vessels. They occur with diabetes, hypertension, subacute bacterial endocarditis, lupus and papillo-oedema of any cause. Hard exudates are numerous small yellow-white spots, having distinct edges and a smooth, solid-looking surface. They often form a circular pattern, clustered around a venous microinfarction. They also may form a linear or star pattern. (This is in contrast with drusen, which have a scattered haphazard location (see Figure 14.33).)

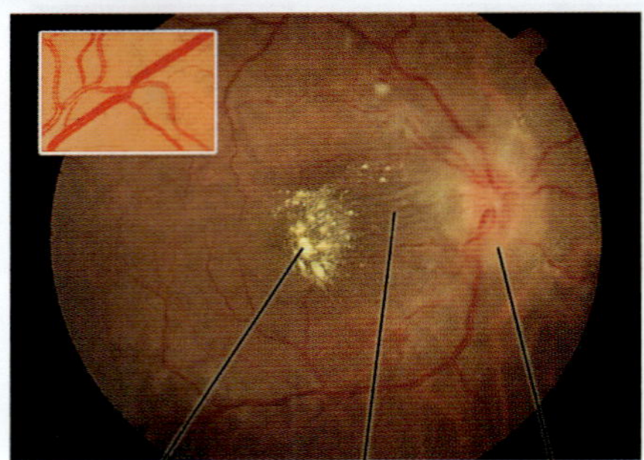

Arteriovenous crossing (nicking)

Inset shows arteriovenous crossing with interruption of blood flow. When vein is occluded, it dilates distal to crossing. This person also has disc oedema and *hard exudates* in a macular star pattern that occur with acutely elevated (malignant) hypertension. With hypertension, the arteriole wall thickens and becomes opaque so that no blood is seen inside it (silver-wire arteries).

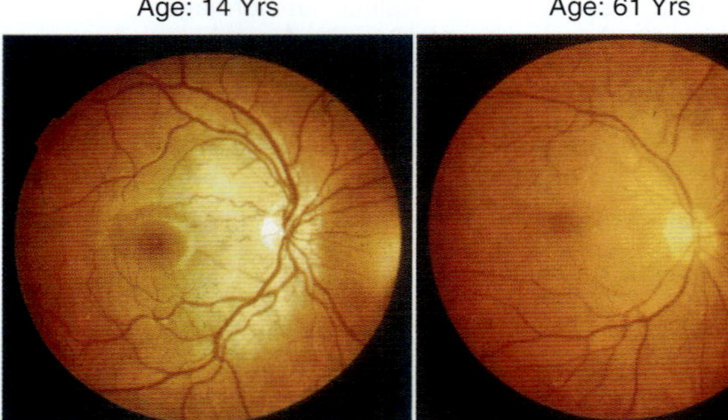

Narrow (attenuated) arteries

Narrow arteries indicate a generalised decrease in arteriole diameter. The light reflex also narrows. It occurs with severe hypertension (shown above on right) and with occlusion of the central retinal artery and retinitis pigmentosa.

BIBLIOGRAPHY

Anstice NS, Thomson B. The measurement of visual acuity in children: An evidence-based update. Clin Exp Optom 2014;29:3–11.

Australian Institute of Health and Welfare (AIHW). Eye health among Australian children, Cat. no. PHE 105. Canberra: AIHW; 2008.

Australian Institute of Health and Welfare (AIHW). Australia's health, Cat. no. AUS 122. Canberra: AIHW; 2016.

Australian Institute of Health and Welfare (AIHW). Indigenous eye health measures. Canberra: AIHW; 2017.

Boudville A, Anjou M, Taylor H. Eye health promotion to improve awareness and prevent vision loss among Indigenous Australians. Health Promot J Austr 2013;24:76–7.

Centre for Community Child Health. National children's vision screening project. Final report. Melbourne: Centre for Community Child Health; 2009.

Deloitte Access Economics. Eyes to the future. A clear outlook on age-related macular degeneration. Canberra: Deloitte Access Economics; 2011.

Department of Health and Ageing (DOHA). Third progress report on the implementation of the national framework for action to promote eye health and prevent avoidable blindness and vision loss. Canberra: DOHA, Commonwealth of Australia; 2015. Available at: https://health.gov.au/internet/main/publishing.nsf/Content/8F3A179870AE7DC2CA258035007E09C1/$File/3rd%20Progress%20report%20under%20National%20Framework%20for%20Eye%20Health.pdf.

Dirani M. Out of sight. A report into diabetic eye disease in Australia. Melbourne: Baker IDI Heart and Diabetes Institute and Centre for Eye Research Australia; 2013.

Dirani M, Keel S, Foreman J, et al. Prevalence of trachomatous trichiasis in Australia: the national eye health survey. Clin Exp Ophthalmol 2017;46(1):13–17. doi:10.1111/ceo.13003.

Findlay Q, Reid K. Dry eye disease: when to treat and when to refer. Aust Prescr 2018;41(5):160–3.

Foreman J, Keel S, Xie J, et al. The national eye health survey. Melbourne: Vision 2020 Australia; 2016.

Foreman J, Xie J, Keel S, et al. The prevalence and causes of vision loss in Indigenous and non-Indigenous Australians. Ophthalmology 2017;124(12):1743–52.

Harper R. Basic ophthalmology. 9th ed. San Francisco: American Academy of Ophthalmology; 2010.

Harvey N. Sensory perception. In Berman A, Snyder SJ, Kozier B, et al, editors. Kozier and Erb's fundamentals of nursing. Frenchs Forest, NSW: Pearson; 2010.

Jonas JB, Aung T, Bourne RR, et al. Glaucoma. Lancet 2017;390: 2083–93.

Kanski JJ, Bowling B. Clinical ophthalmology. A systematic approach. 7th ed. Oxford: Elsevier Saunders; 2011.

Lechner J, O'Leary O, Stitt A. The pathology associated with diabetic retinopathy. Vision Res 2017;139:7–14. doi:10.1016/j.visres.2017.04.003

Macular Disease Foundation of Australia, Amsler grid. 2020 Available at: https://www.mdfoundation.com.au/content/testing-amsler-grid.

Marieb EM, Keller SM. Essentials of human anatomy and physiology. 12th Global ed. New York: Pearson; 2018.

Marsden, J. Ophthalmic care. 2nd ed. London: M&K Publishing; 2017.

Mitchell P, Liew G, Gopinath B, et al. Age-related macular degeneration. Lancet 2018;392:1147–59.

Morcos A, Wright M: Department of Health and Ageing. National children's vision screening project—Final report. Melbourne: DOHA; 2009. Available at: www.rch.org.au/ccch/resources_and_publications/Reports_and_Discussion_Papers/.

New Zealand Ministry of Health. Diabetes, 2018. Available at: www.health.govt.nz/your-health/conditions-and-treatments/diseases-and-illnesses/diabetes.

Pai AS, Rose KA, Leone JF, et al. Amblyopia prevalence and risk factors in Australian preschool children. Ophthalmology 2012;119(1):138–44. doi:10.1016/j.ophtha.2011.06.024.

Razavi H, Burrow S, Trzesinki A. Review of eye health among Aboriginal and Torres Strait Islander people. Australian Indigenous Health Bulletin 2018.

Rosner M, Fabian ID. Basal Cell Carcinoma. In: Pe'er J, Singh A, editors. Clinical ophthalmic oncology. Berlin: Springer; 2014.

Smith SC, Neely S, Twyford K. Nursing assessment: visual and auditory systems. In: Brown D, Edwards H, Lewis SL, et al, editors. Lewis's medical–surgical nursing. 3rd ed. Chatswood, NSW: Mosby Elsevier; 2012.

Statistics New Zealand. Disability survey: 2014. Tatauranga: Statistics New Zealand; 2014.

Talley NJ, O'Connor S. Clinical examination: a systematic guide to physical diagnosis. 8th ed. Chatswood: Elsevier; 2018.

Taylor P, Mapp K. Clear focus – the economic impact of vision loss in New Zealand in 2009. Canberra: Access Economics; 2010. Available at: https://bf-website-uploads-production.s3.amazonaws.com/uploads/2016/04/Cost_of_vision_loss_in_NZ_report_27_September.pdf.

Taylor HR, Burton MJ, Haddad D, et al. Trachoma. Lancet 2014;384:2142–52. doi:10.1016/S0140-6736(13)62182-0

White SLJ, Wood JM, Black AA, et al. Vision screening outcomes of Grade 3 children in Australia: differences in academic achievement. Int J Educ Res 2017;83:154–9.

World Health Organisation. Blindness and vision impairment. 2019. Available at: https://www.who.int/news-room/fact-sheets/detail/blindness-and-visual-impairment.

Chapter Fifteen
Ear assessment

Written by Carolyn Jarvis
Adapted by Suzanne Sharrad

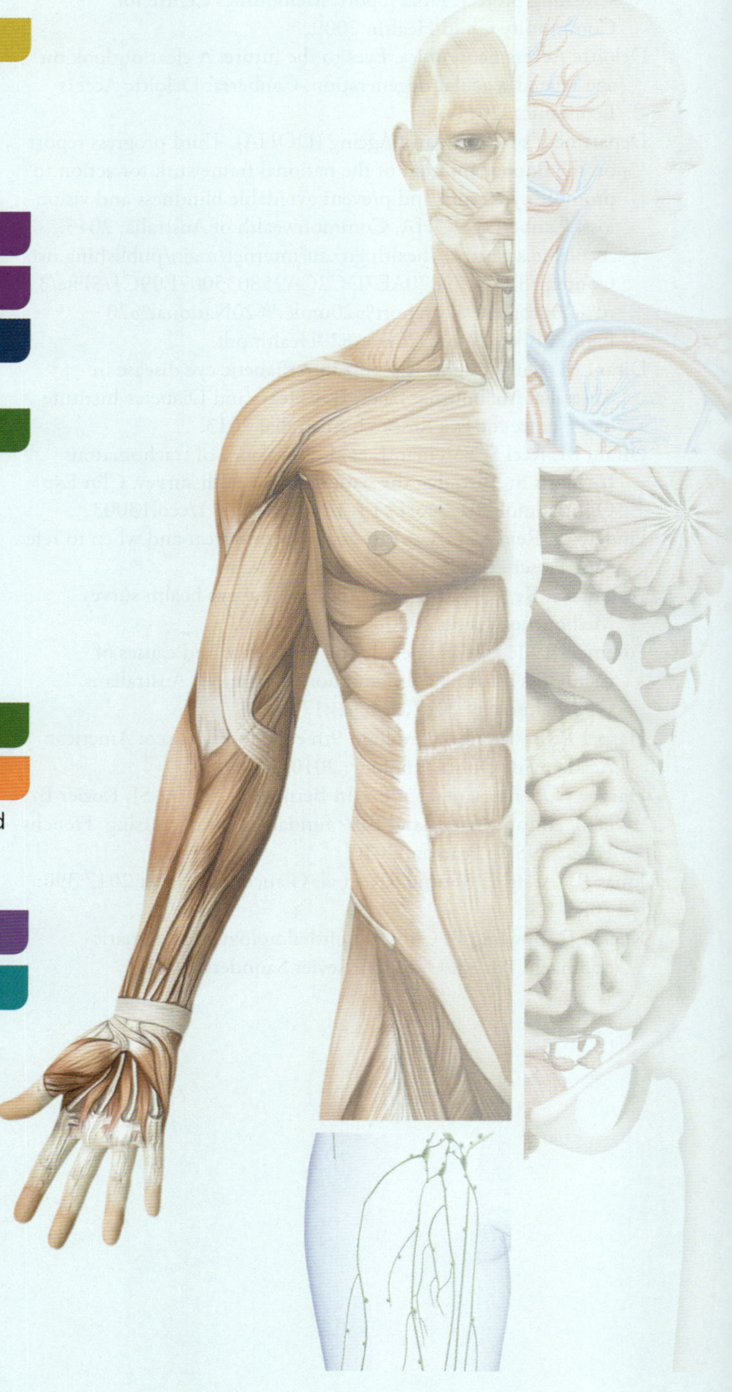

INTRODUCTION

The ear is the sensory organ for hearing and maintaining equilibrium. In this chapter the structure and function of the external and internal ear are reviewed. Additionally, the chapter provides direction about how to conduct a comprehensive ear assessment and respond to its findings. However, as changes in neurological function can affect hearing, it is advisable to also review the relevant sections in Chapter 12.

Structure and function

The ear has three parts: the external, middle and inner ear. The external ear is called the **auricle** or **pinna** and consists of movable cartilage and skin (Figure 15.1). Note the landmarks of the auricle and use these terms to describe any assessment findings. Note, too, that although the mastoid process, the bony prominence behind the lobule, is not part of the ear, it remains an important landmark.

EXTERNAL EAR

The external ear has a characteristic shape and serves to funnel sound waves into its opening, the **external auditory canal** (Figure 15.2). The canal is a cul-de-sac 2.5–3 cm long in the adult and terminates at the eardrum, or tympanic membrane. It is lined with glands that secrete cerumen (commonly referred to as earwax), a yellow waxy material that lubricates and protects the ear. It does this by repelling water and trapping dust and stopping small particles from entering and damaging the ear. Ordinarily cerumen migrates out to the meatus by the movements of chewing and talking. The presence of cerumen can press against the eardrum and occlude the auditory canal and impair hearing. Cerumen can be either grey and flaky or described as 'wet' in which case it is honey brown to dark brown in colour and moist in consistency. The presence and composition of cerumen are not related to poor hygiene.

The outer one-third of the canal is made up of cartilage that is covered by skin; the inner two-thirds consist of bone also covered by thin sensitive skin. The canal has a slight S-curve in the adult. The outer third curves up and towards the back of the head, whereas the inner two-thirds angles down and forwards towards the nose.

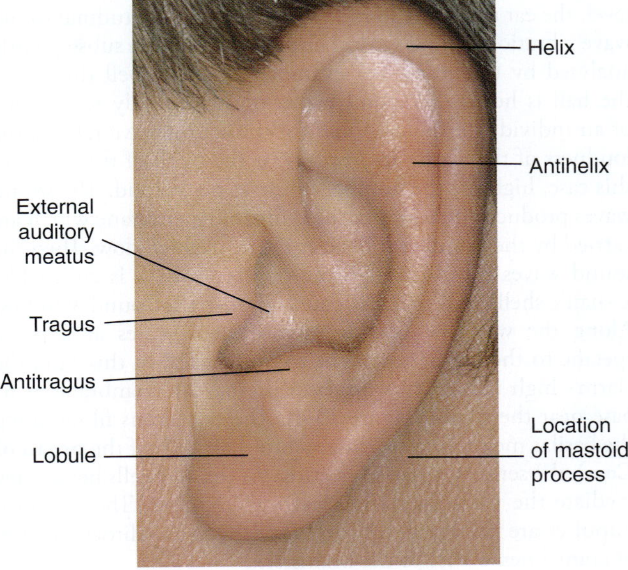

Figure 15.1
Parts of the ear.

The **tympanic membrane**, or **eardrum**, separates the external and middle ear and is tilted obliquely to the ear canal, facing downwards and somewhat forwards. It is a translucent membrane, pearly grey in colour and with a prominent cone of light in the anteroinferior quadrant, which is the reflection of the otoscope light (Figure 15.3). The drum is oval and slightly concave, pulled in at its centre by one of the middle ear ossicles, the **malleus**. The parts of the malleus show through the translucent drum; these are the **umbo**, the **manubrium** (handle) and the **short process**. The small, slack, superior section of the tympanic membrane is called the **pars flaccida**. The remainder of the drum, which is thicker and tauter, is the **pars tensa**. The **annulus** is the outer fibrous rim of the drum.

Lymphatic drainage of the external ear flows to the parotid, mastoid and superficial cervical nodes.

MIDDLE EAR

The middle ear is a tiny air-filled cavity inside the temporal bone (see Figure 15.2). It contains tiny ear bones, or auditory ossicles: the **malleus**, **incus** and **stapes**. In the middle ear, several openings are present. The opening of the middle ear to the outer ear is covered by the tympanic membrane. The openings to the inner ear are the oval window at the end of the stapes, and the round window. Another opening is the **Eustachian tube**, which connects the middle ear with the nasopharynx and allows the passage of air. The tube is normally closed, but it opens with swallowing or yawning.

The middle ear has three functions: (1) it conducts sound vibrations from the outer ear to the central hearing apparatus in the inner ear, (2) it protects the inner ear by reducing the amplitude of loud sounds and (3) its Eustachian tube allows equalisation of air pressure on each side of the tympanic membrane so that the membrane does not rupture (e.g. during altitude changes in an aeroplane).

INNER EAR

The inner ear contains the **bony labyrinth**, which holds the sensory organs for equilibrium and hearing. Within the bony labyrinth, the **vestibule** and the **semicircular canals** compose the vestibular apparatus, and the **cochlea** (Latin for 'snail shell') contains the central hearing apparatus. Although the inner ear is not accessible to direct examination, its functions can be assessed.

HEARING

The auditory system can be divided into three levels when concerned with the function of hearing. They include the peripheral, brainstem and cerebral cortex. At the peripheral

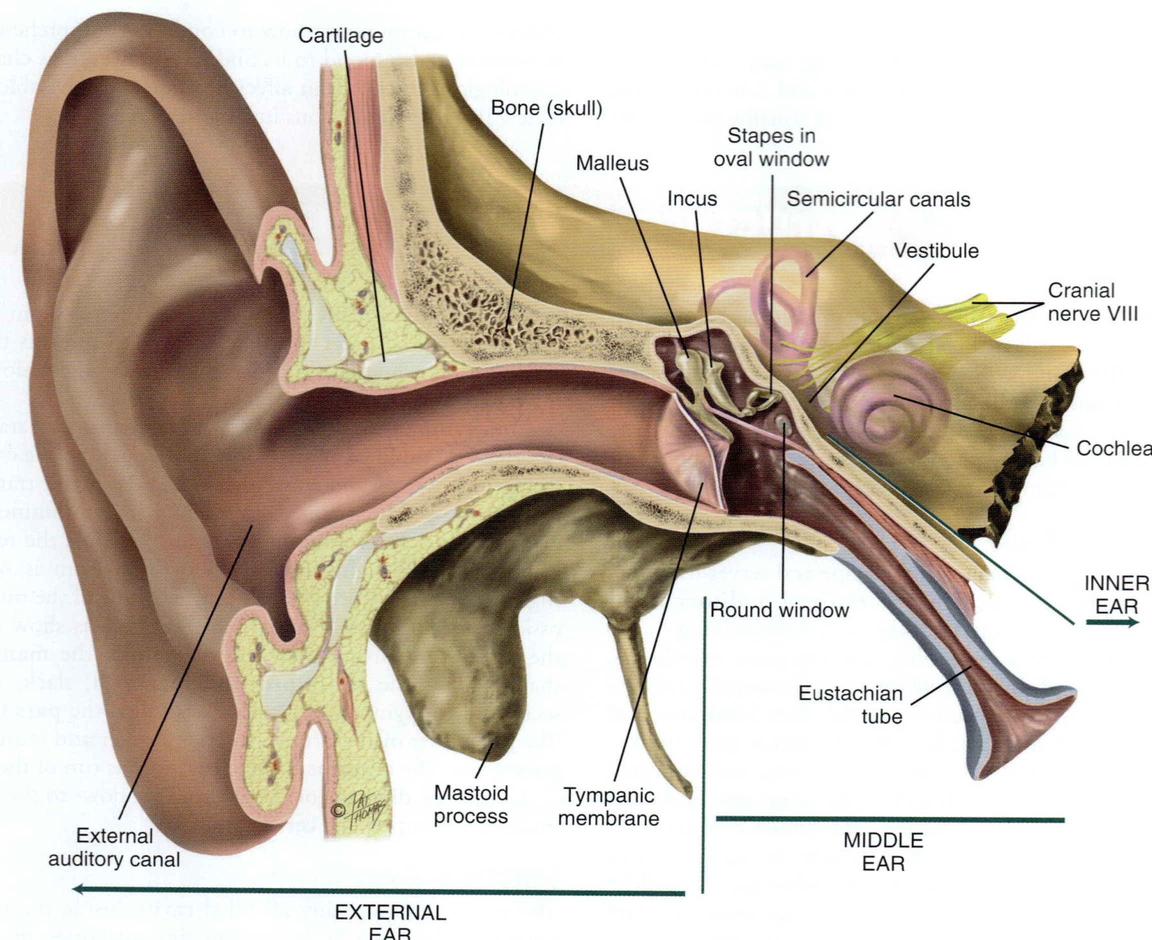

Figure 15.2
External ear and middle ear structures.

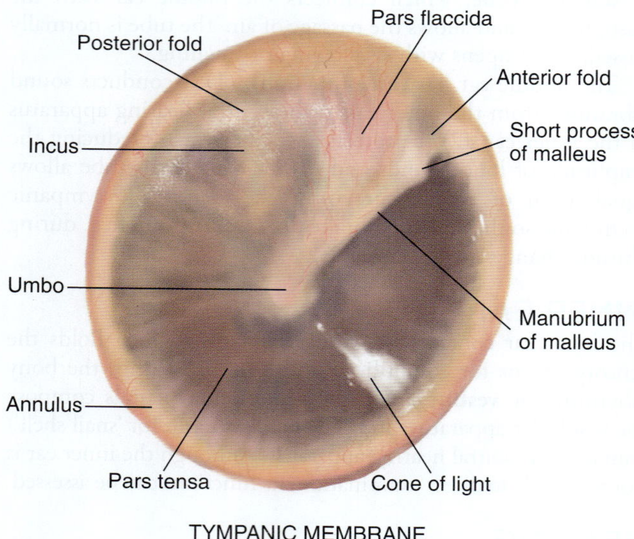

Figure 15.3
Tympanic membrane.

level, the ear transmits sound by converting longitudinal sound wave vibrations into electrical impulses, which are subsequently analysed by the brain. For example, an alarm bell ringing in the hall is heard. Its sound waves travel instantly to the ears of an individual. The *amplitude* of the sound wave reflects the loudness of the alarm; its *frequency* is the pitch of the wave (in this case, high) or the number of cycles per second. The sound waves produce vibrations of the tympanic membrane which are carried by the middle ear ossicles to the oval window. Then the sound waves travel through the cochlea (which is coiled like a snail's shell) and are dissipated against the round window. Along the way, the **basilar membrane** vibrates at a point specific to the frequency of the sound. Again, in this case, the alarm's high frequency stimulates the basilar membrane at its base near the stapes (Figure 15.4). The numerous fibres along the basilar membrane are the receptor hair cells of the **organ of Corti**, the sensory organ of hearing. As the hair cells bend, they mediate the vibrations into electrical impulses. The electrical impulses are subsequently conducted by the auditory portion of cranial nerve VIII to the brainstem.

The function at the brainstem level is *binaural interaction*, in which the sound is identified and the sound direction is determined. How does this occur? Each ear is actually one half

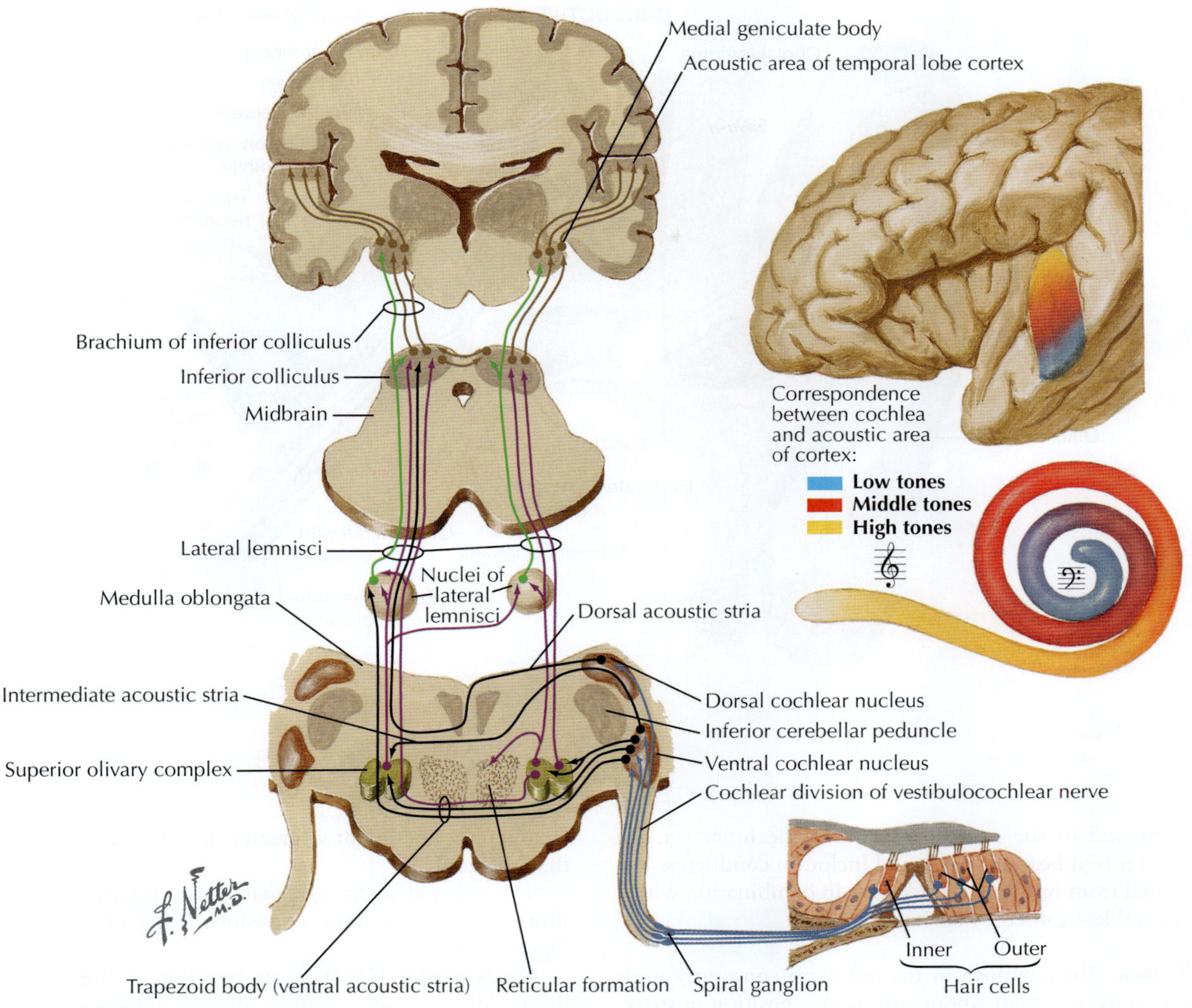

Figure 15.4
Pathways of hearing.

of the total sensory organ. As the ears are located on each side of a movable head, the cranial nerve VIII from each ear sends signals to both sides of the brainstem. Areas in the brainstem are sensitive to differences in intensity and timing of the messages from the two ears, depending on the way the head is turned.

Finally, the function of the cortex is to interpret the meaning of the sound and begin the appropriate response. Incredibly, all this happens in the split second it takes for an individual to react to the alarm.

Pathways of hearing. The normal pathway of hearing is air conduction described above. It is the most efficient pathway. An alternative route of hearing is by bone conduction. Here, the bones of the skull vibrate. These vibrations are transmitted directly to the inner ear and to cranial nerve VIII.

Hearing loss. Obstruction to the transmission of sound caused by a problem in the outer, middle or inner hearing pathway or auditory nerve pathway can cause hearing loss. Hearing loss may be mild, moderate, severe or profound. Hearing loss is classified as conductive or sensorineural, or congenital or acquired (Eggermont 2017). A conductive hearing loss involves a mechanical dysfunction of the external or middle ear (Figure 15.5). It is a partial loss because an individual will be able to hear if the sound amplitude is increased enough to reach normal nerve elements in the inner ear. Conductive hearing loss may be caused by impacted cerumen, foreign bodies, a perforated tympanic membrane, pus or serum in the middle ear and otosclerosis (a decrease in mobility of the ossicles).

Sensorineural (or perceptive) **loss** signifies pathology of the inner ear, cranial nerve VIII or the auditory areas of the cerebral cortex. A simple increase in amplitude may not enable an individual to understand words. Sensorineural hearing loss may be caused by *presbycusis*, a gradual nerve degeneration that occurs with advancing years of age, and by ototoxic drugs, which affect the hair cells in the cochlea.

A third type of hearing loss can be caused by a combination of conductive and sensorineural hearing loss in the same ear. This is known as a **mixed hearing loss**. It is caused by problems in the conductive pathways of the ear, that is, in the outer or

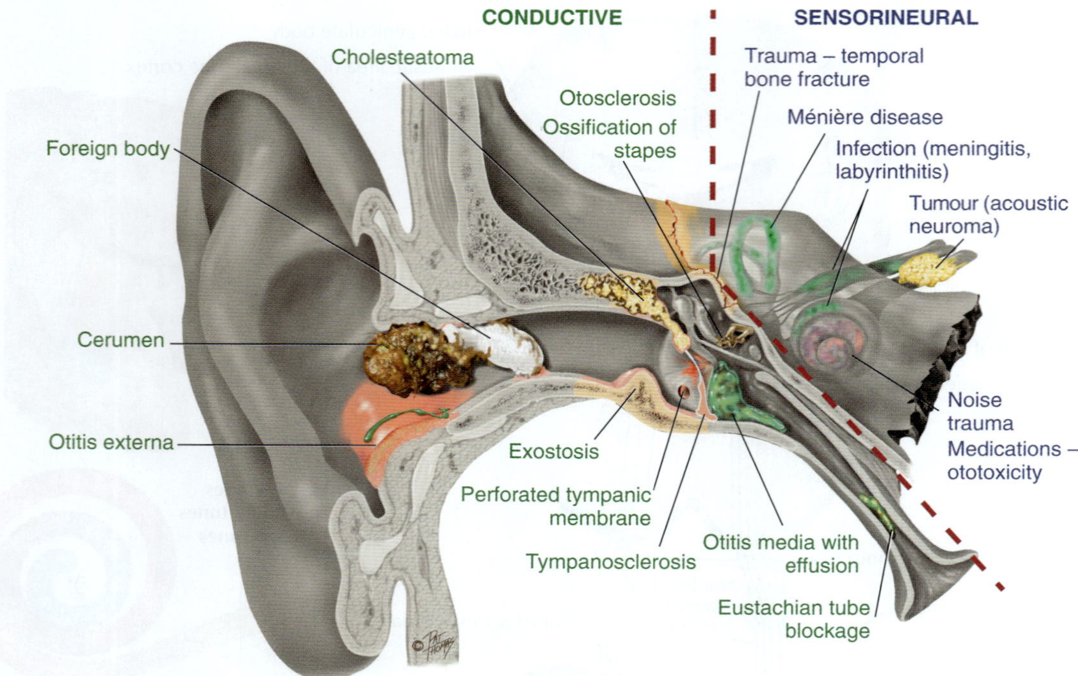

Figure 15.5
Hearing loss.

middle ear and in the nerve pathways of the inner ear. An example of mixed hearing loss would include a conductive loss that resulted from middle ear infections in combination with a sensorineural loss caused by ageing.

Equilibrium. The labyrinth in the inner ear constantly feeds information to your brain about your body's position in space. It works like a plumb line to determine verticality or depth. The ear's plumb lines register the angle of your head in relation to gravity. If the labyrinth ever becomes inflamed, it feeds the wrong information to the brain, creating a staggering gait and a strong, spinning, whirling sensation called *vertigo*.

DEVELOPMENTAL CONSIDERATIONS

Infants and children

The inner ear starts to develop early in the fifth week of gestation. In early development, the ear is posteriorly rotated and low set; later it ascends to its normal placement around eye level. A child may be born with hearing loss (pre-lingual) putting the child at risk for delayed speech and social development and learning deficit. For example, if maternal rubella infection occurs during the first trimester, it can damage the organ of Corti and impair hearing. Post-lingual hearing loss develops **after** the acquisition of speech and language, usually **after** the age of six years.

The infant's Eustachian tube is relatively shorter and wider and its position is more horizontal than the adult's. At this stage, it is easier for pathogens from the nasopharynx to migrate through to the middle ear (Figure 15.6). The lumen is surrounded by lymphoid tissue, which increases during childhood; thus, the lumen can be easily occluded. These factors place the infant at greater risk of middle ear infections than the adult.

The external auditory canal of the infant and toddler is shorter and has a slope opposite to that of the adult's (see Figure 15.6).

Otitis media (OM) is an infection or inflammation of the middle ear and can affect all ages. Infection ascends into the middle ear cavity via the throat and causes swelling of the lining and blockage of the Eustachian tube and reduction of airflow (Coleman & Cervin 2019). A lack of ventilation, resulting from obstruction of the Eustachian tube or passage of nasopharyngeal secretions into the middle ear, leads to an accumulation of fluid. This fluid may be serous, as in acute otitis media, or purulent, as occurs in suppurative otitis media and causes the tympanic membrane to bulge. Persistent otitis media and fluid in the middle ear may lead to effusion and hearing loss, placing the child at risk of delayed cognitive development (Coleman & Cervin 2019).

The incidence of otitis media is also increased in premature infants, in those with Trisomy 21 (Down syndrome) and in babies fed by bottle in a supine position. In the supine position, the effects of gravity and sucking tend to draw the nasopharyngeal contents directly into the middle ear (Chonmaitree et al 2016).

The adult

Otosclerosis is a common cause of conductive hearing loss in the early adult years between the ages of 20 and 40 years. It is a gradual hardening that causes the foot plate of the stapes to become fixed in the oval window, impeding the transmission of sound and causing progressive deafness.

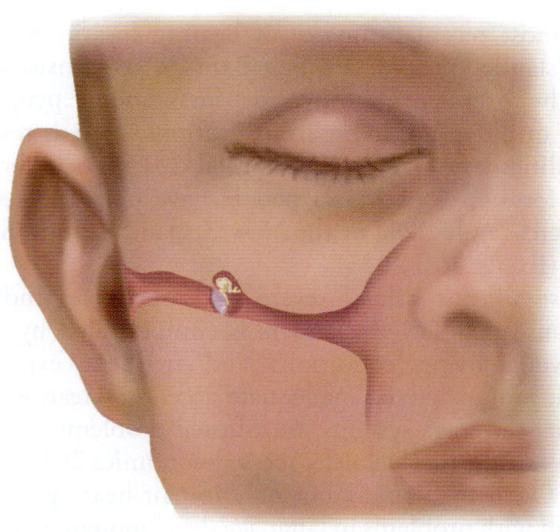

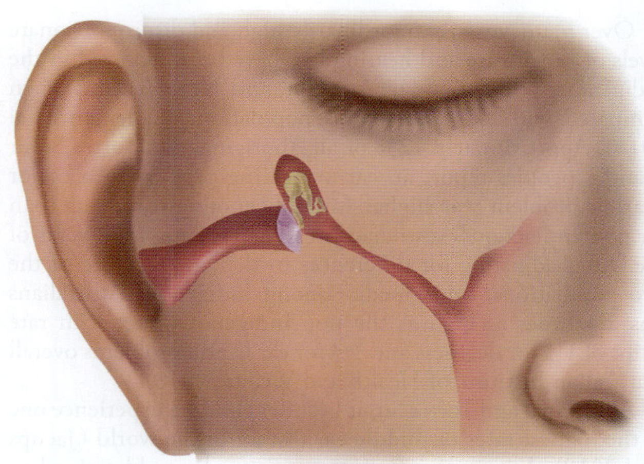

Figure 15.6
Infant and adult Eustachian tubes.

Late adulthood (65+ years)

In an individual over 65 years, cilia lining the ear canal can become coarse and stiff. This change may cause decreased hearing because it impedes sound waves travelling towards the tympanic membrane. It also causes cerumen to accumulate and oxidise, which greatly reduces hearing. The cerumen itself is drier because of atrophy of the apocrine glands. Also, a life history of frequent ear infections may result in scarring of the tympanic membrane.

Impacted cerumen is a common but reversible cause of hearing loss in people over 65 years. After removal of cerumen, most people have significantly improved hearing ability. Improvement of the hearing health of people over 65 years can be achieved by the routine performance of otoscopic examinations and irrigation of the ear canal when impacted cerumen occurs.

A person living in a noise-polluted area (e.g. near an airport or a busy highway) has a greater risk of hearing loss due to damage to the inner ear cells located in the cochlea. But **presbycusis** is a type of hearing loss that occurs with ageing, even in people living in a quiet environment. It is a gradual sensorineural loss caused by nerve degeneration in the inner ear or auditory nerve. Its onset usually occurs in the fifth decade, after which it slowly progresses. The person first notices a high-frequency tone loss; it is harder to hear consonants (high-pitched components of speech) than vowels. This makes words sound garbled. The ability to localise sound is impaired also. This communication dysfunction is accentuated when unfavourable background noise is present (e.g. with music, with dishes clattering or at a large noisy party).

The auditory reaction time increases after age 70 years; that is, there is a delay in receiving and sending nerve impulses associated with hearing in an ageing adult (Jamaa et al 2018).

CULTURAL AND SOCIAL CONSIDERATIONS

In today's society, the most significant cause of hearing loss is noise-induced hearing loss. Other causes include accidents, the effects of ototoxic drugs or chemicals and normal ageing.

Noise-induced hearing loss results from damage to the hearing cells of the cochlea of the inner ear. The damage, which results from either exposure to very loud noise or long-term exposure to 'reasonably loud noise', can often be attributed to prolonged employment in high-noise industries. Any noise louder than 85 decibels (dB) has potential to cause hearing loss. Hearing loss in children is associated with lifelong negative consequences of language development, socialisation, education (including numeracy and literacy), social and emotional wellbeing and self-esteem, training and employment opportunities, mental health and self-harm and domestic violence (Jervis-Bardy et al 2017). People of all ages with hearing loss are at risk of feeling isolated and frustrated (Deloitte Access Economics 2017a, 2017b, 2017c). A recently published study by Wang et al (2019) found that in Australia, across middle age, there is high and rising prevalence of slight and mild hearing loss which implies Australia has an opportunity to prevent progression of hearing loss in significant numbers of its population to reduce the profound later burden of age-related hearing loss. For younger age groups, the great concern about the use of digital devices remains (World Health Organization 2019a) (see 'Promoting a healthy lifestyle' below).

In New Zealand, the prevalence of hearing loss was estimated to be 18.9% of all New Zealanders. Prevalence is higher amongst males than females and it increases with age such that it is believed that most people will have mild hearing loss in their old age (90+ year old) (Deloitte Access Economics 2017a, 2017b, 2017c). Hearing loss is a major cause of disability and compensation (Deloitte Access Economics 2017a, 2017b, 2017c).

Over many years, extraordinarily high and disproportionate levels of ear disease and hearing loss have been reported in the Indigenous populations of Australia and New Zealand when compared with non-Indigenous populations (Coleman et al 2018). Approximately 12% of all Aboriginal and Torres Strait Islander peoples report an ear or hearing problem. An ear or hearing problem was higher for Indigenous Australians than for non-Indigenous Australians in all age groups 0–54 years of age. After adjusting for differences in the age structure of the two populations, otitis media among Indigenous Australians was 2.4 times as high as the non-Indigenous rate, with rate ratios of 1:4 for deafness and 1:3 for ear health problems overall (Australian Institute of Health and Welfare 2018).

Aboriginal and Torres Strait Islander children experience one of the highest rates of middle ear disease in the world (Jacups et al 2018). A recent inquiry into otitis media and hearing loss among Aboriginal and Torres Strait Islander children revealed that while only 7% of one-year-old children had bilaterally normal ears, half (51%) of the children investigated had 'glue ear', and 41% had bulging or perforated ear drums (Leach & Morris 2017). It was noted that parents reported that the children were not experiencing pain. Perhaps even more alarming are the results of the birth cohort study of almost 400 Aboriginal and Torres Strait Islander infants recruited at one month of age and reviewed again at 2, 4, 6, 12, 18 and 36 months of age. In this study it was reported that only one baby had normal ears at every visit to age 7 months, whereas 40% of one-month-old infants had otitis media in one ear, and 95% had bilateral otitis media. Chronic suppurative otitis media was seen in 5% of infants at 4 months of age and 27% at 36 months of age. By the time the infants in this study were one month of age, 50% had multiple bacteria colonisations of the nasopharynx (Leach & Morris 2017).

The most recent estimates of hearing loss in Māori and Pacific Islander peoples are based on 2001 Census data, in which the prevalence of hearing loss among people aged 15 years or older, not living in institutions, such as residential care facilities, was 7.5% (Exeter et al 2015). In reference to hearing loss, 43% of Māori people have permanent hearing loss, whereas only 22% of the New Zealand Europeans are so affected (Exeter et al 2015).

The significant risk of severe otitis media in Indigenous Australians and New Zealanders is compounded by poverty, overcrowded living conditions and frequent exposure to nonpathogenic bacteria, inadequate access to clean water and functional sewerage systems, nutritional problems and lack of access to healthcare (Deloitte Access Economics 2017a, 2017b, 2017c). Otitis media may not only impair hearing but is also associated with problems in language development, educational outcomes and reduced employment opportunities.

In Australia, funding has been provided for ear health initiatives aiming to give Aboriginal and Torres Strait Islander children a better start to education and to reduce the number of people experiencing avoidable hearing loss (Australian Institute of Health and Welfare 2018). In New Zealand, the Ministry of Health provides services via the National Screening Unit (Ministry of Health NZ 2019). Strategies implemented by the Australian and New Zealand governments include: the development of agencies such as Hearing Australia and The National Foundation for the Deaf Inc., to provide quality hearing resources to all people with hearing loss; conducting inquiries into hearing health; conducting research; providing national codes of practice and initiating screening programs for all children.

Subjective data

Determining what an individual feels or experiences in both recent and past times contributes subjective data to the assessment of ear health. Questions are focused on presence of pain, infection, discharge, hearing loss, vertigo, the environmental circumstances and how the individual cares for their ears. As you read this section, think critically about each assessment finding and its clinical significance. It is important that you adjust your assessment techniques if the person is hearing impaired.

1. Presenting concern
2. Earaches
3. Infections
4. Discharge
5. Hearing loss
6. Environmental noise
7. Tinnitus
8. Vertigo
9. Health and lifestyle management

Practice note: Before you commence the assessment, introduce yourself to the person, confirm the person's identity, discuss the purpose and scope of the assessment, clarify any questions the person may have and obtain verbal consent from the person to perform the assessment.

ASSESSMENT GUIDELINES	CLINICAL SIGNIFICANCE AND CLINICAL ALERTS
1. Presenting concern	
• Do you have any problems concerning your hearing or your ears? It is important to ascertain the person's perception of their presenting health concern. • If the person does perceive a problem—ask how does this impact on their quality of life?	**Note:** During history taking, the following clues from normal conversation indicate possible hearing loss: • Person lip reading or watching your face and lips closely rather than your eyes • Frowning or straining forwards to hear • Posturing of head to catch sounds with better ear • Misunderstanding your questions or frequently asking you to repeat • Irritability or showing startle reflex when you raise your voice (recruitment) • Speech sounds garbled, possibly with vowel sounds distorted • Inappropriately loud voice • Flat, monotonous tone of voice.
2. Presence, location and characteristics of earache	
Are you experiencing any earache or other pain in ears? • Location—does the pain feel close to the surface or deep in the head? • Does it hurt when you push on the ear or pull on the earlobe? • Assess the character of the earache or pain—ask the person to describe the pain; for example, dull, aching or sharp, stabbing? Is it constant or does it come and go? Is it affected by changing position of head? Ever had this kind of pain before?	**Otalgia**—ear pain—may be directly due to ear disease or may be referred pain from a problem in teeth or oropharynx. Pain that occurs when the person puts pressure on the ear or pulls the earlobe may indicate the presence of an inner ear infection. The character of the pain may indicate the severity of the ear problem. ***Clinical alert:*** People with severe or persistent earache should be referred to a medical practitioner.
• Presence of any accompanying cold symptoms or sore throat? Have there been any problems with sinuses or teeth? • Do you have any allergies?	Virus/bacteria from upper respiratory tract infections may migrate up the Eustachian tube to involve middle ear. **Allergic rhinitis** can commonly occur alongside otitis media. The inflammation and oedema of the nasopharynx can lead to Eustachian tube obstruction. If the obstruction persists for long enough, pressure in the middle ear results in development of middle ear fluid by transudation.
• Past or recent trauma of the ear area; for example, have you ever been hit on the ear or on the side of the head, or had any sports injury? Ever had any trauma from a foreign body?	Trauma may rupture the tympanic membrane.
• What have you done to try to relieve the earache/pain?	Assess effect of coping strategies or self-initiated interventions.
3. Presence or history of infections	
Have you experienced any ear infections? As an adult, or in childhood? • How frequent were they? How were they managed?	A history of chronic ear problems suggests possible sequelae.

ASSESSMENT GUIDELINES	CLINICAL SIGNIFICANCE AND CLINICAL ALERTS
4. Presence or history of discharge from the ear	
Has there been ever been any discharge from your ears?	Discharge (**otorrhoea**) suggests an infected canal or a perforated eardrum. For example:
• Colour—Does it look like pus or is it bloody?	**External otitis media**—purulent, sanguineous or watery discharge. **Acute otitis media with perforation**—purulent discharge.
• Odour—Is there any odour/smell to the discharge?	**Cholesteatoma**—dirty yellow/grey discharge, which is malodorous.
• Is there any relationship between the discharge and the ear pain?	Typically with perforation—ear pain occurs first, yet stops with a popping sensation then drainage occurs.
5. Presence or history of hearing loss	
Ever had any trouble hearing? • Onset—Did the loss come on slowly or all at once?	**Presbycusis** is gradual onset over years, whereas hearing loss resulting from trauma is often sudden. ***Clinical alert:*** Refer any sudden loss in one or both ears *not* associated with upper respiratory tract infection (URTI) for further investigation.
• Character—Has all your hearing decreased, or just on hearing certain sounds?	
• In what situations do you notice the loss: conversations, using the telephone, listening to TV or at a party?	Loss is apparent when competition from background noise is present, as at a party.
• Do people seem to shout at you?	**Recruitment**—a marked loss when sound is at low intensity, but sound actually becomes painful when repeated in a loud voice.
• Do ordinary sounds seem hollow, as if you are hearing in a barrel or under water? • Have you recently travelled by aeroplane? • Is there any family history of hearing loss? • Have you tried to treat the hearing loss with a hearing aid or other device? Have you tried anything to help with your hearing?	Character of hearing loss when cerumen expands and becomes impacted, for example, after swimming or showering.
• Assess the person's coping strategies. How does the loss affect your daily life? Any job problem? Feel embarrassed? Frustrated? How do your family, friends react?	Hearing loss can cause social isolation and can lessen pleasure of leisure activities.
6. Environmental noise	
• Any loud noises at home or on the job? For example, do you live in a noise-polluted area, near an airport or busy traffic area? Now or in the past?	Old trauma to hearing initially goes unnoticed but results in further decibel loss in later years.
• Are you near other noises such as heavy machinery or a loud persistent noise or loud music?	
• Assess the person's coping strategies. Have you taken any steps to protect your ears, such as headphones or ear plugs?	

ASSESSMENT GUIDELINES	CLINICAL SIGNIFICANCE AND CLINICAL ALERTS
7. Tinnitus	
• Have you ever felt ringing, crackling or buzzing in your ears? • When did this occur?	**Tinnitus** originates within the person; it accompanies some hearing or ear disorders.
• Does this seem louder at night?	Tinnitus seems louder with no competition from environment noise.
• Are you taking any medications?	Many medications have ototoxic sequelae: aspirin, aminoglycosides (streptomycin, gentamicin, kanamycin, neomycin), ethacrynic acid, frusemide, indomethacin, naproxen, quinine, vancomycin.
8. Vertigo	
• Ever felt vertigo, that is, the room spinning around or yourself spinning? (Vertigo is a true twirling motion.)	True rotational spinning occurs with dysfunction of labyrinth. **Objective vertigo**—feels like room spins. **Subjective vertigo**—person feels as if they are spinning. Dizziness and lightheadedness is likely to be due to changes in blood pressure. See Chapter 12.
• Ever felt dizzy, like you are not quite steady, like falling or losing your balance? Giddy, lightheaded?	Distinguish true vertigo from dizziness or lightheadedness. People who experience vertigo are at risk of falling or injury.
9. Health and lifestyle management	
• How do you clean your ears?	Assess potential trauma from invasive instruments. Cotton-tipped applicators can impact cerumen, causing hearing loss.
• When was the last time you had your hearing checked? • If a hearing loss was noted, did you obtain a hearing aid? How long have you had it? Do you wear it? How does it work? Any trouble with upkeep, cleaning, changing batteries?	Prescribe frequency of hearing assessment according to person's age or risk factors.
Additional history for infants and children (questions for parents or guardians)	
Ear infections. At what age was the child's first episode? How many ear infections in the last 6 months? How many in total? How were these managed? • Assess the child's feeding type, e.g. bottle or breast fed? What is the child's usual position during feeding? • Has the child had any surgery, such as insertion of tympanoplasty tubes/ventilation tubes (commonly called grommets) or removal of tonsils?	Bottle feeding, particularly in the supine position, is a risk factor for the development of ear infections in infants and younger children. A first episode occurring within 3 months of life increases the risk of recurrent otitis media. Recurrent otitis media is three episodes in past 6 months but more likely in the presence of otitis media with effusions (Kaur et al 2017).
• Are the infections increasing in frequency, in severity or staying the same?	
• Does anyone in the home smoke cigarettes or a pipe?	Passive and gestational smoke is a risk factor for otitis media (Vanker et al 2017).
• Does your child receive childcare outside your home? In a daycare centre or someone else's home? How many children in the group being cared for?	Attendance at daycare and bottle feeding (as opposed to breastfeeding) are also risk factors for otitis media (Megged et al 2017).

SUBJECTIVE DATA

ASSESSMENT GUIDELINES	CLINICAL SIGNIFICANCE AND CLINICAL ALERTS
Does the child seem to be hearing well? • Have you noticed that the infant startles with loud noise? Did the infant babble around 6 months? Do they talk? At what age did talking start? Was the speech intelligible? • Ever had the child's hearing tested? If there was a hearing loss, did it follow any diseases in the child, or in the mother during pregnancy?	Children at risk for hearing deficit include those exposed to maternal rubella, syphilis, cytomegalovirus or toxoplasmosis or to maternal ototoxic drugs in utero; premature infants; low birth weight infants; trauma or hypoxia at birth; and infants with congenital liver or kidney disease. In children, the incidence of meningitis, measles, mumps, otitis media and any illness with persistent high fever may increase risk of hearing deficit (Hockenberry et al 2016). ***Clinical alert:*** It is important to identify any problem early, because a child with hearing loss is at risk for delayed speech and social development and learning deficit.
Does the child tend to put objects in the ears? Is the older child or adolescent active in contact sports?	These children are at increased risk for trauma.

OBJECTIVE DATA

Objective data

The focus of ear examination includes screening for hearing loss and assessing for other ear problems such as ear pain, discharge, lumps or the presence of foreign objects. A nurse will be able to detect problems in the ear canal or tympanic membrane. Signs of infection, excessive cerumen or foreign objects will clearly be seen.

Collecting objective data is an important part of any ear assessment. The objective ear assessment is used for screening infants and children for hearing loss, investigating symptoms such as ear pain, pressure and fullness, checking for excessive cerumen or other objects in the ear canal and locating the site of an ear infection. Objective data collection also enables a nurse to monitor the effectiveness of a treatment plan for an ear problem.

Changes in the objective data have significant implications. Infants and children with ear problems have been known to be irritable, display signs of stress and anxiety and be socially isolated. Social isolation is also a common consequence for adolescents, adults and older adults (Peelle & Wingfield 2016). As the adult ages, changes in ear function can result in risk of injury due to dizziness or hearing loss.

Preparation

Position the adult sitting up straight with their head at your eye level. Occasionally, the ear canal is partially filled with cerumen, which obstructs your view of the tympanic membrane. In this case, the person should be referred to a medical practitioner for further assessment.

Equipment needed

Otoscope with bright light (fresh batteries give off white—not yellow—light)

Hand hygiene solution

PROCEDURES AND NORMAL FINDINGS	ABNORMAL FINDINGS AND CLINICAL ALERTS
General inspection	
You will have already noted the ability of the person to hear your instructions and questions during subjective data collection. Make a note of your findings.	
Inspect and palpate the external ear	
Size and shape	
The ears are of equal size bilaterally with no swelling or thickening. Ears of unusual size and shape may be a normal familial trait with no clinical significance.	**Microtia**—ears smaller than 4 cm vertically. **Macrotia**—ears larger than 10 cm vertically. Oedema.

PROCEDURES AND NORMAL FINDINGS	ABNORMAL FINDINGS AND CLINICAL ALERTS
Skin condition	
The skin is intact, with no lumps or lesions. On some people you may note **Darwin's tubercle**, a small painless nodule at the helix. This is a congenital variation and is not significant (see Table 15.2).	Reddened, excessively warm skin indicates inflammation (see Table 15.1). Crusts and scaling occur with otitis externa, eczema, contact dermatitis, seborrhoea. Enlarged tender lymph nodes in the region indicate inflammation of the pinna or mastoid process. Red-blue discolouration indicates frostbite. Tophi, sebaceous cyst, chondrodermatitis, keloid, carcinoma (see Table 15.2).
Tenderness	
Move the pinna and push on the tragus. They should feel firm and movement should produce no pain. Palpating the mastoid process should also produce no pain.	Pain with movement occurs with otitis externa and furuncle (infection of a hair follicle). Pain at the mastoid process may indicate mastoiditis or lymphadenitis of the posterior auricular node.
The external auditory meatus	
Note the size of the opening to direct your choice of speculum for the otoscope. No swelling, redness or discharge should be present.	**Atresia**—absence or closure of the ear canal. A sticky yellow discharge accompanies otitis externa or may indicate otitis media if the drum has ruptured. A ruptured tympanic membrane will be detected on otoscopic examination.
	Clinical alert: Frank blood or clear, watery drainage (cerebrospinal fluid (CSF)) after trauma suggests basal skull fracture. The person should be referred for urgent medical review.
Some cerumen is usually present. The colour varies from grey-yellow to light brown and black, and the texture varies from moist and waxy to dry and desiccated. A large amount of cerumen obscures visualisation of the canal and drum.	Impacted cerumen is a common cause of conductive hearing loss.
Inspect with the otoscope	
As you inspect the external ear, note the size of the auditory meatus. Then choose the largest speculum that will fit comfortably in the ear canal and attach it to the otoscope. Tilt the person's head slightly away from you towards the opposite shoulder. This method brings the obliquely sloping eardrum into better view.	
Pull the pinna up and back on a pre-adolescent child or adult; this helps straighten the S-shape of the canal (Figure 15.7). Hold the pinna gently but firmly. Do not release traction on the ear until you have finished the examination and the otoscope is removed.	Pulling on the pinna may cause and increase pain if the person has otitis media.

PROCEDURES AND NORMAL FINDINGS	ABNORMAL FINDINGS AND CLINICAL ALERTS
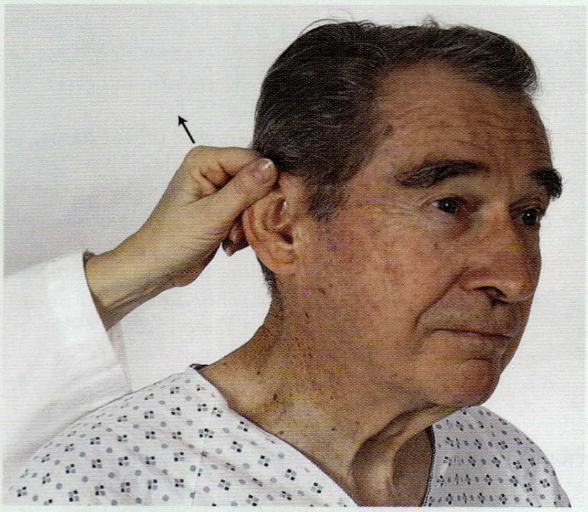 **Figure 15.7** Pulling on adult pinna.	
Hold the otoscope 'upside down' along your fingers and have the dorsa (back) of your hand along the person's cheek braced to steady the otoscope (Figure 15.8). This position feels awkward to you only at first. It soon will feel natural and you will find it useful to prevent forceful insertion. Also, your stabilising hand acts as a protecting lever if the person suddenly moves their head. 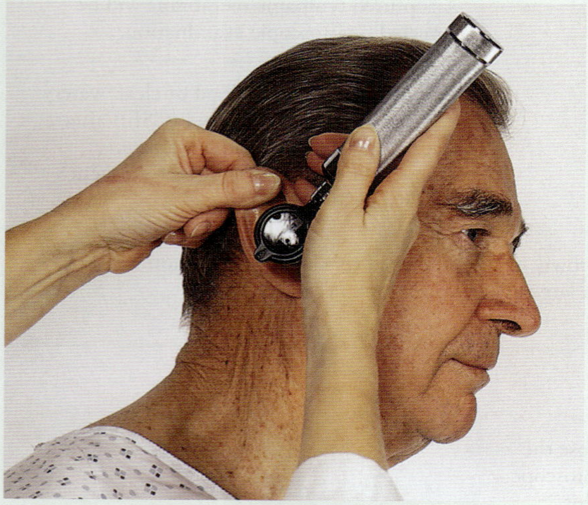 **Figure 15.8** Holding the otoscope.	
Insert the speculum slowly and carefully along the axis of the canal. Watch the insertion; then put your eye up to the otoscope. Avoid touching the inner 'bony' section of the canal wall, which is covered by a thin epithelial layer and is sensitive to pain. Sometimes you cannot see anything but canal wall. If so, try to reposition the person's head, apply more traction on the pinna and re-angle the otoscope to look forwards towards the person's nose.	

PROCEDURES AND NORMAL FINDINGS	ABNORMAL FINDINGS AND CLINICAL ALERTS
Once it is in place, you may need to rotate the otoscope slightly to visualise the entire eardrum; do this gently. Lastly, perform the otoscopic examination before you test hearing; ear canals with impacted cerumen give the erroneous impression of pathological hearing loss. See Table 15.3.	
The external canal	
Note any redness and swelling, lesions, foreign bodies or discharge. If any discharge is present, note the colour and odour. (Also, clean any discharge from the speculum before examining the other ear to avoid contamination with possibly infectious material.) For a person with a hearing aid, note any irritation on the canal wall from poorly fitting hearing aid ear moulds.	Redness and swelling occur with otitis externa; canal may be completely closed with swelling. This condition clearly will induce temporary unilateral hearing loss and has implications for communication. Purulent otorrhoea suggests otitis externa or otitis media if the drum has ruptured. Foreign body, polyp, furuncle, exostosis (see Table 15.3).
The tympanic membrane	
Colour and characteristics. Systematically explore its landmarks (Figure 15.9). The normal eardrum is shiny and translucent, with a pearl-grey colour. The cone-shaped light reflex is prominent in the anteroinferior quadrant (at 5 o'clock in the right drum and 7 o'clock in the left drum). This is the reflection of your otoscope light. Sections of the malleus are visible through the translucent drum: the umbo, manubrium and short process. (Infrequently, you also may see the incus behind the drum; it shows as a whitish haze in the upper posterior area.) At the periphery the annulus looks whiter and denser.	Yellow–amber drum colour occurs with otitis media with effusion (serous). Red colour occurs with acute otitis media. Absent or distorted landmarks. Air/fluid level or air bubbles behind drum indicate otitis media with effusion (see Table 15.4).
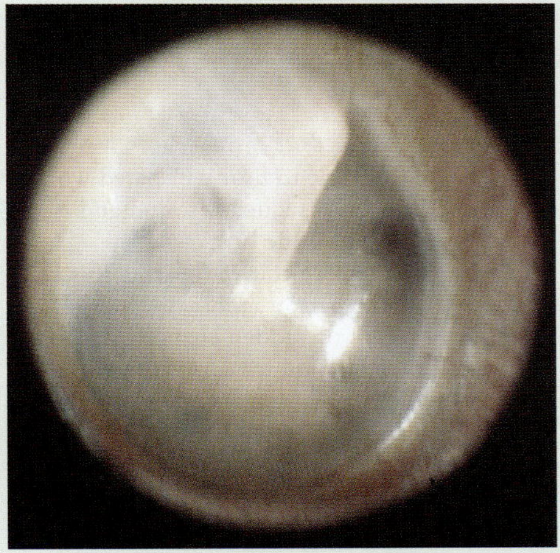 **Figure 15.9** Tympanic membrane.	
Position. The eardrum is flat, slightly pulled in at the centre and flutters when the person performs the Valsalva manoeuvre or holds the nose and swallows (insufflation). You may elicit these manoeuvres to assess drum mobility. Avoid them with an ageing person because they may disrupt equilibrium. Also, avoid middle ear insufflation in a person with upper respiratory infection because it could propel infectious matter into the middle ear.	Retracted drum resulting from vacuum in middle ear with obstructed Eustachian tube. Bulging drum from increased pressure in otitis media. Drum hypomobility is an early sign of otitis media (see Table 15.4).

OBJECTIVE DATA

PROCEDURES AND NORMAL FINDINGS	ABNORMAL FINDINGS AND CLINICAL ALERTS
Integrity of membrane. Inspect the eardrum and the entire circumference of the annulus for perforations. The normal tympanic membrane is intact. Some adults may show scarring, which is a dense white patch on the drum. This is a sequela of repeated ear infections. Refer to Table 15.5 below.	Perforation shows as a dark oval area or as a larger opening on the drum. Vesicles on drum (see Table 15.4).

TABLE 15.5 Abnormal views seen on otoscopy

APPEARANCE OF EARDRUM	INDICATES	SUGGESTED CONDITION
Yellow-amber colour	Serum or pus	Otitis media with effusion (OME) or chronic otitis media
Prominent landmarks	Retraction of drum	Vacuum in middle ear from obstructed Eustachian tube
Air/fluid level or air bubbles	Serous fluid	Otitis media with effusion
Absent or distorted light reflex	Bulging of eardrum	Acute otitis media
Bright red colour	Infection in middle ear	Acute otitis media
Blue or dark red colour	Blood behind drum	Trauma, skull fracture
Dark, round or oval areas	Perforation	Drum rupture
White dense areas	Scarring	Sequelae of infections
Diminished or absent landmarks	Thickened drum	Chronic otitis media
Black or white dots on drum or canal	Colony of growth	Fungal infection

Test hearing acuity

Whispered voice test

PROCEDURES AND NORMAL FINDINGS	ABNORMAL FINDINGS AND CLINICAL ALERTS
Test one ear at a time while masking hearing in the other ear to prevent sound transmission around the head. This is done by placing one finger on the tragus and rapidly pushing it in and out of the auditory meatus. Shield your lips so the person cannot compensate for a hearing loss (consciously or unconsciously) by lip reading or using the 'good' ear. With your head 30–60 cm from the person's ear, exhale and whisper slowly some two-syllable words, such as Tuesday, armchair, football and fourteen. Normally, the person repeats each word correctly after you say it.	The person is unable to hear whispered words. A whisper is a high-frequency sound and is used to detect high-tone loss. If the whisper test is positive (hearing loss indicated) or the person reports deafness or significant recent or sudden change in hearing they should be referred for formal hearing testing (audiometry) (Talley & O'Connor 2018).

The vestibular apparatus

PROCEDURES AND NORMAL FINDINGS	ABNORMAL FINDINGS AND CLINICAL ALERTS
The **Romberg test** assesses the ability of the vestibular apparatus in the inner ear to help maintain standing balance. The Romberg test also assesses intactness of the cerebellum and proprioception, and therefore it is also discussed in Chapter 12 (see Figure 12.28).	

Additional objective data for infants and children

Hearing acuity

PROCEDURES AND NORMAL FINDINGS	ABNORMAL FINDINGS AND CLINICAL ALERTS
Newborn—startle (Moro) reflex, acoustic blink reflex **3–4 months**—acoustic blink reflex, infant stops movement and appears to 'listen', halts sucking, quiets if crying, cries if quiet	Absence of alerting behaviour may indicate congenital deafness.
6–8 months—infant turns head to localise sound, responds to own name	Failure to localise sound.

OBJECTIVE DATA

PROCEDURES AND NORMAL FINDINGS	ABNORMAL FINDINGS AND CLINICAL ALERTS
Preschool and school-age child—child must be screened with audiometry Note that a young child may be unaware of a hearing loss because the child does not know how one 'ought' to hear.	No intelligible speech by 2 years of age. Note these behavioural manifestations of hearing loss: • The child is inattentive in casual conversation. • The child reacts more to movement and facial expression than to sound. • The child's facial expression is strained or puzzled. • The child frequently asks to have statements repeated. • The child confuses words that sound alike. • The child has an accompanying speech problem: speech is monotonous or garbled; the child mispronounces or omits sounds. • The child appears shy and withdrawn and 'lives in a world of their own'. • The child frequently complains of earaches. • The child hears better at times when the environment is more conducive to hearing.
	Clinical alert: If the child has any symptoms of hearing difficulty they should be referred for formal hearing testing (audiometry) (Talley & O'Connor 2018).
Inspect external ear structure	
Examination of the external ear is similar to that described for the adult, with the addition of examination of position and alignment on head. Note the ear position. The top of the pinna should match an imaginary line extending from the corner of the eye to the occiput. Also, the ear should be positioned within 10 degrees of vertical (Figure 15.10). Low-set ears or deviation in alignment may be associated with some congenital syndromes.	

10°

Normal alignment

> 10°

Low-set ears and deviation in alignment

Figure 15.10
Ear alignment.

OBJECTIVE DATA

PROCEDURES AND NORMAL FINDINGS	ABNORMAL FINDINGS AND CLINICAL ALERTS
Otoscopic examination	
Eardrum assessment is mandatory for any infant or child requiring care for illness or fever. For the infant or young child, the timing of the otoscopic examination is best towards the end of the complete examination. Many young children protest vigorously during this procedure no matter how well you prepare, and it is difficult to re-establish cooperation afterwards. Save the otoscopic examination until last. Then the parent/caregiver can hold and comfort the child.	
To help prepare the child, let the child hold your funny-looking 'torch', that is the otoscope. You may wish to have the child look in the parent's/caregivers' ear as you hold the otoscope (Figure 15.11). **Figure 15.11** Child preparation.	
Positioning of the child is important. You need a clear view of the canal. Avoid harsh restraint, but you must protect the eardrum from injury in case of sudden head movement. Enlist the aid of a cooperative parent/caregiver. Prop an infant upright against the adult's chest or shoulder, with the adult's arm around the upper part of the head (Figure 15.12). A toddler can be held in the parent's/caregiver's lap or may lie on the examining table with their arms secured (Figure 15.13). In each case, the child's head is stabilised to avoid movement against the otoscope.	

PROCEDURES AND NORMAL FINDINGS	ABNORMAL FINDINGS AND CLINICAL ALERTS

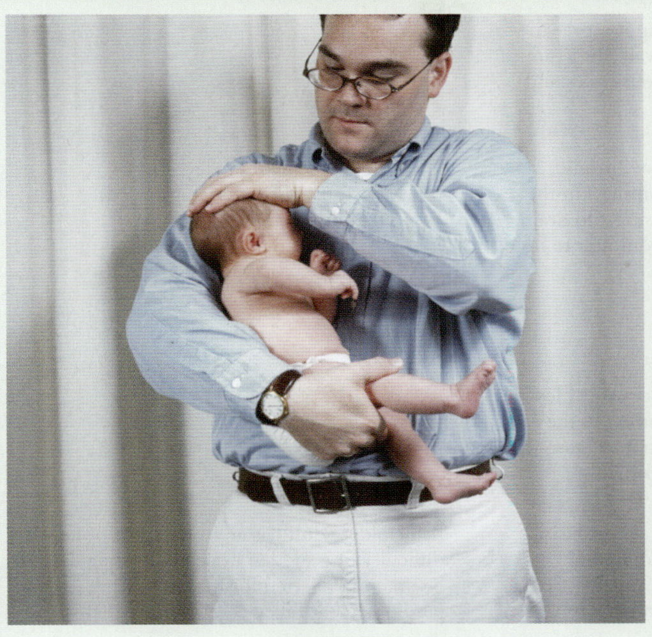

Figure 15.12
Holding infant.

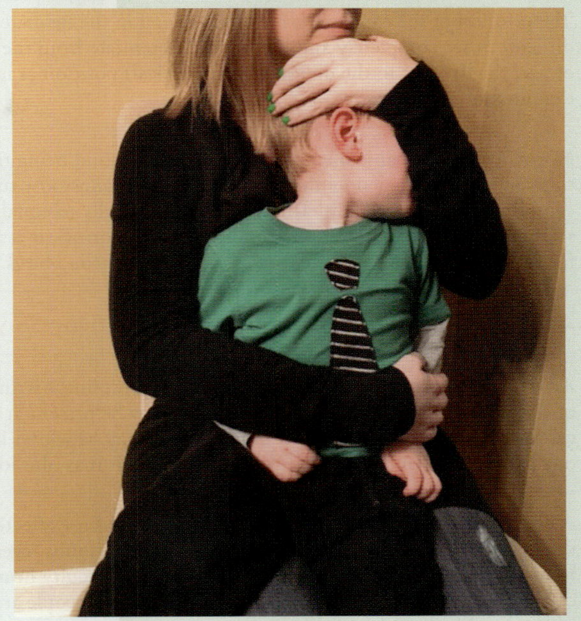

Figure 15.13
Positioning of child.

Remember to pull the pinna straight down on an infant or a child under 3 years old. This method will match the slope of the ear canal (Figure 15.14).

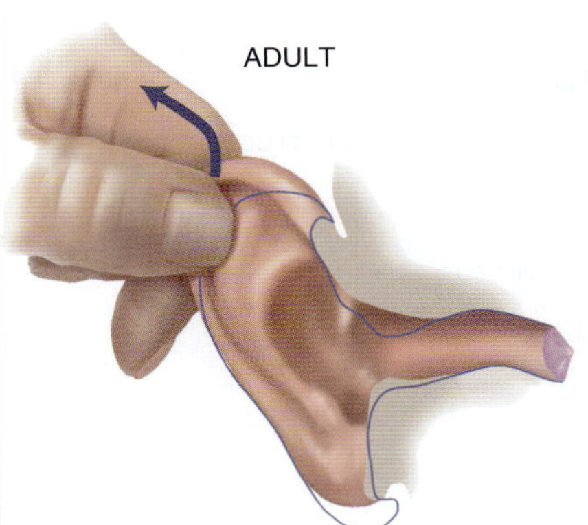

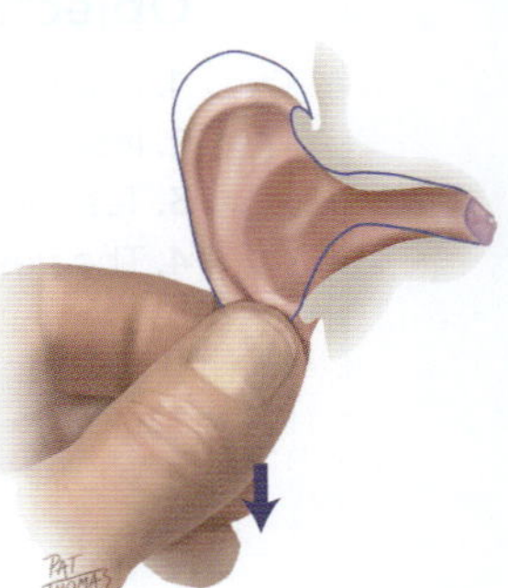

Figure 15.14
Pulling of pinna.

At birth the patency of the ear canal is determined, but the otoscopic examination is not performed because the canal is filled with amniotic fluid and vernix caseosa. After a few days the tympanic membrane is examined. During the first few days, the tympanic membrane often looks thickened and opaque. It may look 'injected' and have a mild redness from increased vascularity. The eardrum also looks injected in infants after crying.

PROCEDURES AND NORMAL FINDINGS	ABNORMAL FINDINGS AND CLINICAL ALERTS
The position of the eardrum is more horizontal in the neonate, making it more difficult to see completely and harder to differentiate from the canal wall. By 1 month of age, the drum is in the oblique (more vertical) position as in the older child, and examination is a bit easier.	
Normally the tympanic membrane is intact. In a child being treated for chronic otitis media, you may note the presence of a tympanostomy tube (grommet) in the central part of the eardrum. This is inserted surgically to equalise pressure and drain secretions. Finally, although the condition is not normal, it is not uncommon to note a foreign body in a child's canal, such as a small stone or a bead.	**Chronic otitis media** relieved by tympanostomy tubes (see Table 15.4). Foreign body (see Table 15.3).
Additional objective data for the adult over 65 years	
An older person may have pendulous earlobes with linear wrinkling because of loss of elasticity of the pinna. Coarse, wiry hairs may be present at the opening of the ear canal. During otoscopy the eardrum normally may be whiter in colour and more opaque, duller than in the early or middle adult. It may also look thickened.	
A high-tone frequency hearing loss is apparent for those affected with presbycusis, the hearing loss that occurs with ageing. This condition is revealed in difficulty hearing whispered words in the voice test and in difficulty hearing consonants during conversational speech. The older adult may feel that 'people are mumbling' and feels isolated in family or friendship groups.	If the older adult has any symptoms of hearing difficulty or a sudden hearing loss they should be urgently referred for formal hearing testing (audiometry) (Talley & O'Connor 2018).

Summary Checklist

EAR ASSESSMENT

Subjective data

1. Presenting concern
2. Earaches
3. Infections
4. Discharge
5. Hearing loss
6. Environmental noise
7. Tinnitus
8. Vertigo
9. Health and lifestyle management

Objective data

1. Inspect and palpate external ear structures
2. Inspect with otoscope
3. Test hearing acuity
4. The vestibular apparatus

PROMOTING A HEALTHY LIFESTYLE

THE MODERN WORLD: EARBUDS/HEADPHONES, LOUD MUSIC AND HEARING LOSS

The World Health Organization (WHO) estimates that 1.1 billion young people globally (aged between 12 and 35 years) are at risk of hearing loss due to exposure to noise in recreational settings. One in five teenagers have some form of hearing loss because of headphone/ear bud use (WHO 2019a, 2019b). In the teenage group, that's an alarming 30% increase since the 1990s (WHO 2019a, 2019b).

Many of us are wearing headphones/ear buds all day, every day, as we listen to music or podcasts on our commute to school or work, while exercising or relaxing or merely to drown out other environmental noise. Earphones are placed over the ear and earbuds are placed directly in the ear canal; both result in the sound being placed closer to the eardrum. Listening with earbuds boosts sound signals. An increase of 10 dB increases the impact of the sound tenfold. Sound at 70 dB transmits 1000 times as much energy as sound at 40 dB. Normal conversation takes place at about 60 dB, whereas a chainsaw typically records at 100 dB and a rock concert at 110 dB (WHO 2019b).

Further, because the sound is digital, there is virtually no distortion, no matter how loud the volume with most earbud wearers not necessarily aware of the sound levels they're exposing themselves to (Scott & Armitage 2018). Most significantly, because digital music devices can hold thousands of songs and play for hours without the need for recharging, users tend to listen continuously for hours at a time. In this example, hearing loss occurs slowly and often goes unnoticed until it is quite extensive. It is feared that exposure to audio played directly into our ears will lead to a prematurely deaf generation of Australians (Scott & Armitage 2018). It has also been established that 40% of 12–35 year olds are subject to 'binge listening' by being exposed to potentially damaging sound levels at clubs, dance parties, discotheques and bars (WHO 2019d). In such venues, patrons are exposed to very loud noises for a period of up to 3–5 hours.

Hearing loss as a result of loud sounds cannot be reversed (Eggermont 2017). However, while it is often difficult to explain the risks to young people who tend not to worry about future damage, nurses can raise awareness of the problem and provide information about appropriate preventative measures. Deciding how much noise is too much can be understood by the concept of a 'noise dose' which refers to the relationship between the level of noise and the time of exposure. Many experts suggest that digital music players should be designed either to prevent playing of music above 85 dB or to be limited to a maximum volume of 100 dB.

Early prevention is the key to preventing hearing loss due to an excessive noise dose. To maintain a safe level of hearing it is recommended that:

- the time of exposure is halved for every increase of 3 dB of noise level above 85 dB.
- people use larger headphones that rest over the ear opening or noise-cancelling headphones that eliminate background noise so that listeners do not have to increase the volume so high.

Refer the person to *A toolkit for safe listening devices and systems* (WHO and International Telecommunications Union 2019c) which provides the necessary practical guidance for the implementation of the global standard for safe listening devices.

ELECTRONIC CIGARETTES (E-CIGARETTES) USE AND HEARING LOSS

While the e-cigarette was initially designed as a smoking cessation device, instead it is rapidly being favoured as an electronic device for delivery of nicotine (Song et al 2018). The device is used to inhale solutions of nicotine, flavourings and other chemicals. The added solution is turned into an aerosol by the battery operated device which is then inhaled into the lungs. The amount of nicotine in individual solutions is variable. Vaping occurs when the user inhales and exhales the aerosol, often referred to as vapour, which is produced by an e-cigarette. The efficacy as a smoking cessation device has not been investigated (Ferkol et al 2018). However, research into the effect on the upper airway or middle ear found that e-cigarette use affected the viability of middle ear epithelial cells potentially leading to hearing loss (Song et al 2018). Nurses must be alert to the impending problems associated with e-cigarettes and inform users about the risks.

OBJECTIVE DATA

Documentation and critical thinking

FOCUSED ASSESSMENT: CLINICAL CASE STUDY 1

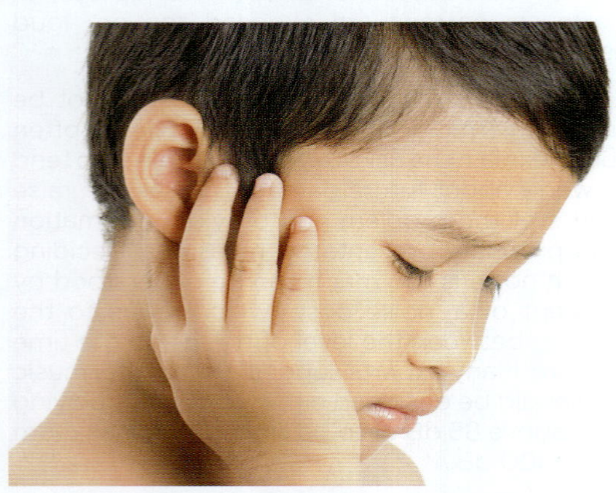

Context

The registered nurse works as a practice nurse in a busy local multidisciplinary health clinic. This role includes screening assessments for clients who attend.

Subjective

Matthew Williams is a 4-year-old child who was brought into the local health clinic by his mother after he had been crying for most of the night and was difficult to settle. The only sleep the child had was when he was held upright against his mother's chest, but he slept for short periods only. The child feels warm to touch.

History: Matthew is the second child born to Mr. and Mrs. Williams. He was born at term. The pregnancy, labour and delivery were uncomplicated. Matthew is up to date with all childhood immunisations and has no significant previous medical history. His mother reports that Matthew has recently had a mild cold.

Social history: Matthew and his parents live in a small two-bedroom house approximately 40 km north of the central business district. He shares a bedroom with his older sister who is aged 6 years. Matthew's father works at the local council undertaking park and garden maintenance and Matthew's mother works as a receptionist in a community centre. The children are cared for by their maternal grandmother. The grandmother also cares for two other grandchildren every day. Both parents and Matthew's grandmother smoke up to 10 cigarettes each per day.

Yesterday, Matthew's grandmother put him to bed for his afternoon nap. He did not sleep very long before he awoke crying and clearly tugging at his right ear. He would have a small drink but refused to eat solid food. His mother measured his temperature later in the day when she had taken him home. Matthew's temperature was measured at 38°C (tympanic). Matthew has been fussing and crying most of the night. His mother has not tried to give him any medication.

Objective

T 38.4°C (tympanic), HR 100, R 20.

Alert, developmentally appropriate for age.

Skin: Warm and dry, no rashes or lesions.

Eyes: No exudate, conjunctivae clear, sclerae white.

Ears: Left tympanic membrane is intact and pearly grey in appearance. Right tympanic membrane dull red and bulging, no light reflex.

Nose: snuffly breathing with small amount of clear nasal discharge

Mouth/throat: Oral mucosa pink, no lesions or exudate, tonsils 1+

Lungs: Breath sounds clear and equal bilaterally, unlaboured

Collaborative problem

Probable acute otitis media—needs referral to the general practitioner for review and management strategies

Problem statements/nursing diagnoses

Pain related to inflammation in right tympanic membrane

Risk for chronic ear infection injury related to risk factors

Discomfort related to high temperature

Knowledge deficit for parents and guardians about risk factors and aspects of care

FOCUSED ASSESSMENT: CLINICAL CASE STUDY 2

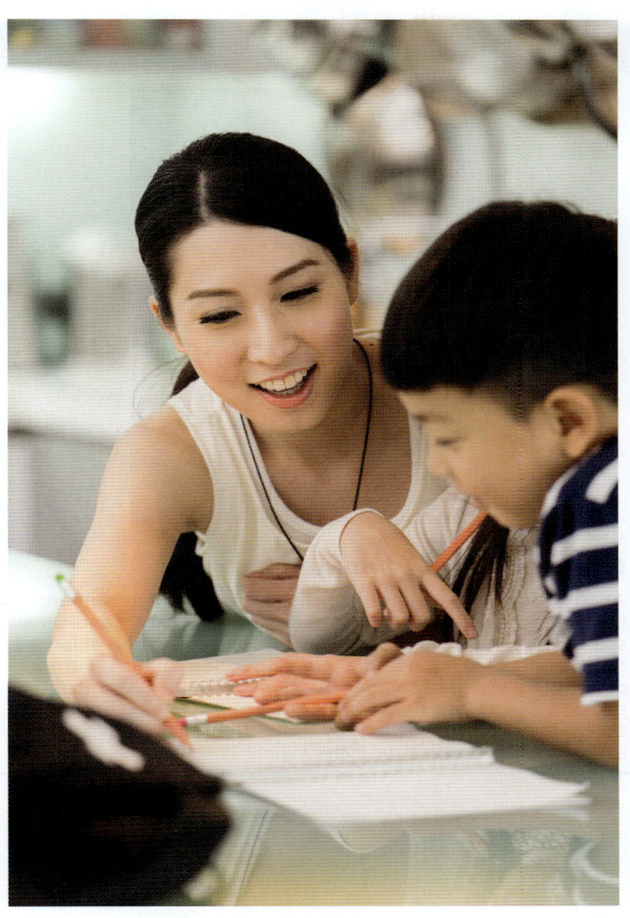

Context

The registered nurse works as a practice nurse in a busy local multidisciplinary health clinic. This role includes screening assessments for clients who attend.

Subjective

Julia Chong is a 35-year-old single woman. She is employed as a teacher in a local primary school, teaching children who are in year 2. She has presented to the health clinic complaining of 'ringing in her ears' that she has felt since attending a concert on Saturday night and being unable to hear the children clearly when they spoke to her over the last couple of days at school.

She reports that in her early twenties she went out to local bands or nightclubs almost every weekend. Over the period of the last year or so she has found it hard to hear when she is in the company of a group of people or if there is background noise. She has been frustrated when she can't participate in the conversation and is left feeling isolated.

She also states she has had intermittent periods of tinnitus that did not bother her and which she did not seek medical attention for.

Objective

T 37°C oral, HR 72, BP 120/70.

Ears: Right and left tympanic membranes are intact and pearly grey in appearance. Small amount of yellow cerumen in left ear canal.

Nose: Able to breath effectively through both nostrils.

Throat: Moist and pink. Tonsils present.

Hearing: Whisper test—reduced hearing in right and left ear.

Collaborative problem

Probable noise-induced hearing loss—requires referral for testing of auditory function and to general practitioner for examination and management.

Problem statements/nursing diagnoses

Disturbed sensory perception related to ringing in ears and hearing impairment

Risk of impaired verbal communication related to hearing loss and its implications on personal and professional life

Lack of knowledge related to preventative measures and management strategies.

Abnormal findings

TABLE 15.1 Abnormalities of the external ear

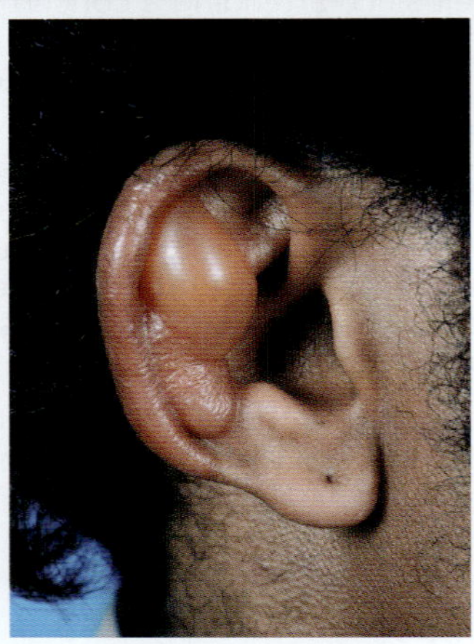

Frostbite

Reddish blue discolouration and swelling of auricle after exposure to extreme cold. Vesicles or bullae may develop, the person feels pain and tenderness and ear necrosis may ensue.

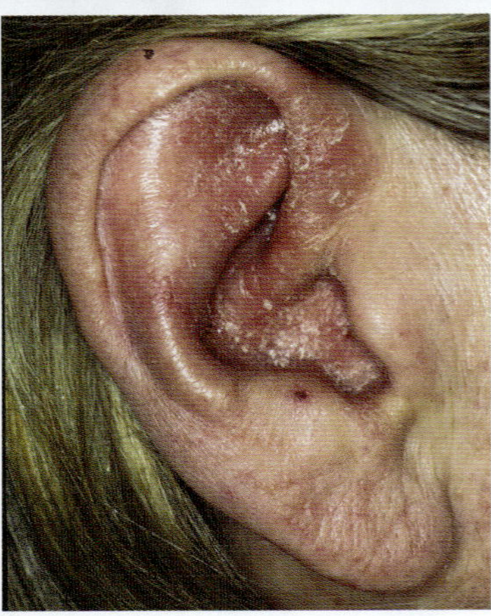

Otitis externa (swimmer's ear)

An infection of the outer ear, with severe painful movement of the pinna and tragus, redness and swelling of pinna and canal, scanty purulent discharge, scaling, itching, fever and enlarged tender regional lymph nodes. Hearing is normal or slightly diminished. More common in hot humid weather. Swimming causes canal to become waterlogged and swell; skinfolds are set up for infection. Prevent by using rubbing alcohol or 2% acetic acid eardrops after every swim.

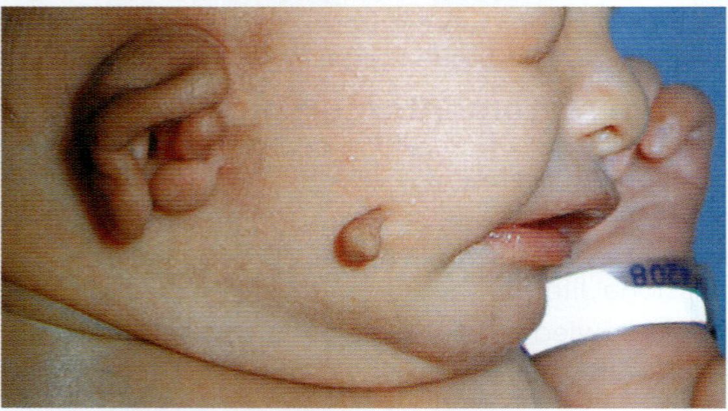

Branchial remnant and ear deformity

A facial remnant or leftover of the embryological branchial arch usually appears as a skin tag, in this case one containing cartilage. They occur most often in the preauricular area, in front of the tragus. When bilateral, there is increased risk of renal anomalies.

TABLE 15.2 Lumps and lesions on the external ear

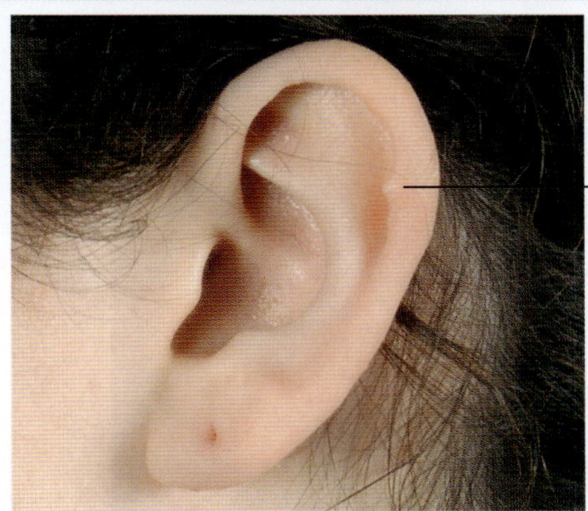

Darwin's tubercle

Small painless nodule at the helix. It is a congenital variation and is not significant. Distinguish this condition from tophus.

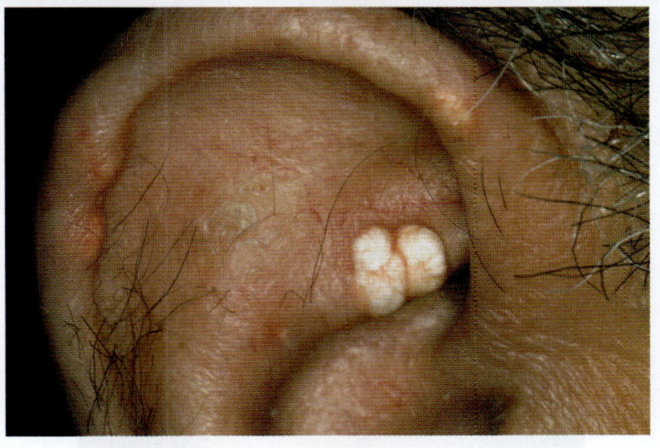

Tophi

Small, whitish-yellow, hard, nontender nodules in or near helix or antihelix; contain greasy, chalky material of uric acid crystals and are a sign of gout.

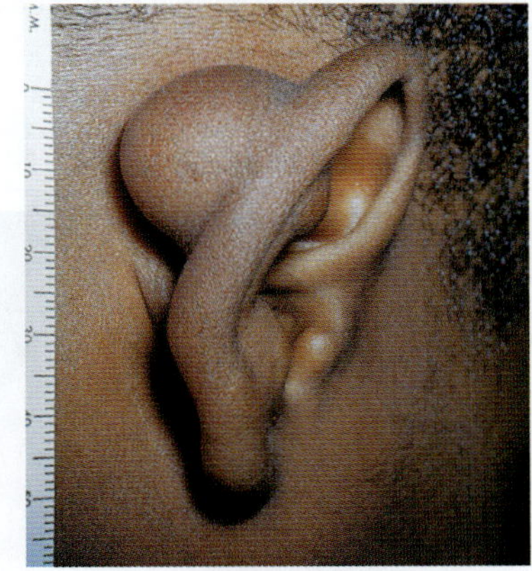

Sebaceous cyst

Location is commonly behind lobule, in the postauricular fold. A nodule with central black punctum indicates blocked sebaceous gland. It is filled with waxy sebaceous material and is painful if it becomes infected. Often are multiple.

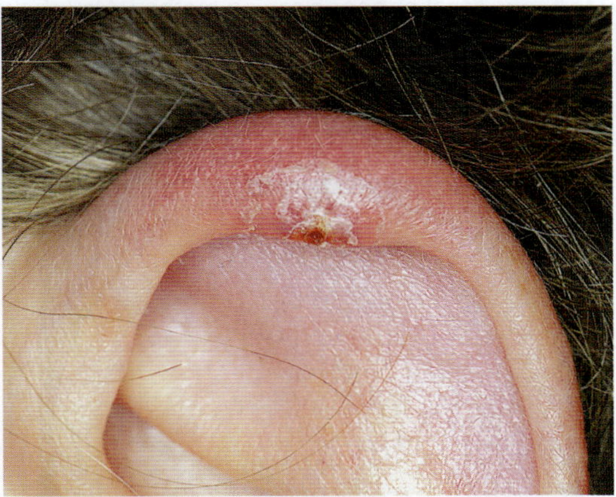

Chondrodermatitis nodularis helicus

Painful nodules develop on the rim of the helix (where there is no cushioning subcutaneous tissue) as a result of repetitive mechanical pressure or environmental trauma (sunlight). They are small, indurated, dull red, poorly defined and very painful.

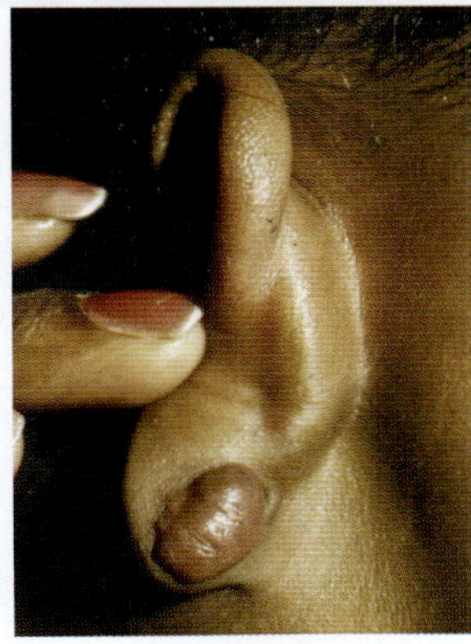

Keloid

Overgrowth of scar tissue, which invades original site of trauma. It is more common in dark-skinned people. In the ear it is most common at lobule at the site of a pierced ear. Overgrowth shown here is unusually large.

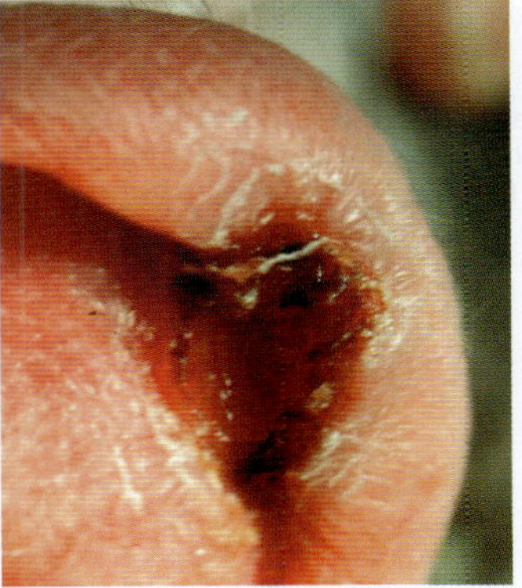

Carcinoma

Ulcerated crusted nodule with indurated base that fails to heal. Bleeds intermittently. Must refer for biopsy. Usually occurs on the superior rim of the pinna, which has the most sun exposure. May occur also in ear canal and show chronic discharge that is either serosanguineous or sanguineous.

TABLE 15.3 Abnormalities in the ear canal

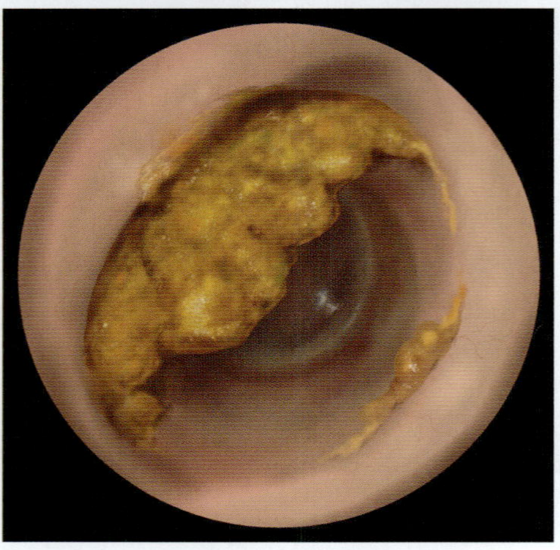

Excessive cerumen

Excessive cerumen is produced or is impacted because of narrow tortuous canal or poor cleaning method. May show as round ball partially obscuring drum or totally occluding canal. Even when canal is 90–95% blocked, hearing stays normal. But when last 5–10% is totally occluded (when cerumen expands after swimming or showering), person has ear fullness and sudden hearing loss.

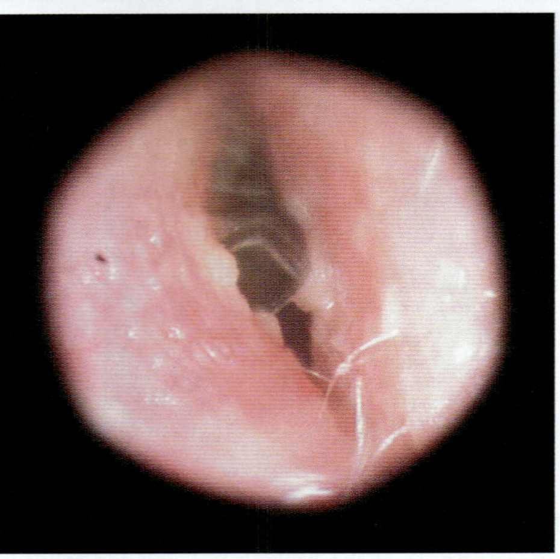

Otitis externa

Severe swelling of canal, inflammation, tenderness. Here canal lumen is narrowed to one-quarter normal size. (See complete description in Table 15.2.)

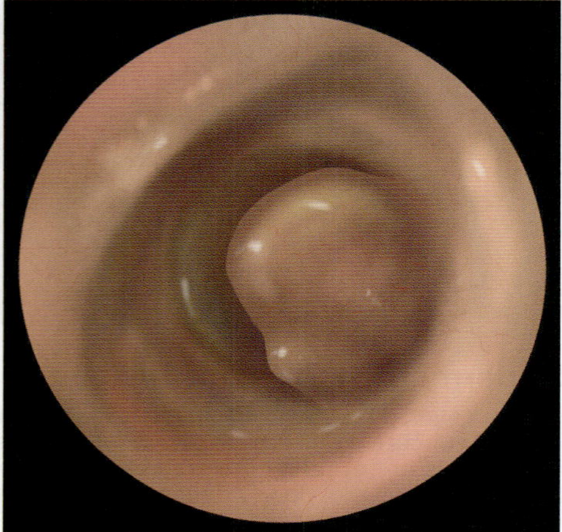

Osteoma

Single, stony hard, rounded nodule that obscures the drum; nontender; overlying skin appears normal. Attached to inner third, the bony part, of canal. Benign, but refer for removal.

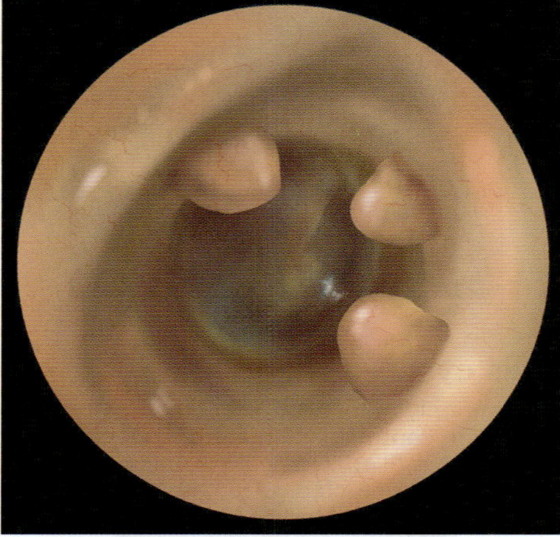

Exostosis

More common than osteoma. Small, bony hard, rounded nodules of hypertrophic bone, covered with normal epithelium. They arise near the drum but usually do not obstruct the view of the drum. They are usually multiple and bilateral. They may occur more frequently in cold-water swimmers. The condition needs no treatment, although it may cause accumulation of cerumen, which blocks the canal.

TABLE 15.3 Abnormalities in the ear canal—cont'd

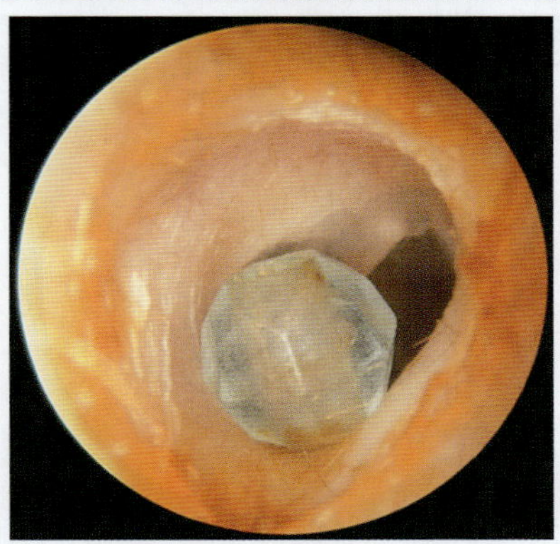

Foreign body

Usually it is children who place a foreign body in the ear (here, a stone completely occludes the canal), which is later noted on routine examination. Common objects are beans, corn, breakfast cereals, jewellery beads, small stones, sponge rubber. Cotton is most common in adults and becomes impacted from cotton-tipped applicators. A trapped live insect is uncommon but makes the person especially frantic.

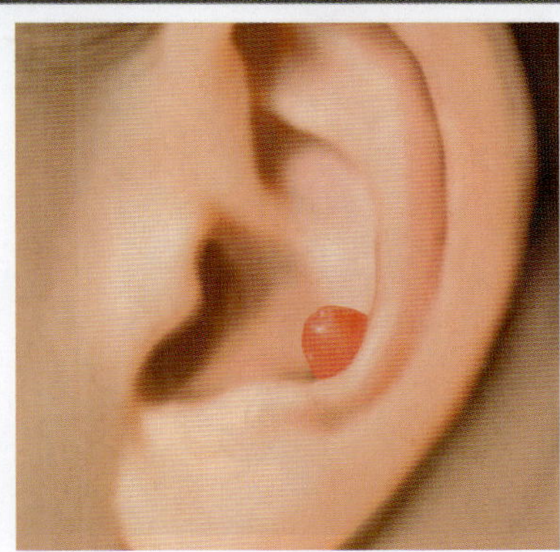

Furuncle

Exquisitely painful, reddened, infected hair follicle. Here, it occurs on the tragus but also may be on cartilaginous part of ear canal. Regional lymphadenopathy often accompanies a furuncle.

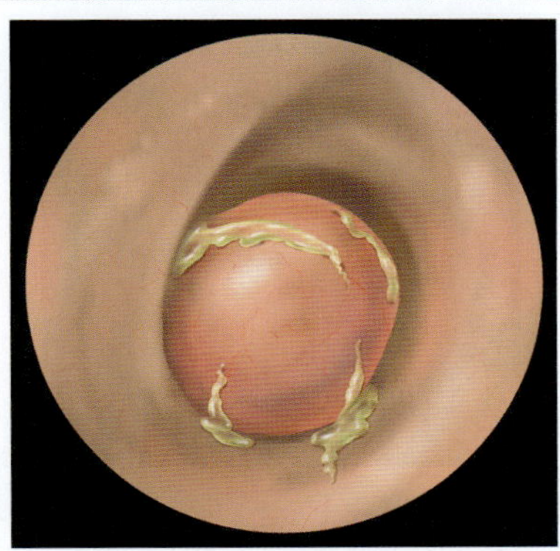

Polyp

Arises in canal from granulomatous or mucosal tissue; redder than surrounding skin and bleeds easily; bathed in foul purulent discharge; indicates chronic ear disease. Benign, but refer for excision.

TABLE 15.4 Abnormalities of the tympanic membrane

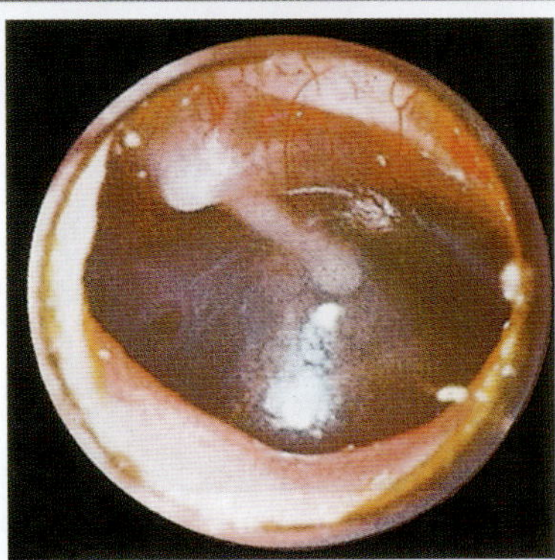

Retracted drum

Landmarks look more prominent and well defined. Malleus handle looks shorter and more horizontal than normal. Short process is very prominent. Light reflex is absent or distorted. The drum is dull and lustreless and does not move. These signs indicate negative pressure and middle ear vacuum from obstructed Eustachian tube and serous otitis media.

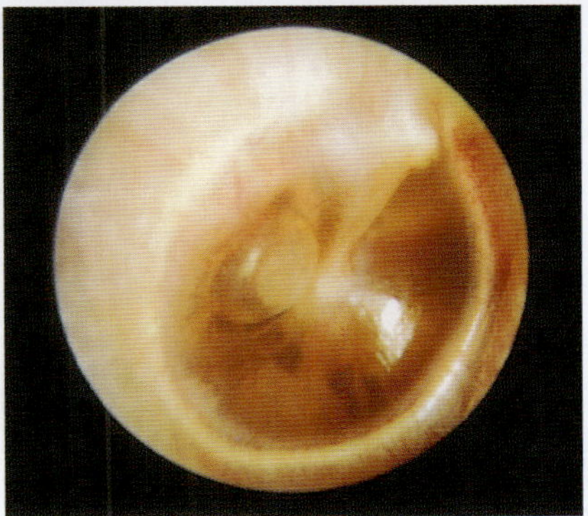

Otitis media with effusion (OME)

An amber-yellow drum suggests serum in middle ear that transudates to relieve negative pressure from the blocked Eustachian tube. You may note an air-fluid level with fine black dividing line or air bubbles visible behind drum. Symptoms are feeling of fullness, transient hearing loss, popping sound with swallowing. Also called serous otitis media, glue ear.

(Continued)

TABLE 15.4 Abnormalities of the tympanic membrane—cont'd

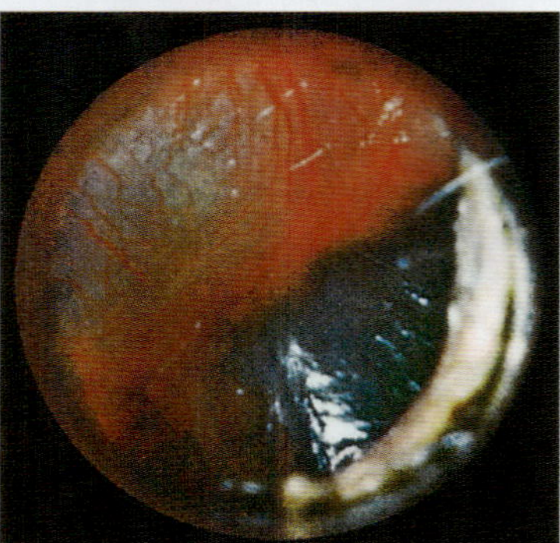

Early stage

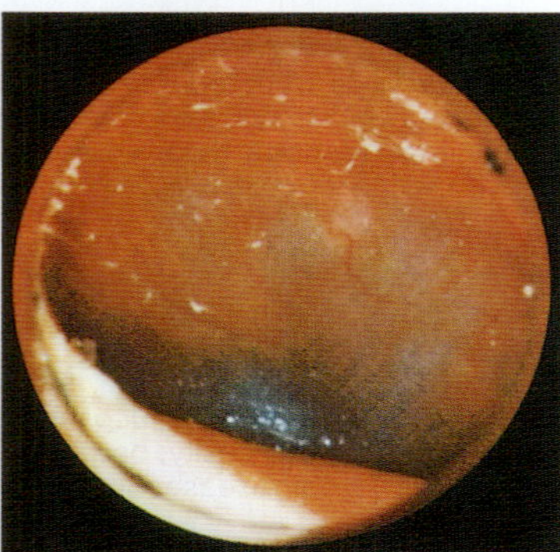

Later stage

Acute (purulent) otitis media

This results when the middle ear fluid is infected. An absent light reflex from increasing middle ear pressure is an early sign. Redness and bulging are first noted in superior part of drum (pars flaccida), along with earache and fever. Then fiery red bulging of entire drum occurs; deep throbbing pain; fever and transient hearing loss. Pneumatic otoscopy reveals drum hypomobility.

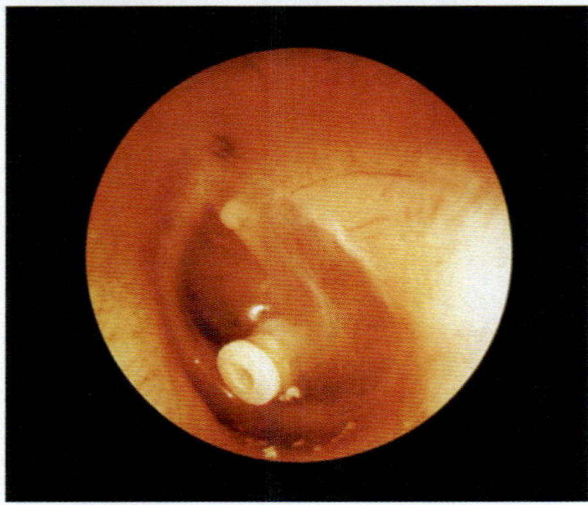

Insertion of tubes (grommets)

Polyethylene tubes are inserted surgically into the eardrum to relieve middle ear pressure and promote drainage of chronic or recurrent middle ear infections. Number of acute infections tends to decrease because of improved aeration. Tubes extrude spontaneously in 12 to 18 months. In Australia and New Zealand these tubes are called ventilation tubes or grommets.

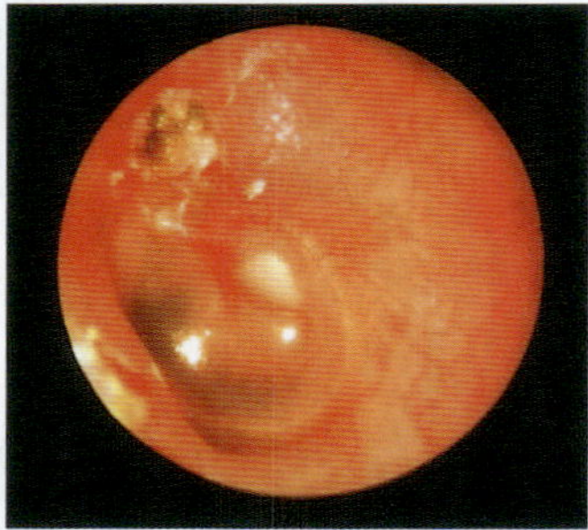

Cholesteatoma

An overgrowth of epidermal tissue in the middle ear or temporal bone may result over the years after a marginal TM perforation. It has a pearly white, cheesy appearance. Growth of cholesteatoma can erode bone and produce hearing loss. Early signs include otorrhoea, unilateral conductive hearing loss and tinnitus.

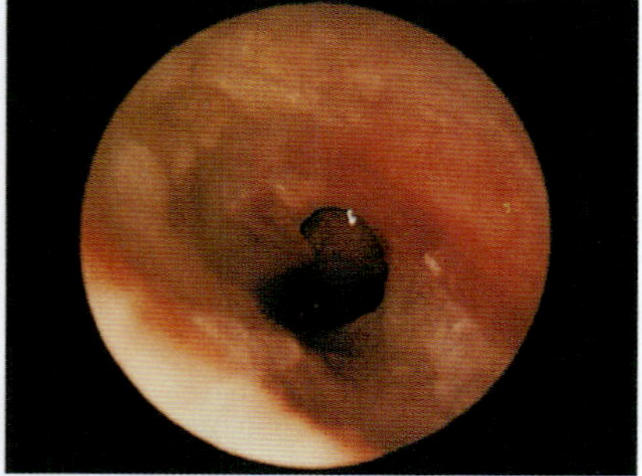

Perforation

If the acute otitis media is not treated, the drum may rupture from increased pressure. Perforations also occur from trauma (e.g. a slap on the ear). Usually the perforation appears as a round or oval darkened area on the drum, but in this photo the perforation is very large. *Central* perforations occur in the pars tensa. *Marginal* perforations occur at the annulus. Marginal perforations are called *attic perforations* when they occur in superior part of the drum, the pars flaccida.

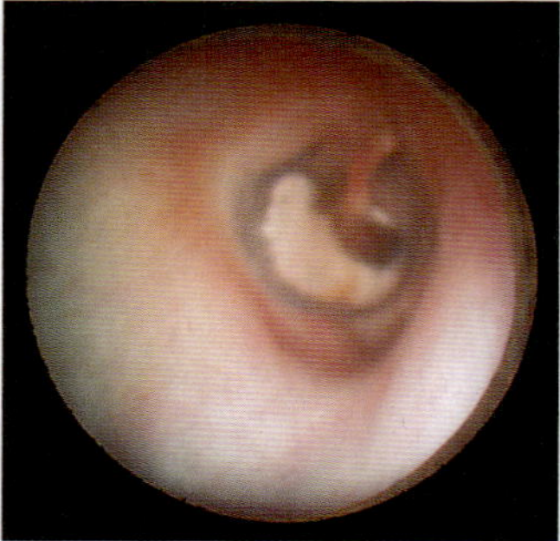

Scarred drum

Dense white patches on the eardrum are sequelae of repeated ear infections. They do not necessarily affect hearing.

TABLE 15.4 Abnormalities of the tympanic membrane—cont'd

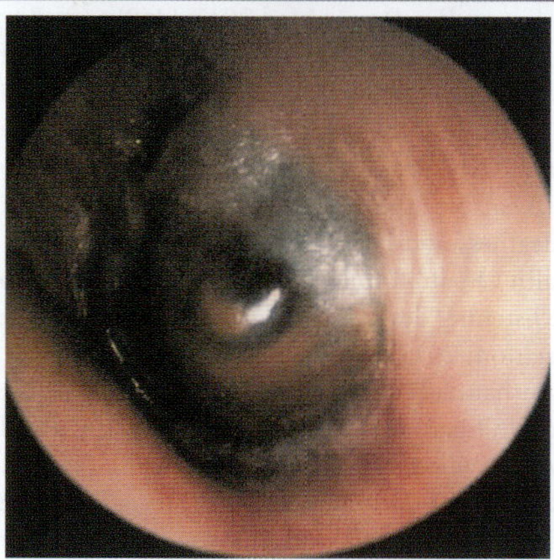

Blue drum (haemotympanum)

This indicates blood in the middle ear, as in trauma resulting in skull fracture.

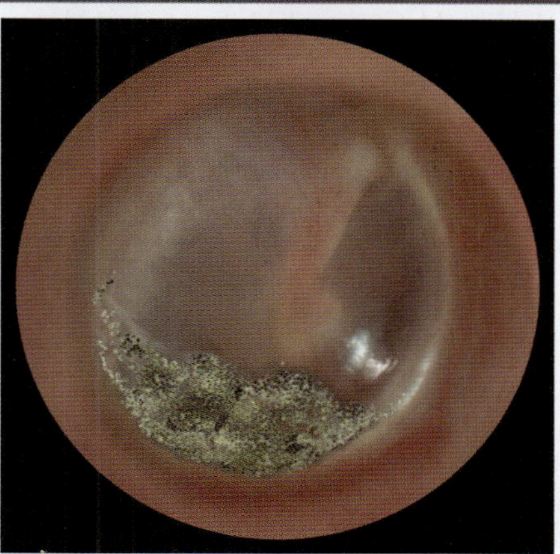

Fungal infection (otomycosis)

Colony of black or white dots on drum or canal wall suggests a yeast or fungal infection.

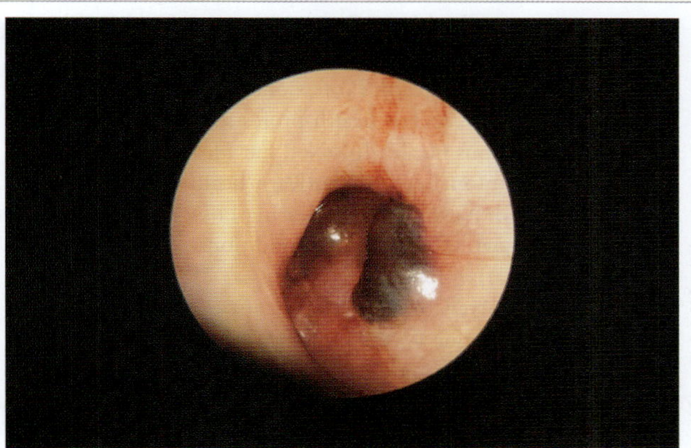

Bullous myringitis

Small vesicles containing blood on the drum; accompany mycoplasma pneumonia and virus infections. May have blood-tinged discharge and severe otalgia.

BIBLIOGRAPHY

Australian Institute of Health and Welfare. Aboriginal and Torres Strait Islander Health Performance Framework (HPF) report. Canberra: Australian Government; 2018.

Australian Medical Association. AMA report card on Indigenous health: a national strategic approach to ending chronic otitis media and its lifelong impacts in Indigenous communities. Canberra: Australian Medical Association; 2017.

Chonmaitree T, Trujillo R, Jennings K, et al. Acute otitis media and other complications of viral respiratory infection. Pediatrics 2016;137(4):e20153555.

Coleman A, Cervin A. Probiotics in the treatment of otitis media. The past, the present and the future. Int J Pediatr Otorhinolaryngol 2019;116:135–40.

Coleman A, Wood A, Bialasiewicz S, et al. The unsolved problem of otitis media in indigenous populations: a systematic review of upper respiratory and middle ear microbiology in indigenous children with otitis media. (Report). Microbiome 2018;6(1).

Deloitte. Access Economics. Listen Hear! New Zealand. Social and economic costs of hearing loss in New Zealand. Final report. Canberra Airport ACT: Deloitte Access Exonomics Pty. Ltd.; 2017a.

Deloitte. Access Economics. The social and economic cost of hearing loss in Australia. Canberra Airport ACT, Hearing Care Industry Association; 2017b.

Deloitte. Access Economics. Social and economic costs of hearing loss in New Zealand. The National Foundation for the Deaf 2017c.

Department of Health. Hearing Services Program Canberra: Australian Government. Available at: http://www.hearingservices.gov.au/wps/portal/hso/site/HSOHome.

Eggermont JJ. Hearing loss: causes, prevention, and treatment. London: Academic Press/Elsevier; 2017.

Exeter DJ, Wu B, Lee AC, et al. The projected burden of hearing loss in New Zealand (2011–2061) and the implications for the hearing health workforce. N Z Med J 2015;128(149):12–21.

Ferkol TW, Farber HJ, La Grutta S, et al. Electronic cigarette use in youths: a position statement of the Forum of International Respiratory Societies. Eur Respir J. 2018;51(5):1800278.

Hockenberry MJ, Wilson D, Rodgers CC. Wong's essentials of pediatric nursing. 10th ed. St Louis: Elsevier; 2016.

Jacups SP, Kinchin I, McConnon KM. Ear, nose, and throat surgical access for remote living indigenous children: What is the least costly model? (Report). J Eval Clin Pract 2018;24(6):1330.

Jemaa AB, Irato G, Zanela A, et al. Congruent auditory display and confusion in sound localization: Case of elderly drivers. Transportation Research Part F: Traffic Psychology and Behaviour 2018;59:524–34.

Jervis-Bardy J, Carney AS, Duguid R, et al. Microbiology of otitis media in Indigenous Australian children. J Laryngol Otol 2017;131(S2):S2–11.

Kaur R, Morris M, Pichichero ME. Epidemiology of acute otitis media in the postpneumococcal conjugate vaccine era. Pediatrics 2017;140(3):e20170181.

Leach A, Morris P. Otitis media and hearing loss among Aboriginal and Torres Strait Islander children: A research summary. Gold Coast Centre of Research Excellence in Ear and Hearing Health of Aboriginal and Torres Strait Islander children. Media ISoRAoO 2017.

Megged O, Abdulgany S, Bar-Meir M. Does acute otitis media in the first month of life increase the risk for recurrent otitis? Clin Pediatr 2017;57(1):89–92.

Ministry of Health New Zealand. National screening unit. 2019. Available at: https://www.nsu.govt.nz/.

Peelle JE, Wingfield A. The Neural Consequences of Age-Related Hearing Loss. Trends in Neurosciences 2016;39(7):486–97.

Scott S, Armitage R. Are headphones making you deaf? ABC News; 2018. Available at: https://www.abc.net.au/news/2018-06-06/headphones-could-be-causing-permanent-hearing-damage/9826294.

Song JJ, Go YY, Mun JY, et al. Effect of electronic cigarettes on human middle ear. Int J Pediatr Otorhinolaryngol 2018;109:67–71.

Talley NJ, O'Connor, S. Talley and O'Connor's clinical examination: A systematic guide to physical diagnosis. 8th ed. Chatswood: Elsevier; 2018.

Vanker A, Gie RP, Zar HJ. The association between environmental tobacco smoke exposure and childhood respiratory disease: A review. Expert Rev Respir Med 2017;11(8):661–73.

Wang J, Sung V, le Clercq CMP, et al. High prevalence of slight and mild hearing loss across mid-life: a cross-sectional national Australian study. Public Health 2019;168:26–35.

World Health Organization (WHO). Deafness and hearing loss. 2019a. Available at: https://www.who.int/news-room/fact-sheets/detail/deafness-and-hearing-loss.

World Health Organization (WHO). WHO-ITU global standard for safe listening devices and systems. Geneva: World Health Organization; 2019b. Available at: https://apps.who.int/iris/bitstream/handle/10665/280086/9789241515283-eng.pdf.

World Health Organisation. Safe listening. 2019c. Available at: https://www.who.int/news-room/q-a-detail/deafness-prevention.

World Health Organization (WHO). Hearing loss due to recreational exposure to loud sounds: a review. Geneva: World Health Organization; 2019d.

Websites

Australian Government, Department of Human Services, Hearing Services Program. Available at: https://www.humanservices.gov.au/organisations/health-professionals/services/medicare/hearing-services-program.

Australian Hearing for Health Professionals. Available at: https://www.hearing.com.au/For-health-professionals.

Australian Indigenous Health InfoNet, Ear Health. Available at: https://healthinfonet.ecu.edu.au/learn/health-topics/ear-health/.

Ministry of Health New Zealand, Hearing Loss. Available at: https://www.health.govt.nz/your-health/conditions-and-treatments/disabilities/hearing-loss.

The Deaf Society. Available at: https://deafsociety.org.au/.

The National Foundation for the Deaf Inc. Available at: www.nfd.org.nz.

World Health Organisation Deafness and Hearing Loss. Available at: https://www.who.int/news-room/fact-sheets/detail/deafness-and-hearing-loss.

Assessing cardiovascular function

Unit 4

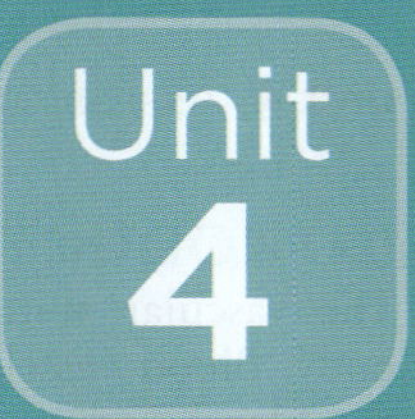

Chapter Sixteen
Peripheral vascular assessment

Written by Carolyn Jarvis
Adapted by Maria Murphy

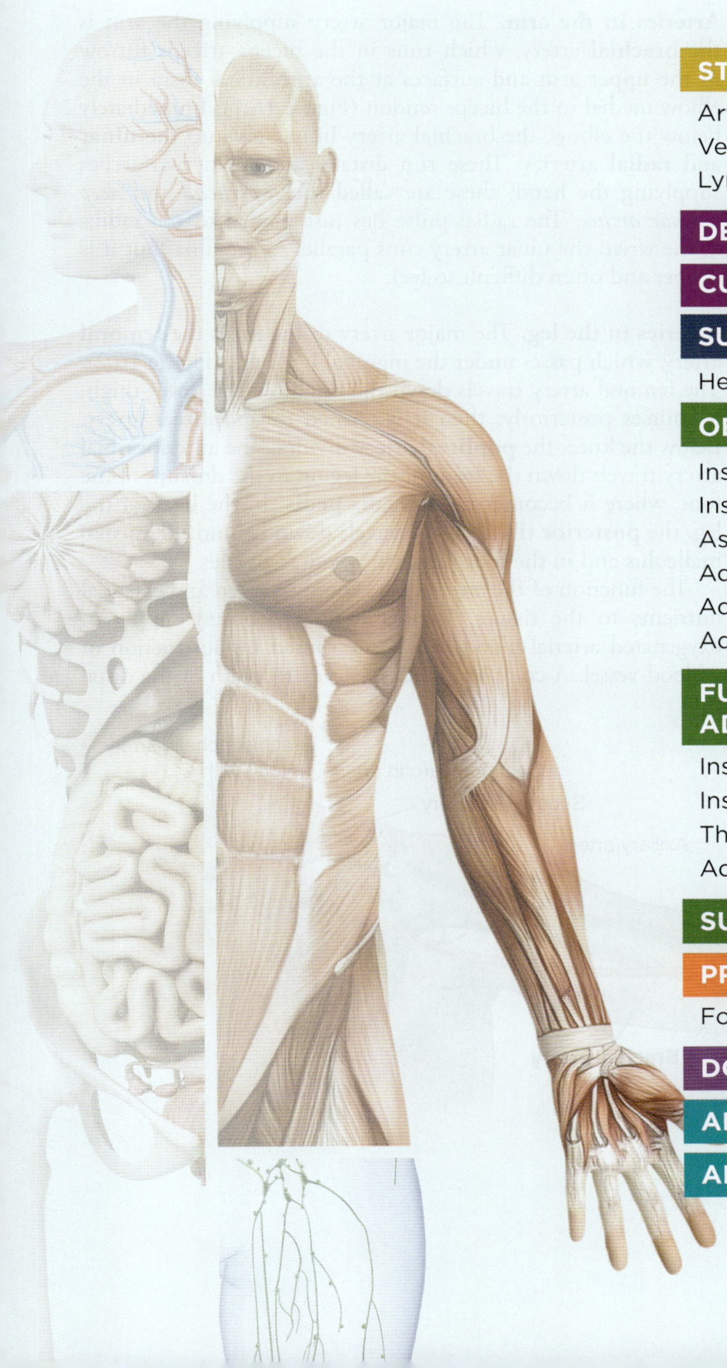

STRUCTURE AND FUNCTION
- Arteries
- Veins
- Lymphatics

DEVELOPMENTAL CONSIDERATIONS

CULTURAL AND SOCIAL CONSIDERATIONS

SUBJECTIVE DATA
- Health history questions

OBJECTIVE DATA
- Inspect and palpate the arms
- Inspect and palpate the legs
- Assess peripheral pulses using the Doppler
- Additional objective data for infants and children
- Additional objective data for the pregnant woman
- Additional objective data for the adult over 65 years

FURTHER OBJECTIVE ASSESSMENT FOR ADVANCED PRACTICE
- Inspect and palpate the arms
- Inspect and palpate the legs
- The ankle–brachial index
- Additional objective data for infants and children

SUMMARY CHECKLIST

PROMOTING A HEALTHY LIFESTYLE
- Foot care

DOCUMENTATION AND CRITICAL THINKING

ABNORMAL FINDINGS

ABNORMAL FINDINGS FOR ADVANCED PRACTICE

INTRODUCTION

The vascular system consists of the blood vessels of the body. Blood vessels are tubes for transporting fluid, such as the blood or lymph. Arteries carry oxygenated blood from the heart to the peripheries. Arterial walls stretch during systole and recoil during diastole resulting in a palpable pulse. Veins carry deoxygenated blood to the heart. Because veins are low pressure vessels they do not usually produce pulsations. The exceptions are large veins such as the right internal carotid vein. Veins distend when there is an increase in intravascular volume. Any disease in the vascular system creates problems with delivery of oxygen and nutrients to the tissues or elimination of waste products from cellular metabolism. The lymphatic system consists of lymph nodes that filter lymphatic fluid. Body tissue fluids are drained first to lymphatic vessels then to lymphatic channels that empty into the bloodstream through lymphatic ducts in the thorax. Any disease in the lymphatic system results in tissue swelling which results from obstruction to lymph flow. Infection may cause enlarged, painful lymph nodes. Neoplasms may result in enlarged lymph nodes. In order to appreciate the impact of disease and trauma to these complex and dynamic systems you are advised to first review the structure and function of the cardiovascular system.

Structure and function

ARTERIES

The heart pumps freshly oxygenated blood through the arteries to all body tissues. The pumping heart makes this a high-pressure system. The artery walls are strong, tough and tense to withstand pressure demands. Arteries contain elastic fibres, which allow their walls to stretch with systole and recoil with diastole. Arteries also contain muscle fibres (vascular smooth muscle), which control the amount of blood delivered to the tissues. The vascular smooth muscle contracts or dilates, which changes the diameter of the arteries to control the rate of blood flow.

Each heartbeat creates a pressure wave, which makes the arteries expand then recoil. It is the recoil that propels blood through like a wave. All arteries have this pressure wave, or **pulse**, throughout their length, but you can feel it only at body sites where the artery lies close to the skin and over a bone. The arteries described in the following sections are accessible to examination.

Temporal artery. The temporal artery is palpated in front of the ear.

Carotid artery. The carotid artery is palpated in the groove between the sternocleidomastoid muscle and the trachea and is covered in Chapter 17 with the great vessels.

Arteries in the arm. The major artery supplying the arm is the **brachial** artery, which runs in the biceps–triceps furrow of the upper arm and surfaces at the antecubital fossa in the elbow medial to the biceps tendon (Figure 16.1). Immediately below the elbow, the brachial artery bifurcates into the **ulnar** and **radial** arteries. These run distally and form two arches supplying the hand; these are called the *superficial* and *deep palmar arches*. The radial pulse lies just medial to the radius at the wrist; the ulnar artery runs parallel to the ulna, but it is deeper and often difficult to feel.

Arteries in the leg. The major artery to the leg is the **femoral** artery, which passes under the inguinal ligament (Figure 16.2). The femoral artery travels down the thigh. At the lower thigh, it courses posteriorly; then it is termed the **popliteal** artery. Below the knee, the **popliteal** artery divides. The anterior tibial artery travels down the front of the leg on to the dorsum of the foot, where it becomes the **dorsalis pedis**. In the back of the leg, the **posterior tibial** artery travels down behind the medial malleolus and in the foot forms the plantar arteries.

The function of the arteries is to supply oxygen and essential nutrients to the tissues. **Ischaemia** is a deficient supply of oxygenated arterial blood to a tissue caused by obstruction of a blood vessel. A complete blockage leads to death of the distal

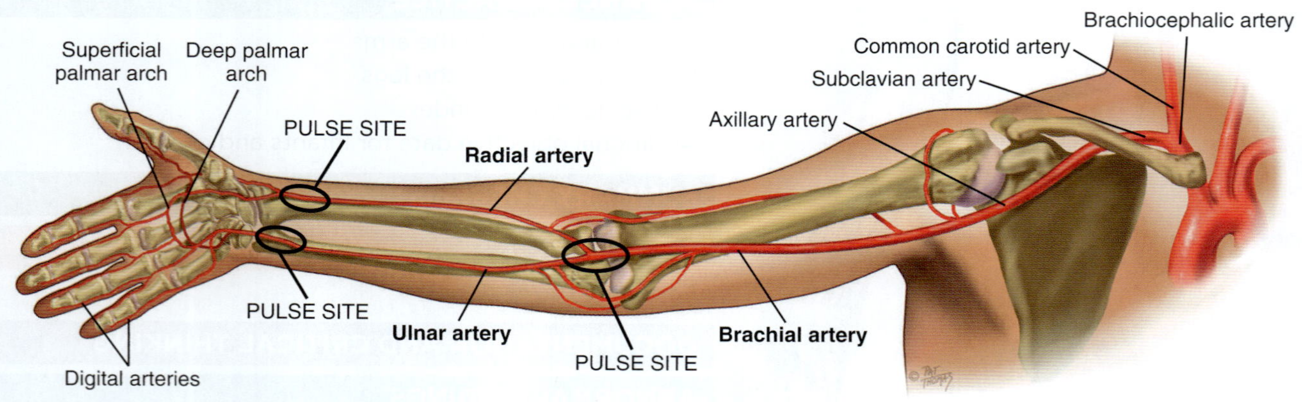

Figure 16.1

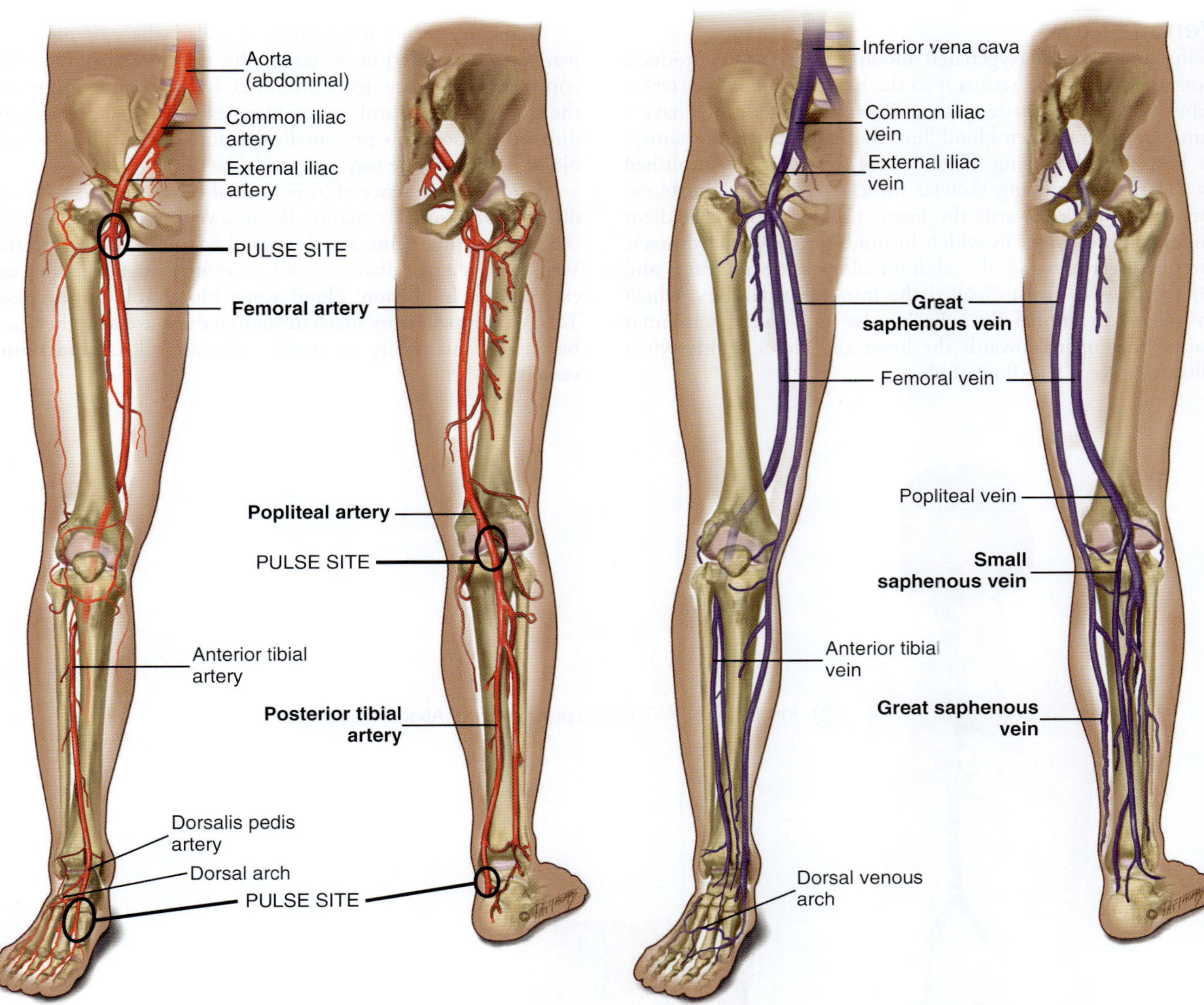

Figure 16.2
Arteries in the leg. © Pat Thomas, 2010

Figure 16.3
Veins in the leg. © Pat Thomas, 2010

tissue. A partial blockage creates an insufficient blood supply and the ischaemia may be apparent only at exercise when oxygen needs increase. Peripheral artery disease (PAD) affects non-coronary arteries and usually refers to arteries in the limbs. It is usually caused by atherosclerosis and less commonly by embolism, arterial dissection or other injury to the major arteries.

VEINS

The course of veins parallels that of arteries, but the body has more veins, and they lie closer to the skin surface. The following veins are accessible to examination.

Jugular veins. Assessment of the jugular veins is presented in Chapter 17.

Veins in the arm. Each arm has two sets of veins: superficial and deep. The superficial veins are in the subcutaneous tissue and are responsible for most of the venous return.

Veins in the leg. The legs have three types of veins (Figure 16.3):

1. The **deep veins** run alongside the deep arteries and conduct most of the venous return from the legs. These are the **femoral** and **popliteal** veins. As long as these veins remain intact, the superficial veins can be excised without harming the circulation.
2. The **superficial veins** are the **great** and **small saphenous** veins. The great saphenous vein, inside the leg, starts at the medial side of the dorsum of the foot. You can see it ascend in front of the medial malleolus; then it crosses the tibia obliquely and ascends along the medial side of the thigh. The small saphenous vein, outside the leg, starts on the lateral side of the dorsum of the foot, ascends behind the lateral malleolus, up the back of the leg, where it joins the popliteal vein.
3. **Perforators** (not illustrated) are connecting veins that join the two sets. They also have one-way valves that direct blood from the superficial into the deep veins.

Venous flow

Veins drain the deoxygenated blood and its waste products from the tissues and return it to the heart. Unlike the arteries, veins are a low-pressure system. Because veins do not have a pump to generate their blood flow, the veins need a mechanism to keep blood moving (Figure 16.4). This is accomplished by (1) the contracting skeletal muscles that milk the blood proximally, back towards the heart; (2) the pressure gradient caused by breathing, in which inspiration makes the thoracic pressure decrease and the abdominal pressure increase; and (3) the one-way valves, called the intraluminal valves, which ensure unidirectional flow. Each valve is a paired semilunar pocket that opens towards the heart and closes tightly when filled to prevent backflow of blood.

In the legs, this mechanism is called the *calf pump*, or *peripheral heart*. While walking, the calf muscles alternately contract (systole) and relax (diastole). In the contraction phase, the gastrocnemius and soleus muscles squeeze the veins and direct the blood flow proximally. Because of the valves, venous blood flows just one way—towards the heart.

Besides the presence of intraluminal valves, venous structure differs from arterial structure. Because venous pressure is lower, the walls of the veins are thinner than those of the arteries. Veins have a larger diameter and are more distensible; they can expand and hold more blood when blood volume increases. This is a compensatory mechanism to reduce stress on the heart. Because of this ability to stretch, veins are called **capacitance vessels**.

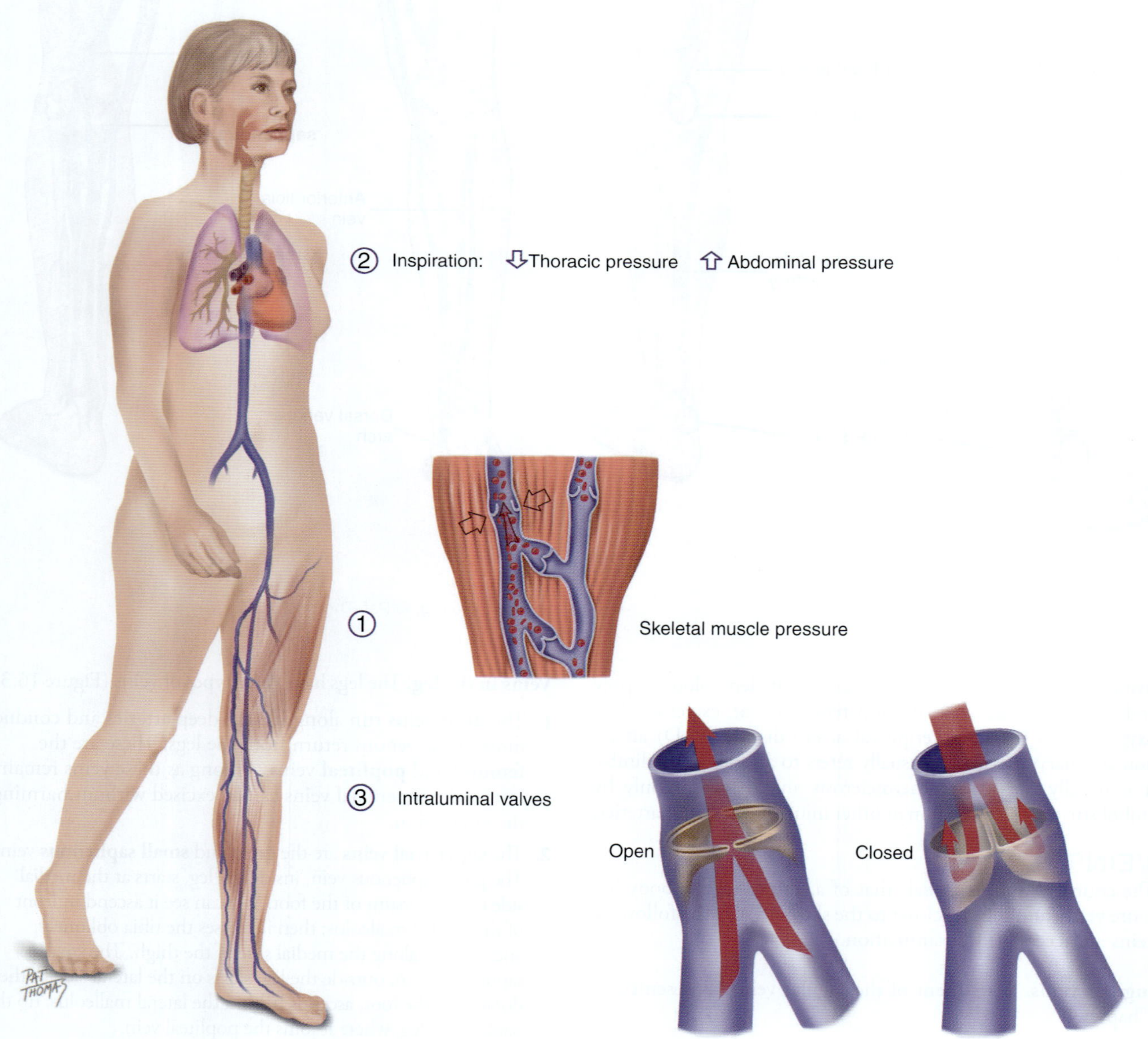

Figure 16.4
Mechanisms of venous flow.

Efficient venous return is dependent on contracting skeletal muscles, competent valves in the veins and a patent lumen. Problems with any of these three elements lead to venous stasis. At risk for venous disease are people who undergo prolonged standing, sitting or bed rest because they do not benefit from the milking action that walking accomplishes. Hypercoagulable states and vein wall trauma are other factors that increase risk for venous disease. Also, dilated and tortuous (varicose) veins create **incompetent valves**, wherein the lumen is so wide the valve cusps cannot approximate. This condition increases venous pressure, which further dilates the vein. Some people have a genetic predisposition to varicose veins, but obesity and pregnancy are increased risk factors.

LYMPHATICS

The lymphatics form a completely separate vessel system, which retrieves excess fluid from the tissue spaces and returns it to the bloodstream (Figure 16.5). During circulation of the blood, somewhat more fluid leaves the capillaries than the veins can absorb. Without lymphatic drainage, fluid would build up in the interstitial spaces and produce oedema.

The vessels drain into two main trunks, which empty into the venous system at the subclavian veins (see Figure 16.6):

1. The **right lymphatic duct** empties into the right subclavian vein. It drains the right side of the head and neck, right arm, right side of thorax, right lung and pleura, right side of the heart and right upper section of the liver.
2. The **thoracic duct** drains the rest of the body. It empties into the left subclavian vein.

The functions of the lymphatic system are (1) to conserve fluid and plasma proteins that leak out of the capillaries, (2) to form a major part of the immune system that defends the body against disease and (3) to absorb lipids from the intestinal tract.

The processes of the immune system are complicated and not fully understood. The immune system detects and eliminates microorganisms that could be harmful to the body (pathogens), both those that come in from the environment and those arising from inside (abnormal or mutant cells). It accomplishes this by phagocytosis (digestion) of the substances by neutrophils and monocytes/macrophages and by production of specific antibodies or specific immune responses by the lymphocytes.

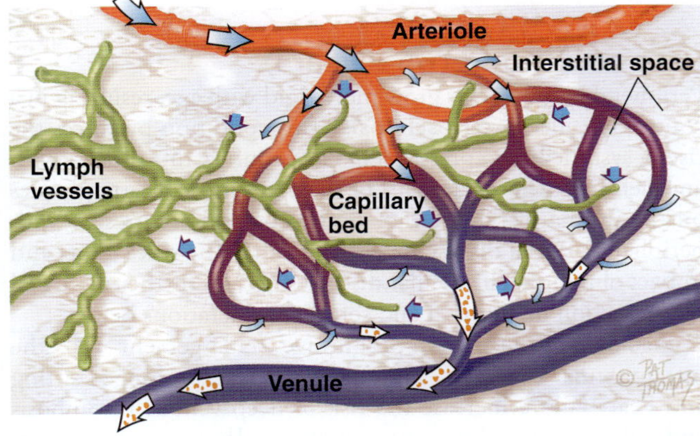

Figure 16.5
© Pat Thomas, 2014

The lymphatic vessels have a unique structure. Lymphatic capillaries start as microscopic open-ended tubes, which siphon interstitial fluid. The capillaries converge to form vessels. The vessels, like veins, drain into larger ones. The vessels have valves, so flow is one way from the tissue spaces into the bloodstream. The many valves make the vessels look beaded. The flow of lymph is slow compared with that of the blood. Lymph flow is propelled by contracting skeletal muscles, by pressure changes secondary to breathing and by contraction of the vessel walls themselves.

Lymph nodes are small oval clumps of lymphatic tissue located at intervals along the vessels. Most nodes are arranged in groups, both deep and superficial, in the body. Nodes filter the fluid before it is returned to the bloodstream and filter out pathogens. The pathogens are exposed to lymphocytes in the lymph nodes. The lymphocytes mount an antigen-specific response to eliminate the pathogens. With local inflammation, the nodes in that area become swollen and tender.

The superficial groups of nodes are accessible to inspection and palpation and give clues to the status of the lymphatic system:

- **Cervical nodes** drain the head and neck and are described in Chapter 18.
- **Axillary nodes** drain the breast and upper arm. They are described in Chapter 28.
- The **epitrochlear node** is in the antecubital fossa and drains the hand and lower arm.
- The **inguinal nodes** in the groin drain most of the lymph from the legs, the external genitalia and the anterior abdominal wall.

Related organs

The spleen, tonsils and thymus aid the lymphatic system (Figure 16.7). The **spleen** is located in the left upper quadrant of the abdomen. It has four functions: (1) to destroy old red blood cells, (2) to produce antibodies, (3) to store red blood cells and (4) to filter microorganisms from the blood.

The **tonsils** (palatine, adenoid and lingual) are located in the throat at the entrance to the respiratory and gastrointestinal tracts and respond to local inflammation.

The **thymus** is the flat, pink-grey gland located in the superior mediastinum behind the sternum and in front of the aorta. It is relatively large in the fetus and young child and atrophies after puberty. It is important in developing the T lymphocytes of the immune system in children, but it serves no function in adults. The T and B lymphocytes originate in the bone marrow and mature in the lymphoid tissue.

DEVELOPMENTAL CONSIDERATIONS

Infants and children

The lymphatic system has the same function in children as in adults. It is well developed at birth and grows rapidly until age 10 or 11 years. By age 6 years, the lymphoid tissue reaches adult size; it surpasses adult size by puberty, then it slowly atrophies. It is possible that the excessive antigen stimulation in children causes the early rapid growth.

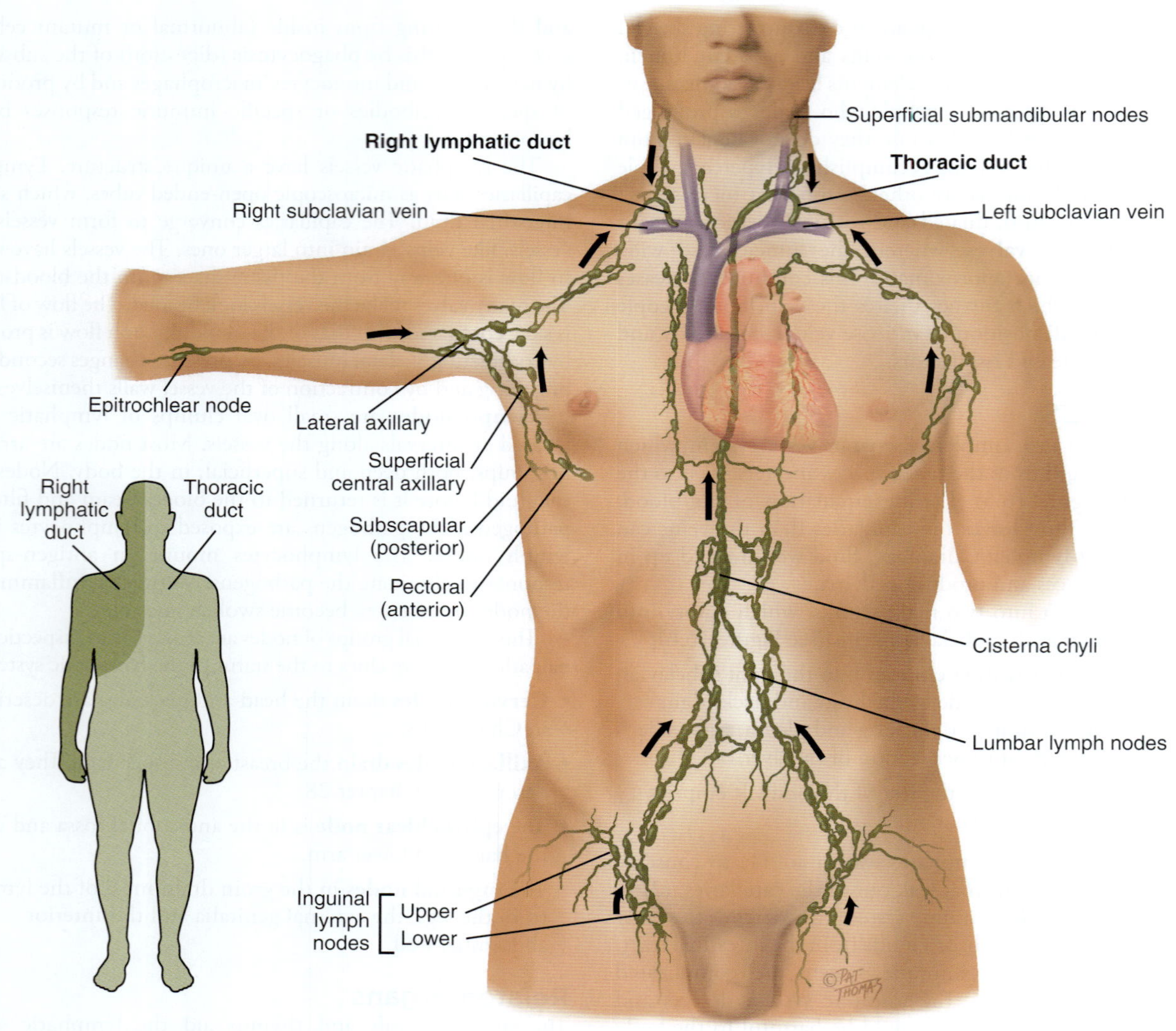

Figure 16.6
Lymphatic ducts and drainage patterns. © Pat Thomas, 2010

Lymph nodes are relatively large in children, and the superficial ones are often palpable even when the child is healthy. With infection, excessive swelling and hyperplasia occur. Enlarged tonsils are familiar signs in respiratory infections. The excessive lymphoid response may also account for the common childhood symptom of abdominal pain with seemingly unrelated problems such as upper respiratory infections (URTI). It is possible that the inflammation of mesenteric lymph nodes produce the abdominal pain.

The pregnant woman

Hormonal changes cause vasodilatation and the resulting drop in blood pressure described in Chapter 27. The growing uterus obstructs drainage of the iliac veins and the inferior vena cava. This condition causes low blood flow and increases venous pressure. This, in turn, causes dependent oedema, varicosities in the legs and vulva and haemorrhoids.

Late adulthood (65+ years)

Peripheral blood vessels grow more rigid with age, resulting in a condition called **arteriosclerosis**. This condition produces the rise in systolic blood pressure. Do not confuse this process with another one, **atherosclerosis**, or the deposition of fatty plaques on the intima of the arteries. Both processes are present with peripheral arterial disease in ageing adults. The risk factors and impact of peripheral vascular disease (PVD) is further discussed in the section on cultural and social considerations below.

Ageing produces a progressive enlargement of the intramuscular calf veins. Prolonged bed rest, prolonged sitting and heart failure increase the risk of deep venous thrombosis and subsequent pulmonary embolism. These conditions are common in ageing and also occur after myocardial infarction (MI). The care for person after MI includes early mobilisation and low-dose anticoagulant medication, which reduce the risk of pulmonary embolism.

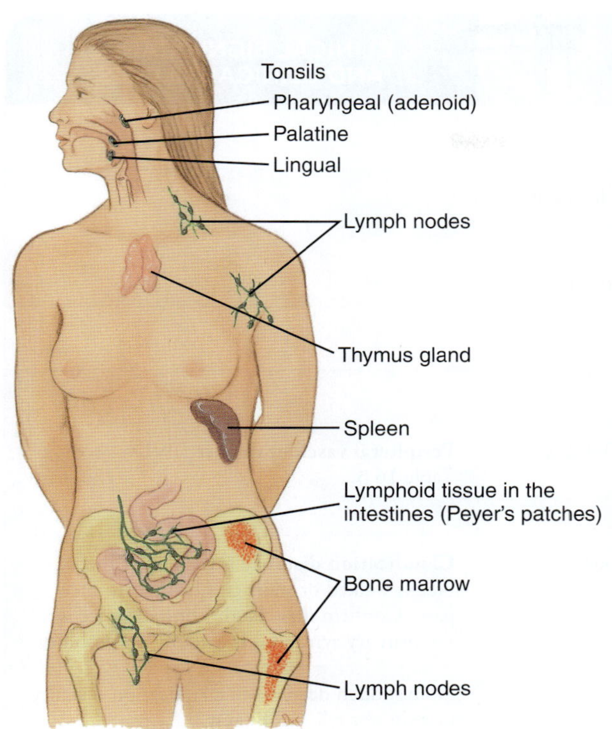

Figure 16.7
Related organs in the immune system.

Loss of lymphatic tissue leads to fewer numbers of lymph nodes and a decrease in the size of remaining nodes in people over 65.

CULTURAL AND SOCIAL CONSIDERATIONS

Peripheral vascular health issues can have profound impact on the person and their family. Peripheral arterial disease (PAD) is an indicator of systemic artherosclerosis; yet it is underdiagnosed and undertreated and a significant cause of morbidity (painful walking, poor wound healing) and mortality in Australia (Si et al 2019). Peripheral arterial disease affects 15% of the Australian population with approximately 50% of these people having no symptoms (Conte & Vale 2018). The Heart Association of Australia and the Heart Foundation of New Zealand consider peripheral arterial disease a coronary artery disease risk equivalent; thus, screening and treatment are important. The ankle-brachial index (ABI) test (see later in this chapter) is a relatively simple non-invasive screening tool for peripheral arterial disease. Questionnaires are additional measures to record the impact of the vascular condition on the person's overall health. The Edinburgh Claudication Questionnaire (ECQ) and the Peripheral Artery Questionnaire (PAQ) are two assessment tools with published versions for use for people who speak a language other than English. The merit of questionnaires as part of the health assessment of the condition allows for the person to advise of the impact the health condition may have over a range of health domains such as physical function, quality of life and social limitations.

Advancing age, male sex, cigarette smoking, hypertension, diabetes, dyslipidaemia, obesity and the presence of other cardiovascular diseases account for the majority of the risk factors for peripheral arterial disease (Song et al 2019). Similar to coronary artery disease, vascular disease progression can be modified by pharmacological and lifestyle interventions that address the person's risk factors. One single site study in Australia reported a comparison of the presenting characteristics and clinical outcomes of indigenous Australians and non-Indigenous Australians with peripheral arterial disease (PAD) (Singh et al 2018). Current smoking status and diabetes were recorded as more prevalent in the indigenous study participants. The longitudinal follow up in the study by Singh and colleagues suggests indigenous study participants present at a younger age with PAD vascular risk factors and poorer clinical outcomes compared to non-Indigenous Australians. There are currently no Australian or New Zealand guidelines recommending routine screening for peripheral vascular disease, although screening should be considered in people over 50 years of age with a history of smoking or diabetes (Conte & Vale 2018). There is further discussion of the major modifiable risk factors in Chapter 17.

Subjective data

As you work through assessment of peripheral vascular function you need to keep in mind that this area is usually assessed in connection with assessment of cardiac function. An accurate assessment requires the nurse to obtain a careful history of the symptoms experienced which will guide clinical examination. This subjective data has been grouped under the following headings:

1. Presenting concern
2. Leg pain or cramps
3. Skin changes on arms or legs
4. Swelling
5. Health and lifestyle management

Practice note: Before you commence the assessment, introduce yourself to the person, confirm the person's identity, discuss the purpose and scope of the assessment, clarify any questions the person may have and obtain verbal consent from the person to perform the assessment.

SUBJECTIVE DATA

ASSESSMENT GUIDELINES	CLINICAL SIGNIFICANCE AND CLINICAL ALERTS
1. Presenting concern	
Do you feel that you have any problem with the circulation in your legs, feet, arms or hands? It is important to ascertain the person's perception of their circulation. • If they do perceive a problem—how does this impact on their quality of life?	
2. Leg pain or cramps	
Any leg pain (cramps)? Where?	
• Describe the type of pain; is it burning, aching, cramping, stabbing? Did this come on gradually or suddenly? • Is it aggravated by activity, walking?	**Peripheral vascular disease** (PVD)—see Table 16.3.
• How far can you walk (blocks/stairs/to your letter box)? What stops you?	**Claudication distance** is the number of blocks walked or stairs climbed to produce pain. Confirm that claudication distance is the primary symptom impacting on mobility.
• Has this amount changed recently? • Is the pain worse with elevation? Worse with cool temperatures?	Note sudden decrease in claudication distance or pain not relieved by rest.
• Does the pain wake you up at night?	Night leg pain is not uncommon in ageing adults. It may indicate the ischaemic rest pain of PVD, severe night muscle cramping (usually the calf) or the restless leg syndrome.
• Any recent change in exercise, a new exercise, increasing exercise?	Pain of musculoskeletal origin rather than vascular. Musculoskeletal pain can be made worse with walking and relieved by rest.
• What relieves this pain: dangling, walking, rubbing? Is the leg pain associated with any skin changes?	Location and interventions that relieve the pain help identify the cause. Foot pain relieved by the intervention of dangling, walking or rubbing the foot relieves an ischaemic pain as insufficient blood flow to the foot is assisted by gravity which supports blood flowing to the ischaemic foot area. Leg cramps reported up and down the lower limb and relieved by rest can occur with diabetes.
• Is it associated with any change in sexual function (males)?	**Aortoiliac occlusion** is associated with impotence (Leriche's syndrome). This is an important sign that the man should be referred for further medical assessment as erectile dysfunction has a strong association with cardiovascular disease.
• Any history of vascular problems, heart problems, diabetes, obesity, pregnancy, smoking, trauma, prolonged standing or bed rest?	Risk factors for PVD include diabetes and cigarette smoking.
3. Skin changes on arms or legs	
Any skin changes in arms or legs? What colour: redness, pallor, blueness, brown discolourations? Hyperpigmentation?	Hyperpigmentation, pallor/cyanosis and oedema are associated with venous stasis.
• Any change in temperature—excess warmth or coolness? • Absence of hair over tibiae? Any numbness?	Coolness, pallor and hair loss are associated with arterial disease.

ASSESSMENT GUIDELINES	CLINICAL SIGNIFICANCE AND CLINICAL ALERTS
• Do your leg veins look bulging and crooked? How have you treated these? Do you use support hose?	**Varicose veins.** Support hose are graduated compression stockings that help to reduce swelling as they are designed to increase blood flow return by compression of the deep venous system.
• Any leg sores or ulcers? Where on the leg? Any pain with the leg ulcer?	Leg ulcers occur with chronic arterial and chronic venous disease (see Table 16.4).
4. Swelling in the arms or legs	
Swelling in one or both legs? When did this swelling start? • What time of day is the swelling at its worst: morning, or after you have been up most of the day? • Does the swelling come and go, or is it constant? • What seems to bring it on: trauma, standing all day, sitting? • What relieves swelling: elevation, support hose? • Is swelling associated with pain, heat, redness, ulceration, hardened skin?	**Oedema** is bilateral when caused by a systemic problem such as heart failure or unilateral when the result of a local obstruction or inflammation.
5. Health and lifestyle management	
• Medications. What medications are you taking (e.g. oral contraceptives, hormone replacement)? • Nutrition: Please describe your usual daily diet. (Note if this diet is representative of the basic food groups, the amount of kilojoules, cholesterol and any additives such as salt.) • Weight: What is your usual weight? Has there been any recent change?	**Thrombophlebitis** may occur as an adverse reaction when taking supplemented oestrogen
• Smoking: Do you smoke cigarettes or other tobacco? At what age did you start? How many packs per day? For how many years have you smoked this amount? Have you ever tried to quit? If so, how did this go? • Alcohol: How much alcohol do you usually drink each week, or each day? Beer/wine/spirits? When was your last drink? What was the number of drinks that episode? Have you ever been told you had a drinking problem? • Exercise: What is your usual amount of exercise each day or week? What stops you? E.g. fatigue, leg pains, other (specify). What type of exercise (state type or sport)? If a sport, what is your usual amount (light, moderate, heavy)?	Tobacco constricts arteries, increases coagulability, injures endothelium and promotes inflammation. Smoking is the strongest risk factor for peripheral arterial disease

Objective data

The focus of the objective data collection is to examine the person for clinical signs that support or are in addition to their report of symptoms. In particular, assessment of the peripheral vascular system is aimed at finding out risk factors for skin breakdown, pain, immobility and changes to everyday activity. Preparation is the essential first step.

Preparation

During a complete physical examination, examine the arms at the very beginning when you are checking the vital signs—the person is sitting. Examine the legs directly after the abdominal examination while the person is still supine. Then have the person stand up to evaluate the leg veins.

Examination of the arms and legs includes peripheral vascular characteristics (described below), the skin (Chapter 22), musculoskeletal findings (Chapter 20) and neurological findings (Chapter 12).

Use inspection and palpation. Compare your findings with the opposite extremity.

Equipment needed

Hand hygiene solution
Occasionally needed:
- Tape measure
- Tourniquet or blood pressure cuff
- Stethoscope
- Doppler

PROCEDURES AND NORMAL FINDINGS	ABNORMAL FINDINGS AND CLINICAL ALERTS
Inspect and palpate the arms	
Lift both of the person's hands in your hands. Inspect, then turn the person's hands over, noting colour of skin and nailbeds; temperature, texture and turgor of skin; and the presence of any lesions, oedema or clubbing. Use the **profile sign** (viewing the finger from the side) to detect early clubbing. The normal nail bed angle is 160°. (See Chapter 22 for a full discussion of skin colour, lesions and clubbing.)	Flattening of angle and **clubbing** (diffuse enlargement of terminal phalanges) occur with congenital cyanotic heart disease and cardiopulmonary disease.
With the person's hands near the level of their heart, check **capillary refill**. This is an index of peripheral perfusion and cardiac output. Depress and blanch the nail beds; release and note the time for colour return. Usually, the vessels refill within a fraction of a second. Consider it normal if the colour returns in less than 1 or 2 seconds. Note conditions that can skew your findings: a cool room, decreased body temperature, cigarette smoking, peripheral oedema and anaemia.	Refill lasting more than 1 or 2 seconds signifies vasoconstriction or decreased cardiac output (hypovolaemia, heart failure, shock). The hands are cold, clammy and pale.
The two arms should be symmetrical in size.	**Oedema** of upper extremities occurs when lymphatic drainage is obstructed, which may occur after breast surgery (see Table 16.4).
Note the presence of any scars on hands and arms. Many occur normally with usual childhood abrasions or with occupations involving hand tools.	Needle tracks occur with IV drug use; linear scars in wrists may signify past self-inflicted injury.
Palpate upper limb pulses	
Palpate both **radial pulses**, noting rate, rhythm, elasticity of vessel wall and equal force (Figure 16.8). Grade the strength on a three-point scale.	Pulses may be more difficult to palpate in an obese person.
3+, increased, full, bounding 2+, **normal** 1+, weak 0, absent 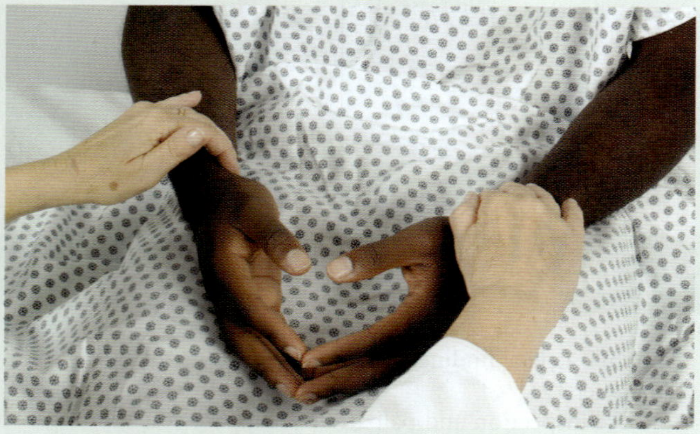 Figure 16.8	**Full, bounding pulse** (3+) occurs with hyperkinetic states (exercise, anxiety, fever), anaemia and hyperthyroidism. **Weak, 'thready' pulse** (1+) occurs with shock and peripheral arterial disease. See Table 16.1 for illustrations of these and irregular pulse rhythms.
It is not usually necessary to palpate the **ulnar pulses.** If indicated, palpate along the medial side of the inner forearm (Figure 16.9), although the ulnar pulses are often not palpable in the normal person.	The ulnar arterial pulses are palpated when a radial artery has been harvested for coronary artery bypass graft surgery.

OBJECTIVE DATA

PROCEDURES AND NORMAL FINDINGS	ABNORMAL FINDINGS AND CLINICAL ALERTS
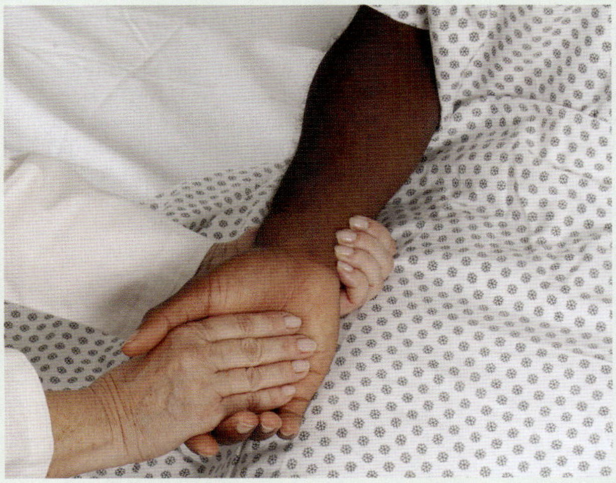 Figure 16.9	
Palpate the **brachial pulses**—their strength should be equal bilaterally (Figure 16.10). 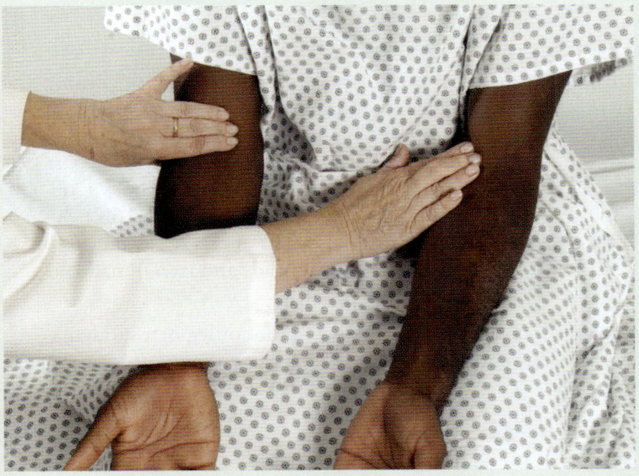 Figure 16.10	

Inspect and palpate the legs

Uncover the legs while keeping the genitalia draped. Inspect both legs together, noting skin colour, hair distribution, venous pattern, size (swelling or atrophy) and any skin lesions or ulcers.	**Pallor** with vasoconstriction; **erythema** with vasodilatation; **cyanosis**.
Normally hair covers the legs. Even if leg hair is shaved, you will still note hair on the dorsa of the toes.	**Malnutrition:** thin, shiny atrophic skin, thick-ridged nails, loss of hair, ulcers, gangrene. Malnutrition, pallor and coolness occur with arterial insufficiency.
The venous pattern is normally flat and barely visible. Note obvious varicosities, although these are best assessed while standing.	The one-way valves in the venous system return blood to the heart. When standing, there is also the additional effect of gravity. Valves that close properly prevent this backflow from occurring.

PROCEDURES AND NORMAL FINDINGS	ABNORMAL FINDINGS AND CLINICAL ALERTS
Both legs should be symmetrical in size without any swelling or atrophy. If the lower legs look asymmetrical or if deep venous thrombosis is suspected, measure the calf circumference with a tape measure (Figure 16.11). Measure at the widest point, taking care to measure the other leg in exactly the same place, i.e. the same number of centimetres down from the patella or other landmark. If lymphoedema is suspected, measure also at the ankle, knee and thigh. Record your findings in centimetres. 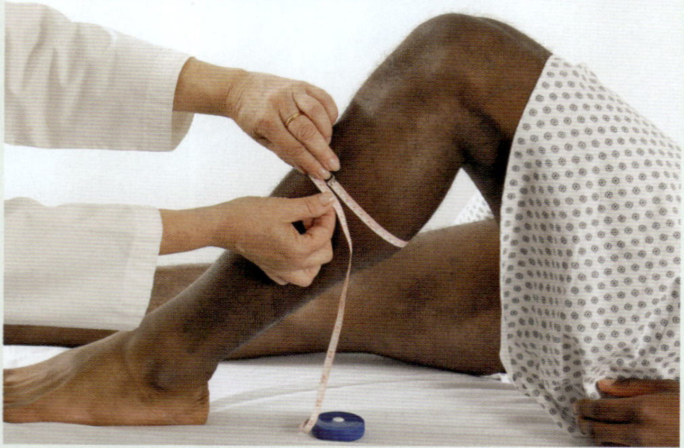 **Figure 16.11**	Diffuse bilateral oedema occurs with systemic illnesses. ***Clinical alert:*** Acute, unilateral, painful swelling and asymmetry of calves of 1 cm or more is abnormal; refer the person to a medical practitioner to determine whether deep venous thrombosis is present. Asymmetry of 1–3 cm occurs with mild lymphoedema; 3–5 cm with moderate lymphoedema; and more than 5 cm with severe lymphoedema (see Table 16.4).
In the presence of skin discolouration, skin ulcers or gangrene, note the size and the exact location.	Brown discolouration occurs with chronic venous stasis due to haemosiderin deposits from red blood cell degradation. Venous ulcers occur usually at medial malleolus because of bacterial invasion of poorly drained tissues (see Table 16.2). With arterial deficit, ulcers occur on tips of toes, metatarsal heads and lateral malleoli.
Palpate for temperature along the legs down to the feet, comparing symmetrical spots (Figure 16.12). The skin should be warm and equal bilaterally. Bilateral cool feet may be due to environmental factors such as cool room temperature, apprehension and cigarette smoking. If any increase in temperature is present higher up the leg, note if it is gradual or abrupt. 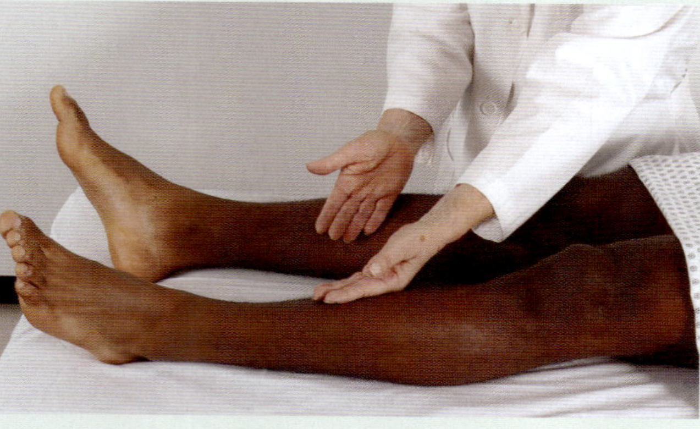 **Figure 16.12**	A unilateral cool foot or leg or a sudden temperature drop as you move down the leg occurs with arterial deficit.

PROCEDURES AND NORMAL FINDINGS	ABNORMAL FINDINGS AND CLINICAL ALERTS
Flex the person's knee, then gently compress the gastrocnemius (calf) muscle anteriorly against the tibia; no tenderness should be present.	***Clinical alert:*** If tenderness on flexion of calf causes pain, do not continue with palpation. Pain can be a sign of deep vein thrombosis, superficial phlebitis, Achilles tendinitis, gastrocnemius and plantar muscle injury and lumbosacral disorders. Where there is any concern that the person could have a deep vein thrombosis they should be referred to a medical practitioner for further assessment.
Palpate peripheral pulses	
Palpate these peripheral arteries in both legs: femoral, popliteal, dorsalis pedis and posterior tibial. Grade the strength on the 4-point scale. Locate the **femoral arteries** just below the inguinal ligament halfway between the pubis and anterior superior iliac spines (Figure 16.13). The simplest method of locating the femoral artery is to recall that the femoral artery is always located at a 45° angle to the person's umbilicus. Press firmly and then slowly release, noting the pulse tap under your fingertips. To differentiate the Femoral Artery from the adjacent Femoral Vein and Nerve, we can use the acronymn: NAVY. Starting from the periphery and moving medially on both the left and right side is the Femoral Nerve/Artery/Vein/Y where the groin meets the two lower limbs. 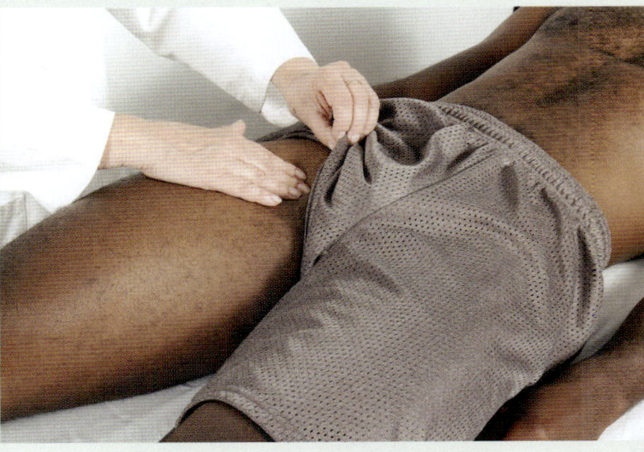 **Figure 16.13**	The femoral artery in a healthy person is palpable. Atherosclerosis may be evident if this pulse is not palpable.
The **popliteal pulse** is a more diffuse pulse and can be difficult to localise. With the leg extended but relaxed, anchor your thumbs on the knee, and curl your fingers around into the popliteal fossa (Figure 16.14). Press your fingers forwards hard to compress the artery against the bone (the lower edge of the femur or the upper edge of the tibia). Often it is just lateral to the medial tendon. 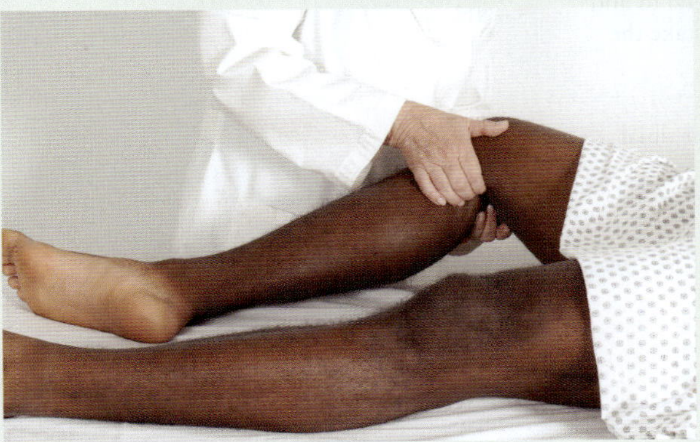 **Figure 16.14**	

OBJECTIVE DATA

PROCEDURES AND NORMAL FINDINGS	ABNORMAL FINDINGS AND CLINICAL ALERTS
If you have difficulty, turn the person prone and lift up the lower leg (Figure 16.15). Let the leg relax against your arm and press in deeply with your two thumbs. Often a normal popliteal pulse is impossible to palpate. 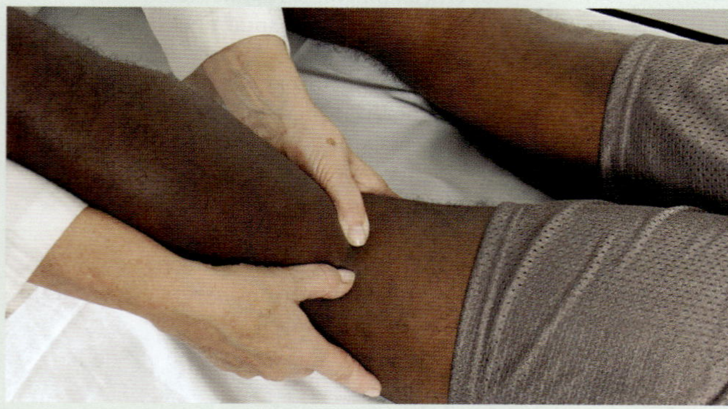 Figure 16.15	
For the **posterior tibial** pulse, curve your fingers around the medial malleolus (Figure 16.16). You will feel the tapping right behind it in the groove between the malleolus and the Achilles tendon. If you cannot, try passive dorsiflexion of the foot to make the pulse more accessible. 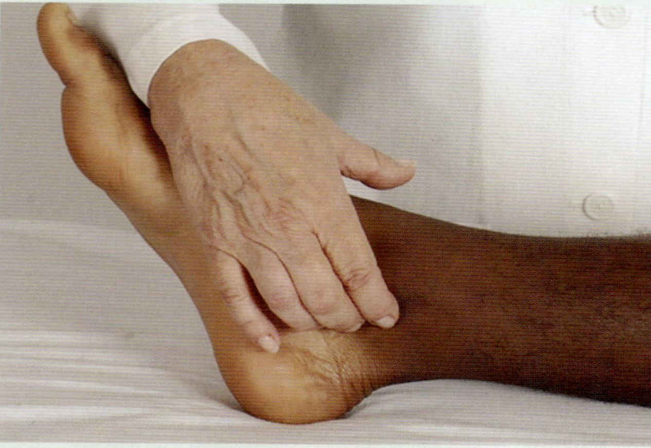 Figure 16.16	
The **dorsalis pedis** pulse requires a very light touch. Normally it is just lateral to and parallel with the extensor tendon of the big toe (Figure 16.17). Do not mistake the pulse in your own fingertips for that of the person.	
In adults over 45 years, occasionally either the dorsalis pedis or the posterior tibial pulse may be hard to find, but not both on the same foot.	

PROCEDURES AND NORMAL FINDINGS	ABNORMAL FINDINGS AND CLINICAL ALERTS
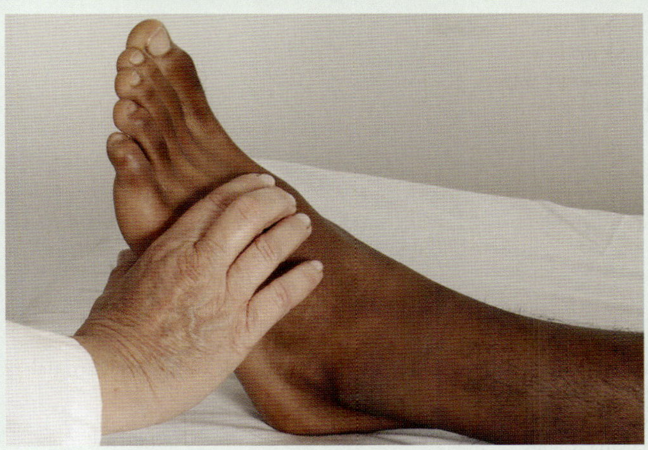 **Figure 16.17**	
Pretibial oedema	
Check for pretibial oedema. Firmly depress the skin over the tibia or the medial malleolus for 5 seconds and release (Figure 16.18A). Normally, your finger should leave no indentation, although a pit is commonly seen if the person has been standing all day or during pregnancy. 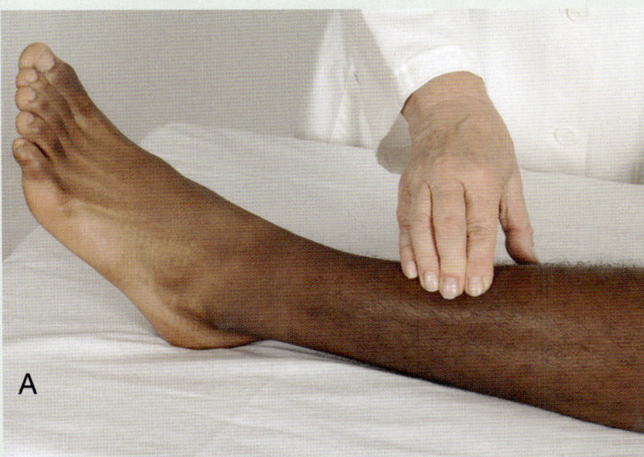 **Figure 16.18A** Check pretibial oedema.	Bilateral, dependent, pitting oedema occurs with heart failure, diabetic neuropathy and hepatic cirrhosis (Figure 16.18B). 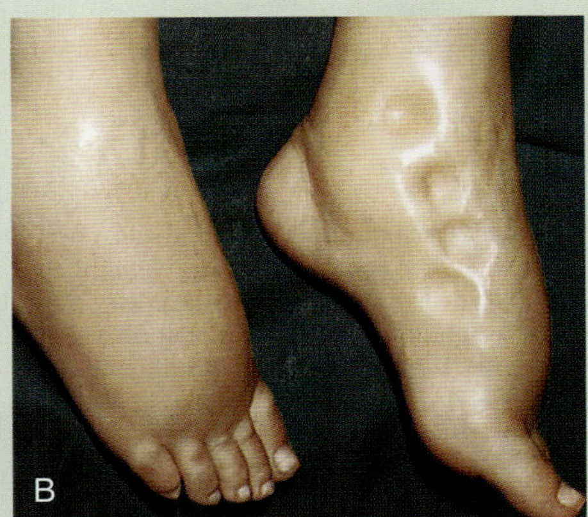 **Figure 16.18B** Pitting oedema.
If pitting oedema is present, grade it on the following scale: 1+ **Mild pitting,** slight indentation, no perceptible swelling of the leg 2+ **Moderate pitting,** indentation subsides rapidly 3+ **Deep pitting,** indentation remains for a short time, leg looks swollen 4+ **Very deep pitting,** indentation lasts a long time, leg is very swollen.	Unilateral oedema occurs with occlusion of a deep vein (see Table 16.5). Unilateral or bilateral oedema occurs with lymphatic obstruction. With these factors, it is 'brawny' or nonpitting and feels hard to the touch.
However, this scale has not been established to be reliable although it is commonly used clinically. The amount of pressure used is arbitrary, as is the judgement of the depth and rate of pitting. Clinicians need a standard quantified scale to ensure consistent clinical measurements and management. Many classify the oedema by measuring the depth of the pitting in centimetres (1+ = 1 cm, 2+ = 2 cm, etc.)	

PROCEDURES AND NORMAL FINDINGS	ABNORMAL FINDINGS AND CLINICAL ALERTS
Ankle circumference is more reliable using a non-stretchable tape at a point 7 cm proximal to the midpoint of the medial malleolus. Because peripheral oedema is a common clinical sign, it is important to detect true changes in the most accurate way available. Check with your own institution to conform to a consistently used scale.	
Leg veins	
Ask the person to stand so that you can assess the venous system. Note any visible, dilated and tortuous veins.	Varicosities occur in the saphenous veins (see Table 16.2).
Skin colour changes	
If you suspect an arterial deficit, raise the legs about 30 cm off the table and ask the person to wag the feet for about 30 seconds to drain off venous blood (Figure 16.19). The skin colour now reflects only the contribution of arterial blood. A light-skinned person's feet normally will look a little pale but still should be pink. A dark-skinned person's feet are more difficult to evaluate, but the soles should reveal extreme colour change. 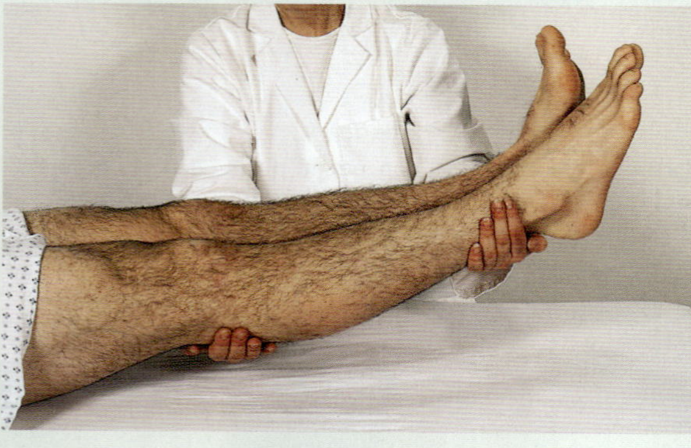 Figure 16.19	Elevational pallor (marked) indicates arterial insufficiency.
Now have the person sit up with the legs over the side of the table (Figure 16.20A). Compare the colour of both feet. Note the time it takes for colour to return to the feet. Normally, this is 10 seconds or less. Note also the time it takes for the superficial veins around the feet to fill—the normal time is about 15 seconds. This test is unreliable if the person has concomitant venous disease with incompetent valves. 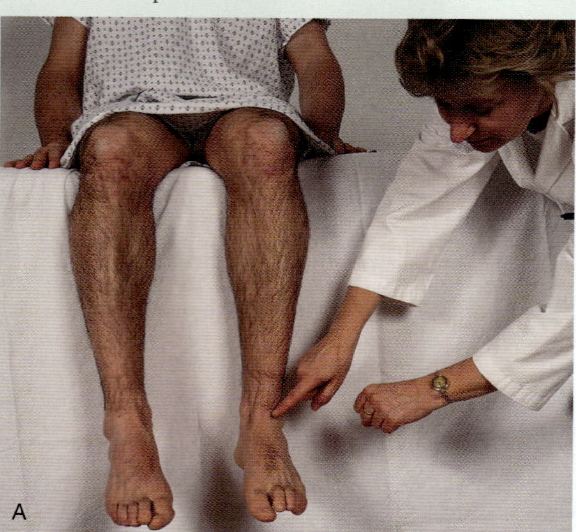 Figure 16.20A	**Dependent rubor** (deep blue-red colour) occurs with severe arterial insufficiency (Figure 16.20B). Chronic hypoxia produces a loss of vasomotor tone and a pooling of blood in the veins. Delayed venous filling occurs with arterial insufficiency. 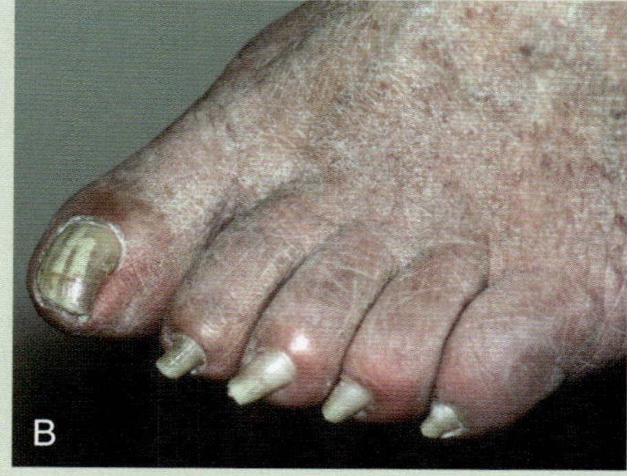 Figure 16.20B

PROCEDURES AND NORMAL FINDINGS	ABNORMAL FINDINGS AND CLINICAL ALERTS
Lower leg strength and sensation	
Test the lower legs for strength (see Chapter 12). Test the lower legs for sensation (see Chapter 12).	Motor loss occurs with severe arterial deficit. Sensory loss occurs with arterial deficit, especially diabetes.
Assessing peripheral pulses using a Doppler	
Use this device to detect a weak peripheral pulse, to monitor blood pressure in infants or children or to measure a low blood pressure or blood pressure in a lower extremity (Figure 16.21). The Doppler magnifies pulsatile sounds from the heart and blood vessels. Position the person supine, with the legs externally rotated so you can reach the medial ankles easily. Place a drop of coupling gel on the end of the handheld transducer. Place the transducer over a pulse site, swivelled at a 45° angle. Apply very light pressure; locate the pulse site by the swishing, whooshing sound. 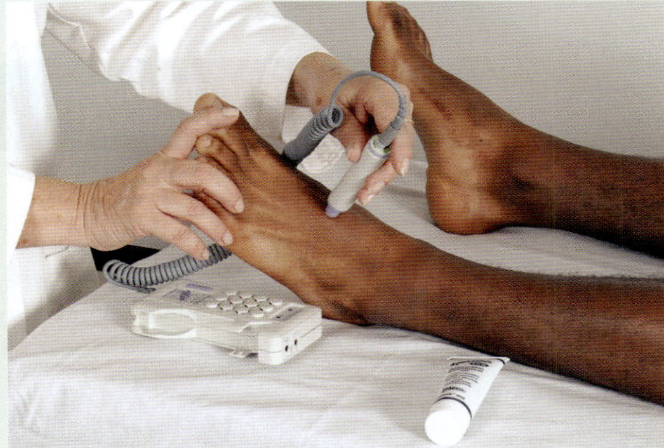 **Figure 16.21**	
Additional objective data for infants and children	
Transient acrocyanosis and skin mottling at birth are discussed in Chapter 22. The pulse strength should be strong and symmetrical. The pulse strength should also be the same in the upper and lower extremities.	**Acrocyanosis** is a vasomotor condition characterised by persistent, painless, usually symmetrical cyanosis of the distal parts of the body (the hands, feet or, rarely, the face) caused by vasospasm of the small vessels of the skin in response to cold (Dean 2018). Weak pulses occur with vasoconstriction of diminished cardiac output. Full, bounding pulses occur with patent ductus arteriosus as a result of the large left-to-right shunt. Diminished or absent femoral pulses while upper extremity pulses are normal suggest coarctation of aorta.
Additional objective assessment data for the pregnant woman	
Expect diffuse bilateral pitting oedema in the lower extremities, especially at the end of the day and into the third trimester. Varicose veins in the legs are also common in the third trimester.	***Clinical alert:*** Generalised oedema with hypertension is a sign of preeclampsia, a serious obstetric health issue. The woman should be referred to her midwife or medical practitioner for further assessment.

PROCEDURES AND NORMAL FINDINGS	ABNORMAL FINDINGS AND CLINICAL ALERTS
Additional objective assessment data for the adults over 65 years	
The dorsalis pedis and posterior tibial pulse may become more difficult to find. Trophic changes associated with arterial insufficiency (thin, shiny skin, thick-ridged nails, loss of hair on lower legs) also occur normally with ageing.	

Further objective assessment for advanced practice

The assessments that are described in the following sections require advanced skill and scope of practice. Nurses working in specialist cardiac units and nurses working in community centres may need to develop these skills. See Chapter 15 for reference.

PROCEDURES AND NORMAL FINDINGS	ABNORMAL FINDINGS AND CLINICAL ALERTS
Inspect and palpate the arms	
Lymph nodes	
Check the epitrochlear lymph node in the depression above and behind the medial condyle of the humerus. Do this by 'shaking hands' with the person and reaching your other hand under the person's elbow to the groove between the biceps and triceps muscles, above the medial epicondyle (Figure 16.22). This node is not normally palpable. **Figure 16.22**	An enlarged epitrochlear node occurs with infection of the hand or forearm.
In addition to the techniques related to inspection and palpation of the arms described previously, the modified Allen test will give you additional data on peripheral circulation of the arms.	

OBJECTIVE DATA

PROCEDURES AND NORMAL FINDINGS	ABNORMAL FINDINGS AND CLINICAL ALERTS
The Allen test	
The **modified Allen test** is used to evaluate the adequacy of collateral circulation prior to cannulating the radial artery (Figure 16.23). **A**, Firmly occlude both the ulnar and the radial arteries of one hand while the person makes a fist several times. This causes the hand to blanch. **B**, Ask the person to open the hand without hyperextending it; then release pressure on the ulnar artery while maintaining pressure on the radial artery. Adequate circulation is suggested by a return to the hand's normal colour in approximately 2–5 seconds. The modified Allen test is a valid tool in primary screening (Sivaharini et al 2018).	**C**, Pallor persists or a sluggish return to colour suggests occlusion of the collateral arterial flow. Avoid radial artery cannulation until adequate circulation is shown.

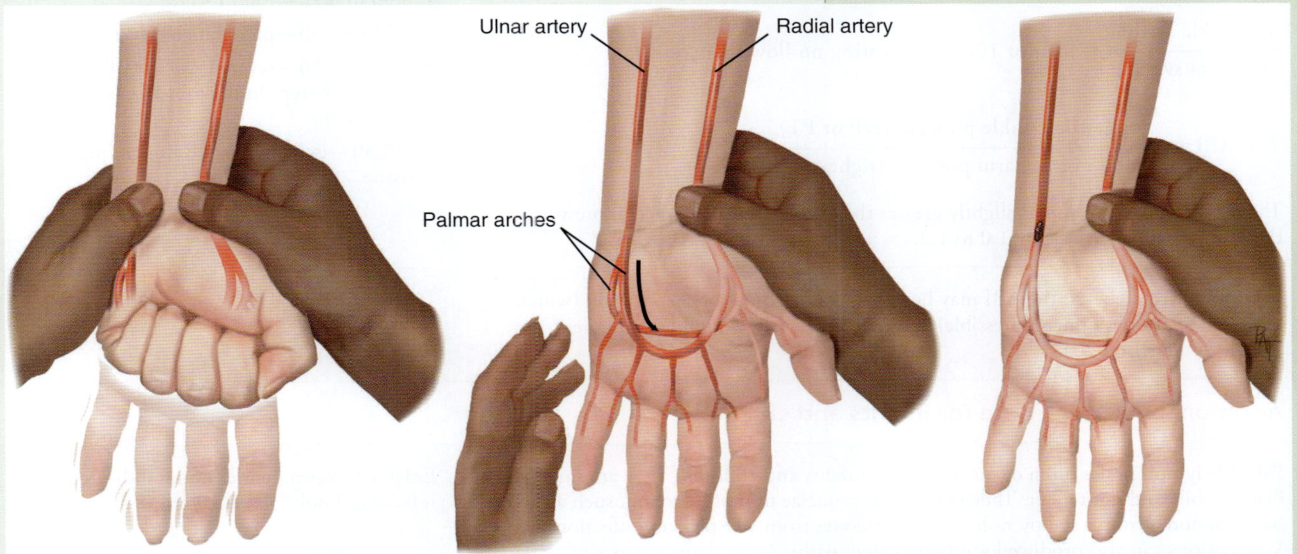

Figure 16.23

PROCEDURES AND NORMAL FINDINGS	ABNORMAL FINDINGS AND CLINICAL ALERTS
Inspect and palpate the legs	
In addition to the techniques related to inspection and palpation of the legs described previously, palpation of inguinal lymph nodes will extend assessment data for the advanced practice nurse. The manual compression test and the ankle brachial index will give you additional data on peripheral circulation of the legs.	
Palpate the inguinal lymph nodes. It is not unusual to find palpable nodes that are small (1 cm or less), movable and nontender.	Enlarged nodes, tender or fixed in area.
The ankle-brachial index (ABI)	
Use of the Doppler stethoscope is a highly specific, noninvasive and readily available way to determine the extent of peripheral arterial disease. The person is lying flat with the head and heels fully supported. Confirm no smoking within 2 hours of the measurement and allow a 5–10-min rest period supine before measurement. Choose the correct cuff width for the arm and the ankle; width should be 40% of limb circumference. Position the ankle cuff just above the malleoli with straight wrapping.	

PROCEDURES AND NORMAL FINDINGS	ABNORMAL FINDINGS AND CLINICAL ALERTS
Use the Doppler probe for both brachial and ankle measurements. In all sites, locate the pulse by Doppler and inflate the cuff 20 mmHg above disappearance of flow signal; then deflate slowly to detect reappearance of flow signal (Organ & Harrison 2017). Measure each site twice and use the average as the recorded pressure. Moving counterclockwise, measure: right arm, right posterior tibial (PT), right dorsalis pedis (DP), left PT, left DP, left arm. Calculate both ABI using this formula: $\text{Right ABI} = \frac{\text{highest right average ankle pressure (DP or PT)}}{\text{Highest average arm pressure (right or left)}}$ For example: $\frac{\text{132 ankle systolic}}{\text{124 arm systolic}} = 1.06$ or 106%, indicating no flow reduction $\text{Left ABI} = \frac{\text{highest left ankle pressure (DP or PT)}}{\text{highest average arm pressure (right or left)}}$ The normal ankle pressure is slightly greater than or equal to the brachial pressure; thus, a normal ABI is usually 1.0 to 1.2.	An ABI of 0.91 to 1.0 is borderline for cardiovascular risk (Aboyans et al 2012). An ABI of 0.91 or less indicates the presence of peripheral arterial disease (PAD): • 0.90 to 0.70—mild PAD • 0.71 to 0.40—moderate to severe PAD • 0.41 to 0.30—severe PAD, usually with rest pain except in the presence of diabetic neuropathy • <0.30—ischaemia, with impending loss of tissue.
In people with diabetes, the ABI may be less reliable because of calcification (which makes their arteries noncompressible) and may give a falsely high measurement (Organ & Harrison 2017).	
Additional objective data for infants and children	
Palpable lymph nodes often occur in healthy infants and children. They are small, firm, mobile and nontender. They may be the sequelae of past infection, such as inguinal nodes from a nappy rash or cervical nodes from a respiratory infection. Vaccinations can also produce local lymphadenopathy. Note characteristics of any palpable nodes and whether they are local or generalised.	Enlarged, warm, tender nodes indicate current infection. Look for source of infection.

OBJECTIVE DATA

Summary Checklist

PERIPHERAL VASCULAR ASSESSMENT

Subjective data

1. Presenting concern
2. Leg pain or cramps
3. Skin changes on arms or legs
4. Swelling in the arms or legs
5. Health and lifestyle management

Objective data

1. Inspect and palpate the arms
2. Inspect and palpate the legs
3. Assessing peripheral pulses using the Doppler

PROMOTING A HEALTHY LIFESTYLE

FOOT CARE

Take care of your feet!

Foot problems often herald more serious health conditions such as arthritis, diabetes and nerve or circulatory disorders. Healthcare providers should not only remember to examine the feet for common foot problems but also be prepared to explain what 'good' foot care really means. Too often healthcare providers will advise good foot care but do not take the time to explain what 'good' foot care entails.

'Good' foot care entails the following:

1. Checking your feet every day.
2. If individuals are unable to see the bottoms of their feet, they need to be instructed to use a mirror or to ask someone to help them.
3. Each foot should be examined for red spots or sensitive areas, discolouration of skin or nails, ingrown nails, pain, cuts, swelling or blisters. A good time to examine feet is after a shower or bath. Feet should be dried carefully, especially between the toes.
4. Toenails should be kept trimmed, straight across, and filed at the edges with an emery board or nail file.
5. Although freshly applied nail polish does not increase the number of bacteria, chipped nail polish may support the growth of larger numbers of organisms on nails. This is especially important for individuals who are already at risk for infection.
6. Keeping the blood flowing to your feet. It is important to keep blood circulating to your feet. This is accomplished by increasing activity. Walking is one of the best exercises for overall circulation.
7. When an individual is not able to walk, putting the feet up when sitting or lying down, stretching, wiggling toes, having a gentle foot massage or warm foot bath are great alternatives.
8. Do not cross legs for long periods of time.
9. Do not smoke.
10. Wear shoes that fit and are comfortable. Wear comfortable shoes that fit well. The size of our feet changes as we age, so it is important to be measured each time we buy new shoes. The best time to measure feet is towards the end of the day, when feet tend to be the largest.
11. Another thing to remember is that most individuals have one foot that is larger than the other. It is recommended that shoes are selected to fit to the larger foot. Further, just as we have different body shapes, our feet have different shapes too.
12. It is important to select shoes that are shaped like your feet. The ball of the foot should fit comfortably into the widest part of the shoe and toes should not be crowded.
13. For women, low-heeled shoes are safer and less damaging than high-heeled shoes.
14. Keeping skin soft and smooth.
15. A thin coat of skin lotion over the tops and bottoms of your feet helps to keep skin soft and smooth. However, this extra moisture should not go between toes.
16. Use mild soap.
17. Be careful about adding oils to bath water. They can make your feet and the bathtub both very slippery.

For more information on foot care:

Australian Orthopaedic Foot and Ankle Society: www.aofas.org.au

Australian Podiatry Association: www.podiatry.org.au

New Zealand Society of Podiatrists: www.podiatry.org.nz

OBJECTIVE DATA

Documentation and critical thinking

FOCUSED ASSESSMENT: CLINICAL CASE STUDY

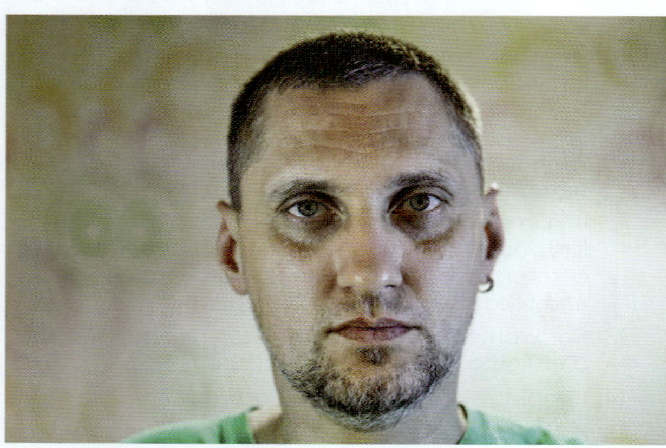

Context

Mr James Kerrigan is a 43-year-old local council employee, admitted to hospital today for 'bypass surgery tomorrow to fix my aorta and these dark-coloured toes'.

Subjective

6 years ago: motorcycle accident with handlebars jammed into groin. Treated and discharged from local hospital. No apparent injury, although the cardiac surgeon now thinks accident may have precipitated present stenosis of aorta.

1 year ago: radiating pain in right calf on walking 0.5 km. Pain relieved with rest.

3 months ago: began experiencing erectile dysfunction, unable to maintain erection during intercourse.

1 month ago: leg pain present after walking two blocks. Numbness and tingling in right foot and calf. Tips of three toes on right foot look dusky in colour. Referred to a surgeon.

Present: leg pain at rest, constant and severe, worse at night, partially relieved by dangling legs over side of bed.

History: no history of heart or vessel disease or hypertension or diabetes or obesity.

Current smoker: 1 packet per day. History of 69 pack years.

Walking is part of occupation, although has been driving the local council truck last 3 months due to leg pain. Not currently on medication.

Social: is married with two young children. Supportive family. Wife will be taking leave from work to care for him when he is discharged home.

Objective

Inspection: Lower extremity size equal bilaterally with no swelling or atrophy. No varicosities. Colour L leg pink, R leg pink when supine, but marked pallor to R foot on elevation. Gangrene at tips of R 2nd, 3rd, 4th toes. Leg hair present but absent on involved toes.

Palpation: R foot cool and temperature progressively warms on palpation up R leg.

Pulses: Femorals, both 1+; popliteals, both 0; posterior tibial, both 0 but present with Doppler; dorsalis pedis both 0, but left dorsalis pedis is present with Doppler, and right is not present with Doppler.

Diagnostic studies: showed stenosis of abdominal aorta below kidneys.

Collaborative problem

Ineffective tissue perfusion related to interruption of flow resulting from injury

Problem statements/nursing diagnoses

Ischaemic rest pain in right leg related to poor blood flow

Impaired tissue integrity in the right toes related to altered circulation

Risk of skin breakdown related to altered circulation

Activity intolerance related to leg pain

Potential for anxiety related to uncertain outcome of surgery and possible need for amputation of toes

Abnormal findings

TABLE 16.1 Variations in arterial pulse

DESCRIPTION	ASSOCIATED WITH
Weak, 'thready' pulse—1+ Hard to palpate, need to search for it, may fade in and out, easily obliterated by pressure	Decreased cardiac output; peripheral arterial disease; aortic valve stenosis

TABLE 16.1 Variations in arterial pulse—cont'd

DESCRIPTION	ASSOCIATED WITH
Full, bounding pulse—3+ Easily palpable, pounds under your fingertips	Hyperkinetic states (exercise, anxiety, fever), anaemia, hyperthyroidism
Water-hammer (Corrigan's) pulse—3+ Greater than normal strength, then collapses suddenly	Aortic valve regurgitation; patent ductus arteriosus
Pulsus bigeminus Rhythm is coupled, every other beat comes early, or normal beat followed by premature beat. The strength of the premature beat is decreased because of shortened cardiac filling time	Conduction disturbance (e.g. premature ventricular contraction, premature atrial contraction)
Pulsus alternans Rhythm is regular, but the strength varies with alternating beats of large and small amplitude	Heart failure
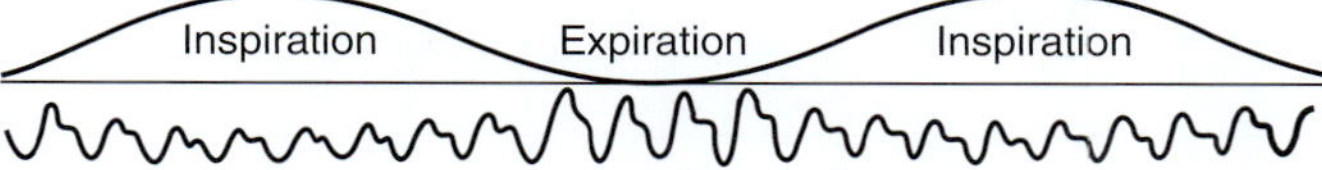 **Pulsus paradoxus** Beats have weaker amplitude with inspiration, stronger with expiration. Best determined during blood pressure measurement; reading decreases (>10 mmHg) during inspiration and increases with expiration	Any condition that blocks venous return to the right side of the heart, or blocks left ventricular filling (e.g. cardiac tamponade; constrictive pericarditis, pulmonary embolism)
 **Pulsus bisferiens** Each pulse has two strong systolic peaks, with a dip in between. Best assessed at the carotid artery	Aortic valve stenosis plus regurgitation

Abnormal findings for advanced practice

TABLE 16.2 Peripheral vascular disease in the legs

CHRONIC ARTERIAL INSUFFICIENCY

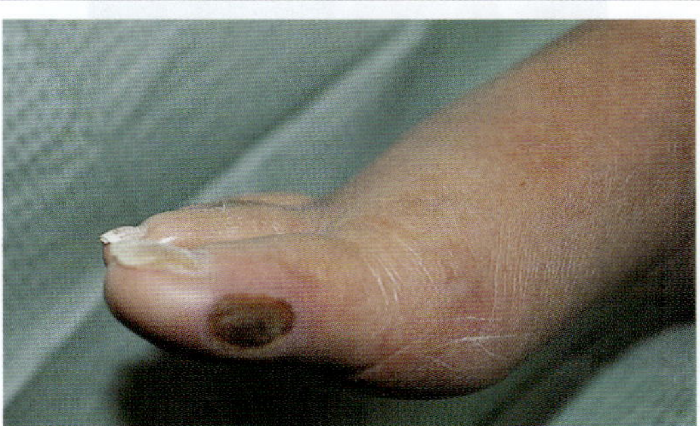

Arteriosclerosis—ischaemic ulcer

Build-up of fatty plaques on inner layer (intima) (atherosclerosis) plus hardening and calcification of arterial wall (arteriosclerosis). The person is likely to report deep muscle pain in calf or foot, claudication (pain with walking), pain at rest indicates worsening of condition. Physical examination is likely to reveal coolness, pallor, elevational pallor and dependent rubor; diminished pulses; systolic bruits; trophic skin; signs of malnutrition (thin, shiny skin, thick-ridged nails, absence of hair, atrophy of muscles); xanthoma formation; distal gangrene.

Ulcers occur at toes, metatarsal heads, heels, lateral ankle and are characterised by pale ischaemic base, well-defined edges and no bleeding

(Continued)

TABLE 16.2 Peripheral vascular disease in the legs—cont'd

<table>
<tr><th colspan="2">CHRONIC VENOUS INSUFFICIENCY</th></tr>
<tr><td>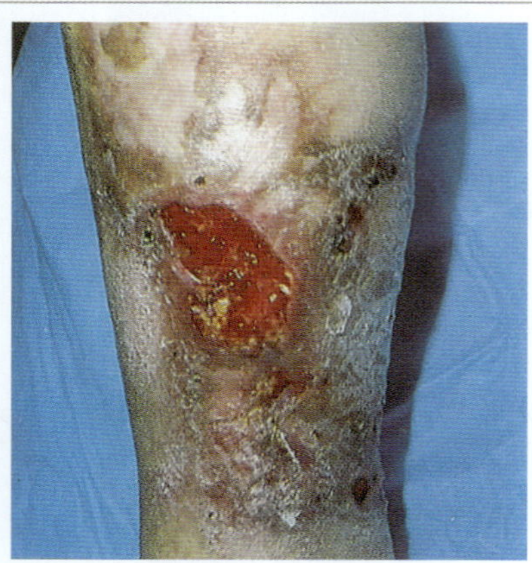
Venous (stasis) ulcer
Venous ulcers account for 80% of lower leg ulcers. The person may report aching pain in calf or lower leg, which is worse at end of the day, and worse with prolonged standing or sitting. Itching with stasis ulcers. There is likely to be lower leg oedema that does not resolve with diuretic therapy; coarse, thickened skin; pulses normal; brown pigment discolouration; petechiae; dermatitis. Venous stasis causes increased venous pressure, which then causes red blood cells (RBCs) to leak out of veins and into the skin. As these RBCs break down, they leave haemosiderin (iron deposits) which are the visible brown pigment deposits.
Ulcers occur at medial malleolus and are characterised by bleeding, uneven edges.</td>
<td>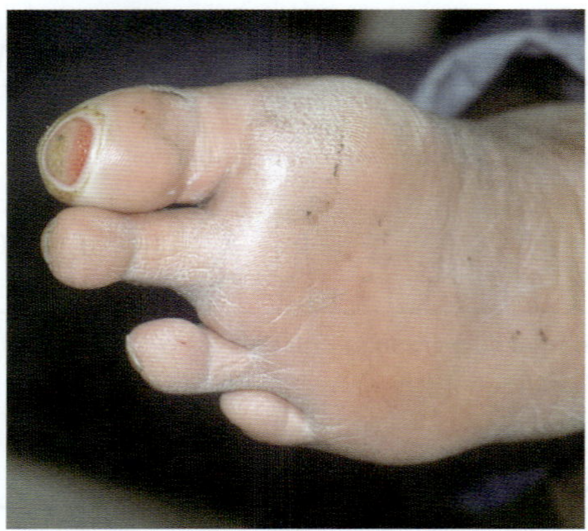
Diabetic (neuropathic) related foot ulcer
Diabetes hastens changes described with arterial ischaemic ulcer, with generalised dysfunction in all arterial areas (peripheral, coronary, cerebral, retinal and renal). A peripheral diabetic ulcer has its pathogenesis in sensory neuropathy with loss of protective sensation, autonomic neuropathy with decreased sweating and dry skin and motor neuropathy with foot deformity. Ulcers then occur with repetitive stress over these at risk areas.</td></tr>
<tr><th>CHRONIC VENOUS DISEASE</th><th>ACUTE VENOUS DISEASE</th></tr>
<tr><td>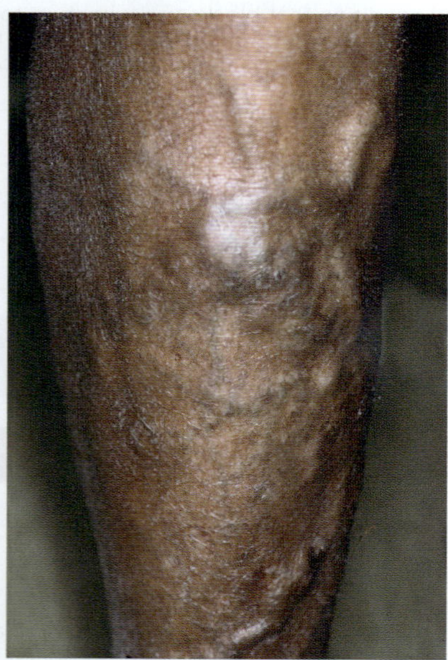
Superficial varicose veins
Incompetent valves permit reflux of blood, producing dilated, tortuous veins. Unremitting hydrostatic pressure causes distal valves to be incompetent and causes worsening of the varicosity. Over age 45 years, occurrence is three times more common in women than in men. The person may report aching, heaviness in calf, easy fatiguability, night leg or foot cramps. Physical examination may reveal dilated, tortuous veins.</td>
<td>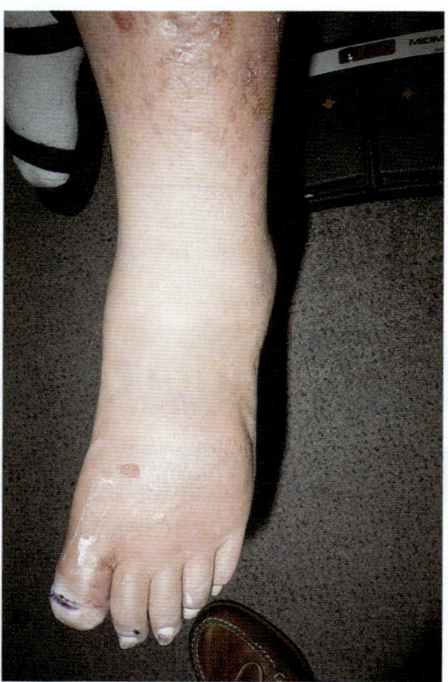
Deep vein thrombophlebitis
A deep vein is occluded by a thrombus, causing inflammation, blocked venous return, cyanosis and oedema.
The person may report sudden onset of intense, sharp, deep muscle pain, may increase with sharp dorsiflexion of foot. Physical examination may reveal increased warmth; swelling (to compare swelling, observe the usual shoe size as in above photo); redness; dependent cyanosis is mild or may be absent; tender to palpation.</td></tr>
</table>

TABLE 16.3 History profiles of pain of peripheral vascular disease

SYMPTOM ANALYSIS	CHRONIC ARTERIAL SYMPTOMS	ACUTE ARTERIAL SYMPTOMS
Location	Deep muscle pain, usually in calf, but may be lower on leg or dorsum of foot	Varies, distal to occlusion, may involve entire leg
Character	Intermittent claudication, feels like 'cramp', 'numbness and tingling', 'feeling of cold'	Throbbing
Onset and duration	Chronic pain, onset gradual after exertion	Sudden onset (within 1 hour)
Aggravating factors	Activity (walking, stairs) 'Claudication distance' is specific number of blocks, stairs it takes to produce pain Elevation (rest pain indicates severe involvement)	
Relieving factors	Rest (usually within 2 min (e.g. lying) Dangling (severe involvement)	
Associated symptoms	Cool, pale skin	Six Ps: pain, pallor, pulselessness, paraesthesia, poikilothermia (coldness), paralysis (indicates severe)
Those at risk	Adults over 65 years, more males than females, inherited predisposition, history of hypertension, smoking, diabetes, hypercholesterolaemia, obesity, vascular disease	History of vascular surgery; arterial invasive procedure; abdominal aneurysm (emboli) (see Table 16.5); trauma, including injured arteries, chronic atrial fibrillation
	CHRONIC VENOUS SYMPTOMS	ACUTE VENOUS SYMPTOMS
Location	Calf, lower leg	Calf
Character	Aching, tiredness, feeling of fullness	Intense, sharp; deep muscle tender to touch
Onset and duration	Chronic pain, increases at end of day	Sudden onset (within 1 hour)
Aggravating factors	Prolonged standing, sitting	Pain may increase with sharp dorsiflexion of foot
Relieving factors	Elevation, lying, walking	
Associated symptoms	Oedema, varicosities, weeping ulcers at ankles	Red, warm, swollen leg
Those at risk	Job with prolonged standing or sitting; obesity; pregnancy; prolonged bed rest; history of heart failure, varicosities or thrombophlebitis; veins crushed by trauma or surgery	

TABLE 16.4 Peripheral vascular disease in the arms

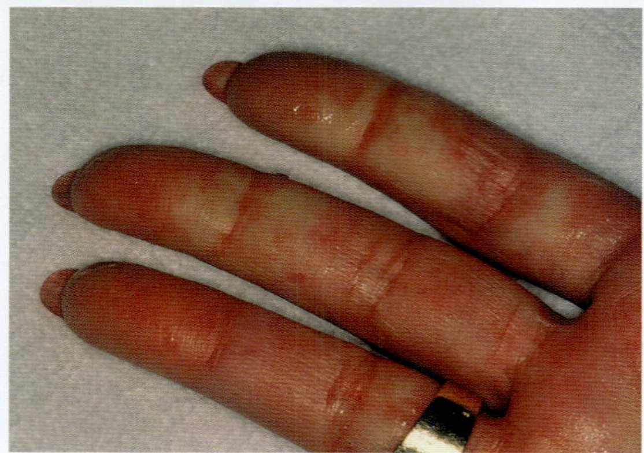

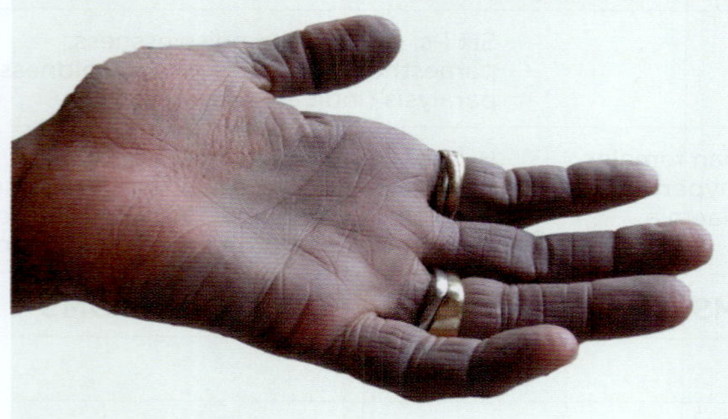

Raynaud's phenomenon

Episodes of abrupt progressive tricolour change of the fingers in response to cold, vibration or stress: first white (pallor) from arteriospasm and resulting deficit in supply; then blue (cyanosis) from slight relaxation of the spasm that allows a slow trickle of blood through the capillaries and increased oxygen extraction of haemoglobin; finally red (rubor) due to return of blood into the dilated capillary bed or reactive hyperaemia.

May have cold, numbness or pain along with pallor or cyanosis stage; then burning, throbbing pain, swelling along with rubor. Lasts minutes to hours; occurs bilaterally.

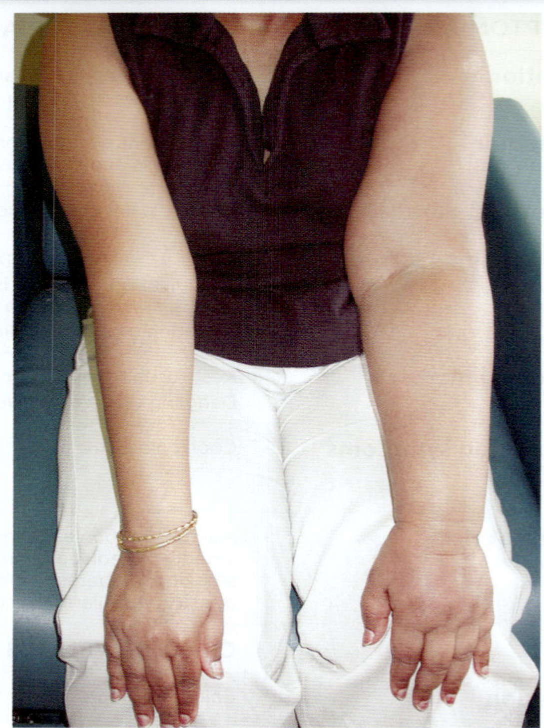

Lymphoedema

Removal of lymph nodes with breast surgery, or damage to lymph nodes and channels with radiation therapy for breast cancer; can impede drainage of lymph. Protein-rich lymph builds up in the interstitial spaces, which further raises local colloid oncotic pressure and promotes more fluid leakage. Stagnant lymphatic fluid can lead to infection, delayed wound healing, chronic inflammation and fibrosis of surrounding tissue. Chronic lymphoedema is unilateral, non-pitting 'brawny' oedema, with overlying skin indurated. This condition is psychologically demoralising as it is perceived as a threat to body image and a constant reminder of the cancer.

TABLE 16.5 Other vascular abnormalities

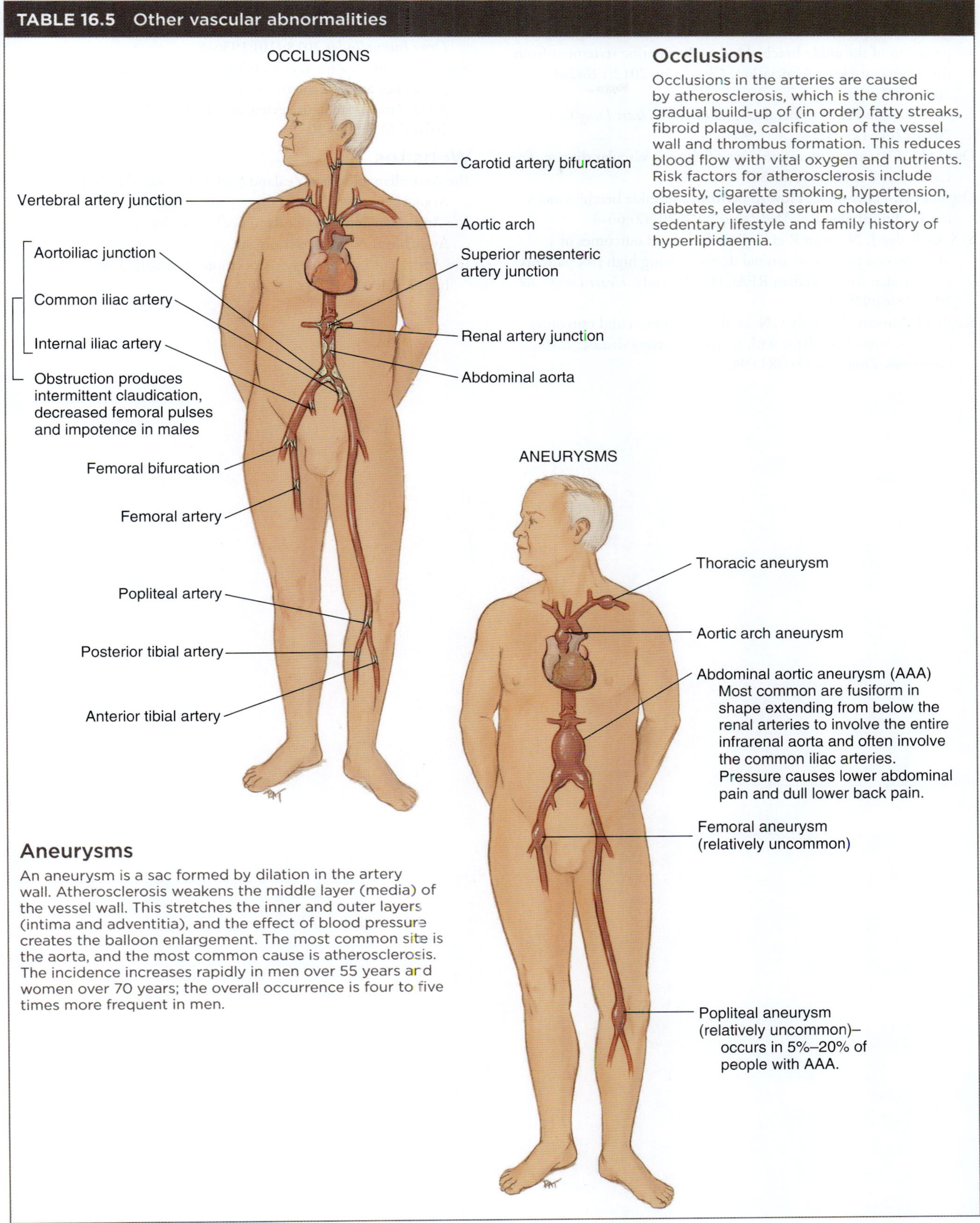

Occlusions

Occlusions in the arteries are caused by atherosclerosis, which is the chronic gradual build-up of (in order) fatty streaks, fibroid plaque, calcification of the vessel wall and thrombus formation. This reduces blood flow with vital oxygen and nutrients. Risk factors for atherosclerosis include obesity, cigarette smoking, hypertension, diabetes, elevated serum cholesterol, sedentary lifestyle and family history of hyperlipidaemia.

Aneurysms

An aneurysm is a sac formed by dilation in the artery wall. Atherosclerosis weakens the middle layer (media) of the vessel wall. This stretches the inner and outer layers (intima and adventitia), and the effect of blood pressure creates the balloon enlargement. The most common site is the aorta, and the most common cause is atherosclerosis. The incidence increases rapidly in men over 55 years and women over 70 years; the overall occurrence is four to five times more frequent in men.

BIBLIOGRAPHY

Aboyans V, Criqui MH, Abraham P, et al. Measurement and interpretation of the ankle-brachial index: A scientific statement from the American Heart Association. *Circulation* 2012;126(24): 2890–909.

Conte SM, Vale PR. Peripheral arterial disease. *Heart Lung Circ* 2018;27(4):427–32.

Dean SM. Cutaneous manifestations of chronic vascular disease. *Prog Cardiovasc Dis* 2018;60(6):567–79.

Organ NM, Harrison C. How to perform the ankle brachial index test in clinical practice. *Med J Aust* 2017;207(2):60–1.

Si S, Golledge J, Norman P, et al. Prevalence and outcomes of undiagnosed peripheral arterial disease among high risk patients in Australia: An Australian REACH Sub-Study. *Heart Lung Circ* 2019;28(6):939–45.

Singh TP, Moxon JV, Healy GN, et al. Presentation and outcomes of indigenous Australians with peripheral artery disease. *BMC Cardiovasc Disord* 2018;18(1):94.

Sivaharini S, Babu KY, Mohanraj KG. Comparative analysis of Allen's test with modified Allen's test and its clinical importance. *Drug Invent Today* 2018;(10):1936–8.

Song P, Rudan D, Zhu Y, et al. Global, regional, and national prevalence and risk factors for peripheral artery disease in 2015: An updated systematic review and analysis. *Lancet Glob Health* 2019;7(8):e1020–30.

Websites

The Australian and New Zealand Society for Vascular Nursing. Available at: www.anzsvn.org.

The Australian and New Zealand Society for Vascular Surgery. Available at: www.anzsvs.org.au.

The Australian Lymphology Association. Available at: www.lymphoedema.org.au.

Chapter Seventeen
Cardiac assessment

Written by Carolyn Jarvis
Adapted by Maria Murphy

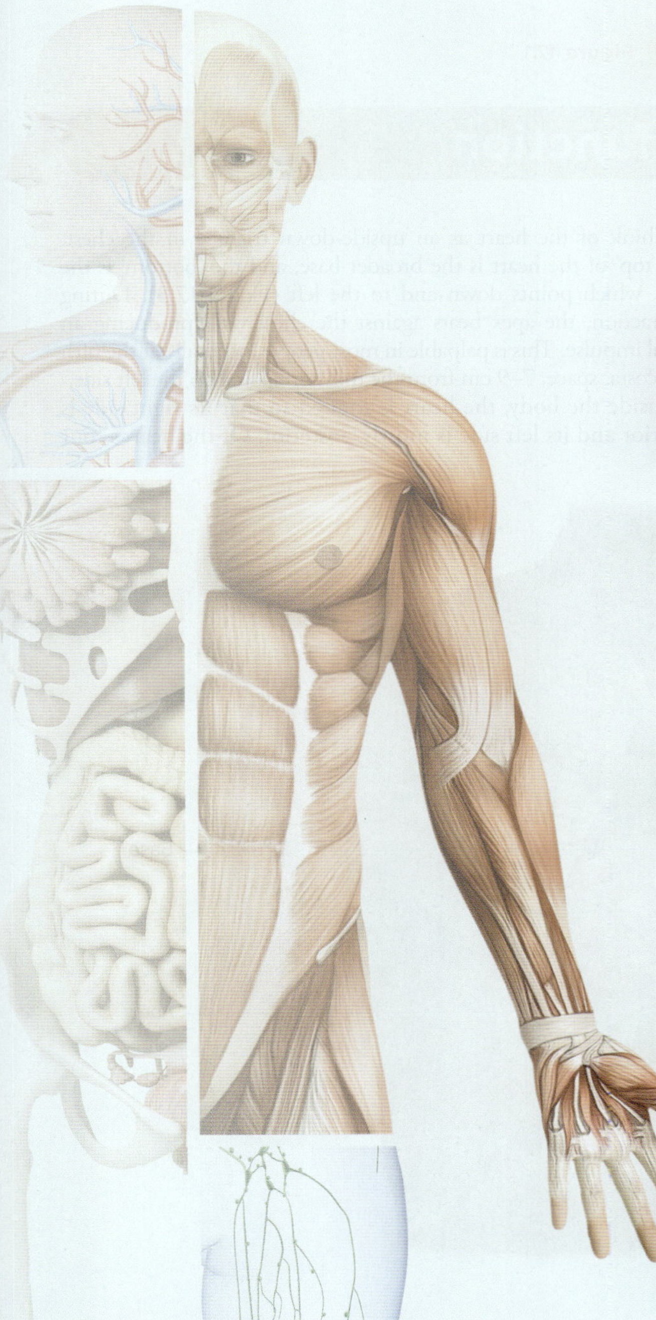

INTRODUCTION

The cardiovascular system consists of the **heart**, a muscular pump, and the **blood vessels**. The blood vessels are arranged in two continuous loops, the pulmonary circulation and the systemic circulation (Figure 17.1). When the heart contracts, it pumps blood simultaneously into both loops. In order to appreciate the impact of disease and trauma to this complex and dynamic system you are advised to first review the structure and function of the cardiovascular system.

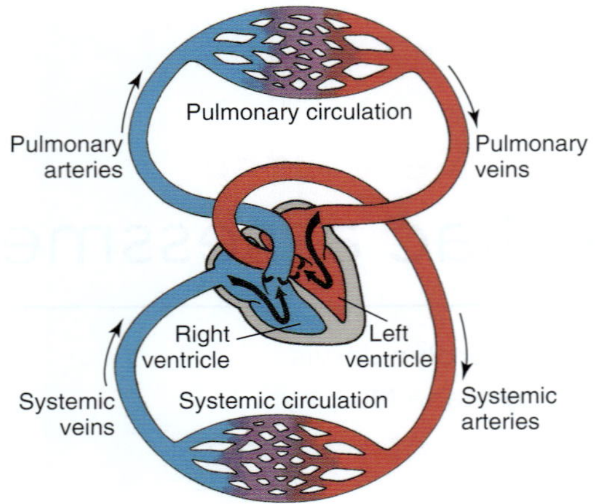

Figure 17.1

Structure and function

POSITION AND SURFACE LANDMARKS

The **praecordium** is the area on the anterior chest overlying the heart and great vessels (Figure 17.2). The great vessels are the major arteries and veins connected to the heart. The heart and the great vessels are located between the lungs in the middle third of the thoracic cage, called the **mediastinum**. The heart extends from the second to the fifth intercostal space and from the right border of the sternum to the left midclavicular line.

Think of the heart as an upside-down triangle in the chest. The 'top' of the heart is the broader base, and the 'bottom' is the apex, which points down and to the left (Figure 17.3). During contraction, the apex beats against the chest wall, producing an apical impulse. This is palpable in most people, normally at the fifth intercostal space, 7–9 cm from the midsternal line on the left side.

Inside the body, the heart is rotated so that its right side is anterior and its left side is mostly posterior. Of the heart's four

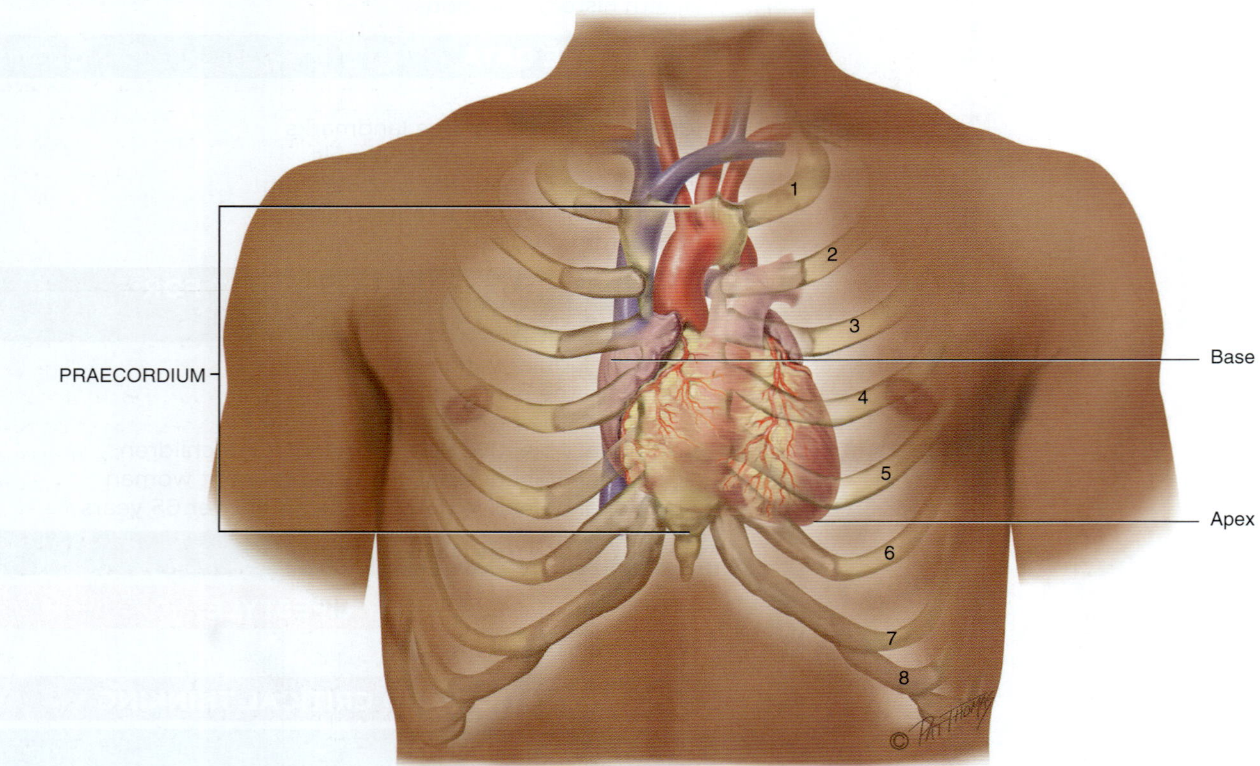

Figure 17.2

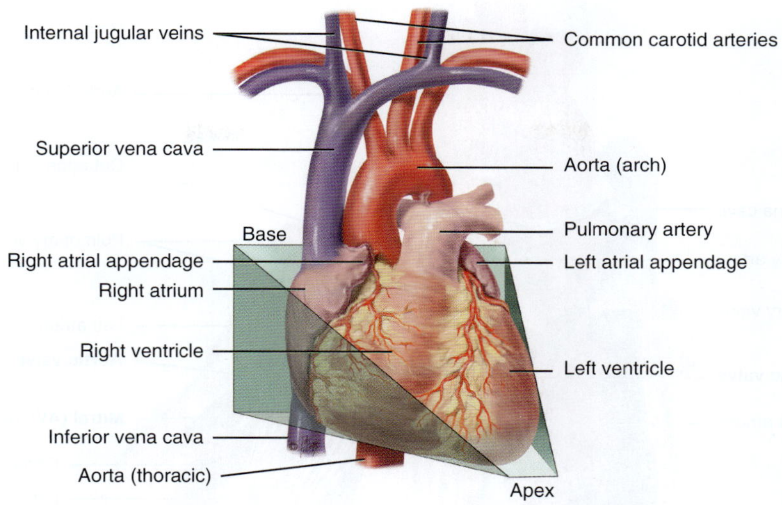

Figure 17.3
©Pat Thomas, 2006

chambers, the right ventricle forms the greatest area of anterior cardiac surface. The left ventricle lies behind the right ventricle and forms the apex and slender area of the left border. The right atrium lies to the right and above the right ventricle and forms the right border. The left atrium is located posteriorly, with only a small portion, the left atrial appendage, showing anteriorly.

The **great vessels** lie bunched above the base of the heart. The **superior** and **inferior vena cava** return deoxygenated venous blood to the right side of the heart. The **pulmonary artery** leaves the right ventricle, bifurcates and carries the venous blood to the lungs. The **pulmonary veins** return the freshly oxygenated blood to the left side of the heart, and the aorta carries it out to the body. The aorta ascends from the left ventricle, arches back at the level of the sternal angle and descends behind the heart.

HEART WALL, CHAMBERS AND VALVES

The **heart wall** has three layers. The **pericardium** is a tough, fibrous, double-walled sac that surrounds and protects the heart (see its cut edge in Figure 17.4). It has two layers that contain 10–30 mL of serous pericardial fluid. This ensures smooth, friction-free movement of the heart muscle. The pericardium is adherent to the great vessels, oesophagus, sternum and pleurae and is anchored to the diaphragm. The **myocardium** is the muscular wall of the heart; it does the pumping. The **endocardium** is the thin layer of endothelial tissue that lines the inner surface of the heart chambers and valves.

The common metaphor is to think of the heart as a pump. But consider that the heart is actually two pumps; the right side of the heart pumps blood into the lungs, and the left side of the heart simultaneously pumps blood into the body. The two pumps are separated by an impermeable wall, the septum. Each side has an **atrium** and a **ventricle**. The atrium (Latin for 'anteroom') is a thin-walled reservoir for holding blood, and the thick-walled ventricle is the muscular pumping chamber. (It is common to use the following abbreviations to refer to the chambers: RA, right atrium; RV, right ventricle; LA, left atrium; and LV, left ventricle.)

The four **chambers** are separated by swinging-door-like structures, called valves, whose main purpose is to prevent backflow of blood. The valves are unidirectional; they can only open one way. The valves open and close passively in response to pressure gradients in the moving blood.

There are four **valves** in the heart (see Figure 17.4). The two **atrioventricula**r (AV) valves separate the atria and the ventricles. The right AV valve is the **tricuspid**, and the left AV valve is the bicuspid or **mitral** valve (so named because it resembles a bishop's mitred cap). The valves are thin leaflets that are anchored by collagenous fibres (**chordae tendineae**) to papillary muscles embedded in the ventricle floor. The AV valves open during the heart's filling phase, or **diastole**, to allow the ventricles to fill with blood. During the pumping phase, or **systole**, the AV valves close to prevent regurgitation of blood back up into the atria. The papillary muscles contract at this time, so that the valve leaflets meet and unite to form a perfect seal without turning themselves inside out.

The **semilunar** (SL) valves are set between the ventricles and the arteries. Each valve has three cusps that look like half-moons. The SL valves are the **pulmonic** valve in the right side of the heart and the **aortic** valve in the left side of the heart. They open during pumping, or **systole**, to allow blood to be ejected from the heart.

Note: There are no valves present between the vena cava and the right atrium, nor between the pulmonary veins and the left atrium. For this reason, abnormally high pressure in the left side of the heart gives a person symptoms of pulmonary congestion, and abnormally high pressure in the right side of the heart shows in the neck veins and abdomen.

DIRECTION OF BLOOD FLOW

Think of a deoxygenated red blood cell being drained downstream into the vena cava. It is swept along with the flow of venous blood and follows the route illustrated in Figure 17.5.

1. From liver to right atrium (RA) through inferior vena cava
   Superior vena cava drains venous blood from the head and upper extremities

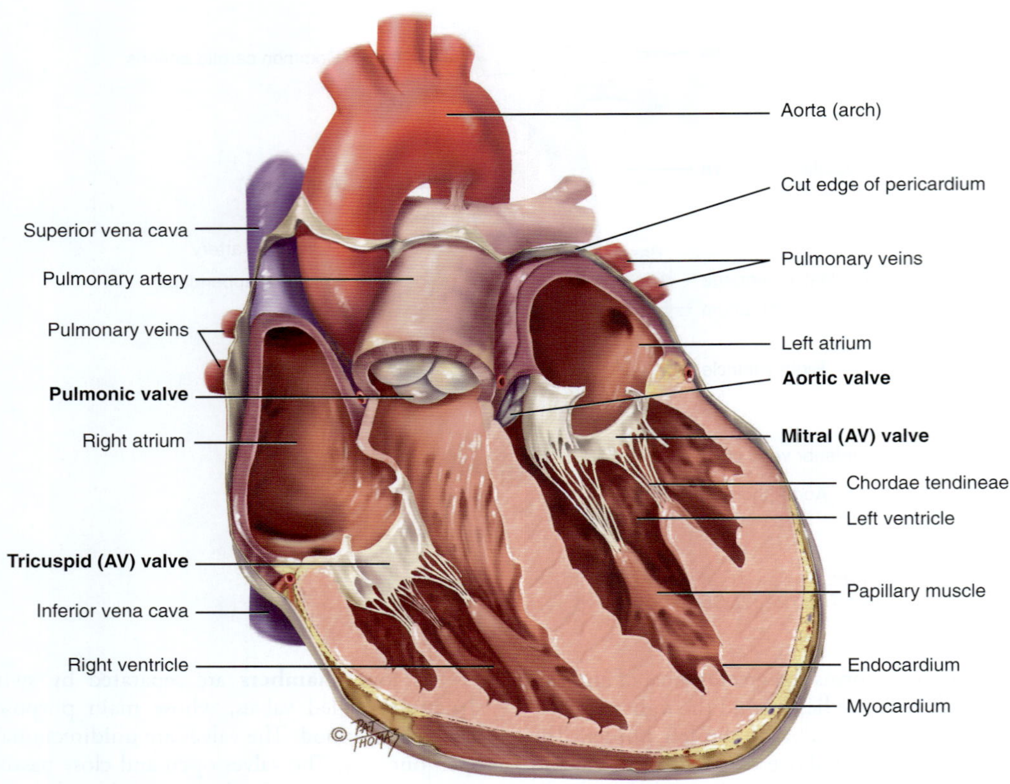

Figure 17.4
©Pat Thomas, 2006

From RA, venous blood travels through tricuspid valve to right ventricle (RV)

2. From RV, venous blood flows through pulmonic valve to pulmonary artery
   Pulmonary artery delivers deoxygenated blood to lungs
3. Lungs oxygenate blood
   Pulmonary veins return oxygenated blood to LA
4. From LA, arterial blood travels through mitral valve to LV
5. LV ejects blood through aortic valve into aorta
6. Aorta delivers oxygenated blood to body.

Remember that the circulation is a continuous loop. The blood is kept moving along by continually shifting pressure gradients. The blood flows from an area of higher pressure to one of lower pressure.

CARDIAC CYCLE

The rhythmic movement of blood through the heart is the **cardiac cycle**. It has two phases, **diastole** and **systole**. In diastole, the ventricles relax and fill with blood. This takes up two-thirds of the cardiac cycle. The heart's contraction is systole. During systole, blood is pumped from the ventricles and fills the pulmonary and systemic arteries. This is one-third of the cardiac cycle.

Diastole. In diastole, the ventricles are relaxed, and the AV valves (i.e. the tricuspid and mitral) are open (Figure 17.6). (Opening of the normal valve is acoustically silent.) The pressure in the atria is higher than that in the ventricles, so blood pours rapidly into the ventricles. This first passive filling phase is called **early** or **protodiastolic filling**.

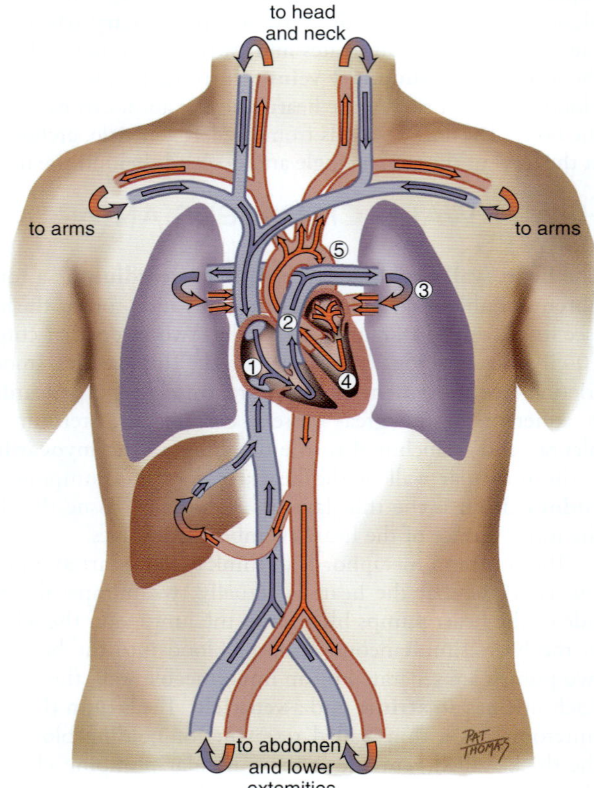

Figure 17.5

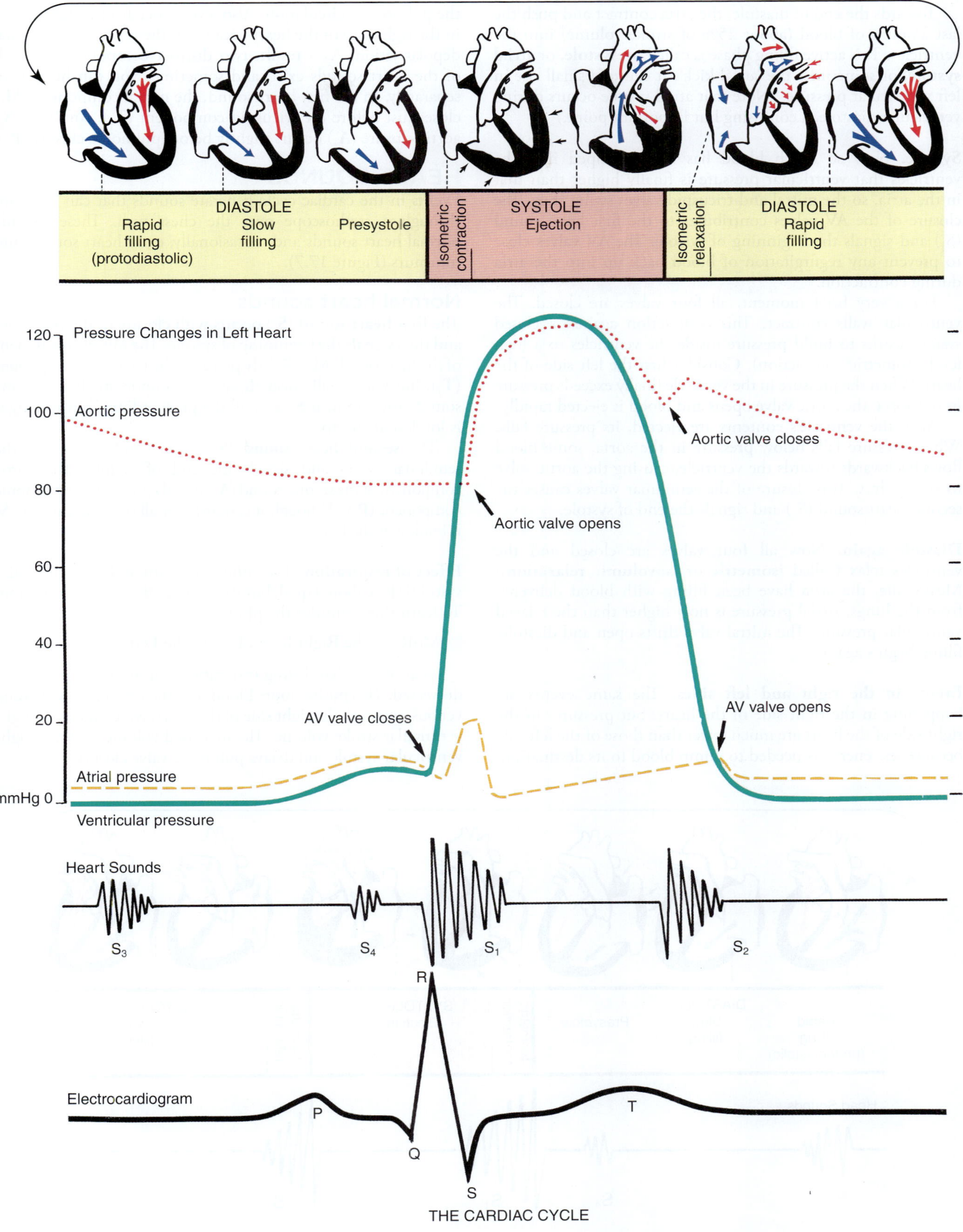

DIASTOLE
Rapid filling (protodiastolic)
Slow filling
Presystole
Isometric contraction
SYSTOLE
Ejection
Isometric relaxation
DIASTOLE
Rapid filling
Pressure Changes in Left Heart
120
100
80
60
40
20
mmHg 0
Aortic pressure
Aortic valve opens
Aortic valve closes
AV valve closes
AV valve opens
Atrial pressure
Ventricular pressure
Heart Sounds
S_3
S_4
S_1
S_2
Electrocardiogram
P
Q
R
S
T
THE CARDIAC CYCLE

Figure 17.6

Towards the end of diastole, the atria contract and push the last amount of blood (about 25% of stroke volume) into the ventricles. This active filling phase is called **presystole**, or **atrial systole**, or sometimes the 'atrial kick'. It causes a small rise in left ventricular pressure. (Note that atrial systole occurs during ventricular diastole, a confusing but important point.)

Systole. Now so much blood has been pumped into the ventricles that ventricular pressure is finally higher than that in the atria, so the mitral and tricuspid valves swing shut. The closure of the AV valves contributes to the first heart sound (S_1) and signals the beginning of systole. The AV valves close to prevent any regurgitation of blood back up into the atria during contraction.

For a very brief moment, all four valves are closed. The ventricular walls contract. This contraction against a closed system works to build pressure inside the ventricles to a high level (isometric contraction). Consider first the left side of the heart. When the pressure in the ventricle finally exceeds pressure in the aorta, the aortic valve opens and blood is ejected rapidly.

After the ventricle's contents are ejected, its pressure falls. When pressure falls below pressure in the aorta, some blood flows backwards towards the ventricle, causing the aortic valve to swing shut. This closure of the semilunar valves causes the second heart sound (S_2) and signals the end of systole.

Diastole again. Now all four valves are closed and the ventricles relax (called **isometric** or **isovolumic relaxation**). Meanwhile, the atria have been filling with blood delivered from the lungs. Atrial pressure is now higher than the relaxed ventricular pressure. The mitral valve drifts open and diastolic filling begins again.

Events in the right and left sides. The same events are happening in the right side of the heart, but pressures in the right side of the heart are much lower than those of the left side because less energy is needed to pump blood to its destination, the pulmonary circulation. Also, events occur just slightly later in the right side of the heart because of the route of myocardial depolarisation. As a result, two distinct components to each of the heart sounds exist, and sometimes you can hear them separately. In the first heart sound, the mitral component (**M_1**) closes just before the tricuspid component (**T_1**). And with **S_2**, aortic closure (**A_2**) occurs slightly before pulmonic closure (**P_2**).

HEART SOUNDS

Events in the cardiac cycle generate sounds that can be heard through a stethoscope over the chest wall. These include normal heart sounds and, occasionally, extra heart sounds and murmurs (Figure 17.7).

Normal heart sounds

The **first heart sound** (**S_1**) occurs with closure of the AV valves and thus signals the beginning of systole. The mitral component of the first sound (**M_1**) slightly precedes the tricuspid component (**T_1**), but you usually hear these two components fused as one sound. You can hear S_1 over all the praecordium, but usually it is loudest at the apex.

The **second heart sound** (**S_2**) occurs with closure of the semilunar valves and signals the end of systole. The aortic component of the second sound (**A_2**) slightly precedes the pulmonic component (**P_2**). Although it is heard over all the praecordium, **S_2** is loudest at the base.

Effect of respiration. The volume of right and left ventricular systole is just about equal, but this can be affected by respiration. To learn this, consider the phrase:

Mo**R**e to the **R**ight heart, **L**ess to the **L**eft

That means that during inspiration, intrathoracic pressure is decreased. This pushes more blood into the vena cava, increasing venous return to the right side of the heart, which increases right ventricular stroke volume. The increased volume prolongs right ventricular systole and delays pulmonic valve closure.

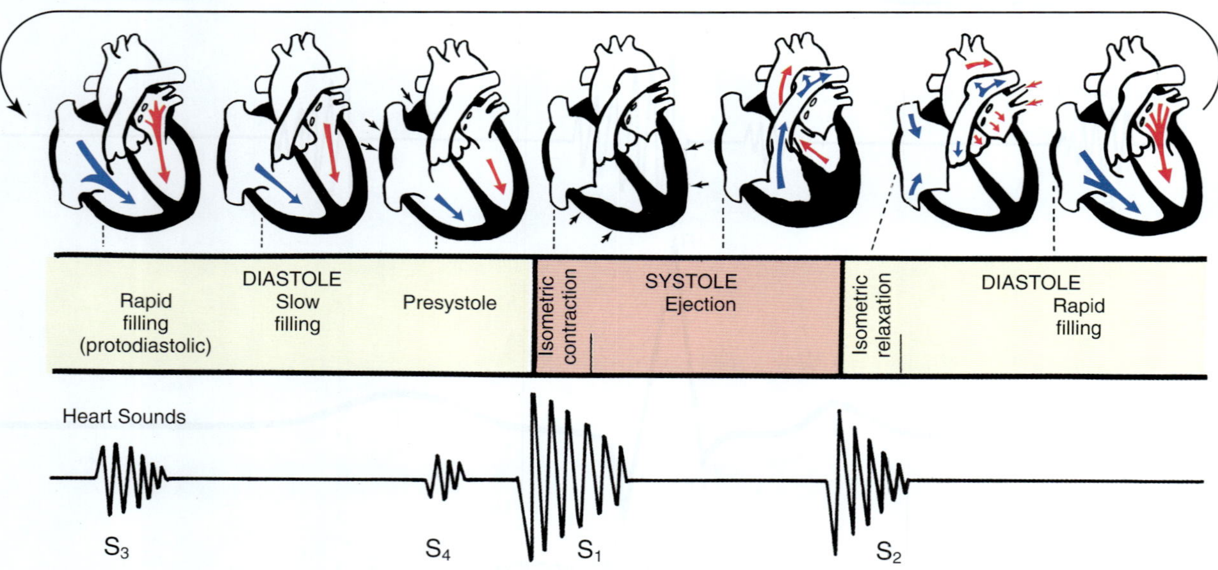

Figure 17.7

Meanwhile, on the left side, a greater amount of blood is sequestered in the lungs during inspiration. This momentarily decreases the amount returned to the left side of the heart, decreasing left ventricular stroke volume. The decreased volume shortens left ventricular systole and allows the aortic valve to close a bit earlier. When the aortic valve closes significantly earlier than the pulmonic valve, you can hear the two components separately. This is a *split* $\mathbf{S_2}$.

Extra heart sounds

Third heart sound ($\mathbf{S_3}$). Normally diastole is a silent event. However, in some conditions, ventricular filling creates vibrations that can be heard over the chest. These vibrations are $\mathbf{S_3}$. The $\mathbf{S_3}$ occurs when the ventricles are resistant to filling during the early rapid filling phase (protodiastole). This occurs immediately after $\mathbf{S_2}$, when the AV valves open and atrial blood first pours into the ventricles. (See a complete discussion of $\mathbf{S_3}$ in Table 17.8.)

Fourth heart sound ($\mathbf{S_4}$). The $\mathbf{S_4}$ occurs at the end of diastole, at presystole, when the ventricle is resistant to filling. The atria contract and push blood into a noncompliant ventricle. This creates vibrations that are heard as $\mathbf{S_4}$. The $\mathbf{S_4}$ occurs just before $\mathbf{S_1}$.

Murmurs

Blood circulating through normal cardiac chambers and valves usually makes no noise. However, some conditions create turbulent blood flow and collision currents. These result in a murmur, much like a pile of stones or a sharp turn in a stream creates a noisy water flow. A murmur is a gentle, blowing, swooshing sound that can be heard on the chest wall. Conditions resulting in a murmur are as follows:

1. Velocity of blood increases (flow murmur) (e.g. in exercise, thyrotoxicosis)
2. Viscosity of blood decreases (e.g. in anaemia)
3. Structural defects in the valves (narrowed valve, incompetent valve) or unusual openings occur in the chambers (dilated chamber, wall defect).

Characteristics of sound

All heart sounds are described by:

1. Frequency (pitch)—heart sounds are described as high pitched or low pitched, although these terms are relative because all are low-frequency sounds, and you need a good stethoscope to hear them
2. Intensity (loudness)—loud or soft
3. Duration—very short for heart sounds; silent periods are longer
4. Timing—systole or diastole.

CONDUCTION

Of all organs, the heart has a unique ability—automaticity. The heart can contract by itself, independent of any signals or stimulation from the body. The heart contracts in response to an electrical current conveyed by a conduction system (Figure 17.8). Specialised cells in the sinoatrial (SA) node near the superior vena cava initiate an electrical impulse. (Because the SA node has an intrinsic rhythm, it is the 'pacemaker'.) The current flows in an orderly sequence, first across the atria to the AV node low in the atrial septum. There, it is delayed slightly so that the atria have time to contract before the ventricles are stimulated. Then, the impulse travels to the bundle of His, the right and left bundle branches, then through the ventricles.

The electrical impulse stimulates the heart to do its work, which is to contract. A small amount of electricity spreads to

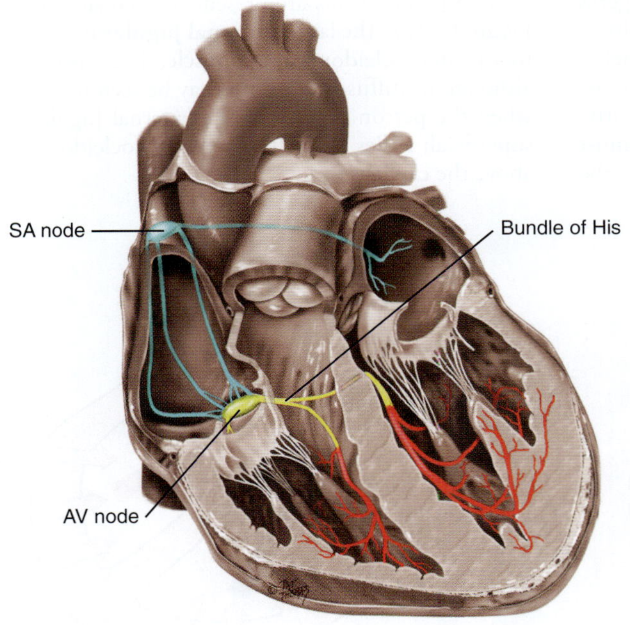

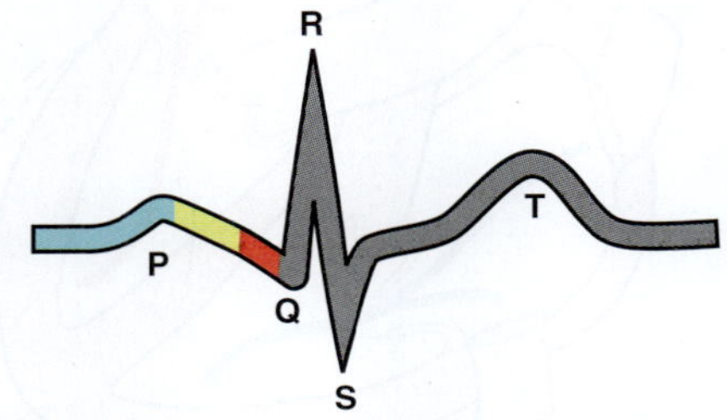

Figure 17.8
©Pat Thomas, 2006

the body surface, where it can be measured and recorded on the electrocardiograph (ECG). The ECG waves are arbitrarily labelled PQRST, which stand for the following elements:
P wave—depolarisation of the atria

PR interval—from the beginning of the P wave to the beginning of the QRS complex (the time necessary for atrial depolarisation plus time for the impulse to travel through the AV node to the ventricles)
QRS complex—depolarisation of the ventricles
T wave—repolarisation of the ventricles.

Electrical events slightly precede the mechanical events in the heart. The ECG juxtaposed on the cardiac cycle is illustrated in Figure 17.6.

PUMPING ABILITY

In the resting adult, the heart normally pumps between 4 and 6 L of blood per min throughout the body. This **cardiac output** equals the volume of blood in each systole (called the stroke volume) times the number of beats per min (heart rate). This is described as:

$$CO = SV \times HR$$

The heart can alter its cardiac output to adapt to the metabolic needs of the body. Preload and afterload affect the heart's ability to increase cardiac output.

Preload is the venous return that builds during diastole. It is the length to which the ventricular muscle is stretched at the end of diastole just before contraction (Figure 17.9).

When the volume of blood returned to the ventricles is increased (as when exercise stimulates skeletal muscles to contract and force more blood back to the heart), the muscle bundles are stretched beyond their normal resting state to accommodate. The force of this switch is the preload. According to the Frank-Starling law, the greater the stretch, the stronger is the heart's contraction. This increased contractility results in an increased volume of blood ejected (increased stroke volume).

Afterload is the opposing pressure the ventricle must generate to open the aortic valve against the higher aortic pressure. It is the resistance against which the ventricle must pump its blood. Once the ventricle is filled with blood, the ventricular end diastolic pressure is 5–10 mmHg, whereas that in the aorta is 70–80 mmHg. To overcome this difference, the ventricular muscle tenses (isovolumic contraction). After the aortic valve opens, rapid ejection occurs.

THE NECK VESSELS

Cardiovascular assessment includes the survey of vascular structures in the neck—the carotid artery and the jugular veins (Figure 17.10). These vessels reflect the efficiency of cardiac function.

The carotid artery pulse

The pulse can be described as a pressure wave generated by each systole pumping blood into the aorta. The carotid artery is a central artery—that is, it is close to the heart. Its timing closely coincides with ventricular systole. (Assessment of the peripheral pulses is found in Chapter 16, and blood pressure assessment is found in Chapter 10.)

The **carotid artery** is located in the groove between the trachea and the sternocleidomastoid muscle, medial to and alongside that muscle. Note the characteristics of its waveform (Figure 17.11): a smooth rapid upstroke, a summit that is rounded and smooth and a downstroke that is more gradual and that has a dicrotic notch caused by closure of the aortic valve (marked D in the figure).

Jugular venous pulse and pressure

The **jugular veins** empty deoxygenated blood directly into the superior vena cava. Because no cardiac valve exists to separate the superior vena cava from the right atrium, the jugular veins give information about activity on the right side of the heart. Specifically, they reflect filling pressure and volume changes. Because volume and pressure increase when the right side of the heart fails to pump efficiently, the jugular veins expose this.

Two jugular veins are present in each side of the neck (see Figure 17.10). The larger **internal jugular** lies deep and medial to the sternocleidomastoid muscle. It is usually not visible, although its diffuse pulsations may be seen in the sternal notch when the person is supine. The external jugular vein is more superficial; it lies laterally to the sternocleidomastoid muscle, above the clavicle.

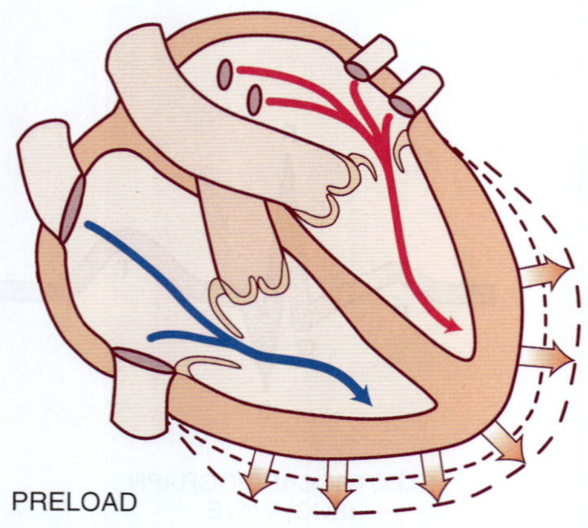

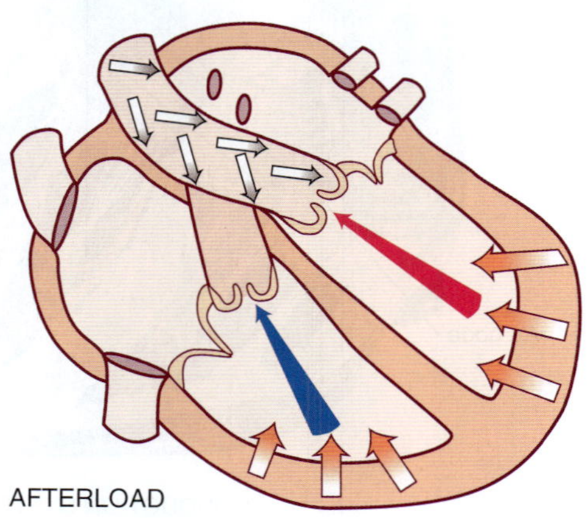

Figure 17.9
©Pat Thomas, 2006

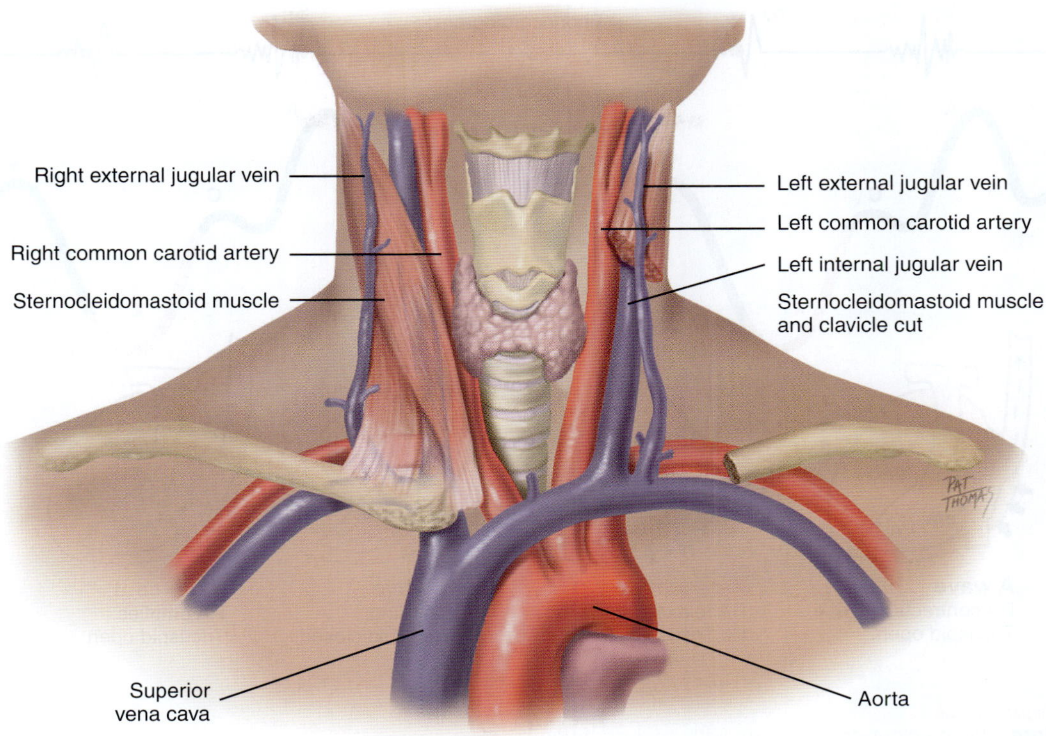

Figure 17.10

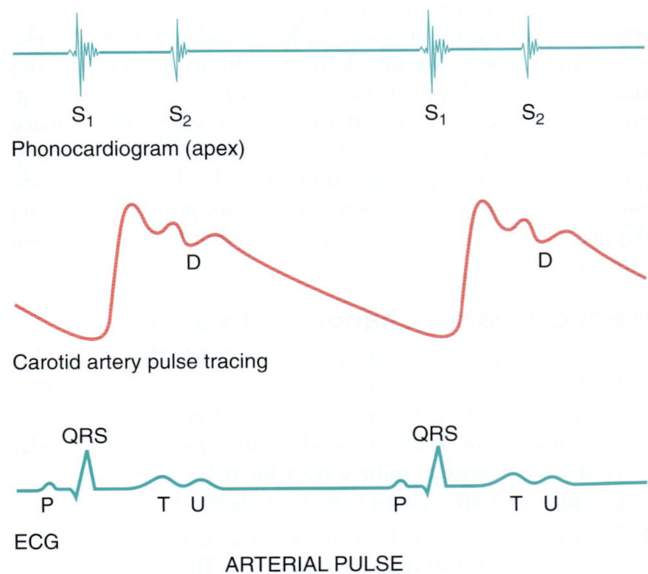

Figure 17.11

Although an arterial pulse is caused by forward propulsion of blood, the jugular pulse is different. The jugular pulse results from a backwash, a waveform moving backwards caused by events upstream. The jugular pulse has five components, as shown in Figure 17.12.

The five components of the jugular venous pulse occur because of events in the right side of the heart. The A wave reflects atrial contraction because some blood flows backwards to the vena cava during right atrial contraction. The C wave, or ventricular contraction, is backflow from the bulging upwards of the tricuspid valve when it closes at the beginning of ventricular systole (not from the neighbouring carotid artery pulsation). Next, the X descent shows atrial relaxation when the right ventricle contracts during systole and pulls the bottom of the atria downwards. The V wave occurs with passive atrial filling because of the increasing volume in the right atria and increased pressure. Finally, the Y descent reflects passive ventricular filling when the tricuspid valve opens and blood flows from the RA to the RV.

DEVELOPMENTAL CONSIDERATIONS

Infants and children

The fetal heart functions early; it begins to beat at the end of 3 weeks' gestation. The lungs are nonfunctional, but the fetal circulation compensates for this (Figure 17.13). Oxygenation takes place at the placenta, and the arterial blood is returned to the right side of the heart. There is no point in pumping all this freshly oxygenated blood through the lungs, so it is rerouted in two ways. First, about two-thirds of it is shunted through an opening in the atrial septum, the **foramen ovale**, into the left side of the heart, where it is pumped out through the aorta. Second, the rest of the oxygenated blood is pumped

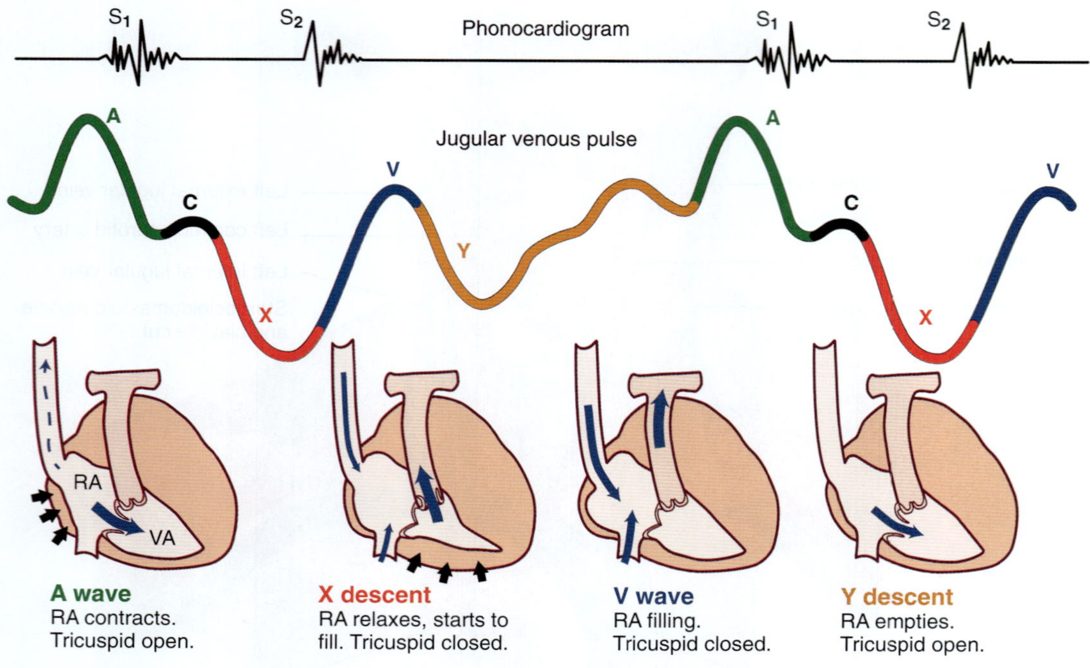

Figure 17.12
Note: Match colour on waveform with its description.

by the right side of the heart out through the pulmonary artery, but it is detoured through the **ductus arteriosus** to the aorta. Because they are both pumping into the systemic circulation, the right and left ventricles are equal in weight and muscle wall thickness.

Inflation and aeration of the lungs at birth produces circulatory changes. Now the blood is oxygenated through the lungs rather than through the placenta. The foramen ovale closes within the first hour because of the new lower pressure in the right side of the heart than in the left side. The ductus arteriosus closes later, usually within 10–15 hours of birth. Now, the left ventricle has the greater workload of pumping into the systemic circulation, so that when the baby has reached 1 year of age, the left ventricle's mass increases to reach the adult ratio of 2:1, left ventricle to right ventricle.

The heart's position in the chest is more horizontal in the infant than in the adult; thus the apex is higher, located at the fourth left intercostal space (Figure 17.14). It reaches the adult position when the child reaches age 7 years.

The pregnant woman

The cardiovascular system adapts to ensure adequate blood supply to the uterus and placenta, to deliver oxygen and nutrients to the fetus and to allow the mother to function normally during the pregnancy. Blood volume increases by 30–40% during pregnancy, with the most rapid expansion occurring during the second trimester. This creates an increase in stroke volume and cardiac output and an increased pulse rate of 10–15 beats per min. The heart rate rises in the first trimester, peaks in the third trimester and returns to baseline within the first 10 postpartum days. Despite the increased cardiac output, arterial blood pressure decreases in pregnancy as a result of peripheral vasodilatation. The blood pressure drops to its lowest point during the second trimester, and then rises after that.

Late adulthood (65+ years)

It is difficult to isolate the 'ageing process' of the cardiovascular system per se because it is so closely interrelated with lifestyle, habits and diseases. We now know that lifestyle is a modifying factor in the development of cardiovascular disease; smoking, diet, alcohol use, exercise patterns and stress have an influence on coronary artery disease. Lifestyle also affects the ageing process; cardiac changes once thought to be due to ageing are partially due to the sedentary lifestyle accompanying ageing (Figure 17.15). What is left to be attributed to the ageing process alone?

Haemodynamic changes with ageing

1. With ageing, there is a rise in the systolic BP. This is caused by thickening and stiffening of the large arteries which, in turn, is caused by collagen and calcium deposits in the vessel walls and loss of elastic fibres. This stiffening (arteriosclerosis) creates an increase in pulse wave velocity because the less compliant arteries cannot store the volume ejected.
2. The overall size of the heart does not increase with age but left ventricular wall thickness increases. This is an adaptive mechanism to accommodate the vascular stiffening mentioned earlier that creates an increased workload on the heart.
3. Diastolic BP may decrease after the sixth decade of life. A rising systolic pressure with a relatively constant diastolic pressure increases the pulse pressure (the difference between the two).
4. No change in resting heart rate occurs with ageing.

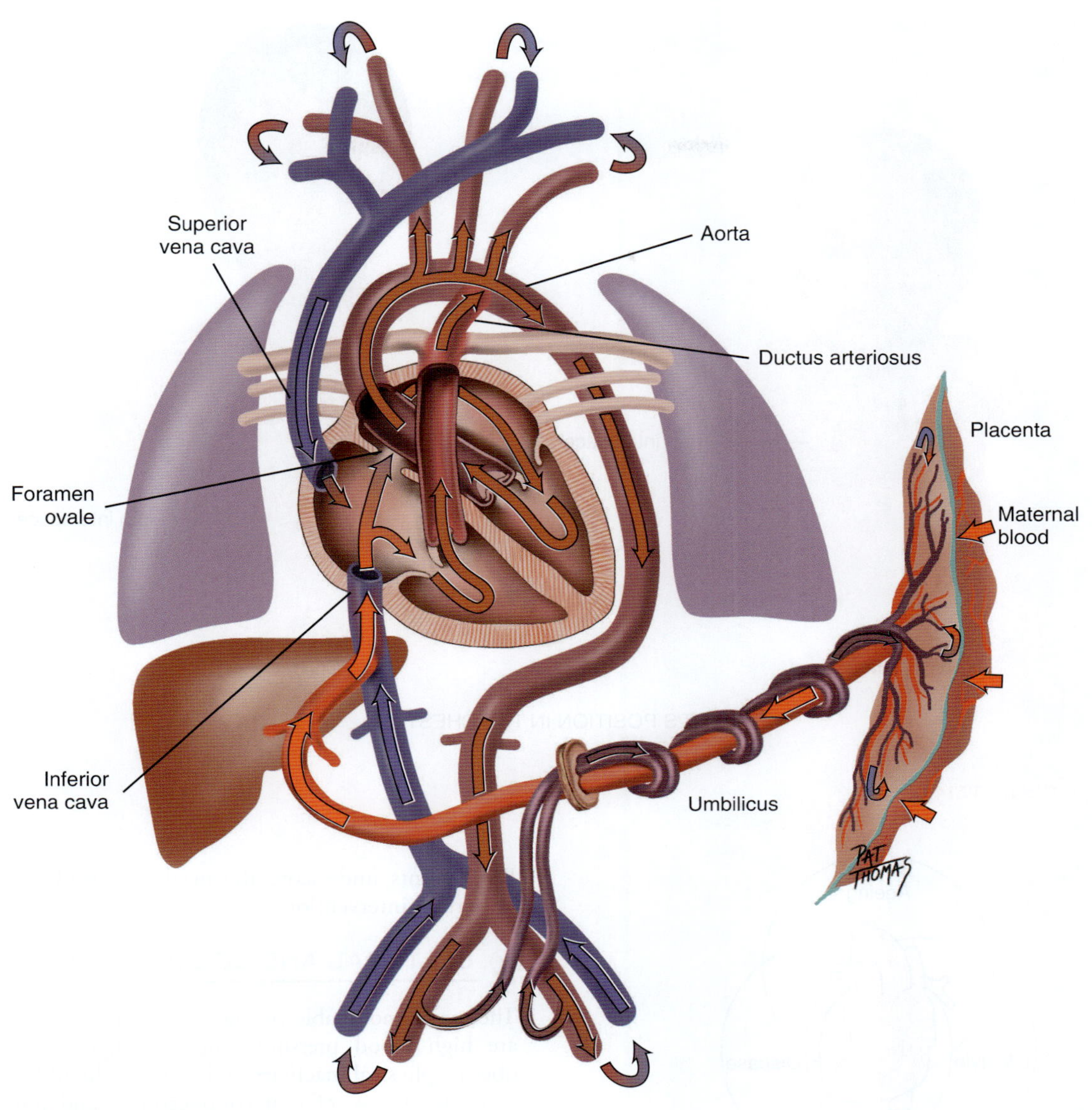

Figure 17.13

5. Cardiac output at rest is not changed with ageing.
6. There is a decreased ability of the heart to augment cardiac output with exercise. This is shown by a decreased maximum heart rate with exercise and diminished sympathetic response. Non-cardiac factors also cause a decrease in maximum work performance with ageing: decrease in skeletal muscle performance, increase in muscle fatigue and increased sense of dyspnoea. However, aerobic exercise conditioning will modify many of the ageing changes in cardiovascular function (Bonow et al 2018).

Dysrhythmias. The presence of supraventricular and ventricular dysrhythmias increases with age. Ectopic beats are common in ageing people; although these are usually asymptomatic in healthy older people, they may compromise cardiac output and blood pressure when disease is present.

Tachyarrhythmias may not be tolerated as well in older people. The myocardium is thicker and less compliant, and early diastolic filling is impaired at rest due to the structural changes that occur in ageing (Nanayakkara et al 2018). Thus, a tachycardia may not be well tolerated because of shortened diastole. Tachyarrhythmias may further compromise a vital organ whose function has already been affected by ageing or disease and significantly increases mortality in people with heart failure (Zhang et al 2018).

Electrocardiograph (ECG). Age-related changes in the ECG occur as a result of histological changes in the conduction system. These changes include:

1. Prolonged P-R interval (first-degree AV block) and prolonged Q-T interval, but the QRS interval is unchanged

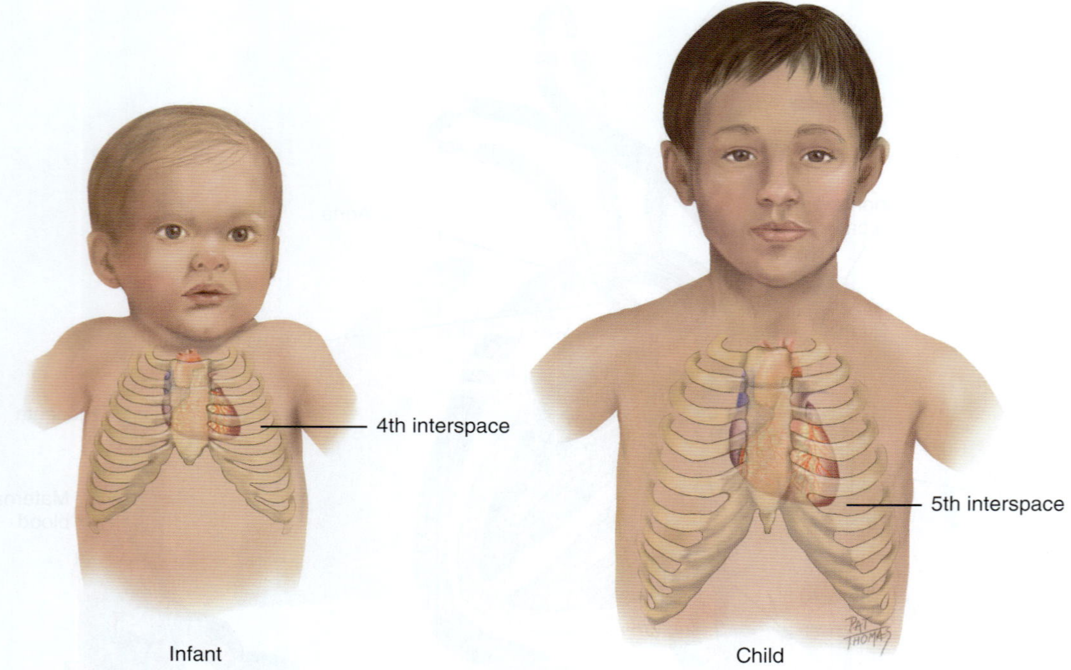

Figure 17.14

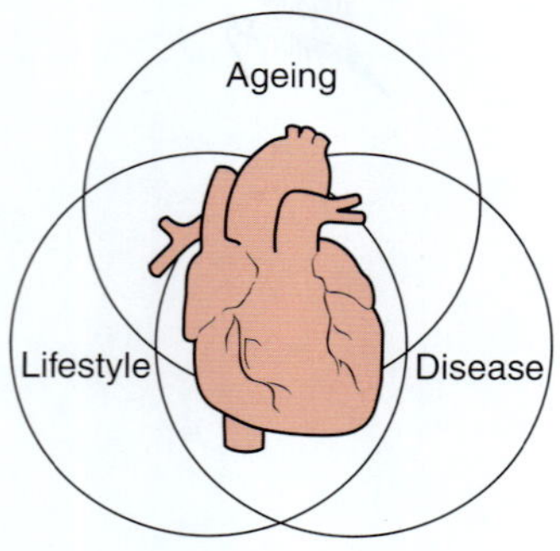

Figure 17.15

2. Left axis deviation from age-related mild LV hypertrophy and fibrosis in left bundle branch
3. Increased incidence of bundle branch block.

Although the haemodynamic changes associated with ageing alone do not seem severe or portentous, the fact remains that the incidence of cardiovascular disease increases with age. The incidence of coronary artery disease increases sharply with advancing age, and accounts for about half of the deaths of people over 65. Hypertension (systolic >140 mmHg and diastolic >90 mmHg) and heart failure also increase with age. Certainly, lifestyle habits (smoking, chronic alcohol use, lack of exercise, diet) play a significant role in the acquisition of heart disease. Also, increasing the physical activity of older adults—even at a moderate level—is associated with a reduced risk of death from cardiovascular diseases and respiratory illnesses. Both points underscore the need for health teaching as an important intervention.

CULTURAL AND SOCIAL CONSIDERATIONS

The major modifiable risk factors for heart disease and stroke are high blood pressure, smoking, high cholesterol levels, obesity, physical inactivity and diabetes. In addition, for some women, the use of oral contraceptives and postmenopausal hormones is a risk factor.

Hypertension. Hypertension causes heart disease by decreasing vascular compliance which results in stiff, inelastic blood vessels and initiates endothelial injury. This process causes a cascade of events accelerating the development of atherosclerosis (Tortora & Derrickson 2019). Untreated hypertension risks damage to heart, main blood vessels, heart valves, brain and kidneys and can cause cardiac arrhythmias including atrial fibrillation (Kjeldsen 2018). The most current report identified 34% of Australians have hypertension (Australian Institute of Health & Welfare (AIHW) 2018a). Indigenous Australians experience hypertension at a 1.2 times higher rate than non-Indigenous Australians (Australian Health Ministers Advisory Council 2017). In New Zealand, it is estimated that approximately 15.8% of adult males and 17.2% of adult females are receiving medication for hypertension. Māori and Pacific adults are 1.4–1.47 times more likely to have measured high blood pressure than other New Zealanders (Ministry of Health NZ 2019).

Because hypertension and the organ damage it causes can be asymptomatic, identifying people most at risk and BP screening is important. Blood pressure can easily be measured in a clinic situation by a health professional although many people will have a raised BP simply due to their anxiety of being examined. Intermittent BP measurements by a health professional or by the person in their home can be performed with more accuracy, however continuous ambulatory blood pressure measurement over a 24–48-hour period has been found to be accurate and cost effective. It also gives the clinician insight into changes in BP over time including when the person is sleeping (Beyhaghi & Viera 2019).

Smoking. Tobacco smoking and exposure to environmental tobacco smoke (sometimes referred to as passive smoking) causes atherosclerosis by impairing endothelial function in blood vessels, increasing arterial stiffness, promoting an inflammatory response and increasing low density lipoprotein (LDL) deposition, and reducing high density lipoprotein levels (DiGiacomo et al 2019). In Australia, one in seven adults (12.4%) smoke daily (Australian Bureau of Statistics (ABS) 2019), and most are over 40 years of age. Rates of smoking are higher in areas of most disadvantage, rural and remote communities, homosexual or bisexual people, people with mental illness and people who are unemployed or unable to work (AIHW 2018b, Ministry of Health NZ 2019). The rate of tobacco smoking in Aboriginal and Torres Strait Islander adults is 2.8 times that of non-Indigenous Australians (AIHW 2018b). Similar prevalence data is reported in New Zealand, with 14.9% of adults currently smoking. Of these, it is estimated that 2.8 times more Māori and 1.47 times more Pacific Islander people currently smoke than other New Zealanders (Ministry of Health NZ 2019).

An Australian study by Banks and colleagues (2019) found that tobacco smokers have double the risk of developing serious cardiovascular disease and five times the risk of developing peripheral vascular disease compared with people who have never smoked. Even 'low' levels of smoking, 4–6 cigarettes per day, had around double the risk of dying from cardiovascular disease than non-smokers. However, stopping smoking before the age of 35–44 years reduces the risk for cardiovascular disease by 90% (Banks et al 2019). All people need to be reminded to quit smoking for the sake of their health on each presentation to a health service. 'Quit' services are government funded and printed information is available in many languages.

Abnormal lipid profile. The lipid profile is comprised of a number of components including total cholesterol, high density lipoproteins (the 'good' cholesterol), low density lipoproteins and triglycerides. While it is essential for many bodily functions, too much of most of the components can lead to cardiovascular disease. Approximately 6.1% of Australians had high cholesterol (ABS 2018). In New Zealand, 13% of adult males and 8.9% of adult females are taking lipid-lowering medication. Of these, it is estimated that 1.2 times more Māori and 1.52 times more Pacific Islander people are currently taking lipid lowering medication than other New Zealanders (Ministry of Health NZ 2019).

Obesity. Body mass index (BMI) is the usual measure used to define and classify obesity. A body mass index (BMI) of 25 kg/m^2 or higher is considered to be overweight, and a BMI of 30 kg/m^2 or higher is considered to be obese. The World Health Organization (WHO 2020) has reported that obesity is reaching epidemic proportions. In Australia, almost 63% of the non-Indigenous population are considered to be overweight or obese (AIHW 2018b). Indigenous females are 1.7 times as likely to be obese as non-Indigenous females, and Indigenous males are 1.4 times as likely to be obese as non-Indigenous males (AIHW 2018b). In New Zealand, the prevalence of obesity in adults is variable, with 65% of Pacific Islander people, 47.5% of Māori, 30.7% of European/other descent and 15.1% of Asian descent being obese (Ministry of Health NZ 2019). Obesity compounds any health problem and increases the incidence of many diseases including cardiovascular disease, diabetes, musculoskeletal disorders and some cancers.

Type 2 diabetes. Diabetes increases the risk of microvascular dysfunction and increases the risk of coronary artery disease, especially in women (Haas et al 2019). The incidence of diabetes is rising internationally; 6.6% of Australian adults have diabetes (AIHW 2018c). This is attributed to increasing rates of obesity, insufficient physical activity, unhealthy diet, tobacco smoking and an ageing population. It is known that there is a higher incidence of diabetes in Indigenous populations, those living in lower socioeconomic areas, those born overseas and living in regional or remote areas of Australia (AIHW 2018c). Within the New Zealand population, the prevalence of diabetes in Māori is 1.95 times and Pacific populations are 3.39 times higher than among other New Zealanders (Ministry of Health NZ 2019). The complications of diabetes are well recognised and include cardiovascular disease, chronic renal disease and blindness.

Rheumatic heart disease. Rheumatic heart disease usually begins in childhood after an episode of acute rheumatic fever which is an abnormal immune response to Group A streptococcal throat infection (Abouzeid et al 2019). Rheumatic heart disease is caused by one or several episodes of acute rheumatic fever, where the heart has become inflamed; the heart valves remain scarred and normal coronary blood flow is interrupted (Rheumatic Heart Disease Australia 2019). It is a treatable and preventable disease (AIHW 2019). However, rheumatic heart disease is described as a disease of poverty, overcrowding, poor access to health services and social disadvantage (Abouzeid et al 2019). It is not surprising therefore that 89% of Australians with acute rheumatic fever and/or rheumatic heart disease are Indigenous Australians; of these, 69% were female and 41% were 5–14 years of age when diagnosed for the first time (AIHW 2019). In New Zealand, Pacific Islander peoples have 158 times, and Māori have 5 times, the first-time incidence rate of rheumatic fever than other New Zealanders (Ministry of Health NZ, Institute of Environmental Science and Research 2018).

In addition to addressing the social and economic factors that contribute to the development of acute rheumatic fever and/or rheumatic heart disease, preventing recurrences of acute rheumatic fever by using prophylactic treatment with antibiotics is therefore critical to controlling the incidence of rheumatic heart disease. See the list of websites at the end of this chapter for information on prevention in Australia and New Zealand. People with rheumatic heart disease may require heart valve replacement surgery or experience a reduced life span due to this health condition.

Subjective data

As you work through assessment of cardiac function you need to keep in mind that this area is usually conducted in connection with assessment of peripheral vascular and respiratory function. An accurate assessment requires the nurse to obtain a careful history of the symptoms the individual experiences and then undertake the relevant clinical examination.

These symptoms have been grouped under the following headings:

1. Presenting concern
2. Chest pain
3. Dyspnoea
4. Orthopnoea
5. Cough
6. Fatigue
7. Cyanosis or pallor
8. Oedema
9. Nocturia
10. Cardiac history
11. Family cardiac history
12. Health and lifestyle management

Practice note: Before you commence the assessment, introduce yourself to the person, confirm the person's identity, discuss the purpose and scope of the assessment, clarify any questions the person may have and obtain verbal consent from the person to perform the assessment.

ASSESSMENT GUIDELINES	CLINICAL SIGNIFICANCE AND CLINICAL ALERTS
1. Presenting concern	
Do you feel that you have any problem/s with your heart and your ability to exercise and go about your daily activities? It is important to ascertain the person's perception of their cardiac function. • If they do perceive a problem—how does this impact on their quality of life?	The person's response to this question will guide areas to focus on in further subjective and objective data collection.
2. Chest pain	
Any chest pain, tightness or heaviness? • Onset: When did it start? How long have you had it *this* time? Had this type of pain before? How often? • Location: Where did the pain start? Does the pain radiate to any other spot? • Character: How would you describe it? Crushing, stabbing, burning, vice-like? (Allow the person to offer adjectives before you suggest them.) (Note if the person uses clenched fist to describe pain.)	**Angina**, an important cardiac symptom, occurs when the heart's vascular supply cannot keep up with metabolic demand. Chest pain also may also be of pulmonary, musculoskeletal or gastrointestinal origin; it is important to differentiate. Typical descriptors of cardiac chest pain are central location, tight heavy sensation, crushing sensation, may radiate to the jaw or left arm. Some people may describe a dull aching sensation or discomfort particularly with angina on exertion (Talley & O'Connor 2018).
• Pain brought on by: activity—what type; rest; emotional upset; after eating; during sexual intercourse; with cold weather?	
• Any associated symptoms: sweating, ashen grey or pale skin, heart skips beat, shortness of breath, nausea or vomiting, racing of heart, extreme fatigue?	Note that the presence of chest pain and/or a squeezing sensation in the chest and the associated symptoms described here are typical of serious cardiac circulatory insufficiency.
• Pain made worse by moving the arms or neck, breathing, lying flat? • Pain relieved by rest or glyceryl trinitrate? How many tablets/sprays?	Try to differentiate pain of cardiac versus non-cardiac origin. See Table 17.2 for differential diagnosis of chest pain ***Clinical alert:*** if the person has taken more than 3 glyceryl trinitrate tablets/sprays in 30 min without relief they must be urgently referred for further assessment and treatment by a medical practitioner.

ASSESSMENT GUIDELINES	CLINICAL SIGNIFICANCE AND CLINICAL ALERTS
3. Dyspnoea	
Any shortness of breath? • What type of activity and how much brings on shortness of breath? How much activity brought it on 6 months ago? • Onset: does the shortness of breath come on unexpectedly? • Duration: constant or does it come and go? • Seem to be affected by position: lying down? • Awaken you from sleep at night?	**Dyspnoea** (shortness of breath (SOB)) • Paroxysmal • Constant or intermittent • Recumbent **Dyspnoea on exertion** (shortness of breath on exertion (SOBOE))—quantify exactly (e.g. after walking two level blocks) **Paroxysmal nocturnal dyspnoea** (PND) occurs with heart failure. Lying down increases volume of intrathoracic blood, and the weakened heart cannot accommodate the increased load. Classically, the person awakens after 2 hours of sleep with the perception of needing fresh air.
• Does the shortness of breath interfere with activities of daily living? If so, what does your shortness of breath prevent you from doing?	
4. Orthopnoea	
How many pillows do you use when sleeping or lying down?	**Orthopnoea** is the need to assume a more upright position to breathe. Note the exact number of pillows used.
5. Cough	
Do you have a cough? • Duration: How long have you had it? • Frequency: Is it related to time of day? • Type: dry, hacking, barking, hoarse or congested?	
• Do you cough up mucus? Colour? Any odour? Blood tinged?	Sputum production, mucoid or purulent. **Haemoptysis** (blood in sputum) is often a pulmonary disorder but also occurs with mitral stenosis.
• Associated with: activity, position (lying down), anxiety, talking? • Shortness of breath on exertion (SOBOE): what activities make it better or worse (sit, walk, exercise)? • Relieved by rest or medication?	
6. Fatigue	
Do you seem to tire easily? Able to keep up with your family and co-workers? • Onset: When did fatigue start? Sudden or gradual? Has any *recent* change occurred in energy level?	
• Fatigue related to time of day: all day, morning, evening?	**Fatigue** from decreased cardiac output is worse in the evening, whereas fatigue from anxiety or depression occurs all day or is worse in the morning.
• How have these symptoms (chest pain, fatigue, breathlessness) affected your life?	

ASSESSMENT GUIDELINES	CLINICAL SIGNIFICANCE AND CLINICAL ALERTS
7. Cyanosis or pallor	
Ever noted that your facial skin turns blue or ashen?	**Cyanosis or pallor** occurs with myocardial infarction or low cardiac output states as a result of decreased tissue perfusion.
8. Oedema	
Any swelling of your feet and legs? • Onset: When did you first notice this? • Any recent change?	**Oedema** is dependent when caused by heart failure.
• What time of day does the swelling occur? Do your shoes feel tight at the end of day? • How much swelling would you say there is? Are both legs equally swollen? • Does the swelling go away with: rest, elevation, after a night's sleep? • Any associated symptoms, such as shortness of breath? If so, does the shortness of breath occur before leg swelling or after?	**Cardiac oedema** is worse in the evening and less so in the morning after elevating legs all night.
9. Nocturia	
Do you awaken at night needing to urinate? If so, how many times do you get up to urinate? How long has this been occurring? Any recent change?	**Nocturia**—recumbency at night promotes fluid reabsorption and excretion; this occurs with heart failure in the person who is ambulatory during the day. See also Chapter 24 for assessment related to urinary function.
10. Cardiac history	
Any history of: hypertension, elevated cholesterol, heart murmur, congenital heart disease, rheumatic fever or unexplained joint pains as a child or youth, recurrent tonsillitis, anaemia? • Ever had heart disease? When was this? Treated by medication, percutaneous intervention or heart surgery? • Last ECG, stress test, serum cholesterol measurement, other heart tests?	
11. Family cardiac history	
Any family history of: hypertension, obesity diabetes, coronary artery disease (CAD), sudden death at younger age, i.e. <60 years?	A family history of heart disease is a significant alert that the client's symptoms are cardiac in origin.
12. Health and lifestyle management	
(Identify risk factors for cardiovascular disease) • **Nutrition:** Please describe your usual daily diet. (Note: If this diet is representative of the basic food groups, the number of kilojoules, cholesterol and any additives such as salt.) • **Weight:** What is your usual weight? Has there been any recent change? • **Exercise:** What is your usual amount of exercise each day or week? What stops you? E.g. fatigue, leg pains, other (specify). What type of exercise (state type or sport)? If a sport, what is your usual amount (light, moderate, heavy)? • Do you take any **medications** for your illness such as digitalis, beta-blockers? Aware of side effects? Have you recently stopped taking your medication? Why? Are you taking any complementary therapies? If so, what are you taking and for how long? • **Smoking:** Do you smoke cigarettes or other tobacco? At what age did you start? How many packs per day? For how many years have you smoked this amount? Have you ever tried to quit? If so, how did this go? • **Alcohol:** How much alcohol do you usually drink each week, or each day? Beer/wine/spirits? When was your last drink? What was the number of drinks that episode? Have you ever been told you had a drinking problem?	

ASSESSMENT GUIDELINES	CLINICAL SIGNIFICANCE AND CLINICAL ALERTS
Additional subjective data for infants (questions for parents or guardians)	
• How was the mother's health during pregnancy: any unexplained fever, rubella first trimester, other infection, hypertension, medications taken? • Have you noted any cyanosis while feeding, crying? Is the baby able to eat, suckle or complete feed without tiring?	To screen for heart disease in infants, note fatigue during feeding. An infant with heart failure takes small amounts at each feed; becomes dyspnoeic with sucking; may be diaphoretic, then falls into exhausted sleep; awakens after a short time hungry again.
• Growth: Has the baby grown as expected by growth charts and about the same as siblings or peers? • Activity: Were this baby's developmental milestones achieved as expected? Is the baby able to play without tiring? How many sleeps does the baby take each day? How long does a sleep last?	Poor weight gain is an indicator of heart abnormalities.
Additional subjective data for children (questions for parents or guardians)	
• Growth: Has the child grown as expected by growth charts? • Activity: Is this child able to keep up with siblings or age mates? Is the child willing or reluctant to go out to play? Is the child able to climb stairs, ride a bike? Does the child squat to rest during play or to watch television, or assume a knee–chest position while sleeping? Have you noted 'blue spells' during daily activities? • Has the child had any unexplained joint pains or unexplained fever? • Does the child have frequent headaches, nosebleeds? • Does the child have frequent respiratory infections? How many per year? How are they treated? Have any of these proved to be streptococcal infections? • Family history: Does the child have a sibling with a heart defect? Is anyone in the child's family known to have chromosomal abnormalities, such as Down syndrome?	Fatigue. Record specific limitations. Cyanosis is a serious indication of heart or lung dysfunction.
Additional subjective data for the pregnant woman	
Blood pressure • Have you had high blood pressure during this or earlier pregnancies? – What was your usual blood pressure level before pregnancy? How has your blood pressure been monitored during pregnancy? – If high blood pressure, what treatment has been started?	
• Any associated symptoms: weight gain, protein in urine, swelling in feet, legs or face?	***Clinical alert:*** Hypertension, proteinuria and oedema are signs of pre eclampsia, a serious condition that can occur during pregnancy, placing the mother and fetus at risk. Those pregnant with these symptoms should be referred to their medical practitioner or midwife.
• Have you had any faintness or dizziness with this pregnancy?	
Additional subjective data for the adult over 65 years	
History of heart or lung disease • Hypertension, coronary artery disease or chronic obstructive pulmonary disease? – What efforts to treat this have been started? – Usual symptoms changed recently? Does your illness interfere with activities of daily living?	
Medications • Do you take any medications for your illness such as digitalis, beta-blockers? Aware of side effects? Have you recently stopped taking your medication? Why? **Environment** • Does your home have any stairs? How often do you need to climb them? Does this have any effect on activities of daily living?	Not taking medication may be related to side effects or lack of understanding of the chronic nature of heart disease.

SUBJECTIVE DATA

Objective data

The focus of the clinical examination is to examine the person for clinical signs that support or are in addition to their report of symptoms. In particular, assessment of cardiac function is aimed at assessing risk factors, pain, fatigue, dyspnoea, risk of falling and the impact of symptoms on the person's usual activities of daily living.

Preparation

When performing an assessment of the carotid arteries, the person can be sitting up. To assess the jugular veins and the praecordium, the person should be supine with the head and chest slightly elevated.

Stand on the person's right side; this will facilitate your hand placement and auscultation of the praecordium.

The room must be warm—chilling makes the person uncomfortable, and shivering interferes with heart sounds. Where possible, try to conduct the assessment in a quiet room; heart sounds are very soft, and any ambient room noise masks them.

Ensure the female's privacy by keeping her breasts draped. The female's left breast overrides part of the area you will need to examine. Gently displace the breast upwards, or ask the woman to hold it out of the way.

When performing a regional cardiovascular assessment, use this order:

1. Pulse and blood pressure (Chapter 10)
2. Peripheral circulation (Chapter 16)
3. Neck vessels
4. Praecordium.

The logic of this order is that you will begin observations peripherally and move in towards the heart.

Equipment needed

Stethoscope with diaphragm and bell endpieces
Alcohol wipe (to clean endpiece)
Hand hygiene solution

PROCEDURES AND NORMAL FINDINGS	ABNORMAL FINDINGS AND CLINICAL ALERTS
General inspection	
During collection of subjective data you will have noticed the colour of the person's skin and mucous membranes, ease of breathing, height to weight ratio, level of hygiene and grooming and general demeanor. All of these factors provide clues to the functioning of the cardiovascular system.	
Identify surface landmarks	
Identify position of clavicles, sternum, ribs and apex of heart (5th intercostal space, midclavicular line)	
Inspect and palpate the neck vessels	
Palpate the carotid artery	
Located central to the heart, the carotid artery yields important information on cardiac function.	
Palpate each carotid artery medial to the sternocleidomastoid muscle in the neck (Figure 17.16). Avoid excessive pressure on the carotid sinus area higher in the neck; excessive vagal stimulation here could slow down the heart rate, especially in adults over 65. Take care to palpate gently. Palpate only one carotid artery at a time to avoid compromising arterial blood to the brain.	**Carotid sinus hypersensitivity** is the condition in which pressure over the carotid sinus leads to a decreased heart rate, decreased BP and cerebral ischaemia with syncope. This may occur in older adults with hypertension or occlusion of the carotid artery.

PROCEDURES AND NORMAL FINDINGS	ABNORMAL FINDINGS AND CLINICAL ALERTS
Figure 17.16	
Feel the rate, rhythm and strength of the pulse. Normally the pulse is easy to palpate and the normal strength is 2+ or moderate (Chapter 16). Your findings should be the same bilaterally.	Diminished pulse feels small and weak (decreased stroke volume). Increased pulse feels full and strong (hyperkinetic states) (see Table 16.1).
Inspect the jugular venous pulse	
From the jugular veins you can assess the central venous pressure (CVP) and thus judge the heart's efficiency as a pump. Although the external jugular vein is easier to see, the internal (especially the right) jugular vein is attached more directly to the superior vena cava and is thus more reliable for assessment. You cannot see the internal jugular vein itself, but you can see its pulsation. The person should be placed in the supine position anywhere from a 30 to a 45 degree angle, wherever you can best see the pulsations. In general, the higher the venous pressure is, the higher the position you need. Remove the pillow to avoid flexing the neck; the head should be in the same plane as the trunk. Turn the person's head slightly away from the examined side, and direct a strong light tangentially onto the neck to highlight pulsations and shadows.	
Note the external jugular veins overlying the sternocleidomastoid muscle. In some people, the veins are not visible at all, whereas in others they are full in the supine position. As the person is raised to a sitting position, these external jugulars flatten and disappear, usually at 45 degrees.	Unilateral distension of external jugular veins is due to local cause (kinking or aneurysm). Full distended external jugular veins above 45 degrees signify increased CVP as with heart failure.
Now look for pulsations of the internal jugular veins in the area of the suprasternal notch or around the origin of the sternocleidomastoid muscle around the clavicle. You must be able to distinguish internal jugular vein pulsation from that of the carotid artery. It is easy to confuse them because they lie close together. Use the guidelines shown in Table 17.1.	

OBJECTIVE DATA

PROCEDURES AND NORMAL FINDINGS	ABNORMAL FINDINGS AND CLINICAL ALERTS

TABLE 17.1 Characteristics of jugular versus carotid pulsations

	INTERNAL JUGULAR PULSE	CAROTID PULSE
1 Location	Lower, more lateral, under or behind the sternocleidomastoid muscle	Higher and medial to this muscle
2 Quality	Undulant and diffuse, two visible waves per cycle	Brisk and localised, one wave per cycle
3 Respiration	Varies with respiration; its level descends during inspiration when intrathoracic pressure is decreased	Does not vary
4 Palpable	No	Yes
5 Pressure	Light pressure at the base of the neck easily obliterates	No change
6 Position of person	Level of pulse drops and disappears as the person is brought to a sitting position	Unaffected

Inspect and palpate the praecordium

Inspect the anterior chest

Arrange tangential lighting to accentuate any flicker of movement.

Pulsations. You may or may not see the **apical impulse**, the pulsation created as the left ventricle rotates against the chest wall during systole. When visible, it occupies the fourth or fifth intercostal space, at or inside the midclavicular line. It is easier to see in children and in those with thinner chest walls.

A **heave** or **lift** is a sustained forceful thrusting of the ventricle during systole. It occurs with ventricular hypertrophy as a result of increased workload. A right ventricular heave is seen at the sternal border; a left ventricular heave is seen at the apex (see Table 17.9).

Palpate the apical impulse

Localise the apical impulse precisely by using one finger pad (Figure 17.17A). Asking the person to 'exhale and then hold it' aids the examiner in locating the pulsation. You may need to roll the person midway to the left to find it; note that this also displaces the apical impulse further to the left (Figure 17.17B).

The point at which you can palpate the apical impulse is the point at which you place your stethoscope to auscultate the apical heart sounds.

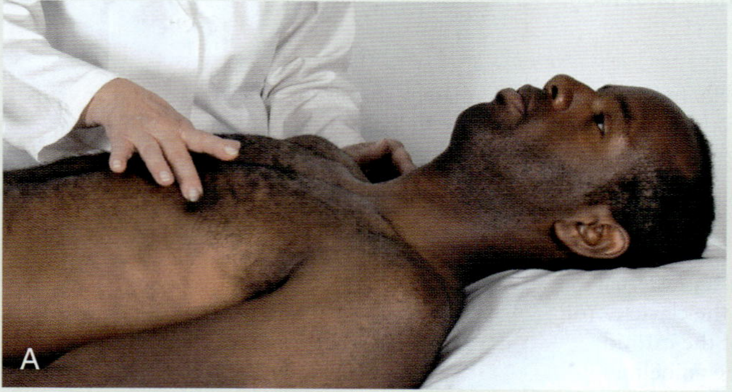

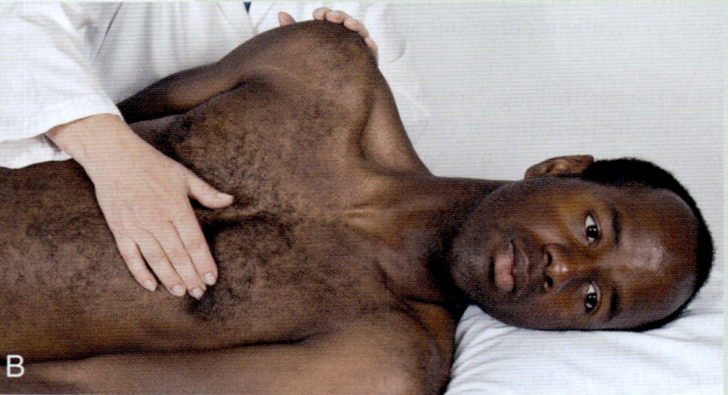

Figure 17.17A, B
The apical impulse.

PROCEDURES AND NORMAL FINDINGS	ABNORMAL FINDINGS AND CLINICAL ALERTS
Note: • *Location*—The apical impulse should occupy only one interspace, the fourth or fifth, and be at or medial to the midclavicular line • *Size*—Normally 1 cm × 2 cm • *Amplitude*—Normally a short, gentle tap • *Duration*—Short, normally occupies only first half of systole	Cardiac enlargement: • Left ventricular dilatation (volume overload) displaces impulse down and to left and increases size more than one space. • Increased force and duration but no change in location occurs with left ventricular hypertrophy and no dilatation (pressure overload) (see Table 17.9).
The apical impulse is easily palpated in most adults. It is not palpable in obese persons or in persons with thick chest walls. With high cardiac output states (anxiety, fever, hyperthyroidism, anaemia), the apical impulse increases in amplitude and duration.	Not palpable with chronic obstructive pulmonary disease due to hyperinflated lungs.

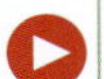

Auscultation of the apical (mitral) area

PROCEDURES AND NORMAL FINDINGS	ABNORMAL FINDINGS AND CLINICAL ALERTS
In most situations, the generalist registered nurse will only need to perform the skill of auscultation of the two heart sounds at the apex of the heart. To do this, you will use both endpieces of your stethoscope when auscultating heart sounds. Although all heart sounds are low frequency, the diaphragm is for relatively higher pitched sounds, and the bell is for relatively lower pitched ones. Locate the fifth intercostal space at the left midclavicular line—mitral valve area. Before you begin, alert the person: 'I always listen to the heart in a number of places on the chest. Just because I am listening a long time does not necessarily mean that something is wrong'. After you place the stethoscope, try closing your eyes briefly to tune out any distractions. Concentrate, and listen selectively to ***one sound at a time***. Consider that at least two, and perhaps three or four, sounds may be happening in less than 1 second. You cannot process everything at once. Begin with the diaphragm endpiece and use the following routine: (1) note the rate and rhythm, (2) identify S_1 and S_2 and (3) assess S_1 and S_2 separately.	
Note the rate and rhythm. The rate ranges normally from 60 to 100 beats per min. (Review the full discussion of the pulse in Chapter 10 and the normal rates across age groups.) The rhythm should be regular, although **sinus arrhythmia** occurs normally in young adults and children. With sinus arrhythmia, the rhythm varies with the person's breathing, increasing at the peak of inspiration and slowing with expiration. Note any other irregular rhythm. If one occurs, check if it has any pattern, or if it is totally irregular.	**Premature beat**—an isolated beat is early, or a pattern occurs in which every third or fourth beat sounds early. **Irregularly irregular**—no pattern to the sounds; beats come rapidly and at random intervals.
When you notice any irregularity, check for a **pulse deficit** by auscultating the apical beat while simultaneously palpating the radial pulse. Count a serial measurement (one after the other) of apical beat and radial pulse. Normally, every beat you hear at the apex should perfuse to the periphery and be palpable. The two counts should be identical. When different, subtract the radial rate from the apical and record the remainder as the pulse deficit. • $\mathbf{S_1}$ is louder than $\mathbf{S_2}$ at the apex; $\mathbf{S_2}$ is louder than $\mathbf{S_1}$ at the base. • $\mathbf{S_1}$ coincides with the carotid artery pulse. Feel the carotid gently as you auscultate at the apex; the sound you hear as you feel each pulse is $\mathbf{S_1}$ (Figure 17.18).	A **pulse deficit** signals a weak contraction of the ventricles; it occurs with atrial fibrillation, premature beats and heart failure.

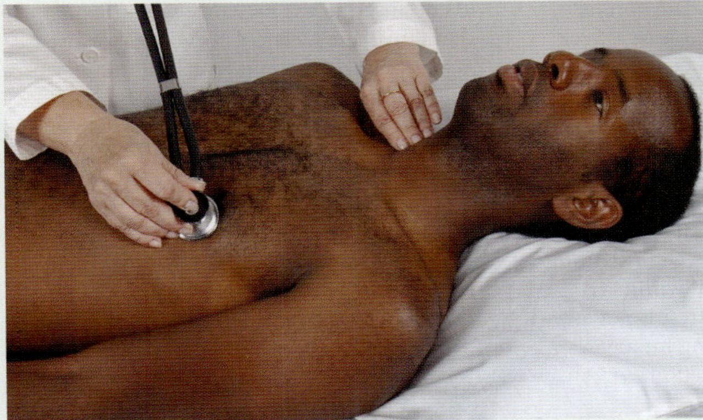

Figure 17.18

PROCEDURES AND NORMAL FINDINGS	ABNORMAL FINDINGS AND CLINICAL ALERTS
• S_1 coincides with the R wave (the upstroke of the QRS complex) if the person is on an ECG monitor. • **Listen to S_1 and S_2 separately.** Note whether each heart sound is normal, accentuated, diminished or split. Inch your diaphragm across the chest as you do this.	
First heart sound (S_1). Caused by closure of the AV valves, S_1 signals the beginning of systole. You can hear it over the entire praecordium, although it is loudest at the apex (Figure 17.19). (Sometimes the two sounds are equally loud at the apex, because S_1 is lower pitched than S_2.) S_1 S_2 APEX LUB — dup **Figure 17.19**	Causes of accentuated or diminished S_1 (see Table 17.4). Both heart sounds are diminished with conditions that place an increased amount of tissue between the heart and your stethoscope: chronic obstructive pulmonary disease (hyperinflated lungs), obesity, pericardial fluid.
You can hear S_1 with the diaphragm with the person in any position and equally well in inspiration and expiration. **Second heart sound (S_2).** The S_2 is associated with closure of the semilunar valves. You can hear it with the diaphragm, over the entire praecordium, although S_2 is loudest at the base (Figure 17.20). S_1 S_2 BASE lub — DUP **Figure 17.20**	Accentuated or diminished S_2 (see Table 17.5).
Laboratory studies	
There are many relevant specialist laboratory tests done to assess heart function. We have listed the most common tests that are undertaken as part of clinical assessment. Reference values may vary by healthcare service depending on the laboratory testing procedures.	***Clinical alert:*** Notify medical practitioner of any abnormal results.
Troponin I or T: Troponin levels are very sensitive and specific for myocardial damage. Increased amounts of troponin are released into the circulating blood with myocardial damage. This blood test helps confirm a clinical diagnosis. The normal levels rise within a few hours of onset of pain and remain elevated for at least a week. Levels vary according to a specific laboratory, however an example of a cut-off for elevation (> 99th percentile of a reference population) is (Aroney & Cullen 2016): • high sensitivity troponin T (hsTnT; Roche Elec-sys) level of 14 ng/L • high sensitivity troponin I (hsTnI; Abbott Architect) level of 26 ng/L	Elevated troponin levels confirm the diagnosis of myocardial infarction (MI). If a MI occurred in the previous week, then an alternative test such as CK-MB will be used as the original troponin levels will not have returned to baseline.
Creatine kinase: CK is an enzyme found in the heart, brain and skeletal muscle. CK-MB is more specific to heart muscle damage. CK-MB serum levels will rise from 4 hours after the onset of chest pain. The serum level returns to normal within 48 hours (Royal College of Pathologists Australia (RCPA) 2019). This test is not as sensitive as troponin testing and is more likely to be used when assessing for a new myocardial reinfarction within 10–14 days of the last myocardial infarction. Reference interval (RCPA 2019): • 0–10 U/L; 0–5% of the total CK (enzyme activity) • 0–6 mg/L (immunoassay)	

OBJECTIVE DATA

PROCEDURES AND NORMAL FINDINGS	ABNORMAL FINDINGS AND CLINICAL ALERTS
Potassium: K^+ is an intracellular ion and is an essential ion for cardiac function. The test becomes abnormal within 12 hours of commencement of pain and remains abnormal for about 7 days. Reference interval (RCPA 2019): • 3.5–5.2 mmol/L (adults)	**Hypokalaemia** is commonly associated with tissue destruction or high stress. Variation in potassium levels may be evident on the 12-lead ECG.
Haemoglobin (Hb): This test is part of a full blood count and is used to exclude anaemia. People with anaemia may report fatigue. Insufficient haemoglobin may be a trigger for activation of angina symptoms. Haemoglobin levels vary by gender, with adult, pregnant, child or a newborn age range. Values will also increase in high altitudes. Levels vary according to a specific laboratory however an example reference interval is (Australian Red Cross Blood Service 2019): • Non-pregnant women (15+ years of age)—120–160 g/L • Men (15+ years of age)—130–180 g/L	Interpretation requires consideration of baseline haemoglobin levels and presenting symptoms.
Brain-type natriuretic peptide (BNP): BNP levels rise with the severity of heart failure. When pressure in the ventricles rises, BNP levels become elevated. The serum levels can rise before the person becomes symptomatic with heart failure. This test can be ordered when the person reports fatigue or dyspnoea and it assists in generating a clinical diagnosis. Reference interval (RCPA 2019): • BNP < 100 ng/L Congestive heart failure (CHF) unlikely • BNP 100–500 ng/L Equivocal range • BNP > 500 ng/L Consistent with the diagnosis of CHF	BNP levels are elevated in the presence of heart failure.

Further objective assessment for advanced practice

The assessments that are described in the following section require advanced skill and scope of practice. Nurses working in specialist cardiac care units, intensive care units as well as community health centres may need to develop these skills. Advanced assessment for infants and children is performed by specialist neonatal and paediatric nurses, some midwives and maternal and child health nurses.

Equipment

Rulers

PROCEDURES AND NORMAL FINDINGS	ABNORMAL FINDINGS AND CLINICAL ALERTS
Estimate the jugular venous pressure	
As a follow-on from inspecting the jugular venous pulse, think of the jugular veins as a CVP manometer attached directly to the right atrium. You can 'read' the CVP at the highest level of pulsations (Figure 17.21). Use the angle of Louis (sternal angle) as an arbitrary reference point and compare it with the highest level of venous pulsation. Hold a vertical ruler on the sternal angle. Align a straight edge on the ruler like a T-square and adjust the level of the horizontal straight edge to the level of pulsation. Read the level of intersection on the vertical ruler; normal jugular venous pulsation is 2 cm or less above the sternal angle. Also state the person's position, for example, 'internal jugular vein pulsations 3 cm above sternal angle when elevated 30 degrees'.	Elevated pressure is a level of pulsation that is more than 3 cm above the sternal angle while at 45 degrees. This occurs with heart failure.

PROCEDURES AND NORMAL FINDINGS	ABNORMAL FINDINGS AND CLINICAL ALERTS
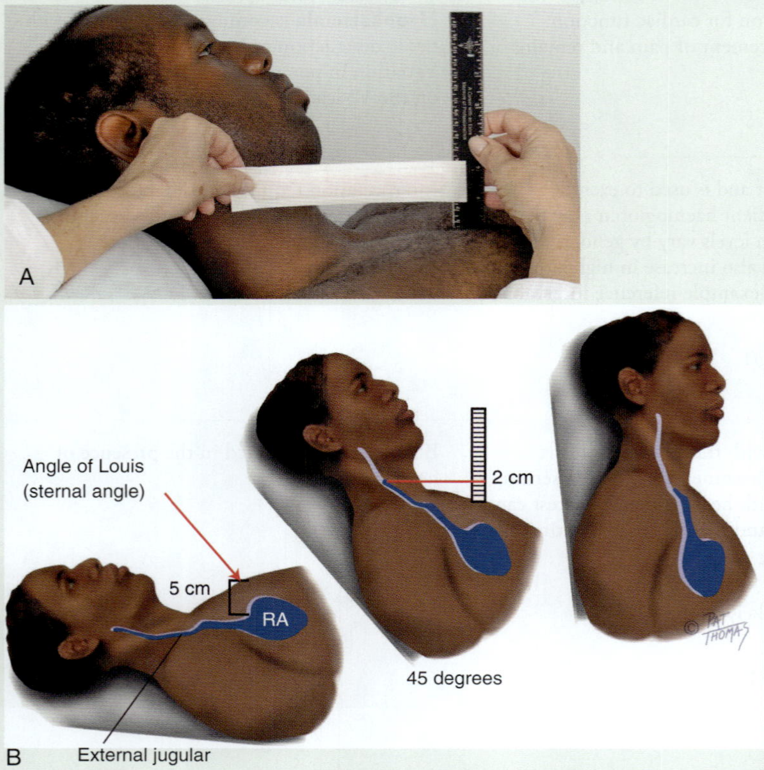 Figure 17.21A, B If you cannot find the internal jugular veins, use the external jugular veins and note the point where they look collapsed. Be aware that the technique of estimating venous pressure is difficult and is not always a reliable predictor of CVP. Consistency in grading among examiners is difficult to achieve.	
If venous pressure is elevated, or if you suspect heart failure, perform **hepatojugular reflux** (Figure 17.22). Position the person comfortably supine and instruct them to breathe quietly through an open mouth. Hold your right hand on the right upper quadrant of the person's abdomen just below the rib cage. Watch the level of jugular pulsation as you push in with your hand. Exert firm sustained pressure for 30 seconds. This empties venous blood out of the liver sinusoids and adds its volume to the venous system. If the heart is able to pump this additional volume (i.e. if no elevated CVP is present), the jugular veins will rise for a few seconds, then recede to the previous level. 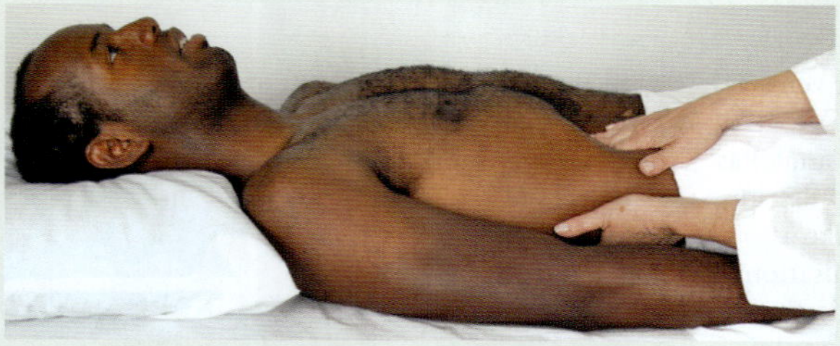 Figure 17.22 Hepatojugular reflux.	If heart failure is present, the jugular veins will elevate and stay elevated as long as you push.

PROCEDURES AND NORMAL FINDINGS	ABNORMAL FINDINGS AND CLINICAL ALERTS
Percussion is used to outline the heart's borders, but often it has been displaced by the chest X-ray or echocardiogram. These are much more accurate in detecting heart enlargement. When the right ventricle enlarges, it does so in the anteroposterior diameter, which is better seen on X-ray film. Also, percussion is of limited usefulness with the female breast tissue or in an obese person or a person with a muscular chest wall.	
However, there are times when your percussing hands are the only tools you have with you, such as in an outpatient setting, extended care facility or the person's home. When you need to search for cardiac enlargement, place your stationary finger in the person's fifth intercostal space over on the left side of the chest near the anterior axillary line. Slide your stationary hand towards yourself, percussing as you go, and note the change of sound from resonance over the lung to dull (over the heart). Normally, the left border of cardiac dullness is at the midclavicular line in the fifth interspace and slopes in towards the sternum as you progress upwards, so that by the second interspace the border of dullness coincides with the left sternal border. The right border of dullness normally matches the sternal border.	Cardiac enlargement is due to increased ventricular volume or wall thickness; it occurs with hypertension, CAD, heart failure and cardiomyopathy.
Ausculate the carotid artery	
For persons middle-aged or older, or who show symptoms or signs of cardiovascular disease, follow on from inspection of the neck vessels and auscultate each carotid artery for the presence of a **bruit** (pronounced bru'-ee) (Figure 17.23). This is a blowing, swishing sound indicating blood flow turbulence; normally none is present. 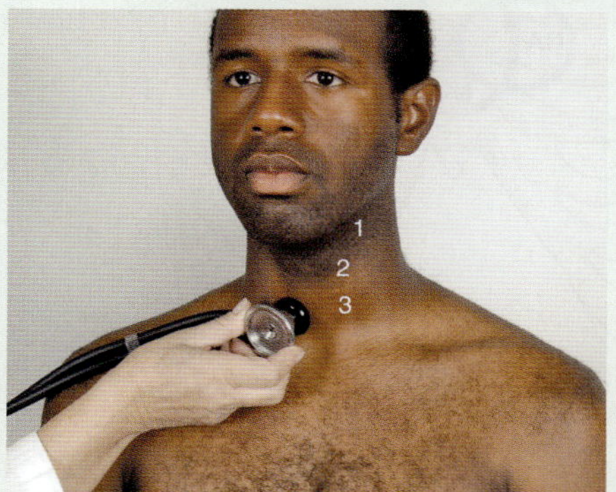 Figure 17.23	A **bruit** indicates turbulence due to a local vascular cause, such as atherosclerotic narrowing.
Keep the neck in a neutral position. Lightly apply the bell of the stethoscope over the carotid artery at three levels: (1) the angle of the jaw, (2) the midcervical area and (3) the base of the neck (see Figure 17.23). Avoid compressing the artery because this could create an artificial bruit, and it could compromise circulation if the carotid artery is already narrowed by atherosclerosis. Ask the person to take a breath, exhale and hold it briefly while you listen so that tracheal breath sounds do not mask or mimic a carotid artery bruit. (Holding the breath on inhalation will also tense the levator scapulae muscles, which makes it hard to hear the carotids.) Sometimes you can hear normal heart sounds transmitted to the neck; do not confuse these with a bruit.	A **carotid bruit** is audible when the lumen is occluded by half to two-thirds. Bruit loudness increases as the atherosclerosis worsens until the lumen is occluded by two-thirds. After that, bruit loudness decreases. When the lumen is completely occluded, the bruit disappears. Thus, absence of a bruit does not ensure absence of a carotid lesion. A **murmur** sounds much the same but is caused by a cardiac disorder. Some aortic valve murmurs (aortic stenosis) radiate to the neck and must be distinguished from a local bruit.

PROCEDURES AND NORMAL FINDINGS	ABNORMAL FINDINGS AND CLINICAL ALERTS

Auscultate the praecordium

In addition to auscultation at the apical area, some advanced practice nurses need to develop skills in auscultation across the praecordium. First you need to identify the auscultatory areas where you will listen. These include the four traditional valve 'areas' (Figure 17.24). The valve areas are not over the actual anatomical locations of the valves but are the sites on the chest wall where sounds produced by the valves are best heard. The sound radiates with the direction of blood flow. The valve areas are:

- Second right interspace—aortic valve area
- Second left interspace—pulmonic valve area
- Left lower sternal border—tricuspid valve area
- Fifth interspace at around left midclavicular line—mitral valve area.

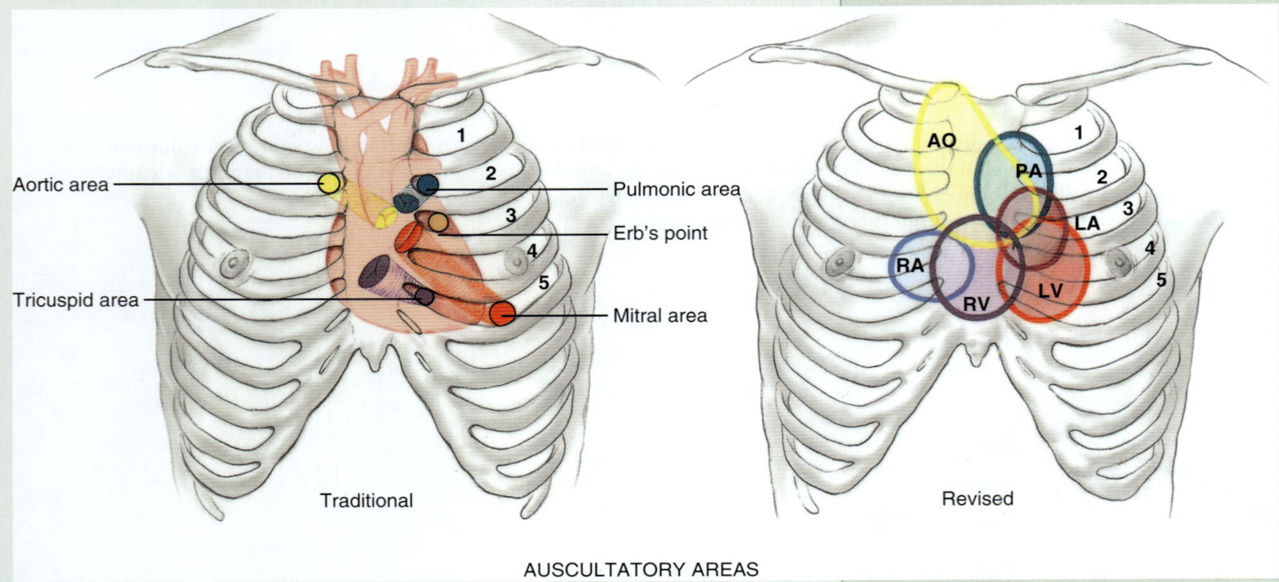

Figure 17.24

Do not limit your auscultation to only four locations. Sounds produced by the valves may be heard all over the praecordium. (For this reason, many experts even discourage the naming of the valve areas.) Thus, learn to inch your stethoscope in a rough **Z** pattern, from the base of the heart across and down, then over to the apex. Or start at the apex and work your way up. Include the sites shown in Figure 17.24.

After you place the stethoscope, try closing your eyes briefly to tune out any distractions. Concentrate, and listen selectively to ***one sound at a time***. Consider that at least two, and perhaps three or four, sounds may be happening in less than 1 second. You cannot process everything at once. Begin with the diaphragm endpiece and use the following routine: (1) note the rate and rhythm, (2) identify $\mathbf{S_1}$ and $\mathbf{S_2}$, (3) assess $\mathbf{S_1}$ and $\mathbf{S_2}$ separately, (4) listen for extra heart sounds and (5) listen for murmurs.

PROCEDURES AND NORMAL FINDINGS	ABNORMAL FINDINGS AND CLINICAL ALERTS

A split S_1 is normal, but it occurs rarely. A split S_1 means you are hearing the mitral and tricuspid components separately. It is audible in the tricuspid valve area, the left lower sternal border. The split is very rapid, with the two components only 0.03 second apart.

Splitting of S_2. A split S_2 is a normal phenomenon that occurs towards the end of inspiration in some people. Recall that closure of the aortic and pulmonic valves is nearly synchronous. Because of the effects of respiration on the heart described earlier, inspiration separates the timing of the two valves' closure, and the aortic valve closes 0.06 second before the pulmonic valve. Instead of one DUP, you hear a split sound—T-DUP (Figure 17.25). During expiration, synchrony returns, and the aortic and pulmonic components fuse together. A split S_2 is heard only in the pulmonic valve area, the second left interspace.

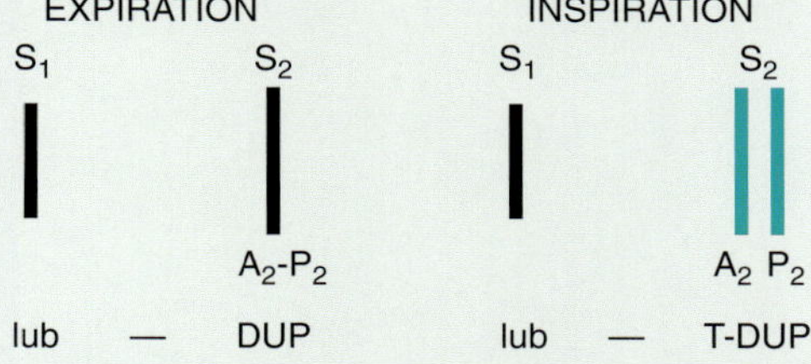

Figure 17.25

When you first hear the split S_2, do *not* be tempted to ask the person to hold their breath so that you can concentrate on the sounds. Breath holding will only equalise ejection times in the right and left sides of the heart and cause the split to go away. Instead, concentrate on the split as you watch the person's chest rise up and down with breathing. The split S_2 occurs about every fourth heartbeat, fading in with inhalation and fading out with exhalation.

Focus on systole, then on diastole, and listen for any extra heart sounds. Listen with the diaphragm, then switch to the bell, covering all auscultatory areas (Figure 17.26). Usually, these are silent periods. When you do detect an extra heart sound, listen carefully to note its timing and characteristics. During systole, the **midsystolic click** (which is associated with mitral valve prolapse) is the most common extra sound (see Table 17.7). The third and fourth heart sounds occur in diastole; either may be normal or abnormal (see Table 17.8).

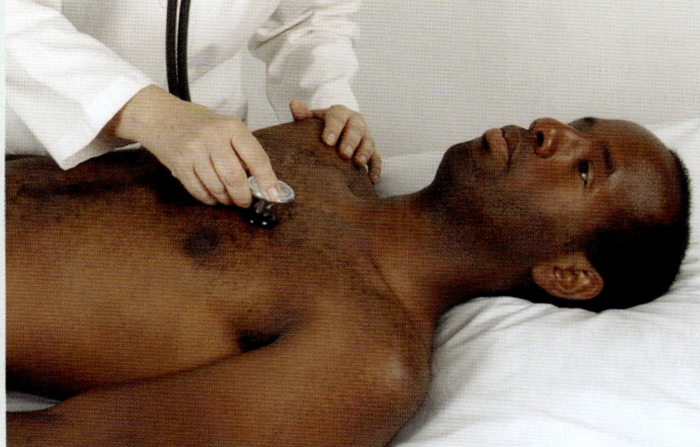

Figure 17.26

A **fixed split** is unaffected by respiration; the split is always there.

A **paradoxical split** is the opposite of what you would expect; the sounds fuse on inspiration and split on expiration (see Table 17.6).

A pathological S_3 (ventricular gallop) occurs with heart failure and volume overload; a pathological S_4 (atrial gallop) occurs with CAD (see Table 17.8 for a full description).

PROCEDURES AND NORMAL FINDINGS	ABNORMAL FINDINGS AND CLINICAL ALERTS
Listen for murmurs. A murmur is a blowing, swooshing sound that occurs with turbulent blood flow in the heart or great vessels. Except for the innocent murmurs described, murmurs are abnormal. If you hear a murmur, describe it by indicating these following characteristics:	Murmurs may be due to congenital defects and acquired valvular defects. Study Tables 17.10 and 17.11 for a complete description.
Timing. It is crucial to define the murmur by its occurrence in systole or diastole. You must be able to identify $\mathbf{S_1}$ and $\mathbf{S_2}$ accurately to do this. Try to further describe the murmur as being in early, mid- or late systole or diastole; throughout the cardiac event (termed pansystolic or holosystolic/pandiastolic or holodiastolic); and whether it obscures or muffles the heart sounds.	A **systolic murmur** may occur with a normal heart or with heart disease; a **diastolic murmur** always indicates heart disease.
Loudness. Describe the intensity in terms of six 'grades'. For example, record a grade ii murmur as 'ii/vi'. *Grade i*—Barely audible, heard only in a quiet room and then with difficulty *Grade ii*—Clearly audible, but faint *Grade iii*—Moderately loud, easy to hear *Grade iv*—Loud, associated with a thrill palpable on the chest wall *Grade v*—Very loud, heard with one corner of the stethoscope lifted off the chest wall *Grade vi*—Loudest, still heard with entire stethoscope lifted just off the chest wall **Pitch**. Describe the pitch as high, medium or low. The pitch depends on the pressure and the rate of blood flow producing the murmur. **Pattern.** The intensity may follow a pattern during the cardiac phase, growing louder (crescendo), tapering off (decrescendo) or increasing to a peak and then decreasing (crescendo–decrescendo, or diamond shaped). Because the whole murmur is just milliseconds long, it takes practice to diagnose any pattern.	
Quality. Describe the quality as musical, blowing, harsh or rumbling. **Location**. Describe the area of maximum intensity of the murmur (where it is best heard) by noting the valve area or intercostal spaces. **Radiation**. The murmur may be transmitted downstream in the direction of blood flow and may be heard in another place on the praecordium, the neck, the back or the axilla. **Posture**. Some murmurs disappear or are enhanced by a change in position. Some murmurs are common in healthy children or adolescents and are termed *innocent* or *functional.* **Innocent** indicates having no valvular or other pathological cause; **functional** is due to increased blood flow in the heart (e.g. in anaemia, fever, pregnancy, hyperthyroidism). The contractile force of the heart is greater in children. This increases blood flow velocity. The increased velocity plus a smaller chest measurement makes an audible murmur. The innocent murmur is generally soft (grade ii), midsystolic, short, crescendo–decrescendo and with a vibratory or musical quality ('vooot' sound like violin strings). Also, the innocent murmur is heard at the second or third left intercostal space and disappears with sitting, and the young person has no associated signs of cardiac dysfunction. Although it is important to distinguish innocent murmurs from pathological ones, it is best to suspect all murmurs as pathological until they are proved otherwise. Diagnostic tests such as ECG, phonocardiogram and echocardiogram are needed to establish an accurate diagnosis.	The murmur of mitral stenosis is rumbling, whereas that of aortic stenosis is harsh (see Table 17.11).
Change position. After auscultating in the supine position, roll the person towards their left side. Listen with the bell at the apex for the presence of any diastolic filling sounds (i.e. the $\mathbf{S_3}$ or $\mathbf{S_4}$) (Figure 17.27).	$\mathbf{S_3}$ and $\mathbf{S_4}$ and the murmur of mitral stenosis sometimes may be heard only when on the left side.

OBJECTIVE DATA

PROCEDURES AND NORMAL FINDINGS	ABNORMAL FINDINGS AND CLINICAL ALERTS
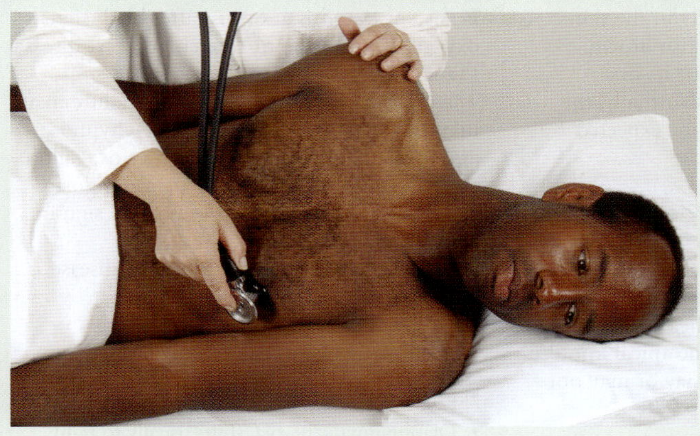 Figure 17.27	
Ask the person to sit up, lean forwards slightly and exhale. Listen with the diaphragm firmly pressed at the base, right and left sides. Check for the soft, high-pitched, early diastolic murmur of aortic or pulmonic regurgitation (Figure 17.28). 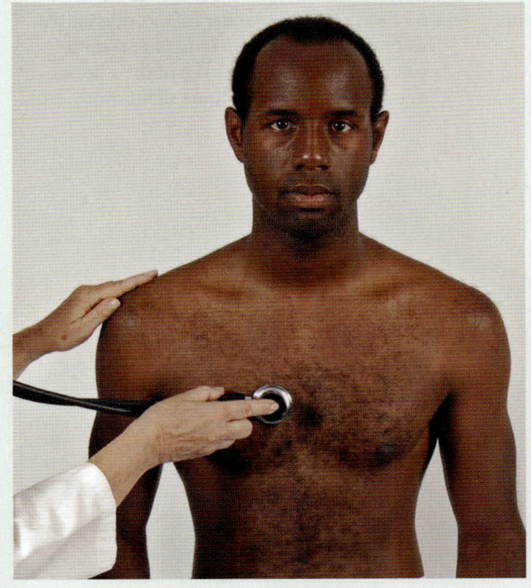 Figure 17.28	Murmur of aortic regurgitation sometimes may be heard only when the person is leaning forwards in the sitting position.
Additional objective data for infants	
The transition from fetal to pulmonic circulation occurs in the immediate newborn period. Fetal shunts normally close within 10 to 15 hours but may take up to 48 hours. Thus, you should assess the cardiovascular system during the first 24 hours and again in 2–3 days.	Failure of shunts to close (e.g. **patent ductus arteriosus (PDA), atrial septal defect (ASD)**): see Table 17.10.

PROCEDURES AND NORMAL FINDINGS	ABNORMAL FINDINGS AND CLINICAL ALERTS
Note any extra cardiac signs that may reflect cardiac status particularly in the skin, liver size and respiratory status. The skin colour should be pink to pinkish brown, depending on the infant's genetic heritage. If cyanosis occurs, determine its first appearance—at or shortly after birth versus after the neonatal period. Normally, the liver is not enlarged, and the respirations are not laboured. Also, note the expected parameters of weight gain throughout infancy.	Persistent cyanosis at or just after birth signals oxygen desaturation of congenital heart disease (Table 17.10). The most important signs of heart failure in an infant are persistent tachycardia, tachypnoea and liver enlargement. Engorged veins, gallop rhythm and pulsus alternans are also signs. Respiratory crackles are an important sign in adults but not in infants. Failure to thrive occurs with cardiac disease.
Palpate the apical impulse to determine the size and position of the heart. Because the infant's heart has a more horizontal placement, expect to palpate the apical impulse at the fourth intercostal space just lateral to the midclavicular line. It may or may not be visible.	The apex is displaced with: • Cardiac enlargement, shifts to the left • Pneumothorax, shifts away from affected side • Diaphragmatic hernia, shifts usually to right because this hernia occurs more often on the left • Dextrocardia, a rare anomaly in which the heart is located on right side of chest.
The heart rate is best auscultated because radial pulses are hard to count accurately. Use the small (paediatric size) diaphragm and bell (Figure 17.29). The heart rate may range from 70 to 190 per min immediately after birth, then stabilise to an average of 120 per min. Infants normally have wide fluctuations with activity, from 170 per min or more with crying or being active to 70–90 per min with sleeping. Variations are greatest at birth and are even more so with premature babies (see Table 10.1). 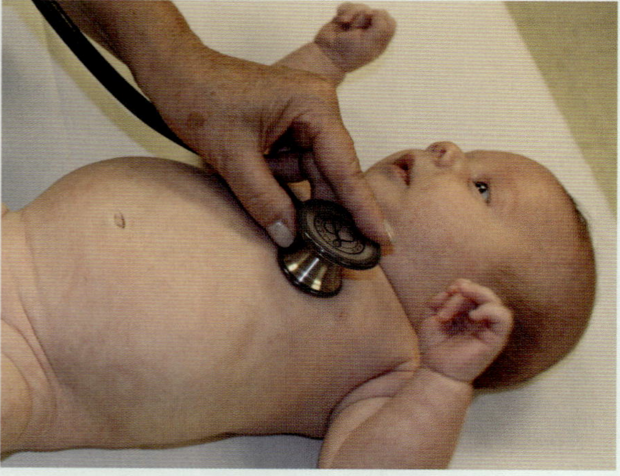 **Figure 17.29**	Persistent tachycardia is >200 beats per min in newborns, or >150 beats per min in infants. Bradycardia is <90 beats per min in newborns or <60 beats per min in older infants or children. This causes a serious drop in cardiac output because the small muscle mass of their hearts cannot increase stroke volume significantly.
Expect the **heart rhythm** to have sinus arrhythmia, the phasic speeding up or slowing down with the respiratory cycle. Rapid rates make it more challenging to evaluate heart sounds. Expect heart sounds to be louder in infants than in adults because of the infant's thinner chest wall. Also, $\mathbf{S_2}$ has a higher pitch and is sharper than $\mathbf{S_1}$. Splitting of $\mathbf{S_2}$ just after the height of inspiration is common, not at birth, but beginning a few hours after birth.	Investigate any irregularity except sinus arrhythmia. Fixed split $\mathbf{S_2}$ indicates atrial septal defect (see Table 17.10).
Murmurs in the immediate newborn period do not necessarily indicate congenital heart disease. Murmurs are relatively common in the first 2–3 days because of fetal shunt closure. These murmurs are usually grade i or ii, are systolic, accompany no other signs of cardiac disease and disappear in 2–3 days. The murmur of PDA is a continuous machinery murmur, which disappears by 2–3 days. On the other hand, absence of a murmur in the immediate newborn period does not ensure a perfect heart; congenital defects can be present that are not signalled by an early murmur. It is best to listen frequently and to note and describe any murmur according to the characteristics listed above.	Persistent murmur after 2–3 days, holosystolic murmurs or those that last into diastole, and those that are loud—all warrant further evaluation.

PROCEDURES AND NORMAL FINDINGS	ABNORMAL FINDINGS AND CLINICAL ALERTS
Additional objective data for children	
Note any **extracardiac or cardiac signs** that may indicate heart disease: poor weight gain, developmental delay, persistent tachycardia, tachypnoea, dyspnoea on exertion, cyanosis and clubbing. Note that clubbing of fingers and toes usually does not appear until late in the first year, even with severe cyanotic defects.	
The apical impulse is sometimes visible in children with thin chest walls. Note any obvious bulge or any heave—these are not normal.	A praecordial bulge to the left of the sternum with a hyperdynamic praecordium signals cardiac enlargement. The bulge occurs because the cartilaginous rib cage is more compliant. A substernal heave occurs with right ventricular enlargement, and an apical heave occurs with left ventricular hypertrophy.
Palpate the apical impulse: in the fourth intercostal space to the left of the midclavicular line until age 4 years; at the fourth interspace at the midclavicular line from age 4 to 6 years; and in the fifth interspace to the right of the midclavicular line at age 7 years (Figure 17.30). 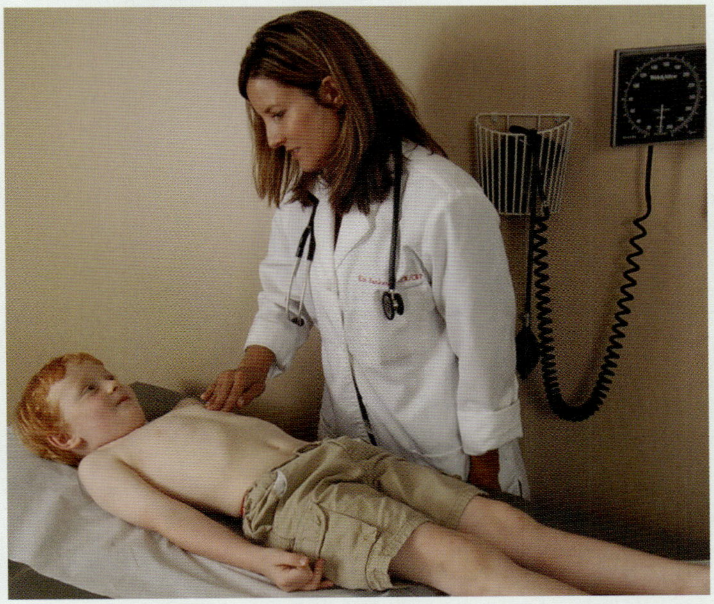 Figure 17.30	The apical impulse moves laterally with cardiac enlargement. Thrill (palpable vibration).
The average heart rate slows as the child grows older, although it is still variable with rest or activity (see Table 10.1). The heart rhythm remains characterised by sinus arrhythmia. Physiological S_3 is common in children (see Table 17.8). It occurs in early diastole, just after S_2, and is a dull soft sound that is best heard at the apex. A **venous hum**—due to turbulence of blood flow in the jugular venous system—is common in healthy children and has no pathological significance. It is a continuous, low-pitched, soft hum that is heard throughout the cycle, although it is loudest in diastole. Listen with the bell over the supraclavicular fossa at the medial third of the clavicle, especially on the right, or over the upper anterior chest.	

PROCEDURES AND NORMAL FINDINGS	ABNORMAL FINDINGS AND CLINICAL ALERTS
The venous hum is not usually affected by respiration, may sound louder when the child stands and is easily obliterated by occluding the jugular veins in the neck with your fingers.	This latter manoeuvre helps differentiate the venous hum from other cardiac murmurs (e.g. PDA).
Heart murmurs that are innocent (or functional) in origin are very common through childhood. Some authors say they have a 30% occurrence, and some authors say nearly all children may demonstrate a murmur at some time. Most innocent murmurs have these characteristics: soft, relatively short systolic ejection murmur; medium pitch; vibratory; best heard at the left lower sternal or midsternal border, with no radiation to the apex, base or back. For the child whose murmur has been shown to be innocent, it is very important that the parents understand this completely. They need to believe that this murmur is just a 'noise' and has no pathological significance. Otherwise, the parents may become overprotective and limit activity for the child, which may result in the child developing a negative self-concept.	Distinguish innocent murmurs from pathological ones. This may involve referral to another examiner or the performance of diagnostic tests such as the ECG or ultrasonography.
Additional objective data for the pregnant woman	
The **vital signs** usually yield an increase in resting pulse rate of 10–15 beats per min and a drop in blood pressure from the normal pre-pregnancy level. The BP decreases to its lowest point during the second trimester and then slowly rises during the third trimester. The BP varies with position. It is usually lowest in left lateral recumbent position, a bit higher when supine and highest when sitting. **Inspection of the skin** often shows a mild hyperaemia in light-skinned women because the increased cutaneous blood flow tries to eliminate the excess heat generated by the increased metabolism. Palpation of the apical impulse is higher and lateral compared with the normal position, as the enlarging uterus elevates the diaphragm and displaces the heart up and to the left and rotates it on its long axis. **Auscultation of the heart sounds** shows changes caused by the increased blood volume and workload: Heart sounds • Exaggerated splitting of S_1 and increased loudness of S_1 • A loud, easily heard S_3 **The ECG** has no changes except for a slight left axis deviation and T wave inversion in the lateral leads and lead III due to the change in the heart's position (upward movement of the diaphragm due to size of the uterus and fetus) (Mockridge & Maclennan 2019).	Suspect pregnancy-induced hypertension with a sustained rise of 30 mmHg systolic or 15 mmHg diastolic under basal conditions.
Additional objective data for the adult over 65 years	
A gradual rise in systolic blood pressure is common with ageing; the diastolic blood pressure stays fairly constant with a resulting widening of pulse pressure. Some adults over 65 experience **orthostatic hypotension**, a sudden drop in blood pressure when rising to sit or stand. Use caution in palpating and auscultating the carotid artery. Avoid pressure in the carotid sinus area, which could cause a reflex slowing of the heart rate. Also, pressure on the carotid artery could compromise circulation if the artery is already narrowed by atherosclerosis. When measuring jugular venous pressure, view the right internal jugular vein. The aorta stiffens, dilates and elongates with ageing, which may compress the left neck veins and obscure pulsations on the left side.	
The chest often increases in anteroposterior diameter with ageing. This makes it more difficult to palpate the apical impulse and to hear the splitting of $\mathbf{S_2}$. The $\mathbf{S_4}$ often occurs in people over 65 with no known cardiac disease. Systolic murmurs are common, occurring in over 50% of such people. Occasional premature ectopic beats are common and do not necessarily indicate underlying heart disease. When in doubt, obtain an ECG. However, consider that the ECG only records for one isolated min in time and may need to be supplemented by a test of 24-hours ambulatory heart monitoring.	The $\mathbf{S_3}$ is associated with heart failure and is always abnormal over age 35 years (see Table 17.8).

OBJECTIVE DATA

Summary Checklist

CARDIAC ASSESSMENT

Subjective data

1. Presenting concern
2. Chest pain
3. Dyspnoea
4. Orthopnoea
5. Cough
6. Fatigue
7. Cyanosis or pallor
8. Oedema
9. Nocturia
10. Past cardiac history
11. Family cardiac history
12. Health and lifestyle management

Objective Data

1. General inspection
2. Identify relevant surface landmarks
3. Inspect and palpate neck vessels
4. Inspect and palpate the praecordium
5. Auscultation of apical (mitral) area
6. Laboratory studies

PROMOTING A HEALTHY LIFESTYLE

WOMEN AND HEART ATTACKS

When someone complains of chest pain or pain radiating down the left arm, almost everyone thinks heart attack. After all, these are the symptoms that typically occur. Aren't they? Well, yes and no. They are the most 'typical' symptoms men get, but not women. For women, the symptoms can be quite different or atypical. These 'atypical' symptoms may be one of the reasons that more women than men are dying from heart disease these days.

Women are more likely to feel angina as a hot or cold burning sensation, or even as a tenderness to touch, in their back, shoulders, arms or jaw. They often have no chest discomfort or pain at all. Women's symptoms of heart attacks frequently include nausea, vomiting, indigestion, shortness of breath or extreme fatigue but, again, no chest pain. All of these symptoms are easy to attribute to something else other than the heart and are often ignored. Scientific evidence now shows that women tend to minimise their symptoms of cardiac disease. However, part of this may be due to a lack of awareness.

Women's not so 'atypical' symptoms of cardiovascular disease or a heart attack include:

- Pain, discomfort, deep ache, pressure or throbbing 'above the waist'—including the back, shoulders, arms, stomach, jaw and, sometimes, the chest
- Breathlessness or inability to catch the breath—with or without exertion or when waking up
- Clammy sweating and dizziness—what some refer to as a 'cold sweat'
- Anxiety—feelings of impending doom or unusual nervousness
- Oedema or swelling, usually in ankles or lower legs
- Nausea and indigestion
- Sleep disturbance
- Unusual fatigue or weakness.

Cardiovascular disease is the number one cause of death in women. Women should be made aware of and pay attention to the particular symptoms and seek immediate care if they occur. The following resources have up to date information for women about heart disease

The Heart Foundation (Australia): https://www.heartfoundation.org.au/your-heart/women-and-heart-disease

The Heart Foundation (New Zealand): https://www.heartfoundation.org.nz/your-heart/women-and-heart-disease

Documentation and critical thinking

FOCUSED ASSESSMENT: CLINICAL CASE STUDY

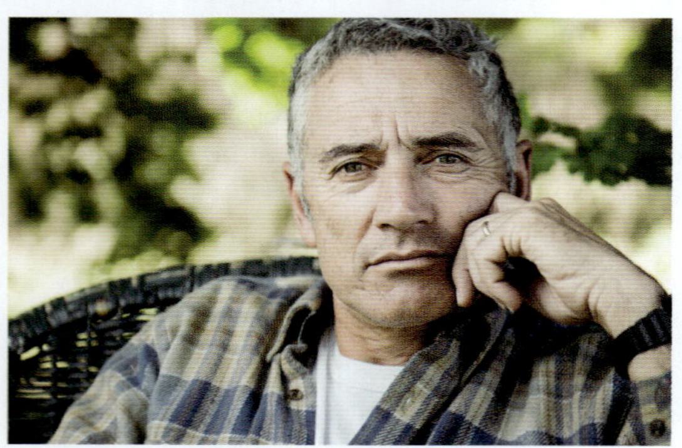

Context

Mr Neil Andrews is a 53-year-old male who runs his own building company and was admitted to the cardiac ward with chest pain for investigation. The registered nurse is completing an admission assessment.

Subjective

One year ago, Mr Andrews was admitted to hospital with crushing substernal chest pain, radiating to left shoulder, accompanied by nausea, vomiting and diaphoresis.

At that time, he was diagnosed as having an acute coronary syndrome, with no cardiac enzyme elevation and minor 12-lead ECG irregularities of T wave flattening in leads V5, V6, I and AVL. Mr Andrews was hospitalised for 4 days. During this time, he was commenced on antiplatelet therapy (aspirin), underwent serial 12-lead ECG and cardiac enzyme testing for 24 hours and scheduled for an inpatient percutaneous coronary angiogram. The angiogram identified a narrowing in his right coronary artery <50% in diameter and he was commenced on medication to slow down his disease progression.

Since that hospital admission, Mr Andrews has continued to work. He had occasional fleeting episodes of chest pain with exercise, relieved by rest.

One day ago—had increasing frequency of chest pain, about every 2 hours, lasting a few min, saw pain as warning to visit local doctor.

Day of admission—severe substernal chest pain ('like someone sitting on my chest') unrelieved by rest. Went to see his GP, while in office had episode of chest pain same as last year, accompanied by diaphoresis, no nausea and vomiting or shortness of breath, relieved by 2 glyceryl trinitrate sprays. Transferred to hospital by ambulance. No further pain since presentation to the emergency department 4 hours ago. No new 12-lead ECG changes since last admission.

Current chest pain: 2/10 central with no radiation.

Family hx—mother died of AMI at age 38 years.

Health and life style management—smoked 1½ pack cigarettes daily × 34 years (51 (CHECK) pack years), quit 1 year ago, no alcohol, diet—trying to limit fat and fried food, still high in added salt.

Objective

General inspection: Appears anxious. Appears overweight for height.

Extremities: Skin pink, no cyanosis. Upper extremities—capillary refill sluggish, no clubbing. Lower extremities—no oedema, no hair growth 10 cm below knee bilaterally.

Pulses: carotid, brachial, radial, femoral – 2+; popliteal and posterior tibial – 0; dorsalis pedis – 1+. All equal bilaterally.

B/P R arm = L arm 104/66 mmHg

Praecordium: Inspection. Apical impulse visible 5th ICS, 7 cm left of midsternal line.

Palpation: Apical impulse palpable in 5th and 6th ICS.

Auscultation: Apical rate 92 regular, S_1–S_2 are normal, not diminished or accentuated.

Height: 182 cm; **Weight:** 101 kg; **BMI:** 30.5

Collaborative problems

Chest pain related to reduction in cardiac blood flow

Ineffective tissue perfusion related to interruption in cardiovascular blood flow

Decreased cardiac output related to reduction in stroke volume

Problem statements/nursing diagnoses

Chest pain related to reduction in cardiac blood flow

Fatigue related to reduced cardiac output

Anxiety and fear related to new cardiac episode and uncertainty about diagnosis

Knowledge deficit about reducing cardiac risk factors

Abnormal findings

TABLE 17.2 Differential diagnosis of chest pain

	COMMON PAIN DESCRIPTION	LOCATION/RADIATION	POSSIBLE ASSOCIATED SYMPTOMS
Cardiovascular (ischaemic)			
Angina pectoris: stable (no change in pain pattern within last 60 days)	Pressure-like discomfort (e.g. tightness, squeezing, burning, heaviness that lasts 3–5 min precipitated by activity and often resolves with rest)	Generalised substernal or retrosternal: can radiate to teeth, jaw, neck, one or both arms or shoulders; or there may be no pain and only associated symptoms	Diaphoresis, nausea, vomiting, dyspnoea
Prinzmetal or variant angina	Pressure-like discomfort often occurring at rest and early morning hours	Retrosternal: can radiate to jaw, neck, left arm or shoulder	Palpitations, syncope or feelings of syncope
Acute coronary syndrome (unstable angina, myocardial infarction)	Heaviness; vice-like, squeezing, crushing, tightness; vague, burning, constricting or pressure; poorly localised pain lasting 20–30 min to hours and does not resolve with rest	Generalised substernal or retrosternal: can radiate to teeth, jaw, neck, one or both arms or shoulders; or there may be no pain and only associated symptoms	Indigestion-like feeling, nausea, vomiting, dizziness, flushing, perspiration, palpitations, dyspnoea
Cardiovascular (nonischaemic)			
Pericarditis	Sudden sharp and stabbing pain relieved often by sitting or leaning forwards and worsens by lying down or with inspiration	Substernal, which can radiate to trapezius muscle region	Dry cough, muscle and joint aches, fever
Mitral valve prolapse	Sharp pain not associated with activity	Chest pain without radiation	Fatigue, light-headedness, dyspnoea, irregular heartbeat, palpitations, exercise intolerance
Aortic dissection	Sudden severe pain with change in location and/or tearing sensation lasting for hours	Anterior chest pain with radiation to the neck, jaw, or intrascapular region of the back	Mental status changes, limb pain and weakness, dyspnoea
Pulmonary hypertension (secondary)	Cardiac-like chest pain with exertion	Chest region	Dyspnoea, lower-extremity oedema, fatigue
Pulmonary			
Pulmonary embolism	Sharp, stabbing pain worsening with deep breaths	Pain can be experienced in chest, back, shoulder or upper abdomen	Dyspnoea, haemoptysis, cough
Pneumonia	Sharp or stabbing pain associated with cough	Mostly generalised to one side of chest but can have upper abdominal pain	Cough, fever, dyspnoea, chills, sputum, myalgia, malaise
Pneumothorax	Acute/sudden and sharp	Lateral region of the chest but can have referred pain to shoulder	Acute dyspnoea, cough
Gastrointestinal			
Gastro-oesophageal reflux	May be angina-like; however, usually burning sensation with eating large meals reproduced by lying down and relieved by sitting up	Retrosternal region	Cough, regurgitation of food, abdominal pain
Oesophageal spasm	Crushing chest pain	Substernal	Dysphagia, sensation of object in throat or oesophagus
Cholecystitis	Sudden onset of pain that crescendos and can last for up to 20 min, usually after eating a fatty meal	Epigastrium or right upper abdomen that can radiate to right intrascapular region, shoulder or back	Nausea, vomiting, anorexia, fever

(Continued)

TABLE 17.2 Differential diagnosis of chest pain—cont'd			
	COMMON PAIN DESCRIPTION	LOCATION/RADIATION	POSSIBLE ASSOCIATED SYMPTOMS
Pancreatitis	Sudden dull, boring, steady pain unrelieved by lying supine; leaning forwards or the fetal position may ease pain	Epigastrium or periumbilical pain radiating to back	Nausea, vomiting, anorexia, and sometimes diarrhoea
Dermatological			
Herpes zoster	Unilateral, burning, bore-like pain	Chest region in dermatome distribution	Tingling, itching, burning
Musculoskeletal/Neurological			
Costochondritis	Sharp, pleuritic-type pain worsens with deep breathing, palpation or movement	Area from 2nd through to 5th intercostal spaces; can radiate to arm, depending on where initial inflammation occurs	Chest tightness, warmth at area of pain
Chest wall muscle strain	Sharp pain with moving, stretching or pushing movements of the arms; palpation of area reproduces the pain	Area around the strained muscle, sternum or ribs	Muscle spasm, crepitation, swelling, loss of strength
Psychogenic			
Depression	Heaviness	Chest region	Fatigue, restlessness, withdrawal, weight gain or loss, depressed mood
Anxiety	Sharp pain	Chest region	Palpitations, dizziness, sweating, shaking, restlessness, fatigue, irritability

Adapted from Zitkus BS. Take chest pain to heart, *Nurse Practitioner*, 35(9):41–47, 2010.

TABLE 17.3 Clinical portrait of heart failure

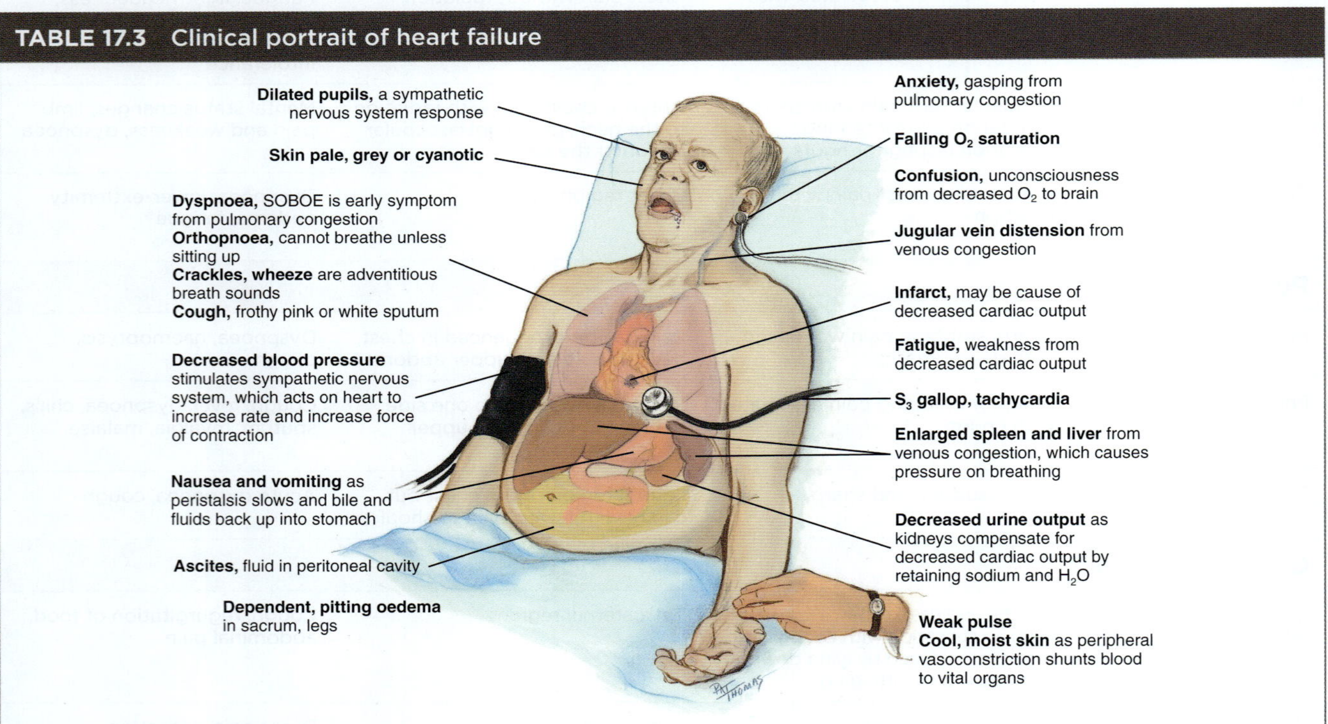

Decreased cardiac output occurs when the heart fails as a pump, and the circulation becomes backed up and congested.

Signs and symptoms of heart failure come from two basic mechanisms: (1) the heart's inability to pump enough blood to meet the metabolic demands of the body, and (2) the kidney's compensatory mechanisms of abnormal retention of sodium and water to compensate for the decreased cardiac output. This increases blood volume and venous return, which causes further congestion.

Onset of heart failure may be: (1) acute, as following a myocardial infarction when direct damage to the heart's contracting ability has occurred; or (2) chronic, as with hypertension, when the ventricles must pump against chronically increased pressure.

Abnormal findings for advanced practice

TABLE 17.4 Variations in S_1

The intensity of S_1 depends on three factors: (1) position of AV valve at the start of systole, (2) structure of the valve leaflets and (3) how quickly pressure rises in the ventricle.

	FACTOR	EXAMPLES
Loud (Accentuated) S_1		
S_1 S_2	1. Position of AV valve at start of systole—wide open and no time to drift together 2. Change in valve structure—calcification of valve, needs increasing ventricular pressure to close the valve against increased atrial pressure	Hyperkinetic states where blood velocity is increased: exercise, fever, anaemia, hyperthyroidism Mitral stenosis with leaflets still mobile
Faint (Diminished) S_1		
S_1 S_2	1. Position of AV valve—delayed conduction from atria to ventricles. Mitral valve drifts shut before ventricular contraction closes it 2. Change in valve structure—extreme calcification, which limits mobility	First-degree heart block (prolonged PR interval) Mitral insufficiency
	3. More forceful atrial contraction into noncompliant ventricle; delays or diminishes ventricular contraction	Severe hypertension—systemic or pulmonary
Varying intensity of S_1		
S_1 S_2 S_1 S_2	1. Position of AV valve varies before closing from beat to beat 2. Atria and ventricles beat independently	Atrial fibrillation—irregularly-irregular rhythm Complete heart block with changing PR interval
Split S_1		
S_1 S_2 T M	Mitral and tricuspid components are heard separately	Normal but uncommon

TABLE 17.5 Variations in S_2

	CONDITION	EXAMPLE
Accentuated S_2		
S_1 S_2	1. Higher closing pressure 2. Exercise and excitement increase pressure in aorta 3. Pulmonary hypertension 4. Semilunar valves calcified but still mobile	Systemic hypertension, ringing or booming S_2 Mitral stenosis, heart failure Aortic or pulmonic stenosis
Diminished S_2		
S_1 S_2	1. A fall in systemic blood pressure causes a decrease in valve strength 2. Semilunar valves thickened and calcified, with decreased mobility	Shock Aortic or pulmonic stenosis

TABLE 17.6 Variations in split S_2

	Diagram	CONDITION	EXAMPLE
Normal splitting	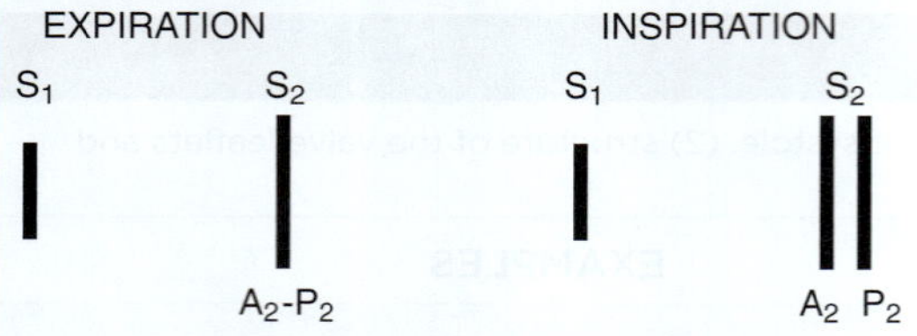 EXPIRATION: S_1, S_2 (A_2-P_2); INSPIRATION: S_1, S_2 (A_2 P_2)		
Fixed split	EXPIRATION: S_1, S_2 (A_2 P_2); INSPIRATION: S_1, S_2 (A_2 P_2)	A fixed split is unaffected by respiration; the split is always there.	Atrial septal defect Right ventricular failure
Paradoxical split 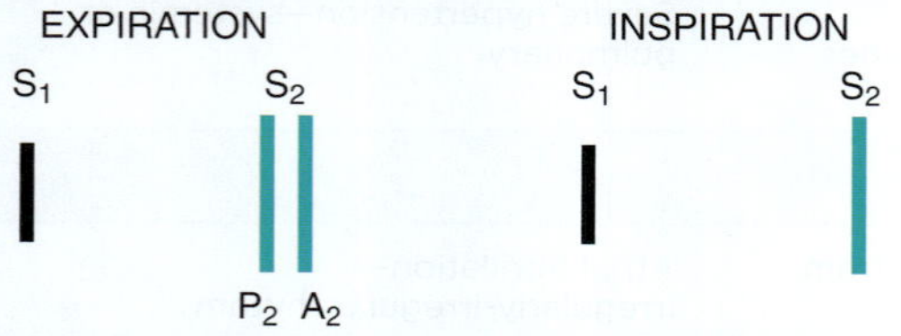	EXPIRATION: S_1, S_2 (P_2 A_2); INSPIRATION: S_1, S_2	Conditions that delay aortic valve closure cause the opposite of a normal split. In inspiration, $\mathbf{P_2}$ is normally delayed so with a paradoxical split, the sounds fuse. In expiration you hear the split, in the order of $\mathbf{P_2A_2}$.	Aortic stenosis Left bundle branch block Patent ductus arteriosus
Wide split 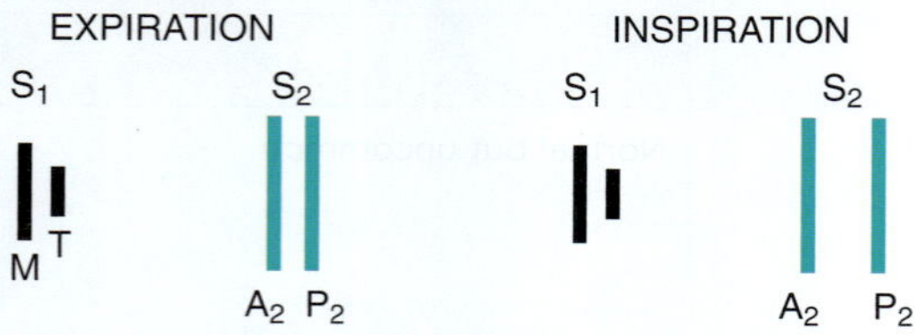	EXPIRATION: S_1 (M T), S_2 (A_2 P_2); INSPIRATION: S_1, S_2 (A_2 P_2)	When the right ventricle has delayed electrical activation, the split is very wide on inspiration and is still there on expiration.	Right bundle branch block (which delays $\mathbf{P_2}$)

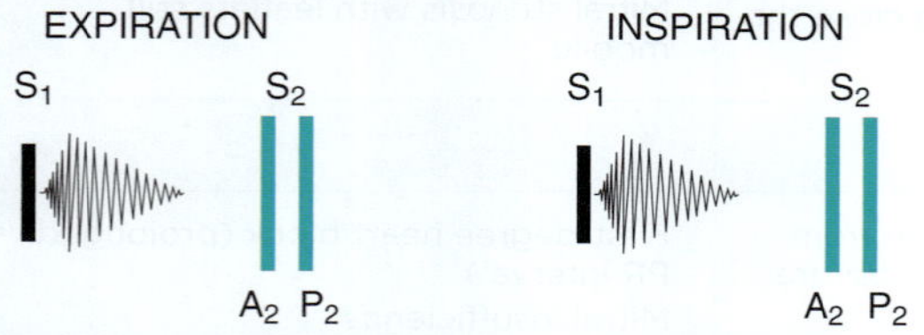

TABLE 17.7 Systolic extra sounds

Early systolic Ejection click Aortic prosthetic valve sounds	Mid-/late systolic Midsystolic (mitral) click

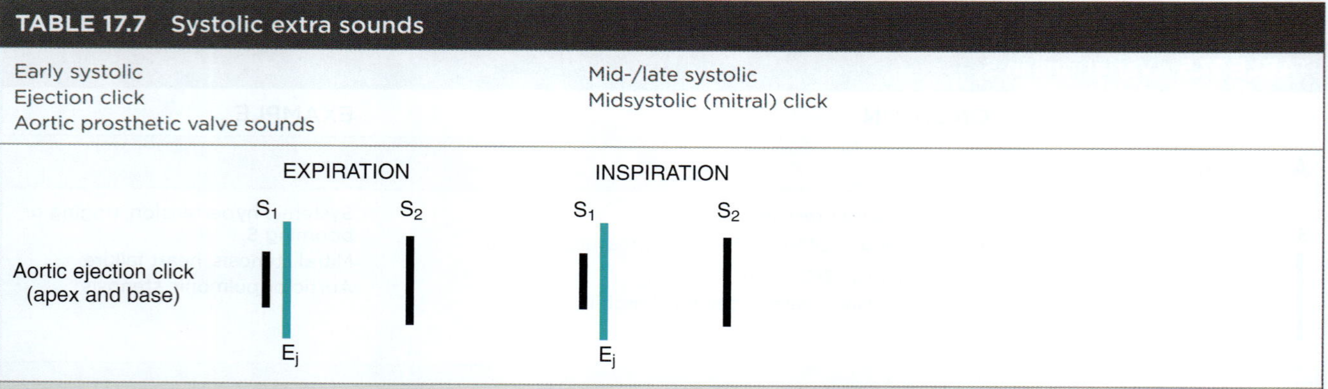

Ejection click

The ejection click occurs early in systole at the start of ejection because it results from opening of the semilunar valves. Normally, the SL valves open silently, but in the presence of stenosis (e.g. aortic stenosis, pulmonic stenosis) their opening makes a sound. It is short and high pitched, with a click quality, and is heard better with the diaphragm.

The aortic ejection click is heard at the second right interspace and apex and may be loudest at the apex. Its intensity does not change with respiration. The pulmonic ejection click is best heard in the second left interspace and often grows softer with inspiration.

TABLE 17.7 Systolic extra sounds—cont'd

'Ball-in-cage'
AO = aortic opens
AC = aortic closes

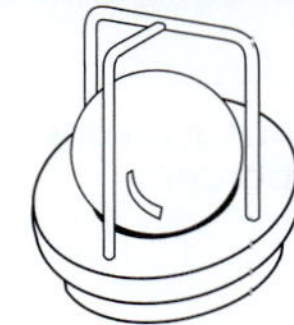

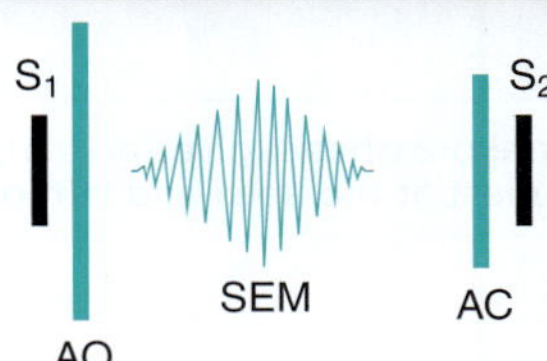

Aortic prosthetic valve sounds

As a sequela of modern technological intervention for heart problems, some people now have *iatrogenically* induced heart sounds. The opening of an aortic ball-in-cage prosthesis (e.g. Starr-Edwards prosthesis) produces an early systolic sound. This sound is less intense with a tilting disk prosthesis (e.g. Bjork-Shiley prosthesis) and is absent with a tissue prosthesis (e.g. porcine).

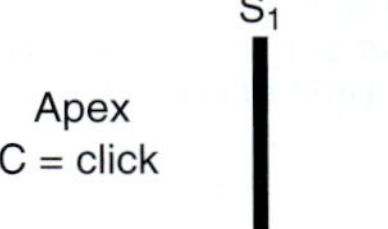

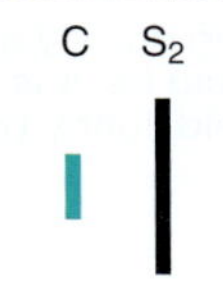

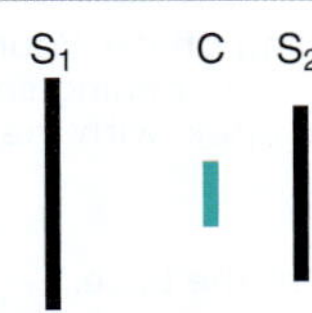

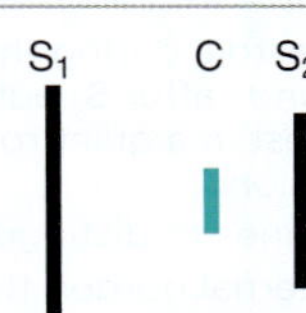

Midsystolic click

Although it is systolic, this is not an ejection click. It is associated with **mitral valve prolapse**, in which the mitral valve leaflets not only close with contraction but balloon back up into the left atrium. During ballooning, the sudden tensing of the valve leaflets and the chordae tendineae creates the click.

The sound occurs in mid- to late systole and is short and high pitched, with a click quality. It is best heard with the diaphragm, at the apex, but also may be heard at the left lower sternal border. The click is usually followed by a systolic murmur. The click and murmur move with postural change; when the person assumes a squatting position, the click may move closer to $\mathbf{S_2}$, and the murmur may sound louder and delayed. The Valsalva manoeuvre also moves the click closer to $\mathbf{S_2}$.

TABLE 17.8 Diastolic extra sounds

Early diastole	Mid-diastole	Late diastole
Opening snap	Third heart sound	Fourth heart sound
Mitral prosthetic valve sound	Summation sound ($\mathbf{S_3}$ + $\mathbf{S_4}$)	Pacemaker-induced sound

EXPIRATION

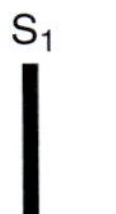

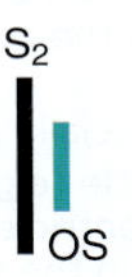

INSPIRATION

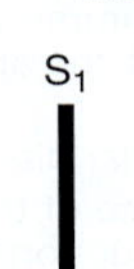

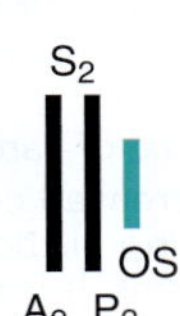

Opening snap

Normally the opening of the AV valves is silent. In the presence of stenosis, increasingly higher atrial pressure is required to open the valve. The deformed valve opens with a noise: the opening snap. It is sharp and high pitched, with a snapping quality. It sounds after $\mathbf{S_2}$ and is best heard with the diaphragm at the third or fourth left interspace at the sternal border, less well at the apex.

The opening snap is usually not an isolated sound. As a sign of mitral stenosis, the opening snap usually ushers in the low-pitched diastolic rumbling murmur of that condition.

'Ball-in-cage'

MO = mitral prosthesis opens
MC = S_1

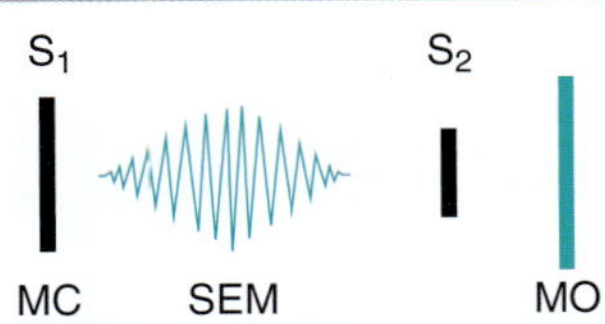

(Continued)

TABLE 17.8 Diastolic extra sounds—cont'd

Mitral prosthetic valve sound

An iatrogenic sound, the opening of a ball-in-cage mitral prosthesis, gives an early diastolic sound: an opening click just after $\mathbf{S_2}$. It is loud, is heard over the whole praecordium and is loudest at the apex and left lower sternal border.

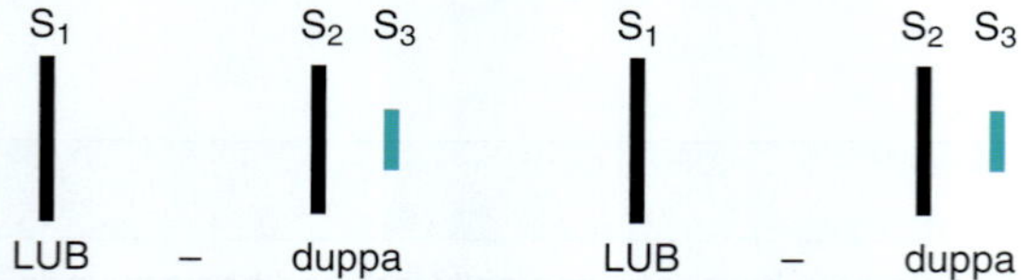

Third heart sound

The $\mathbf{S_3}$ is a ventricular filling sound. It occurs in early diastole during the rapid filling phase. Your hearing quickly accommodates to the $\mathbf{S_3}$, so it is best heard when you listen initially. It sounds after $\mathbf{S_2}$ but later than an opening snap would be. It is a dull, soft sound, and it is low pitched, like 'distant thunder'. It is heard best in a quiet room, at the apex, with the bell held lightly (just enough to form a seal), and with the person in the left lateral position.

The $\mathbf{S_3}$ can be confused with a split $\mathbf{S_2}$. Use these guidelines to distinguish the $\mathbf{S_3}$:

- *Location*—The $\mathbf{S_3}$ is heard at the apex or left lower sternal border; the split $\mathbf{S_2}$ at the base.
- *Respiratory variation*—The $\mathbf{S_3}$ does not vary in timing with respirations; the split $\mathbf{S_2}$ does.
- *Pitch*—The $\mathbf{S_3}$ is lower pitched; the pitch of the split $\mathbf{S_2}$ stays the same.

The $\mathbf{S_3}$ may be normal (physiological) or abnormal (pathological). The **physiological** $\mathbf{S_3}$ is heard frequently in children and young adults; it occasionally may persist after age 40 years, especially in women. The normal $\mathbf{S_3}$ usually disappears when the person sits up.

In adults, the $\mathbf{S_3}$ is usually abnormal. The **pathological** $\mathbf{S_3}$ is also called a **ventricular gallop** or an $\mathbf{S_3}$ gallop, and it persists when sitting up. The $\mathbf{S_3}$ indicates decreased compliance of the ventricles, as in heart failure. The $\mathbf{S_3}$ may be the earliest sign of heart failure. The $\mathbf{S_3}$ may originate from either the left or the right ventricle; a left-sided $\mathbf{S_3}$ is heard at the apex in the left lateral position, and a right-sided $\mathbf{S_3}$ is heard at the left lower sternal border with the person supine and is louder in inspiration.

The $\mathbf{S_3}$ occurs also with conditions of volume overload, such as mitral regurgitation and aortic or tricuspid regurgitation. The $\mathbf{S_3}$ is also found in high cardiac output states in the absence of heart disease, such as hyperthyroidism, anaemia and pregnancy. When the primary condition is corrected, the gallop disappears.

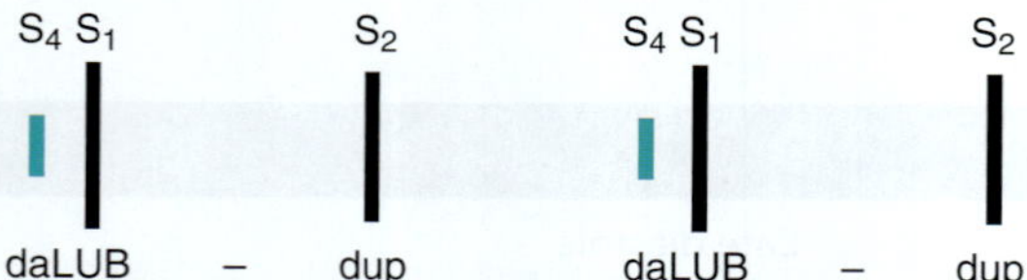

Fourth heart sound

The $\mathbf{S_4}$ is a ventricular filling sound. It occurs when the atria contract late in diastole. It is heard immediately before $\mathbf{S_1}$. This is a very soft sound, of very low pitch. You need a good bell, and you must listen for it. It is heard best at the apex, with the person in left lateral position.

A **physiological** $\mathbf{S_4}$ may occur in adults older than 40 or 50 years with no evidence of cardiovascular disease, especially after exercise.

A **pathological** $\mathbf{S_4}$ is termed an **atrial gallop** or an $\mathbf{S_4}$ gallop. It occurs with decreased compliance of the ventricle (e.g. coronary artery disease, cardiomyopathy) and with systolic overload (afterload), including outflow obstruction to the ventricle (aortic stenosis) and systemic hypertension. A left-sided $\mathbf{S_4}$ occurs with these conditions. It is heard best at the apex, in the left lateral position.

A right-sided $\mathbf{S_4}$ is less common. It is heard at the left lower sternal border and may increase with inspiration. It occurs with pulmonary stenosis or pulmonary hypertension.

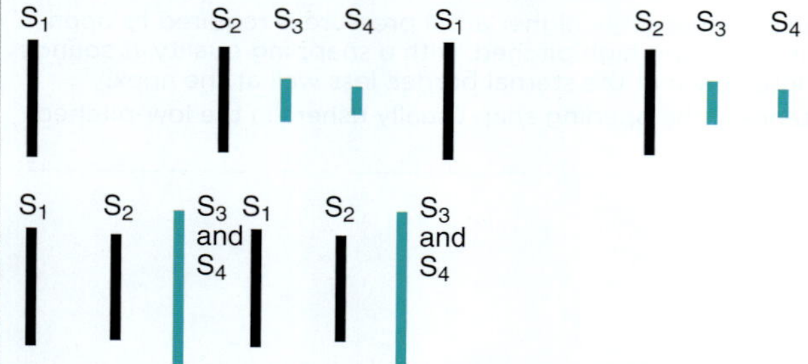

Summation sound

When both the pathological $\mathbf{S_3}$ and $\mathbf{S_4}$ are present, a quadruple rhythm is heard. Often, in cases of cardiac stress, one response is tachycardia. During rapid rates, the diastolic filling time shortens and the $\mathbf{S_3}$ and $\mathbf{S_4}$ move closer together. They sound superimposed in mid-diastole, and you hear one loud, prolonged, summated sound, often louder than either $\mathbf{S_1}$ or $\mathbf{S_2}$.

TABLE 17.8 Diastolic extra sounds—cont'd

EXTRACARDIAC SOUNDS

Pericardial friction rub

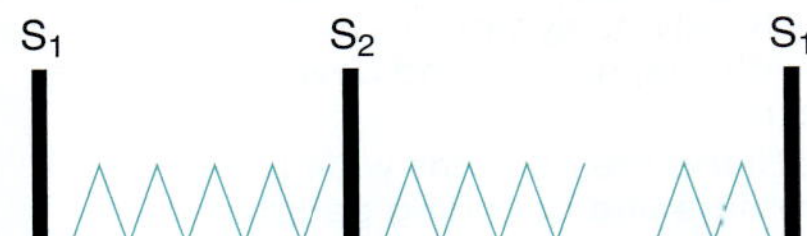

Inflammation of the praecordium gives rise to a friction rub. The sound is high pitched and scratchy, like sandpaper being rubbed. It is best heard with the diaphragm, with the person sitting up and leaning forwards, and with the breath held in expiration.

A friction rub can be heard at any place on the praecordium but is usually best heard at the apex and left lower sternal border, places where the pericardium comes in close contact with the chest wall. Timing may be systolic and diastolic. The friction rub of pericarditis is common during the first week after a myocardial infarction and may last only a few hours.

TABLE 17.9 Abnormal pulsations on the praecordium

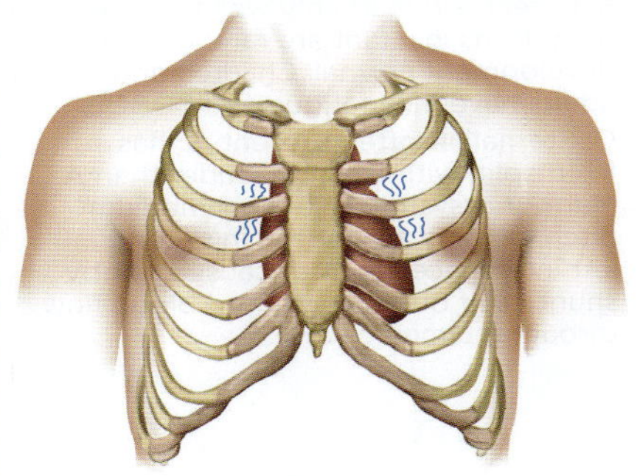

Base

A **thrill** in the second and third right interspaces occurs with severe aortic stenosis and systemic hypertension.

A **thrill** in the second and third left interspaces occurs with pulmonic stenosis and pulmonic hypertension.

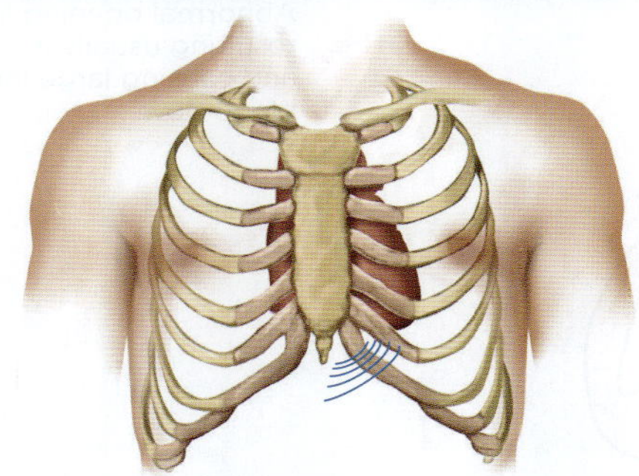

Left sternal border

A **lift (heave)** occurs with right ventricular hypertrophy, as found in pulmonic valve disease, pulmonic hypertension and chronic lung disease. You feel a diffuse lifting impulse during systole at the left lower sternal border. It may be associated with retraction at the apex because the left ventricle is rotated posteriorly by the enlarged right ventricle.

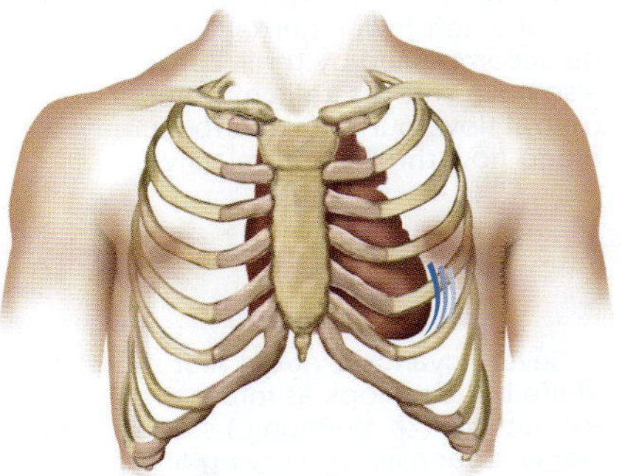

Apex

Cardiac enlargement displaces the apical impulse laterally and over a wider area when left ventricular hypertrophy and dilatation are present. This is **volume overload**, as in mitral regurgitation, aortic regurgitation and left-to-right shunts.

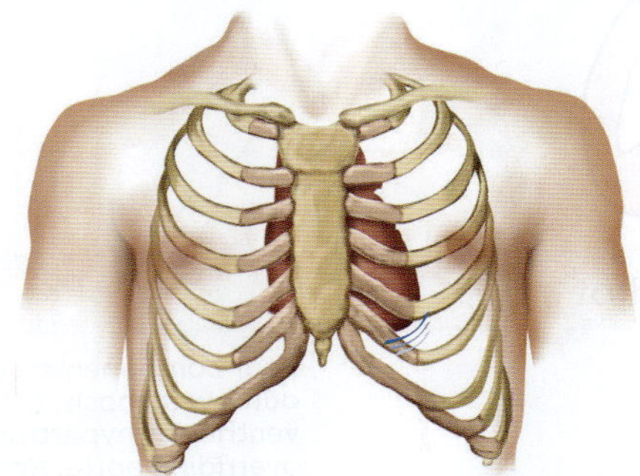

Apex

The apical impulse is increased in force and duration but is not necessarily displaced to the left when left ventricular hypertrophy occurs alone without dilatation. This is **pressure overload**, as found in aortic stenosis or systemic hypertension.

TABLE 17.10 Congenital heart defects

	DESCRIPTION	CLINICAL DATA
Patent ductus arteriosus (PDA)		
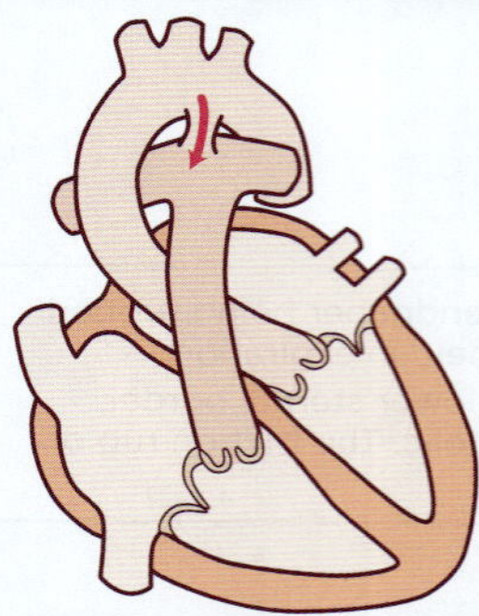	Persistence of the channel joining left pulmonary artery to aorta. This is normal in the fetus and usually closes spontaneously within hours of birth.	S: Usually no symptoms in early childhood; growth and development are normal. O: Blood pressure has wide pulse pressure and bounding peripheral pulses from rapid runoff of blood into low-resistance pulmonary bed during diastole. Thrill often palpable at left upper sternal border. The continuous murmur heard in systole and diastole is called a machinery murmur.
Atrial septal defect (ASD)		
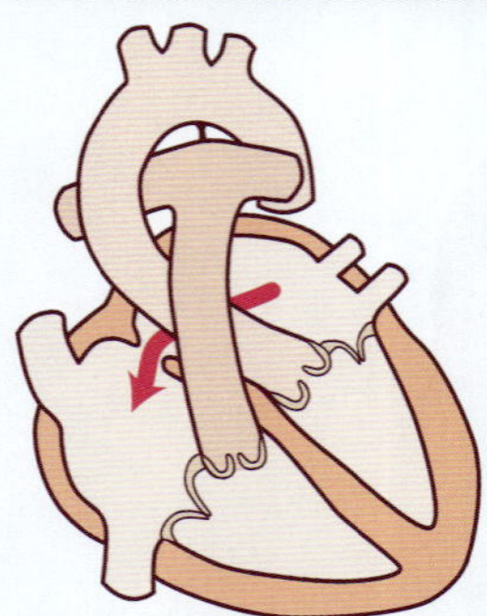	Abnormal opening in the atrial septum, resulting usually in left-to-right shunt and causing large increase in pulmonary blood flow.	S: Defect is remarkably well tolerated. Symptoms in infant are rare; growth and development normal. Children and young adults have mild fatigue and SOBOE. O: Sternal lift often present. $\mathbf{S_2}$ has fixed split, with $\mathbf{P_2}$ often louder than $\mathbf{A_2}$. Murmur is systolic, ejection, medium pitch, best heard at base in second left interspace. Murmur caused not by shunt itself but by increased blood flow through pulmonic valve.
Ventricular septal defect (VSD)		
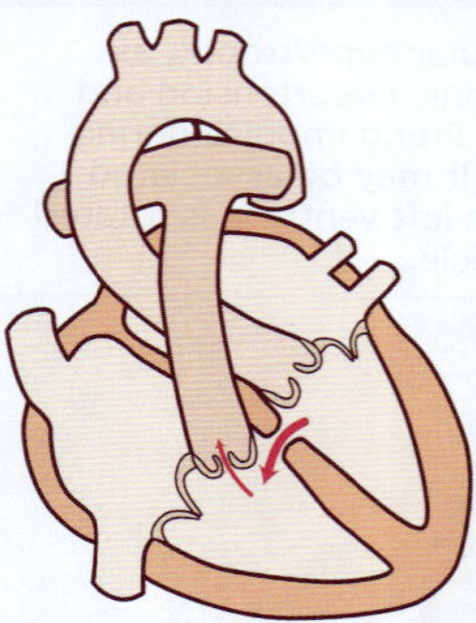	Abnormal opening in septum between the ventricles, usually subaortic area. The size and exact position vary considerably.	S: Small defects are asymptomatic. Infants with large defects have poor growth, slow weight gain; later look pale, thin and delicate. May have feeding problems; SOBOE; frequent respiratory infections; and, when the condition is severe, heart failure. O: Loud, harsh holosystolic murmur, best heard at left lower sternal border, may be accompanied by thrill. Large defects also have soft diastolic murmur at apex (mitral flow murmur) due to increased blood flow through mitral valve.
Tetralogy of Fallot		
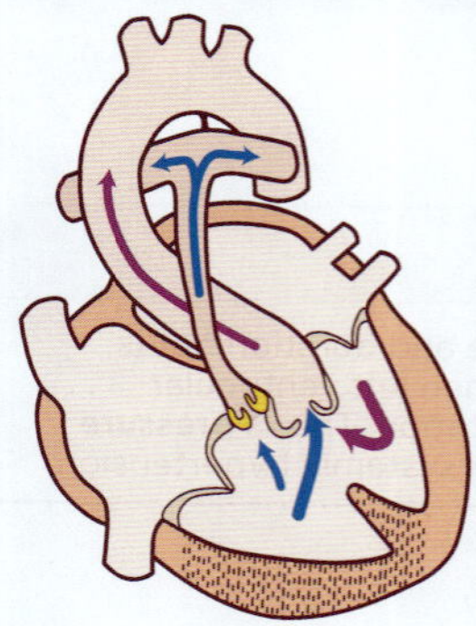	Four components: (1) right ventricular outflow stenosis, (2) VSD, (3) right ventricular hypertrophy and (4) overriding aorta. *Result*: shunts a lot of venous blood directly into aorta away from pulmonary system, so blood never gets oxygenated.	S: Severe cyanosis, not in first months of life but develops as infant grows and RV outflow (i.e. pulmonic) stenosis gets worse. Cyanosis with crying and exertion at first, then at rest. Uses squatting posture after starts walking. SOBOE common. Development is slowed. O: Thrill palpable at left lower sternal border. $\mathbf{S_1}$ normal; $\mathbf{S_2}$ has $\mathbf{A_2}$ loud and $\mathbf{P_2}$ diminished or absent. Murmur is systolic, loud, crescendo-decrescendo.

TABLE 17.10 Congenital heart defects—cont'd

Coarctation of the aorta

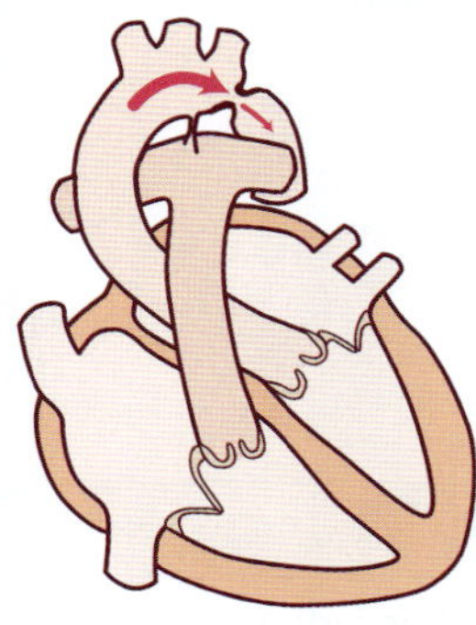	Severe narrowing of descending aorta, usually at the junction of the ductus arteriosus and the aortic arch, just distal to the origin of the left subclavian artery. Results in increased workload on left ventricle. Associated with defects of aortic valve in most cases, as well as associated patent ductus arteriosus; and associated ventricular septal defect.	S: In infants with associated lesions or symptoms, diagnosis occurs in first few months as symptoms of heart failure develop. For asymptomatic children and adolescents, growth and development are normal. Diagnosis usually accidental due to blood pressure findings. Adolescents may complain of vague lower extremity cramping that is worse with exercise. O: Upper extremity hypertension over 20 mmHg higher than lower extremity measures is a hallmark of coarctation. Another important sign is absent or greatly diminished femoral pulses. A systolic murmur is heard best at the left sternal border, radiating to the back.

TABLE 17.11 Murmurs due to valvular defects

Midsystolic ejection murmurs

Due to forward flow through semilunar valves

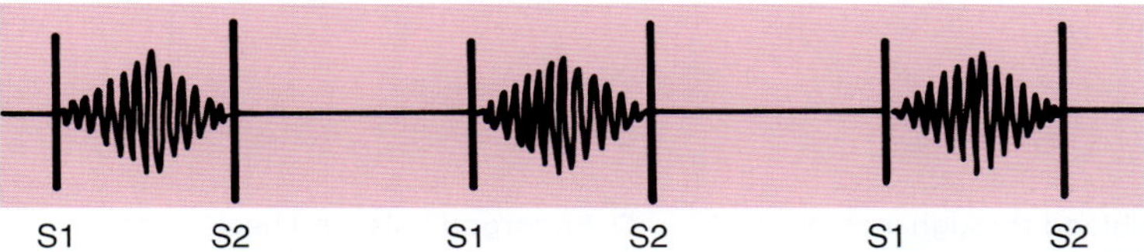

	DESCRIPTION	CLINICAL DATA
Aortic stenosis		
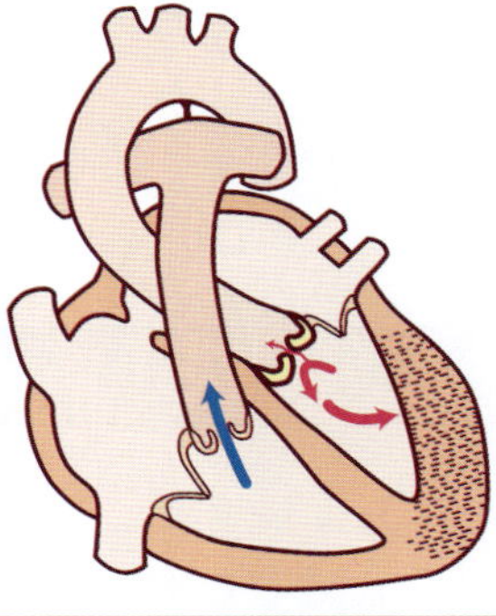	Calcification of aortic valve cusps restricts forward flow of blood during systole; LV hypertrophy develops.	S: Fatigue, SOB, SOBOE, palpitation, dizziness, fainting, anginal pain. O: Pallor, slow diminished radial pulse, low blood pressure and auscultatory gap are common. Apical impulse sustained and displaced to left. Thrill in systole over second and third right interspaces and right side of neck. **S_1** normal, often ejection click present, often paradoxical split **S_2**, **S_4** present with LV hypertrophy. Murmur: loud, harsh, midsystolic, crescendo-decrescendo, loudest at second right interspace, radiates widely to side of neck, down left sternal border, or apex.
Pulmonic stenosis		
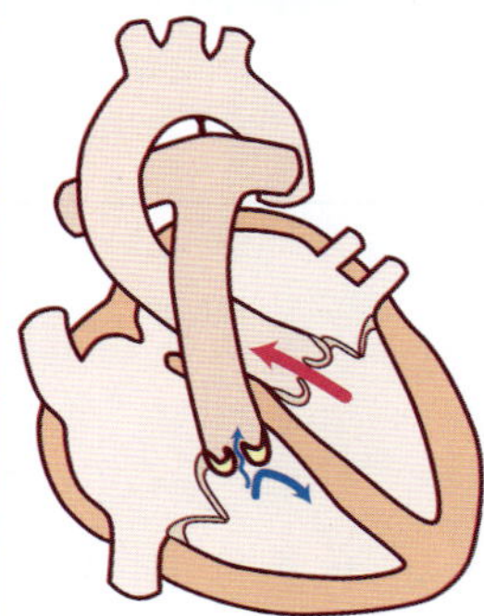	Calcification of pulmonic valve restricts forward flow of blood.	O: Thrill in systole at second and third left interspace, ejection click often present after **S_1**, diminished **S_2** and usually with wide split, **S_4** common with RV hypertrophy. Murmur: systolic, medium pitch, coarse, crescendo-decrescendo (diamond shape), best heard at second left interspace, radiates to left and neck.

(Continued)

TABLE 17.11 Murmurs due to valvular defects—cont'd

Pansystolic regurgitant murmurs		
Due to backward flow of blood from area of higher pressure to one of lower pressure 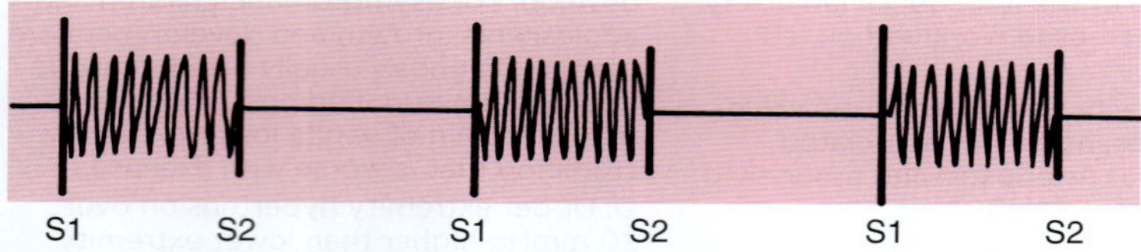 		
Mitral regurgitation		
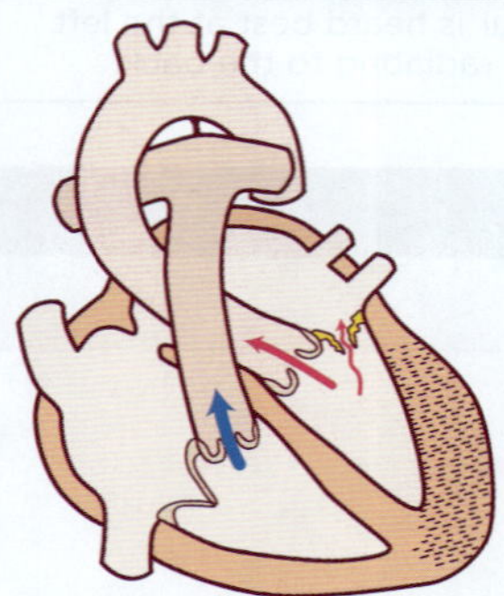	Stream of blood regurgitates back into LA during systole through incompetent mitral valve. In diastole, blood passes back into LV again along with new flow; results in LV dilatation and hypertrophy.	S: Fatigue, palpitation, orthopnoea, PND. O: Thrill in systole at apex. Lift at apex. Apical impulse displaced down and to left. **S**$_1$ diminished, **S**$_2$ accentuated, **S**$_3$ at apex often present. Murmur: pansystolic, often loud, blowing, best heard at apex, radiates well to left axilla.
Tricuspid regurgitation		
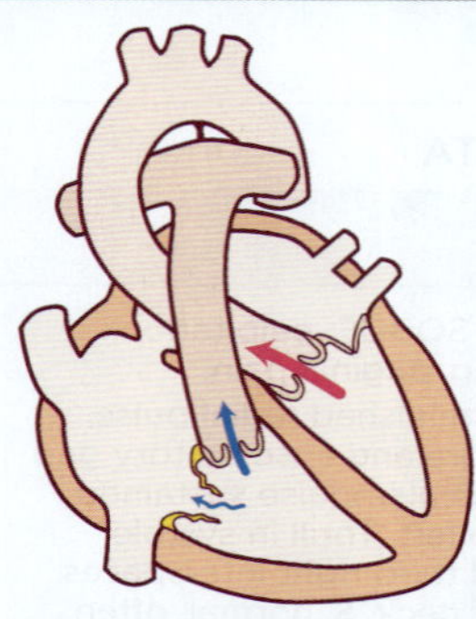	Backflow of blood through incompetent tricuspid valve into RA.	O: Engorged pulsating neck veins, liver enlarged. Lift at sternum if RV hypertrophy present, often thrill at left lower sternal border. Murmur: soft, blowing, pansystolic, best heard at left lower sternal border, increases with inspiration.
Diastolic rumbles of AV valves		
Filling murmurs at low pressures, best heard with bell lightly touching skin 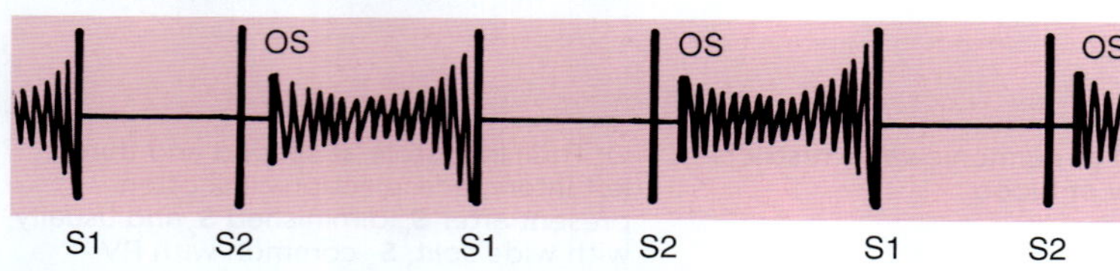 		

TABLE 17.11 Murmurs due to valvular defects—cont'd

Mitral stenosis

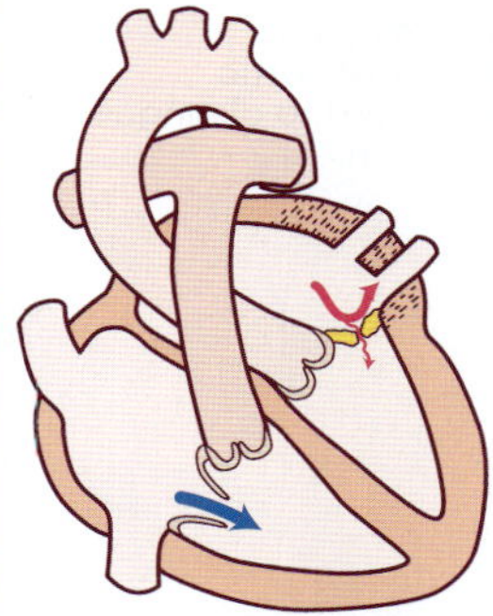

Calcified mitral valve will not open properly, impedes forward flow of blood into LV during diastole. Results in LA enlarged and LA pressure increased.

S: Fatigue, palpitations, SOBOE, orthopnoea, occasional PND or pulmonary oedema.

O: Diminished, often irregular arterial pulse. Lift at apex, diastolic thrill common at apex. $\mathbf{S_1}$ accentuated; opening snap after $\mathbf{S_2}$ heard over wide area of praecordium, followed by murmur.

Murmur: low-pitched diastolic rumble, best heard at apex, with person in left lateral position; does not radiate.

Tricuspid stenosis

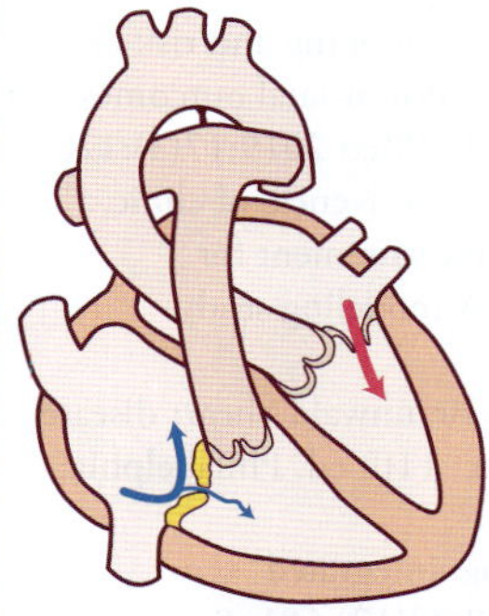

Calcification of tricuspid valve impedes forward flow into RV during diastole.

O: Diminished arterial pulse, jugular venous pulse prominent.

Murmur: diastolic rumble; best heard at left lower sternal border; louder in inspiration.

Early diastolic murmurs

Due to SL valve incompetence

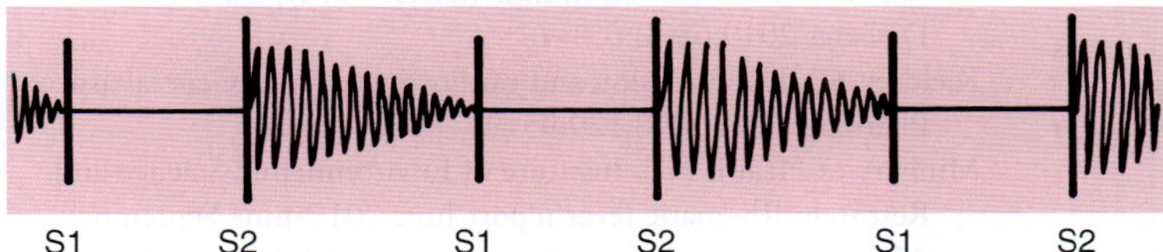

Aortic regurgitation

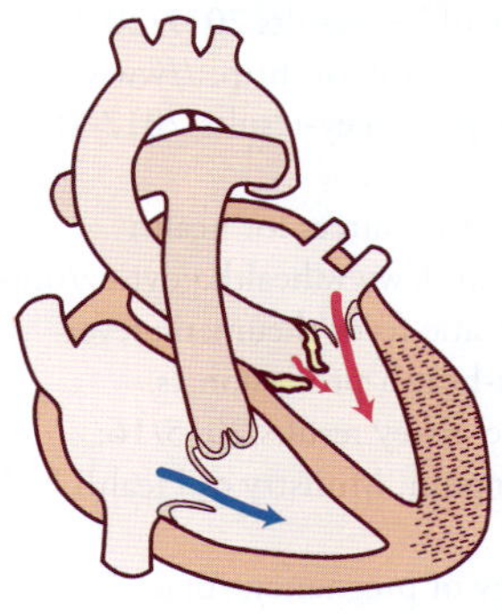

Stream of blood regurgitates back through incompetent aortic valve into LV during diastole. LV dilatation and hypertrophy due to increased LV stroke volume. Rapid ejection of large stroke volume into poorly filled aorta, then rapid runoff in diastole as part of blood pushed back into LV.

S: Only minor symptoms for many years, then rapid deterioration: SOBOE, PND, angina, dizziness.

O: Bounding 'water-hammer' pulse in carotid, brachial and femoral arteries. Blood pressure has wide pulse pressure. Pulsations in cervical and suprasternal area, apical impulse displaced to left and down, apical impulse feels brief.

Murmur starts almost simultaneously with $\mathbf{S_2}$: soft high pitched, blowing diastolic, decrescendo, best heard at third left interspace at base, as person sits up and leans forwards, radiates down.

(Continued)

TABLE 17.11 Murmurs due to valvular defects—cont'd

Pulmonic regurgitation		
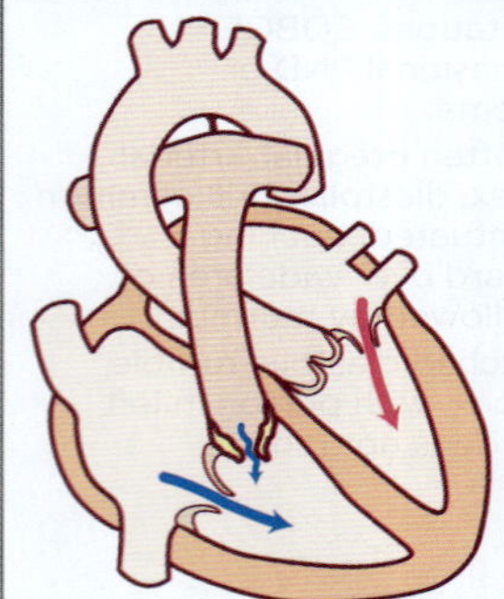	Backflow of blood through incompetent pulmonic valve, from pulmonary artery to RV.	Murmur has same timing and characteristics as that of aortic regurgitation, and is hard to distinguish on physical examination.

BIBLIOGRAPHY

Abouzeid M, Wyber R, La Vincente S, et al. Time to tackle rheumatic heart disease: data needed to drive global policy dialogues. Glob Public Health 2019 Mar 4;14(3):456–68.

Aroney CN, Cullen L. Appropriate use of serum troponin testing in general practice: a narrative review. Med J Aust 2016 Jul;205(2):91–4.

Australian Bureau of Statistics (ABS). National health survey: First results 2017–2018—High cholesterol, Cat No. 4364.0.55.001. 2018. Available at: https://www.abs.gov.au/ausstats/abs@.nsf/Lookup/by%20Subject/4364.0.55.001~2017-18~Main%20Features~High%20cholesterol~45.

Australian Bureau of Statistics (ABS). National health survey: First results 2017–2018—Smoking, Cat No. 4364.0.55.001. 2019. Available at: https://www.abs.gov.au/ausstats/abs@.nsf/Lookup/by%20Subject/4364.0.55.001~2017-18~Main%20Features~Smoking~85.

Australian Health Ministers' Advisory Council. Aboriginal and Torres Strait Islander health performance framework 2017 Report. Canberra: AHMAC; 2017. Available at: https://www.pmc.gov.au/resource-centre/indigenous-affairs/health-performance-framework-2017-report.

Australian Institute of Health & Welfare. Cardiovascular disease snapshot. Catalogue number CVD83. Canberra: AIHW; 2018a. Available at: https://www.aihw.gov.au/reports/heart-stroke-vascular-disease/cardiovascular-health-compendium/contents/how-many-australians-have-cardiovascular-disease.

Australian Institute of Health and Welfare (AIHW). Australia's health 2018. Canberra: AIHW, Australia's health series no. 16. AUS 221. 2018b. Available at: https://www.aihw.gov.au/reports/australias-health/australias-health-2018/contents/table-of-contents.

Australian Institute of Health & Welfare. Diabetes snapshot. Catalogue number CVD82. Canberra: AIHW; 2018c. Available at: https://www.aihw.gov.au/reports/diabetes/diabetes-snapshot/contents/how-many-australians-have-diabetes.

Australian Institute of Health & Welfare. Acute rheumatic fever and rheumatic heart disease in Australia, Web report, Cat. No: CVD86. 2019. Available at: https://www.aihw.gov.au/reports/indigenous-australians/acute-rheumatic-fever-rheumatic-heart-disease/contents/summary.

Australian Red Cross Blood Service. Anaemia. 2019. Available at: https://mytransfusion.com.au/reasons-transfusion/anaemia.

Banks E, Joshy G, Korda RJ, et al. Tobacco smoking and risk of 36 cardiovascular disease subtypes: fatal and non-fatal outcomes in a large prospective Australian study. BMC Med 2019;17(1):128.

Beyhaghi H, Viera AJ. Comparative cost-effectiveness of clinic, home, or ambulatory blood pressure measurement for hypertension diagnosis in US adults: A modeling study. Hypertension 2019;73(1):121–31.

Bonow R, Mann D, Tomaselli G, editor. Braunwald's heart disease: a textbook of cardio-vascular medicine. 11th ed. Philadelphia: Saunders; 2018.

Brennan EJ. Chronic heart failure nursing: integrated multidisciplinary care. Br J Nurs 2018;27(12):681–8.

DiGiacomo SI, Jazayeri MA, Barua RS, et al. Environmental tobacco smoke and cardiovascular disease. Int J Environ Res Public Health 2019;16(1):96.

Haas AV, Rosner BA, Kwong RY, et al. Sex differences in coronary microvascular function in individuals with type 2 diabetes. Diabetes 2019;68(3):631–6.

Kjeldsen SE. Hypertension and cardiovascular risk: General aspects. Pharmacol Res 2018;129:95–9.

Ministry of Health NZ, Institute of Environmental Science and Research: Rhematic fever report June 2017-June September 2018. Available at: https://surv.esr.cri.nz/PDF_surveillance/RheumaticFever/RheumaticfeverbI-annualreportJuly2017-June2018.pdf.

Ministry of Health NZ. Annual update of key results 2017/2018: New Zealand health survey. 2019. Available at: https://www.health.govt.nz/publication/annual-update-key-results-2017-18-new-zealand-health-survey.

Ministry of Health NZ. Rheumatic fever resources for health professionals. 2017. Available at: https://www.health.govt.nz/our-work/diseases-and-conditions/rheumatic-fever/rheumatic-fever-resources/rheumatic-fever-resources-health-professionals.

Ministry of Health NZ. Annual update of key results 2015/16: New Zealand Health Survey. Wellington: Ministry of Health NZ; 2016.

Mockridge A, Maclennan K. Physiology of pregnancy. Anaesth Intens Care Med 2019. Available at: https://doi.org/10.1016/j.mpaic.2019.05.001.

Nanayakkara S, Marwick TH, Kaye DM. The ageing heart: the systemic and coronary circulation. Heart 2018;104(5):370–6.

Rheumatic Heart Disease Australia. Available at: https://www.rhdaustralia.org.au

Royal College of Pathologists Australia (RCPA). RCPA manual of use and interpretation of pathology tests. 2019. Available at: https://www.rcpa.edu.au/Manuals/RCPA-Manual.

Talley NJ, O'Connor S. Clinical examination: a systematic guide to physical diagnosis. 8th ed. Chatswood, NSW: Elsevier; 2018.

Tortora GJ, Derrickson BH. Principles of anatomy and physiology. 2nd Asia-Pacific ed. Melbourne: Wiley; 2019.

World Health Organisation. 2020. Obesity and overweight. Available at: https://www.who.int/en/news-room/fact-sheets/detail/obesity-and-overweight

Zhang D, Tu H, Wadman MC, et al. Substrates and potential therapeutics of ventricular arrhythmias in heart failure. Eur J Pharmacol 2018;833:349–56.

Zipes DP, Libby P, Bonow RO, et al. Braunwald's heart disease: a textbook of cardiovascular medicine. Philadelphia: Elsevier Saunders; 2018.

Websites

Australasian Cardiovascular Nursing College. Available at: www.acnc.net.au

Australian Institute of Health & Welfare. Available at: www.aihw.gov.au

Cardiac Society of Australia & New Zealand. Available at: www.csanz.edu.au

Cardiomyopathy Association of Australia. Available at: www.cmaa.org.au

Heart Foundation (Australia). Available at: https://www.heartfoundation.org.au

Heart Foundation New Zealand. Available at: www.heartfoundation.org.nz

Indigenous HeartInfoNet web resource. Available at: healthinfonet.ecu.edu.au/learn/health-topics/cardiovascular-health

Rheumatic Heart Disease Australia. Available at: https://www.rhdaustralia.org.au

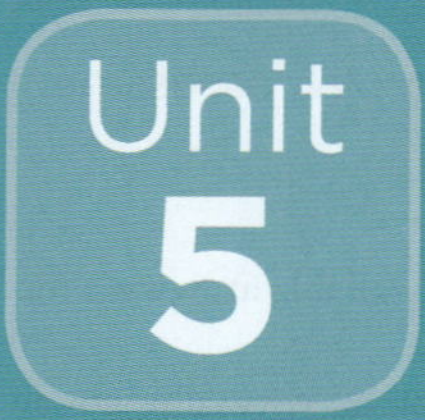

Unit 5

Assessing respiratory function

Chapter Eighteen

Upper airways assessment

Written by Carolyn Jarvis
Adapted by Amy Johnston

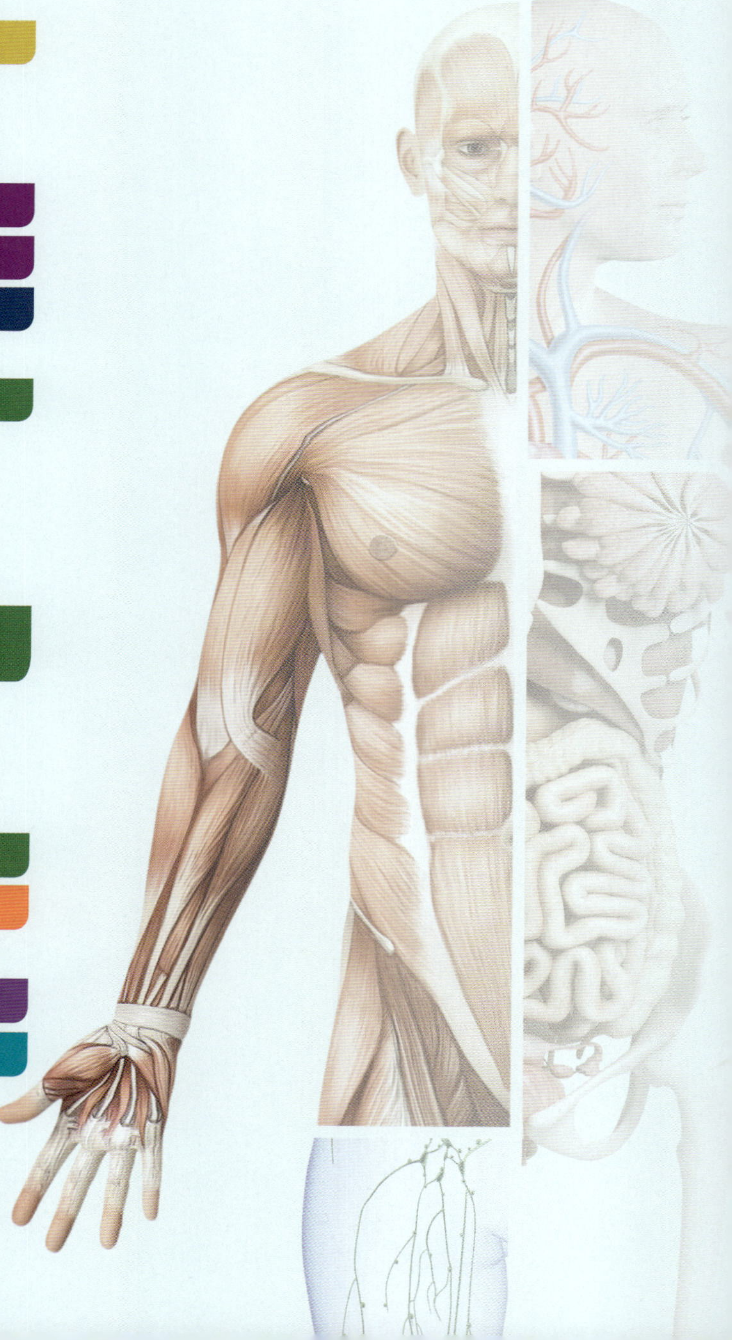

INTRODUCTION

The upper airways, including the nose and throat, are especially important when considering a person's respiratory and olfactory function. To appreciate the impact of disease, trauma and/or alteration in the function of these intricate structures you are advised to review the structure and function of the nose and throat and the relationships to each other in light of the primary digestive function of the mouth (Chapter 21).

Structure and function

NOSE

The **nose** is the first segment of the respiratory system. It warms, moistens and filters the inhaled air, and it is a key sensory organ for chemical senses, including smell. The external nose is shaped like a triangle with one side attached to the face (Figure 18.1). On its leading edge, the superior part is the *bridge* and the free corner is the *tip*. The oval openings of the nose are the *nares* (nostrils); just inside, each naris widens into the *vestibule*. The *columella* divides the two nares and is continuous inside with the nasal septum. The *ala* is the lateral outside wing of the nose on either side. The support for the upper third of the external nose is made up of bone; the nasal bone, medially and the frontal processes of the maxillary bones laterally. The lower two-thirds of the support structure for the nose is made up of the septal and alar cartilages.

The space inside the **nasal cavity** is much larger than the external nose suggests (Figure 18.2). Nasal space extends back inside the skull over the roof of the mouth. The anterior edge of the cavity is lined with numerous coarse nasal hairs, or vibrissae. The cavity is lined with a blanket of ciliated mucous membrane. The nasal hairs filter the coarsest matter from inhaled air, including insects and other floating debris, helping to block the entry of very large particles into the airway. The ciliated mucous blanket, the respiratory mucosa, further inside the nasal space traps smaller particles such as dust and bacteria, enhancing air filtration to limit particle movement into the lower respiratory spaces. Nasal mucosa appears redder than oral mucosa because of the richer blood supply present, used to warm and humidify inhaled air and ensure ongoing mucous production.

The nasal cavity is divided medially by the **septum** into two slit-like air passages. The anterior part of the septum holds a rich vascular network, *Kiesselbach's plexus* or *Little's area*, the most common origin of nosebleeds. In many people, the nasal septum is not absolutely straight and may deviate towards one or the other passage. This deviation may contribute to poor airflow and snoring.

The lateral walls of each nasal cavity contain three parallel bony projections—the superior, middle and inferior **turbinates**. They increase the surface area inside the nasal passages so that more blood vessels and ciliated mucous membranes are available to warm, humidify and filter the inhaled air. They also provide an area across which olfactory (smell) receptors can be located. Underlying each turbinate is a cleft, the **meatus**, which is named for the turbinate above. The sinuses drain into the middle meatus, and tears from the nasolacrimal duct drain into the inferior meatus.

The olfactory receptors lie embedded in the olfactory mucosa on the roof of the nasal cavity and in the upper one-third of the septum. The neurons associated with these receptors for smell merge to form the olfactory nerve, cranial nerve I, which moves through the sieve-like cribriform plate of the ethmoid bone and transmit to the temporal lobe of the brain. While smell is not considered necessary for human survival, loss of the sense of smell can decrease food enjoyment and potentially impact on food choices and kilojoule intake (Schwartz et al 2018). Increasingly, smell is used as a marker of possible neural degeneration as it decays in people with many neurodegenerative conditions such as Alzheimer's disease and schizophrenia prior to the onset of other neurological symptoms (Marin et al 2018). Olfactory neurons are special in that in healthy persons, they regenerate throughout life. Stem cells that give rise to olfactory cells are present in the olfactory mucosa (Boody et al 2019).

The **paranasal sinuses** are air-filled pockets within the cranial bones of the skull (Figure 18.3). They communicate with the nasal cavity and are lined with the same type of ciliated mucous membrane. They lighten the weight of the skull bones, serve

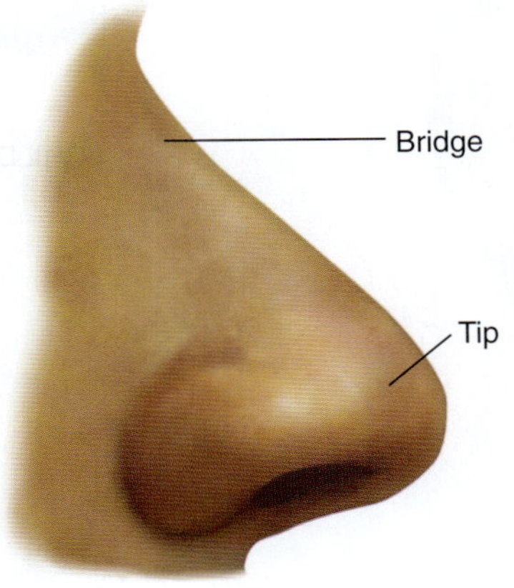

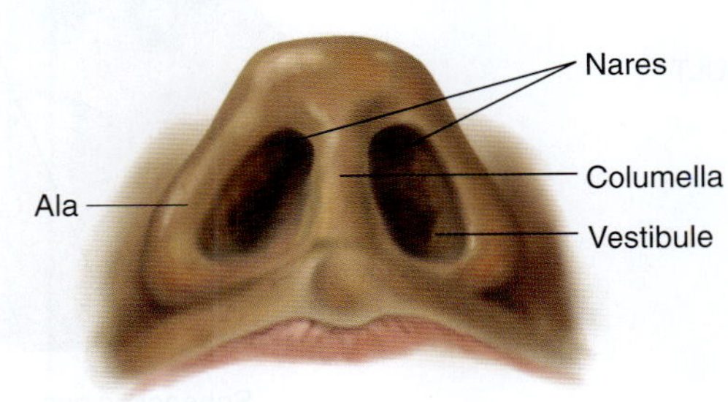

Figure 18.1
Nasal structures.

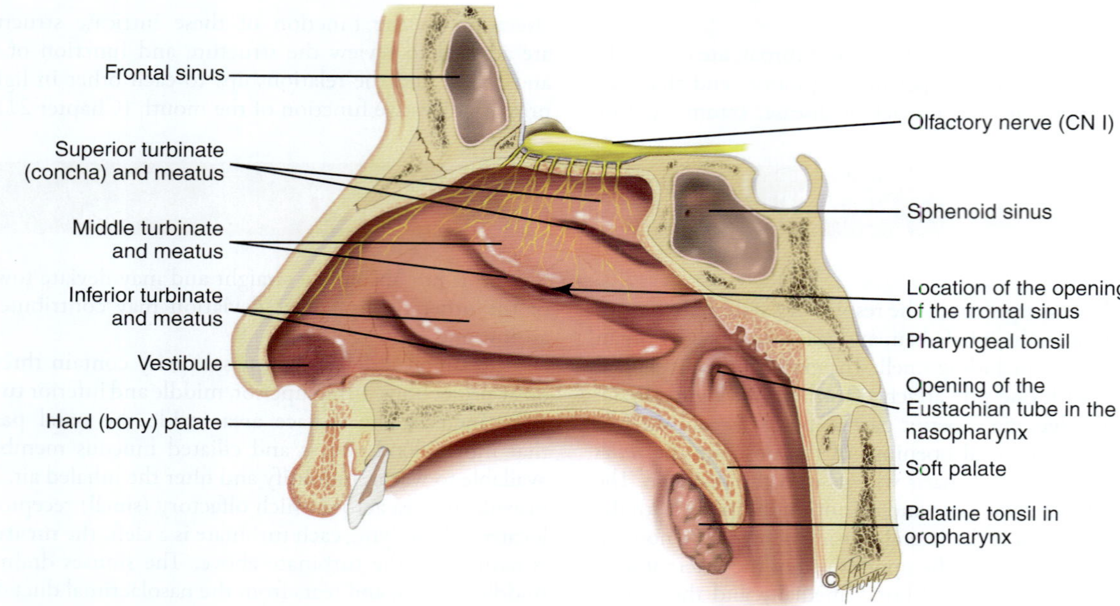

Figure 18.2

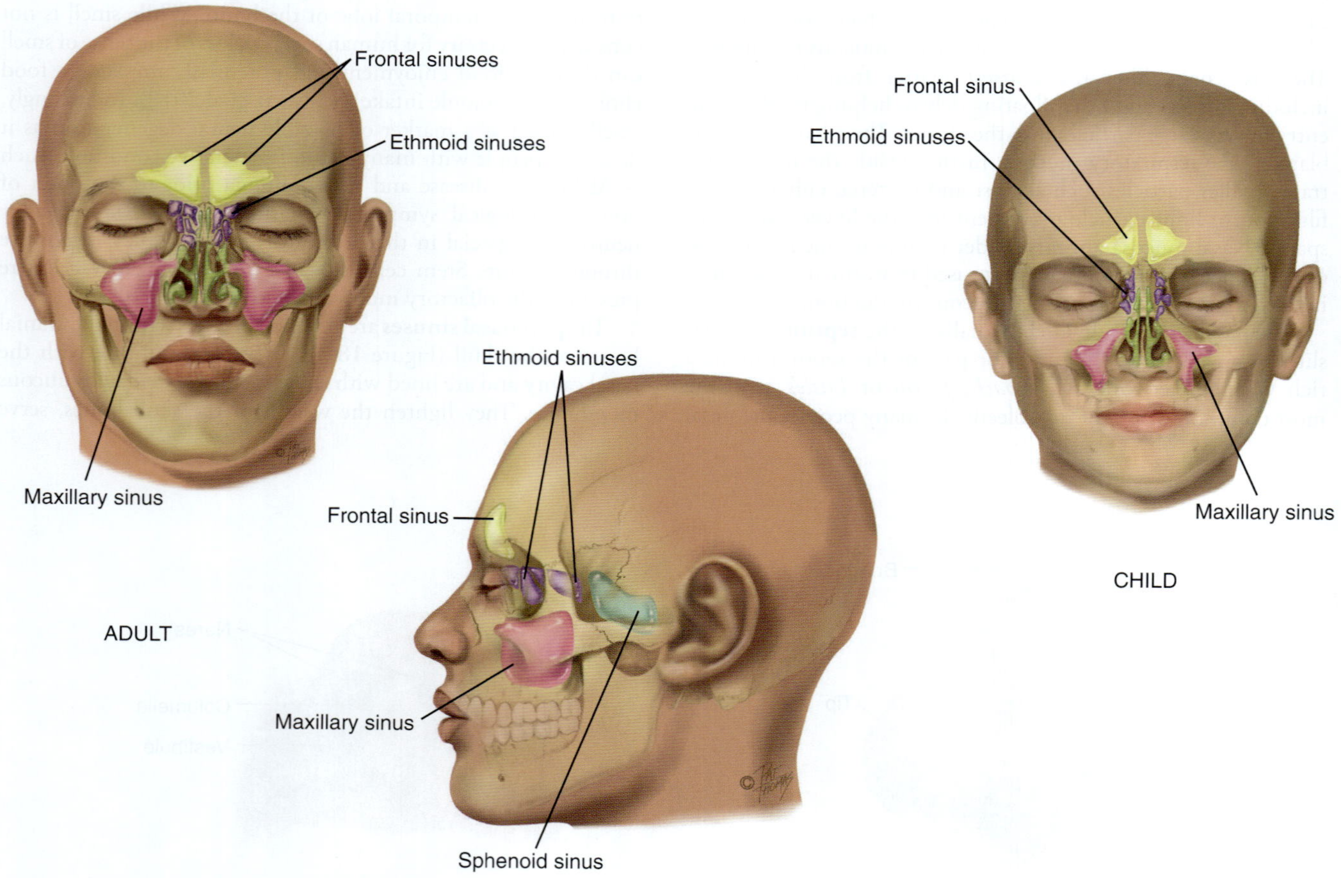

Frontal sinuses
Ethmoid sinuses
Maxillary sinus
ADULT
Ethmoid sinuses
Frontal sinus
Maxillary sinus
Sphenoid sinus
Frontal sinus
Ethmoid sinuses
Maxillary sinus
CHILD

Figure 18.3
Paranasal sinuses.

as resonators for sound production and provide mucus which drains into the nasal cavity. The sinus openings are narrow and easily occluded, which may cause pressure build-up, discomfort and enhanced/associated inflammation or sinusitis.

Two pairs of sinuses are accessible to examination: the **frontal** sinuses in the frontal bone above and medial to the orbits and the **maxillary** sinuses in the maxilla (cheekbone) along the side walls of the nasal cavity. The other two sets are smaller and deeper: the **ethmoid** sinuses between the orbits and the **sphenoid** sinuses deep within the skull in the sphenoid bone. Sinuses support the humidification and warming of inspired air and the trapping of moisture and warmth in the body during exhalation.

Only the maxillary and ethmoid sinuses are present at birth. The maxillary sinuses reach full size after all permanent teeth have erupted. The ethmoid sinuses grow rapidly between 6 and 8 years of age and after puberty. The frontal sinuses are absent at birth, are fairly well developed between 7 and 8 years of age and reach full size after puberty. The sphenoid sinuses are minute at birth and develop after puberty.

THROAT

The throat, or pharynx, is the area of the upper airway behind or posterior to the mouth and nose. The most superior section of the pharynx, directly behind the nose, is the nasopharynx. The pharyngeal tonsils (adenoids) and the pharyngotympanic (Eustachian) tube openings are located in the nasopharyngeal region (see Figure 19.1). Inferior to, but continuous with, the nasopharynx is the **oropharynx**. The **oropharynx** is separated from the mouth by a fold of tissue on each side, the anterior tonsillar pillar. Behind the folds are the palatine and lingual **tonsils**, each a mass of lymphoid tissue. The tonsils are the same colour as the surrounding mucous membrane, although they look more granular, and their surface shows deep crypts. Tonsillar tissue enlarges during childhood until puberty and then involutes. The posterior pharyngeal wall is seen behind these structures. Some small blood vessels may be visible.

The **nasopharynx** is continuous with the oropharynx, although it is above the oropharynx and behind the nasal cavity. The pharyngeal tonsils (adenoids) and the Eustachian tube openings are located here (see Figure 18.2). The section of the pharynx below the level of the epiglottis is known as the laryngopharyngeal region: the entry to the larynx (voice box) and the trachea (lower section of the upper airway).

LYMPHATICS

The lymphatic system is an extensive vessel system, which is separate from the cardiovascular system. The lymphatics are a major part of the immune system, whose function is to detect and eliminate foreign substances from the body. The vessels allow the flow of clear, watery fluid (lymph) from the tissue spaces into the lymphatic and then back into the cardiovascular circulation. Lymph nodes are small, oval clusters of lymphatic tissue that are set at intervals along the lymph vessels like beads on a string (Figure 18.4). The nodes filter the lymph and engulf pathogens, limiting potentially harmful substances from entering the circulation. Nodes are located throughout the body but are accessible to palpation examination only in four areas: head and neck, arms, axillae and inguinal region. The oral cavity and throat have a rich lymphatic network (Figure 18.5). Although sources differ as to their nomenclature, one commonly used system is given here. Note that their labels correspond to adjacent structures.

- *Preauricular*, in front of the ear
- *Posterior auricular* (mastoid), superficial to the mastoid process
- *Occipital*, at the base of the skull

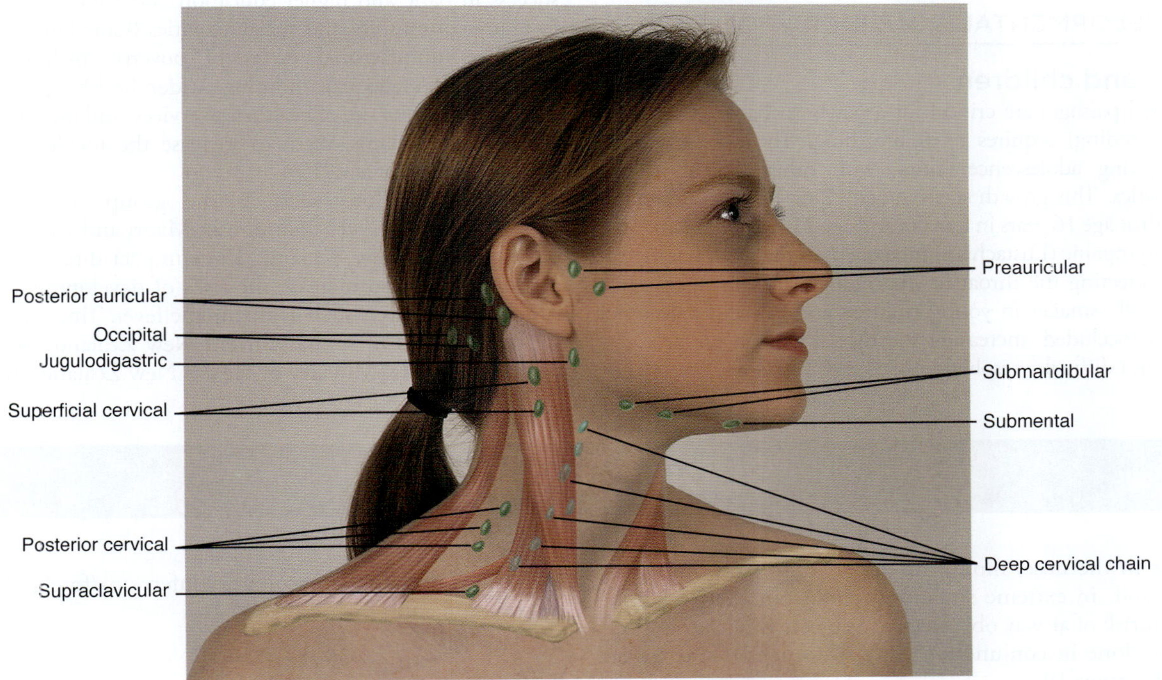

Figure 18.4

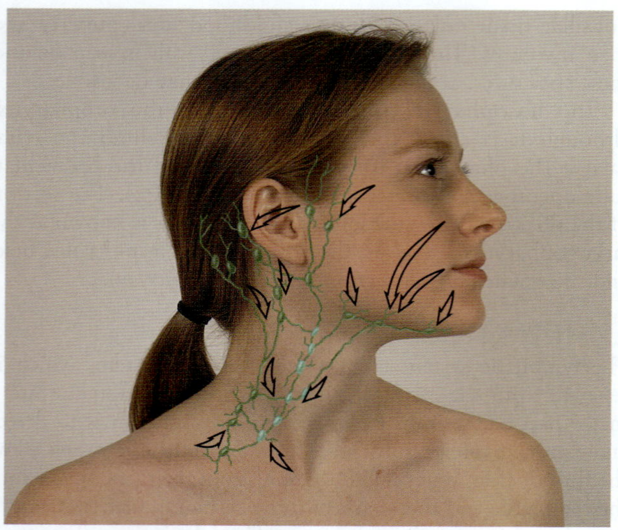

Figure 18.5

- *Submental*, midline, behind the tip of the mandible
- *Submandibular*, halfway between the angle and the tip of the mandible
- *Jugulodigastric*, under the angle of the mandible
- *Superficial cervical*, overlying the sternocleidomastoid muscle
- *Deep cervical*, deep under the sternocleidomastoid muscle
- *Posterior cervical*, in the posterior triangle along the edge of the trapezius muscle
- *Supraclavicular*, just above and behind the clavicle, at the sternocleidomastoid muscle.

DEVELOPMENTAL CONSIDERATIONS

Infants and children

Patent nasal passages are critical for a newborn baby, as effective suckling (feeding) requires nasal breathing. The nose develops further during adolescence, along with other secondary sex characteristics. This growth starts at age 12 or 13 years, reaching full growth at age 16 years in females and age 21 years in males. The pharyngotympanic (Eustachian) tube opens in the nasopharyngeal region connecting the throat to the middle ear. This opening is proportionally smaller in young children and can easily become blocked or occluded, increasing the risk of middle ear pressure variation and difficulty resolving middle ear infections.

The upper sections of the trachea (subglottic region) tend to be proportionally narrower in young children with a very vascular and loosely attached mucosal lining. This increases the risks of partial and even total occlusion of the airway with infection and inflammation, particularly associated with high risk conditions such as epiglottitis.

The pregnant woman

Nasal stuffiness and epistaxis may occur during pregnancy because of increased vascularity in the upper respiratory tract. The gums may be hyperaemic and softened, and may bleed with normal toothbrushing.

Late adulthood (65+ years)

A gradual loss of subcutaneous fat starts during later middle adult years, making the nose appear more prominent in some people. The nasal hairs grow coarser and stiffer and may not filter the air as well. The hairs may protrude and cause itching and sneezing. Many older people clip these hairs, thinking them unsightly, but this practice may increase the risk of infection and airway irritation. Olfaction, or the sense of smell, may diminish for many reasons, including underlying neurodegenerative disorders.

CULTURAL AND SOCIAL CONSIDERATIONS

Ear, nose and throat infections remain almost twice as high in the Australian Indigenous population as in the remainder of the population, contributing to the potentially preventable hospitalisation rates in Indigenous Australians (AIHW 2019). These infections contribute to burden of disease in the Australian Indigenous population (Azzopardi et al 2018). The hearing impairment resulting from un/poorly treated otitis media has been recognised to reduce engagement with written and aural media, success in basic and higher education and ability to participate in many community and social activities (Graydon et al 2019). Ongoing multifactorial cycles of poverty, malnourishment, overcrowded inadequate housing, wider health ignorance and lack of access to or use of healthcare services, and thus poor health and living standards, seem to increase the incidence of otitis media (Banham et al 2019).

Throat infections such as the group A streptococcal infections are also very common in Māori and Pacific Islander populations in New Zealand. These impact directly on health outcomes and also increase the risks of development of acute systemic conditions such as rheumatic fever. Thus, strep throat forms the focus of several current New Zealand government health initiatives (Ministry of Health New Zealand 2017).

Subjective data

Disorders in the nose, mouth or throat cause pain, impaired function and, in extreme situations, could put the person at significant risk of airway obstruction. Subjective data collection should be done in conjunction with assessment of the lower airways (Chapter 19).

1. Presenting concern
2. Nasal discharge
3. Blocked nose (upper respiratory infections/foreign body/ common cold)
4. Sinus pain
5. Trauma
6. Epistaxis (nosebleeds)
7. Allergies

8. Altered smell
9. Pain in mouth or throat
10. Sores or lesions in mouth or throat
11. Hoarseness or change in voice
12. Lumps or swelling in the neck, mouth or throat
13. Health and lifestyle management

Practice note: Before you commence the assessment, introduce yourself to the person, confirm the person's identity, discuss the purpose and scope of the assessment, clarify any questions the person may have and obtain verbal consent from the person to perform the assessment.

SUBJECTIVE DATA

ASSESSMENT GUIDELINES	CLINICAL SIGNIFICANCE AND CLINICAL ALERTS
1. Presenting concern	
Do you feel you have any problem with your nose mouth or throat? It is important to ascertain the person's perception of their health of their upper airways. If a problem is perceived, ask, 'Does this impact on your quality of life, and how?'	
2. Any ear, nose or throat discharge	
Any nasal discharge or runny nose? Continuous? • Is the discharge watery, purulent, mucoid, bloody? • Describe any ear or throat discharge and frequency	**Rhinorrhoea** occurs with colds, allergies, sinus infection, trauma.
3. Blocked nose (upper respiratory infections/foreign body/common cold)	
Any unusually frequent or severe colds (upper respiratory infections)? How often do these occur?	Most people have occasional colds; thus, asking this more precise question yields more meaningful data.
4. Sinus pain	
Any sinus pain or sinusitis? How is this treated? • Do you have chronic postnasal drip?	**Chronic postnasal drip** is a sign of sinusitis.
5. Trauma	
Ever had any trauma or a blow to the nose? • Can you breathe through your nose? Are both sides obstructed, or one?	Trauma may cause deviated septum, which may cause nares to be obstructed.
6. Epistaxis (nosebleeds)	
Any nosebleeds? How often? • How much bleeding—a teaspoonful or does it pour out? • Colour of the blood—red or brown? Clots? • From one nostril or both? • Aggravated by nose-picking or scratching?	**Epistaxis** occurs with trauma, vigorous nose blowing, foreign body.
• How do you treat the nosebleeds? Are they difficult to stop?	Person should sit up with head tilted forwards, pinch nose between thumb and forefinger for 5–15 min.
7. Allergies	
Any **allergies** or hay fever? To what are you allergic (e.g. pollen, dust, pets)? • How was this determined? • What type of environment makes it worse? Can you avoid exposure?	**'Seasonal' rhinitis** if due to pollen; 'perennial' if allergen is dust.
• Do you use inhalers, nasal spray, nose drops? How often? Which type? • How long have you used this?	Misuse of over-the-counter nasal medications may irritate the mucosa, causing rebound swelling, a common problem.

SUBJECTIVE DATA

ASSESSMENT GUIDELINES	CLINICAL SIGNIFICANCE AND CLINICAL ALERTS
8. Altered smell	
Experienced any change in sense of smell or received reports of altered smelling ability from associates?	People are often poor at detecting changes in their smelling ability and often rely on reports from others. Sense of smell may deteriorate with chronic allergy, decreased nasal patency, prolonged cigarette smoking or the development of neurodegenerative conditions such as Alzheimer's, Parkinson's or motor neuron diseases.
9. Pain in mouth or throat	
Do you currently have a **sore throat**? When did it start? How frequently do you get them?	
• Is it associated with cough, fever, fatigue, decreased appetite, headache, postnasal drip or hoarseness?	
• Is it worse when rising? What is the humidity level in the room where you sleep? Any dust or smoke inhaled at work?	
• How have you treated this sore throat: medication, gargling? How effective are these? Have your tonsils or adenoids been taken out?	Untreated **streptococcal infection** of the throat may lead to the complication of acute rheumatic fever.
10. Sores or lesions	
Have you noticed any **sores** or **ulcers** in the mouth, tongue or gums? • How long have you had it? Ever had this before? • Is it single or multiple?	History helps determine whether oral lesions have infectious, traumatic, immunological or malignant aetiology.
• Does it seem to be associated with stress, season change, food?	
• How have you treated the sore? Applied any local medication?	
11. Hoarseness or change in voice	
Do you have any **hoarseness**, voice change? For how long? • Feel like having to clear your throat? Or, like a 'lump in your throat'? • Use your voice a lot at work, recreation? • Does the hoarseness seem associated with a cold, sore throat?	A disorder of the larynx with many causes, such as overuse of the voice, upper respiratory infection, chronic inflammation, lesions or a neoplasm.
12. Lumps, swelling or sore areas in the neck, mouth or throat	
Any **lumps or swelling** in the neck, mouth or throat? • Any recent infection? Any tenderness?	Tenderness suggests acute infection.
• For a lump that persists, how long have you had it? Has it changed in size?	A persistent lump arouses suspicion of malignancy. For those more than 40 years old, suspect malignancy until proven otherwise.

ASSESSMENT GUIDELINES	CLINICAL SIGNIFICANCE AND CLINICAL ALERTS
13. Health and lifestyle management	
Medication use: prescribed and recreational, including smoking. What medications are you taking? If so what and how often? Do you use recreational drugs? If so what and how often? • Do you smoke? Pipe or cigarettes? Nicotine vaporiser? How many packs per day? For how many years?	Chronic tobacco use (smoking and/or chewing) is associated with significant oral and lung disease.
Additional subjective data for infants and children (questions for parents or guardians)	
• Does the child have any mouth lesions or throat infections? How frequently do these occur?	
• Does the child have frequent sore throat, tonsillitis, ear or nasal infections? How often? How are these treated? Have they ever been documented as streptococcal infections?	

Objective data

The purpose of the examination of the upper airways is to assess patterns of pain, or any other abnormalities, and the impact these have on the person's respiratory function. Objective examination should be done in conjunction with assessment of lower airways (Chapter 19).

Preparation

Position the person sitting up straight with their head at your eye level.

Equipment needed

Penlight
Two tongue blades
Hand hygiene solution
Gauze to invert and displace tongue
Can be useful to have access to a suction device, especially for younger children or older adults

PROCEDURES AND NORMAL FINDINGS	ABNORMAL FINDINGS AND CLINICAL ALERTS
General inspection	
During collection of subjective data you will have noticed the colour of the person's skin and mucous membranes, ease of breathing, tone of voice and general demeanor. All of these factors provide clues to the functioning of the upper respiratory system.	
Inspect and palpate the external nose	
Normally, the nose is symmetrical, in the midline and in proportion to other facial features (Figure 18.6A). Inspect for any deformity, asymmetry, deviated septum, inflammation or skin lesions. If an injury is reported or suspected, palpate gently for any pain or break in contour.	A **deviated septum** can cause the person difficulty with breathing through the nose (Figure 18.6B).

PROCEDURES AND NORMAL FINDINGS	ABNORMAL FINDINGS AND CLINICAL ALERTS
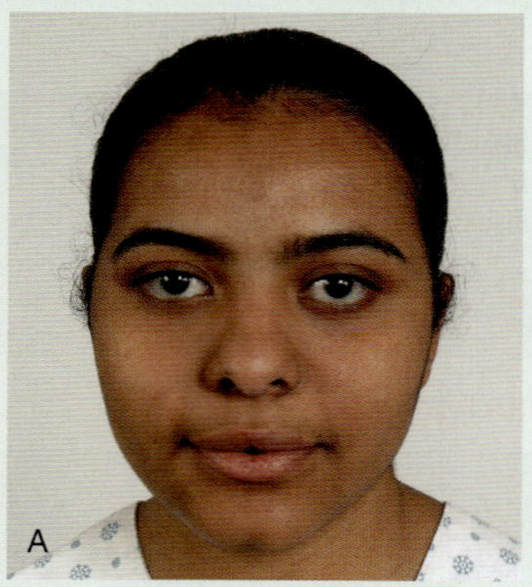 **Figure 18.6A**	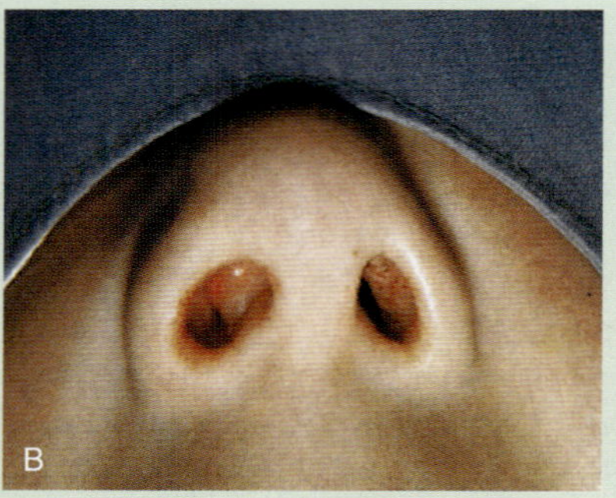 **Figure 18.6B** Deviated septum
Test the patency of the nostrils by pushing each nasal wing shut with your finger while asking the person to sniff inwards through the other naris. This may reveal an obstruction. The sense of smell, mediated by cranial nerve I, is usually not tested in a routine examination. See Chapter 12.	Absence of sniff indicates obstruction (e.g. common cold, nasal polyps, rhinitis).
Inspect the mouth	
Lips and mouth	
Inspect the lips for colour and moisture. Retract the lips and note their inner surface as well (Figure 18.7). Inspect the anterior structures of the mouth and move posteriorly. Use a tongue blade to retract structures and a bright light for optimal visualisation. **Figure 18.7**	**Circumoral pallor** occurs with shock and anaemia; cyanosis (blue tinge) with hypoxaemia and chilling; cherry red lips with carbon monoxide poisoning. ***Clinical alert:*** a significant change in the colour of the lips indicates the need for immediate further assessment.
Tongue	
Check the tongue for presence of swelling.	***Clinical alert:*** While nurses would not normally check for tongue swelling when assessing the upper airways, where there is evidence of anaphylaxis with sudden onset of dyspnoea and/or dysphagia a medical officer must be notified immediately.

OBJECTIVE DATA

PROCEDURES AND NORMAL FINDINGS	ABNORMAL FINDINGS AND CLINICAL ALERTS
Palate	
Observe the uvula; it normally looks like a fleshy pendant hanging in the midline (Figure 18.8). Ask the person to say 'ahhh' and note the soft palate and uvula rise in the midline. This tests one function of cranial nerve X, the vagus nerve. 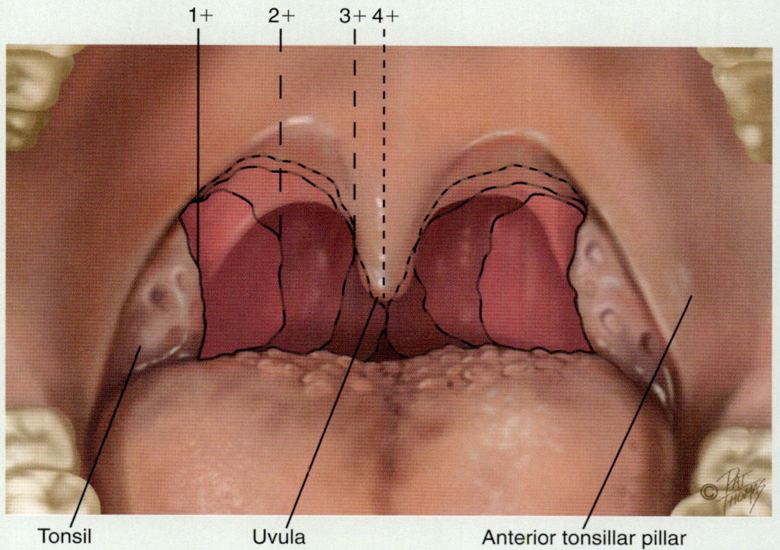 **Figure 18.8**	***Clinical alert*:** Significant oedema may indicate an increased risk of airway compromise and aspiration. Further assessment of swallow and airway patency is required. See Chapter 21 for further information on swallow assessment. See Table 18.2 for abnormalities of the uvula.
Inspect the throat	
With your light, observe the oval, rough-surfaced **tonsils** behind the anterior tonsillar pillar (see Figure 18.8). Their colour is the same pink as the oral mucosa, and their surface is peppered with indentations or crypts. In some people the crypts collect small plugs of whitish cellular debris. This does not indicate infection. However, there should be no exudate on the tonsils. Tonsils are graded in size as follows: **1+** Visible **2+** Halfway between tonsillar pillars and uvula **3+** Touching the uvula **4+** Touching each other You may normally see 1+ or 2+ tonsils in healthy people, especially in children, because lymphoid tissue is proportionately enlarged until puberty.	With an acute infection, tonsils are bright red, swollen and may have exudate or large white spots. See Table 18.2 for abnormalities of the throat. A white membrane covering the tonsils may accompany infectious mononucleosis, leukaemia and diphtheria. Tonsils are enlarged to 2+, 3+ or 4+ with an acute infection.
Enlarge your view of the posterior pharyngeal wall by depressing the tongue with a tongue blade (Figure 18.9). Push down halfway back on the tongue. (Some people can lower their own tongue so the tongue blade is not needed.) Scan the posterior wall for colour, exudate or lesions. When finished, discard the tongue blade.	

PROCEDURES AND NORMAL FINDINGS	ABNORMAL FINDINGS AND CLINICAL ALERTS
Figure 18.9	
During the examination, notice any breath odour. This is common and usually is due to a local cause, such as poor oral hygiene, heavy smoking. Occasionally it may indicate a systemic disease.	A foul, fetid odour may be noticed as occurs in dental or respiratory infections.
Additional objective data for infants and children	
Because the oral examination is intrusive for the infant or young child, consider playing a game to help prepare the child. Encourage the preschool child to use a tongue blade to look into a puppet's mouth. Or place a mirror so that the child can look into the mouth while you do. The school-age child is usually cooperative and loves to show off missing or new teeth. With some infants and toddlers, you need to be opportunistic with this examination. For example, take advantage of crying episodes to examine the open mouth and oropharynx.	
Ask the parent to help position the child. Place the infant supine on the table/bed, with the arms restrained (Figure 18.10). The older infant and toddler may be held on the parent's lap with one of the parent's hands holding the arms down and the other hand securing the child's head against the parent's chest.	
Figure 18.10	

OBJECTIVE DATA

PROCEDURES AND NORMAL FINDINGS	ABNORMAL FINDINGS AND CLINICAL ALERTS
Nose. There should be no nasal flaring or narrowing with breathing. It is essential to determine the patency of the nares in the immediate newborn period because most newborns are nose breathers. When inspection of the nares is indicated, gently push up the tip of the nose with your thumb while using your other hand to shine the light into the naris. With a toddler, be alert for the possible foreign body lodged in the nasal cavity (see Table 18.1).	**Nasal flaring** in the infant indicates respiratory distress and the need for further assessment. A transverse ridge across the nose occurs in a child with chronic allergy from wiping the nose upwards with palm. Nasal narrowing on inhalation is seen with chronic nasal obstruction and mouth breathing.
On the palate, **Epstein pearls** are a normal finding in newborns and infants (Figure 18.11). They are small, whitish, glistening, pearly papules along the median raphe of the hard palate and on the gums, where they look like teeth. They are small retention cysts and disappear in the first few weeks. **Figure 18.11** Epstein pearls.	A high-arched palate is usually normal in the newborn, but a very narrow or high arch also occurs with Turner's syndrome, Ehlers-Danlos syndrome, Marfan's syndrome and Treacher Collins syndrome, or develops in the mouth-breather in chronic allergies.
The tonsils are not visible in the newborn. They gradually enlarge during childhood, remaining proportionately larger until puberty. Tonsils appear still larger if the infant is crying or gagging. Normally the newborn can produce a strong, lusty cry.	

Further objective assessment for advanced practice

The assessments that are described in the following sections require advanced skill and scope of practice. Nurses working in specialist units and some community nurses need to develop these skills.

Equipment

Nasal speculum

PROCEDURES AND NORMAL FINDINGS	ABNORMAL FINDINGS AND CLINICAL ALERTS
Inspect the nasal cavity	
Inspect the turbinates, the bony ridges curving down from the lateral walls. The superior turbinate will not be in your view, but the middle and inferior turbinates appear the same light red colour as the nasal mucosa. Note any swelling but do not try to push the speculum past it. Turbinates are quite vascular and tender if touched.	Turbinates swell marginally in a cyclical manner, thus apparent abnormalities, particularly asymmetries, need to be repeatedly assessed over time.
Note any polyps, benign growths that accompany chronic allergy, and distinguish them from the normal turbinates.	Polyps are smooth, pale grey, avascular, mobile, nontender (see Table 18.1).

PROCEDURES AND NORMAL FINDINGS	ABNORMAL FINDINGS AND CLINICAL ALERTS
Palpate the sinus areas	
Using your thumbs, press over the frontal sinuses below the eyebrows (Figure 18.12A) and over the maxillary sinuses below the cheekbones (Figure 18.12B). Take care not to press directly on the eyeballs. The person should feel firm pressure but no pain. 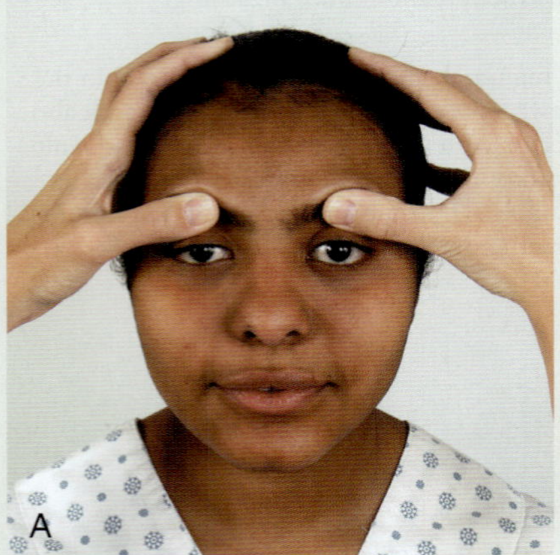 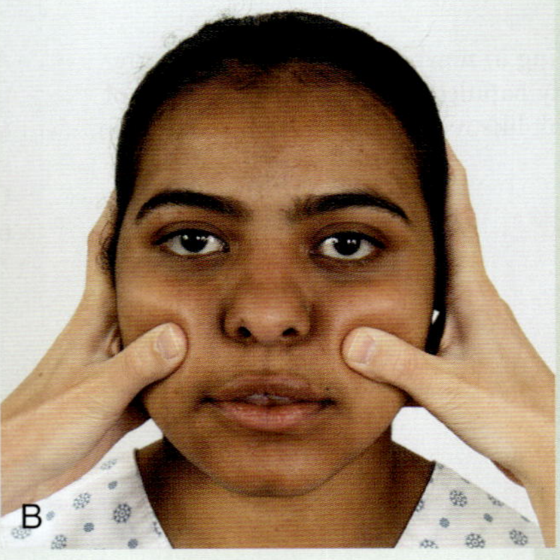 Figure 18.12 A, B	Sinus areas are tender to palpation in persons with chronic allergies and acute infection (**sinusitis**).
Palpate the trachea	
Normally, the trachea is midline; palpate for any tracheal shift. Place your index finger on the trachea in the sternal notch, and slip it off to each side (Figure 18.13). The space should be symmetrical on both sides. Note any deviation from the midline. 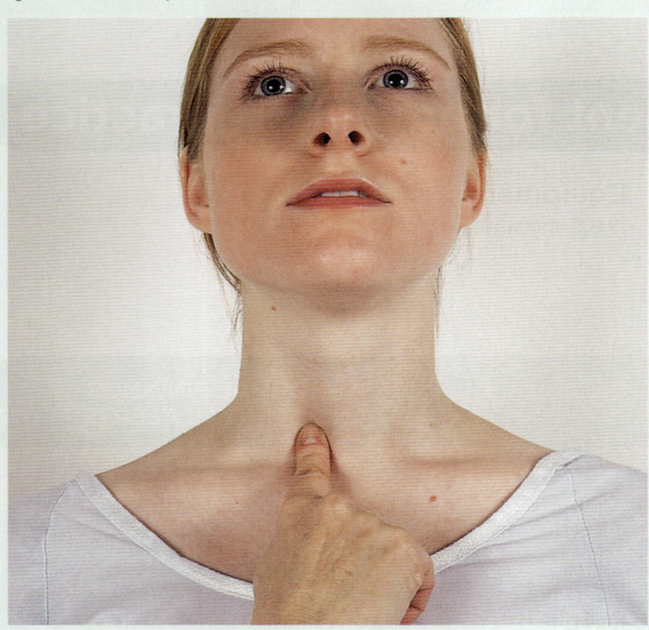 Figure 18.13	Conditions of tracheal shift: • The trachea may be *pushed to the unaffected* (or healthy) side with a pneumothorax, aortic aneurysm, a tumour or unilateral thyroid lobe enlargement. • The trachea is *pulled towards the affected* (diseased) side with significant atelectasis, pleural adhesions or fibrosis. • **Tracheal tug** is a rhythmic downwards pull that is synchronous with systole and occurs with aortic arch aneurysm.

OBJECTIVE DATA

PROCEDURES AND NORMAL FINDINGS	ABNORMAL FINDINGS AND CLINICAL ALERTS
Begin with anterior structures and move posteriorly. Use a tongue blade to retract structures and a bright light for optimal visualisation.	

Palpate the lymph nodes in the neck area

PROCEDURES AND NORMAL FINDINGS	ABNORMAL FINDINGS AND CLINICAL ALERTS
Using a gentle circular motion of your fingerpads, palpate the lymph nodes (Figure 18.14). When symptoms warrant, check for parotid tenderness by palpating in a line from the outer corner of the eye to the lobule of the ear. Beginning with the preauricular lymph nodes in front of the ear, palpate the 10 groups of lymph nodes in a routine order. Many nodes are closely packed, so you must be systematic and thorough in your examination. Once you establish your sequence, do not vary or you may miss some small nodes.	The parotid is swollen with mumps (see Table 21.12).

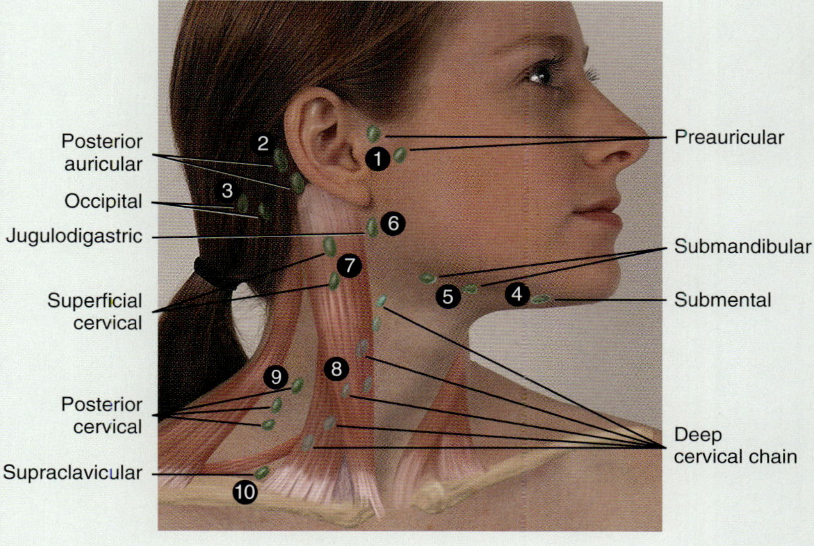

Figure 18.14

PROCEDURES AND NORMAL FINDINGS	ABNORMAL FINDINGS AND CLINICAL ALERTS
Use gentle pressure because strong pressure could push the nodes into the neck muscles. It is usually most efficient to palpate with both hands, comparing the two sides symmetrically. However, the submental gland under the tip of the chin is easier to explore with one hand. When you palpate with one hand, use your other hand to position the person's head. For the deep cervical chain, tip the person's head towards the side being examined to relax the ipsilateral muscle (Figure 18.15). Then you can press your fingers under the muscle. Search for the supraclavicular node by having the person hunch the shoulders and elbows forwards (Figure 18.16); this relaxes the skin. The inferior belly of the omohyoid muscle crosses the posterior triangle here; do not mistake it for a lymph node.	

PROCEDURES AND NORMAL FINDINGS	ABNORMAL FINDINGS AND CLINICAL ALERTS
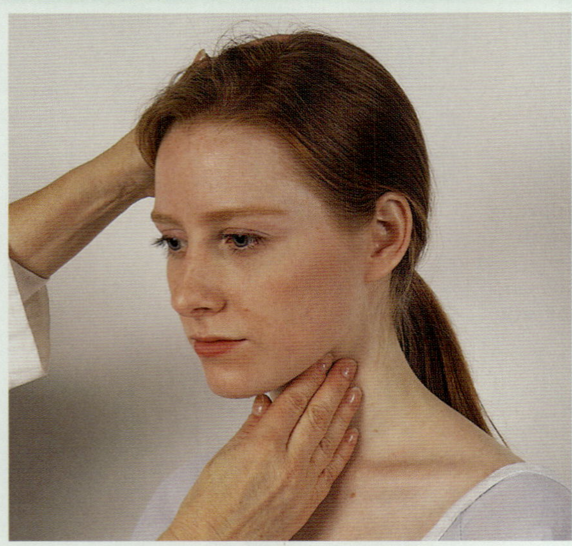 Figure 18.15 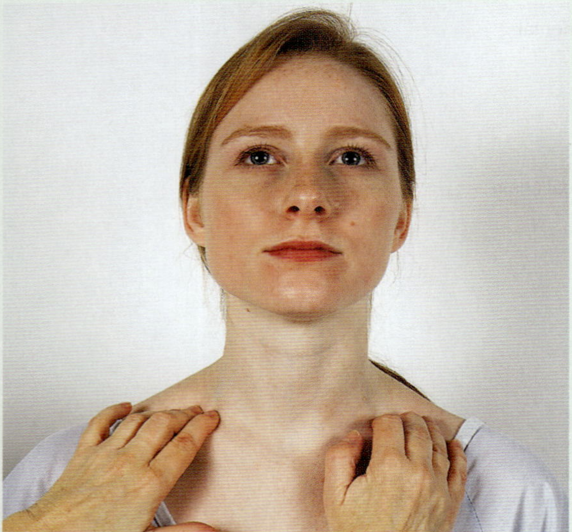 Figure 18.16	
If nodes are enlarged or tender, check the area they drain for the source of the problem. For example, those in the upper cervical or submandibular area often relate to inflammation or a neoplasm in the head and neck. Follow up on or refer your findings. An enlarged lymph node, particularly when you cannot find the source of the problem, deserves prompt attention.	The following criteria are common clues but are not definitive in all circumstances. • **Acute infection**—nodes are bilateral, enlarged, warm, tender and firm but freely movable. • **Chronic inflammation** (e.g. in tuberculosis the nodes are clumped). • **Cancerous nodes** are hard, unilateral, nontender and fixed. • A single, enlarged, nontender, hard, left supraclavicular node (Virchow's node) may indicate neoplasm in thorax or abdomen. • Painless, rubbery, discrete nodes that gradually appear occur with Hodgkin's lymphoma.

OBJECTIVE DATA

Summary Checklist

UPPER AIRWAYS ASSESSMENT

Subjective

1. Presenting concern
2. Ear, nose or throat discharge
3. Blocked nose
4. Sinus pain
5. Trauma
6. Epistaxis
7. Allergies
8. Altered smell
9. Pain in mouth or throat
10. Sores or lesions
11. Hoarseness or change in voice
12. Lumps or swelling in the neck
13. Health and lifestyle management

Objective data

1. General inspection
2. Inspect and palpate the external nose
3. Inspect the mouth
4. Inspect the throat

PROMOTING A HEALTHY LIFESTYLE

OUR AMAZING SMELLING ABILITY: PURPOSE AND PREDICTION

The sense of smell in humans is an important 'safety' sensory system, even though it may not be as well developed at detecting airborne chemicals as in other mammals. People use their sense of smell every day in a number of ways. For example, smell enables people to help determine the safety of food before they eat it, ensuring detection of spoiled food which could induce gastric upset, nausea and vomiting. It also is an important contributor to food flavour which is thought to increase kilojoule intake and thus to help maintain good nutritional status, particularly in older people. Smell can alert people to the presence of dangerous chemicals such as solvents like petrol or gas and also to fire and smoke. Smell can alert people who are predisposed to skin and soft tissue ulceration and other peripheral wound formation, such as people with chronic diabetes, to the presence of poorly cared for or mismanaged wounds. Detecting and identifying smells is an essential part of many people's professional duties, including that of clinical nurses, alerting nurses to the presence of infection, gangrene and other disease states such as diabetic ketoacidosis. Finally, a functioning sense of smell can support and assist patients in maintaining social connections, by helping to ensure basic personal hygiene.

Tests of smell

With the re/introduction of school nurses and the increasing importance of nurses in clinics and GP practices to conduct basic health screening, it is increasingly important for nurses to be aware of the various tests of sensory function, including smell (Lafreniere & Parham 2019). There are a number of specialist tests used to assess smell in adults. These are currently rarely used in standard clinical practice, but can accurately detect smelling ability and loss of smelling ability. The Pennsylvania Scratch'n'Sniff test is a test in which small cards are impregnated with odours that are released when the surface is scratched (Morley et al 2018).

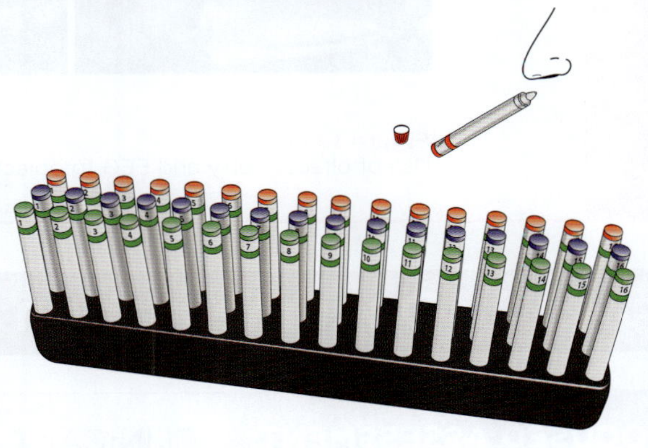

Figure 18.17
'Sniffin' Sticks' test.

When a person has scratched the card and smelt the odour, they are asked to identify the odour from one of four possible options written on the page, in a multiple choice test. This test is easy to administer and has been shown to be an excellent test of odour identification in the clinic.

Other tests of smelling ability can be more detailed and time-consuming, but are typically more informative. For example, the 'Sniffin' Sticks' test (Figure 18.17) requires people to sniff the barrel of a felt-tipped pen which contains different amounts (concentrations) of one of many different specific odorants (Besser et al 2019). These tests enable assessment of various aspects of our ability to smell including odour identification, discrimination (identifying the differences between smells) and detection threshold in various cultural groups and age groups. These tests come with 'picture' (visual) selection options for people with verbal dysfunction or reduced cognitive abilities.

The most objective test of smell requires an olfactometer, a machine which delivers warmed and humidified air together with specific concentrations of odour directly to a person's nose. Simultaneous EEG recordings enable clinicians to record brain activity associated with smell detection (Figure 18.18).

Why test for smell?

Smell is also a unique system because olfactory nerves (neurons), unlike those in any other human sensory system, continue to regenerate throughout life. Decrement or loss of smell often occurs prior to other clinical symptoms of such degenerative conditions, alerting clinicians to the need for medication or other clinical intervention. Thus, increasingly, loss of smell is being used as part of the screening tools applied to older people to detect neurological damage (Marin et al 2018). With increasingly aged populations, the need to screen effectively for neurodegeneration, often via relatively simple, nursing-applied tests, is also growing.

Exciting future possibilities

The presence of 'stem cells' ready to make new neurons in the human adult brain offers hope of transplantation therapies to reduce the impact and severity of many neurological dysfunctions in the future (Boody et al 2019). Australian scientists are already harvesting stem cells from the olfactory mucosa of people to grow new nerve cells (Alizadeh et al 2019) . It has been shown that non-neural cells such as heart, liver and kidney can also be grown from stem cells collected from the olfactory mucosa (Child et al 2018).

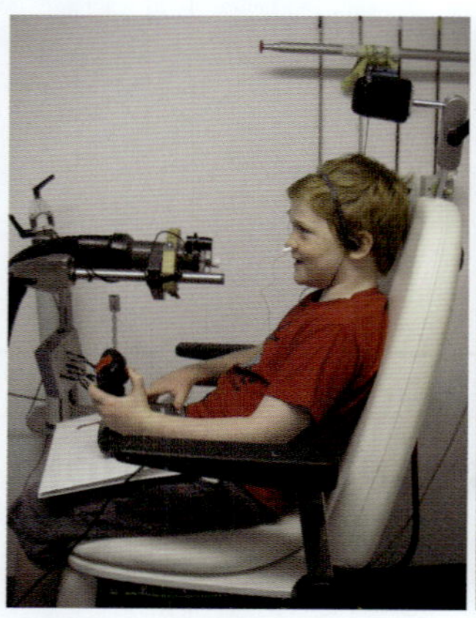

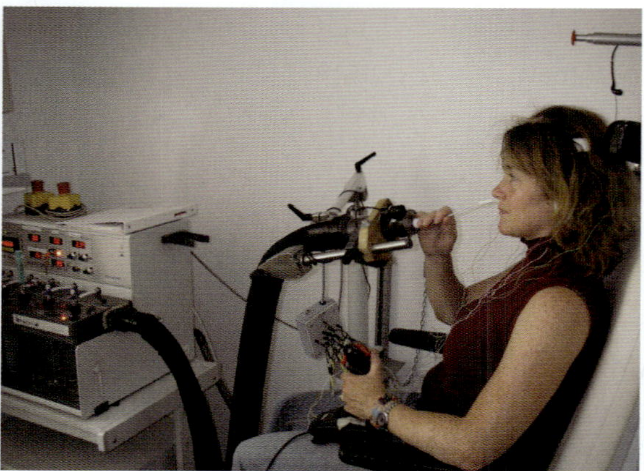

Figure 18.18
Use of olfactometry and EEG to objectively assess smelling ability.

Documentation and critical thinking

FOCUSED ASSESSMENT: CLINICAL CASE STUDY

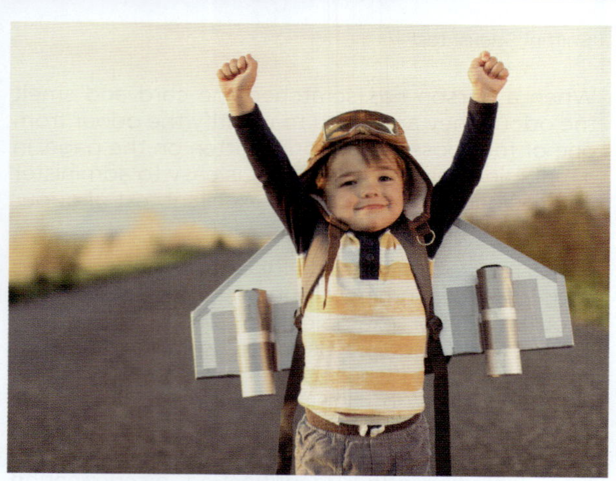

Context

Nurse practitioner in an emergency department performing an assessment following an initial triage assessment of a foreign body in the nose.

Subjective

A 3-year-old boy, Liam Crawford, is brought into hospital by his distressed parents. Liam was observed pushing a small plastic bead up his nose this morning. They encouraged Liam to blow his nose but the bead is still stuck. Liam has no other significant health problems.

Objective

Liam is relaxed and cooperative but says his nose is sore and reports a lack of sense of smell (anosmia). Liam's parents are visibly anxious.

Nose: (L) naris patent. (R) naris: reddened distal mucosa with no nasal discharge observed. The foreign body is lodged high in the airway obstructing airflow. No pain with light palpation.

Collaborative problem

Foreign body in nose.

Problem statement/nursing diagnosis

Obstructed nasal airway related to presence of foreign body.

Abnormal findings

TABLE 18.1 Abnormalities of the nose

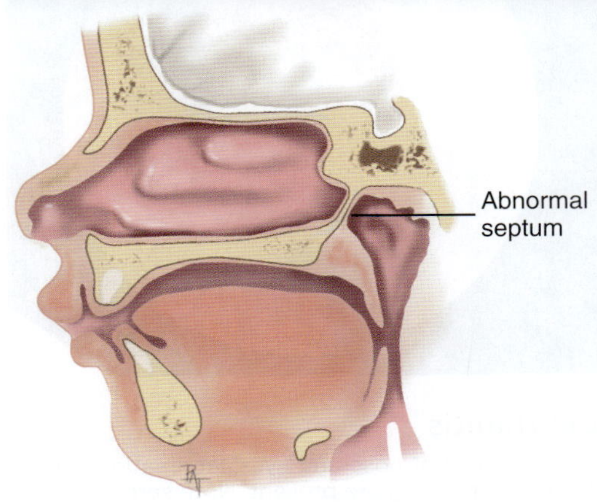

Choanal atresia

A bony or membranous septum between the nasal cavity and the pharynx of the newborn. When the condition is bilateral, it requires the immediate insertion of an oral airway to prevent asphyxia because most newborns are obligate nose breathers. When the condition is unilateral, the infant may be asymptomatic until the onset of the first respiratory infection.

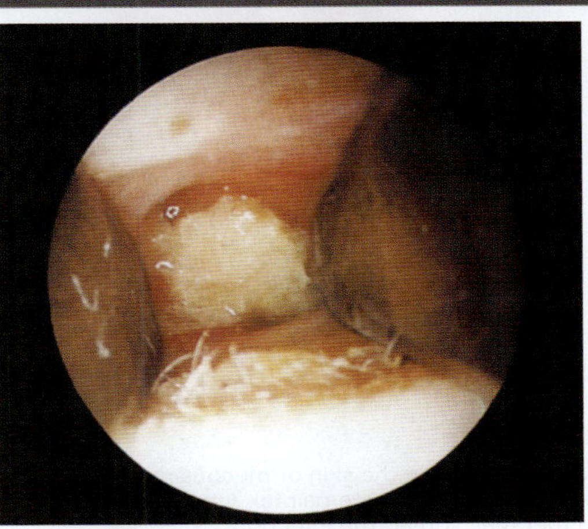

Foreign body

Children particularly are apt to put an object up the nose (here, yellow plastic foam), producing unilateral mucopurulent drainage and foul odour. Because some risk for aspiration exists, removal should be prompt.

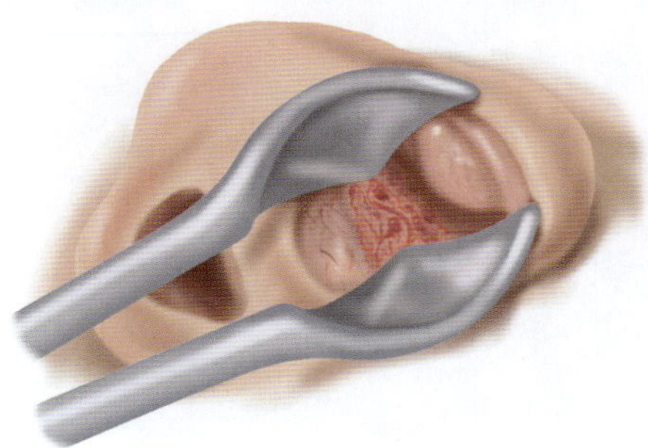

Epistaxis

The most common site of a nosebleed is Kiesselbach's plexus in the anterior septum. It may be spontaneous from a local cause or a sign of underlying illness. Causes include nose picking, forceful coughing or sneezing, fracture, foreign body, rhinitis, heavy exertion or a coagulation disorder. Bleeding from the anterior septum is easily controlled and rarely severe. A posterior haemorrhage is less common (<10%) but is more profuse, harder to manage and more serious.

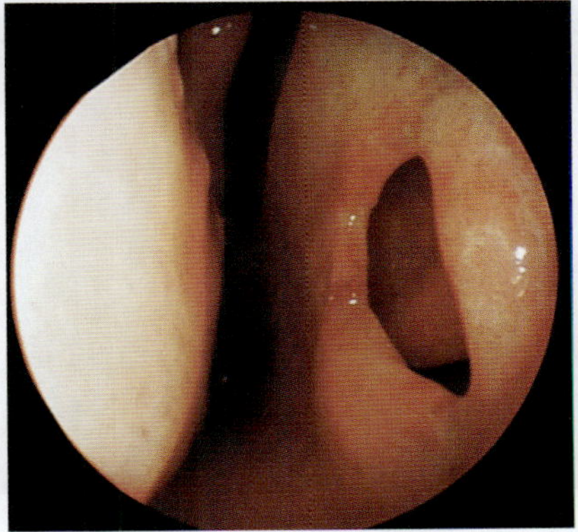

Perforated septum

A hole in the septum, usually in the cartilaginous part, may be caused by snorting cocaine, chronic infection, trauma from continual picking of crusts or nasal surgery. It is seen directly, or as a spot of light when the penlight is directed into the other naris.

(Continued)

TABLE 18.1 Abnormalities of the nose—cont'd

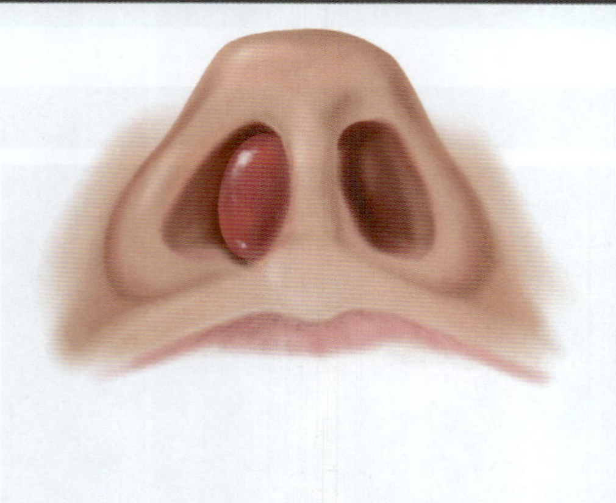

Furuncle

A small boil located in the skin or mucous membrane; appears red and swollen and is quite painful. Avoid any manipulation or trauma that may spread the infection.

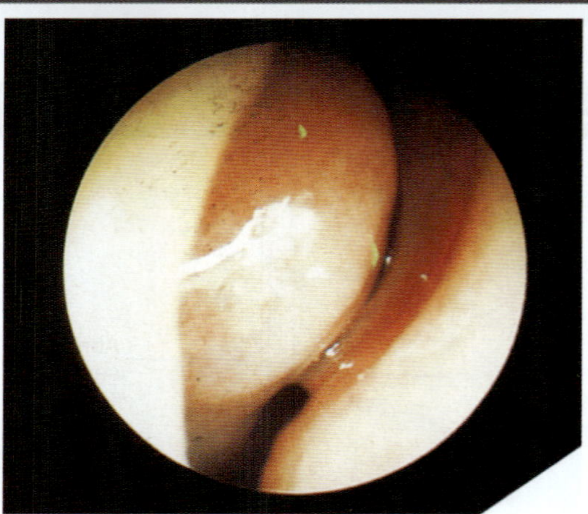

Allergic rhinitis

Rhinorrhoea, itching of nose and eyes, lacrimation, nasal congestion and sneezing are present. Note serous oedema and swelling of turbinates to fill the air space. Turbinates are usually pale (although may appear violet), and their surface looks smooth and glistening. May be seasonal or perennial, depending on allergen. Individual has a strong family history of seasonal allergies.

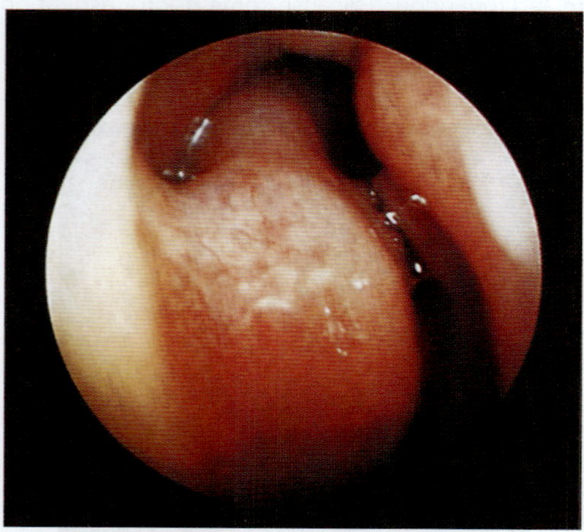

Acute rhinitis

The first sign is a clear, watery discharge, rhinorrhoea, which later becomes purulent. This is accompanied by sneezing and swollen mucosa, which causes nasal obstruction. Turbinates are dark red and swollen.

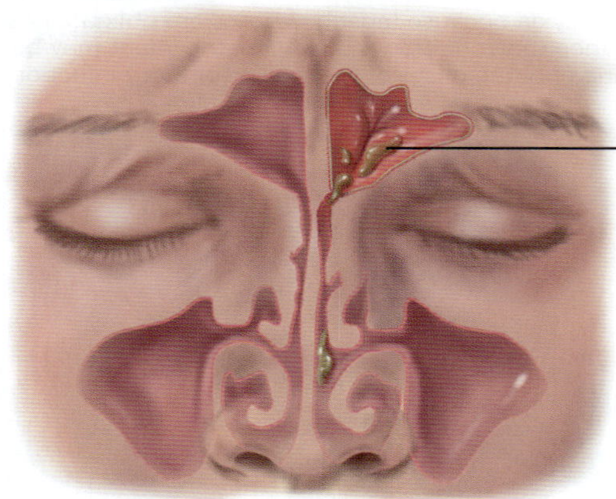

Sinusitis

Facial pain, after upper respiratory infection; signs include red swollen nasal mucosa, swollen turbinates and purulent discharge. Person also has fever, chills, malaise. With maxillary sinusitis, dull throbbing pain occurs in cheeks and teeth on the same side, and pain with palpation is present. With frontal sinusitis, pain is above the supraorbital ridge.

TABLE 18.1 Abnormalities of the nose—cont'd

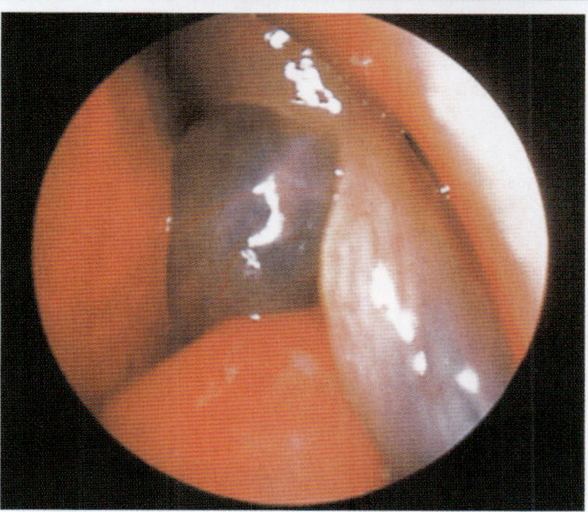

Nasal polyps

Smooth, pale grey nodules, which are overgrowths of mucosa, most commonly caused by chronic allergic rhinitis. May be stalked. A common site is protrusion from the middle meatus. Often multiple, they are mobile and nontender in contrast to turbinates. They may obstruct air passageways as they get larger. Symptoms include the absence of a sense of smell and a 'valve that moves' in the nose as the person breathes.

TABLE 18.2 Abnormalities of the oropharynx

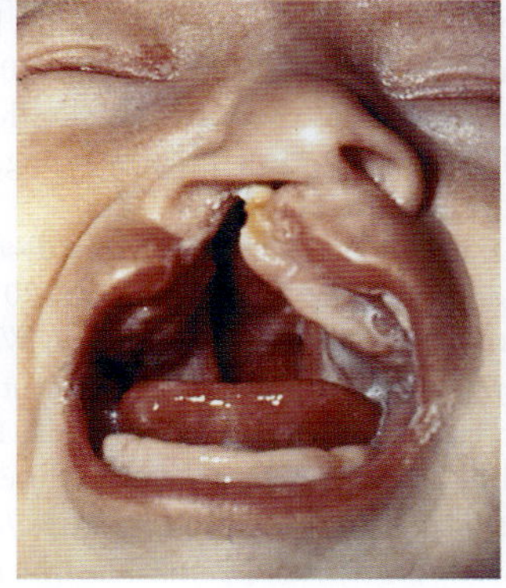

Cleft palate

A congenital defect, the failure of fusion of the maxillary processes. Wide variation occurs in the extent of cleft formation, from upper lip only, palate only, uvula only, to cleft of the nostril and the hard and soft palates.

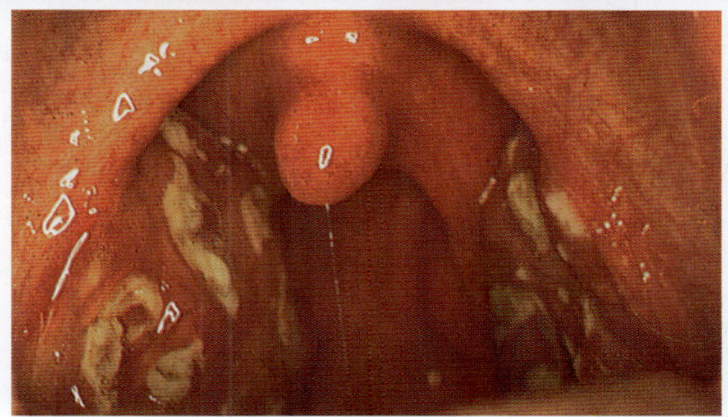

Peritonsillar abcess

(Continued)

TABLE 18.2 Abnormalities of the oropharynx—cont'd

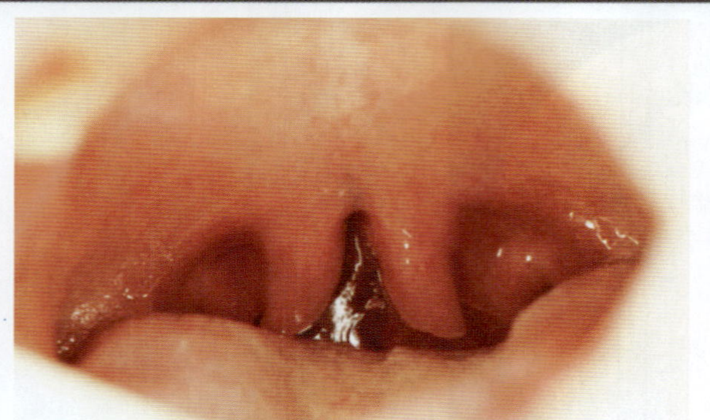 **Bifid uvula** The uvula looks partly severed. May indicate a submucous cleft palate, which feels like a notch at the junction of the hard and soft palates. The submucous cleft palate may affect speech development because it prevents necessary air trapping.	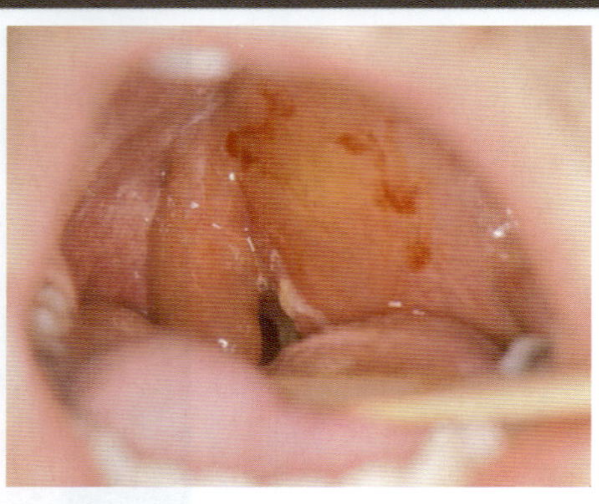 **Acute tonsillitis and pharyngitis** Bright red throat; swollen tonsils; white or yellow exudates on tonsils and pharynx; swollen uvula; and enlarged, tender anterior cervical and tonsillar nodes. Accompanied by severe sore throat, painful swallowing, fever >38°C of sudden onset. **Caution:** One cannot discriminate bacterial from viral infection on clinical data alone; all sore throats need a throat culture. Bacterial pharyngitis caused by group A β-haemolytic *Streptococcus*, if untreated, may lead to the complication of rheumatic fever. This is a serious complex illness characterised by fever, malaise, swollen joints, rash and scarring on the heart valves.

BIBLIOGRAPHY

Alizadeh R, Kamrava SK, Bagher Z, et al. Human olfactory stem cells: As a promising source of dopaminergic neuron-like cells for treatment of Parkinson's disease. Neurosci Lett 2019;696:52–9.

Australian Institute of Health and Welfare (AIHW). Potentially preventable hospitalisations in Australia by small geographic areas. Cat. no. HPF 36. Canberra: AIHW; 2019. Available at: www.aihw.gov.au/reports/primary-health-care/potentially-preventable-hospitalisations/contents/overview.

Azzopardi PS, Sawyer SM, Carlin JB, et al. Health and wellbeing of indigenous adolescents in Australia: a systematic synthesis of population data. Lancet 2018;391(10122):766–82.

Banham D, Karnon J, Lynch. Health related quality of life (HRQoL) among aboriginal South Australians: a perspective using survey-based health utility estimates. Health Qual Life Outcomes 2019;17(1):39.

Besser G, Jobs L, Liu DT, et al. The Sniffin' Sticks Odor discrimination memory test: a rapid, easy-to-use, reusable procedure for testing olfactory memory. Ann Otol Rhinol Laryngol 2019;128(3):227–32.

Boody BS, Sharma R, Bronson WH, et al. Update on stem cell applications in spine surgery. Contemp Spine Surg 2019;20(3):1–7.

Child KM, Herrick DB, Schwob JE, et al. The neuroregenerative capacity of olfactory stem cells is not limitless: implications for aging. J Neurosci 2018;38(31):6806–24.

Graydon K C, Miller WH, Gunasekera H. Global burden of hearing impairment and ear disease. J Laryngol Otol 2019;133(1):18–25.

Lafreniere D, Parham K. Sensory health and healthy aging: Hearing and smell. In: Coll P, editor. Healthy Aging. Champaign, IL: Springer; 2019. pp. 145–58.

Marin C, Vilas D, Langdon C, et al. Olfactory dysfunction in neurodegenerative diseases. Curr Allergy Asthm R 2018;18(2):42.

McCuaig R, Wong D, Gardiner FW, Rawlinson W, Dahlstrom JE, Robson S. Periodontal pathogens in the placenta and membranes in term and preterm birth. Placenta 2018 Aug 1;68:40-3.

Ministry of Health, New Zealand. Rheumatic fever resources for health professionals. 2017. Available at: https://www.health.govt.nz/our-work/diseases-and-conditions/rheumatic-fever/rheumatic-fever-resources/rheumatic-fever-resources-health-professionalspega.

Morley JF, Cohen J, Silveira-Moriyama L, et al. Optimizing olfactory testing for the diagnosis of Parkinson's disease: item analysis of the university of Pennsylvania smell identification test. NPJ Parkinsons Dis 2018;4(1):2.

Schwartz C, Vandenberghe-Descamps M, Sulmont-Rossé C, et al. Behavioral and physiological determinants of food choice and consumption at sensitive periods of the life span, a focus on infants and elderly. Innov Food Sci Emerg Technol 2018;46:91–106.

Chapter Nineteen

Lower airways assessment

Written by Carolyn Jarvis
Adapted by Josh Allen

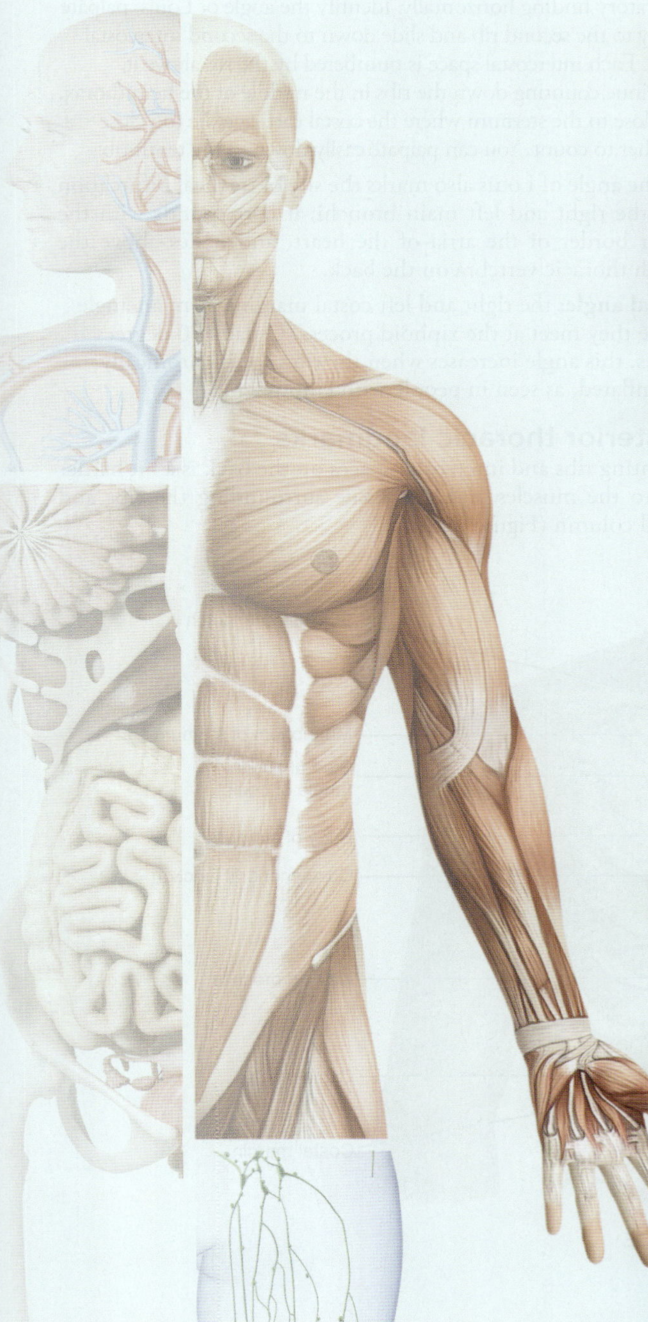

INTRODUCTION

The respiratory system is an important system responsible for the supply of oxygen, removal of carbon dioxide and maintenance of acid–base balance of arterial blood through hypoventilation and hyperventilation. In order to appreciate the impact of disease and trauma to this complex and dynamic system, you are advised to first review the structure and function of the thoracic cage, the lungs and tracheo-bronchial tree and the respiratory centre in the brainstem.

Structure and function

POSITION AND SURFACE LANDMARKS

The **thoracic cage** is a bony structure with a conical shape, which is narrower at the top (Figure 19.1). It is defined by the **sternum**, 12 pairs of **ribs** and 12 thoracic **vertebrae**. Its 'floor' is the **diaphragm**, a musculotendinous septum that separates the thoracic cavity from the abdomen. The first seven ribs attach directly to the sternum via their costal cartilages: ribs 8, 9 and 10 attach to the costal cartilage above, and ribs 11 and 12 are 'floating', with free palpable tips. The **costochondral junctions** are the points at which the ribs join their cartilages. They are not palpable.

Anterior thoracic landmarks

Surface landmarks on the thorax are signposts for underlying respiratory structures. Knowledge of landmarks will help you localise a finding and will facilitate communication of your findings to others.

Suprasternal notch: feel this hollow **U**-shaped depression just above the sternum, in between the clavicles.

Sternum: the 'breastbone' has three parts: the manubrium, the body and the xiphoid process. Walk your fingers down the manubrium a few centimetres until you feel a distinct bony ridge, the manubriosternal angle.

Manubriosternal angle: often called the sternal angle or the 'angle of Louis', this is the articulation of the manubrium and body of the sternum, and it is continuous with the second rib. The angle of Louis is a useful place to start counting ribs, which helps localise a respiratory finding horizontally. Identify the angle of Louis, palpate lightly to the second rib and slide down to the second intercostal space. Each intercostal space is numbered by the rib above it. Continue counting down the ribs in the middle of the hemithorax, not close to the sternum where the costal cartilages lie too close together to count. You can palpate easily down to the tenth rib.

The angle of Louis also marks the site of tracheal bifurcation into the right and left main bronchi; it corresponds with the upper border of the atria of the heart, and it lies above the fourth thoracic vertebra on the back.

Costal angle: the right and left costal margins form an angle where they meet at the xiphoid process. Usually 90 degrees or less, this angle increases when the rib cage is chronically overinflated, as seen in people with emphysema.

Posterior thoracic landmarks

Counting ribs and intercostal spaces on the back is a bit harder due to the muscles and soft tissue surrounding the ribs and spinal column (Figure 19.2).

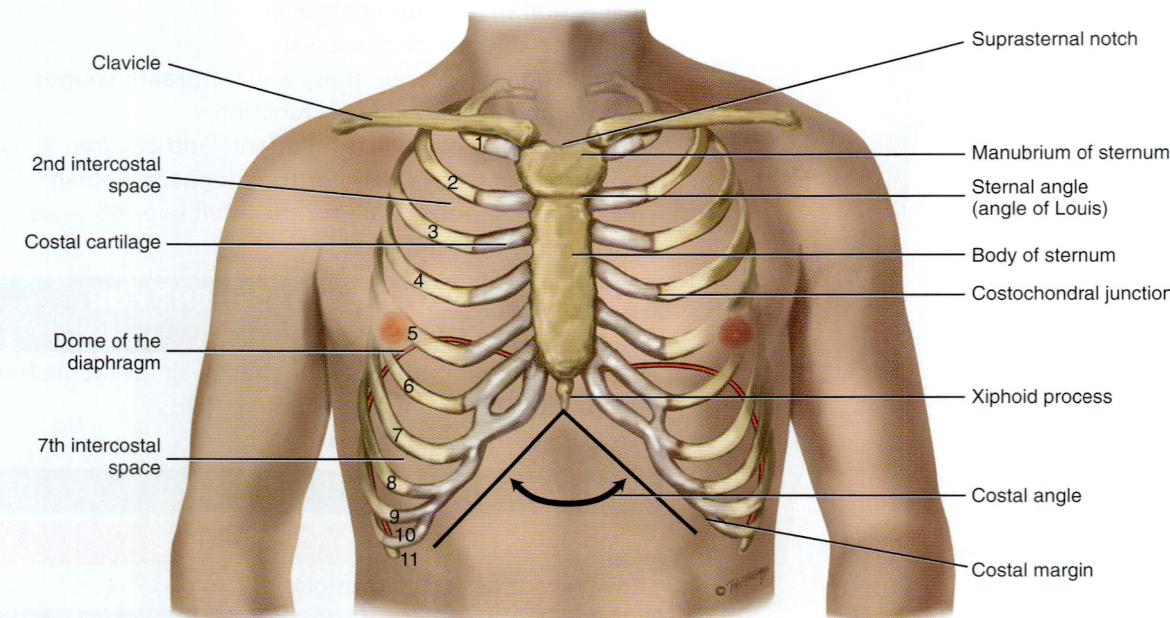

Figure 19.1

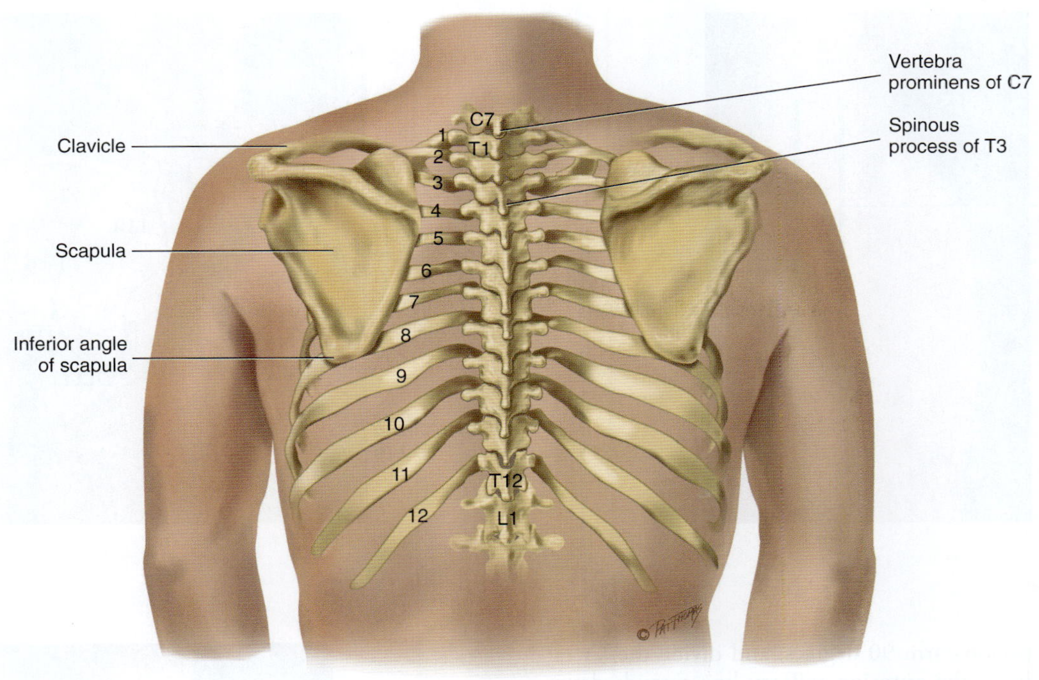

Figure 19.2
© Pat Thomas, 2010

Vertebra prominens: start here. Flex your head and feel for the most prominent bony spur protruding at the base of the neck. This is the spinous process of C7. If two bumps seem equally prominent, the upper one is C7 and the lower one is T1.
Spinous processes: count down these knobs on the vertebrae, which stack together to form the spinal column. Note that the spinous processes align with their same numbered ribs only down to T4. After T4, the spinous processes angle downwards from their vertebral body and overlie the vertebral body and rib below.
Inferior border of the scapula: the scapulae are located symmetrically in each hemithorax. The lower tip is usually at the seventh or eighth rib.
Twelfth rib: palpate midway between the spine and the person's side to identify its free tip.

Reference lines

Use the reference lines to pinpoint a finding vertically on the chest. On the anterior chest, note the **midsternal** line and the **midclavicular** line. The midclavicular line bisects the centre of each clavicle at a point halfway between the palpated sternoclavicular and acromioclavicular joints (Figure 19.3).

The posterior chest wall has the **vertebral** (or midspinal) line and the **scapular** line, which extends through the inferior angle of the scapula when the arms are at the sides of the body (Figure 19.4).

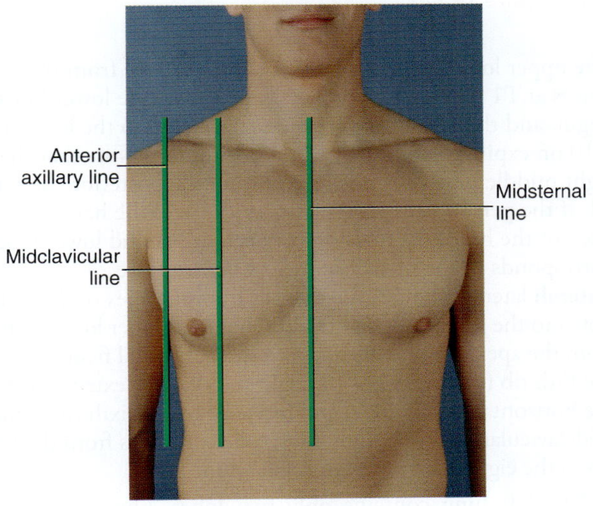

Figure 19.3

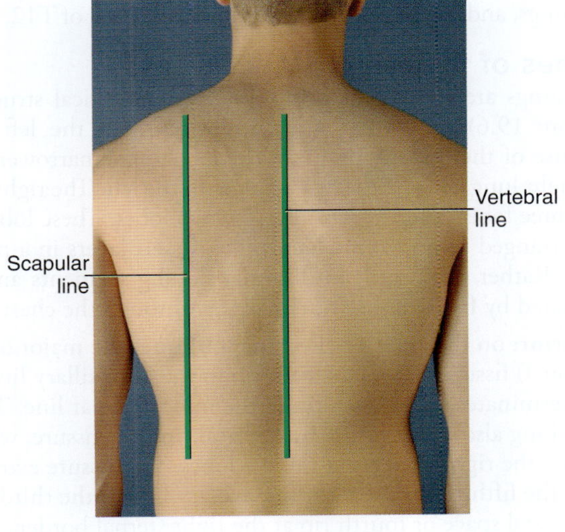

Figure 19.4

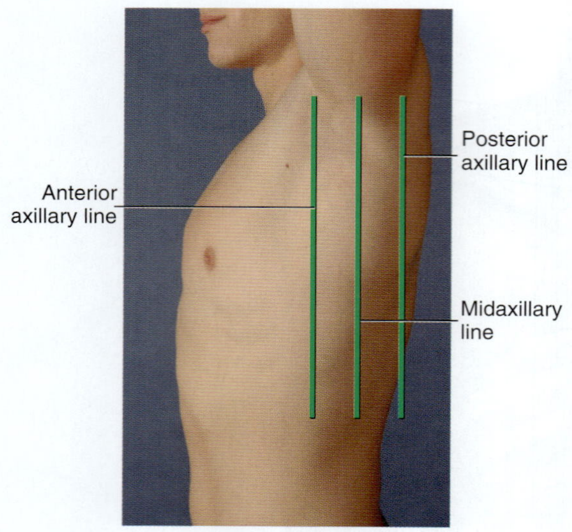

Figure 19.5

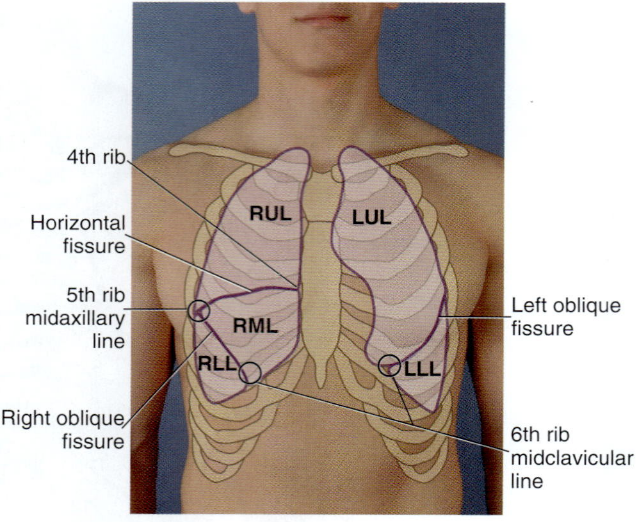

Figure 19.6

Lift up the person's arm 90 degrees, and divide the lateral chest by three lines: the **anterior axillary** line extends down from the anterior axillary fold where the pectoralis major muscle inserts; the **posterior axillary** line continues down from the posterior axillary fold where the latissimus dorsi muscle inserts; and the **midaxillary** line runs down from the apex of the axilla and lies between and parallel to the other two (Figure 19.5).

THE THORACIC CAVITY

The **mediastinum** is the middle section of the thoracic cavity containing the oesophagus, trachea, heart and great vessels. The right and left **pleural cavities**, on either side of the mediastinum, contain the lungs.

Lung borders: in the anterior chest, the **apex**, or highest point, of lung tissue is 3 or 4 cm above the inner third of the clavicles. The **base**, or lower border, rests on the diaphragm at about the sixth rib in the midclavicular line. Laterally, lung tissue extends from the apex of the axilla down to the seventh or eighth rib. Posteriorly, the location of C7 marks the apex of lung tissue, and T10 usually corresponds to the base. Deep inspiration expands the lungs, and their lower border drops to the level of T12.

Lobes of the lungs

The lungs are paired but not precisely symmetrical structures (Figure 19.6). The right lung is shorter than the left lung because of the underlying liver. The left lung is narrower than the right lung because the heart bulges to the left. The right lung has three lobes, and the left lung has two lobes. These lobes are not arranged in horizontal bands like dessert layers in a parfait glass. Rather, they stack in diagonal sloping segments and are separated by **fissures** that run obliquely through the chest.

Anterior: on the anterior chest, the **oblique** (the major or diagonal) fissure crosses the fifth rib in the midaxillary line and terminates at the sixth rib in the midclavicular line. The right lung also contains the **horizontal** (minor) fissure, which divides the right upper and middle lobes. This fissure extends from the fifth rib in the right midaxillary line to the third intercostal space or fourth rib at the right sternal border.
Posterior: the most remarkable point about the posterior chest is that it is almost all lower lobe (Figure 19.7).

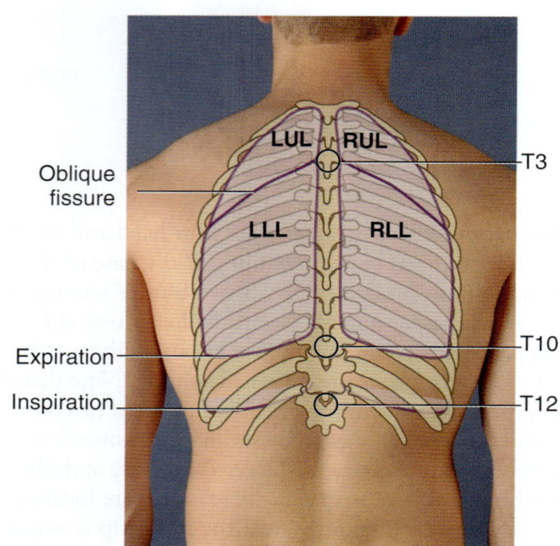

Figure 19.7

The upper lobes occupy a smaller band of tissue from their apices at T1 down to T3 or T4. At this level, the lower lobes begin, and their inferior border reaches down to the level of T10 on expiration and to T12 on inspiration. Note that the right middle lobe does not project onto the posterior chest at all. If the person abducts the arms and places the hands on the back of the head, the division between upper and lower lobes corresponds to the medial border of the scapulae.
Lateral: laterally, lung tissue extends from the apex of the axilla down to the seventh or eighth rib. The right upper lobe extends from the apex of the axilla down to the horizontal fissure at the fifth rib (Figure 19.8). The right middle lobe extends from the horizontal fissure down and forwards to the sixth rib at the midclavicular line. The right lower lobe continues from the fifth rib to the eighth rib in the midaxillary line.

The left lung contains only two lobes, upper and lower (Figure 19.9). These are seen laterally as two triangular areas separated by the oblique fissure. The left upper lobe extends

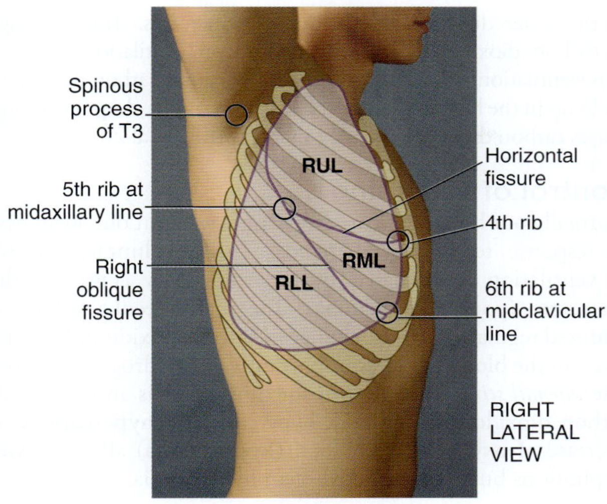

Figure 19.8

Figure 19.9

from the apex of the axilla down to the fifth rib at the midaxillary line. The left lower lobe continues down to the eighth rib in the midaxillary line.

Using these landmarks, take a marker and try tracing the outline of each lobe on a willing partner. Take special note of the three points that commonly confuse beginning examiners:

1. The left lung has no middle lobe.
2. The anterior chest contains mostly upper and middle lobe with very little lower lobe.
3. The posterior chest contains almost all lower lobe.

Pleurae

The thin, slippery **pleurae** form an envelope between the lungs and the chest wall (Figure 19.10). The **visceral** pleura lines the outside of the lungs, dipping down into the fissures. It is continuous with the **parietal** pleura lining the inside of the chest wall and diaphragm.

The inside of the envelope, the pleural cavity, is a potential space filled with only a few millilitres of lubricating fluid. It normally has a vacuum, or negative pressure, which holds the lungs tightly against the chest wall. The lungs slide smoothly and noiselessly up and down during respiration, lubricated by

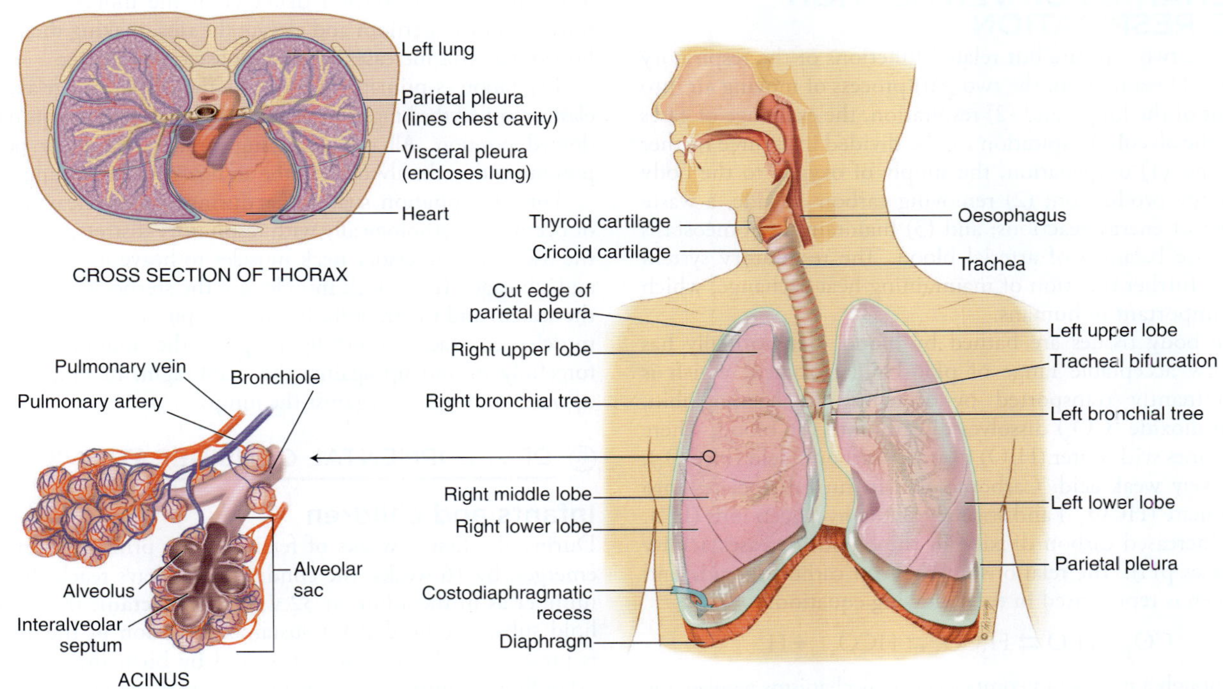

Figure 19.10

a few millilitres of fluid. Think of this as similar to two glass slides with a drop of water between them; although it is difficult to separate the slides, they slide smoothly back and forth. The pleurae extend about 3 cm below the level of the lungs, forming the **costodiaphragmatic recess**. This is a potential space: when it abnormally fills with air or fluid, it compromises lung expansion.

Trachea and bronchial tree

The **trachea** lies anterior to the oesophagus and is 10–11 cm long in the adult. It begins at the level of the cricoid cartilage in the neck and bifurcates just below the sternal angle into the right and left main bronchi. Posteriorly, tracheal bifurcation is at the level of T4 or T5. The right main bronchus is shorter, wider and more vertical than the left main bronchus.

The **trachea** and **bronchi** transport gases between the environment and the lung parenchyma. They constitute the *anatomical dead space*, or space that is filled with air but is not available for gaseous exchange. This is about 150 mL in the adult. The goblet cells and cilia that line the bronchial tree also help to protect alveoli from small particulate matter in the inhaled air. The goblet cells secrete mucus that entraps the particles, while the cilia sweep particles upwards where they can be swallowed or expelled.

An **acinus** is a functional respiratory unit that consists of the bronchioles, alveolar ducts, alveolar sacs and the alveoli. Gaseous exchange occurs across the respiratory membrane in the alveolar duct and in the millions of alveoli. Note how the alveoli are clustered like grapes around each alveolar duct (Figure 19.10). This creates millions of interalveolar septa (walls) that increase tremendously the working space available for gas exchange. This bunched arrangement creates a surface area for gas exchange that is as large as a tennis court.

MECHANICS OF VENTILATION AND RESPIRATION

There are two separate but related functions of the respiratory system: (1) ventilation, the two-part process of moving air into and out of the lungs; and (2) respiration, the exchange of gases across the alveoli. Respiration can be divided into three further functions: (1) oxygenation, the supply of oxygen to the body for energy production; (2) removing carbon dioxide, a waste product of energy reactions; and (3) maintaining homeostasis (acid–base balance) of arterial blood. The respiratory system has one further function of maintaining heat exchange, which is less important in humans.

The body tissues are bathed by blood that normally has a narrow acceptable range of pH. Unlike oxygen, which is predominantly transported by attaching to haemoglobin, carbon dioxide (CO_2) dissolves directly into the blood, where it combines with water (H_2O) to create carbonic acid (H_2CO_3), a relatively weak acid. Carbonic acid in turn dissociates into bicarbonate (HCO_3^-) and strongly acidic hydrogen ions (H^+). Thus, increased carbon dioxide in the blood increases acidity (decreases pH). The relationship between carbon dioxide and hydrogen is represented in the following equation:

$$CO_2 + H_2O \rightleftarrows H_2CO_3 \rightleftarrows HCO_3^- + H^+$$

Although a number of compensatory mechanisms regulate the pH, the lungs help to maintain the balance by eliminating excess carbon dioxide through the process of respiration across the alveoli. When carbon dioxide is exhaled, the equation above moves back in the other direction, and blood pH increases. The exchange of carbon dioxide is highly dependent on ventilation. That is, hypoventilation (slow, shallow breathing) causes carbon dioxide to build up in the blood, and hyperventilation (rapid, deep breathing) causes carbon dioxide to be blown off (Tortora et al 2019).

Control of breathing

Normally our breathing pattern changes without our awareness in response to cellular demands. This involuntary control of ventilation is mediated by the respiratory centre in the brainstem (pons and medulla). The major feedback loop is humoral regulation, or the change in carbon dioxide and oxygen levels in the blood and, less importantly, the hydrogen ion level. The *normal stimulus to breathe* for most of us is an increase of carbon dioxide in the blood, hypercarbia or **hypercapnia**. A decrease of oxygen in the blood (**hypoxaemia**) also increases respirations but is less effective than hypercapnia.

Changing chest size

Ventilation is the physical act of breathing: air rushes into the lungs as the chest size increases (inspiration) and is expelled from the lungs as the chest recoils (expiration). The mechanical expansion and contraction of the chest cavity alters the size of the thoracic container in two dimensions: (1) the vertical diameter lengthens or shortens, which is accomplished by downwards or upwards movement of the diaphragm; and (2) the anteroposterior diameter increases or decreases, which is accomplished by elevation or depression of the ribs (Figure 19.11).

In inspiration, increasing the size of the thoracic container creates a slightly negative pressure relative to the atmosphere, so air rushes in to fill the partial vacuum. The major muscle responsible for this is the diaphragm. During inspiration, contraction of the bell-shaped diaphragm causes it to descend and flatten. This lengthens the vertical diameter of the thorax. Intercostal muscles lift the sternum and elevate the ribs, making them more horizontal. This increases the anteroposterior diameter.

Expiration is primarily passive. As the diaphragm relaxes, the elastic recoil of the lungs and rib cage cause it to return to its natural domed position. All this squeezing creates a relatively positive pressure within the alveoli, and the air flows out of the lungs.

Forced inspiration, such as that during and after heavy exercise or occurring pathologically with respiratory distress, commands the use of the accessory neck muscles to heave up the sternum and rib cage. These neck muscles are the sternocleidomastoids, the scaleni and the trapezii. In forced expiration, the abdominal muscles contract powerfully to push the abdominal viscera forcefully in and up against the diaphragm, making it dome upwards and squeeze against the lungs.

DEVELOPMENTAL CONSIDERATIONS

Infants and children

During the first 5 weeks of fetal life, the primitive lung bud emerges; by 16 weeks, the conducting airways reach the same number as in the adult; at 32 weeks, **surfactant**, the complex lipid substance needed for sustained inflation of the air sacs, is present in adequate amounts; and by birth the lungs have 70 million primitive alveoli ready to start the job of respiration.

When the newborn inhales the first breath, the lusty cry that follows reassures straining parents that their baby is all right (Figure 19.12). The baby's body systems all develop in

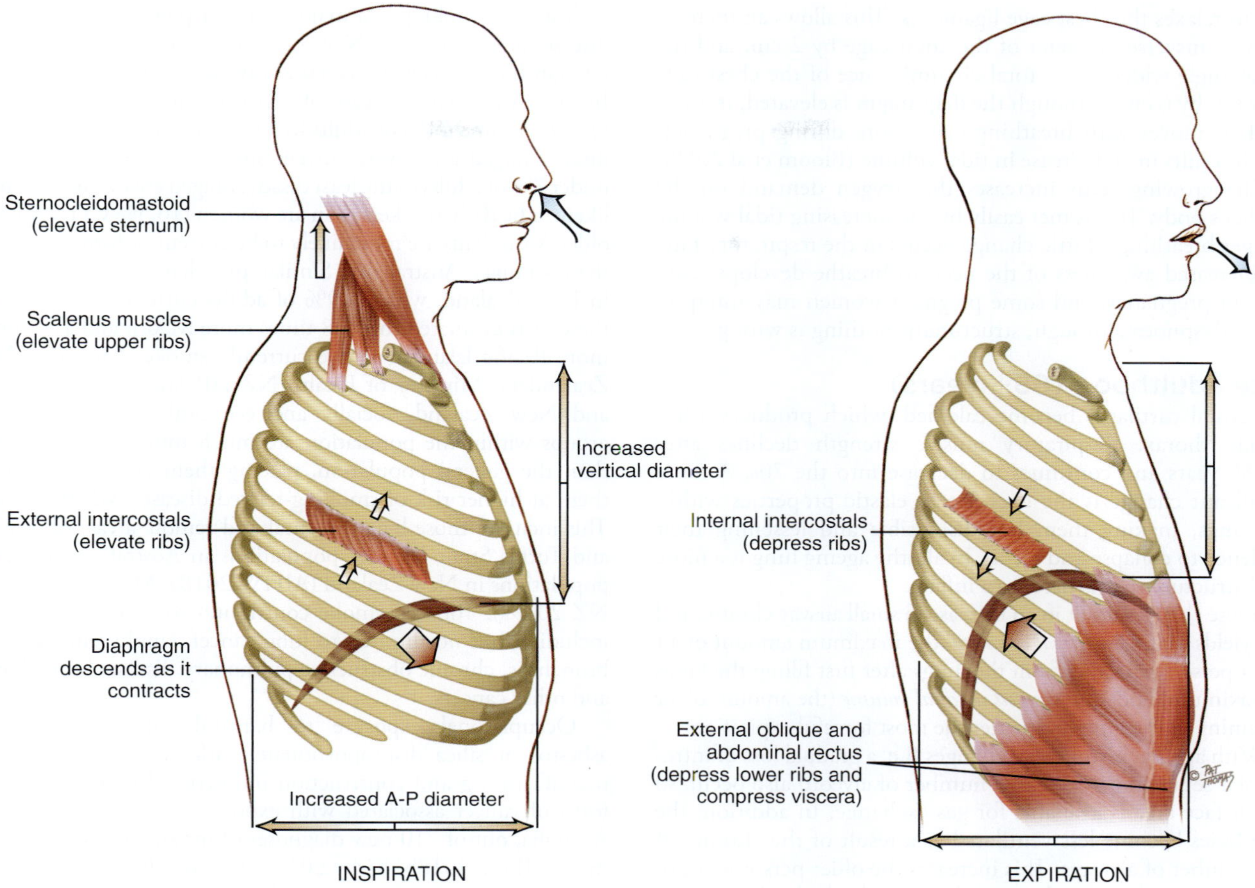

Sternocleidomastoid (elevate sternum)

Scalenus muscles (elevate upper ribs)

External intercostals (elevate ribs)

Diaphragm descends as it contracts

Increased vertical diameter

Increased A-P diameter

INSPIRATION

Internal intercostals (depress ribs)

External oblique and abdominal rectus (depress lower ribs and compress viscera)

EXPIRATION

Figure 19.11

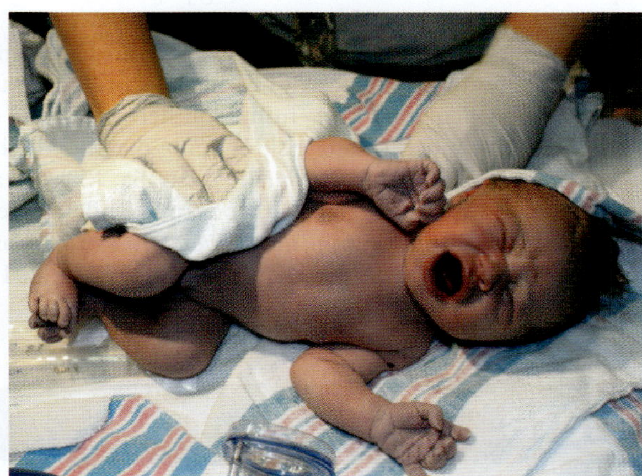

Figure 19.12

utero, but the respiratory system alone does not function until birth. Birth demands its instant performance.

When the umbilical cord is clamped and the blood flow between the baby and the placenta is disrupted, blood gushes into the baby's pulmonary circulation. Relatively less resistance exists in the pulmonary arteries than in the aorta, so the foramen ovale in the heart closes just after birth. (See the discussion of fetal circulation in Chapter 17.) The ductus arteriosus (linking the pulmonary artery and the aorta) contracts and closes some hours later, and pulmonary and systemic circulation are functional.

Respiratory development continues throughout childhood, with increases in diameter and length of airways, and increases in size and number of alveoli, reaching the adult range of 300 million by adolescence.

In the presence of older caregivers who smoke, the relatively smaller size and immaturity of children's pulmonary systems results in enormous vulnerability and increased risks to child health. Prenatal exposure results in chronic hypoxia and low birth weight. Postnatal exposure to environmental tobacco smoke is linked to increased rates of otitis media, respiratory tract infections and childhood asthma (Zhang et al 2019). Other conditions associated with exposure to tobacco smoke include sudden infant death syndrome (SIDS), negative behavioural and cognitive functioning and increased rates of adolescent smoking.

The pregnant woman

The enlarging uterus elevates the diaphragm 4 cm during pregnancy. This decreases the vertical diameter of the thoracic cage, but this decrease is compensated for by an increase in the horizontal diameter. The increased production of the hormone relaxin relaxes the chest cage ligaments. This allows an increase in the transverse diameter of the chest cage by 2 cm, and the costal angle widens. The total circumference of the chest cage increases by 6 cm. Although the diaphragm is elevated, it is not fixed. It moves with breathing even more during pregnancy, which results in an increase in tidal volume (Bloom et al 2018).

The growing fetus increases the oxygen demand on the mother's body. This is met easily by the increasing tidal volume (deeper breathing). Little change occurs in the respiratory rate. An increased awareness of the need to breathe develops, even early in pregnancy, and some pregnant women may interpret this as dyspnoea although, structurally, nothing is wrong.

Late adulthood (65+ years)

The costal cartilages become calcified, which produces a less mobile thorax. Respiratory muscle strength declines after age 50 years and continues to decrease into the 70s. A more significant change is the decrease in elastic properties within the lungs, making them less distensible and lessening their tendency to collapse and recoil. In all, the ageing lung is a more rigid structure that is harder to inflate.

These changes result in an increase in small airway closure, and that yields a *decreased vital capacity* (the maximum amount of air that a person can expel from the lungs after first filling the lungs to maximum) and an *increased residual volume* (the amount of air remaining in the lungs even after the most forceful expiration).

With ageing, histological changes (i.e. a gradual loss of intra-alveolar septa and a decreased number of alveoli) also occur, so less surface area is available for gas exchange. In addition, the lung bases become less ventilated as a result of the closing off of a number of airways. This increases the older person's risk of dyspnoea with exertion beyond their usual workload.

The histological changes also increase the older person's risk of postoperative pulmonary complications. That is, the older person has a greater risk of postoperative atelectasis and infection from a decreased ability to cough, a loss of protective airway reflexes and increased secretions.

CULTURAL AND SOCIAL CONSIDERATIONS

Respiratory diseases associated with exposure to harmful substances or infectious organisms disproportionately affect particular groups within Australian and New Zealand society. Lifestyle factors such as tobacco smoking, occupational exposure to asbestos or silica and environmental exposure to air pollutants or infectious diseases are each associated with particular groups within society.

Tobacco smoking is a major cause of preventable death and disease in Australia and New Zealand. There is a strong inverse relationship between tobacco use and socio-economic indicators. In the Australian Bureau of Statistics health survey report (2019), around 21% of adults living in the most socio-economic disadvantaged areas were current smokers, compared with just under 7% of adults in the least disadvantaged areas. Men are more likely to be daily smokers than are women (16.5% v 11.1%), and older Australians are more likely to be current or former smokers than younger Australians. Similar prevalence data is reported in New Zealand, with 14.9% of adults currently smoking. Of these, it is estimated that 2.8 times more Māori, and 1.47 times more Pacific Islander people currently smoke than other New Zealanders (Ministry of Health NZ 2019a). In both Australia and New Zealand, socially and economically disadvantaged groups within the population are much more likely to smoke than the general population, placing them and those around them at higher risk of smoking-related disease (AIHW 2018a). This includes those living in rural and remote areas, Aboriginal and Torres Strait Islander populations in Australia, and Māori populations in New Zealand (AIHW 2018a, Ministry of Health NZ 2019a). Tobacco smoke contributes to a range of diseases including but not limited to lung cancer, emphysema, chronic bronchitis, chronic obstructive pulmonary disease, heart disease and other cancers.

Occupational exposure to harmful substances such as asbestos or silica disproportionately affects males working in manufacturing and construction industries. Mesothelioma is a form of cancer associated with exposure to asbestos fibres. In Australia, out of 710 new diagnoses of mesothelioma, 592 were men (AIHW 2018b, Kirby 2019). The so-called 'third-wave' of asbestos-related disease is expected to see a shift in from industrial exposure to exposure that occurs in the setting of home-renovations (Soeberg et al 2018). Similarly, silicosis arising from occupational exposure to the silica contained in manufactured stone products has increased with the rising popularity of home renovations (Hoy et al 2018, Leso et al 2019).

Finally, while both Australia and New Zealand have some of the lowest rates of tuberculosis (TB) in the world, migrant communities, particularly those from Southern, Central or Eastern Asia are at much greater risk of being diagnosed with TB than the rest of the population. In Australia, 87% of all TB notifications were in foreign-born persons, while in New Zealand, 78% of all TB notifications were in foreign-born persons (Australian Government Department of Health 2019, Ministry of Health NZ 2019b).

Subjective data

Subjective data relating to the respiratory system can give important clues as to an individual's respiratory health and function as well as indicators of risk for development of lung disorders. Gathering information about respiratory function is also important in determining an individual's ability to perform activities of living.

1. Presenting concern
2. Shortness of breath
3. Chest pain with breathing
4. Cough
5. History of respiratory infections
6. Smoking history
7. Environmental exposure
8. Health and lifestyle management

Practice note: Before you commence the assessment, introduce yourself to the person, confirm the person's identity, discuss the purpose and scope of the assessment, clarify any questions the person may have and obtain verbal consent from the person to perform the assessment.

ASSESSMENT GUIDELINES	CLINICAL SIGNIFICANCE AND CLINICAL ALERTS
1. Presenting concern	
Do you feel you have any problem with your lungs or your breathing? It is important to ascertain the person's perception of the health of their lungs. If a problem is perceived ask 'How does this impact on your quality of life?'	
2. Shortness of breath	
Have you ever had any **shortness of breath**, difficulty breathing or difficulty catching your breath? What brings it on? How severe is it? How long does it last?	**Dyspnoea** Determine how much activity precipitates the shortness of breath (SOB)—state specific number of blocks walked, number of stairs.
• Is it affected by position, such as lying down? How many pillows do you sleep on at night?	**Orthopnoea** is difficulty breathing when supine. Several pillows may be needed to achieve comfort (e.g. 'two-pillow orthopnoea'). This is a common symptom of pulmonary oedema, often as a result of heart failure. Changes in sleep pattern may affect activities of living due to fatigue during the day.
• Does it occur at any specific time of day or night?	**Paroxysmal nocturnal dyspnoea** is awakening from sleep with SOB and needing to be upright to achieve comfort.
• Shortness of breath episodes associated with night sweats?	**Diaphoresis** is profuse sweating. Although associated with many conditions, nocturnal diaphoresis can indicate the presence of a respiratory infection or malignancy and should be investigated.
• Or cough, chest pain or bluish colour around lips or nails? Wheezing or other sound?	**Cyanosis** is the bluish discolouration of the skin resulting from a lack of oxygen. Peripheral cyanosis (nails) is most often due to circulatory causes and should be investigated further. Central cyanosis (lips) is always due to a gross lack of oxygen and should be considered an emergency. Any wheeze (lower airway) or stridor (upper airway) that you can hear during the interview should prompt you to cease the interview and seek assistance.
• Episodes seem to be related to food, pollen, dust, animals, season or emotion?	**Asthma** attacks may be associated with a specific allergen or extreme cold, anxiety.
• What do you do when having difficulty breathing? Take a special position, or use pursed-lip breathing? Use any oxygen, inhalers or medications?	Assess effect of coping strategies and the need for more teaching.
• How does the shortness of breath affect your work or home activities? Getting better or worse or staying about the same?	Assess effect on activities of daily living.
3. Chest pain with breathing	
Any **chest pain with breathing**? Please point to the exact location.	**Chest pain** with pulmonary origin may be a late sign of pulmonary disease.
• When did it start? Constant or does it come and go?	

SUBJECTIVE DATA

SUBJECTIVE DATA

ASSESSMENT GUIDELINES	CLINICAL SIGNIFICANCE AND CLINICAL ALERTS
• Describe the pain: burning, stabbing?	
• Brought on by respiratory infection, coughing or trauma? Is it associated with fever, deep breathing, unequal chest inflation?	
• What have you done to treat it? Medication or heat application?	
4. Cough	
Do you have a **cough**? When did it start? Gradual or sudden? • How long have you had it? • How often do you cough? At any special time of day or just on arising? Cough wake you up at night?	Some conditions have a characteristic timing of a cough: Continuous throughout day—acute illness (e.g. respiratory infection) Afternoon/evening—may reflect exposure to irritants at work or during the day Night—postnasal drip, sinusitis, asthma Early morning—chronic bronchial inflammation or smoking.
• Do you cough up any phlegm or sputum? How much? What colour is it?	Chronic bronchitis is characterised by a history of productive cough for 3 months of the year for 2 years in a row. Non-productive coughs are associated with upper respiratory tract infections or early heart failure.
• Cough up any blood? Does this look like streaks or frank blood? Does the sputum have a foul odour?	**Haemoptysis.** Some conditions have characteristic sputum production: white or clear mucoid—colds, bronchitis, viral infections; yellow or green—bacterial infections; rust coloured—tuberculosis, pneumococcal pneumonia; pink, frothy—pulmonary oedema, some sympathomimetic medications have a side effect of pink-tinged mucus.
• How would you describe your cough: hacking, dry, barking, hoarse, congested, bubbling?	Some conditions have a characteristic cough: mycoplasma pneumonia—hacking; heart failure—dry; croup—barking; colds, bronchitis, pneumonia—congested.
• Does the cough seem to occur with: activity, position (lying), fever, congestion, talking, anxiety?	
• Does activity make it better or worse?	
• What treatment have you tried? Prescription or over-the-counter medications, traditional or complementary medicine, vaporiser, rest, position change?	Consider whether the problem can be attributed to adverse medication effects; for example, angiotensin converting enzyme (ACE) inhibitors are associated with the side effect of a persistent cough. For people with a frequent productive cough and/or a long smoking history, use the following questionnaire (Figure 19.13). This is a simple, short tool to identify persons who will need spirometry testing to confirm the diagnosis of COPD.
• Is the cough associated with any other symptoms: chest pain, ear pain? Is it tiring? Are you concerned about it?	

ASSESSMENT GUIDELINES	CLINICAL SIGNIFICANCE AND CLINICAL ALERTS

Lung Function Questionnaire

Do you suffer from breathing problems and/or frequent cough?

These questions ask about your breathing problems and/or frequent cough. As you answer these questions, think about how you feel physically when you experience these symptoms. For each question, choose the one answer that best describes your symptoms. Share the answers with your healthcare provider.

Step 1: Answer each question and write the score in the box next to it.
Step 2: Add together the scores in each box to get your total score.
Step 3: Take the test to your provider to talk about your score.

Question	5	4	3	2	1	SCORE
1. How often do you cough up mucus?	Never	Rarely	Sometimes	Often	Very often	☐
2. How often does your chest sound noisy (wheezy, whistling, rattling) when you breathe?	Never	Rarely	Sometimes	Often	Very often	☐
3. How often do you experience shortness of breath during physical activity (walking up a flight of stairs or walking up an incline without stopping to rest)?	Never	Rarely	Sometimes	Often	Very often	☐
4. How many years have you smoked?	Never smoked	10 years or less	11-20 years	21-30 years	More than 30 years	☐
5. What is your age?	Less than 40 years	40-49 years	50-59 years	60-69 years	70 years or older	☐
						TOTAL ☐

Step 4: If your score is 18 or less, you may be at risk for Chronic Obstructive Pulmonary Disease (COPD). COPD includes chronic bronchitis, emphysema, or both.

Figure 19.13

5. History of respiratory infections

ASSESSMENT GUIDELINES	CLINICAL SIGNIFICANCE AND CLINICAL ALERTS
Any **past history** of breathing trouble or lung diseases such as bronchitis, emphysema, asthma, pneumonia?	Consider sequelae after these conditions.
• Any unusually frequent or unusually severe colds?	Because most people have had some colds, it is more meaningful to ask about excess number or severity.
• Any family history of allergies, tuberculosis or asthma?	

6. Smoking history

ASSESSMENT GUIDELINES	CLINICAL SIGNIFICANCE AND CLINICAL ALERTS
Do you **smoke** cigarettes, cigars or ecigarettes? At what age did you start? How many packs per day do you smoke now? For how long? Have you ever smoked? If so, for how long, when did you quit?	
• Have you ever tried to quit? What helped? Why do you think it did not work? What activities do you associate with smoking? Would you like to speak to someone about trying to quit again now? • Live with someone who smokes?	Most people already know they should quit smoking. Instead of admonishing, assess smoking behaviour and ways to modify daily smoking activities. Current smoking cessation practice is to offer brief, non-judgemental smoking cessation support at every opportunity.

7. Environmental exposure

ASSESSMENT GUIDELINES	CLINICAL SIGNIFICANCE AND CLINICAL ALERTS
Are there any **environmental conditions** that may affect your breathing? Where do you work? At a factory, chemical plant, coal mine, farming, outdoors in a heavy traffic area? Any recent overseas travel?	Farmers may be at risk for grain inhalation, pesticide inhalation.
• Do you do anything to protect your lungs, such as wear a mask or have the ventilatory system checked at work? Do you do anything to monitor your exposure? Have periodic examinations, pulmonary function tests, X-ray examination?	

SUBJECTIVE DATA

ASSESSMENT GUIDELINES	CLINICAL SIGNIFICANCE AND CLINICAL ALERTS
• Do you know what specific symptoms to note that may signal breathing problems?	General symptoms: cough, shortness of breath. Some gases produce specific symptoms: carbon monoxide—dizziness, headache, fatigue; sulfur dioxide—cough, congestion.
8. Health and lifestyle management	
What medications are you taking?	
Are you up to date with influenza immunisation, pneumococcal immunisation?	
Additional subjective data for infants and children (questions for parents or guardians)	
• Has the child had any frequent or very severe colds?	4 to 6 uncomplicated upper respiratory infections per year is expected in early childhood.
• Is there any history of allergy in the family?	
– (For child under 2 years of age): At what age were new foods introduced? Was the child breast fed or bottle fed?	Consider new foods or formula as possible allergens.
• Does the child have a cough? Seem congested? Have noisy breathing or wheezing? (Further questions similar to those listed in the section on adults.)	Screen for onset and follow course of childhood chronic respiratory problems: asthma, bronchitis.
• What measures have you taken to child-proof your home? Yard? Is there any possibility of the child inhaling or swallowing toxic substances?	Young children are at risk for accidental aspiration, poisoning and injury.
– Has anyone taught you emergency care measures in case of accidental choking?	
• Any smokers in the home or in the car with child?	Environmental smoke increases the risk of ear and respiratory infections in children.
Additional subjective data for the adult over 65 years	
• **Shortness of breath.** Have you noticed any shortness of breath or fatigue with your daily activities?	Older adults have a less efficient respiratory system (decreased vital capacity, less surface area for gas exchange), so they have less tolerance for activity.
• **Physical activity.** Tell me about your usual amount of physical activity.	May have reduced capacity to perform exercise because of pulmonary function deficits of ageing. Sedentary or bedridden people are at risk for respiratory dysfunction.
• **History of lung disease.** For those with a history of chronic obstructive pulmonary disease, lung cancer or tuberculosis: How are you getting along each day? Any weight change in the last 3 months? How much?	Individuals with chronic respiratory disease use large amounts of energy just breathing, and may require nutritional support.
– How about energy level? Do you tire more easily? How does your illness affect you at home? At work?	Activities may decrease because of increasing shortness of breath or pain.
• **Chest pain.** Do you have any chest pain with breathing?	Some older adults feel pleuritic pain less intensely than younger adults.
	Precisely localised sharp pain (points to it with one finger)—consider fractured rib or muscle injury.

Objective data

Objective data collection begins at the first contact with the person (observation) for threats to the airway (partial or complete obstruction), difficulty breathing, in particular a very rapid or very slow respiratory rate, or other obvious abnormalities such as cyanosis. The presence of any of these abnormalities should prompt immediate intervention. A thorough assessment will involve collecting data through inspection, palpation and auscultation to evaluate lung function and respiratory health.

Preparation

Ask the person to sit upright and the male to disrobe to the waist. For the female, leave the gown on and open at the back. When examining the anterior chest, lift up the gown and drape it on her shoulders rather than removing it completely. This promotes comfort by giving her the feeling of being somewhat clothed. These provisions will ensure further comfort: a warm room, a warm stethoscope diaphragm endpiece, adequate lighting and privacy.

Perform the inspection, palpation and auscultation on the posterior and lateral thorax. Then move to face the person and repeat the assessment on the anterior chest.

Finally, clean your stethoscope endpiece with antiseptic wipe. Because your stethoscope touches many people, it could be a possible vector for both aerobic and anaerobic bacteria. Cleaning your stethoscope is an essential measure to prevent cross contamination.

Equipment needed

Hand hygiene solution
Stethoscope
Antiseptic wipe

PROCEDURES AND NORMAL FINDINGS	ABNORMAL FINDINGS AND CLINICAL ALERTS
General inspection	
During subjective data collection you will have noticed the colour of the person's skin and mucous membranes, ease of breathing, tone of voice, height to weight ratio, level of hygiene and grooming and general demeanor. All of these factors provide clues to the functioning of the lower respiratory system. Make note of your findings.	
Assess the **level of consciousness**. The level of consciousness should be alert and cooperative.	**Cerebral hypoxia** may be reflected by excessive drowsiness or by anxiety, restlessness, confusion and irritability. These findings should trigger immediate intervention.
Note colour and condition of skin on face, nailbeds, lips and ear lobes, oral mucous membranes. The face, lips, nail beds and ear lobes are free of cyanosis or unusual pallor. The oral mucous membranes should be pink and moist. The nails are of normal configuration. Explore any skin lesions (see Chapter 22).	**Cyanosis** occurs due to lack of oxygenated blood supplying body tissues. Cyanosis can be central, meaning that there is a circulatory or ventilatory problem that leads to poor oxygenation in the lungs. **Peripheral cyanosis** occurs when the blood reaching the periphery is not adequately oxygenated. Peripheral cyanosis occurs as a consequence of arterial obstruction, venous obstruction, exposure to cold weather, reduced cardiac output or those related to the cases of central cyanosis. **Clubbing** of distal phalanx occurs with chronic respiratory disease.
Assess the quality of **breaths**. Normal relaxed breathing is automatic and effortless, regular and even and produces no noise. The chest expands symmetrically with each inspiration. Note any localised lag on inspiration.	Noisy breathing occurs with severe asthma or chronic bronchitis. Unequal chest expansion occurs when part of the lung is obstructed or collapsed, as with pneumonia or when guarding to avoid postoperative incisional pain or pleurisy pain.

PROCEDURES AND NORMAL FINDINGS	ABNORMAL FINDINGS AND CLINICAL ALERTS
Note the person's **facial expression**. The facial expression should be relaxed and benign, indicating an unconscious effort of breathing.	A person with COPD may look tense, strained and tired. They may purse the lips in a whistling position. By exhaling slowly and against a narrow opening, the pressure in the bronchial tree remains positive and fewer airways collapse.
	Cutaneous angiomas (spider naevi) associated with liver disease or portal hypertension may be evident on the chest.
Inspect the posterior chest wall	
Note the **shape and configuration** of the chest wall. **Identify bony landmarks;** scapulae, ribs and spine. The spinous processes should appear in a straight line. The thorax is symmetrical, in an elliptical shape, with downward-sloping ribs, about 45 degrees relative to the spine. The scapulae are placed symmetrically in each hemithorax.	Skeletal deformities may limit thoracic cage excursion: scoliosis, kyphosis (see Table 19.3).
The anteroposterior diameter should be less than the transverse diameter. The ratio of anteroposterior to transverse diameter is from 1:2 to 5:7.	Anteroposterior = transverse diameter, or 'barrel chest'. Ribs are horizontal, chest appears as if held in continuous inspiration. This occurs in chronic emphysema from hyperinflation of the lungs (see Table 19.3).
The neck muscles and trapezius muscles should be developed normally for age and occupation.	Neck muscles are hypertrophied in chronic obstructive pulmonary disease (COPD) from aiding in forced inspiration and expiration.
Note the **position** the person takes to breathe. This includes a relaxed posture and the ability to support one's own weight with arms comfortably at the sides or in the lap. Take note of how freely the person is able to speak in between breaths. The person should be able to communicate in full sentences.	People with COPD often sit in a tripod position, leaning forwards with arms braced against their knees, chair or bed. This gives them leverage so that their accessory neck and shoulder muscles can aid in inspiration. A person who is short of breath may only be able to communicate in phrases or single words.
Assess the **skin colour and condition of the chest wall**. Colour should be consistent with person's genetic background, with allowance for sun-exposed areas on the chest and the back. No cyanosis or pallor should be present. Note any lesions. Inquire as to any change in a naevus on the back, for example, where the person may have difficulty monitoring (see Chapter 22).	Use the ABCD system when assessing lesions and naevi (A–asymmetry, B–border, C–colour, D–diameter). Assessing skin colour of a person with very dark skin can be difficult. The ventral surface of the hand may be more useful than the dorsal when assessing for peripheral cyanosis or pallor. The oral mucosa may be most useful to assess for central cyanosis. Cutaneous angiomas (spider naevi) associated with liver disease or portal hypertension may be evident on the chest.
Palpate the posterior chest wall	
Confirm **symmetrical chest expansion** by placing your warmed hands on the posterolateral chest wall with thumbs at the level of T9 or T10. Slide your hands medially to pinch up a small fold of skin between your thumbs (Figure 19.14).	

PROCEDURES AND NORMAL FINDINGS	ABNORMAL FINDINGS AND CLINICAL ALERTS
Figure 19.14	
Ask the person to take a deep breath. Your hands serve as mechanical amplifiers; as the person inhales deeply, your thumbs should move apart symmetrically. Note any lag in expansion.	Unequal chest expansion occurs with marked atelectasis or pneumonia; with thoracic trauma, such as fractured ribs; or with pneumothorax. Pain accompanies deep breathing when the pleurae are inflamed.
Using the fingers, gently **palpate the entire chest wall**. This enables you to note any areas of tenderness, to note skin temperature and moisture, to detect any superficial lumps or masses and to explore any skin lesions noted on inspection.	**Crepitus** is a coarse crackling sensation palpable over the skin surface. It occurs in subcutaneous emphysema when air escapes from the lung and enters the subcutaneous tissue, as after open thoracic injury or surgery.
Auscultate the posterior chest wall for breath sounds	
The passage of air through the tracheobronchial tree creates a characteristic set of noises that are audible through the chest wall. These noises may also be modified by obstruction within the respiratory passageways or by changes in the lung parenchyma, the pleura or the chest wall.	
Evaluate the presence and quality of **normal breath sounds**. The person is sitting, leaning forwards slightly, with arms resting comfortably across the lap. Instruct the person to breathe through the mouth, a little bit more deeply than usual, but to stop if they begin to feel dizzy. Be careful to monitor the breathing throughout the examination and offer times for the person to rest and breathe normally. The person is usually willing to comply with your instructions in an effort to please you and to be a 'good patient'. Watch that they do not hyperventilate to the point of fainting.	

PROCEDURES AND NORMAL FINDINGS	ABNORMAL FINDINGS AND CLINICAL ALERTS
Use the flat diaphragm endpiece of the stethoscope and hold it firmly on the person's chest wall. Listen to at least one full respiration in each location. Side-to-side comparison is most important.	
Do not confuse background noise with lung sounds. Become familiar with these extraneous noises that may be confused with lung pathology if not recognised: 1. Examiner's breathing on stethoscope tubing 2. Stethoscope tubing bumping together 3. Person shivering 4. Man's hairy chest; movement of hairs under stethoscope sounds like crackles (see Table 19.5)—minimise this by pressing harder or by wetting the hair with a damp cloth 5. Rustling of paper gown or paper drapes.	
While standing behind the person, listen to the following lung areas—posterior from the apices at C7 to the bases (around T10) and laterally from the axilla down to the seventh or eighth rib. Use the sequence illustrated in Figure 19.15. 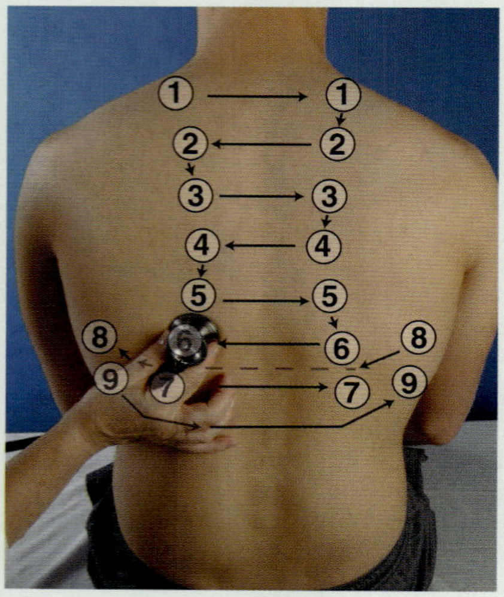 **Figure 19.15**	When assessing a person who is severely short of breath or physically tired and pathology is suspected in the bases or lower lobes, it may be necessary to commence listening at the bases and progress up towards the apices, as well as reduce the number of locations auscultated. This will ensure that the adventitious sounds are heard, while not exacerbating the person's dyspnoea.
Continue to visualise approximate locations of the lobes of each lung so that you correlate your findings to anatomical areas. As you listen, think (1) what AM I hearing over this spot? And (2) what should I EXPECT to be hearing? You should expect to hear three types of normal breath sounds in the adult and older child: **bronchial** (sometimes called tracheal or tubular), **bronchovesicular** and **vesicular**. Study the description of the characteristics of these normal breath sounds in Table 19.1.	

PROCEDURES AND NORMAL FINDINGS	ABNORMAL FINDINGS AND CLINICAL ALERTS

TABLE 19.1 Characteristics of normal breath sounds

	PITCH	AMPLITUDE	DURATION	QUALITY	NORMAL LOCATION
Bronchial (tracheal)	High	Loud	Inspiration < expiration	Harsh, hollow tubular	Trachea and larynx
Bronchovesicular	Moderate	Moderate	Inspiration = expiration	Mixed	Over major bronchi where fewer alveoli are located: posterior, between scapulae especially on right; anterior, around upper sternum in first and second intercostal spaces
Vesicular	Low	Soft	Inspiration = expiration	Rustling, like the sound of the wind in the trees	Over peripheral lung fields where air flows through smaller bronchioles and alveoli

Note the normal location of the three types of breath sounds on the chest wall of the adult and older child (Figures 19.16 and 19.17).

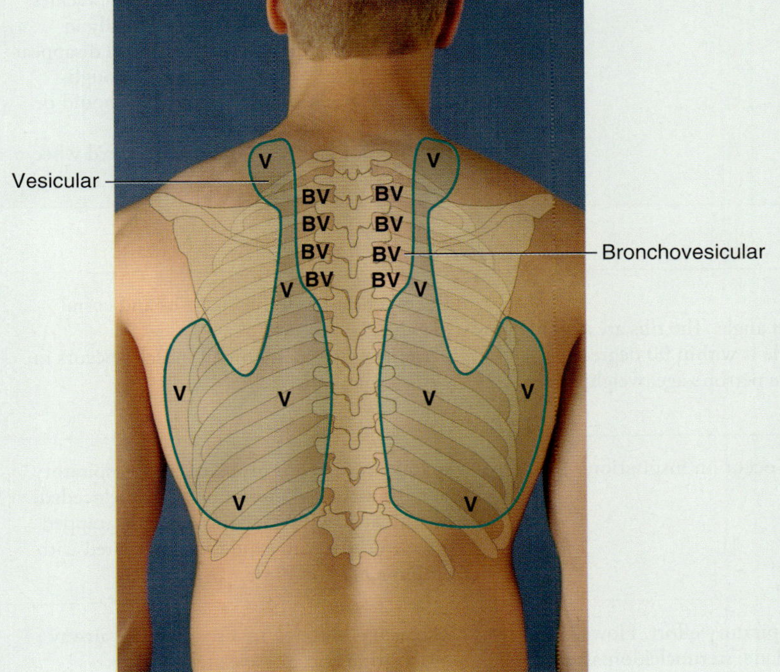

Figure 19.16

Decreased or absent breath sounds occur:

- When the bronchial tree is obstructed at some point by secretions, mucous plug or a foreign body
- In emphysema, air movement is decreased as a result of loss of elasticity in the lung fibres and hyperinflation of the lungs, decreasing the force and noise of inspired air
- When anything obstructs transmission of sound between the lung and your stethoscope, such as pleurisy or pleural thickening, or air (pneumothorax) or fluid (pleural effusion) in the pleural space.

Clinical alert: A silent chest means no air is moving in or out, which is an emergency.

Increased breath sounds mean that sounds are louder than they should be (e.g. bronchial sounds are abnormal when they are heard over an abnormal location, the peripheral lung fields). They have a high-pitched tubular quality, with a prolonged expiratory phase and a distinct pause between inspiration and expiration. They sound very close to your stethoscope, as if they were right *in* the tubing close to your ear. They occur when consolidation (e.g. pneumonia) or compression (e.g. fluid in the intrapleural space) yields a dense lung area that enhances the transmission of sound from the bronchi. When the inspired air reaches the alveoli, it hits solid lung tissue that conducts sound more efficiently to the surface.

PROCEDURES AND NORMAL FINDINGS	ABNORMAL FINDINGS AND CLINICAL ALERTS
Abnormal (adventitious) sounds	
	Note the presence of any abnormal (adventitious) sounds. These are added sounds that are not normally heard in the lungs. If present, they are heard as being superimposed on the breath sounds. They are caused by moving air colliding with secretions in the tracheobronchial passageways or by the popping open of previously deflated airways. Sources differ as to the classification and nomenclature of these sounds (see Table 19.5), but crackles and wheezes are terms commonly used by most examiners. Study Table 19.5 for a complete description of these abnormal adventitious breath sounds.
	One type of adventitious sound, crackles, is sometimes not pathological. These crackles are short, popping, crackling sounds that sound like fine crackles but do not last beyond a few breaths. When sections of alveoli are not fully aerated (as in people who are asleep or in the elderly), they deflate slightly and accumulate secretions. These physiologically 'normal' atelectatic crackles (Table 19.5) are heard when these sections are expanded by a few deep breaths. Crackles are heard only in the periphery, usually in dependent portions of the lungs, and disappear after the first few breaths or after a cough. Crackles which persist beyond this should be considered pathological. During normal tidal flow, high-pitched wheeze occurs with asthma.
Inspect the anterior chest wall	
Note the **shape and configuration** of the chest wall. **Identify bony landmarks;** clavicles, sternum, ribs, costal angle. The ribs are sloping downwards with symmetrical interspaces. The costal angle is within 90 degrees. Development of abdominal muscles is as expected for the person's age, weight and athletic condition.	**Barrel chest** has horizontal ribs and costal angle = 90 degrees. Hypertrophy of abdominal muscles occurs in chronic emphysema.
No retraction or bulging of the intercostal spaces should occur on inspiration.	Retraction suggests obstruction of respiratory tract or increased inspiratory effort is needed, as with atelectasis. Bulging indicates trapped air as in the forced expiration associated with emphysema or asthma.
Normally, accessory muscles are not used to augment respiratory effort. However, with very heavy exercise, the accessory neck muscles (scalene, sternocleidomastoid, trapezius) are used momentarily to enhance inspiration.	**Accessory muscles** are used in acute airway obstruction and massive atelectasis. Rectus abdominis and internal intercostal muscles are used to force expiration in COPD.
The respiratory rate is within normal limits for the person's age (see Table 10.3) and the pattern of breathing is regular. Occasional sighs normally punctuate breathing.	Tachypnoea, bradypnoea, hyperventilation, hypoventilation, periodic breathing (see Table 19.4).

PROCEDURES AND NORMAL FINDINGS	ABNORMAL FINDINGS AND CLINICAL ALERTS
Palpate the anterior chest	
Palpate **symmetrical chest expansion.** Place your hands on the anterolateral wall with the thumbs along the costal margins and pointing towards the xiphoid process (Figure 19.17). 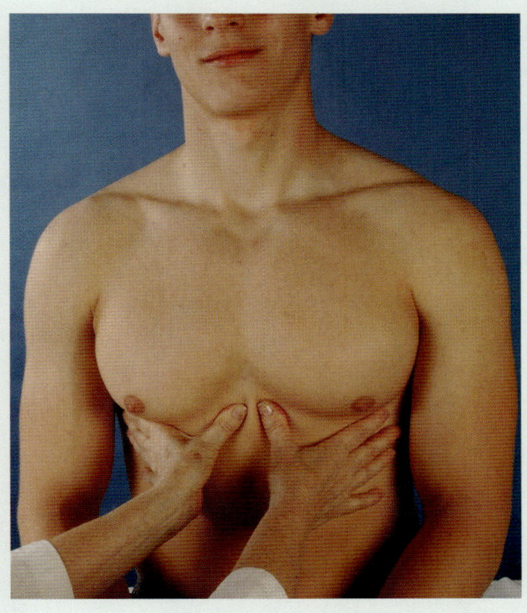 Figure 19.17	Abnormally wide costal angle with little inspiratory variation occurs with emphysema.
Ask the person to take a deep breath. Watch your thumbs move apart symmetrically, and note smooth chest expansion with your fingers. Any limitation in thoracic expansion is easier to detect on the anterior chest because greater range of motion exists with breathing here.	A lag in expansion occurs with atelectasis, pneumonia and postoperative guarding. A palpable grating sensation with breathing indicates pleural friction fremitus (see Table 19.6).
Palpate the anterior chest wall to note any tenderness (normally none is present) and to detect any superficial lumps or masses (again, normally none are present). Note skin mobility and turgor, and note skin temperature and moisture.	
Auscultate the anterior chest wall for breath sounds	
Auscultate the lung fields over the anterior chest from the apices in the supraclavicular areas down to the sixth rib. Progress from side to side as you move downwards, and listen to one full respiration in each location. Do not place your stethoscope directly over the female breast. Displace the breast and listen directly over the chest wall. Use the sequence illustrated in Figure 19.18.	

OBJECTIVE DATA

PROCEDURES AND NORMAL FINDINGS	ABNORMAL FINDINGS AND CLINICAL ALERTS
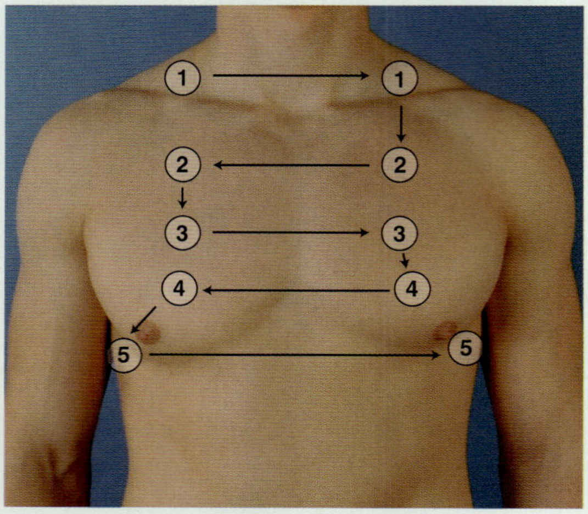 Figure 19.18	
Evaluate normal breath sounds (see Figure 19.19), noting any abnormal breath sounds and any adventitious sounds. If the situation warrants, assess the voice sounds on the anterior chest. 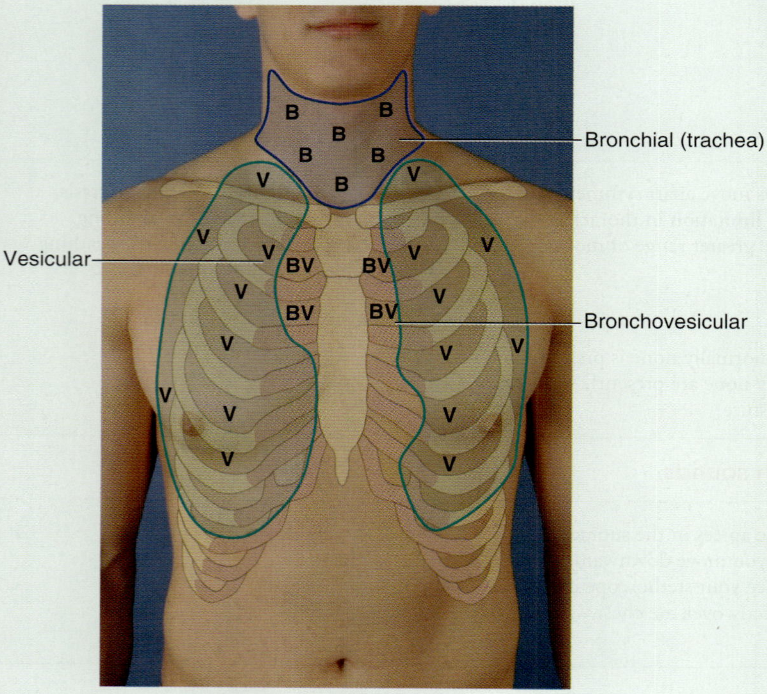 Figure 19.19	Study Table 19.8 for a complete description of abnormal breath sounds.

PROCEDURES AND NORMAL FINDINGS	ABNORMAL FINDINGS AND CLINICAL ALERTS
Measurement of pulmonary function	
The **forced expiratory time** is the number of seconds it takes for the person to exhale from total lung capacity to residual volume. It is a screening measure of airflow obstruction. Although the test is not usually performed in the respiratory assessment, it is useful when you wish to screen for pulmonary function.	
Ask the person to inhale the deepest breath possible and then to blow it all out hard, as quickly as possible, with the mouth open. Listen with your stethoscope over the sternum. The normal time for full expiration is 4 seconds or less.	A forced expiration of 6 seconds or more occurs with obstructive lung disease. Refer this person for more precise pulmonary function studies.
The **pulse oximeter** is a noninvasive method to assess arterial oxygen saturation (SpO_2) and is described in Chapter 10. A healthy person with no lung disease and no anaemia normally has an SpO_2 of 97–98%. However, every SpO_2 result must be evaluated in the context of the person's haemoglobin level, acid–base balance and ventilatory status.	
The **6-min distance (6MD) walk** is a safe, simple, inexpensive, clinical measure of functional status in ageing adults. The 6MD is used as an outcome measure for people in pulmonary rehabilitation because it mirrors conditions that are used in everyday life. Locate a flat-surfaced corridor that has little foot traffic, is wide enough to permit comfortable turns and has a controlled environment. Ensure that the person is wearing comfortable shoes, and equip them with a pulse oximeter to monitor oxygen saturation. Ask the person to set their own pace to cover as much ground as possible in 6 min, and assure the person it is all right to slow down or to stop to rest at any time. Use a stopwatch to time the walk. A person who walks >300 m in 6 min is more likely to engage in activities of daily living.	Ask the person to stop the walk if you measure an SpO_2 below 85% to 88% or if extreme breathlessness occurs.
Additional objective data for infants and children	
To prepare, let the parent hold an infant supported against the chest or shoulder (Figure 19.20). Do not let the usual sequence of the physical examination restrain you; seize the opportunity with a sleeping infant to inspect and then to listen to lung sounds next. This way you can concentrate on the breath sounds before the baby wakes up and possibly cries. Infant crying does not have to be a problem for you, though, because it actually enhances palpation of tactile fremitus and auscultation of breath sounds. Figure 19.20	

PROCEDURES AND NORMAL FINDINGS	ABNORMAL FINDINGS AND CLINICAL ALERTS
A child may sit upright on the parent's lap. Offer the stethoscope and let the child handle it. This reduces any fear of the equipment. Promote the child's participation; school-age children usually are delighted to hear their own breath sounds when you place the stethoscope properly. While listening to breath sounds, ask the young child to take a deep breath and 'blow out' your penlight while you hold the stethoscope with your other hand. Time your letting go of the penlight button so the light goes off after the child blows. Or, ask the child to 'pant like a dog' while you auscultate.	
Inspection. The infant has a rounded thorax with an equal anteroposterior-to-transverse chest diameter (Figure 19.21). By age 6 years, the thorax reaches the adult ratio of 1:2 (anteroposterior-to-transverse diameter). The newborn's chest circumference is 30–36 cm and is 2 cm smaller than the head circumference until 2 years of age. The chest wall is thin with little musculature. The ribs and the xiphoid are prominent; you can see as well as feel the sharp tip of the xiphoid process. The thoracic cage is soft and flexible. 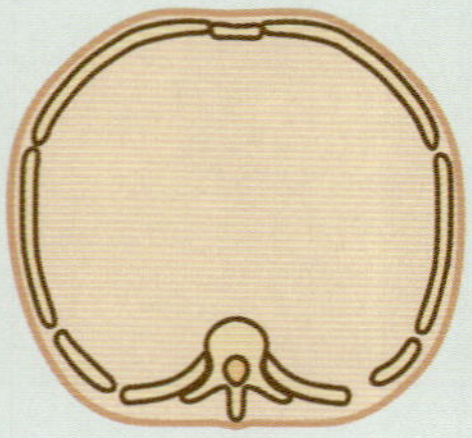 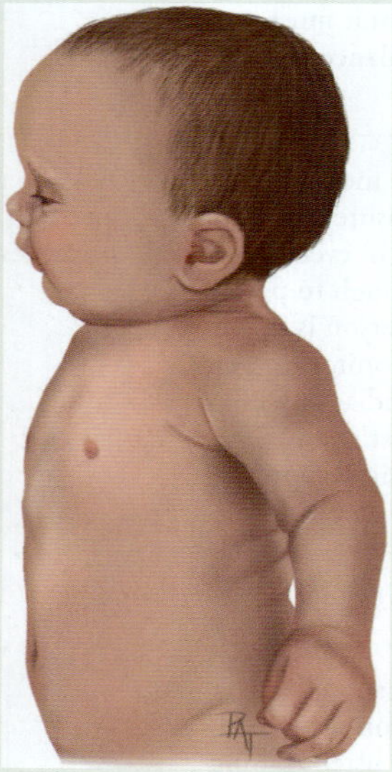 **Figure 19.21**	Note a barrel shape persisting after age 6 years, which may develop with chronic asthma or cystic fibrosis.
In newborn males and females, the breasts may look enlarged by the second or third day from maternal oestrogen. Occasionally a white fluid, sometimes referred to by the slang expression 'witch's milk', can be expressed. This resolves within a week.	
In some children, 'Harrison groove' occurs normally. This is a horizontal groove in the rib cage at the level of the insertion of the diaphragm, extending from the sternum to the midaxillary line.	**Harrison groove** also occurs with rickets from the pull of the diaphragm on weakened ribs.

OBJECTIVE DATA

PROCEDURES AND NORMAL FINDINGS	ABNORMAL FINDINGS AND CLINICAL ALERTS
The newborn's first respiratory assessment is part of the **Apgar scoring system** to measure the successful transition to extrauterine life (Table 19.2). The five standard parameters are scored at 1 min and at 5 min after birth. A 1-min Apgar with a total score of 7–10 indicates a newborn in good condition, needing only suctioning of the nose and mouth and otherwise routine care.	In the immediate newborn period, depressed respirations are due to maternal drugs, interruption of the uterine blood supply or obstruction of the tracheobronchial tree with mucus or fluid. A 1-min Apgar score with a total score of 3–6 indicates a moderately depressed newborn needing more resuscitation and subsequent close observation. A score of 0–2 indicates a severely depressed newborn needing full resuscitation, ventilatory assistance and subsequent intensive care.

TABLE 19.2 Apgar scoring system

	2	1	0
Heart rate	Over 100	Slow (below 100)	Absent
Respiratory effort	Good, sustained cry; regular respirations	Slow, irregular, shallow	Absent
Muscle tone	Active motion, spontaneous flexion	Some flexion of extremities; some resistance to extension	Limp, flaccid
Reflex irritability (response to catheter nares)	Sneeze, cough, cry	Grimace, frown	No response
Colour	Completely pink	Body pink, extremities pale	Cyanotic, pale
			Total score

PROCEDURES AND NORMAL FINDINGS	ABNORMAL FINDINGS AND CLINICAL ALERTS
The infant breathes through the nose rather than the mouth and is an obligate nose breather until 3 months. Slight flaring of the lower costal margins may occur with respirations, but normally no flaring of the nostrils and no sternal retractions or intercostal retractions occur. The diaphragm is the newborn's major respiratory muscle. Intercostal muscles are not well developed. Thus you observe the abdomen bulge with each inspiration but see little thoracic expansion.	Marked **retractions of sternum and intercostal muscles** indicate increased inspiratory effort, as in atelectasis, pneumonia, asthma and acute airway obstruction.
Count the respiratory rate for 1 full min. Normal rates for the newborn are 30–40 breaths per min but may spike up to 60 per min. Obtain the most accurate respiratory rate by counting when the infant is asleep because infants reach rapid rates with very little excitation when awake. The respiratory pattern may be irregular when extremes in room temperature occur or with feeding or sleeping. Brief periods of apnoea less than 10 or 15 seconds are common. This periodic breathing is more common in premature infants.	**Rapid respiratory rates** accompany pneumonia, fever, pain, heart disease and anaemia. In an infant, tachypnoea of 50–100 per min during sleep may be an early sign of heart failure.
Palpation. Palpate symmetrical chest expansion by encircling the infant's thorax with both hands. Further palpation should yield no lumps, masses or crepitus, although you may feel the costochondral junctions in some normal infants.	**Asymmetrical expansion** occurs with diaphragmatic hernia or pneumothorax. **Crepitus** is palpable around a fractured clavicle, which may occur with difficult forceps delivery. **Rachitic rosary**—prominent round knobs at costochondral junctions—is seen in infants with rickets or scurvy.
Auscultation. Auscultation normally yields bronchovesicular breath sounds in the peripheral lung fields of the infant and young child up to age 5–6 years. Their relatively thin chest walls with underdeveloped musculature do not damp off the sound as do the thicker walls of adults, so breath sounds are louder and harsher.	**Diminished breath sounds** occur with pneumonia, atelectasis, pleural effusion or pneumothorax.

PROCEDURES AND NORMAL FINDINGS	ABNORMAL FINDINGS AND CLINICAL ALERTS
Fine crackles are the adventitious sounds commonly heard in the immediate newborn period from opening of the airways and clearing of fluid. Because the newborn's chest wall is so thin, transmission of sounds is enhanced and sound is heard easily all over the chest, making localisation of breath sounds a problem. Even bowel sounds are easily heard in the chest. Try using the smaller paediatric diaphragm endpiece, or place the bell over the infant's interspaces and not over the ribs. Use the paediatric diaphragm on an older infant or toddler.	Persistent **fine crackles** that are scattered over the chest occur with pneumonia, bronchiolitis or atelectasis. Crackles only in upper lung fields occur with cystic fibrosis; crackles only in lower lung fields occur with heart failure. **Expiratory wheezing** occurs with lower airway obstruction (e.g. asthma or bronchiolitis). When unilateral, it may be foreign body aspiration. Persistent peristaltic sounds with diminished breath sounds on the same side may indicate diaphragmatic hernia. **Stridor** is a high-pitched inspiratory crowing sound heard without the stethoscope, occurring with upper airway obstruction (e.g. croup, foreign body aspiration or acute epiglottitis).
Additional objective data for the pregnant woman	
The thoracic cage may appear wider, and the costal angle may feel wider than in the non-pregnant state. Respirations may be deeper, although this can be quantified only with pulmonary function tests.	
Additional objective data for the adult over 65 years	
The rib cage commonly shows an increased anteroposterior diameter, giving a round barrel shape, and **kyphosis** or an outward curvature of the thoracic spine (see Table 19.3). The person compensates by holding the head extended and tilted back. You may palpate marked bony prominences because of decreased subcutaneous fat. Chest expansion may be somewhat decreased with the older person, although it should still be symmetrical. The costal cartilages become calcified with ageing, resulting in a less mobile thorax.	
The frail older person may fatigue easily, especially during auscultation when deep mouth breathing is required. Take care that this person does not hyperventilate and become dizzy. Allow brief rest periods or quiet breathing. If the person does feel faint, holding the breath for a few seconds will restore equilibrium.	
Common diagnostic tests	
Chest X-ray (CXR). A CXR is performed to assess for fractures of the bony thorax (sternum, ribcage, vertebrae) as well as the position and potential pathology associated with the contents of the thorax and mediastinum. In particular, an X-ray can highlight the presence of problems such as pneumonia, pulmonary oedema, pulmonary effusions, atelectasis, pneumothorax or malignancy. In certain circumstances, an abnormal CXR will be followed up with further diagnostic imaging such as a CT or VQ scan or an MRI.	
Sputum microbiology, culture and sensitivity (MC&S). In the presence or suspected presence of a lower respiratory tract infection, a sputum sample will often be used to determine the presence of, type and antibiotic sensitivity of the culprit microorganism.	
Arterial blood gases (ABGs). Performed to evaluate the levels of oxygen and carbon dioxide, as well as the pH and oxygen-carrying capacity of arterial blood. ABGs are routinely used within critical care areas to guide oxygen therapy and ventilator support, but may also be used in the diagnosis of respiratory failure in other areas of healthcare.	Normal values: pH: 7.35–7.45 Oxygen saturation (SaO_2): 94.5–98.2% PaO_2: 80–100 mmHg $PaCO_2$: 35–45 mmHg
Venous blood gases (VBGs). Used more commonly outside of the critical care areas to evaluate the level of carbon dioxide and pH of the venous blood. Unlike ABGs, VBGs are not usually used to guide oxygen therapy. Pulmonary function testing is performed to evaluate the effectiveness of inspiration, expiration, lung capacity and the movement of gases (respiration) across the alveoli.	Normal values: pH: 7.32–7.43 $PvCO_2$: 41–50 mmHg

OBJECTIVE DATA

Further objective assessment for advanced practice

The assessments described in the following section require advanced skill and scope of practice. Nurses working in specialist respiratory units and nurses working in community centres may need to develop these skills.

Equipment

In addition to previously identified equipment Centimetre ruler

PROCEDURES AND NORMAL FINDINGS	ABNORMAL FINDINGS AND CLINICAL ALERTS
Palpate posterior chest wall for tactile fremitus	
Assess **tactile** (or **vocal**) **fremitus**. Fremitus is a palpable vibration. Sounds generated from the larynx are transmitted through patent bronchi and through the lung parenchyma to the chest wall, where you feel them as vibrations. Use either the palmar base (the ball) of the fingers or the ulnar edge of one hand, and touch the person's chest while they repeat the words 'ninety-nine' or 'blue balloon'. These are resonant phrases that generate strong vibrations. Start over the lung apices and palpate from one side to another (Figure 19.22). 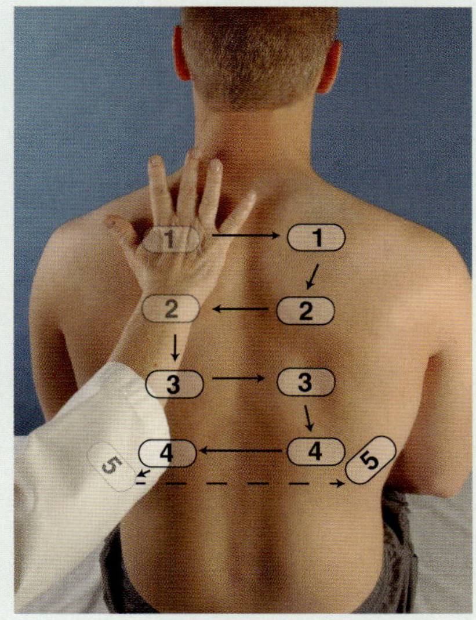 Figure 19.22	**Decreased fremitus** occurs when anything obstructs transmission of vibrations (e.g. obstructed bronchus, pleural effusion or thickening, pneumothorax or emphysema). Any barrier that comes between the sound and your palpating hand will decrease fremitus. **Increased fremitus** occurs with compression or consolidation of lung tissue (e.g. lobar pneumonia). This is present only when the bronchus is patent and when the consolidation extends to the lung surface. Note that only gross changes increase fremitus. Small areas of early pneumonia do not significantly affect fremitus. **Rhonchal fremitus** is palpable with thick bronchial secretions. **Pleural friction fremitus** is palpable with inflammation of the pleura (see Table 19.6).
Fremitus varies among persons but symmetry is most important; the vibrations should feel the same in the corresponding area on each side. However, just between the scapulae, fremitus may feel stronger on the right side than on the left side because the right side is closer to the bronchial bifurcation. Avoid palpating over the scapulae because bone damps out sound transmission. The following factors affect the normal intensity of tactile fremitus: • Relative location of bronchi to the chest wall. Normally, fremitus is most prominent between the scapulae and around the sternum, sites where the major bronchi are closest to the chest wall. Fremitus normally decreases as you progress down because more and more tissue impedes sound transmission. • Thickness of the chest wall. Fremitus feels greater over a thin chest wall than over an obese or heavily muscular one where thick tissue damps the vibration. • Pitch and intensity. A loud, low-pitched voice generates more fremitus than a soft, high-pitched one. Note any areas of abnormal fremitus. Sound is conducted better through a uniformly dense structure than through a porous one, which changes in shape and solidity (as does the lung tissue during normal respiration). Thus, conditions that increase the density of lung tissue make a better conducting medium for sound vibrations and increase tactile fremitus.	

OBJECTIVE DATA

PROCEDURES AND NORMAL FINDINGS	ABNORMAL FINDINGS AND CLINICAL ALERTS

Palpate the anterior chest wall for tactile fremitus

Assess **tactile (vocal) fremitus**. Begin palpating over the lung apices in the supraclavicular areas (Figure 19.23 and Table 19.6). Compare vibrations from one side to the other as the person repeats 'ninety-nine'. Avoid palpating over female breast tissue because breast tissue normally damps the sound.

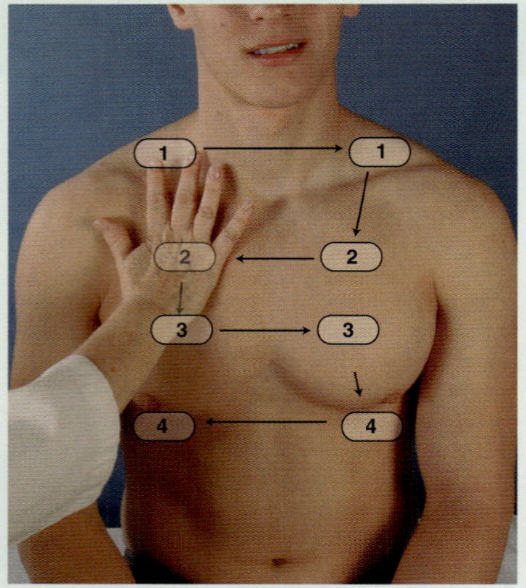

Figure 19.23

Percuss posterior lung fields

Determine the **predominant note over the lung fields**. Start at the apices and percuss the band of normally resonant tissue across the tops of both shoulders (Figure 19.24). Then, percussing in the interspaces, make a side-to-side comparison all the way down the lung region. Percuss at 5-cm intervals. Avoid the damping effect of the scapulae and ribs.

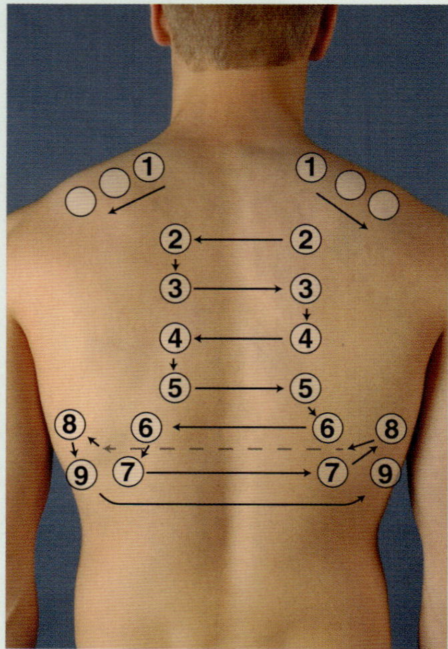

Figure 19.24

OBJECTIVE DATA

PROCEDURES AND NORMAL FINDINGS	ABNORMAL FINDINGS AND CLINICAL ALERTS
Resonance is the low-pitched, clear, hollow sound that predominates in healthy lung tissue in the adult (Figure 19.25). However, resonance is a relative term and has no constant standard. The resonant note may be modified somewhat in the athlete with a heavily muscular chest wall and in the heavily obese adult in whom subcutaneous fat produces scattered dullness. 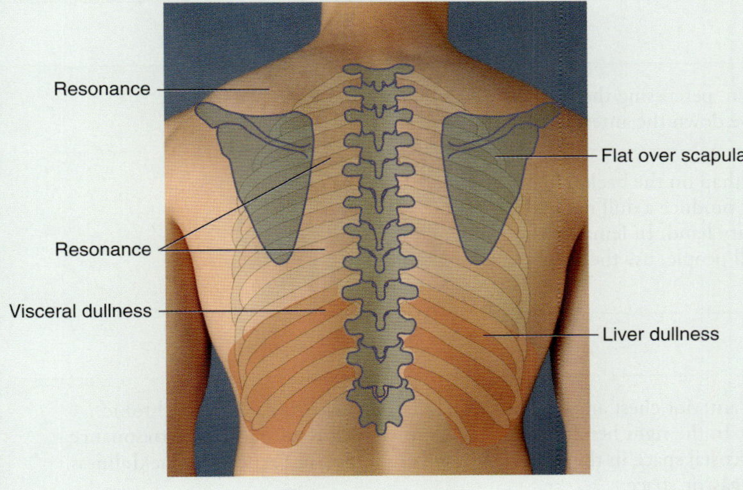 Figure 19.25	**Hyperresonance** is a lower-pitched, booming sound found when too much air is present, as in emphysema or pneumothorax. A **dull** note (soft, muffled thud) signals abnormal density in the lungs, as with pneumonia, pleural effusion, atelectasis or tumour.
The depth of penetration of percussion has limits. Percussion sets into motion only the outer 5–7 cm of tissue. It will not penetrate to reveal any change in density deeper than that. Also, an abnormal finding must be 2–3 cm wide to yield an abnormal percussion note. Lesions smaller than that are not detectable by percussion.	

Diaphragmatic excursion

Determine **diaphragmatic excursion** (Figure 19.26A). Percuss to map out the lower lung border, both in expiration and in inspiration. First, ask the person to 'exhale and hold it' briefly while you percuss down the scapular line until the sound changes from resonant to dull on each side. This estimates the level of the diaphragm separating the lungs from the abdominal viscera. It may be somewhat higher on the right side (about 1–2 cm) because of the presence of the liver. Mark the spot.

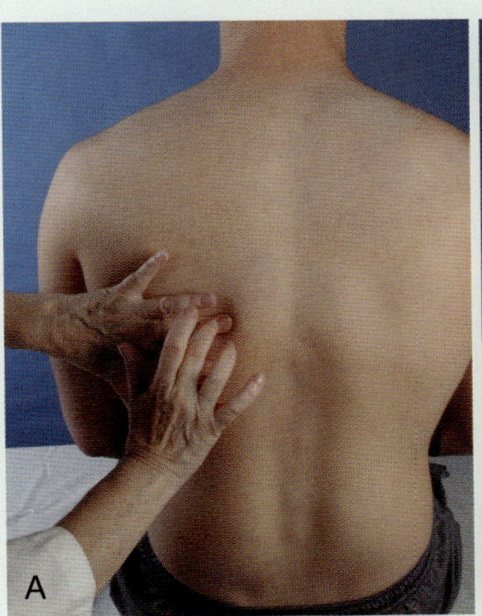

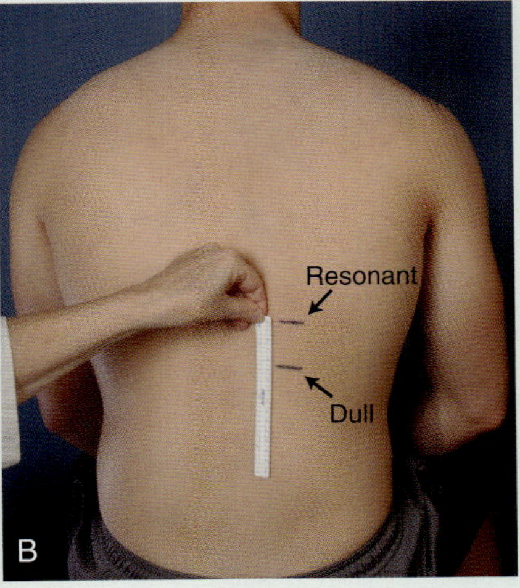

Figure 19.26

PROCEDURES AND NORMAL FINDINGS	ABNORMAL FINDINGS AND CLINICAL ALERTS
Now ask the person to 'take a deep breath and hold it'. Continue percussing down from your first mark and mark the level where the sound changes to dull on this deep inspiration. Measure the difference. This diaphragmatic excursion should be equal bilaterally and measure about 3 to 5 cm in adults, although it may be up to 7–8 cm in well-conditioned people (Figure 19.26B).	Note an abnormally high level of dullness and absence of excursion. These occur with pleural effusion (fluid in the space between the visceral and parietal pleura) or atelectasis of the lower lobes.
Percuss anterior lung fields	
Begin percussing the apices in the supraclavicular areas. Then, percussing the intercostal spaces and comparing one side to the other, move down the anterior chest.	
Intercostal spaces are easier to palpate on the anterior chest than on the back. Do not percuss directly over female breast tissue because this would produce a dull note. Shift the breast tissue over slightly using the edge of your stationary hand. In females with large breasts, percussion may yield little useful data. With all people, use the sequence illustrated in Figure 19.19.	
Sequence for percussion of anterior chest	
Note the borders of cardiac dullness normally found on the anterior chest and do not confuse these with suspected lung pathology (Figure 19.27). In the right hemithorax, the upper border of liver dullness is located in the fifth intercostal space in the right midclavicular line. On the left, tympany is evident over the gastric space. 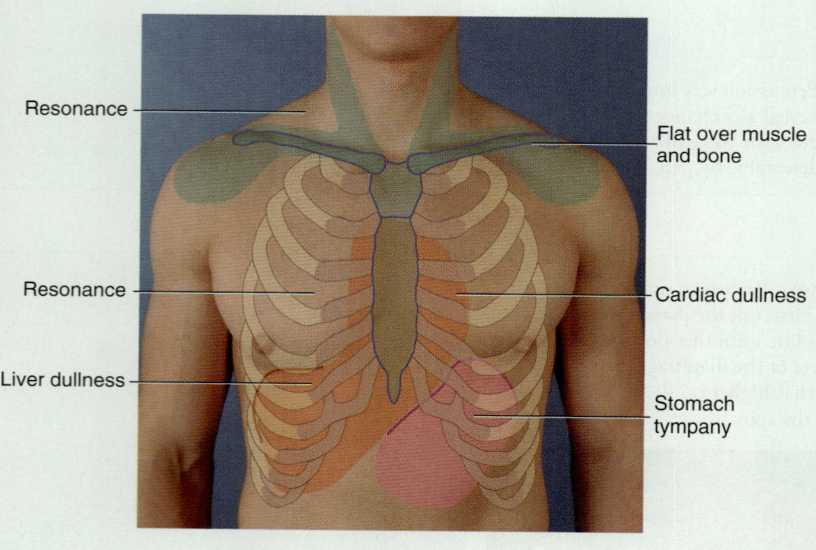 **Figure 19.27**	Lungs are hyperinflated with chronic emphysema, resulting in hyperresonance where you would expect cardiac dullness.
Auscultate for vocal sounds	
Determine the quality of **voice sounds** or **vocal resonance**. The spoken voice can be auscultated over the chest wall just as it can be felt in tactile fremitus. Ask the person to repeat a phrase such as 'ninety-nine' while you listen over the chest wall. Normal voice transmission is soft, muffled and indistinct; you can hear sound through the stethoscope but cannot distinguish exactly what is being said. Pathology that increases lung density enhances transmission of voice sounds.	Consolidation or compression of lung tissue will enhance the voice sounds, making the words more distinct.
Eliciting the voice sounds is not usually done in the routine examination. Rather, these are supplemental manoeuvres that may be used by nurses working in advanced practice roles. When they are performed, the advance practice nurse is assessing for possible presence of **bronchophony**, **egophony** and **whispered pectoriloquy** (Table 19.8).	

OBJECTIVE DATA

Summary Checklist

LOWER AIRWAYS ASSESSMENT

Subjective data

1. Presenting concern
2. Shortness of breath
3. Chest pain
4. Cough
5. History of respiratory infections
6. Smoking history
7. Environmental exposure
8. Health and lifestyle management

Objective data

1. General inspection
2. Inspection of posterior chest wall
3. Palpation of posterior chest wall
4. Auscultation of posterior chest wall for breath sounds
5. Inspection of anterior chest wall
6. Palpation of anterior chest wall
7. Auscultation of anterior chest wall for breath sounds
8. Measurement of pulmonary function

PROMOTING A HEALTHY LIFESTYLE

ENVIRONMENTAL TOBACCO SMOKE (ETS)

Secondhand smoke—there is no risk-free level of exposure!

Secondhand smoke, also referred to as environmental tobacco smoke, is a mixture of *sidestream smoke*, the smoke from the burning end of a cigarette, pipe or cigar, and *mainstream smoke*, the smoke exhaled from the lungs of the individual smoking. The evidence indicates that there is no risk-free level of exposure to secondhand smoke. Exposure to secondhand smoke, which is primarily involuntary, increases our risk for adverse health effects. Further, the general public's exposure to secondhand smoke, regardless of whether they are smokers, is much higher than most people realise. More recently, the rise of e-cigarettes and 'vaping' has raised new questions about the safety of exposure to secondhand vapour. The safety of these alternatives to traditional tobacco smoking is yet to be established, despite their growing popularity.

Secondhand smoke is especially harmful to young children, increasing respiratory infection rates, inner ear infections and aggravation of asthma. There is a causal relationship between maternal smoking during pregnancy and:

- a persistent adverse lung function throughout childhood
- a small reduction in birth weight.

Following birth, infants and children exposed to environmental tobacco smoke face an increased risk of:

- sudden infant death syndrome (SIDS)
- lower level of lung function
- lower respiratory illness
- middle ear infections
- asthma, croup and bronchitis (Campbell et al 2017).

According to the Australian Institute of Health and Welfare (2018a) 4% of children (0–14 years) and 2.8% of all Australians lived in households with at least one regular smoker who smoked indoors, however, the incidence is decreasing. Secondhand smoke contains hundreds of chemicals known to be toxic or carcinogenic, including formaldehyde, benzene, vinyl chloride, arsenic and cyanide. Involuntarily inhaled by nonsmokers, it can linger in the air for hours: long after the cigarette, cigar or pipe has been extinguished.

Exposure to secondhand smoke places nonsmokers at risk for the same diseases as active smoking does. Nonsmokers exposed to secondhand smoke are 25% more likely to have heart disease and 20% more likely to have lung cancer than are those non-smokers who are not exposed to smoke. Separating smokers from nonsmokers, cleaning the air indoors and ventilating buildings do not eliminate the exposure risk to nonsmokers. However, eliminating smoking from indoor spaces does fully protect the nonsmoker.

Documentation and critical thinking

FOCUSED ASSESSMENT: CLINICAL CASE STUDY

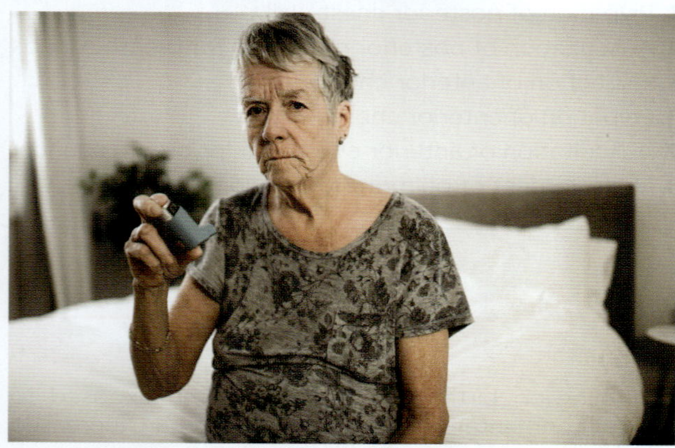

Context

Mrs. Dorothy Smith is a 73-year-old woman who has been admitted for care in your clinical area with an infective exacerbation of chronic obstructive pulmonary disease (COPD).

Subjective

Dorothy reports a history of upper respiratory tract infections over the past two weeks. This has resulted in increased dyspnoea, and decreased ability to independently complete ADLs. Dyspnoea is significantly worse following any exertion. Dorothy tells you that she hasn't been sleeping well and is feeling very tired. Dorothy reports no chest pain, but has had a productive cough, worse in the mornings, producing sputum that is thick and brown coloured. Dorothy has had several other previous admissions for exacerbations of COPD.

She has never smoked tobacco, but her husband was a builder who worked extensively with asbestos containing products. Dorothy was exposed to asbestos dust through shaking out and laundering his dusty clothes every day. Her husband died of cardiac disease several years ago, and Dorothy lives alone. She has two daughters, one of whom lives Interstate. The other daughter has recently moved to be closer to her mother. Dorothy is on regular inhaled medications, including long and short acting beta-agonists, and inhaled corticosteroids.

Objective

General inspection: She is sitting in bed, leaning forward with arms braced against the tray table. She looks tired, and appears anxious and agitated.

Vital signs:

Temperature: 37.8° aurally

HR: 100 bpm

Resp. rate: 28/min, regular, shallow with a prolonged expiration time.

BP: 110/60

SPo_2: 90%

Inspection: Alert and orientated, but only able to speak in short phrases. She is in tripod position and using purse-lipped breathing. Her skin is pale, oral mucous membranes and tongue are dry. No audible wheeze or stridor. Accessory muscle use is noted including neck, shoulder and abdominal muscles. Her thorax is hyper inflated, the sternum is lifted and ribs flared to almost horizontal position.

Palpation: Her skin is cool to touch. Minimal but symmetrical chest expansion. No lumps, masses or tenderness on palpation.

Auscultation: Breath sounds diminished. Quiet continuous wheeze bilaterally, anterior and posterior. No crackles.

Collaborative problem

Probable acute exacerbation of COPD

Problem statements/nursing diagnoses

Impaired gas exchange related to chronic obstructive pulmonary disease

Potential ineffective airway clearance related to chronic obstructive pulmonary disease

Ineffective breathing pattern related to chronic obstructive pulmonary disease

Anxiety related to dyspnoea

Activity intolerance related to dyspnoea

Sleep disturbance related to dyspnoea, cough

Self-care deficit (showering, grooming, dressing, toileting) related to dyspnoea

Abnormal findings

TABLE 19.3 Configurations of the thorax

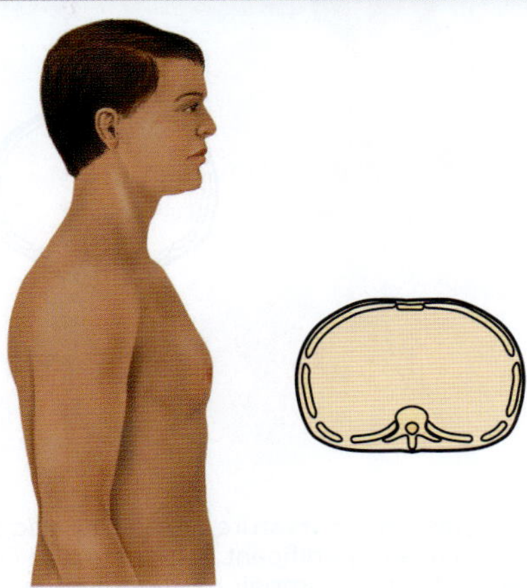

Normal adult (for comparison)

The thorax has an elliptical shape with an anteroposterior-to-transverse diameter of 1:2 or 5:7.

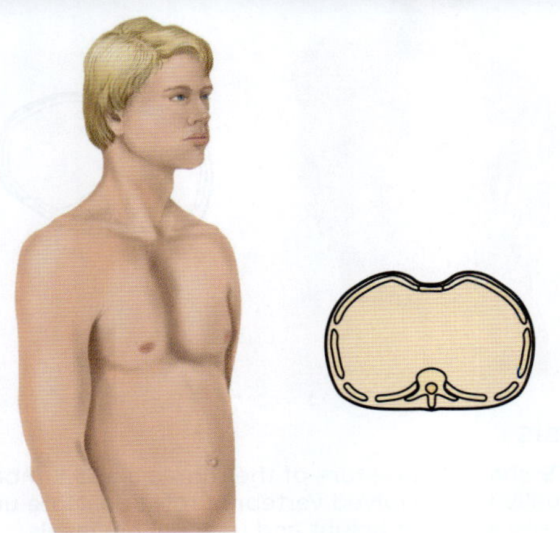

Pectus excavatum

A markedly sunken sternum and adjacent cartilages (also called funnel chest). Depression begins at second intercostal space, becoming depressed most at junction of xiphoid with body of sternum. More noticeable on inspiration. Congenital, usually not symptomatic. When severe, sternal depression may cause embarrassment and a negative self-concept. Surgery may be indicated.

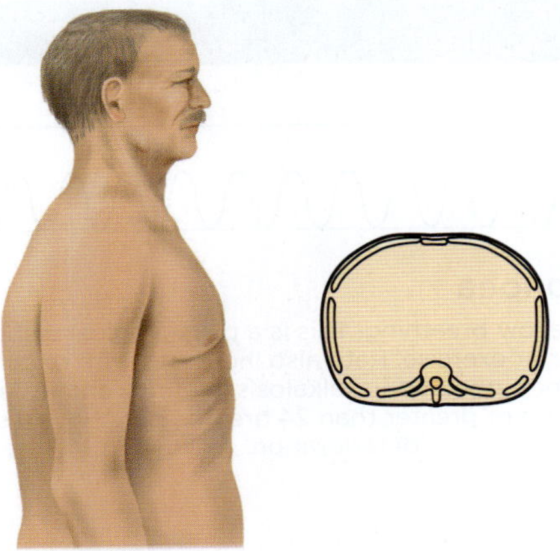

Barrel chest

Note equal anteroposterior-to-transverse diameter and that ribs are horizontal instead of the normal downward slope. This is associated with normal ageing and also with chronic emphysema and asthma as a result of hyperinflation of lungs.

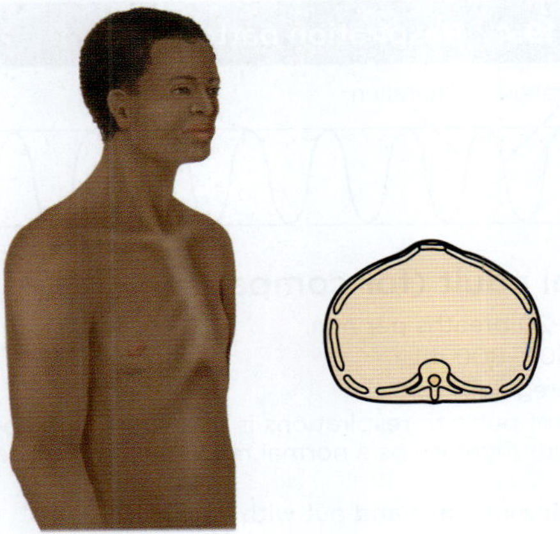

Pectus carinatum

A forward protrusion of the sternum, with ribs sloping back at either side and vertical depressions along costochondral junctions (pigeon chest). Less common than pectus excavatum, this minor deformity requires no treatment. If severe, surgery may be indicated.

(Continued)

TABLE 19.3 Configurations of the thorax—cont'd

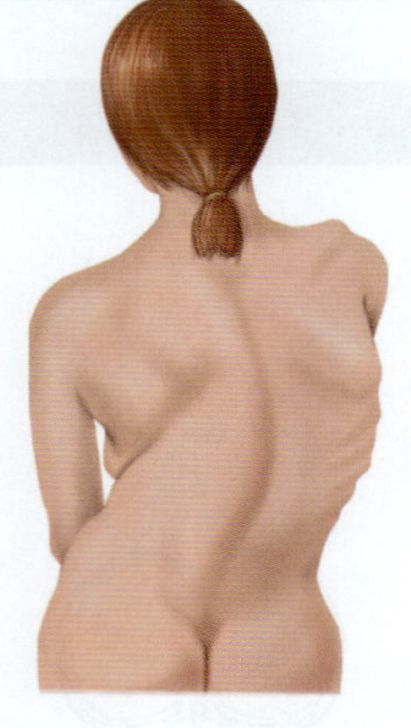
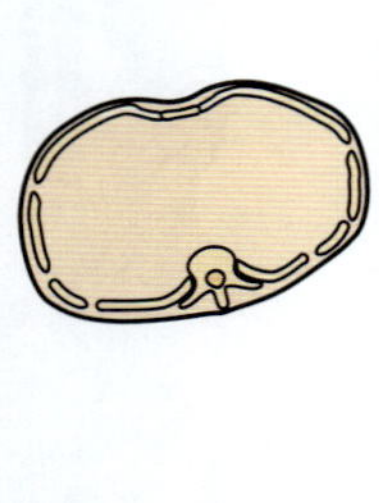

Scoliosis

A lateral **S**-shaped curvature of the thoracic and lumbar spine, usually with involved vertebrae rotation. Note unequal shoulder and scapular height and unequal hip levels, rib interspaces flared on convex side. More prevalent in adolescent age groups, especially girls. Mild deformities are asymptomatic. If severe (>45 degrees) deviation is present, scoliosis may reduce lung volume, then person is at risk for impaired cardiopulmonary function. Primary impairment is cosmetic deformity, negatively affecting self-image. Refer early for treatment, often surgery.

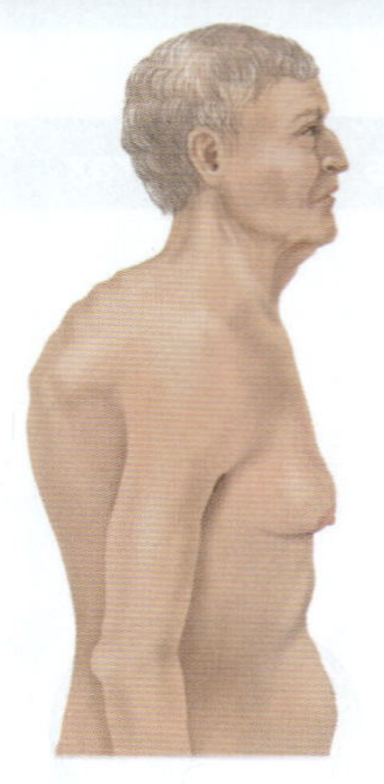
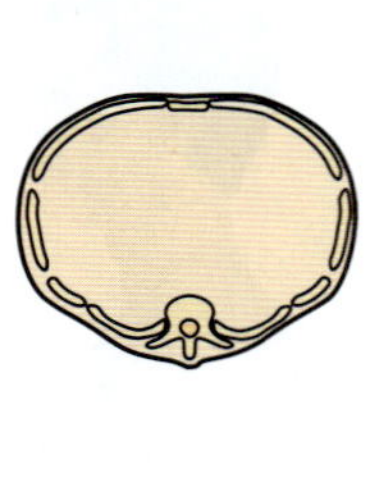

Kyphosis

An exaggerated posterior curvature of the thoracic spine (humpback) that causes significant back pain and limited mobility. Severe deformities impair cardiopulmonary function. If the neck muscles are strong, compensation occurs by hyperextension of head to maintain level of vision.

Kyphosis has been associated with ageing, especially the familiar 'dowager's hump' of postmenopausal osteoporotic women. However, it is common well before menopause. It is related to physical fitness; women with adequate exercise habits are less likely to have kyphosis.

TABLE 19.4 Respiration patterns*

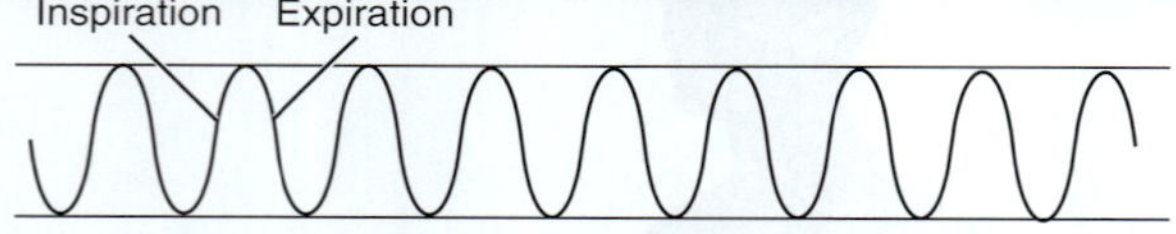

Normal adult (for comparison)

Rate—10–20 breaths per min.

Depth—500–800 mL.

Pattern—regular.

The ratio of pulse to respirations is fairly constant, about 4:1. Both values increase as a normal response to exercise, fear or fever.

Depth—air moving in and out with each respiration.

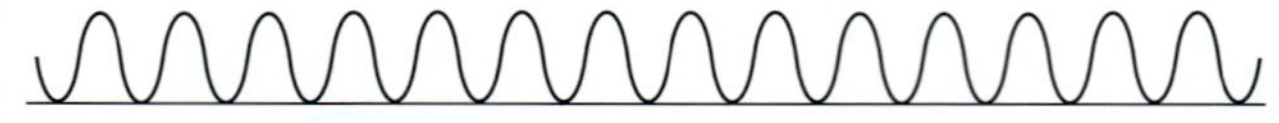

Tachypnoea

Rapid shallow breathing. This is a physiological response to fever, fear or exercise. Rate also increases with respiratory insufficiency, pneumonia, alkalosis, pleurisy and lesions in the pons. A rate of greater than 24 breaths per min is a strong predictor of clinical deterioration.

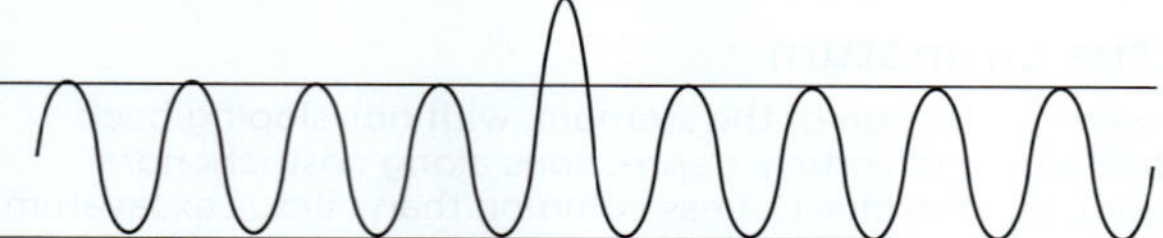

Sigh

Occasional sighs punctuate the normal breathing pattern and are purposeful to expand alveoli. Frequent sighs may indicate emotional dysfunction. Frequent sighs also may lead to hyperventilation and dizziness.

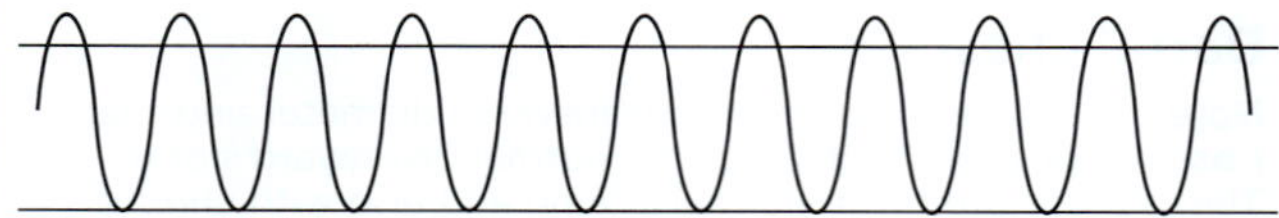

Hyperventilation

Increase in both rate and depth. Normally occurs with extreme exertion, fear or anxiety. Also occurs with diabetic ketoacidosis (Kussmaul's respirations), hepatic coma, salicylate overdose (producing a respiratory alkalosis to compensate for the metabolic acidosis), lesions of the midbrain and alteration in blood gas concentration (either an increase in carbon dioxide or decrease in oxygen). Hyperventilation blows off carbon dioxide, causing a decreased level in the blood (alkalosis).

TABLE 19.4 Respiration patterns*—cont'd

Bradypnoea

Slow breathing. A decreased but regular rate (less than 10 per min), as in drug-induced depression of the respiratory centre in the medulla, increased intracranial pressure and diabetic coma.

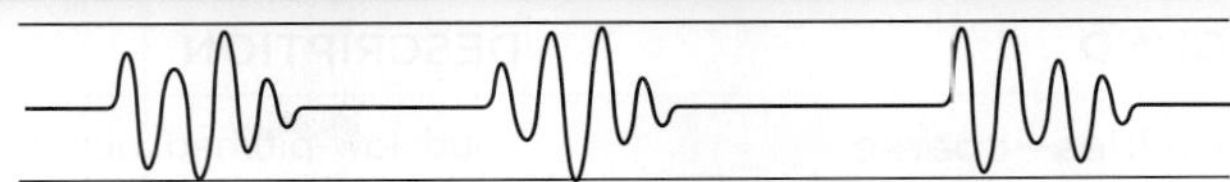

Biot's respiration

Similar to Cheyne-Stokes respiration, except that the pattern is irregular. A series of normal respirations (three to four) is followed by a period of apnoea. The cycle length is variable, lasting anywhere from 10 seconds to 1 min. Seen with head trauma, brain abscess, heat stroke, spinal meningitis and encephalitis.

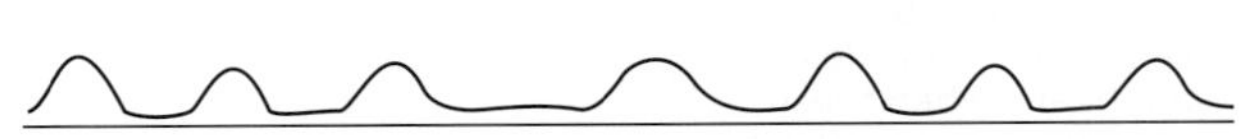

Hypoventilation

An irregular shallow pattern caused by an overdose of narcotics or anaesthetics. May also occur with prolonged bed rest or conscious splinting of the chest to avoid respiratory pain.

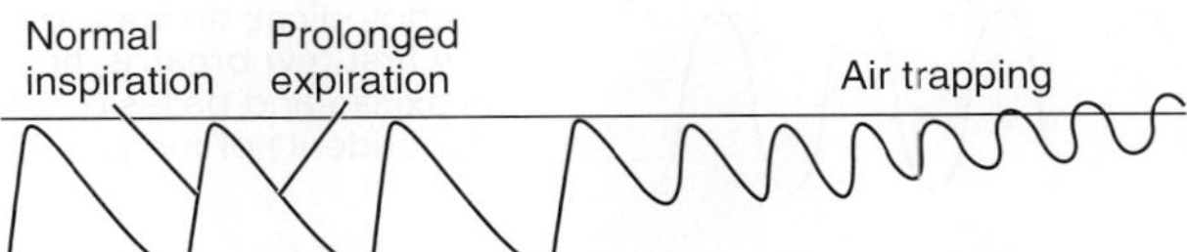

Chronic obstructive breathing

Normal inspiration and prolonged expiration to overcome increased airway resistance. In a person with chronic obstructive lung disease, any situation calling for increased heart rate (exercise) may lead to dyspnoeic episode (air trapping), because then the person does not have enough time for full expiration.

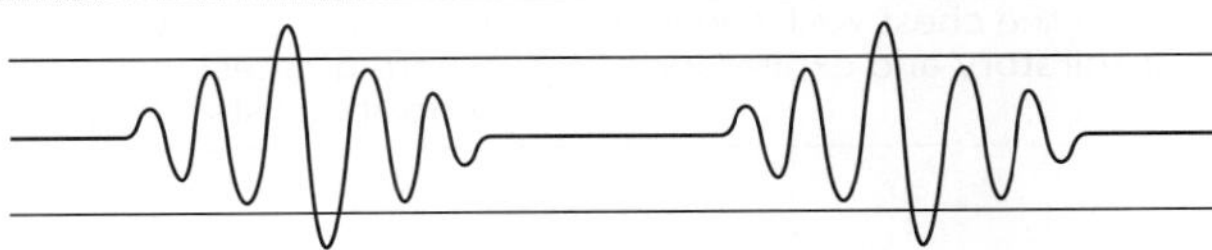

Cheyne-Stokes respiration

A cycle in which respirations gradually wax and wane in a regular pattern, increasing in rate and depth and then decreasing. The breathing periods last 30–45 seconds, with periods of apnoea (20 seconds) alternating the cycle. The most common cause is severe heart failure; other causes are renal failure, meningitis, drug overdose and increased intracranial pressure. Occurs normally in infants and ageing persons during sleep.

*Assess the (1) rate, (2) depth (tidal volume) and (3) pattern.

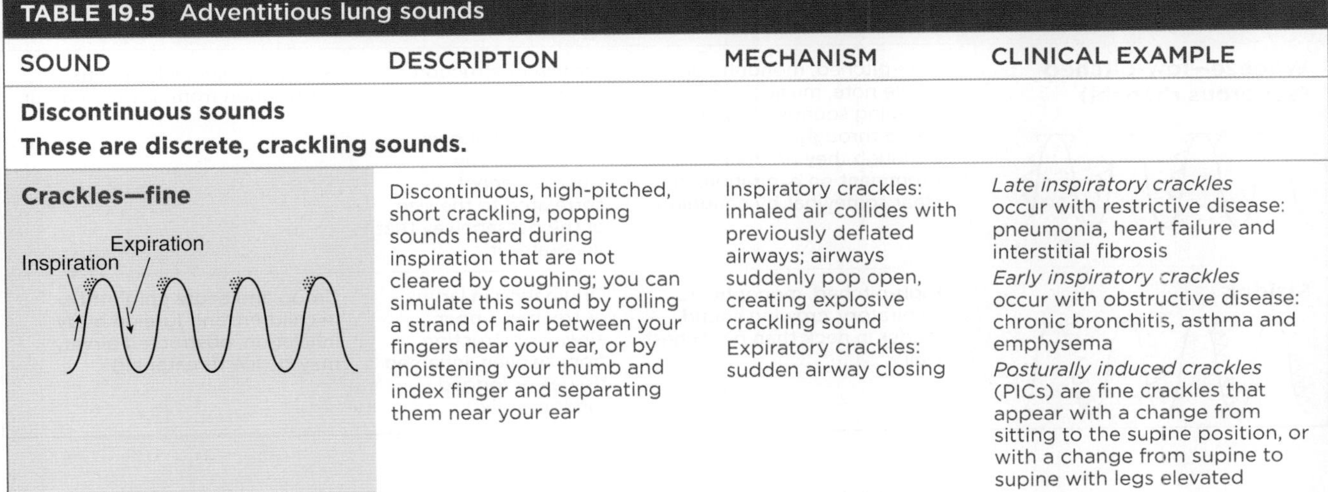

TABLE 19.5 Adventitious lung sounds

SOUND	DESCRIPTION	MECHANISM	CLINICAL EXAMPLE
Discontinuous sounds **These are discrete, crackling sounds.**			
Crackles—fine Expiration Inspiration	Discontinuous, high-pitched, short crackling, popping sounds heard during inspiration that are not cleared by coughing; you can simulate this sound by rolling a strand of hair between your fingers near your ear, or by moistening your thumb and index finger and separating them near your ear	Inspiratory crackles: inhaled air collides with previously deflated airways; airways suddenly pop open, creating explosive crackling sound Expiratory crackles: sudden airway closing	*Late inspiratory crackles* occur with restrictive disease: pneumonia, heart failure and interstitial fibrosis *Early inspiratory crackles* occur with obstructive disease: chronic bronchitis, asthma and emphysema *Posturally induced crackles* (PICs) are fine crackles that appear with a change from sitting to the supine position, or with a change from supine to supine with legs elevated

(Continued)

ABNORMAL FINDINGS

TABLE 19.5 Adventitious lung sounds—cont'd

SOUND	DESCRIPTION	MECHANISM	CLINICAL EXAMPLE
Crackles—coarse	Loud, low-pitched, bubbling and gurgling sounds that start in early inspiration and may be present in expiration; may decrease somewhat by suctioning or coughing but will reappear shortly—sounds like opening a Velcro fastener	Inhaled air collides with secretions in the trachea and large bronchi	Pulmonary oedema, pneumonia, pulmonary fibrosis and the terminally ill who have a depressed cough reflex
Atelectatic crackles	Sound like fine crackles but do not last and are not pathological; disappear after the first few breaths; heard in axillae and bases (usually dependent) of lungs	When sections of alveoli are not fully aerated, they deflate and accumulate secretions. Crackles are heard when these sections re-expand with a few deep breaths	In ageing adults, bedridden persons or in persons just aroused from sleep
Pleural friction rub	A very superficial sound that is coarse and low pitched; it has a grating quality as if two pieces of leather are being rubbed together; sounds just like crackles, but *close* to the ear; sounds louder if you push the stethoscope harder onto the chest wall; sound is inspiratory and expiratory	Caused when pleurae become inflamed and lose their normal lubricating fluid; their opposing roughened pleural surfaces rub together during respiration; heard best in anterolateral wall where greatest lung mobility exists	Pleuritis, accompanied by pain with breathing (rub disappears after a few days if pleural fluid accumulates and separates pleurae)
Continuous sounds These are connected, musical sounds.			
Wheeze—high-pitched (sibilant)	High-pitched, musical squeaking sounds that sound polyphonic (multiple notes as in a musical chord); predominate in expiration but may occur in both expiration and inspiration	Air squeezed or compressed through passageways narrowed almost to closure by collapsing, swelling, secretions or tumours; the passageway walls oscillate in apposition between the closed and barely open positions; the resulting sound is similar to a vibrating reed	Diffuse airway obstruction from acute asthma or chronic emphysema
Wheeze—low-pitched (sonorous rhonchi)	Low-pitched; monophonic single note, musical snoring, moaning sounds; they are heard throughout the cycle, although they are more prominent on expiration; may clear somewhat by coughing	Airflow obstruction as described by the vibrating reed mechanism above; the pitch of the wheeze cannot be correlated to the size of the passageway that generates it	Bronchitis, single bronchus obstruction from airway tumour
Stridor	High-pitched, monophonic, inspiratory, crowing sound, louder in neck than over chest wall	Originating in larynx or trachea, upper airway obstruction from swollen, inflamed tissues or lodged foreign body	Croup and acute epiglottitis in children, and foreign body inhalation, obstructed airway may be life threatening

Abnormal findings for advanced practice

TABLE 19.6 Abnormal tactile fremitus

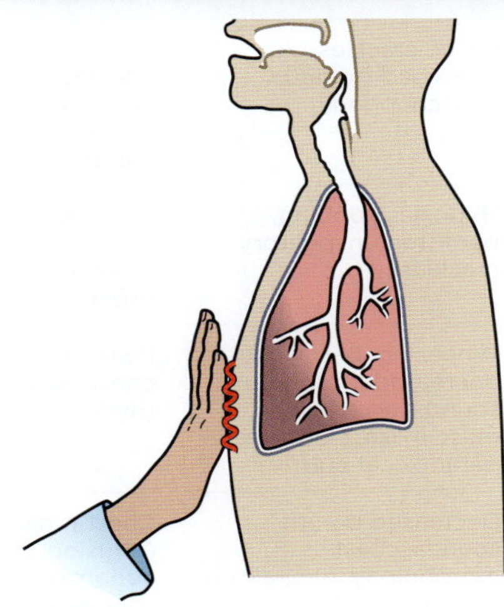

Increased tactile fremitus

Occurs with conditions that increase the density of lung tissue, thereby making a better conducting medium for vibrations (e.g. compression or consolidation (pneumonia)). There must be a patent bronchus and consolidation must extend to lung surface for increased fremitus to be apparent.

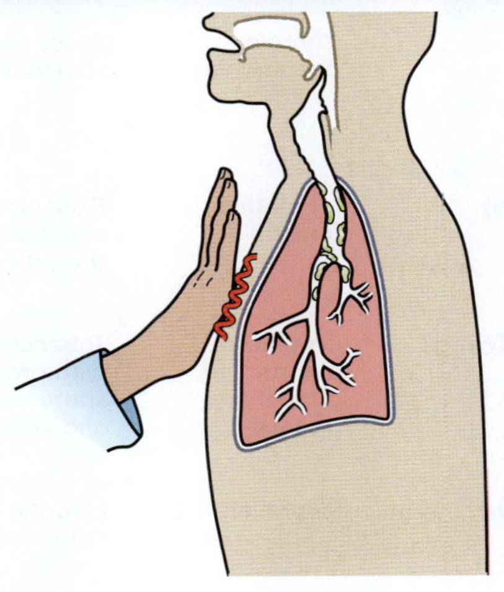

Rhonchal fremitus

Vibration felt when inhaled air passes through thick secretions in the larger bronchi. This may decrease somewhat by coughing.

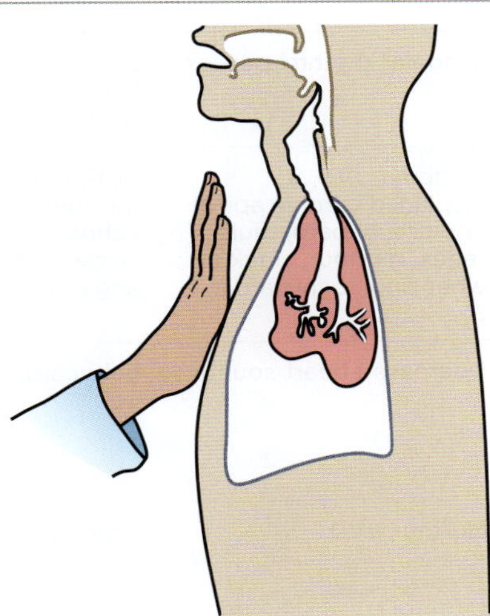

Decreased tactile fremitus

Occurs when anything obstructs transmission of vibrations (e.g. an obstructed bronchus, pleural effusion or thickening, pneumothorax and emphysema). Any barrier that gets in the way of the sound and your palpating hand decreases fremitus.

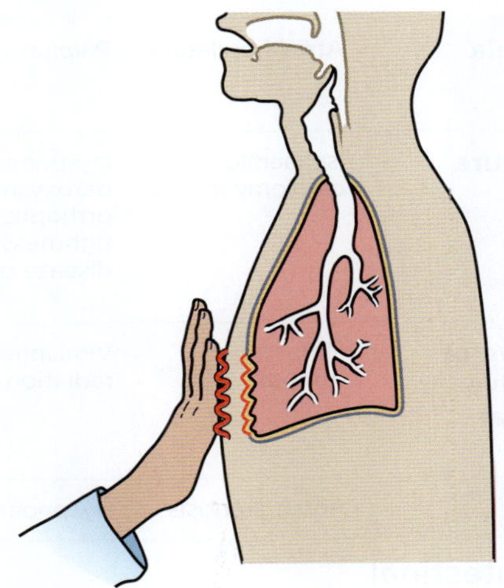

Pleural friction fremitus

Produced when inflammation of the parietal or visceral pleura causes a decrease in the normal lubricating fluid. Then the opposing surfaces make a coarse grating sound when rubbed together during breathing. Although this sound is best detected by auscultation, it may sometimes be palpable and feels like two pieces of leather grating together. It is synchronous with respiratory excursion. Also called a *palpable friction rub*.

TABLE 19.7 Diagnostic clues to chronic dyspnoea and associated systems

SYSTEM/ PHYSIOLOGY	EXAMPLE	HISTORY	EXAMINATION	DIAGNOSTIC STUDY
Pulmonary				
Alveolar	Chronic pneumonia	Fever, productive cough, shortness of breath	Fever, crackles, increased fremitus, bronchophony	Chest radiography, chest CT, bronchoscopy/ bronchoalveolar lavage, culture or biopsy
Interstitial	Idiopathic fibrosis	Exertional dyspnoea, dry cough, malignancy, prescription or illicit drug use, chemical exposures	Hypoxia, clubbing, persistent inspiratory crackles	Chest radiography (fibrosis, interstitial markings), chest CT, bronchoscopy/biopsy
Obstruction of air flow	Chronic obstructive pulmonary disease	Tobacco use, cough, relief with bronchodilator, increased sputum production, haemoptysis and weight loss with malignancy	Wheezing, barrel chest, decreased breath sounds, accessory muscle use, clubbing, paradoxical pulse	Peak flow, spirometry, chest radiography (hyperinflation), PFT
Restrictive	Pleural effusion	Pleuritic chest pain, dyspnoea not improved with oxygen	Decreased breath sounds, chest morphology, pleural rub, basal dullness	Chest radiography (effusion, anatomical abnormality), spirometry, PFT
Vascular	Chronic pulmonary emboli	Fatigue, pleuritic chest pain, prior emboli/deep venous thrombosis, syncope	Wheezing, lower extremity swelling, pleural rub, prominent P_2, murmur, right ventricular heave, JVD	D-dimer, ventilation/ perfusion scan, CT angiography, echocardiography, right heart catheterisation
Cardiac				
Arrhythmia	Atrial fibrillation	Palpitations, syncope	Irregular rhythm, pauses	ECG, event recorder, Holter monitor, stress testing
Heart failure	Ischaemic cardiomyopathy	Dyspnoea on exertion, paroxysmal nocturnal dyspnoea, orthopnoea, chest pain or tightness, prior coronary artery disease or atrial fibrillation	Oedema, JVD, S_3, displaced cardiac apical impulse, hepatojugular reflex, murmur, crackles, wheezing, tachycardia, S_4	ECG, brain natriuretic peptide, echocardiography, stress testing, coronary angiography
Restrictive or constrictive pericardial disease	Metastatic tumour	Viral infection, malignancy, chest radiation, inflammatory diseases	Decreased heart sounds	Echocardiography
Valvular	Aortic stenosis	Dyspnoea on exertion	Murmur, JVD	Echocardiography
Gastrointestinal				
Aspiration	Gastro-oesophageal reflux disease	Postprandial, night cough	Intermittent crackles, wheezes	Chest radiography, oesophagography, oesophageal pH
Neuromuscular				
Respiratory muscle weakness	Phrenic nerve palsy	Known neuromuscular disorders, weakness	Atrophy	Maximal inspiratory and expiratory pressures
Psychological				
—	Anxiety	Anxiety, depression, history of trauma or abuse	Sighing	Normal

Wahls SA: Causes and evaluation of chronic dyspnea, *American Family Physician*, 86(2): 173–180, 2012.

TABLE 19.8 Voice sounds

TECHNIQUE	NORMAL FINDING	ABNORMAL FINDING
Bronchophony Ask the person to repeat 'ninety-nine' while you listen with the stethoscope over the chest wall; listen especially if you suspect pathology	Normal voice transmission is soft, muffled and indistinct; you can hear sound through the stethoscope but cannot distinguish exactly what is being said	Pathology that increases lung density will enhance transmission of voice sounds; you auscultate a clear 'ninety-nine'. The words are more distinct than normal and sound close to your ear
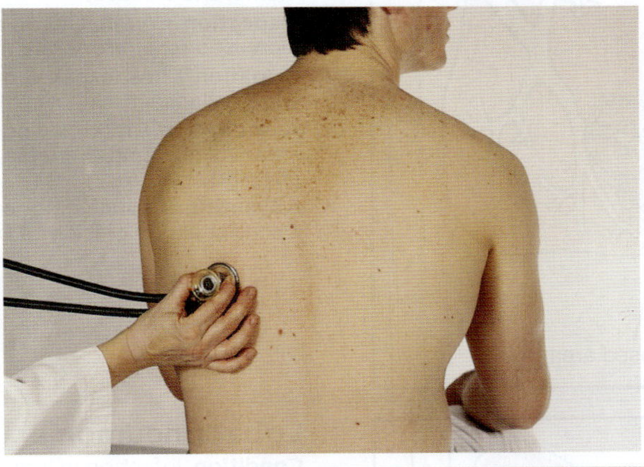		
Egophony (Greek: the voice of a goat) Auscultate the chest while the person phonates a long 'ee-ee-ee-ee' sound	Normally, you should hear 'eeeeeee' through your stethoscope	Over area of consolidation or compression, the spoken 'eeee' sound changes to a bleating long 'aaaaa' sound
Whispered pectoriloquy Ask the person to whisper a phrase like 'one-two-three' as you auscultate	The normal response is faint, muffled and almost inaudible	With only small amounts of consolidation, the whispered voice is transmitted very clearly and distinctly, although still somewhat faint; it sounds as if the person is whispering right into your stethoscope, 'one-two-three'

TABLE 19.9 Assessment of common respiratory conditions

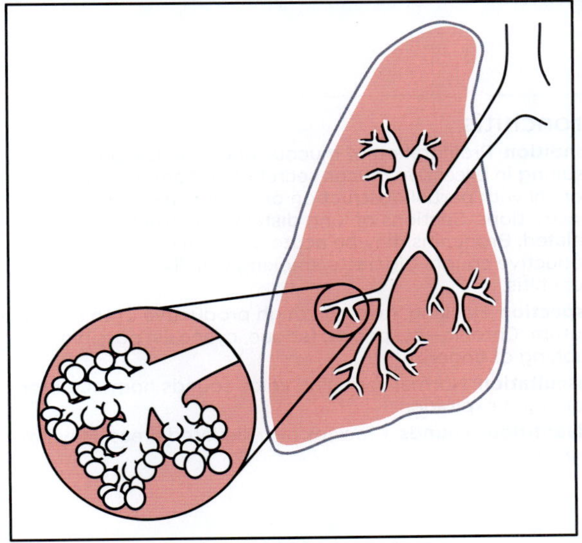

Normal lung (for comparison)

Inspection Anteroposterior < transverse diameter, relaxed posture, normal musculature; rate 10–20 breaths per min, regular, no cyanosis or pallor.

Palpation Symmetrical chest expansion. No lumps, masses or tenderness.

Auscultation Vesicular over peripheral fields. Bronchovesicular parasternally (anterior) and between scapulae (posterior). Infant and young child—bronchovesicular throughout.

Adventitious sounds None.

(Continued)

TABLE 19.9 Assessment of common respiratory conditions—cont'd

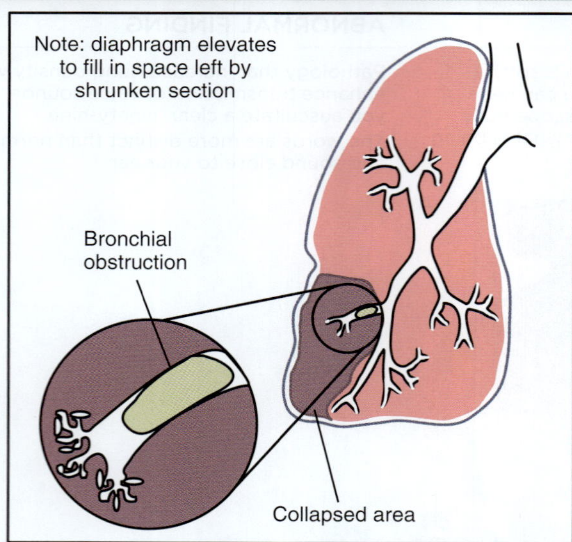

Atelectasis (collapse)

Condition Collapsed shrunken section of alveoli, or an entire lung, as a result of (1) airway obstruction (e.g. the bronchus is completely blocked by thick exudate, aspirated foreign body or tumour), the alveolar air beyond it is gradually absorbed by the pulmonary capillaries and the alveolar walls cave in; (2) compression on the lung; and (3) lack of surfactant (hyaline membrane disease).

Inspection Cough. Lag on expansion on affected side. Increased respiratory rate and pulse. Possible cyanosis.

Palpation Chest expansion decreased on affected side. With large collapse, tracheal shift towards affected side.

Auscultation Breath sounds decreased vesicular or absent over area. Voice sounds variable, usually decreased or absent over affected area.

Adventitious sounds None if bronchus is obstructed. Occasional fine crackles if bronchus is patent.

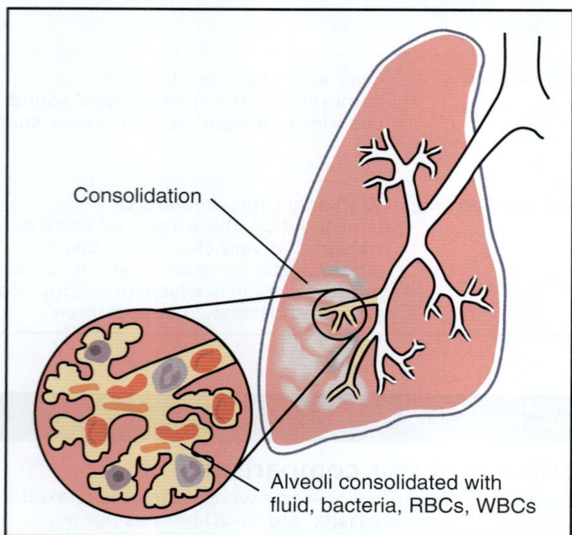

Lobar pneumonia

Condition Infection in lung parenchyma leaves alveolar membrane oedematous and porous, so red blood cells and white blood cells pass from blood to alveoli. Alveoli progressively fill up (become consolidated) with bacteria, solid cellular debris, fluid and blood cells, all of which replace alveolar air. This results in decreased surface area of the respiratory membrane, which causes hypoxaemia.

Inspection Increased respiratory rate. Guarding and lag on expansion on affected side. Children—sternal retraction, nasal flaring.

Palpation Chest expansion decreased on affected side.

Auscultation Breath sounds louder with patent bronchus, as if coming directly from larynx. Voice sounds have increased clarity, bronchophony, egophony, whispered pectoriloquy present. Children—diminished breath sounds may occur early in pneumonia.

Adventitious sounds Crackles, fine to medium.

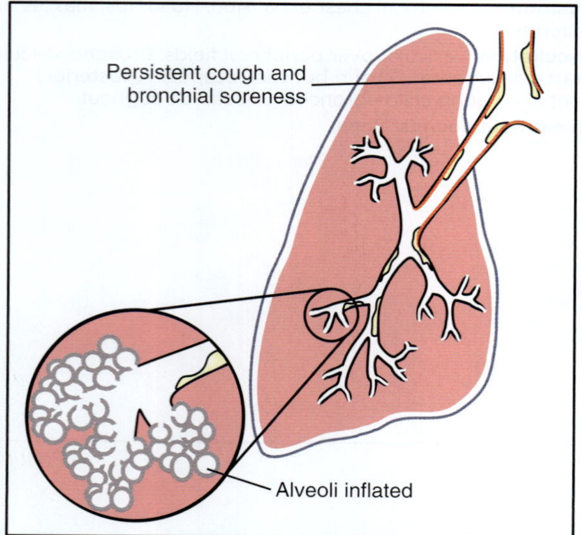

Bronchitis

Condition Proliferation of mucous glands in the passageways, resulting in excessive mucus secretion. Inflammation of bronchi with partial obstruction of bronchi by secretions or constrictions. Sections of lung distal to obstruction may be deflated. Bronchitis may be acute or chronic with recurrent productive cough. Cigarette smoking usually causes chronic bronchitis.

Inspection Hacking, rasping cough productive of thick mucoid sputum. Chronic—dyspnoea, fatigue, cyanosis, possible clubbing of fingers.

Auscultation Normal vesicular. Voice sounds normal. Chronic—prolonged expiration.

Adventitious sounds Crackles over deflated areas. May have wheeze.

TABLE 19.9 Assessment of common respiratory conditions—cont'd

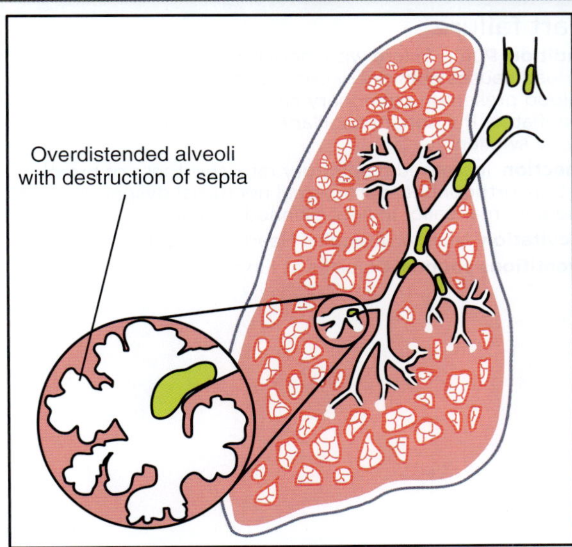

Emphysema

Condition Caused by destruction of pulmonary connective tissue (elastin, collagen); characterised by permanent enlargement of air sacs distal to terminal bronchioles and rupture of interalveolar walls. This increases airway resistance, especially on expiration—producing a hyperinflated lung and an increase in lung volume. Cigarette smoking accounts for 80–90% of cases of emphysema.

Inspection Increased anteroposterior diameter. Barrel chest. Use of accessory muscles to aid respiration. Tripod position. Shortness of breath, especially on exertion. Respiratory distress. Tachypnoea.

Auscultation Decreased breath sounds. May have prolonged expiration. Muffled heart sounds resulting from overdistension of lungs.

Adventitious sounds Usually none; occasionally, wheeze.

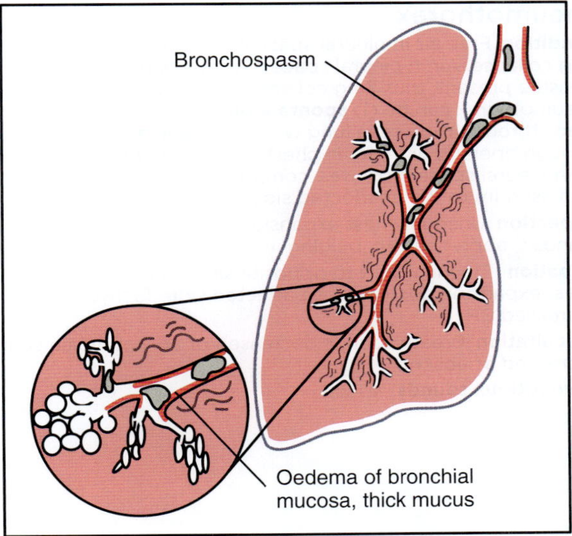

Asthma (reactive airway disease)

Condition An allergic hypersensitivity to certain inhaled allergens (pollen), irritants (tobacco, ozone), microorganisms, stress or exercise that produces a complex response characterised by bronchospasm and inflammation, oedema in walls of bronchioles and secretion of highly viscous mucus into airways. These factors greatly increase airway resistance, especially during expiration, and produce the symptoms of wheezing, dyspnoea and chest tightness.

Inspection During severe attack: increased respiratory rate, shortness of breath with audible wheeze, use of accessory neck muscles, cyanosis, apprehension, retraction of intercostal spaces. Expiration laboured, prolonged. When chronic, may have barrel chest.

Auscultation Diminished air movement. Breath sounds decreased, with prolonged expiration. Voice sounds decreased.

Adventitious sounds Bilateral wheezing on expiration, sometimes inspiratory and expiratory wheezing.

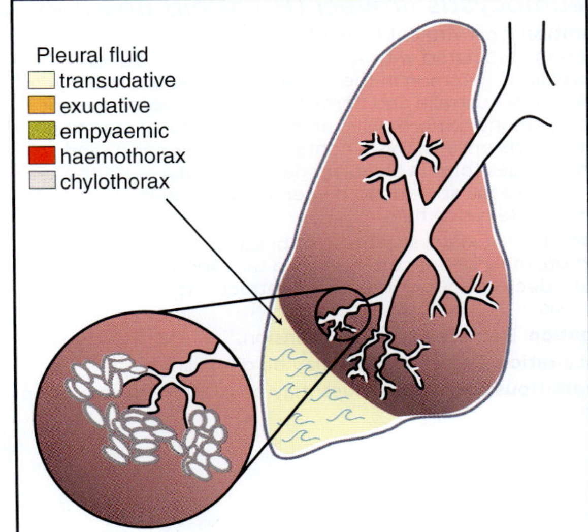

Pleural effusion (fluid) or thickening

Condition Collection of excess fluid in the intrapleural space, with compression of overlying lung tissue. Effusion may contain watery capillary fluid (transudative), protein (exudative), purulent matter (empyaemic), blood (haemothorax) or milky lymphatic fluid (chylothorax). Gravity settles fluid in dependent areas of thorax. Presence of fluid subdues all lung sounds.

Inspection Increased respirations, dyspnoea; may have dry cough, tachycardia, cyanosis, abdominal distension.

Auscultation Breath sounds decreased or absent. Voice sounds decreased or absent. When remainder of lung is compressed near the effusion, may have bronchial breath sounds over the compression along with bronchophony, egophony, whispered pectoriloquy.

Adventitious sounds None.

(Continued)

TABLE 19.9 Assessment of common respiratory conditions—cont'd

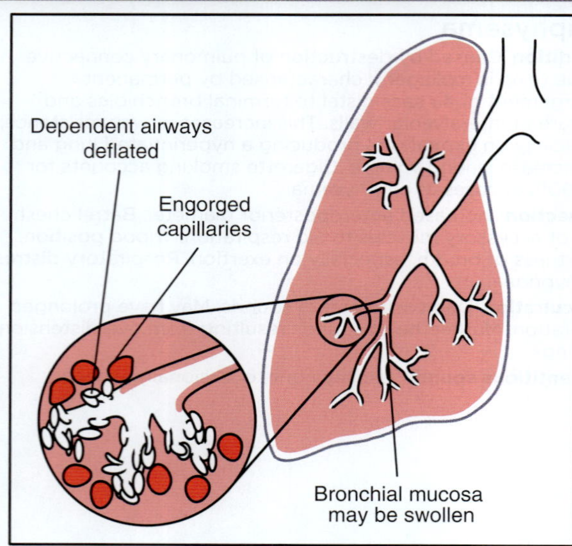

Heart failure

Condition Pump failure with increasing pressure of cardiac overload causes pulmonary congestion or an increased amount of blood present in pulmonary capillaries. Dependent air sacs are deflated. Pulmonary capillaries engorged. Bronchial mucosa may be swollen.

Inspection Increased respiratory rate, shortness of breath on exertion, orthopnoea, paroxysmal nocturnal dyspnoea, nocturia, ankle oedema, pallor in light-skinned people.

Auscultation Normal vesicular. Heart sounds include S_3 gallop.

Adventitious sounds Crackles at lung bases.

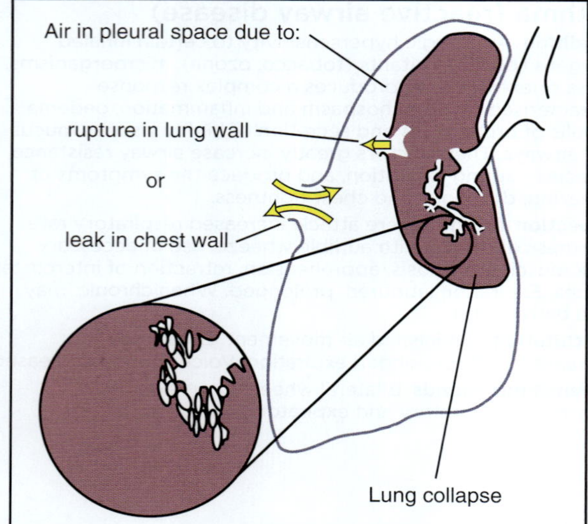

Pneumothorax

Condition Free air in pleural space causes partial or complete lung collapse. Air in pleural space neutralises the usual negative pressure present; thus lung collapses. Usually unilateral. Pneumothorax can be (1) **spontaneous** (air enters pleural space through rupture in lung wall), (2) **traumatic** (air enters through opening or injury in chest wall) or (3) **tension** (trapped air in pleural space increases, compressing lung and shifting mediastinum to the unaffected side).

Inspection Unequal chest expansion. If large, tachypnoea, cyanosis, apprehension, bulging in interspaces.

Palpation Tracheal shift to opposite side (unaffected side). Chest expansion decreased on affected side. Tachycardia, decreased BP.

Auscultation Breath sounds decreased or absent. Voice sounds decreased or absent.

Adventitious sounds None.

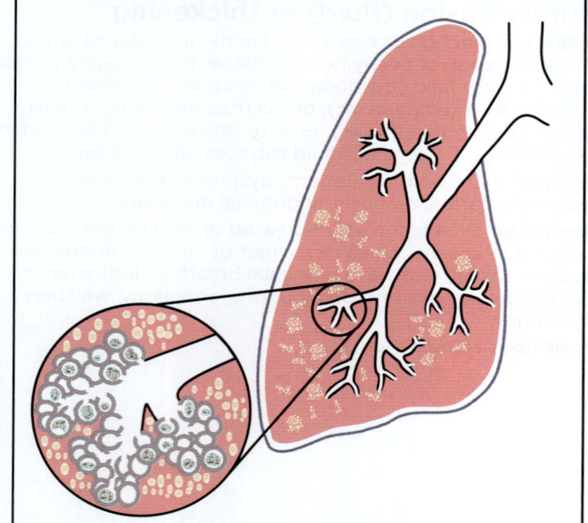

Pneumocystis jiroveci (P. carinii) pneumonia

Condition This virulent form of pneumonia is a protozoal infection associated with AIDS. The parasite *P. jiroveci (P. carinii)* is common in the United States, and relatively common in Australia and harmless to most people, except to the immunocompromised, in whom a diffuse interstitial pneumonitis ensues. Cysts containing the organism and macrophages form in alveolar spaces, alveolar walls thicken and the disease spreads to bilateral interstitial infiltrates of foamy, protein-rich fluid.

Inspection Anxiety, shortness of breath, dyspnoea on exertion, malaise are common; also tachypnoea; fever; a dry, nonproductive cough; intercostal retractions in children; cyanosis.

Palpation Decreased chest expansion.

Auscultation Breath sounds may be diminished.

Adventitious sounds Crackles may be present but are often absent.

TABLE 19.9 Assessment of common respiratory conditions—cont'd

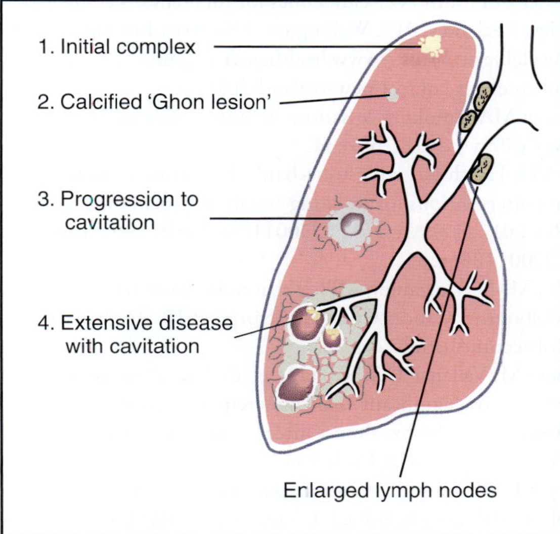

Tuberculosis

Condition Inhalation of tubercle bacilli into the alveolar wall starts: (1) Initial complex is acute inflammatory response—macrophages engulf bacilli but do not kill them. Tubercle forms around bacilli; (2) scar tissue forms, lesion calcifies and shows on X-ray; (3) reactivation of previously healed lesion. Dormant bacilli now multiply, producing necrosis, cavitation and caseous lung tissue (cheese-like); (4) extensive destruction as lesion erodes into bronchus, forming air-filled cavity. Apex usually has the most damage.

Subjective Initially asymptomatic, showing as positive skin test or on X-ray. Progressive tuberculosis involves weight loss, anorexia, easy fatiguability, low-grade afternoon fevers, night sweats. May have pleural effusion, recurrent lower respiratory infections.

Inspection Cough initially nonproductive, later productive of purulent, yellow-green sputum, may be blood tinged. Dyspnoea, orthopnoea, fatigue, weakness.

Palpation Skin moist at night from night sweats.

Auscultation Normal or decreased vesicular breath sounds.

Adventitious sounds Crackles over upper lobes common, persist following full expiration and cough.

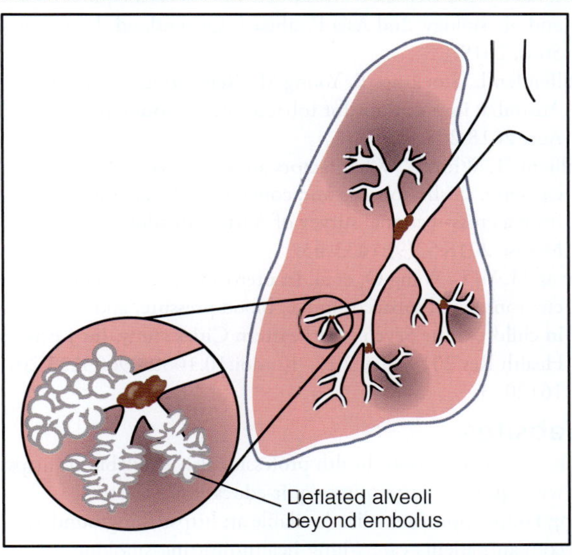

Pulmonary embolism

Condition Pulmonary embolism is the occlusion of one or more pulmonary arteries. Undissolved materials (e.g. thrombus, air bubbles, fat globules) originating elsewhere in the body detach and travel through venous system and right heart before lodging in the pulmonary artery(ies). Over 95% arise from deep vein thrombi in lower legs as a result of stasis of blood, vessel injury or hypercoagulability. Pulmonary embolism results in ischaemia of downstream lung tissue, increased pulmonary artery pressure, decreased cardiac output and hypoxia. Rarely, a saddle embolus in bifurcation of pulmonary arteries leads to sudden death from hypoxia. More often, small to medium pulmonary branches occlude, leading to dyspnoea. These may resolve naturally using the body's own fibrolytic activity or through the administration of fibrinolytics.

Subjective Chest pain, worse on deep inspiration, dyspnoea.

Inspection Apprehensive, restless, anxiety, mental status changes, cyanosis, tachypnoea, cough, haemoptysis, PaO_2 <80 on pulse oximetry. Arterial blood gases show respiratory alkalosis.

Palpation Diaphoresis, hypotension.

Auscultation Tachycardia, accentuated pulmonic component of S_2 heart sound.

Adventitious sounds Crackles, wheezes.

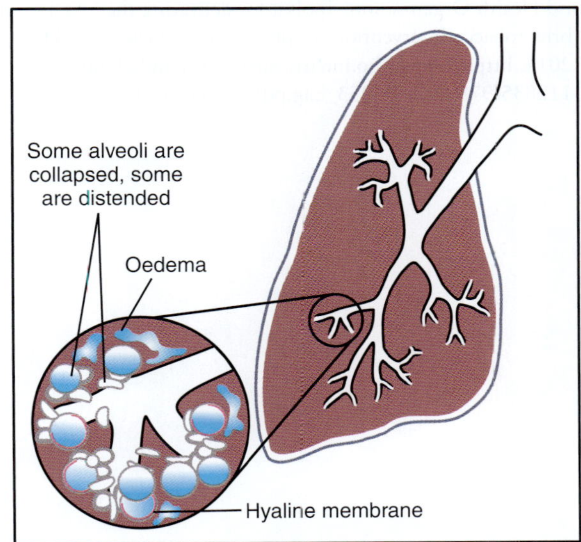

Acute respiratory distress syndrome (ARDS)

Condition An acute pulmonary insult (trauma, gastric acid aspiration, shock, sepsis) damages alveolar capillary membrane, leading to increased permeability of pulmonary capillaries and alveolar epithelium, and to pulmonary oedema. Gross examination (autopsy) would show dark red, firm, airless tissue, with some alveoli collapsed and hyaline membranes lining the distended alveoli.

Subjective Acute onset of dyspnoea, apprehension.

Inspection Restlessness, disorientation, rapid shallow breathing, productive cough, thin frothy sputum, retractions of intercostal spaces and sternum. Decreased PaO_2, blood gases show respiratory alkalosis, X-rays show diffuse pulmonary infiltrates, a late sign is cyanosis.

Palpation Hypotension.

Auscultation Tachycardia.

Adventitious sounds Crackles, rhonchi.

BIBLIOGRAPHY

Australian Bureau of Statistics. Smoking, National Health Survey: First results, 2017–18. 2019. Available at: https://www.abs.gov.au/ausstats/abs@.nsf/Lookup/by%20Subject/4364.0.55.001~2017-18~Main%20Features~Smoking~85.

Australian Government, Department of Health. The strategic plan for control of tuberculosis in Australia, 2016–2020: Towards disease elimination. The national tuberculosis advisory committee for the communicable diseases network of Australia, Vol 43. 2019. Available at: https://www1.health.gov.au/internet/main/publishing.nsf/Content/ohp-ntac-tb-strat-plan.htm.

Australian Indigenous HealthInfoNet. Overview of Aboriginal and Torres Strait Islander health status. Perth, WA: Australian Indigenous HealthInfoNet; 2018. Available at: https://ro.ecu.edu.au/cgi/viewcontent.cgi?article=6912&context=ecuworkspost2013.

Australian Institute of Health and Welfare (AIHW). Australia's health 2018. Australia's health series no. 16. AUS 221. Canberra: AIHW; 2018a.

Australian Institute of Health and Welfare. Media Release: Two new cases of mesothelioma diagnosed every day in Australia, with one of the poorest survival rates of any cancer. 2018b. Available at: https://www.aihw.gov.au/news-media/media-releases/2018/november/mesothelioma-in-australia.

Bloom SL, Cunningham FG, Dashe JS, et al. Williams obstetrics [Internet]. New York: McGraw-Hill Education Medical; 2018. Available at: http://search.ebscohost.com/login.aspx?direct=true&db=cat00097a&AN=deakin.b3899249&authtype=sso&custid=deakin&site=eds-live&scope=site.

Campbell MA, Ford C, Winstanley MH. The health effects of secondhand smoke. 4.17 Health effects of secondhand smoke for infants and children. In: Scollo, MM, Winstanley, MH, editors. Tobacco in Australia: facts and issues. Melbourne: Cancer Council Victoria; 2017. Available at: http://www.tobaccoinaustralia.org.au/chapter-4-secondhand/4-17-health-effects-of-secondhand-smoke-for-infants.

Hoy RF, Baird T, Hammerschlag G, et al. Artificial stone-associated silicosis: a rapidly emerging occupational lung disease. Occup Environ Med 2018;75(1):3–5.

Kirby T. Australia reports on audit of silicosis for stonecutters. Lancet 2019;393(10174):861.

Leso V, Fontana L, Romano R, et al. Artificial stone associated silicosis: a systematic review. Int J Environ Res Public Health 2019;16(4):568. doi.org/10.3390/ijerph16040568.

Ministry of Health NZ. Annual update of key results 2017/2018: New Zealand health survey; 2019a. Available at: https://www.health.govt.nz/publication/annual-update-key-results-2017-18-new-zealand-health-survey.

Ministry of Health NZ. Guidelines for tuberculosis control in New Zealand, 2019. Wellington: Ministry of Health; 2019b. Available at: https://www.health.govt.nz/publication/guidelines-tuberculosis-control-new-zealand-2019.

Rahman MA. Smoking cessation: do nurses have any role? Aust Nurs Midwifery J 2018;26(3):34.

Rice VH, Heath L, Livingstone-Banks J, Hartmann-Boyce J. Nursing interventions for smoking cessation. Cochrane Database Syst Rev 2017;(12):Art. No.: CD001188. doi:10.1002/14651858.CD001188.pub5

Scollo, MM, Winstanley, MH. Tobacco in Australia: facts and issues. Melbourne: Cancer Council Victoria; 2018. Available at: www.TobaccoInAustralia.org.au.

Soeberg M, Vallance DA, Keena V, et al. Australia's ongoing legacy of asbestos: significant challenges remain even after the complete banning of asbestos almost fifteen years ago. Int J Environ Res Public Health 2018;15(2):384.

Talley NJ, O'Connor S. Clinical examination: a systematic guide to physical diagnosis. 8th ed. Chatswood, NSW: Elsevier; 2018.

Tortora, GJ, Derrickson BH, Burkett B, et al. Principles of anatomy and physiology. 2nd Asia Pacific ed. Queensland: John Wiley & Sons; 2019.

Wolfenden L, Stockings E, Yoong SL. Regulating e-cigarettes in Australia: implications for tobacco use by young people. Med J Aust 2018;208(1):89.

Williams T, White V. What factors are associated with electronic cigarette, shisha-tobacco and conventional cigarette use? Findings from a cross-sectional survey of Australian adolescents. Subst Use Misuse 2018;53(9):1433-43.

Zhang H, Yu L, Wang Q, et al. In utero and postnatal exposure to environmental tobacco smoke, blood pressure, and hypertension in children: the Seven Northeastern Cities study. Int J Environ Health Res 2019 May 29:1–12. doi:10.1080/09603123.2019.1612043.

Websites

Quit—Quit education (health professionals). Available at: https://www.quit.org.au/resources/quit-education/

Lung Foundation Australia. Available at: https://lungfoundation.com.au/patients-carers/lung-health/quitting-smoking/

World Health Organisation. Toolkit for delivering the 5A's and 5R's brief tobacco interventions in primary care. Geneva: WHO; 2014. https://apps.who.int/iris/bitstream/handle/10665/112835/9789241506953_eng.pdf?sequence=1.

Assessing musculoskeletal function

Unit 6

Chapter Twenty

Musculoskeletal assessment

Written by Carolyn Jarvis
Adapted by Fran Pearce

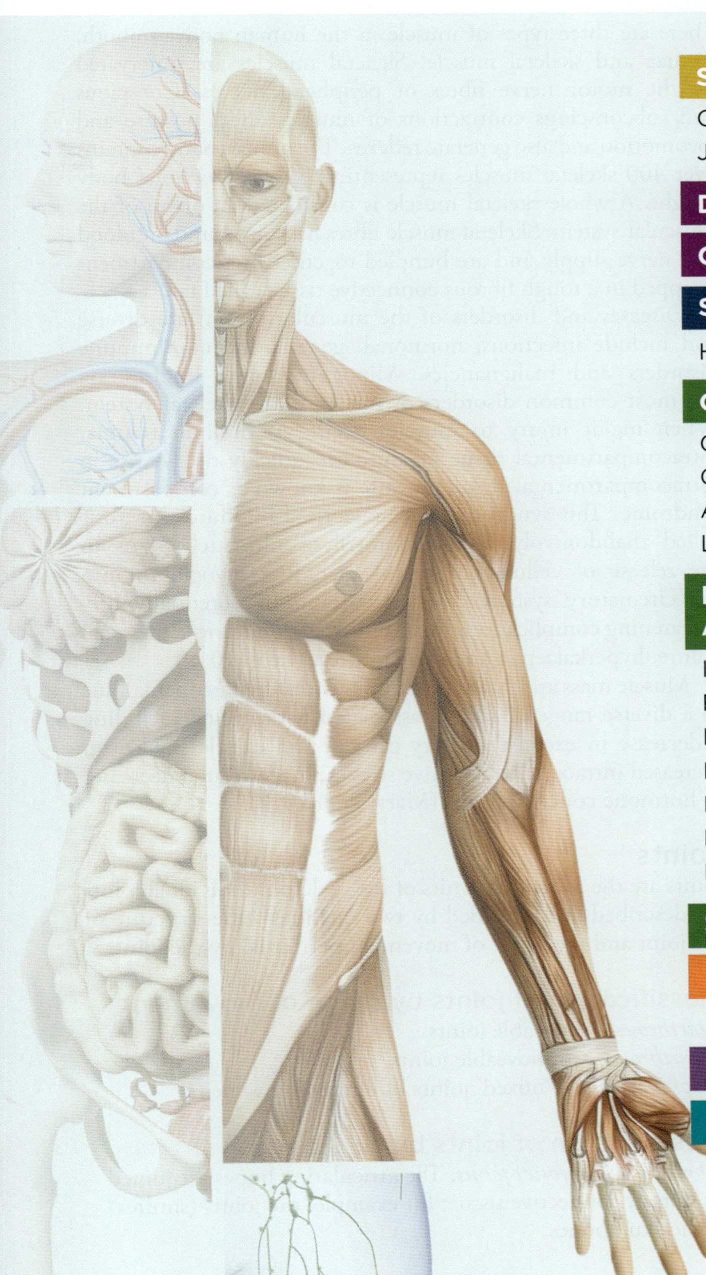

INTRODUCTION

The musculoskeletal system is a vast organ system that provides locomotion, and an upright posture and protection for the body. It is composed of various forms of connective tissue which include bones, skeletal muscle, cartilage, ligaments, tendons and joints. In order to appreciate the impact of disease and trauma to this complex and dynamic system, you are advised to first review the structure and function of bones, skeletal muscle, cartilage, ligaments, tendons and joints.

Structure and function

The musculoskeletal system has both structural and metabolic functions. Its structural function is essential for locomotion, respiration and the protection of internal organs and the central nervous system. The marrow within bones contains critical components of the haematopoietic and immune system. The bone marrow produces B cells, granulocytes and immature thymocytes, in addition to red blood cells and platelets.

Its metabolic function is as a storehouse for calcium, phosphorus and carbonate, and as a buffering system in hydrogen ion concentration. Bone plays a major role in conjunction with the renal system in blood calcium level regulation (Komaba 2018). The enormous mineral surface of the skeleton can also bind toxins and heavy metals, minimising their ability to cause cellular damage.

COMPONENTS OF THE MUSCULOSKELETAL SYSTEM

Bone

Bone is a mineralised connective tissue consisting of cells embedded in a protein matrix of collagen, alkaline phosphatase and osteopontin. This dynamic tissue responds to mechanical stresses through a complex process of remodelling. The remodelling process involves the resorption of micro-damaged bone by osteoclast cells followed by a phase of bone formation by osteoblast cells. In healthy adults, this process is coupled to ensure bone density remains stable. Gonadal steroid hormones, parathyroid hormone and various growth factors have been shown to affect this process, indicating a central regulatory mechanism (Marieb & Keller 2018). When this process becomes uncoupled, normal bone density is altered, leading to a change in the normal architecture of bone seen in diseases such as osteoporosis and Paget's disease (Kravets 2018).

Cartilage

This connective tissue is a firm gel-like substance characterised by resilience and the ability to absorb mechanical forces. The human body contains three major types of cartilage: hyaline cartilage, elastic cartilage and fibrocartilage. Hyaline cartilage is the most common type of cartilage found in parts of the respiratory tract and on joint surfaces. Within joints, articular cartilage protects the joint by distributing applied loads, and by providing a low-friction-bearing surface to maximise movement. Fibrocartilage is found in the intervertebral discs, menisci of the knee joint and the symphysis pubis. Its structure provides resistance to the compression and shearing forces within these joints. All types of cartilage are avascular and aneural, therefore tears in cartilage cannot heal.

Ligaments and tendons

Ligaments and tendons are connective tissues with complex biomechanical properties. Ligaments connect bone to bone and tendons connect muscles to bone. Injury to a ligament or tendon results in a drastic change in structure, resulting in the formation of scar tissue that is biomechanically inferior. For example, repair of the anterior cruciate ligament (ACL) in the knee requires a new piece of tissue graft from a hamstring muscle. The resultant graft does not possess the same qualities of strength and stability as the original ACL.

Muscles

There are three types of muscle in the human body: smooth, cardiac and skeletal muscle. Skeletal muscles are innervated by the motor nerve fibres of peripheral nerves. Conscious and subconscious contractions of muscles affect posture and locomotion and also generate reflexes. The human body contains over 400 skeletal muscles representing 40–50% of total body weight. A whole skeletal muscle is considered an organ of the muscular system. Skeletal muscle fibres have an abundant blood and nerve supply and are bundled together in a compartment wrapped in a tough fibrous connective tissue called fascia.

Diseases and disorders of the muscular system are diverse and include infections, hormonal, genetic and autoimmune disorders and malignancies. Minor traumatic injuries are the most common disorders of the muscular skeletal system. When major injury to muscles occurs as in limb trauma, intracompartmental tissue pressure can quickly rise. A rise in intracompartmental tissue pressure is known as compartment syndrome. This syndrome is characterised by muscle necrosis called rhabdomyolysis. Rhabdomyolysis ultimately leads to the release of cellular contents—including myoglobin into the circulatory system. This may result in potentially life-threatening complications including myoglobinuric acute renal failure, hyperkalaemia and cardiac arrest (Lynn 2019).

Muscle mass and strength declines with age (sarcopenia) due to a diverse range of factors associated with ageing including a decrease in exercise, dietary protein and calorie intake, an increased intracellular oxidative stress and age-related decreases in hormone concentrations (Marty et al 2017).

Joints

Joints are the functional units of the skeleton. Individual joints are described and classified by two qualities—the structure of the joint and the range of movement permitted by the joint.

Classification of joints by range of movement

Diarthroses—moveable joints
Synarthroses—immoveable joints
Amphiarthroses—'mixed' joints of limited movement

Classification of joints by structure

Fibrous (synarthrotic) joints. The articulating bones are joined by fibrous connective tissue; for example, the joints (sutures) of the skull bones.

Cartilaginous (amphiarthrotic) joints. The articulating bones are joined by cartilage; for example, the pubic symphysis. *Synovial (diarthrotic) joints.* These are freely mobile joints characterised by a joint cavity lined with synovial tissue and supported by ligaments, tendons and bursae (Figure 20.1). Synovial joints may be also sub-classified according to the type of movement that they permit; for example, the ball and socket joint of the hip and hinge joint of the knee.

Each joint reflects a compromise between stability and range of motion. The bones of the skull, for example, are stable but immobile, whereas the shoulder joint allows for a full range of motion but is a relatively unstable joint.

Movement of joints involving muscle contraction produces the following patterns of motion (Figure 20.2):

1. Flexion—bending a limb at a joint
2. Extension—straightening a limb at a joint
3. Abduction—moving a limb away from the midline of the body
4. Adduction—moving a limb towards the midline of the body
5. Pronation—turning the forearm so that the palm is down
6. Supination—turning the forearm so that the palm is up
7. Circumduction—moving the arm in a circle around the shoulder
8. Inversion—moving the sole of the foot inwards at the ankle
9. Eversion—moving the sole of the foot outwards at the ankle
10. Rotation—moving the head around a central axis
11. Protraction—moving a body part forwards and parallel to the ground
12. Retraction—moving a body part backwards and parallel to the ground
13. Elevation—raising a body part
14. Depression—lowering a body part.

JOINT ANATOMY

Temporomandibular joint. The temporomandibular joint (TMJ) is the articulation of the mandible and the temporal bone (Figure 20.3). The TMJ permits jaw function for speaking and chewing. The joint allows three motions: (1) hinge action to open and close the jaws, (2) gliding action for protrusion and retraction and (3) gliding for side-to-side movement of the lower jaw.

Spinal column. The **vertebrae** are 33 connecting bones stacked in a vertical column (Figure 20.4). The spinous processes can be palpated as a furrow down the midline of the back. The furrow has paravertebral muscles mounded on either side down to the sacrum, where it flattens. Humans have 7 cervical, 12 thoracic, 5 lumbar, 5 sacral and 3 or 4 coccygeal vertebrae. The following surface landmarks will orient you to their levels:

- The spinous processes of C7 and T1 are prominent at the base of the neck.
- The inferior angle of the scapula normally is at the level of the interspace between T7 and T8.
- An imaginary line connecting the highest point on each iliac crest crosses L4.
- An imaginary line joining the two symmetric dimples that overlie the posterior superior iliac spines crosses the sacrum.

A lateral view shows that the vertebral column has four curves (a double-**S** shape) (Figure 20.5). The cervical and lumbar curves are concave (inwards or anterior), and the thoracic and sacrococcygeal curves are convex (outwards or posterior). The balanced or compensatory nature of these curves, together with the resilient intervertebral discs, allows the spine to absorb a great deal of shock.

The **intervertebral discs** are fibrocartilaginous plates that constitute a quarter of the length of the column (Figure 20.6). Each disc is made up of three basic structures: the nucleus pulposus, the annulus fibrosus and the vertebral end plates. The inner **nucleus pulposus** is the semi-fluid gel centre and has the consistency of toothpaste in the young adult.

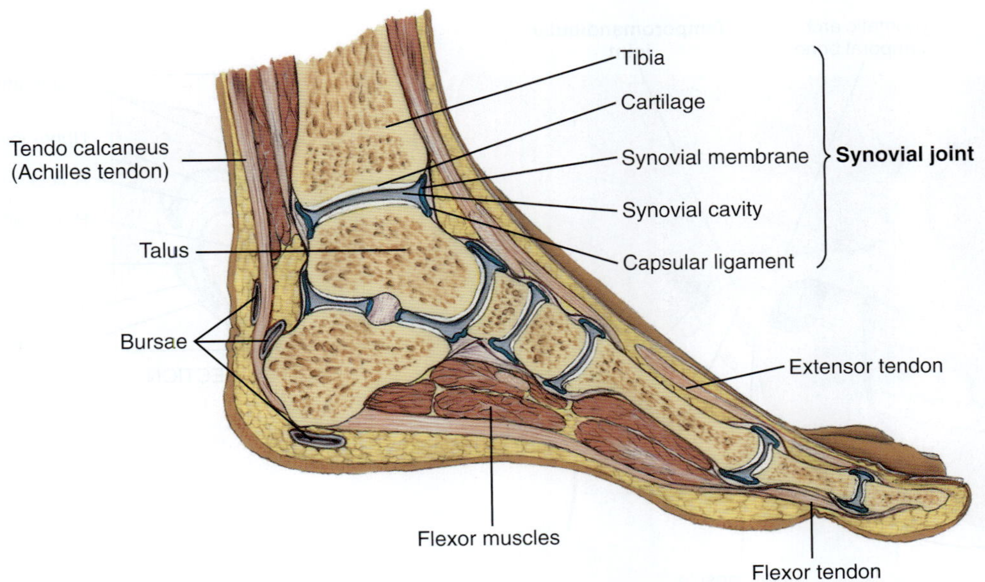

Figure 20.1

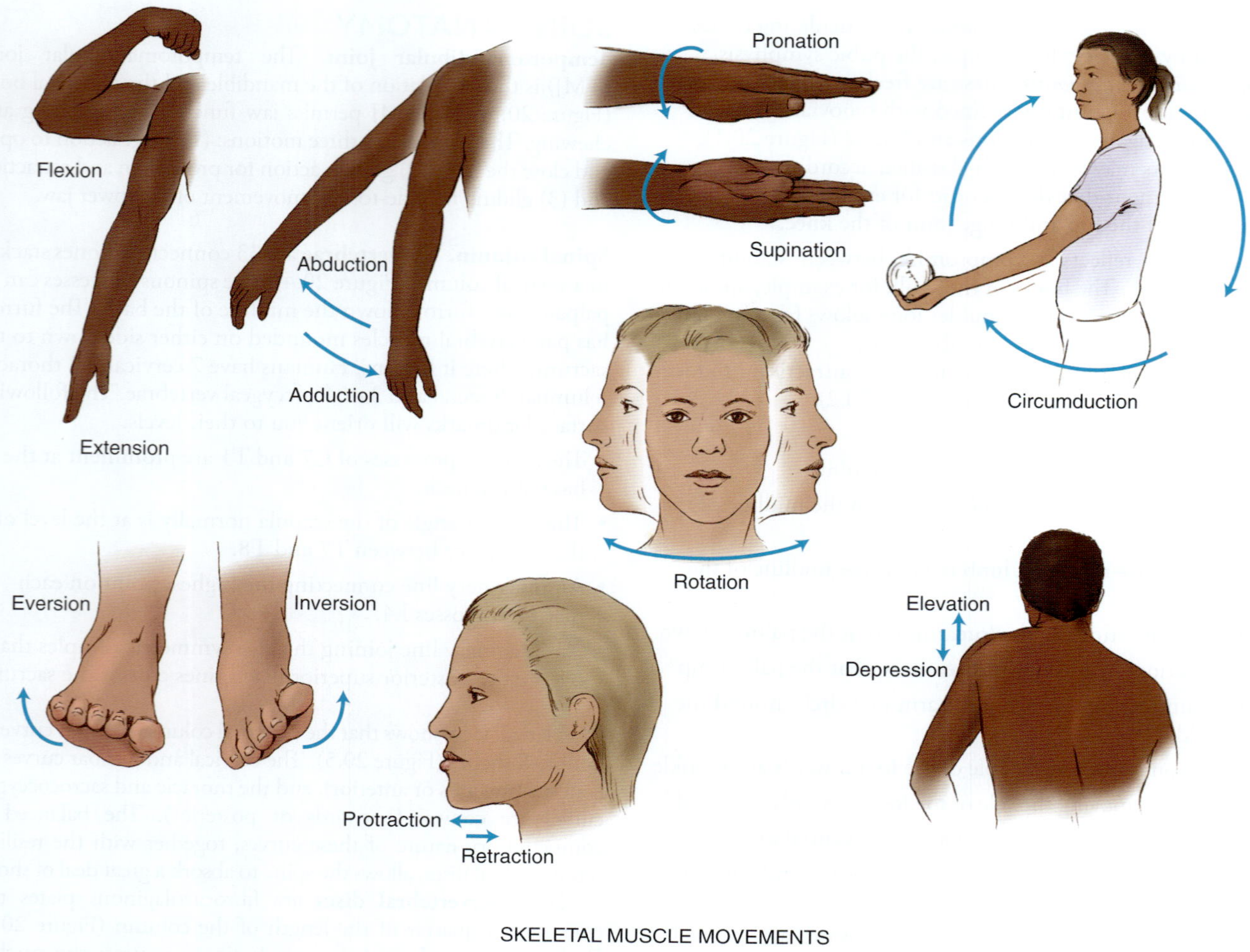

Flexion
Extension
Abduction
Adduction
Pronation
Supination
Circumduction
Rotation
Eversion
Inversion
Protraction
Retraction
Elevation
Depression
SKELETAL MUSCLE MOVEMENTS

Figure 20.2
© Pat Thomas, 2006.

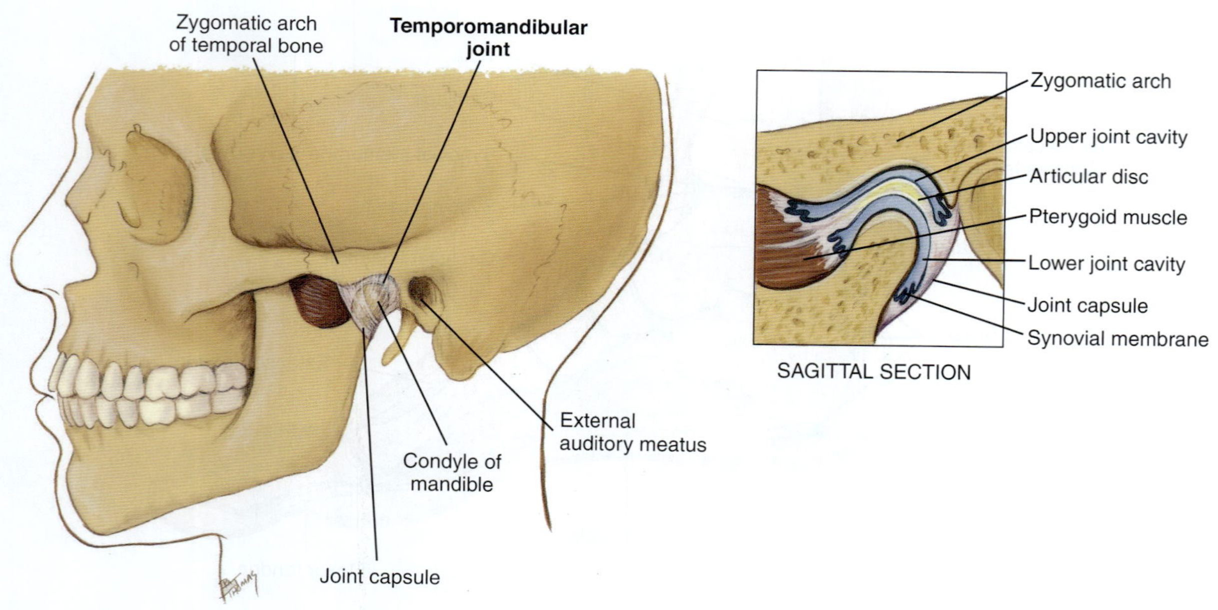

Figure 20.3

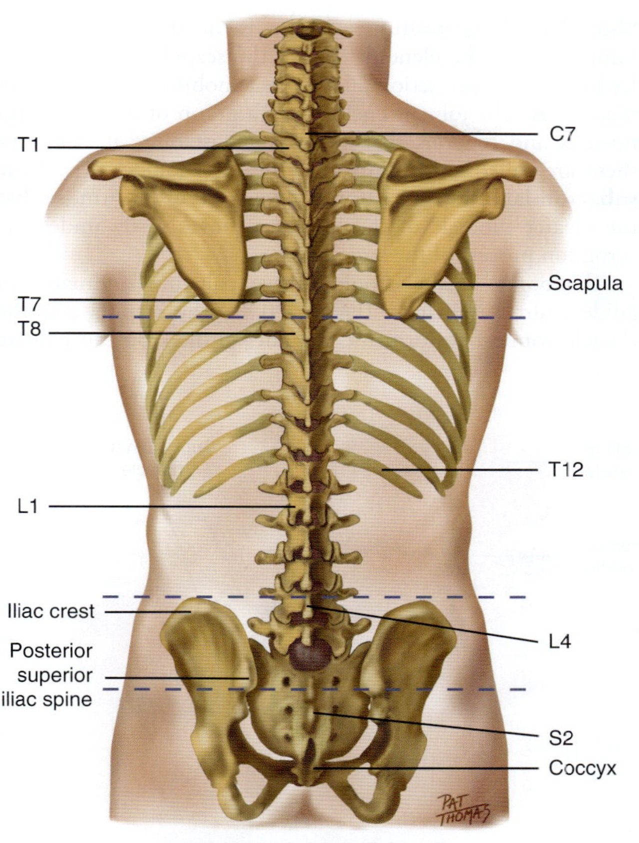

Figure 20.4

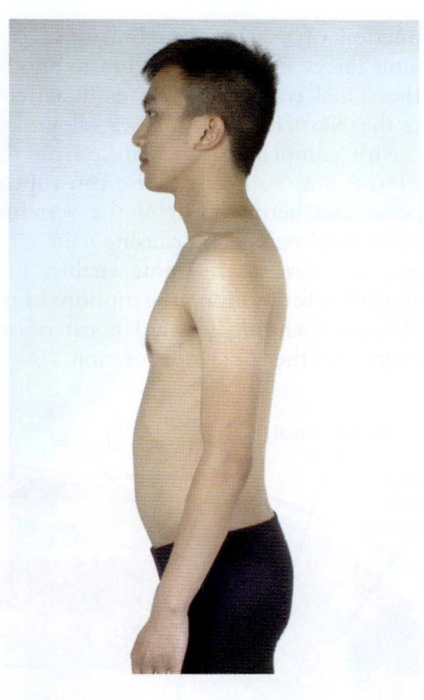

Figure 20.5
Curves of vertebral column.

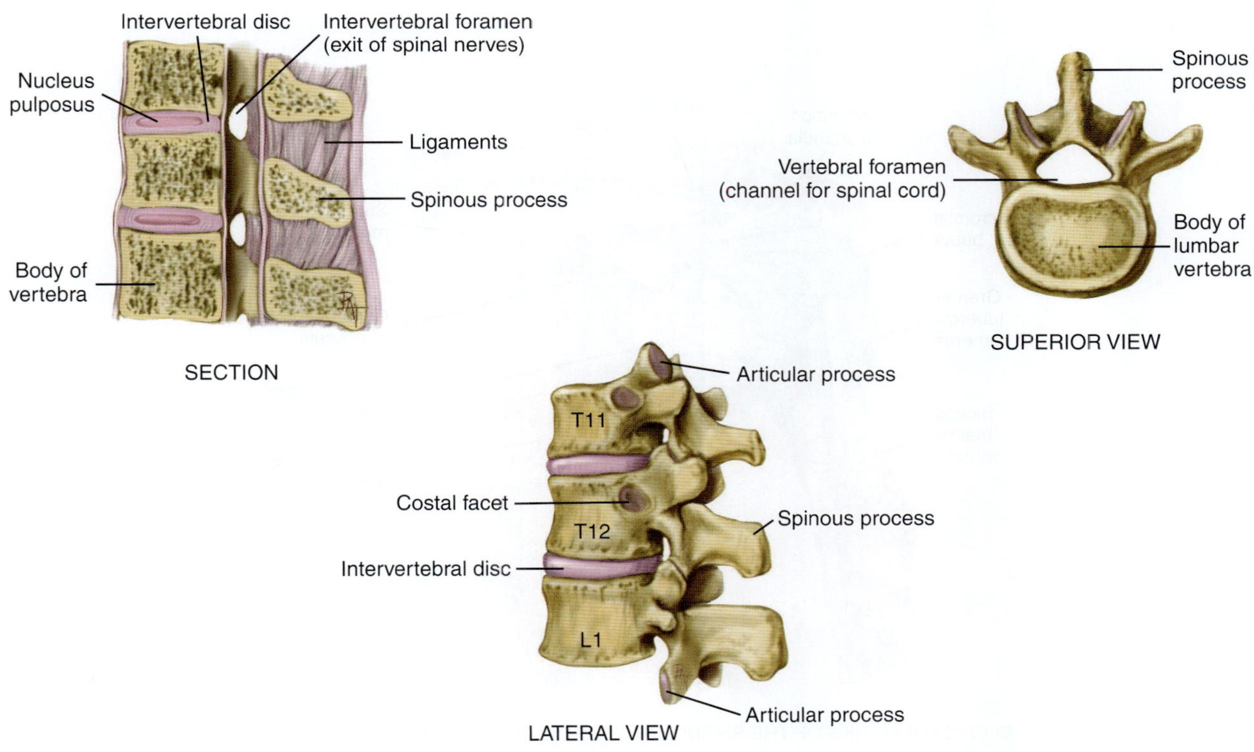

Figure 20.6

The main function of the intervertebral discs is to transfer the compression forces from one vertebra to another as loads are put on the spinal column during daily activities. As the spine moves, the elasticity of the discs allows compression on one side, with compensatory expansion on the other. If compression forces are too great, a disc can rupture and the nucleus pulposus can herniate out of the vertebral column, compressing the spinal nerves and causing pain.

The unique structure of the spine enables both upright posture and flexibility for motion. The motions of the vertebral column are flexion (bending forwards), extension (bending back), abduction (to either side) and rotation.

Shoulder. The **glenohumeral joint** is the articulation of the humerus with the glenoid fossa of the scapula (Figure 20.7). Its ball-and-socket action allows great mobility of the arm on many axes. The joint is enclosed by a group of four powerful muscles and tendons that support and stabilise it. Together these are called the **rotator cuff** of the shoulder. The large **subacromial bursa** helps during abduction of the arm, so that the greater tubercle of the humerus moves easily under the acromion process of the scapula.

The bones of the shoulder have palpable landmarks to guide your examination (Figure 20.8). The scapula and the clavicle connect to form the shoulder girdle. You can palpate

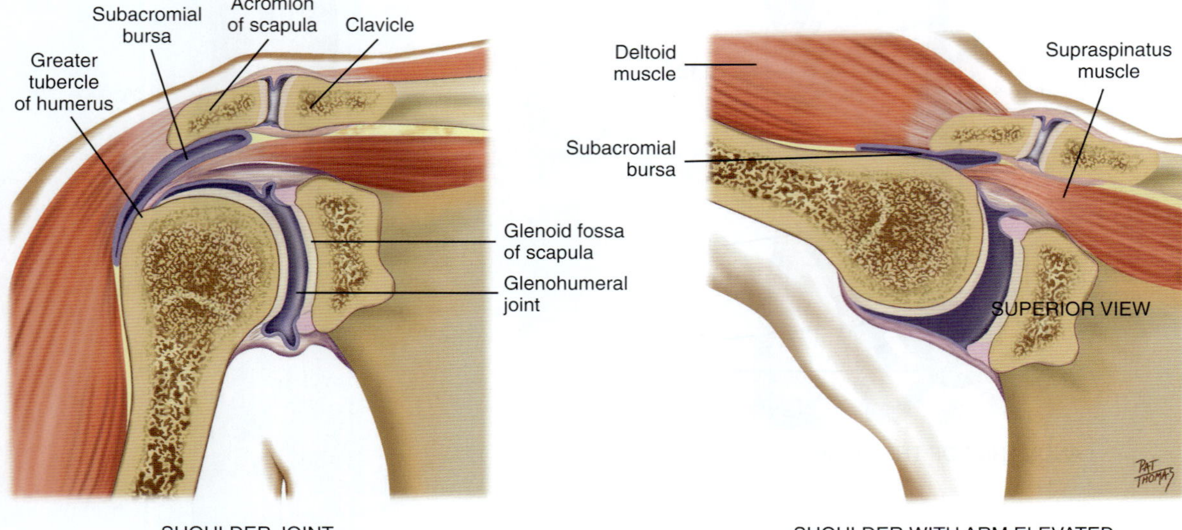

Figure 20.7

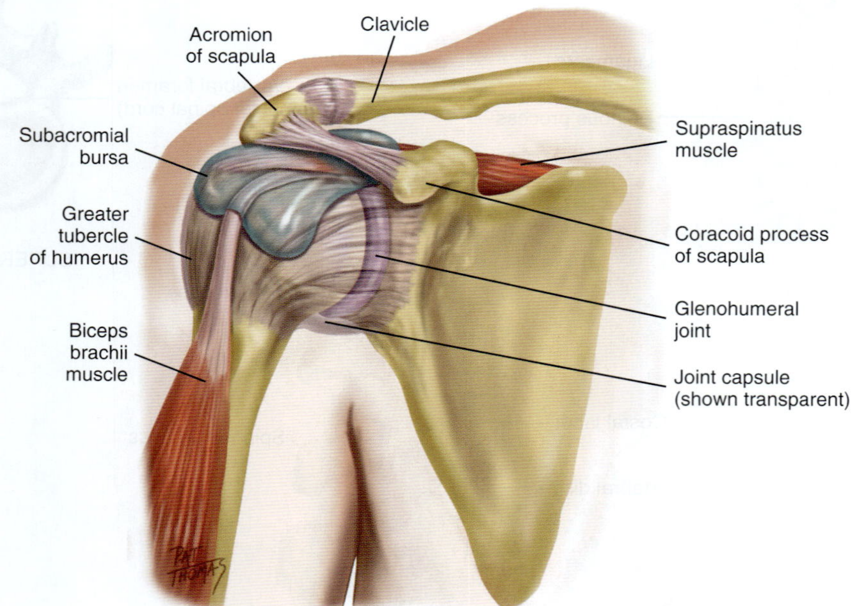

Figure 20.8

the bump of the scapula's **acromion process** at the very top of the shoulder. Move your fingers in a small circle outwards, down and around. The next bump is the **greater tubercle** of the humerus a few centimetres down and laterally, and from that the **coracoid process** of the scapula is a few centimetres medially. These surround the deeply situated joint.

Elbow. The elbow joint contains the three bony articulations of the humerus, radius and ulna of the forearm (Figure 20.9). Its hinge action moves the forearm (radius and ulna) on one plane, allowing flexion and extension. The olecranon bursa lies between the olecranon process and the skin.

Palpable landmarks are the **medial** and **lateral epicondyles** of the humerus and the large **olecranon process** of the ulna in between them. The sensitive ulnar nerve runs between the olecranon process and the medial epicondyle.

The radius and ulna articulate with each other at two radioulnar joints, one at the elbow and one at the wrist. These move together to permit pronation and supination of the hand and forearm.

Wrist and carpals. Of the body's 206 bones, over half are in the hands and feet. The wrist or **radiocarpal joint** is the articulation of the radius (on the thumb side) and a row of carpal bones (Figure 20.10). Its condyloid action permits movement in two planes at right angles: flexion and extension, and side-to-side deviation. The groove of this joint can be palpated on the dorsum of the wrist.

The **midcarpal** joint is the articulation between the two parallel rows of carpal bones. It allows flexion, extension and some rotation. The **metacarpophalangeal** and the **interphalangeal** joints permit finger flexion and extension. The flexor tendons of the wrist and hand are enclosed in synovial sheaths.

Hip. The hip joint is the articulation between the acetabulum and the head of the femur (Figure 20.11). As in the shoulder, ball-and-socket action permits a wide range of motion on many axes. The hip has somewhat less range of motion (ROM) than the shoulder, but it has more stability as befits its weight-bearing function. Hip stability is due to powerful muscles that spread over the joint, a strong fibrous articular capsule and the very deep insertion of the head of the femur. Three bursae facilitate movement.

Palpation of these bony landmarks will guide your examination. You can feel the entire iliac crest, from the **anterior superior iliac spine** to the posterior. The **ischial tuberosity** lies under the gluteus maximus muscle and is palpable when the hip is flexed. The **greater trochanter** of the femur is normally the width of the person's palm below the iliac crest and halfway between the anterior superior iliac spine and the ischial tuberosity. This landmark is best palpated when the person is standing, in a flat depression on the upper lateral side of the thigh.

Knee. The knee joint is the articulation of three bones—the femur, the tibia and the patella (kneecap)—in one common articular cavity (Figure 20.12). It is the largest joint in the body and is complex. It is a hinge joint, permitting flexion and extension of the lower leg, as well as a slight medial and lateral rotation.

The knee's synovial membrane is the largest in the body. It forms a sac at the superior border of the patella, called the **suprapatellar pouch**, which extends up as much as 6 cm behind the quadriceps muscle. Two wedge-shaped cartilages, called the **medial** and **lateral menisci**, cushion the tibia and femur. The joint is stabilised by two sets of ligaments. The **cruciate ligaments** (not shown) crisscross within the knee; they give anterior and posterior stability and help control rotation. The **collateral ligaments** connect the joint at both sides;

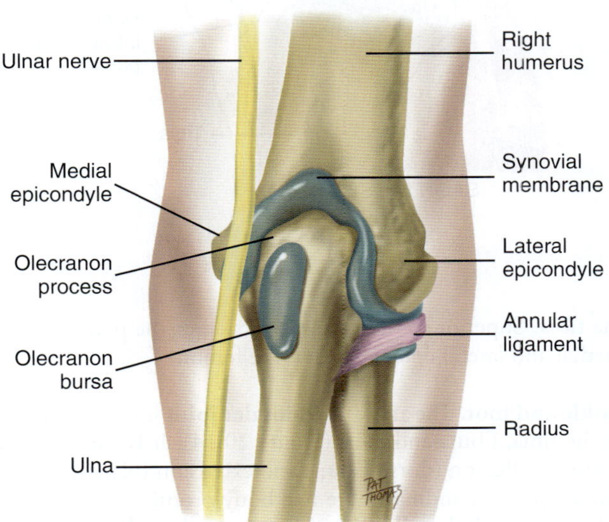

Figure 20.9

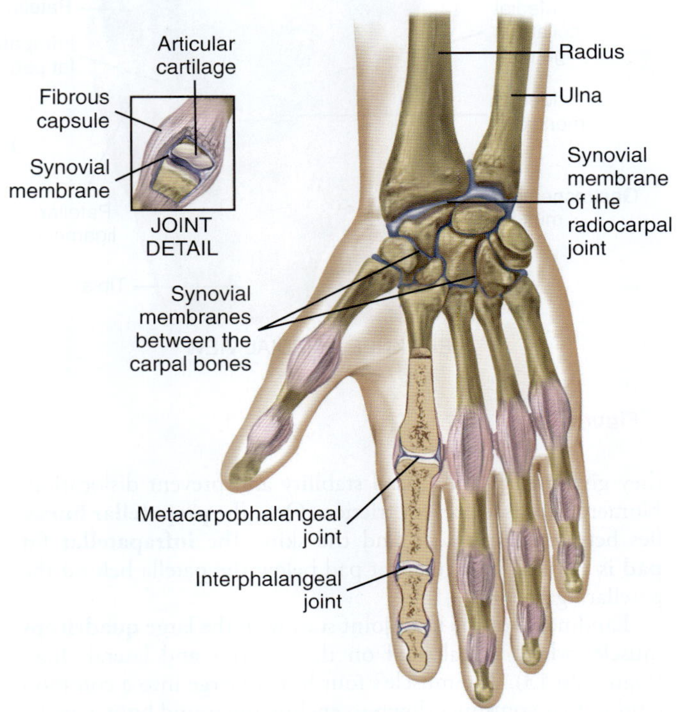

Figure 20.10

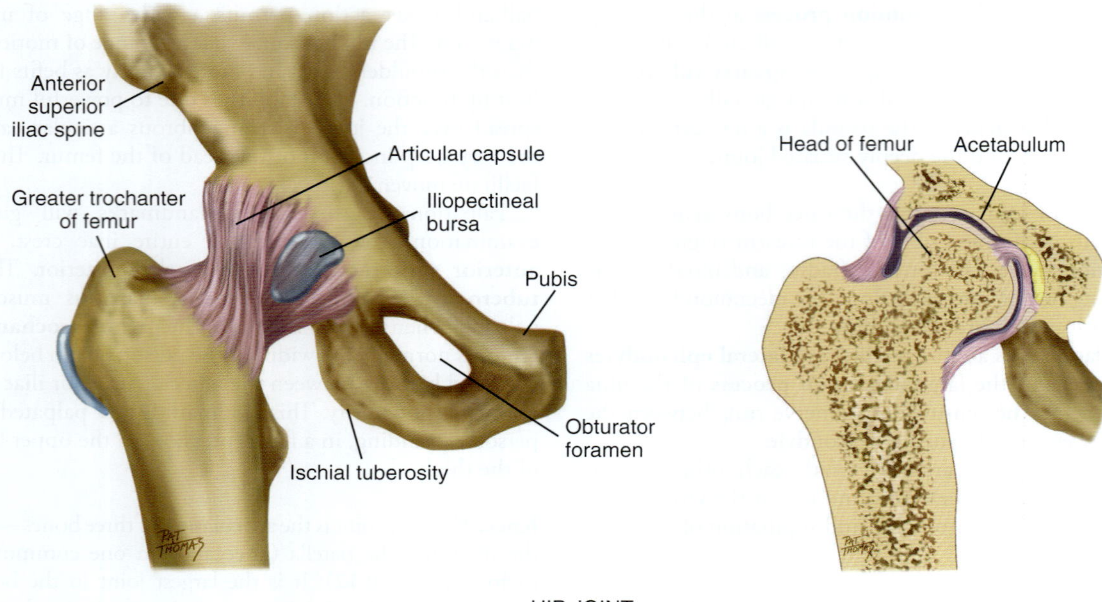

Figure 20.11

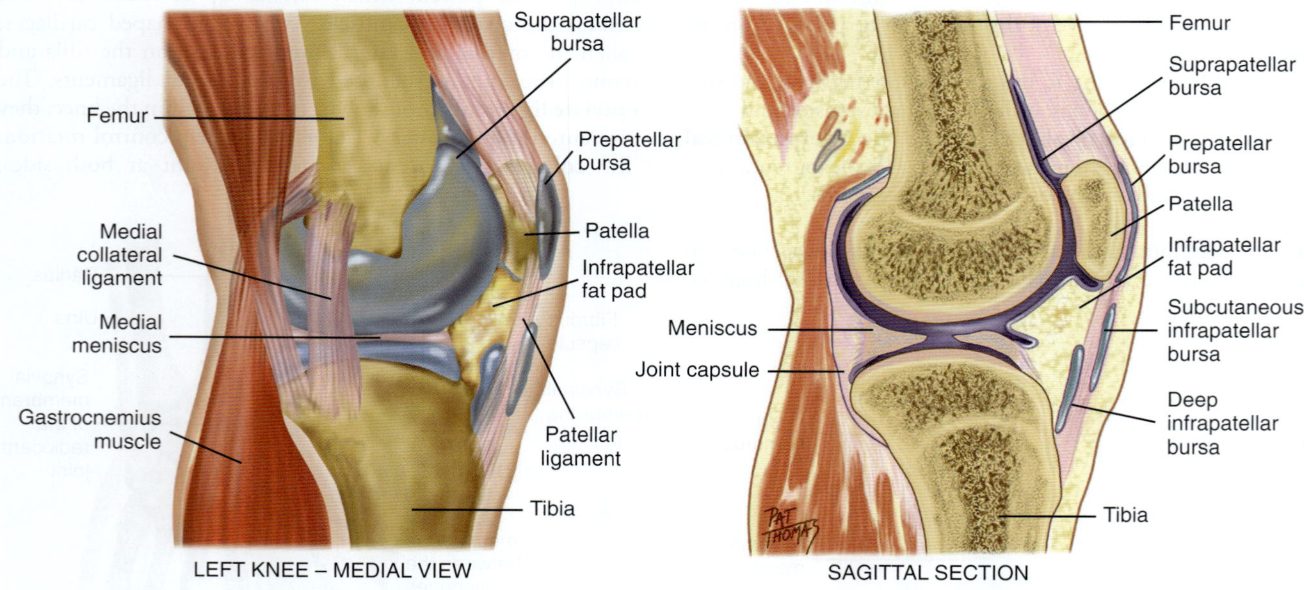

Figure 20.12

they give medial and lateral stability and prevent dislocation. Numerous bursae prevent friction. One, the **prepatellar bursa**, lies between the patella and the skin. The **infrapatellar fat pad** is a small, triangular fat pad below the patella behind the patellar ligament.

Landmarks of the knee joint start with the large **quadriceps** muscle, which is palpated on the anterior and lateral thigh (Figure 20.13). The muscle's four heads merge into a common tendon that continues down to enclose the round bony patella. Then the tendon inserts down on the **tibial tuberosity**, which is palpated as a bony prominence in the midline. Move to the sides and superiorly and note the lateral and medial condyles of the tibia. Superior to these on either side of the patella are the medial and lateral epicondyles of the femur.

Ankle and foot. The ankle or **tibiotalar joint** is the articulation of the tibia, fibula and talus (Figure 20.14). It is a hinge joint, limited to flexion (dorsiflexion) and extension (plantar flexion) on one plane. Landmarks are two bony prominences on either side—the **medial malleolus** and the **lateral malleolus**. Strong, tight medial and lateral ligaments extend from each malleolus onto the foot. These help the lateral stability of the ankle joint, although they may be torn in eversion or inversion sprains of the ankle.

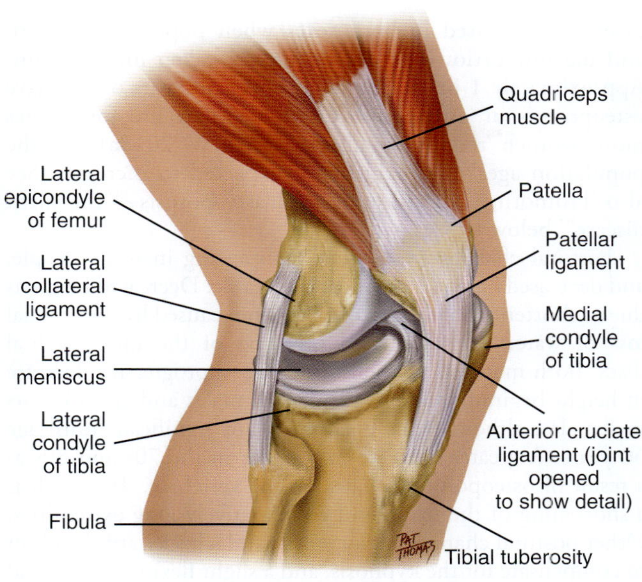

Figure 20.13

Joints distal to the ankle give additional mobility to the foot. The subtalar joint permits inversion and eversion of the foot. The foot has a longitudinal arch, with weight-bearing distributed between the parts that touch the ground—the heads of the metatarsals and the calcaneus (heel).

DEVELOPMENTAL CONSIDERATIONS

Infants and children

By 3 months' gestation, the fetus has formed a 'scale model' of the skeleton that is made up of cartilage. During succeeding months in utero, the cartilage ossifies into true bone and starts to grow. Bone growth continues after birth—rapidly during infancy and then steadily during childhood—until adolescence, when both boys and girls undergo a rapid growth spurt.

Long bones grow in two dimensions. They increase in width or diameter by deposition of new bony tissue around the shafts. Lengthening occurs at the epiphyses, or growth plates. These specialised growth centres are transverse discs located at the ends of long bone. Any trauma or infection at this location puts the growing child at risk for bone deformity. This longitudinal growth continues until closure of the epiphyses; the last closure occurs at about age 20 years.

Skeletal contour changes are apparent at the vertebral column. At birth the spine has a single C-shaped curve. At 3–4 months, raising the baby's head from prone position develops the anterior curve in the cervical neck region. From 1 year to 18 months, standing erect develops the anterior curve in the lumbar region. Musculoskeletal conditions seen in the neonatal period include developmental dysplasia of the hip (DDH), talipes equinovarus (clubfoot) and upper and lower limb development deformities.

The term developmental dysplasia of the hip (DDH) describes a wide range of hip abnormalities found within the neonatal period in which the femoral head has an abnormal relationship to the acetabulum. Variances in these disorders range from stable hips with acetabular dysplasia to complete displacement of the femoral head out of an abnormal acetabulum. The prevalence of DDH varies due to diagnostic criteria, examiner skills and disorder progress. Minor hip dysplasia often resolves spontaneously. The incidence is estimated to be between 1.6 and 28.5 neonates per 1000 births (Studer et al 2016). Successful clinical DDH screening programs within Australia using midwives, maternal child health nurses and primary care clinicians have been created in order to eliminate 'late diagnosed' DDH. Untreated DDH has the potential to cause longterm hip dysplasia and arthritis.

Musculoskeletal conditions, however, are evident throughout childhood, affecting up to 30% of children and adolescents. The majority are self-limiting, and often trauma related. These conditions also include life-threatening disorders such as malignant disease and infection. Chronic musculoskeletal conditions include a spectrum of autoimmune/inflammatory joint and muscle disorders. Juvenile idiopathic arthritis (JIA) relates to the group of heterogeneous diseases which are a

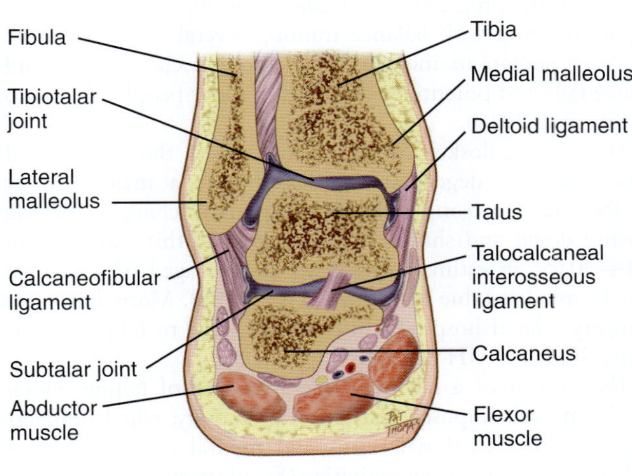

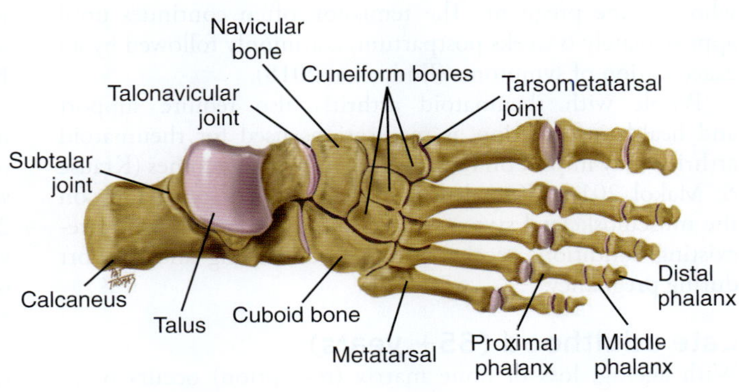

Figure 20.14

feature of chronic inflammatory arthritis of unknown cause lasting longer than 6 weeks with onset before 16 years of age. In Australia, the estimated overall prevalence of JIA is 1 per 1000 children (AIHW 2018c, 2018d). Juvenile arthritis affects the child's growth and musculoskeletal development. The associated disability, chronic pain and growth disturbances impact on all aspects of the child's life and family/social dynamics. Australian studies indicate that joint inflammation relapses are common with up to three quarters requiring ongoing medication at 12 months (Tiller et al 2018).

The pregnant woman

It has been reported that almost all women experience some degree of musculoskeletal discomfort during pregnancy with 25% experiencing pelvic girdle pain and 50–80% of pregnant women experiencing low back pain (Gutke et al 2018). Increased levels of circulating hormones (oestrogen, relaxin from the corpus luteum and corticosteroids) cause increased mobility in the joints. Increased mobility in the sacroiliac, sacrococcygeal and symphysis pubis joints in the pelvis contributes to the noticeable changes in maternal posture. The most characteristic change is progressive lordosis, which compensates for the enlarging fetus; otherwise, the centre of balance would shift forwards. Lordosis compensates by shifting the weight further back on the lower extremities. This shift in balance in turn creates strain on the low back muscles, which in some women is felt as low back pain during late pregnancy.

Anterior flexion of the neck and slumping of the shoulder girdle are other postural changes that compensate for the lordosis. These upper back changes may put pressure on the ulnar and median nerves during the third trimester. Carpal tunnel syndrome in pregnancy is often bilateral and mostly present in the third trimester. The course of carpal tunnel syndrome found in association with pregnancy varies with most women having resolution of symptoms following the birth, although some women will have persistent symptoms (Department of Health 2018).

Effects of pregnancy on preexisting musculoskeletal conditions

Pregnancy and the associated changes in circulating hormones and postural changes impact on a diverse range of preexisting musculoskeletal conditions. Examples include remission rates in up to 75% of women with preexisting rheumatoid arthritis who become pregnant. The remission often continues until approximately 6 weeks postpartum, commonly followed by an exacerbation of symptoms (Eudy et al 2018).

People with rheumatoid arthritis also require support and health information as medications used for rheumatoid arthritis may impact on fertility and on birth outcomes (Krause & Makol 2016). Knowledge of the effects of pregnancy on the musculoskeletal system is vital to ensure people with pre-existing conditions receive effective counselling and support during pregnancy.

Late adulthood (65+ years)

With ageing, loss of bone matrix (resorption) occurs more rapidly than new bone growth (deposition). The net effect is a loss of bone density, or **osteoporosis**. While the age-adjusted incidence of osteoporotic hip fracture in Australia appears to have decreased over recent years, the actual number of cases has increased in both sexes when population growth and the proportion of older people are taken into account. Approximately 1 in 10 Australians over 50 years of age have osteoporosis or osteopenia. Of these, there are four times more women than men affected (AIHW 2018a). As the population ages, the incidence is expected to increase. (See also 'Promoting a healthy lifestyle: osteoporosis—"the silent disease"' below.)

Postural changes are evident with ageing in some people, and decreased height is the most noticeable. Decreased height is due to shortening of the vertebral column caused by the gradual loss of water and associated thinning of the intervertebral discs. Both men and women can expect a progressive decrease in height beginning at age 40 years in males and age 43 years in females, although this decrease is not significant until age 60 years. A greater decrease may occur in the 70s and 80s as a result of osteoporotic collapse of the vertebrae. The result is a shortening of the trunk and comparatively long extremities. Other postural changes are kyphosis, and a backwards head tilt to compensate for the kyphosis, and a slight flexion of hips and knees.

The distribution of subcutaneous fat changes through life. Usually, men and women gain weight in their 40s and 50s. The contour is different, even if the weight is the same as when younger. They begin to lose fat in the face and deposit it in the abdomen and hips. In the 80s and 90s, fat further decreases in the periphery, which is especially noticeable in the forearms and becomes more apparent over the abdomen and hips. Loss of subcutaneous fat leaves bony prominences more marked (e.g. tips of vertebrae, ribs, iliac crests) and body hollows deeper, for example, cheeks and axillae.

An absolute loss in muscle mass occurs with ageing; some muscles decrease in size, and some atrophy, producing weakness, particularly in people with low physical activity levels. The contour of muscles becomes more prominent, and muscle bundles and tendons feel more distinct. This age-related loss of muscle mass and strength termed sarcopenia affects balance and gait, and is correlated to functional decline in some older people (Dhillon & Hasni 2017).

It has become more apparent that lifestyle affects musculoskeletal changes. A sedentary lifestyle hastens the musculoskeletal changes of ageing. Multi-modal exercise incorporating progressive resistance training, weight-bearing impact training with balance training several times per week has been shown to increase bone and muscle strength and reduce falls and potentially fractures in older people (de Souto Barreto et al 2019).

The musculoskeletal changes and the associated musculoskeletal degenerative diseases have a major impact on the older person's safety. Gait pattern changes include slowing down and shorter stride length. Within Australia in 2014–2015, an estimated 111,222 people aged 65 and over were hospitalised due to falls (AIHW 2018b). More than 40% of injury-related hospital admissions are due to falls and falls related injuries (AIHW 2018c).

The impact of a fall may lead to a fear of falling which spirals into self-imposed restriction of activity, which impacts negatively on functional status and mental health reducing both physical and social activities (Seonhye et al 2018). Falls prevention programs are thus widespread at both State and Commonwealth level within Australia.

CULTURAL AND SOCIAL CONSIDERATIONS

Musculoskeletal conditions are the most common chronic conditions in Australia affecting 30% of the Australian population and represent some of the most common causes of pain and disability (AIHW 2018c). The most common musculoskeletal conditions affecting Australians are back pain and problems, osteoarthritis, other forms of arthritis and osteoporosis. Chronic musculoskeletal conditions account for 6.9% of total hospitalisations in Australia (AIHW 2019).

Road trauma represents a leading cause of traumatic musculoskeletal injury worldwide (WHO 2018). Within Australia sequelae include not only functional impairments such as chronic pain and joint disorders but also a range of psychological, social and economic challenges. These often-profound injuries cause a ripple effect of loss and grief that affects their families, friends and their communities (Gane et al 2018).

As a group, Indigenous Australians experience widespread disadvantage and health inequality. Musculoskeletal diseases contribute to over 20% of the non-fatal disease burden in Indigenous Australians aged 45–74 years—Indigenous Australian males are twice as likely to have a hip fracture as other Australian males, whereas Indigenous females are 26% more likely to have a hip fracture than other Australian females. Indigenous Australians are on average much younger than other Australians at the time of their hip fracture, aged 65 years (compared with 81 years) for males and 74 years (compared with 83 years) for females (AIHW 2016). Chronic musculoskeletal diseases and trauma statistics for Indigenous Australians are incomplete.

In Australia, an increasing trend for vitamin D deficiency has been highlighted. Vitamin D deficiency is directly linked to osteomalacia and osteoporosis. The most significant bone health concerns have been highlighted for people born in a country other than Australia or other main English-speaking countries, residing in the southern parts of Australia, being obese, smoking (in women only), having low physical activity levels, not taking Vitamin D or calcium supplements and being tested in winter and spring (Malacova et al 2019).

Subjective data

As noted previously, musculoskeletal disorders cause pain, stiffness and impairment to activities of daily living. A comprehensive musculoskeletal assessment should be integrated into a health assessment as numerous general health issues and prescribed medications affect this system. For example, chronic heart and lung disease impacts on mobility. Visual deficits, hypotension, vitamin B_{12} deficiency and incontinence all increase falls risks.

Musculoskeletal assessment is a systematic process involving application of knowledge of functional anatomy, and the mechanisms of injury and disease across the life span. As nursing roles expand within Australia and New Zealand, it is often the nurse who has the first point of contact with the person in both community and hospital settings.

This assessment process involves initially allowing the person to tell their story, through history taking, of the impact of their joint dysfunction and pain on their lives. Due to the often chronic nature of musculoskeletal disorders it is important to ask about previous complementary therapies, non-prescription medications and remedies. A thorough history will assist in identifying the nature of the musculoskeletal problems; for example, acute injury, degenerative, inflammatory, infective or malignant disorders.

A medical history including current medications is an essential part of musculoskeletal assessment. A variety of endocrine/metabolic disorders, nutritional conditions and medications can impact on bone health. Diseases such as hyperthyroidism, diabetes, renal disease, malabsorption syndromes and glucocorticoids, loop diuretics and aluminium are the most common risk factors. There is also a strong genetic link associated with musculoskeletal health so the person should be asked to discuss any family history of fractures or arthritis.

As musculoskeletal function is linked to neurological function, it is suggested you refer to Chapter 12. As acute and chronic pain is also often associated with musculoskeletal disorders it is suggested you refer to Chapter 13.

The subjective assessment focuses on the following:

1. Presenting concern
2. Gait, arms, legs and spine (GALS) screening assessment
3. Joints
4. Muscles
5. Bones
6. Functional assessment (activities of daily living (ADLs)
7. Health and lifestyle management

Practice note: Before you commence the assessment, introduce yourself to the person, confirm the person's identity, discuss the purpose and scope of the assessment, clarify any questions the person may have and obtain verbal consent from the person to perform the assessment.

ASSESSMENT GUIDELINES	CLINICAL SIGNIFICANCE AND CLINICAL ALERTS
1. Presenting concern	
Do you feel that you have any problem/s with your joints, muscles, bones or walking and moving that affects your ability to exercise and go about your daily activities? It is important to ascertain the person's perception of their musculoskeletal function. • If they do perceive a problem—how does this impact on their quality of life?	The person's response to this question will guide you to areas to focus on in further subjective and objective data collection.

ASSESSMENT GUIDELINES	CLINICAL SIGNIFICANCE AND CLINICAL ALERTS
2. Gait, arms, legs and spine (GALS) screening assessment	
A screening musculoskeletal examination can rapidly identify those people who require comprehensive musculoskeletal assessment. The gait, arms, legs and spine (GALS) screening assessment is a highly sensitive, specific and well-validated screening assessment for the detection of joint abnormalities (Dacre 2019, Doherty et al 1992). Subjective data from this screening assessment involves three core questions. • 'Have you any pain or stiffness in your muscles, joints or back?' • 'Can you dress yourself completely without any difficulty?' and • 'Can you walk up and down stairs without any difficulty?' A positive response to the first question and/or a negative response to the second or third question indicates a detailed history should be taken. A paediatric-specific GALS assessment (pGALS) has also proved highly sensitive, specific and well validated (Dacre 2019, Foster & Jandial 2013).	
3. Joints	
• Any problems with your joints? Tell me about your **pain**?	**Joint pain and loss of function** are the most common musculoskeletal concerns that prompt a person to seek care.
• **Location:** Which joints? On one side or both sides?	**Rheumatoid arthritis (RA)** involves symmetrical joints; other musculoskeletal illnesses and trauma involve isolated or unilateral joints.
• **Quality:** What does the pain feel like: aching, stiff, sharp or dull, shooting? • **Severity:** How strong is the pain? • **Onset:** When did this pain start?	Exquisitely tender felt with acute inflammation. Chronic pain is often associated with degenerative musculoskeletal disorders.
• **Timing:** What time of day does the pain occur? How long does it last? How often does it occur?	RA pain is worse in morning when arising; osteoarthritis is worse later in the day; tendinitis is worse in morning, improves during the day.
• Is the pain aggravated by movement, rest, position, weather? Is the pain relieved by rest, medications, application of heat or ice?	Most joint pain is mechanical except in RA, when deformities restrict movement. Many people have tried prescribed medications, homeopathic remedies, over-the-counter (OTC) medications or combination formulations. These need to be identified and included in your assessment.
• Is the pain associated with chills, fever, recent sore throat, trauma and repetitive activity?	Joint pain 10–14 days after an untreated strep throat suggests rheumatic fever. Joint injury occurs from trauma or repetitive motion.
• Any stiffness in your joints?	RA **stiffness** occurs in morning and after rest periods.
• Any swelling, heat, redness in the joints?	Suggests acute inflammation.
• Any limitation of movement in any joint? Which joint? • Which activities give you problems? (See Functional assessment below.)	**Decreased ROM** may be due to joint disease or to muscle contracture.
4. Muscles	
• Any problems in the muscles, such as any pain or cramping? Which muscles?	**Myalgia** is usually felt as cramping or aching.
• If in calf muscles: Is the pain with walking? Does it go away with rest?	Suggests intermittent claudication (Chapter 16).

ASSESSMENT GUIDELINES	CLINICAL SIGNIFICANCE AND CLINICAL ALERTS
• Are your muscle aches associated with fever, chills, the 'flu'?	Viral illness often includes myalgia.
• Any weakness in muscles? • Location: Where is the weakness? How long have you noticed weakness?	**Weakness** may involve peripheral vascular system or neurological systems (Chapters 12 and 16).
• Do the muscles look different there?	Smaller muscles indicate atrophy. Swelling may indicate haematoma or tumour.
5. Bones	
• Any bone pain? Is the pain affected by movement? • Any deformity of any bone or joint? Is the deformity due to injury or trauma? Does the deformity affect ROM? • Any accidents or trauma ever affected the bones or joints: fractures, joint strain, sprain, dislocation? Which ones?	Trauma causes sharp pain that increases with movement. Other bone pain usually feels 'dull' and 'deep' and is unrelated to movement. Injury to ligaments affects joint kinematics, e.g. whiplash trauma may result in cervical ligament laxity and chronic pain syndromes.
• When did this occur? What treatment was given? Any problems or limitations now as a result?	Previous joint trauma increases risk of degenerative arthritis. Many people with back pain have sought treatments provided by physiotherapists, chiropractors, osteopaths or acupuncturists.
• Any back pain? In which part of your back? Is pain felt anywhere else, like shooting down your leg or arm? • How long have you had this pain?	The aetiology is diverse, e.g. degenerative or traumatic conditions of the spine, fibrositis, inflammatory spondyloarthropathy and metabolic bone conditions are also cited as causes.
• Any numbness and tingling? Any limping?	Spinal nerve-root dysfunction is associated with altered sensory and motor function. See Chapter 12.
6. Functional assessment (ADLs)	
• How do your joint (muscle, bone) problems create any limits on your usual activities of daily living (ADLs)? Which ones? (Note: Ask about each category; if the person answers 'yes', ask specifically about each activity in the category.)	Functional assessment screens the safety of independent living, the need for community supports and quality of life.
• **Bathing**—getting in and out of the shower/bath, turning on taps? Can you wash your back, legs, feet, hair?	Degenerative lower limb joint dysfunction affects mobility and steppage and increases risk of falls. Upper limb nerve compression affects precision and grip, e.g. carpal tunnel syndrome.
• **Toileting**—urinating, moving bowels, able to get self on/off toilet, wipe self?	Altered bowel and bladder function may be an indication of cauda equina syndrome.
• **Dressing**—doing buttons, zipper, fasten opening behind neck, pulling dress or sweater overhead, pulling up pants. Tying shoelaces, getting shoes that fit?	Indicates upper limb dysfunction. Degenerative processes lead to foot deformity, pain and disability. Foot deformities and ill-fitting shoes all increase falls risk.
• **Grooming**—shaving, brushing teeth, brushing or fixing hair, applying make-up?	Indicates upper limb dysfunction or psychosocial issues.
• **Eating**—preparing meals, pouring liquids, cutting up foods, bringing food to mouth, drinking?	Indicates upper limb dysfunction or psychosocial issues.

SUBJECTIVE DATA

ASSESSMENT GUIDELINES	CLINICAL SIGNIFICANCE AND CLINICAL ALERTS
• **Mobility**—walking, walking up or down stairs, getting in/out of bed, getting out of house?	When the person is found to have significant impairment of mobility a falls risk screening must be conducted.
• **Communicating**—talking, using phone, writing?	Indicates upper limb/hand dysfunction. Chronic diseases can cause social isolation and depression.
7. Health and lifestyle management	
• Any **occupational hazards** that could affect the muscles and joints? Does your work involve heavy lifting? Is there any repetitive motion or chronic stress to joints in your work? What measures have you used to alleviate these?	Assess risk for back injury, rotator cuff damage or carpal tunnel syndrome. Where the workplace is identified as contributing to potential injury, the person should undergo a formal workplace assessment.
• Tell me about your **exercise** program. Describe the type of exercise, frequency, the warm-up program.	
• Any pain during exercise? How do you treat it?	
• Has your **weight** changed recently? Please describe your usual daily diet. (Note the person's usual kilojoule intake, all four food groups, daily amount of protein, calcium.)	Weight impacts on joint function. Low calcium and vitamin D together with smoking and excessive alcohol are associated with osteoporosis.
• Are you taking any **medications** for musculoskeletal system: aspirin, anti-inflammatory, muscle relaxant, pain reliever? Are you taking any herbal supplements, vitamins or other 'natural remedies'?	Over-the-counter medications are common first-line treatments for joint pain, e.g. glucosamine. Chronic pain sufferers often use multiple analgesia. Complementary medications have iatrogenic effects and should be included in a health history.
If person has chronic disability and/or severe musculoskeletal dysfunction, how have these symptoms/illness affected: • Your interaction with family and friends • Your employment and leisure activities • The way you view yourself • How you manage your health • The impact on your social life • The impact on your stress levels and coping ability?	Assess for • Self-esteem disturbance • Loss of independence • Body image disturbance • Role performance disturbance • Social isolation/stress and coping • Health management ability. Significant issues in any of these areas may indicate the need for further focused assessment.
Additional subjective data for infants and children (questions for parents or guardians)	
Children with musculoskeletal problems often present to primary care services with traumatic or non-traumatic injuries. The majority of problems are self-limiting; however, the presentation of life-threatening illnesses such as malignancy or septic arthritis will require urgent referrals to specialty services. Chronic illnesses such as juvenile arthritis and the muscular dystrophies also require urgent referrals to improve care outcomes.	Children with growing pains do not limp or experience morning stiffness. **Non-accidental injury (NAI)** can present as unexplained fracture patterns or bruising with incongruity between child's and the carer's/parent's history. Ensuring the child's safety and completing detailed documentation are priorities. Refer to your local State and Territory legislation on non-accidental injury and your local hospital/community guidelines for assessment and treatment plans.

ASSESSMENT GUIDELINES	CLINICAL SIGNIFICANCE AND CLINICAL ALERTS
	The nurse within the emergency department and primary setting requires a comprehensive knowledge of growth and development patterns from neonate to adolescent and the associated disease and injury profiles at different stages. Effective pain management is also essential if a comprehensive and targeted history is to be obtained.
• Were you told about any trauma to infant during labour and delivery? Did the baby's head come first? Was there a need for forceps?	Traumatic delivery increases risk for fractures (e.g. humerus, clavicle) and hip dysplasia.
• Did the baby need resuscitation?	Period of anoxia may result in hypotonia of muscles.
• Were the baby's motor milestones achieved at about the same time as siblings or age mates? Have any of the baby's milestones changed recently?	Pain, joint dysfunction, malaise and fever all impact on activity and learning capacity, hence milestones may be affected. For example, toddler may stop walking, develop enuresis or have sleep disturbances.
• Has your child been well? Any weight loss, fever or malaise?	Recent fever with pain and/or swelling of one joint or bone may indicate an infective or inflammatory process.
• Has your child ever broken any bones? Any bruising or dislocations? Where and how were these treated?	Fractures of the epiphyseal plate may lead to deformity. Immediate pain and swelling following traumatic injury and mechanical dysfunction may indicate a musculoskeletal condition.
• Have you ever noticed any bone deformity? Head tilting or spinal curvature? Unusual shape of toes or feet? At what age? Have you ever sought treatment for any of these?	Gait changes can indicate normal development or undiagnosed hip problems, e.g. DDH, Perthes and slipped upper femoral epiphysis (SUFE). Spinal problems may present as asymmetrical ribs or waist and head tilting.
Additional subjective data for adolescents	
• Involved in any sports at school or after school? How frequently (times per week)?	40% of bone mass accumulates during adolescence. This is achieved through exercise and a healthy diet.
• Do you use any special equipment? Does any training program exist for your sport?	Assess use of safety equipment (e.g. mouth guards, helmets) and safe sporting practices. Use of safety equipment and presence of adult supervision decreases risk of sports injuries.
• What is the nature of your daily warm-up?	Lack of adequate warm-up increases risk of sports injury.
• What do you do if you get hurt?	Students may not report injury or pain for fear of limiting participation in sport.
• Have you ever noticed any bone deformity? Spinal curvature?	Adolescents with scoliosis may report unilateral changes in shoulders, rib cage, hip levels and an uneven waist.
Additional subjective data for adults over 65 years	
The questions you should ask the adult should be focused on functional abilities. The aim is to elicit any loss of function, self-care deficit, or safety risk that may occur as a process of ageing or musculoskeletal illness. Ask questions only where relevant to the person's situation.	

SUBJECTIVE DATA

ASSESSMENT GUIDELINES	CLINICAL SIGNIFICANCE AND CLINICAL ALERTS
• Any change in weakness over the past months or years?	Pain/joint dysfunction impacts on activity and increases weakness and lethargy.
• Any increase in falls or stumbling over the past months or years?	It is essential to focus on exploring all falls risks in a positive manner.
• Do you use any walking aids to help you get around inside your home and outside your home? Where did you purchase these walking aids?	All gait aids should be supplied as part of a comprehensive mobility assessment performed by a physiotherapist.

Objective data

The purpose of the musculoskeletal examination is to assess patterns of pain, joint abnormalities and the impact these have on the person's activities of daily living (ADLs) and psychosocial functioning. Note additional ADL information as the person goes through the motions necessary for an examination: gait, posture, how the person sits in a chair, rises from chair, takes off jacket, manipulates a small object such as a pen and rises from the supine position. It is essential to identify painful joints during the history to ensure these are examined last.

The subjective data will assist in targeting your objective assessment and referral criteria. Musculoskeletal assessment can be challenging for the nurse and the person. It often involves asking intimate questions as well as requiring the person to be partially undressed and therefore vulnerable. You need to ensure the privacy and comfort of the person during musculoskeletal assessment.

Preparation

All forms of musculoskeletal assessment require a systematic approach:

- Head to toe
- Proximal to distal
- Compare corresponding paired joint.

Expect symmetry of structure and function and normal parameters for that joint.

In addition, a neurovascular assessment of upper and lower limbs is a mandatory component for all musculoskeletal assessments (see Chapters 12 and 16 for details of neurological and peripheral vascular assessment).

As you approach this examination, focus on the principles of 'look, feel, then move'.

Look (inspect)—asymmetry of joints, joint swelling, deformity, abnormalities of muscle and soft tissue bulk, erythema, ecchymosis, lesions and rashes, general health of the person.
Feel (palpate)—soft tissue swelling, bony or crystal nodules, tenderness, joint warmth and pain.
Move—active movement first followed by passive movement. Perform painful movements last.

PROCEDURES AND NORMAL FINDINGS	ABNORMAL FINDINGS AND CLINICAL ALERTS
General inspection	
During collection of subjective data you will have noticed ease of movement and breathing, ability to sit and stand, height to weight ratio, level of hygiene and grooming and general demeanor. All of these factors provide clues to the functioning of the musculoskeletal system.	
Gait, arms, legs and spine (GALS) screening assessment	
Gait	
Observe the person walking, turning then walking back. Observe for symmetry and smoothness of gait. Does the person limp? Observe for any reduced muscle bulk in the gluteals. Can the person turn quickly?	**Antalgic gait** is a symptom of pain with weight bearing. The stance phase of the gait is abnormally shortened relative to the swing phase. **Ataxia** is gross lack of coordination of muscle movement. It is a neurological sign (see Chapter 12).

PROCEDURES AND NORMAL FINDINGS	ABNORMAL FINDINGS AND CLINICAL ALERTS

Arms

Shoulder movements (Figures 20.15A and 20.15B)

- Ask the person to place their hands behind their head, with their elbows back. This movement assesses abduction, external rotation of the shoulder and elbow flexion.
- Palpate each shoulder for rotator cuff problems.

Elbow movements and hands

- Ask the person to extend their arms fully and turn their hands over so palms are down (Figure 20.15C).
- Following this ask the person to turn their hands over.
- Observe the elbow and hands for any joint/tissue swelling or deformities.

Grip strength (Figures 20.15D)

- Ask the person to make a fist. Observe the hand and finger movements.
- Ask the person to grip your fingers and assess the degree of grip strength.

Observe for pain

- Squeeze across the second to fifth metacarpal. Observe for pain. (See Figure E).

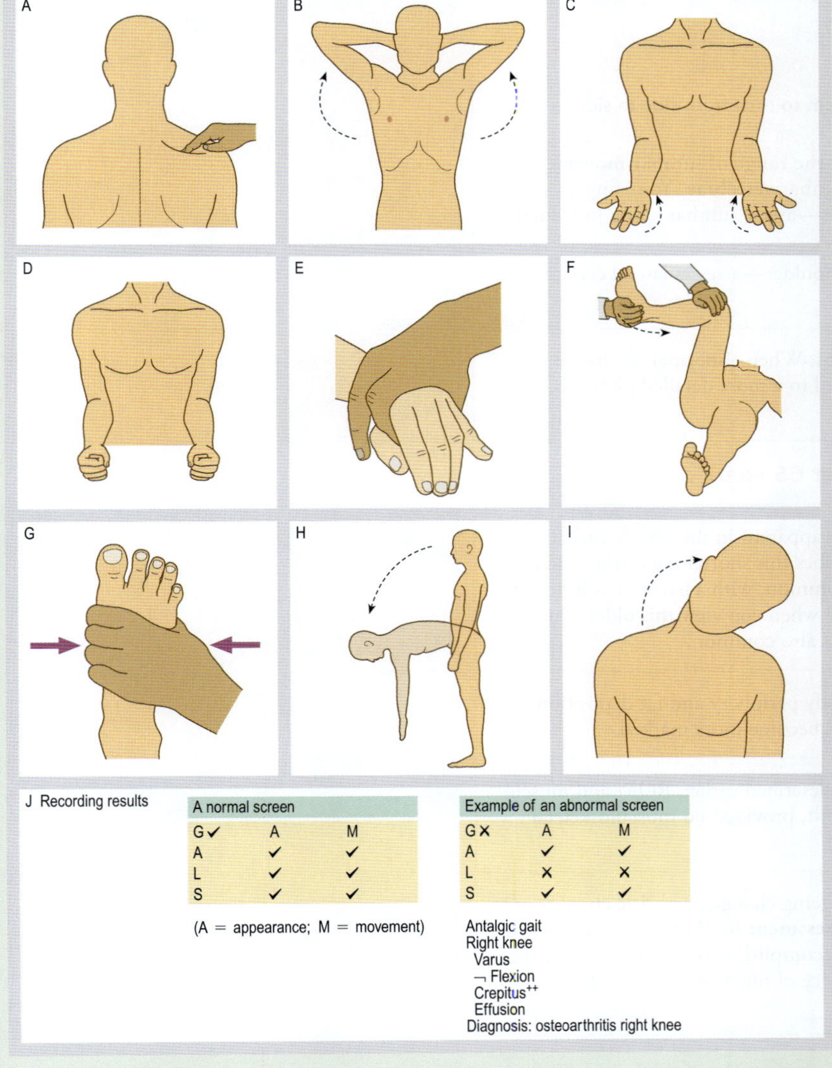

Figure 20.15
The GALS screening assessment.

PROCEDURES AND NORMAL FINDINGS	ABNORMAL FINDINGS AND CLINICAL ALERTS
Legs	
Position the person lying down with upper torso covered. **Hip movement** • Hold the knee and hip flexed to 90 degrees. Assess the degree of internal rotation in each hip (Figure 20.15F). **Knee** • Observe for any reduced muscle bulk especially in quadriceps. • Assess: ask the person to flex and extend both knees. • Palpate the knee for crepitus and warmth. **Inspection of feet and shoes** • Inspect the feet for any swelling, deformity or any callosities (Figure 20.15G). • Look at person's shoes for unequal wear.	
Spine	
Inspect the spinal column for any abnormalities including kyphosis, scoliosis or lordosis. Observe for **symmetry of legs and pelvis.** **Thoracolumbar spine** • Hold the person's pelvis from behind and ask them to turn from side to side—assesses thoracolumbar rotation. • Ask the person to touch their toes. Palpate for the range of lumbar movement (Figure 20.15H). Place two fingers over the lumbar vertebrae. Your fingers should move apart as the person bend forwards—assess lumbar spine movement. **Cervical spine** • Ask the person to bring their ear towards their shoulder—assesses lateral cervical flexion (Figure 20.15I).	
Record results using the framework of Figure 20.15J. When abnormal results are obtained on the screening GALS assessment proceed to a more detailed physical examination.	
Additional objective data for adults over 65 years	
Postural changes include a decrease in height, more apparent in the eighth and ninth decades. 'Lengthening of the arm–trunk axis' describes this shortening of the trunk with comparatively long extremities. Kyphosis is common, with a backwards head tilt to compensate. This creates the outline of a figure 3 when you view this older adult from the left side. Slight flexion of hips and knees is also common.	
Contour changes include a decrease of fat in the body periphery and fat deposition over the abdomen and hips. The bony prominences become more marked.	
For most adults over 65, ROM testing proceeds as described earlier. ROM and muscle strength are much the same as with the younger adult, provided no musculoskeletal illnesses or arthritic changes are present.	
Functional assessment. For those with advanced ageing changes, arthritic changes or musculoskeletal disability, perform a **functional assessment for ADLs.** This applies the ROM and muscle strength assessments to the accomplishment of specific activities. You need to determine adequate and safe performance of functions essential for independent home life.	

PROCEDURES AND NORMAL FINDINGS		ABNORMAL FINDINGS AND CLINICAL ALERTS
Instructions to person	**Common adaptation for ageing changes**	
1. Walk (with shoes on).	Shuffling pattern; swaying; arms out to help balance; broader base of support; person may watch feet.	
2. Climb up stairs.	Person holds hand rail; may haul body up with it; may lead with favoured (stronger) leg.	
3. Walk down stairs.	Holds hand rail, sometimes with both hands. If the person is weak, they may descend sideways, lowering the weaker leg first. If the person is unsteady, they may watch feet.	
4. Pick up object from floor.	Person often bends at waist instead of bending knees; holds furniture to support while bending and straightening.	
5. Rise up from sitting in chair.	Person uses arms to push off chair arms, upper trunk leans forwards before body straightens, feet planted wide in broad base of support.	
6. Rise up from lying in bed.	May roll to one side, push with arms to lift up torso, grab bedside table to increase leverage.	
Laboratory studies		
There are many relevant specialist laboratory tests done to assess musculoskeletal health. We have listed the most common tests.		
Vitamin D: essential for bone and muscle health and regulating the immune system and cell activity. Vitamin D is required for effective absorption of calcium. A serum 25-hydroxyvitamin D (25-OHD) level of ≥ 50 nmol/L at the end of winter (10–20 nmol/L higher at the end of summer) (Royal College of Pathologists Australia (RCPA) 2019).		**Low Vitamin D:** associated with rickets, bone and muscle pain.
Rheumatoid factor: Normal levels are < 30 IU/L (RCPA 2019).		People who have rheumatoid arthritis and a positive rheumatoid factor tend to have more aggressive disease.
Calcium: to detect hyper- or hypocalcaemia. Corrected calcium rather than total calcium levels are used for clinical diagnosis. Reference levels for corrected calcium: 2.10–2.6 mmol/L; total calcium: 2.10–2.60 mmol/L (RCPA 2019).		**Hypercalcaemia** is associated with hyperparathyroidism, malignancy, bony metastases, sarcoidosis, vitamin D or A toxicity. **Hypocalcaemia** is associated with hypopara-thyroidism, renal failure, osteomalacia or rickets.

OBJECTIVE DATA

Further objective assessment for advanced practice

The assessments that are described in the following sections require advanced skill and scope of practice. A complete musculoskeletal examination, as described in the following section, is appropriate for persons with a positive musculoskeletal screening assessment.

Equipment

Goniometer

PROCEDURES AND NORMAL FINDINGS	ABNORMAL FINDINGS AND CLINICAL ALERTS
Inspection of joints	
Note the **size** and **contour** of the joint. Inspect the skin and tissues over the joints for **colour**, **swelling** and any **masses** or **deformity**. Presence of swelling is significant and signals joint irritation.	
Palpation of joints	
Palpate each joint, including its skin for temperature, its muscles, bony articulations and area of joint capsule. Notice any heat, tenderness, crepitus, swelling or masses. Joints are not normally tender to palpation. If any tenderness does occur, try to localise it to specific anatomical structures (e.g. skin, muscles, bursae, ligaments, tendons, fat pads or joint capsule).	Swelling may be excess joint fluid (effusion), thickening of the synovial lining, inflammation of surrounding soft tissue (bursae, tendons) or bony enlargement. Deformities include dislocation (one or more bones in a joint being out of position), **subluxation** (partial dislocation of a joint), **contracture** (shortening of a muscle leading to limited range of motion of joint) or **ankylosis** (stiffness or fixation of a joint).
The synovial membrane is not normally palpable. When thickened, it feels 'doughy' or 'boggy'. A small amount of fluid is present in the normal joint, but it is not palpable.	Palpable fluid is abnormal. Because fluid is contained in an enclosed sac, if you push on one side of the sac, the fluid will shift and cause a visible bulging on another side.
Range of motion (ROM)	
Ask for **active ROM** while stabilising the body area proximal to that being moved. Familiarise yourself with the type of each joint and its normal ROM so that you can recognise limitations. If you see a limitation, gently attempt **passive motion**. Anchor the joint with one hand while your other hand slowly moves it to its limit. The normal ranges of active and passive motion should be the same.	
If any limitation or any increase in ROM occurs, use a goniometer to measure the angles precisely (Figure 20.16). First extend the joint to neutral or 0 degrees. Centre the 0 point of the goniometer on the joint. Keep the fixed arm of the goniometer on the 0 line and use the movable arm to measure; then flex the joint and measure through the goniometer to determine the angle of greatest flexion.	

OBJECTIVE DATA

PROCEDURES AND NORMAL FINDINGS	ABNORMAL FINDINGS AND CLINICAL ALERTS
Figure 20.16	
Joint motion normally causes no tenderness, pain or crepitation. Do not confuse crepitation with the normal discrete 'crack' heard as a tendon or ligament slips over bone during motion, such as when you do a knee bend.	**Crepitation** is an audible and palpable crunching or grating that accompanies movement. It occurs when the articular surfaces in the joints are roughened, as with rheumatoid arthritis (see Table 20.1).
Muscle testing	
Test the strength of the prime mover muscle groups for each joint. Repeat the motions you elicited for active ROM. Now ask the person to flex and hold as you apply opposing force. Muscle strength should be equal bilaterally and should fully resist your opposing force. (Note: Muscle status and joint status are interdependent and should be interpreted together. Chapter 12 discusses the examination of muscles for size and development, tone and presence of tenderness.)	
A wide variability of strength exists among people. You may wish to use a grading system from no voluntary movement to full strength, as shown.	
Temporomandibular joint	
With the person seated, **inspect** the area just anterior to the ear. Place the tips of your first two fingers in front of each ear and ask the person to open and close the mouth. Drop your fingers into the depressed area over the joint, and note smooth motion of the mandible. An audible and palpable snap or click occurs in many healthy people as the mouth opens (Figure 20.17). Then ask the person to:	Swelling looks like a round bulge over the joint, although it must be moderate or marked to be visible. Crepitus and pain occur with temporomandibular joint dysfunction.
Instructions to person / **Motion and expected range** • Open mouth maximally. — Vertical motion. You can measure the space between the upper and lower incisors. Normal is 3–6 cm, or three fingers inserted sideways. • Partially open mouth, side to side — Lateral motion. Normal extent is 1–2 cm. Protrude lower jaw and move it (Figure 20.18). • Stick out lower jaw. — Protrude without deviation.	Lateral motion may be lost earlier and more significantly than vertical.

<table>
<tr><th>PROCEDURES AND NORMAL FINDINGS</th><th>ABNORMAL FINDINGS AND CLINICAL ALERTS</th></tr>
<tr><td>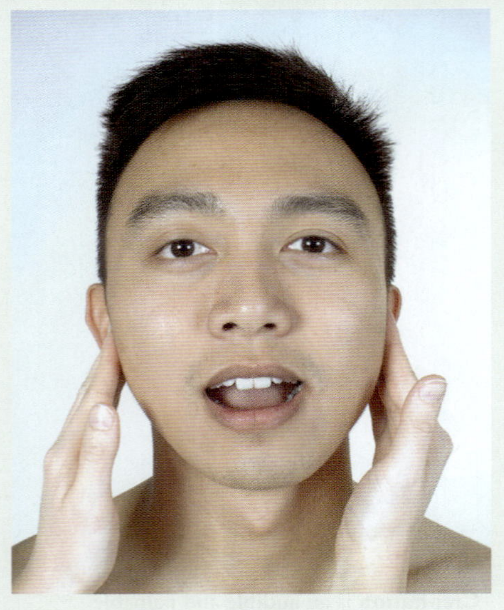
Figure 20.17
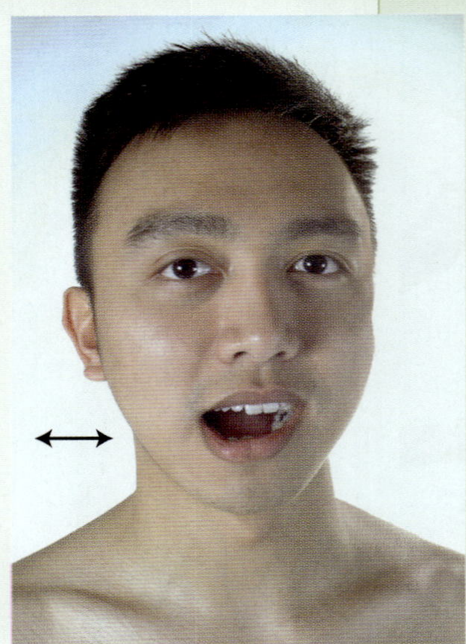
Figure 20.18</td><td></td></tr>
<tr><td>Palpate the contracted temporalis and masseter muscles as the person clenches the teeth. Compare right and left sides for size, firmness and strength. Ask the person to move the jaw forwards and laterally against your resistance, and to open mouth against your resistance. This also tests the integrity of cranial nerve V (trigeminal).</td><td></td></tr>
<tr><td colspan="2">Cervical spine</td></tr>
<tr><td>Inspect the alignment of head and neck. The spine should be straight and the head erect. Palpate the spinous processes and the sternocleidomastoid, trapezius and paravertebral muscles. They should feel firm, with no muscle spasm or tenderness.</td><td>Head tilted to one side.
Asymmetry of muscles.
Tenderness and hard muscles with muscle spasm.</td></tr>
<tr><td>Ask the person to follow these motions (Figure 20.19):
Instructions to person — Motion and expected range
• Touch chin to chest. — Flexion of 45 degrees (Figure 20.19A).
• Lift the chin towards the ceiling. — Hyperextension of 55 degrees.
• Touch each ear towards the corresponding shoulder. — Lateral bending of 40 degrees (Figure 20.19B). Do not lift up the shoulder.
• Turn the chin towards each shoulder. — Rotation of 70 degrees (Figure 20.19C).</td><td>Practice alert—do not examine neck movement where there is any suspicion of neck trauma.
Limited ROM.
Pain with movement.</td></tr>
</table>

PROCEDURES AND NORMAL FINDINGS	ABNORMAL FINDINGS AND CLINICAL ALERTS
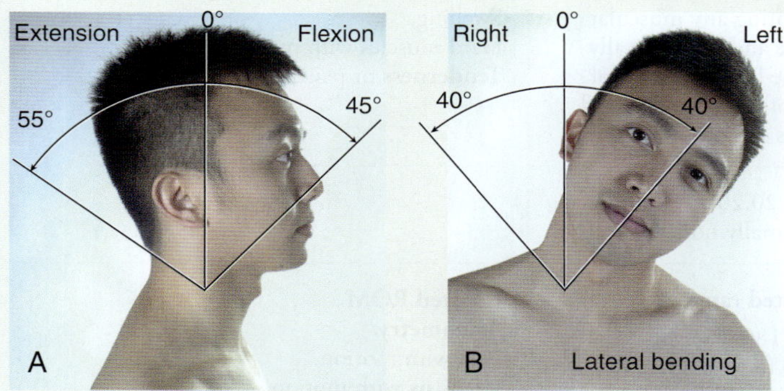 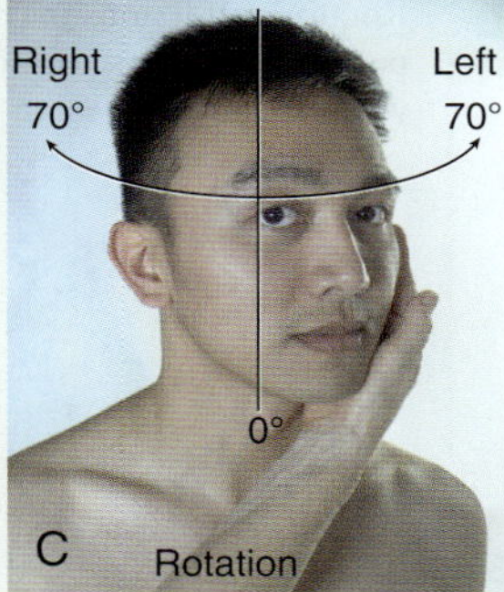 **Figure 20.19**	
Repeat the motions while applying opposing force. The person normally can maintain flexion against your full resistance. This also tests integrity of cranial nerve XI (spinal).	Practice alert—do not examine neck movement where there is any suspicion of neck trauma. Limited ROM. Pain with movement.
Inspect and palpate the upper extremities	
Shoulder	
Inspect and compare both shoulders posteriorly and anteriorly. Check the size and contour of the joint and compare shoulders for equality of bony landmarks. Normally, no redness, muscular atrophy, deformity or swelling is present. Check the anterior aspect of the joint capsule and the subacromial bursa for abnormal swelling.	**Redness.** Inequality of bony landmarks. **Atrophy,** shows as lack of fullness. Dislocated shoulder loses the normal rounded shape and looks flattened laterally.
	Swelling from excess fluid is best seen anteriorly. Considerable fluid must be present to cause a visible distension because the capsule normally is so loose (see Table 20.2).
If the person reports any shoulder pain, ask that they point to the spot with the hand of the unaffected side.	Swelling of subacromial bursa is localised under deltoid muscle and may be accentuated when the person tries to abduct the arm. Be aware that shoulder pain may be from local causes or it may be referred pain from a hiatus hernia or a cardiac or pleural condition, which could be potentially serious. Pain from a local cause is reproducible during the examination by palpation or motion.

PROCEDURES AND NORMAL FINDINGS	ABNORMAL FINDINGS AND CLINICAL ALERTS
While standing in front of the person, **palpate** both shoulders, noting any muscular spasm or atrophy, swelling, heat or tenderness. Start at the clavicle and methodically explore the acromioclavicular joint, scapula, greater tubercle of the humerus, area of the subacromial bursa, the biceps groove and the anterior aspect of the glenohumeral joint. Palpate the pyramid-shaped axilla; no adenopathy or masses should be present.	Swelling. Hard muscles with muscle spasm. **Tenderness** or pain.
Test ROM by asking the person to perform four motions (Figure 20.20). Cup one hand over the shoulder during ROM to note any crepitation; normally none is present.	
Instructions to person / **Motion and expected range** • With arms at sides and elbows extended, move both arms forwards and up in wide vertical arcs, then move them back. — Forward flexion of 180 degrees. Hyperextension up to 50 degrees (Figure 20.20A). • Rotate arms internally behind back, place back of hands as high as possible towards the scapulae. — Internal rotation of 90 degrees (Figure 20.20B). • With arms at sides and elbows extended, raise both arms in wide arcs in the coronal plane. Touch palms together above head. — Abduction of 180 degrees. Adduction of 50 degrees (Figure 20.20C). • Touch both hands behind the head with elbows flexed and rotated posteriorly. — External rotation of 90 degrees head (Figure 20.20D).	**Limited ROM.** **Asymmetry.** Pain with motion. **Crepitus** with motion. Rotator cuff lesions may cause limited ROM, pain and muscle spasm during abduction, whereas forward flexion stays fairly normal.

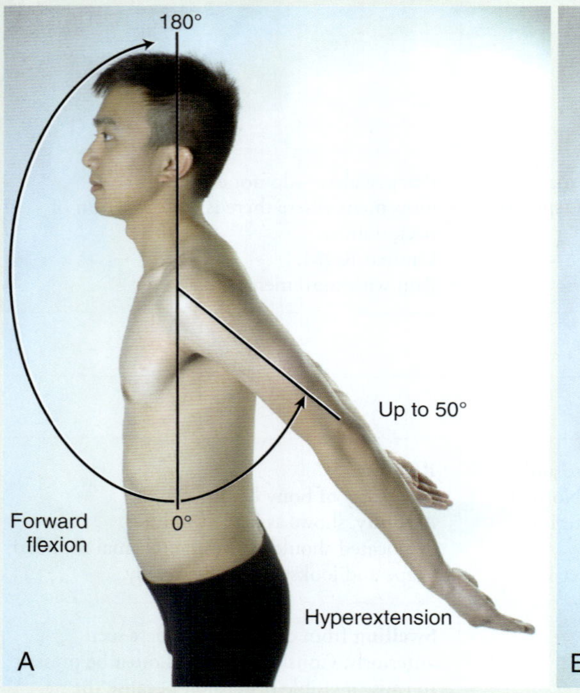

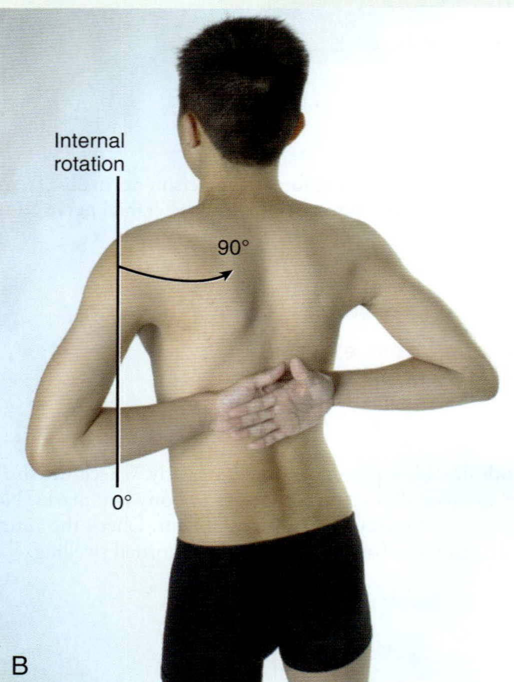

Figure 20.20 A,B

PROCEDURES AND NORMAL FINDINGS	ABNORMAL FINDINGS AND CLINICAL ALERTS
Test the strength of the shoulder muscles by asking the person to shrug the shoulders, flex forwards and up and abduct against your resistance. The shoulder shrug also tests the integrity of cranial nerve XI, the spinal accessory.	

PROCEDURES AND NORMAL FINDINGS	ABNORMAL FINDINGS AND CLINICAL ALERTS

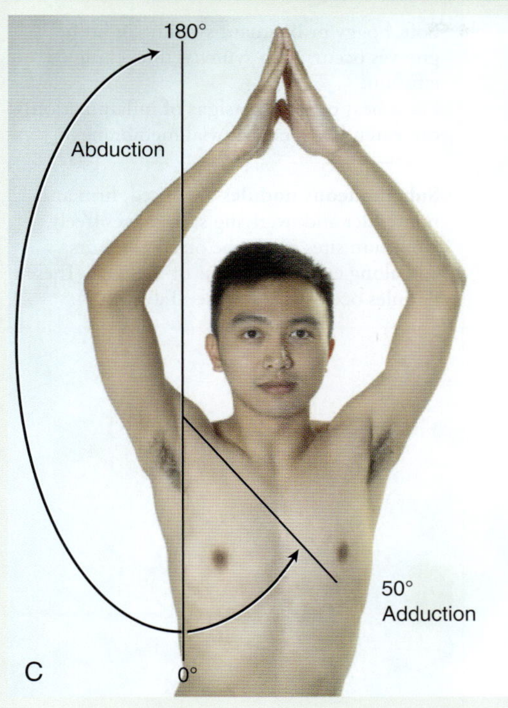

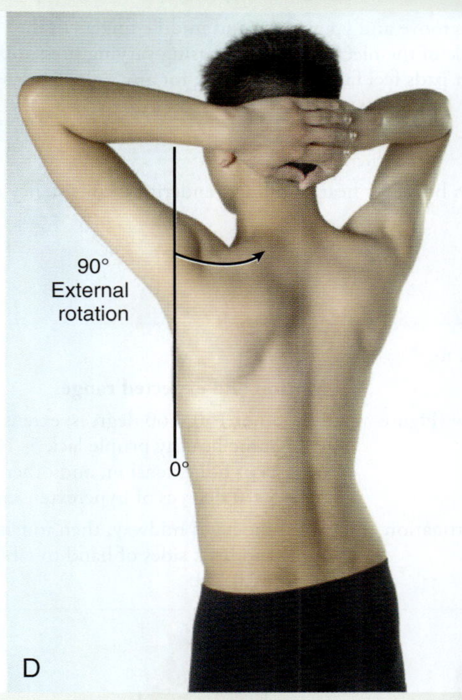

Figure 20.20 C,D

Elbow

PROCEDURES AND NORMAL FINDINGS	ABNORMAL FINDINGS AND CLINICAL ALERTS
Inspect the size and contour of the elbow in both flexed and extended positions. Look for any deformity, redness or swelling. Check the olecranon bursa and the normally present hollows on either side of the olecranon process for abnormal swelling.	**Subluxation** of the elbow shows the forearm dislocated posteriorly. Swelling and redness of olecranon bursa are localised and easy to observe because of the close proximity of the bursa to skin. **Effusion** or synovial thickening shows first as a bulge or fullness in groove on either side of the olecranon process, and it occurs with gouty arthritis.
Palpate with the elbow flexed about 70 degrees and as relaxed as possible (Figure 20.21). Use your left hand to support the person's left forearm and palpate the extensor surface of the elbow—the olecranon process and the medial and lateral epicondyles of humerus—with your right thumb and fingers. 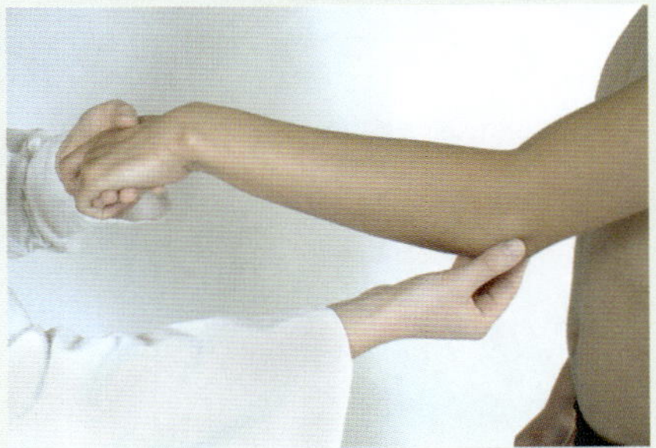 **Figure 20.21** Epicondyles, head of radius and tendons are common sites of inflammation and local tenderness, or 'tennis elbow'.	

PROCEDURES AND NORMAL FINDINGS	ABNORMAL FINDINGS AND CLINICAL ALERTS
With your thumb in the lateral groove and your index and middle fingers in the medial groove, palpate either side of the olecranon process using varying pressure. Normally, present tissues and fat pads feel fairly solid. Check for any synovial thickening, swelling, nodules or tenderness.	Soft, boggy or fluctuant swelling in both grooves occurs with synovial thickening or effusion. Local heat or redness (signs of inflammation) can extend beyond synovial membrane.
Palpate the area of the olecranon bursa for heat, swelling, tenderness, consistency or nodules.	**Subcutaneous nodules** are raised, firm and nontender and overlying skin moves freely. Common sites are in the olecranon bursa and along extensor surface of the ulna. These nodules occur with RA (see Table 20.3).
Test ROM by asking the person to: **Instructions to person** — **Motion and expected range** • Bend and straighten the elbow (Figure 20.22). — Flexion of 150–160 degrees; extension at 0. Some healthy people lack 5–10 degrees of full extension, and others have 5–10 degrees of hyperextension. • Movement of 90 degrees in pronation and supination. — Hold the hand midway; then touch front and back sides of hand to table. (Figure 20.23).	
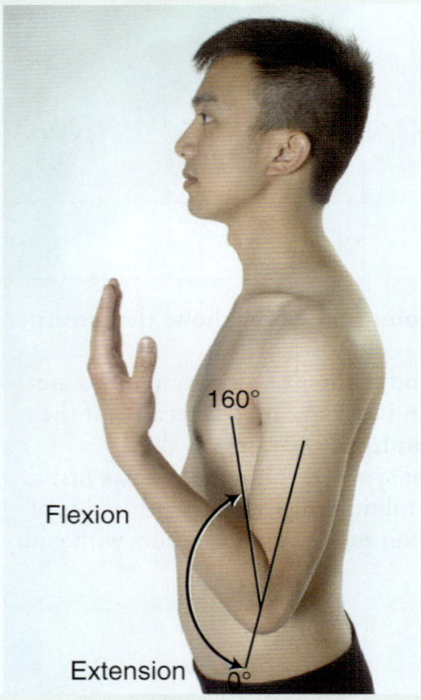 Figure 20.22 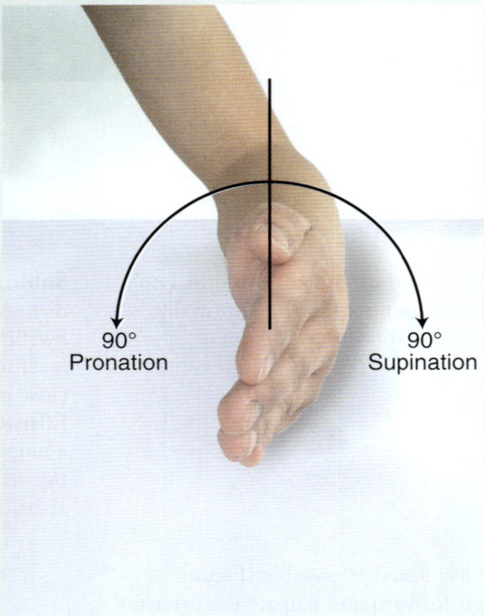 Figure 20.23	
While testing **muscle strength**, stabilise the person's arm with one hand (Figure 20.24). Have the person flex the elbow against your resistance applied just proximal to the wrist. Then ask the person to extend the elbow against your resistance.	

OBJECTIVE DATA

PROCEDURES AND NORMAL FINDINGS	ABNORMAL FINDINGS AND CLINICAL ALERTS
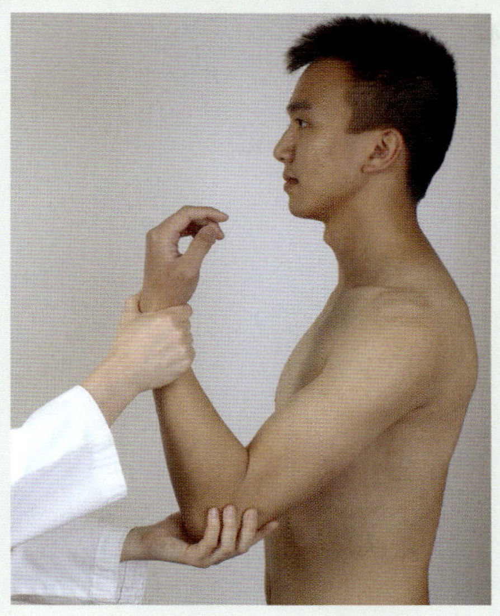 **Figure 20.24**	
Wrist and hand	
Inspect the hands and wrists on the dorsal and palmar sides, noting position, contour and shape. The normal functional position of the hand shows the wrist in slight extension. This way, the fingers can flex efficiently, and the thumb can oppose them for grip and manipulation. The fingers lie straight in the same axis as the forearm. Normally, no swelling or redness, deformity or nodules are present.	**Subluxation** of wrist. **Ulnar deviation;** fingers list to ulnar side. **Ankylosis;** wrist in extreme flexion. Dupuytren's contracture; flexion contracture of finger(s).
The skin looks smooth with knuckle wrinkles present and no swelling or lesions. Muscles are full, with the palm showing a rounded mound proximal to the thumb (the **thenar eminence**) and a smaller rounded mound proximal to the little finger.	Swan-neck or boutonnière deformity in fingers. Atrophy of the thenar eminence (see Table 20.4).
Palpate each joint in the wrist and hands. Facing the person, support the hand with your fingers under it and palpate the wrist firmly with both your thumbs on its dorsum (Figure 20.25). Make sure the person's wrist is relaxed and in straight alignment. Move your palpating thumbs side to side to identify the normal depressed areas that overlie the joint space. Use gentle but firm pressure. Normally, the joint surfaces feel smooth, with no swelling, bogginess, nodules or tenderness. 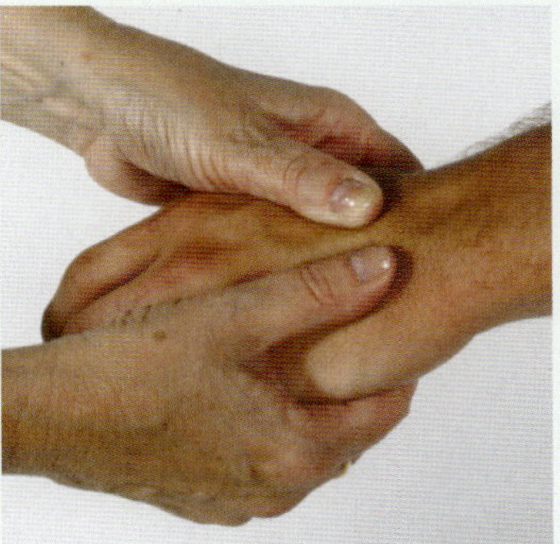 **Figure 20.25**	Ganglion in wrist. Synovial swelling on dorsum. Generalised swelling. Tenderness.

OBJECTIVE DATA

PROCEDURES AND NORMAL FINDINGS	ABNORMAL FINDINGS AND CLINICAL ALERTS
Palpate the metacarpophalangeal joints with your thumbs, just distal to and on either side of the knuckle (Figure 20.26). 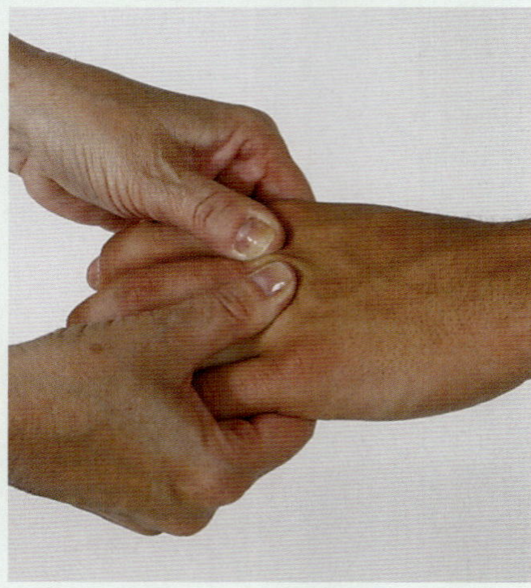 **Figure 20.26**	
Use your thumb and index finger in a pinching motion to palpate the sides of the interphalangeal joints (Figure 20.27). Normally, no synovial thickening, tenderness, warmth or nodules are present. 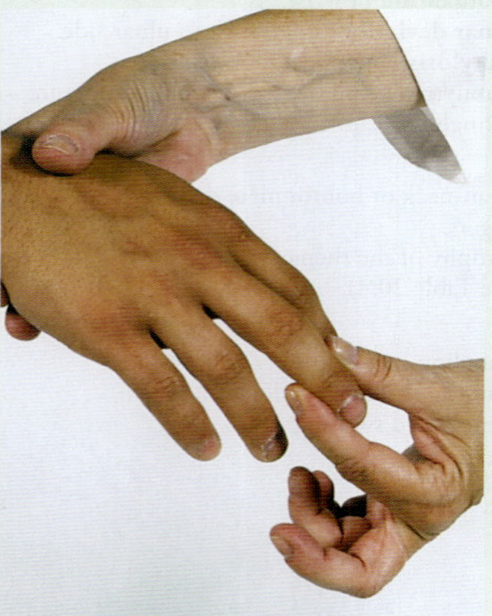 **Figure 20.27**	**Heberden's and Bouchard's nodules** are hard and nontender and occur with osteoarthritis (see Table 20.4).

PROCEDURES AND NORMAL FINDINGS		ABNORMAL FINDINGS AND CLINICAL ALERTS
Test ROM (Figure 20.28) by asking the person to:		**Loss of ROM** here is the most common and most significant functional loss of the wrist. Limited motion. Pain on movement.
Instructions to person	**Motion and expected range**	
• Bend the hand up at the wrist.	Hyperextension of 70 degrees (Figure 20.28A).	
• Bend hand down at the wrist.	Palmar flexion of 90 degrees.	
• Bend the fingers up and down at metacarpophalangeal joints.	Flexion of 90 degrees. Hyperextension of 30 degrees (Figure 20.28B).	
• With palms flat on table, turn them outwards and in.	Ulnar deviation of 50–60 degrees and radial deviation of 20 degrees (Figure 20.28C).	
• Spread fingers apart; make a fist.	Abduction of 20 degrees; fist tight. The responses should be equal bilaterally (Figure 20.28D and E).	
• Touch the thumb to each finger and to the base of little finger.	The person is able to perform, and the responses are equal bilaterally (Figure 20.28F).	

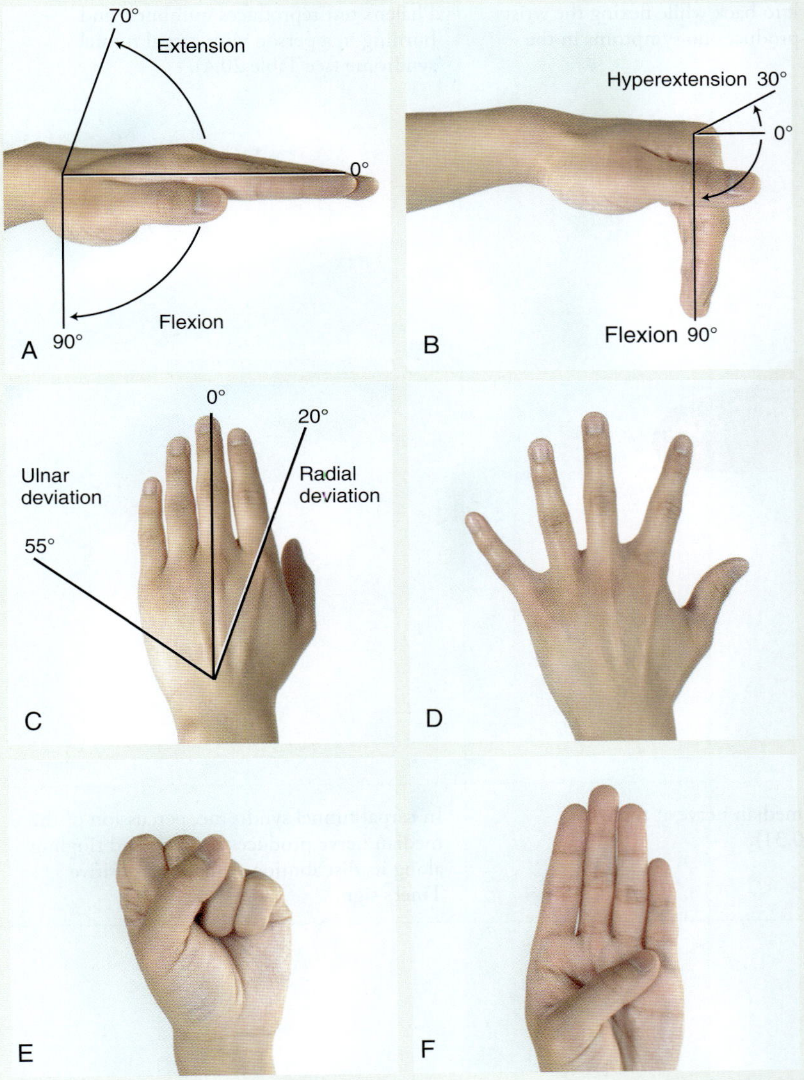

Figure 20.28

PROCEDURES AND NORMAL FINDINGS	ABNORMAL FINDINGS AND CLINICAL ALERTS
For **muscle testing**, position the person's forearm supinated (palm up) and resting on a table (Figure 20.29). Stabilise by holding your hand at the person's midforearm. Ask the person to flex the wrist against your resistance at the palm. 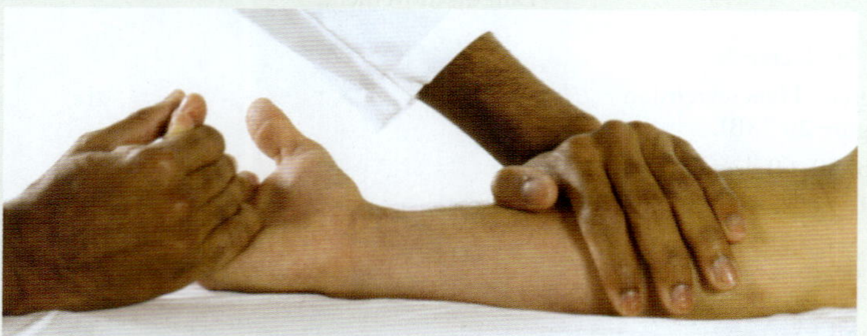 **Figure 20.29**	
Phalen's test. Ask the person to hold both hands back to back while flexing the wrists 90 degrees. Acute flexion of the wrist for 60 seconds produces no symptoms in the normal hand (Figure 20.30). 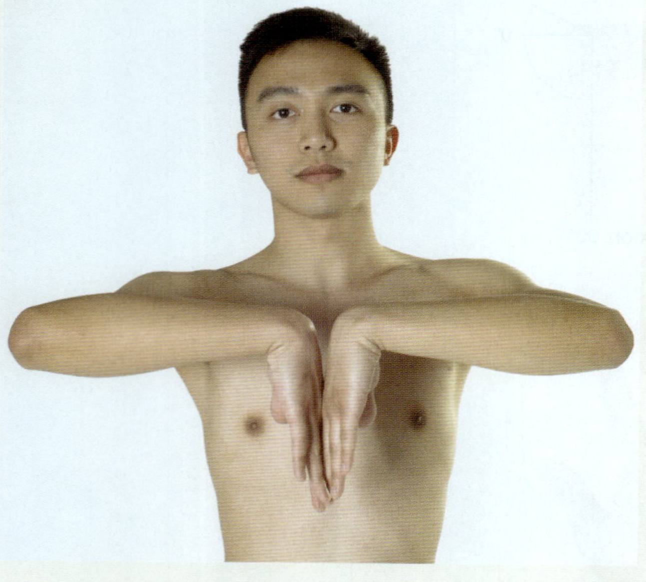 **Figure 20.30** Phalen's test.	Phalen's test reproduces numbness and burning in a person with carpal tunnel syndrome (see Table 20.4).
Tinel's sign. Direct percussion of the location of the median nerve at the wrist produces no symptoms in the normal hand (Figure 20.31).	In carpal tunnel syndrome, percussion of the median nerve produces burning and tingling along its distribution, which is a positive Tinel's sign.

PROCEDURES AND NORMAL FINDINGS		ABNORMAL FINDINGS AND CLINICAL ALERTS

Examiner's hand

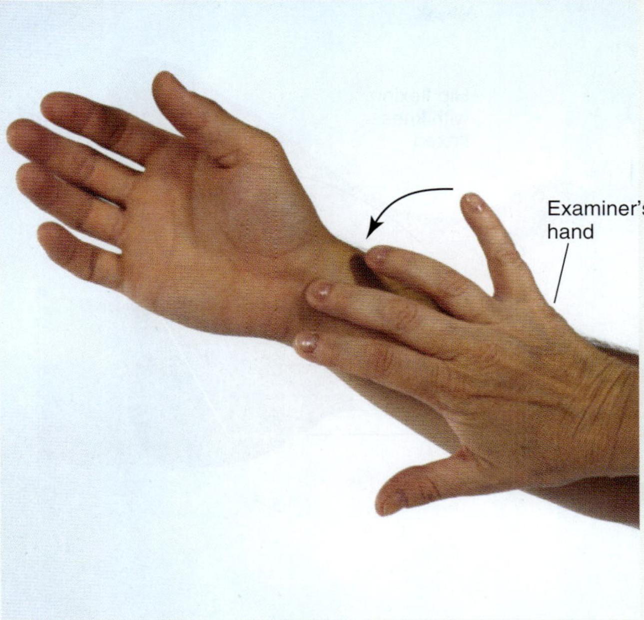

Figure 20.31
Tinel's sign.

Inspect and palpate lower extremities

Hip

PROCEDURES AND NORMAL FINDINGS		ABNORMAL FINDINGS AND CLINICAL ALERTS
Wait to **inspect** the hip joint together with the spine a bit later in the examination as the person stands. At that time, note symmetrical levels of iliac crests, gluteal folds and equally sized buttocks. A smooth, even gait reflects equal leg lengths and functional hip motion.		
Help the person into a supine position and **palpate** the hip joints. The joints should feel stable and symmetrical, with no tenderness or crepitance. **Assess ROM** (Figure 20.32) by asking the person to:		Pain with palpation. Crepitation.
Instructions to person	**Motion and expected range**	
• Raise each leg with knee extended.	Hip flexion of 90 degrees (Figure 20.32A).	Limited motion. Pain with motion.
• Bend each knee up to the chest while keeping the other leg straight.	Hip flexion of 120 degrees. The opposite thigh should remain on the table (Figure 20.32B).	Flexion flattens the lumbar spine; if this reveals a flexion deformity in the opposite hip, it represents a positive *Thomas test*.
• Flex knee and hip to 90 degrees. Stabilise by holding the thigh with one hand and the ankle with the other hand. Swing the foot outwards. Swing the foot inwards. (Foot and thigh move in opposite directions.)	Internal rotation of 40 degrees. External rotation of 45 degrees (Figure 20.32C).	Limited internal rotation of hip is an early and reliable sign of hip disease.
• Swing leg laterally, then medially, with knee straight. Stabilise pelvis by pushing down on the opposite anterior superior iliac spine.	Abduction of 40 to 45 degrees. Adduction of 20–30 degrees (Figure 20.32D).	Limitation of abduction of the hip while supine is the most common motion dysfunction found in hip disease.

Figure 20.32 A,B

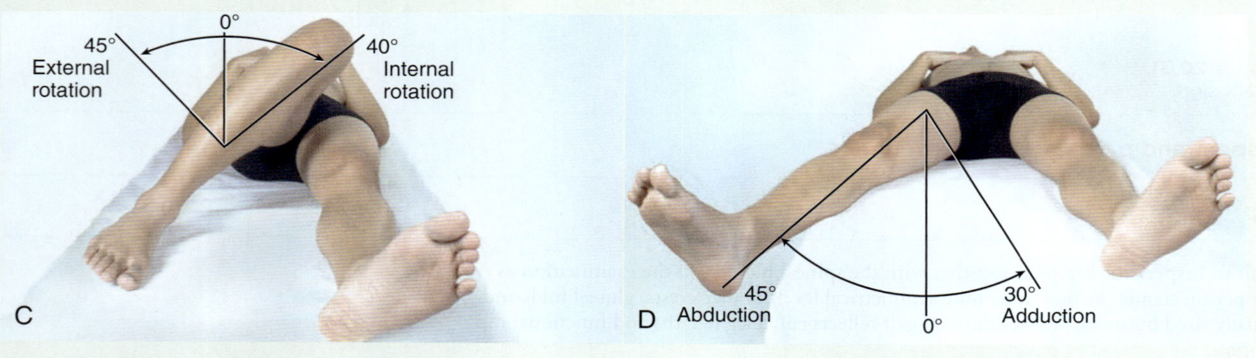

Figure 20.32 C,D

PROCEDURES AND NORMAL FINDINGS		ABNORMAL FINDINGS AND CLINICAL ALERTS
• When standing (later in examination), swing straight leg back behind body. Stabilise pelvis to eliminate exaggerated lumbar lordosis. The most efficient way is to ask person to bend over the table and to support the trunk on the table. Or the person can lie prone on the table.	Hyperextension of 15 degrees when stabilised.	
Knee		
The person should remain supine with legs extended, although some examiners prefer the knees to be flexed and dangling for **inspection**. The skin normally looks smooth, with even colouring and no lesions.		Shiny and atrophic skin. Swelling or inflammation (see Table 20.5). Lesions (e.g. psoriasis).
Inspect lower leg alignment. The lower leg should extend in the same axis as the thigh.		Angulation deformity: • Genu varum (bowlegs) (see below) • Genu valgum (knock knees) • Flexion contracture

OBJECTIVE DATA

PROCEDURES AND NORMAL FINDINGS	ABNORMAL FINDINGS AND CLINICAL ALERTS
Inspect the knee's shape and contour. Normally, distinct concavities, or hollows, are present on either side of the patella. Check them for any sign of fullness or swelling. Note other locations, such as the prepatellar bursa and the suprapatellar pouch, for any abnormal swelling.	Hollows disappear; then they may bulge with synovial thickening or effusion.
Check the quadriceps muscle in the anterior thigh for any atrophy. Because it is the prime mover of knee extension, this muscle is important for joint stability during weight bearing.	Atrophy occurs with disuse or chronic disorders. First, it appears in the medial part of the muscle, although it is difficult to note because the vastus medialis is relatively small.
Enhance **palpation** with the knee in the supine position with complete relaxation of the quadriceps muscle. Start high on the anterior thigh, about 10 cm above the patella. Palpate with your left thumb and fingers in a grasping fashion (Figure 20.33). Proceed down towards the knee, exploring the region of the suprapatellar pouch. Note the consistency of the tissues. The muscles and soft tissues should feel solid, and the joint should feel smooth, with no warmth, tenderness, thickening or nodularity. **Figure 20.33**	Feels fluctuant or boggy with synovitis of suprapatellar pouch.
When swelling occurs, you need to distinguish whether it is due to soft tissue swelling or increased fluid in the joint. The tests for the bulge sign and ballottement of the patella aid this assessment.	
Bulge sign. For swelling in the suprapatellar pouch, the bulge sign confirms the presence of small amounts of fluid as you try to move the fluid from one side of the joint to the other. Firmly stroke up on the medial aspect of the knee two or three times to displace any fluid (Figure 20.34A). Tap the lateral aspect (Figure 20.34B). Watch the medial side in the hollow for a distinct bulge from a fluid wave. Normally, none is present. **Figure 20.34** Bulge sign.	The bulge sign occurs with very small amounts of effusion, 4–8 mL, from fluid flowing across the joint (Figure 20.34C).

PROCEDURES AND NORMAL FINDINGS	ABNORMAL FINDINGS AND CLINICAL ALERTS

Ballottement of the patella. This test is reliable when larger amounts of fluid are present. Use your left hand to compress the suprapatellar pouch to move any fluid into the knee joint. With your right hand, push the patella sharply against the femur. If no fluid is present, the patella is already snug against the femur (Figure 20.35A).

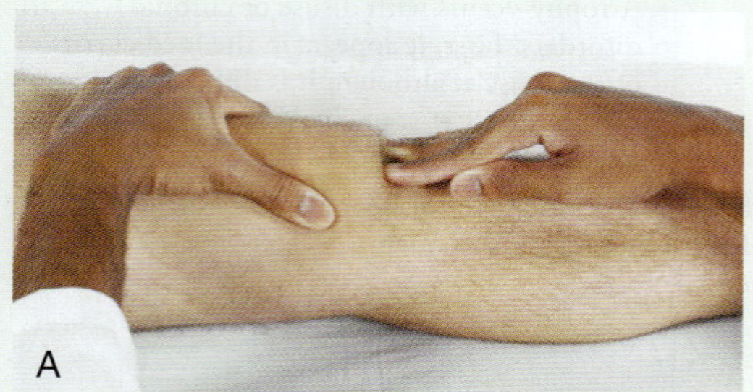

If fluid has collected, your tap on the patella moves it through the fluid, and you will hear a tap as the patella bumps up on the femoral condyles (Figure 20.35B).

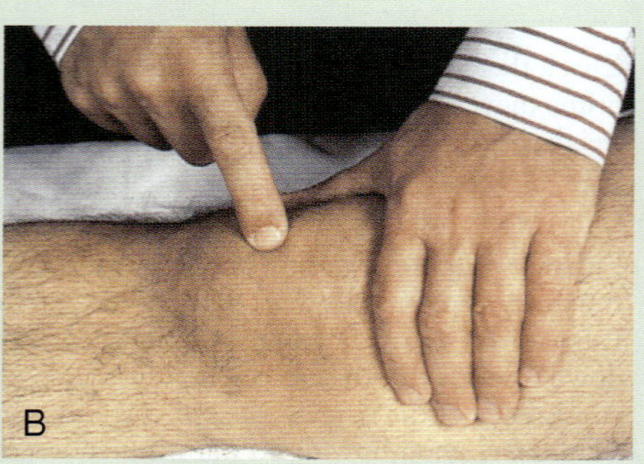

Figure 20.35
Ballottement.

Continue palpation and explore the tibiofemoral joint (Figure 20.36). Note smooth joint margins and absence of pain. Palpate the infrapatellar fat pad and the patella. Check for crepitus by holding your hand on the patella as the knee is flexed and extended. Some crepitus in an otherwise asymptomatic knee is not uncommon.

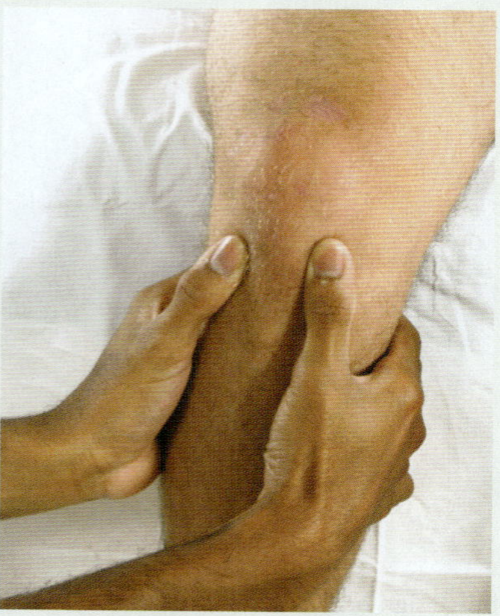

Figure 20.36

Irregular bony margins occur with osteoarthritis.
Pain at joint line.
Pronounced crepitus is significant and it occurs with degenerative diseases of the knee.

Check ROM (Figure 20.37) by asking the person to:

Instructions to person	Motion and expected range
• Bend each knee.	Flexion of 130–150 degrees.
• Extend each knee.	A straight line of 0 degrees in some persons; a hyperextension of 15 degrees in others.
• Check knee ROM during ambulation.	

Limited ROM.
Contracture.
Pain with motion.
Limp.
Sudden locking—the person is unable to extend the knee fully. This usually occurs with a painful and audible 'pop' or 'click'. Sudden buckling, or 'giving way', occurs with ligament injury, which causes weakness and instability.

PROCEDURES AND NORMAL FINDINGS	ABNORMAL FINDINGS AND CLINICAL ALERTS
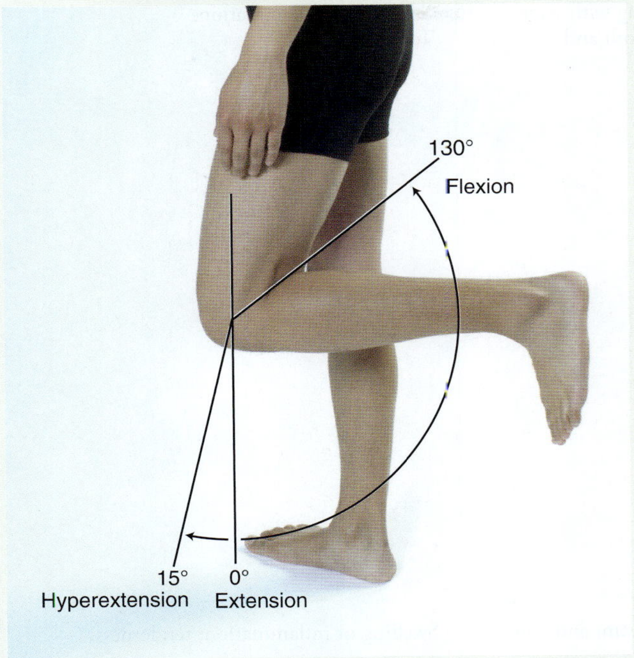 130° Flexion 15° Hyperextension 0° Extension **Figure 20.37**	
Check **muscle strength** by asking the person to maintain knee flexion while you oppose by trying to pull the leg forwards. Muscle extension is demonstrated by the person's success in rising from a seated position in a low chair or by rising from a squat without using the hands for support.	
Special test for meniscal tears. *McMurray's test.* Perform this test when the person has reported a history of trauma followed by locking, giving way or local pain in the knee. Position the person supine as you stand on the affected side. Hold the heel and flex the knee and hip. Place your other hand on the knee with fingers on the medial side. Rotate the leg in and out to loosen the joint. Externally rotate the leg and push a valgus (inwards) stress on the knee. Then slowly extend the knee. Normally the leg extends smoothly with no pain.	If you hear or feel a 'click', McMurray's test is positive for a torn meniscus.
Ankle and foot	
Inspect while the person is in a sitting, non–weight-bearing position, as well as when standing and walking. Compare both feet, noting position of feet and toes, contour of joints and skin characteristics. The foot should align with the long axis of the lower leg; an imaginary line would fall from midpatella to between the first and second toes.	
Weight-bearing should fall on the middle of the foot, from the heel, along the midfoot, to between the second and third toes. Most feet have a longitudinal arch, although that can vary normally from 'flat feet' to a high instep.	
The toes point straight forwards and lie flat. The ankles (malleoli) are smooth bony prominences. Normally the skin is smooth, with even colouring and no lesions. Note the locations of any calluses or bursal reactions because they reveal areas of abnormal friction. Examining well-worn shoes helps assess areas of wear and accommodation.	Hallux valgus (see Table 20.6). Hammertoes. Claw toes. Swelling or inflammation. Calluses. Ulcers.

PROCEDURES AND NORMAL FINDINGS	ABNORMAL FINDINGS AND CLINICAL ALERTS
Support the ankle by grasping the heel with your fingers while palpating with your thumbs (Figure 20.38). Explore the joint spaces. They should feel smooth and depressed, with no fullness, swelling or tenderness. 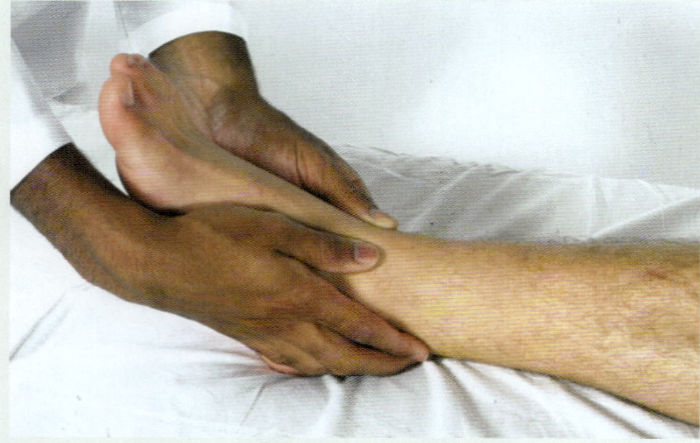 Figure 20.38	Swelling or inflammation. Tenderness.
Palpate the metatarsophalangeal joints between your thumb on the dorsum and your fingers on the plantar surface (Figure 20.39). 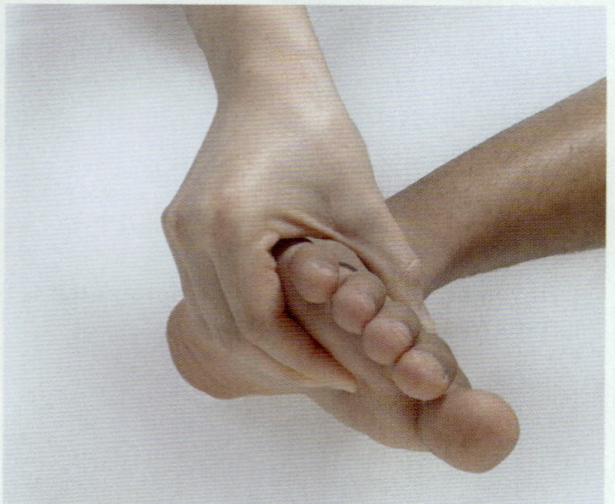 Figure 20.39	Swelling or inflammation; tenderness.
Using a pinching motion of your thumb and forefinger, palpate the interphalangeal joints on the medial and lateral sides of the toes.	
Test ROM (Figure 20.40) by asking the person to: **Instructions to person** / **Motion and expected range** • Point toes towards the floor. — Plantar flexion of 45 degrees. • Point toes towards your nose. — Dorsiflexion of 20 degrees (Figure 20.40A). • Turn soles of feet out, then in. — Eversion of 20 degrees. (Stabilise the ankle with one hand, hold heel with the other to test the subtalar joint.) • Flex and straighten toes. — Inversion of 30 degrees (Figure 20.40B).	Limited ROM. Pain with motion.

PROCEDURES AND NORMAL FINDINGS	ABNORMAL FINDINGS AND CLINICAL ALERTS
Figure 20.40	
Assess **muscle strength** by asking the person to maintain dorsiflexion and plantar flexion against your resistance.	Unable to hold flexion.

Inspect and palpate the spine

PROCEDURES AND NORMAL FINDINGS	ABNORMAL FINDINGS AND CLINICAL ALERTS
The person should be standing, draped in a gown open at the back. Place yourself far enough back so that you can see the entire back. **Inspect** and note whether the spine is straight by following an imaginary vertical line from the head through the spinous processes and down through the gluteal cleft, and by noting equal horizontal positions for the shoulders, scapulae, iliac crests and gluteal folds, and equal spaces between arm and lateral thorax on the two sides (Figure 20.41A). The person's knees and feet should be aligned with the trunk and should be pointing forwards.	A difference in shoulder elevation and in level of scapulae and iliac crests occur with scoliosis (see Table 20.7).
From the side, note the normal convex thoracic curve and concave lumbar curve (Figure 20.41B). An enhanced thoracic curve, or kyphosis, is common in people over 65 years. A pronounced lumbar curve, or lordosis, is common in obese people. 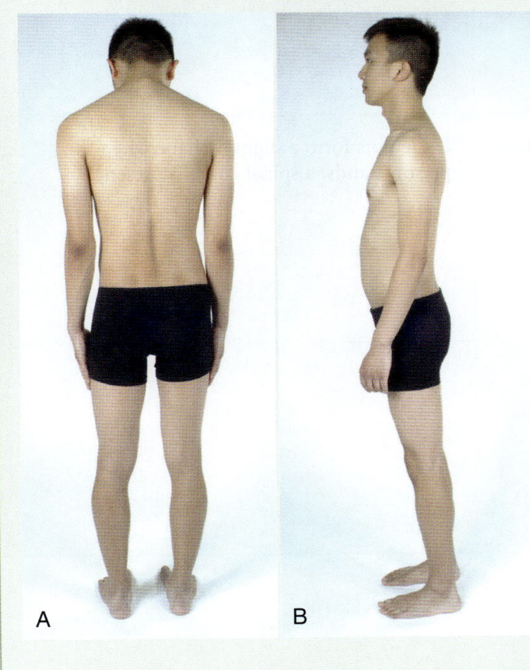 Figure 20.41	Lateral tilting and forward bending occur with a herniated nucleus pulposus (see Table 20.8).

PROCEDURES AND NORMAL FINDINGS	ABNORMAL FINDINGS AND CLINICAL ALERTS
Palpate the spinous processes. Normally they are straight and not tender. Palpate the paravertebral muscles; they should feel firm with no tenderness or spasm.	**Spinal curvature.** **Tenderness. Spasm** of paravertebral muscles.
Check **ROM** of the spine by asking the person to bend forwards and touch the toes (Figure 20.42). Look for flexion of 75–90 degrees and smoothness and symmetry of movement. Note that the concave lumbar curve should disappear with this motion, and the back should have a single convex C-shaped curve. 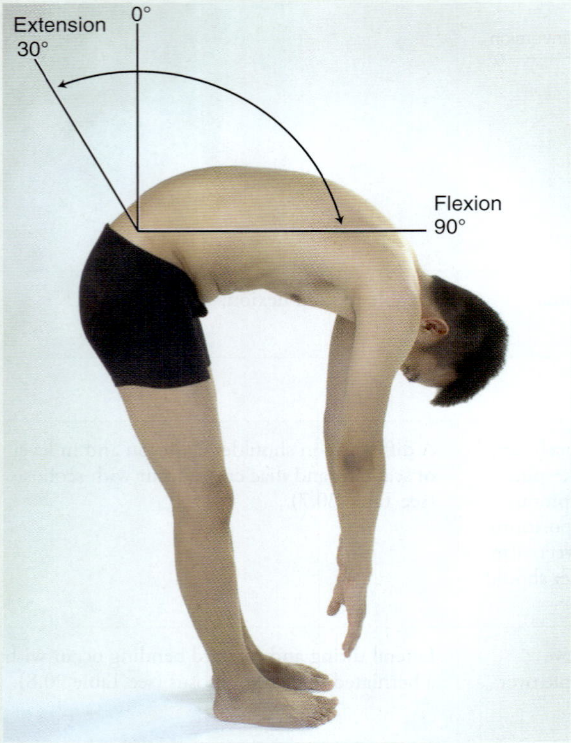 Extension 30° 0° Flexion 90° **Figure 20.42**	
If you suspect a spinal curvature during inspection, this may be more clearly seen when the person touches the toes. While the person is bending over, mark a dot on each spinous process. When the person resumes standing, the dots should form a straight vertical line.	If the dots form a slight S-shape when the person stands, a spinal curve is present.
Stabilise the pelvis with your hands. Check ROM (Figure 20.43) by asking the person to:	
Instructions to person / **Motion and expected range** • Bend sideways. — Lateral bending of 35 degrees (Figure 20.43A). • Bend backwards. — Hyperextension of 30 degrees. • Twist shoulders to one side, bilaterally then the other. — Rotation of 30 degrees (Figure 20.43B).	

OBJECTIVE DATA

PROCEDURES AND NORMAL FINDINGS	ABNORMAL FINDINGS AND CLINICAL ALERTS
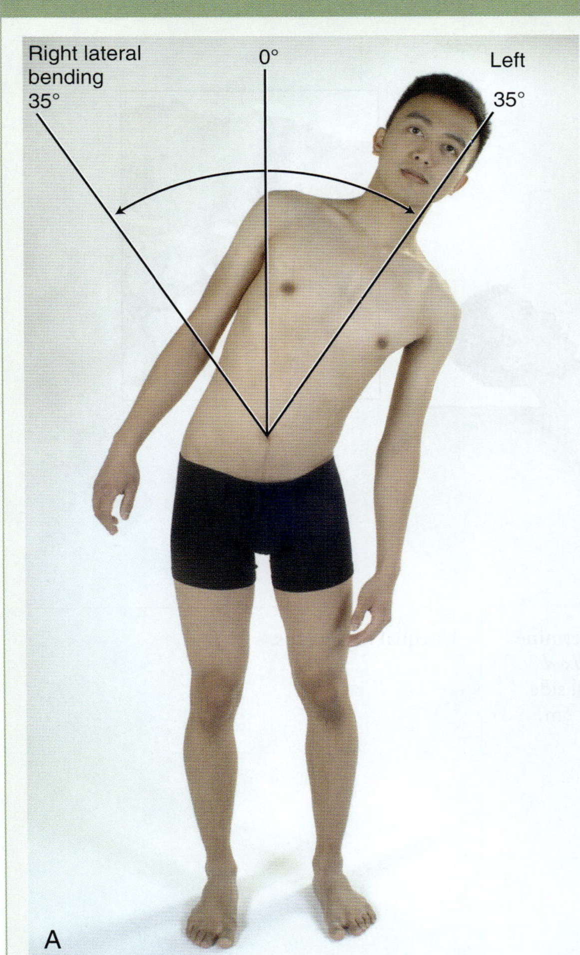 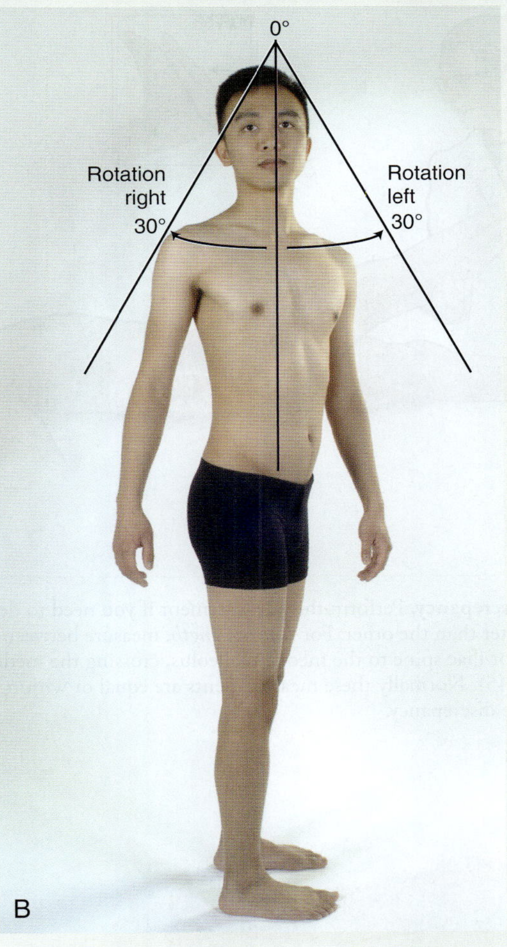 **Figure 20.43**	
These manoeuvres reveal only gross restriction. Movement is still possible even if some spinal fusion has occurred.	
Finally, ask the person to walk on their toes for a few steps; then return walking on the heels.	
Straight leg raising or Lasègue's test. These manoeuvres reproduce back and leg pain and help confirm the presence of a herniated nucleus pulposus. Straight leg raising while keeping the knee extended normally produces no pain. Raise the affected leg just short of the point where it produces pain. Then dorsiflex the foot (Figure 20.44). Raise the unaffected leg while leaving the other leg flat. Inquire about the involved side.	Lasègue's test is positive if it reproduces sciatic pain. If lifting the affected leg reproduces sciatic pain, it confirms the presence of a herniated nucleus pulposus. If lifting the unaffected leg reproduces sciatic pain, it strongly suggests a herniated nucleus pulposus.

OBJECTIVE DATA

PROCEDURES AND NORMAL FINDINGS	ABNORMAL FINDINGS AND CLINICAL ALERTS
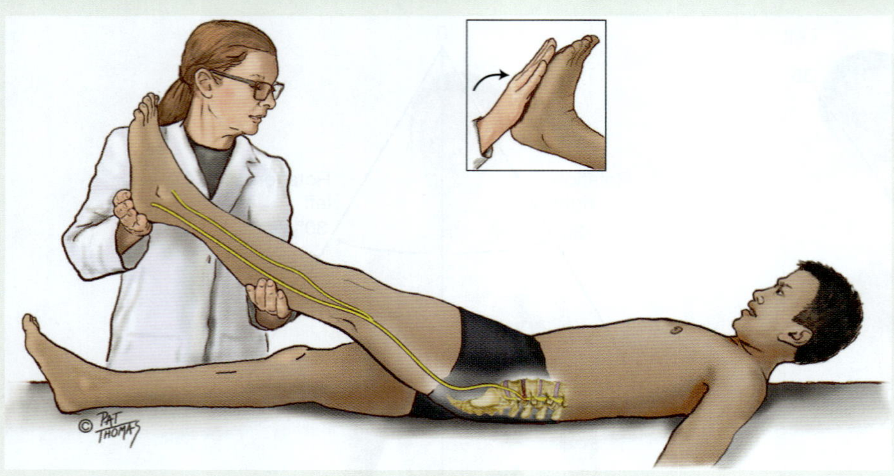 Figure 20.44	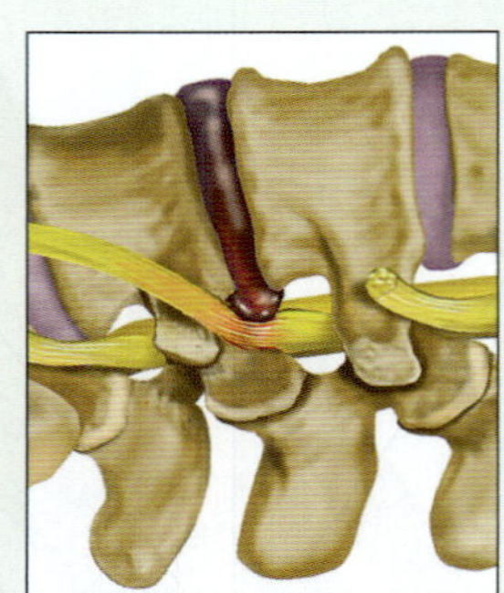
Measure leg length discrepancy. Perform this measurement if you need to determine whether one leg is shorter than the other. For *true leg length*, measure between *fixed* points, from the anterior iliac spine to the medial malleolus, crossing the medial side of the knee (Figure 20.45). Normally these measurements are equal or within 1 cm, indicating no true bone discrepancy. 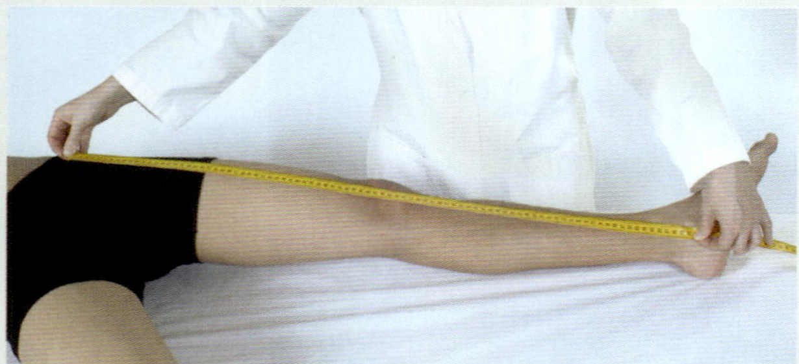 Figure 20.45	Unequal leg lengths.
Sometimes the true leg length is equal, but the legs still look unequal. For *apparent leg length*, measure from a nonfixed point (the umbilicus) to a fixed point (medial malleolus) on each leg.	True leg lengths are equal, but apparent leg lengths unequal—this condition occurs with pelvic obliquity or adduction or flexion deformity in the hip.
Additional objective data for infants	
Review the developmental milestones discussed in Chapter 3. Keep handy a concise chart of the usual sequence of motor development so that you can refer to expected findings for the age of each child you are examining. Use the Denver II test to screen the fine and gross motor skills for the child's age. Because some overlap exists between the musculoskeletal and neurological examinations, assessment of muscle tone, resting posture and motor activity are discussed in Chapter 12.	

PROCEDURES AND NORMAL FINDINGS	ABNORMAL FINDINGS AND CLINICAL ALERTS
Examine the infant fully undressed and lying on the back. Take care to place the newborn on a warming table to maintain body temperature.	
Feet and legs. Start with the feet and work your way up the extremities. Note any *positional deformities*, a residual of fetal positioning. Often the newborn's feet are not held straight but in a varus (apart) or valgus (together) position. It is important to distinguish whether this position is flexible (and thus usually self-correctable) or fixed. Scratch the outside of the bottom of the foot. If the deformity is self-correctable, the foot assumes a normal right angle to the lower leg. Or immobilise the heel with one hand and gently push the forefoot to the neutral position with the other hand. If you can move it to neutral position, it is flexible.	A true deformity is fixed and assumes a right angle only with forced manipulation or not at all.
Note the relationship of the forefoot to the hindfoot. Commonly, the hindfoot is in alignment with the lower leg and just the forefoot angles inwards. This forefoot adduction is *metatarsus adductus.* It is usually present at birth and usually resolves spontaneously by age 3 years.	**Metatarsus varus**—adduction and inversion of forefoot. **Talipes equinovarus** (see Table 20.8).
Check for *tibial torsion*, a twisting of the tibia. Place both feet flat on the table, and push to flex up the knees. With the patella and the tibial tubercle in a straight line, place your fingers on the malleoli. In an infant, note that a line connecting the four malleoli is parallel to the table.	More than 20 degrees of deviation; or if lateral malleolus is anterior to medial malleolus indicates tibial torsion.
Tibial torsion may originate from intrauterine positioning and then may be exacerbated at a later age by continuous sitting in a reverse tailor position, the 'TV squat'. This is sitting with the buttocks on the floor and the lower legs splayed back and out on either side.	
Hips. Check the hips for *developmental hip dysplasia (DDH).* The most reliable method is **Ortolani's manoeuvre**, which should be done at every professional visit until the infant is 1 year old. With the infant supine, flex the knees holding your thumbs on the inner mid-thighs, and your fingers outside on the hips touching the greater trochanters. Adduct the legs until your thumbs touch (Figure 20.46A). Then gently lift and *abduct,* moving the knees apart and down so their lateral aspects touch the table (Figure 20.46B). This normally feels smooth and has no sound.	This test is usually performed by experienced midwives and maternal and child health nurses—not generalist nurses. Hip instability feels like a clunk as the head of the femur pops back into place. This is a *positive Ortolani's sign* and warrants referral and ultrasound investigation.
A B **Figure 20.46** Ortolani's manoeuvre.	
The **Allis test** is also used to check for hip dislocation by comparing leg lengths (Figure 20.47). Place the baby's feet flat on the table and flex the knees up. Scan the tops of the knees; normally they are at the same elevation.	This test is usually performed by experienced midwives and maternal and child health nurses—not generalist nurses. Finding one knee significantly lower than the other is a *positive indication of Allis' sign* and suggests hip dislocation.

OBJECTIVE DATA

PROCEDURES AND NORMAL FINDINGS	ABNORMAL FINDINGS AND CLINICAL ALERTS
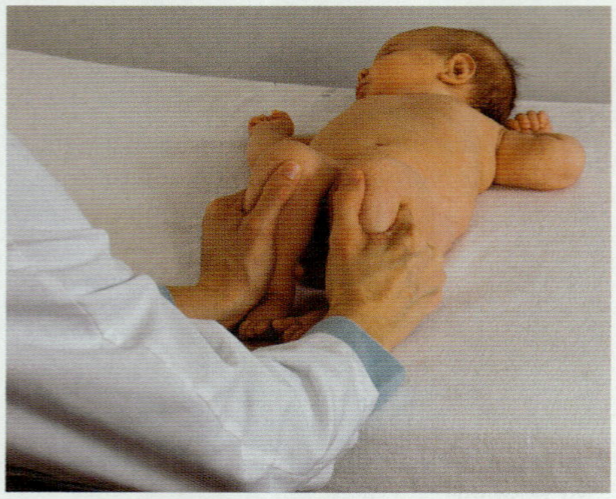 Figure 20.47	
Note the gluteal folds. Normally they are equal on both sides. However, some asymmetry may occur in healthy children.	Unequal gluteal folds may accompany hip dislocation after 2–3 months of age.
Hands and arms. Inspect the hands, noting shape, number and position of fingers and palmar creases.	Polydactyly is the presence of extra fingers or toes. Syndactyly is webbing between adjacent fingers or toes (see Table 20.4).
	A simian crease is a single palmar crease that occurs with Down syndrome, accompanied by short broad fingers, incurving of little fingers and low-set thumbs.
Palpate the length of the clavicles because the clavicle is the bone most frequently fractured during birth. The clavicles should feel smooth, regular and without crepitus. Also note equal ROM of arms during Moro's reflex.	Fractured clavicle: Note irregularity at the fracture site, crepitus and angulation. The site has rapid callus formation with a palpable lump within a few weeks. Observe limited arm ROM and unilateral response to Moro's reflex.
Back. Lift up the infant and examine the back. Note the normal single **C** curve of the newborn's spine (Figure 20.48). By 2 months of age, the infant can lift the head while prone. This builds the concave cervical spinal curve and indicates normal forearm strength. Inspect the length of the spine for any tuft of hair, dimple in midline, cyst or mass. Normally, none are present. 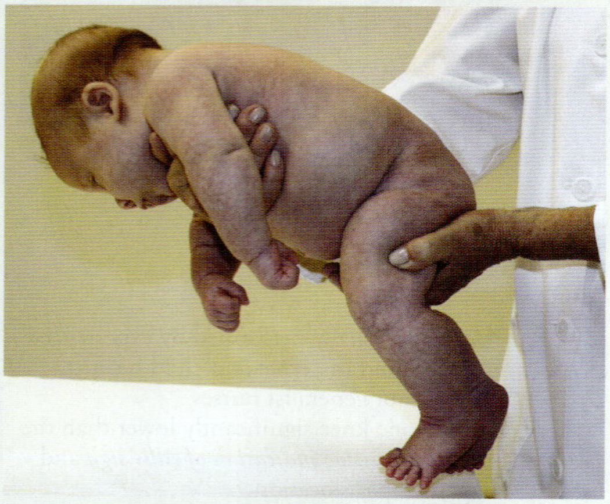 Figure 20.48	A tuft of hair over a dimple in the midline may indicate spina bifida.

PROCEDURES AND NORMAL FINDINGS	ABNORMAL FINDINGS AND CLINICAL ALERTS
	A small dimple in the midline—anywhere from the head to the coccyx—suggests dermoid sinus. Mass, such as meningocele.
Observe ROM through spontaneous movement of extremities.	
Test muscle strength by lifting up the infant with your hands under the axillae (Figure 20.49). A baby with normal muscle strength wedges securely between your hands. 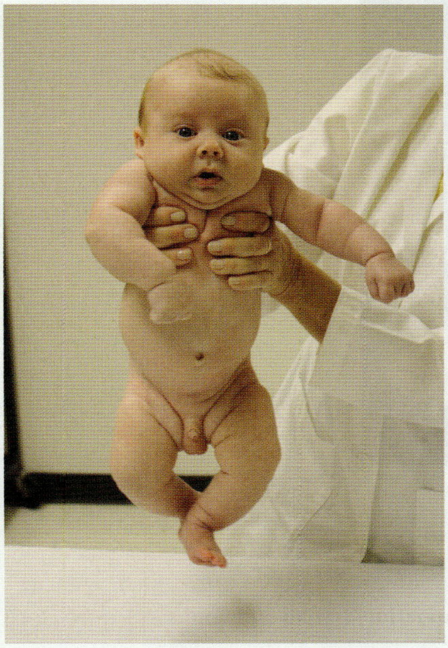 Figure 20.49	A baby who starts to 'slip' between your hands shows weakness of the shoulder muscles.
Additional objective data for preschool and school-age children	
Once the infant learns to crawl and then to walk, the waking hours show perpetual motion. This is convenient for your musculoskeletal assessment; you can observe the muscles and joints during spontaneous play before a table-top examination. Most young children enjoy showing off their physical accomplishments. For specific motions, coax the toddler: 'Show me how you can walk to Mummy' or 'Climb these steps'. Ask the preschooler to hop on one foot or to jump.	
Back. While the child is standing, note the posture. From behind, you should note a 'plumb line' from the back of the head, along the spine, to the middle of the sacrum. Shoulders are level within 1 cm, and scapulae are symmetrical. From the side, lordosis is common throughout childhood, appearing more pronounced in children with a protuberant abdomen.	**Lordosis** is marked with muscular dystrophy and rickets.
Legs and feet. Anteriorly, note the leg position. A 'bowlegged' stance (*genu varum*) is a lateral bowing of the legs (Figure 20.50A). It is present when you measure a persistent space of more than 2.5 cm between the knees when the medial malleoli are together. Genu varum is normal for 1 year after the child begins walking. The child may walk with a waddling gait. This resolves with growth; no treatment is indicated.	**Genu varum** also occurs with rickets.

OBJECTIVE DATA

PROCEDURES AND NORMAL FINDINGS	ABNORMAL FINDINGS AND CLINICAL ALERTS
'Knock knees' (*genu valgum*) are present when there is more than 2.5 cm between the medial malleoli when the knees are together (Figure 20.50B). It occurs normally between 2 and 3½ years of age. Also, treatment is not indicated. (Note: To remember the two conditions, remember to link the Rs and Gs: genu va**r**um—knees apa**r**t; genu val**g**um—knees to**g**ether.)	Genu valgum also occurs with rickets, poliomyelitis and syphilis.

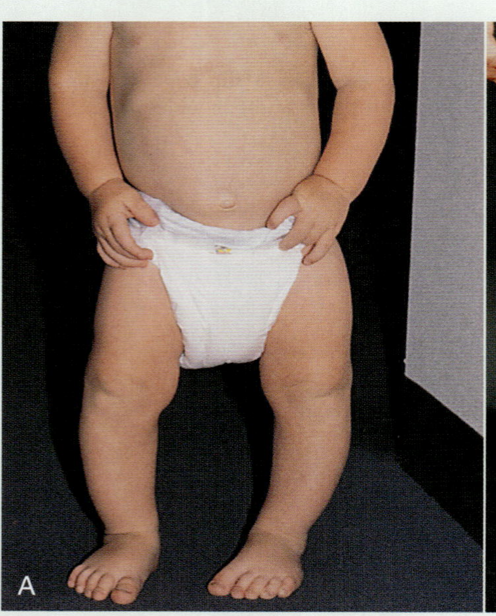
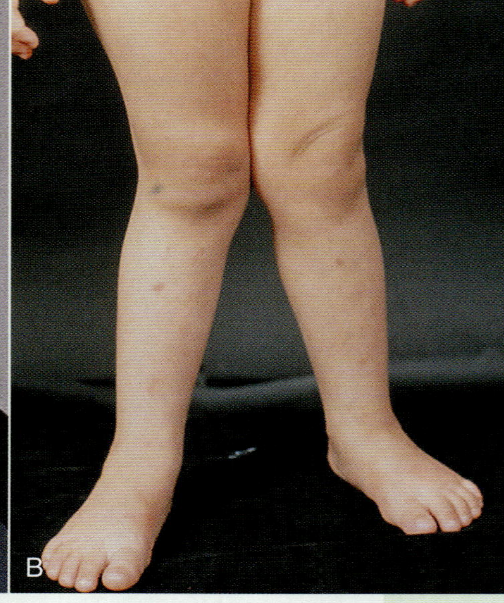

Figure 20.50
A. Genu varum. B. Genu valgum.

PROCEDURES AND NORMAL FINDINGS	ABNORMAL FINDINGS AND CLINICAL ALERTS
Often, parents tell you they are concerned about the child's foot development. The most common questions are about 'flatfeet' and 'pigeon toes'. Flatfoot (*pes planus*) is pronation, or turning in, of the medial side of the foot. The young child may look flatfooted because the normal, longitudinal arch is concealed by a fat pad until age 3 years. When standing begins, the child takes a broad-based stance, which causes pronation. Thus, pronation is common between 12 and 30 months. You can see it best from behind the child, where the medial side of the foot drops down and in.	**Pronation** beyond 30 months.
Pigeon toes, or toeing in, are demonstrated when the child tends to walk on the lateral side of the foot, and the longitudinal arch looks higher than normal. It often starts as a forefoot adduction, which usually corrects spontaneously by age 3 years, as long as the foot is flexible.	Toeing in from forefoot adduction that is fixed, or lasts beyond age 3 years. Toeing in from tibial torsion.
Check the child's gait while walking away from and returning to you. Let the child wear socks, because a cold tile floor will distort the usual gait. From 1 to 2 years of age, expect a broad-based gait, with arms out for balance. Weight-bearing falls on the inside of the foot. From 3 years of age, the base narrows and the arms are closer to the sides. Inspect the shoes for spots of greatest wear to aid your judgement of the gait. Normally the shoes wear more on the outside of the heel and the inside of the toe.	Limp, usually caused by trauma, fatigue or hip disease. Abnormal gait patterns (Chapter 12).
The child may sit for the remainder of the examination. Start with the feet and hands of the child from 2 to 6 years of age because the child is happy to show these off, and proceed through the examination described earlier.	
Particularly, check the arm for full ROM and presence of pain. Look for subluxation of the elbow (head of the radius). This occurs most often between 2 and 4 years of age as a result of forceful removal of clothing or dangling while adults suspend the child by the hands.	Inability to supinate the hand while the arm is flexed, together with pain in elbow, indicates subluxation of the head of the radius.

OBJECTIVE DATA

PROCEDURES AND NORMAL FINDINGS	ABNORMAL FINDINGS AND CLINICAL ALERTS
Palpate the bones, joints and muscles of the extremities as described in the adult examination.	Pain or tenderness in extremities is usually caused by trauma or infection.
	Fractures are usually due to trauma and are exhibited as an inability to use the area, a deformity or an excess of motion in the involved bone with pain and crepitation.
	Enlargement of the tibial tubercles with tenderness suggests Osgood-Schlatter disease (see Table 20.5).
Additional objective data for adolescents	
Proceed with the musculoskeletal examination you provide for the adult, except pay special note to spinal posture. Kyphosis is common during adolescence because of chronic poor posture. Be aware of the risk of sports-related injuries with the adolescent, because sports participation and competition often peak with this age-group. **The National Self-Detection Program for Scoliosis** (Scoliosis Australia). This program entails the distribution of a brochure for the target age group (girls 10–12 years of age) in which the physical signs of scoliosis are described. Advise the person to consult with their family doctor if they have any concerns. The program is endorsed by the Paediatrics and Child Health Division of the Royal Australasian College of Physicians (Scoliosis Australia 2019).	**Scoliosis** is most apparent during the pre-adolescent growth spurt. Asymmetry suggests scoliosis—ribs hump up on one side as child bends forwards, and with unequal landmark elevation (see Table 20.7).
Screen for scoliosis with the *forward bend test* (Figure 20.51). Seat yourself behind the standing child and ask the child to stand with the feet shoulder-width apart and bend forwards slowly to touch the toes. Expect a straight vertical spine while standing and also while bending forwards. Posterior ribs should be symmetrical, with equal elevation of shoulders, scapulae and iliac crests. You may wish to mark each spinous process with a felt marker. The lineup of ink dots highlights even a subtle curve. 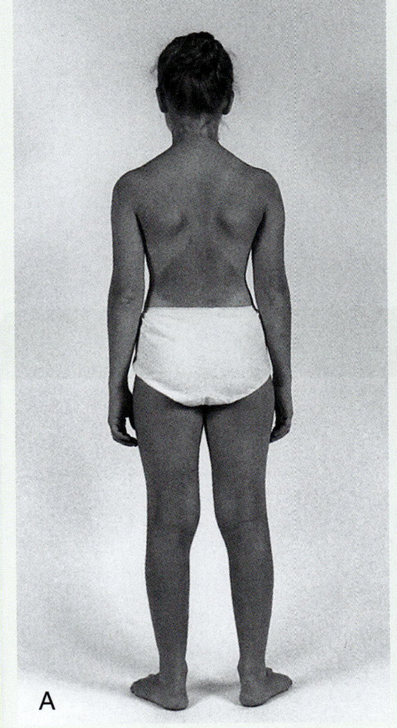 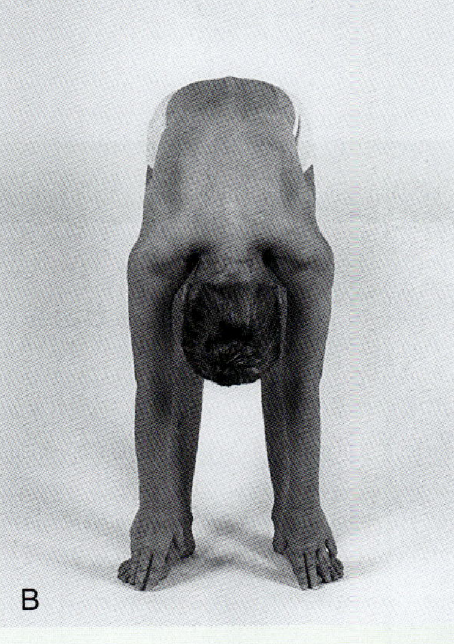 Figure 20.51	

PROCEDURES AND NORMAL FINDINGS	ABNORMAL FINDINGS AND CLINICAL ALERTS
Additional objective data for the pregnant woman	
Proceed through the examination described in the adult section. Expected postural changes in pregnancy include progressive lordosis and, towards the third trimester, anterior cervical flexion, kyphosis and slumped shoulders (Figure 20.52A). When the pregnancy is at term, the protuberant abdomen and the relaxed mobility in the joints create the characteristic 'waddling' gait (Figure 20.52B).	
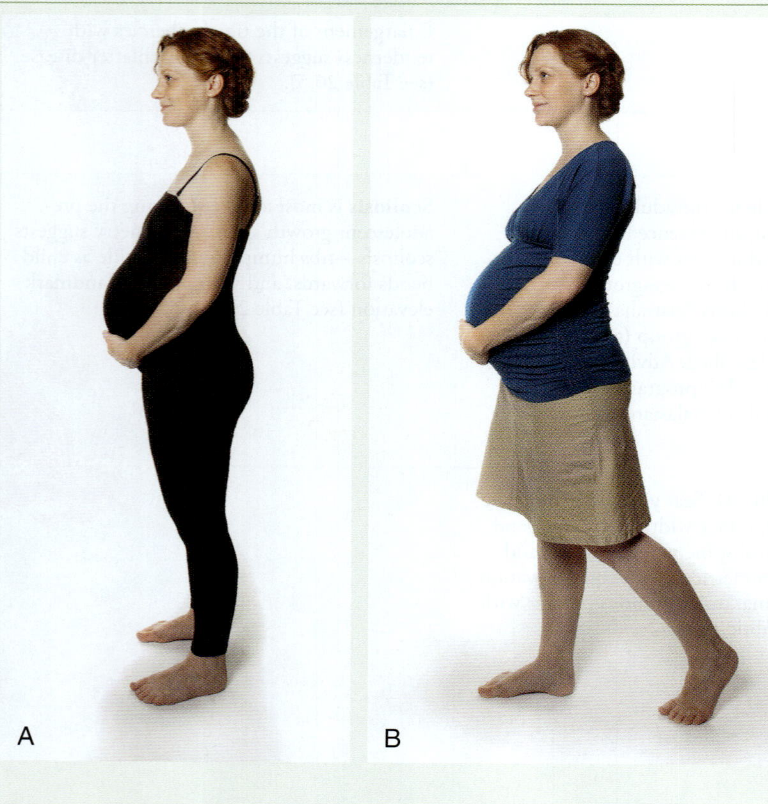 A B **Figure 20.52**	

Summary Checklist

MUSCULOSKELETAL ASSESSMENT

Subjective data

1. Presenting concern
2. Gait, arms, legs and spine (GALS) screening assessment
3. Joints
4. Muscles
5. Bones
6. Functional assessment
7. Health and lifestyle management

Objective data

1. General inspection
2. Gait, arms, legs & spine (GALS) screening assessment
3. Laboratory studies

PROMOTING A HEALTHY LIFESTYLE

OSTEOPOROSIS—'THE SILENT DISEASE'

Bone is a dynamic tissue, which responds to mechanical stresses through a complex process of remodelling. The remodelling process involves the resorption of microdamaged bone by osteoclast cells followed by a phase of bone formation by osteoblast cells. In healthy adults, this process is coupled to ensure bone density remains stable. This process commences in childhood with peak bone mass reached by the end of the second decade of life. Studies suggest that more than 95% of the adult skeleton is formed by the end of adolescence (Marieb & Keller 2018). There is also a direct association between good nutrition and exercise in the development of bone health and bone mass in children and adolescence, emphasising the value of a healthy lifestyle from childhood through to adulthood (McVeigh et al 2019, Rouf et al 2019).

When this bone remodelling process becomes uncoupled, normal bone density is altered, leading to a change in the normal architecture of bone seen in diseases such as osteoporosis. Osteoporosis is a systemic skeletal disorder characterised by decreased bone mass and micro-architectural deterioration of bone tissue, leading to enhanced bone fragility and a consequent increase in fracture risk (Ferrari 2019). The loss of bone occurs 'silently' and progressively. Often there are no symptoms until the first fracture occurs. Fractures associated with osteoporosis are termed low trauma or fragility fractures and occur most frequently in the neck of femur, vertebrae and distal radius (Kanis 2019).

It is estimated that 11% of Australians aged 50 years and over have osteoporosis or osteopenia; females are four times as likely to have osteoporosis than males, but this varies with age (AIHW 2018c). As the population ages, these rates are expected to rise. Osteoporosis has a significant impact on the person in terms of risk of fracture, actual fracture, disability or even death. It also has a huge burden on the health system on the direct costs of treating fracture, rehabilitation and ongoing support (Tatangelo et al 2019).

Risk factors for osteoporosis and fractures include both non-modifiable factors and modifiable factors (RACGP 2017):

1. **Non-modifiable factors:**
   - Family history—especially maternal family history of osteoporotic fracture
2. **Modifiable and lifestyle factors:**
   - Early menopause
   - Multiple falls
   - Low physical activity or immobility
   - Low body weight or obesity
   - Low muscle mass and strength
   - Poor balance
   - Protein or calcium undernutrition
   - Smoking
   - Alcohol (>2 standard drinks per day)
   - Vitamin D deficiency and/or lack of sunlight
3. **Medical conditions** (including malabsorption syndromes, including coeliac disease and inflammatory bowel disease, chronic renal and liver diseases, rheumatoid arthritis, hyperthyroidism)
4. **Medications** (including glucocorticoids, hormone therapy for breast and prostate cancers, antiepileptic therapy, antipsychotic)

Risk assessment includes health and medical history, clinical examination, assessment of bone mineral density and X-ray absorptiometry (DXA) scanning. Nurses should be actively promoting bone health with all people. This includes information concerning the following (RACGP 2017, Rizzoli 2019):

Bone health awareness

- Risk factors for osteoporosis
- The need for screening of risk
- 'Know your bones' - bone health assessment tool

Diet and lifestyle

- Adequate calcium and protein intake
- Adequate but safe exposure to sunlight (Vitamin D)
- Healthy body weight and BMI
- Cessation of smoking
- Follow the national guidelines for alcohol consumption
- Exercise (high impact and strength training for increasing bone mineral density and improving balance 2–3 times per week)

Provide resources

- Know Your Bones: www.knowyourbones.org.au
- Osteoporosis Australia: www.osteoporosis.org.au
- Osteoporosis New Zealand: https://osteoporosis.org.nz

Documentation and critical thinking

FOCUSED ASSESSMENT: CLINICAL CASE STUDY

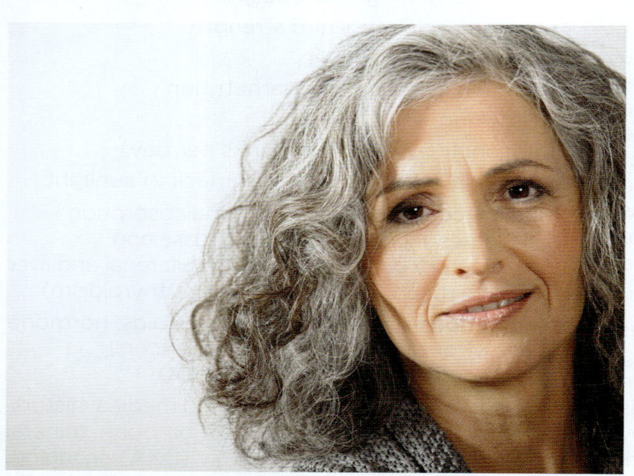

Context

The registered nurse is working as an occupational health nurse in an onsite multidisciplinary health clinic that is part of a large multinational company. The role includes providing first aid treatment, assessing workplace injuries, conducting audiometric assessments and providing occupational health and injury management advice.

Subjective data

Mari Timms is a 45-year-old female office worker with a diagnosis of rheumatoid arthritis 3 years ago, who seeks care now for 'swelling and burning pain in my hands' for 1 day, which is impacting on her ability to complete her normal work tasks and daily activities. She has not been assessed by a rheumatologist since diagnosis and is subsequently not on an effective disease-modifying treatment program.

Ms Timms was diagnosed as having rheumatoid arthritis at age 41 years by a rheumatologist. Since that time, her 'flare-ups' seem to come every 6–8 months. Acute episodes involve hand joints and are treated with aspirin, which gives relief. Typically experiences morning stiffness, lasting ½–1 hour. Joints feel warm, swollen and tender. Has had weight loss of 4 kg over last 4 years and feels fatigued much of the time. States should rest more, but 'I can't take the time'. Daily exercises have been prescribed but she doesn't do them regularly. When she has a flare up, she feels better in a few days and decreases aspirin dose by herself.

Objective data

Joint range of motion within normal limits with exception of joints of the wrist and hands. Radiocarpal, metacarpophalangeal and proximal interphalangeal joints are red, swollen and tender to palpation. Spindle-shaped swelling of proximal interphalangeal joints of third digit right hand and second digit left hand; ulnar deviation of metacarpophalangeal joints.

Collaborative problem

Acute joint pain (especially in hands) related to inflammation from arthritis—referral back to specialist via clinic medical practitioner.

Problem statements/Nursing diagnoses

Impaired physical mobility (in hands) related to arthritis.

Acute joint pain (especially in hands) related to inflammation from arthritis.

Fatigue related to systemic effects of arthritis and pain.

Lack of knowledge about disease and symptom management and need for ongoing follow up.

Abnormal findings for advanced practice

TABLE 20.1 Abnormalities affecting multiple joints

INFLAMMATORY CONDITIONS

Rheumatoid arthritis (RA)

This is a chronic, systemic inflammatory disease of joints and surrounding connective tissue. Inflammation of synovial membrane leads to thickening; then to fibrosis, which limits motion, and finally to bony ankylosis. The disorder is symmetrical and bilateral and is characterised by heat, redness, swelling and painful motion of the affected joints. RA is associated with fatigue, weakness, anorexia, weight loss, low-grade fever and lymphadenopathy. Associated signs are described in the following tables, especially Table 20.4.

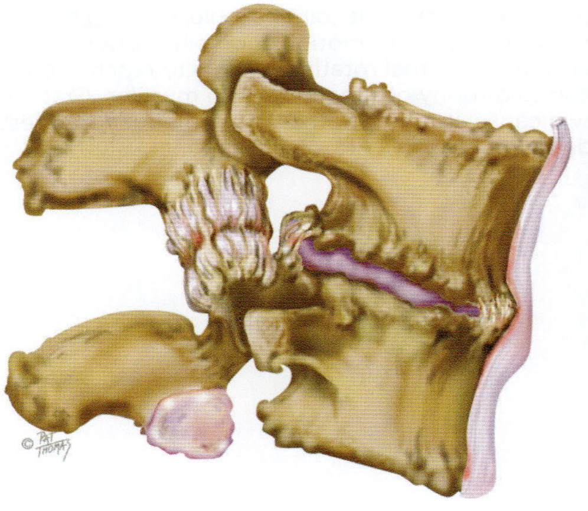

Ankylosing spondylitis

Chronic progressive inflammation of spine, sacroiliac and larger joints of the extremities, leading to bony ankylosis and deformity. A form of RA, this affects primarily men by a 10:1 ratio, in late adolescence or early adulthood. Spasm of paraspinal muscles pulls spine into forward flexion, obliterating cervical and lumbar curves. Thoracic curve exaggerated into single kyphotic rounding. Also includes flexion deformities of hips and knees.

DEGENERATIVE CONDITIONS

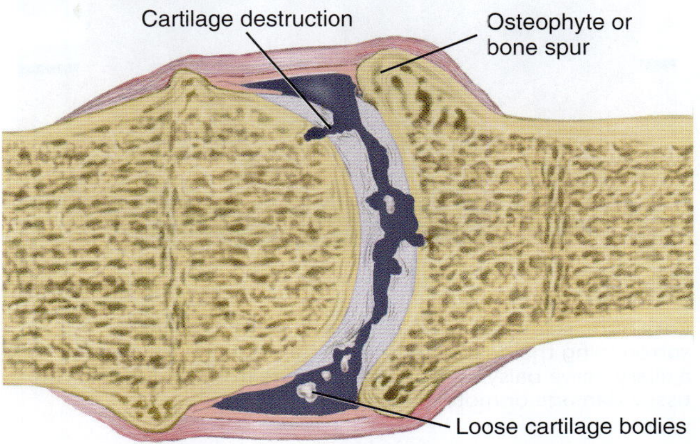

Osteoarthritis (degenerative joint disease)

Noninflammatory, localised, progressive disorder involving deterioration of articular cartilages and subchondral bone and formation of new bone (osteophytes) at joint surfaces. Ageing increases incidence; nearly all adults over 60 years old have some radiographic signs of osteoarthritis. Asymmetrical joint involvement commonly affects hands, knees, hips and lumbar and cervical segments of the spine. Affected joints have stiffness, swelling with hard, bony protuberances, pain with motion and limitation of motion (see Table 20.4).

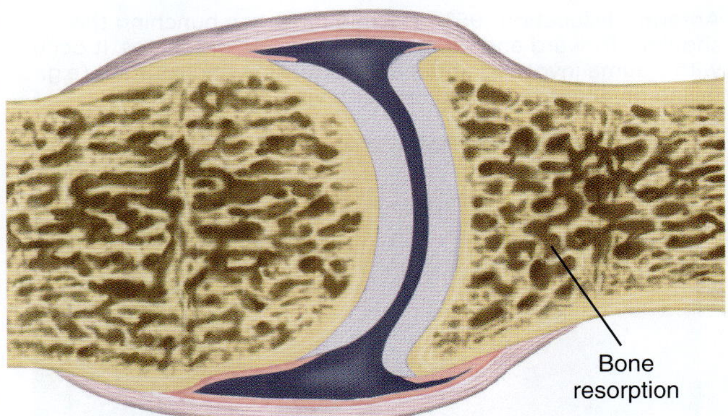

Osteoporosis

Decrease in skeletal bone mass occurring when rate of bone resorption is greater than that of bone formation. The weakened bone state increases risk for stress fractures, especially at wrist, hip and vertebrae. Occurs primarily in postmenopausal women. Osteoporosis risk also is associated with smaller height and weight, younger age at menopause, lack of physical activity and lack of oestrogen replacement therapy.

TABLE 20.2 Abnormalities of the shoulder

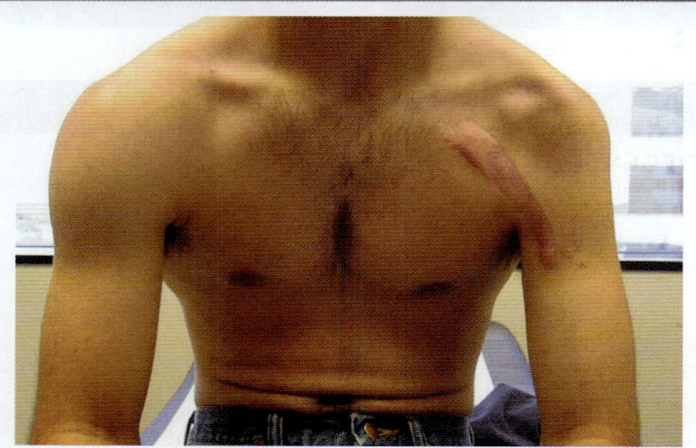

Atrophy

Loss of muscle mass is exhibited as a lack of fullness surrounding the deltoid muscle. In this case, atrophy is due to axillary nerve palsy. Atrophy also occurs from disuse, muscle tissue damage or motor nerve damage.

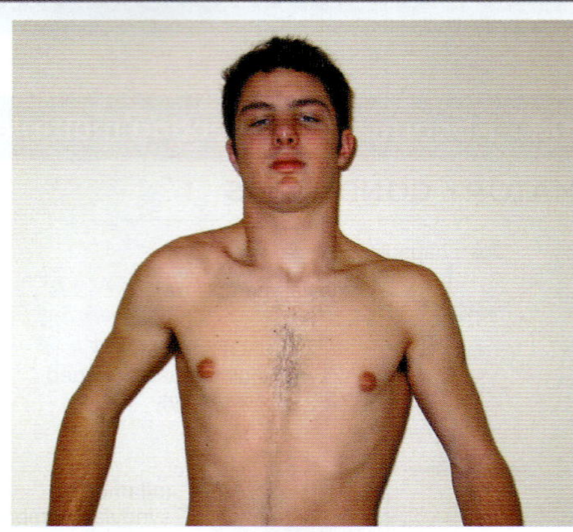

Tear of rotator cuff

Characteristic 'hunched' position and limited abduction of arm. Occurs from traumatic adduction while arm is held in abduction, or from fall on shoulder, throwing or heavy lifting. Positive drop arm test: If the arm is passively abducted at the shoulder, the person is unable to sustain the position and the arm falls to the side.

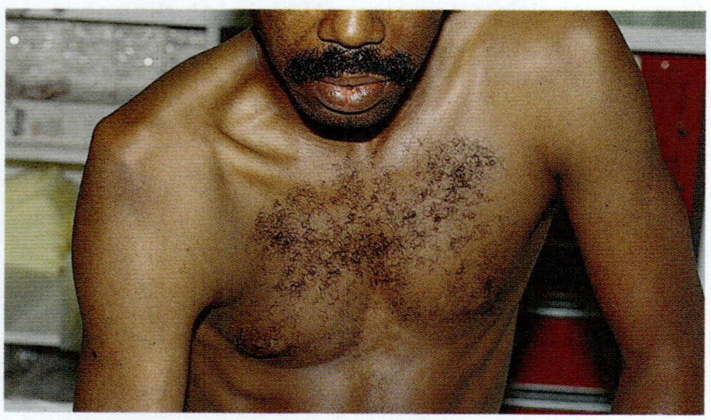

Dislocated shoulder

Anterior dislocation (95%) is exhibited when hunching the shoulder forward and the tip of the clavicle dislocates. It occurs with trauma involving abduction, extension and rotation (e.g. falling on an outstretched arm or diving into a pool).

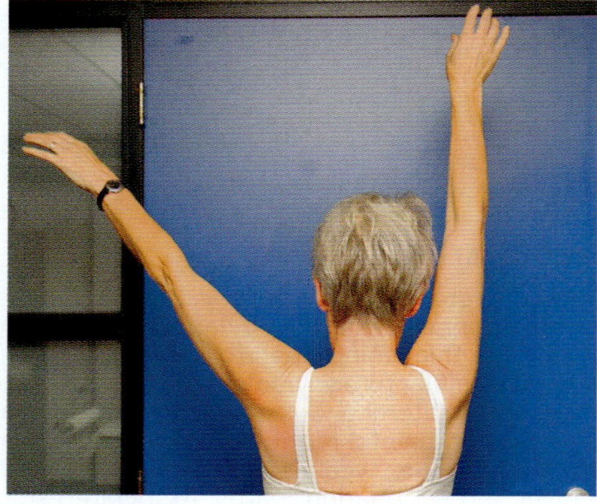

Frozen shoulder—adhesive capsulitis

Fibrous tissues form in the joint capsule, causing stiffness, progressive limitation of motion and pain. Motion limited in abduction and external rotation; unable to reach overhead. It may lead to atrophy of shoulder girdle muscles. Gradual onset; unknown cause. It is associated with prolonged bed rest or shoulder immobility. May resolve spontaneously.

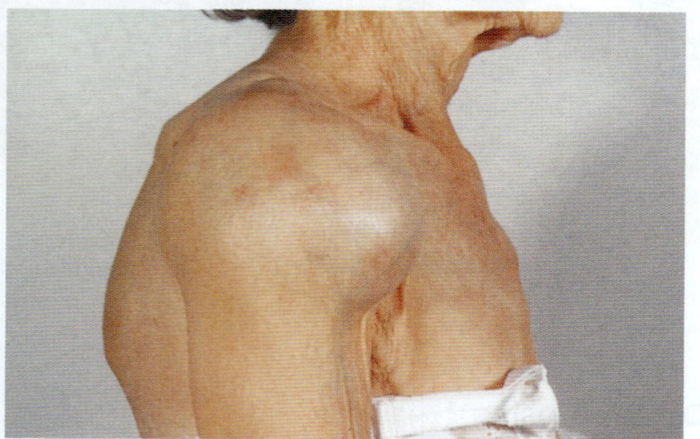

Joint effusion

Swelling from excess fluid in the joint capsule, here from rheumatoid arthritis. Best observed anteriorly. Fluctuant to palpation. Considerable fluid must be present to cause a visible distension because the capsule is normally so loose.

TABLE 20.3 Abnormalities of the elbow

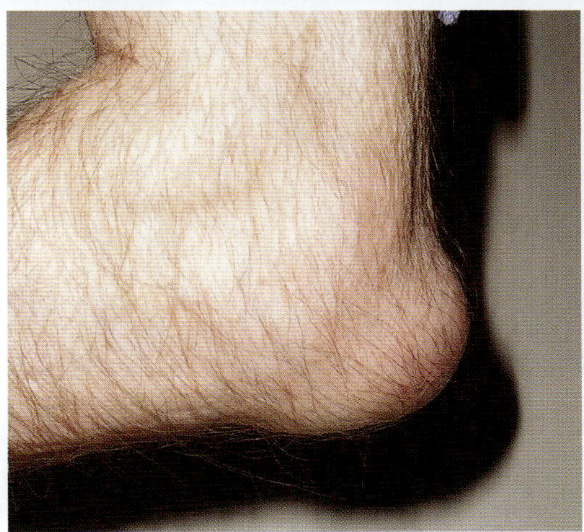

Olecranon bursitis

Large soft knob, or 'goose egg', and redness from inflammation of olecranon bursa. Localised and easy to see because bursa lies just under skin.

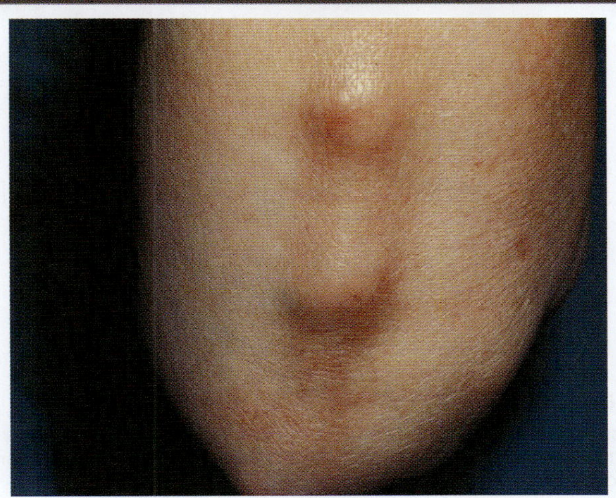

Subcutaneous nodules

Raised, firm, nontender nodules that occur with rheumatoid arthritis. Common sites are in the olecranon bursa and along extensor surface of arm. The skin slides freely over the nodules.

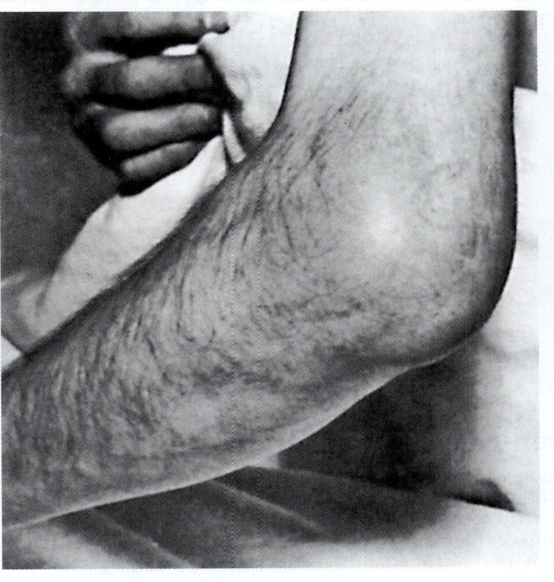

Arthritis

Joint effusion or synovial thickening, seen first as bulge or fullness in grooves on either side of olecranon process. Redness and heat can extend beyond area of synovial membrane. Soft, boggy or fluctuant fullness to palpation. Limited extension of elbow. Occurs with OA, RA, gout and trauma.

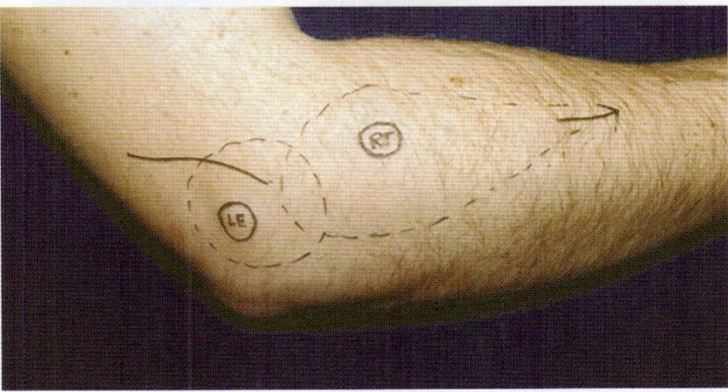

Epicondylitis—tennis elbow

Chronic disabling pain at lateral epicondyle of humerus; radiates down extensor surface of forearm. Pain can be located with one finger. Resisting extension of the hand will increase the pain. Occurs with activities combining excessive pronation and supination of forearm with an extended wrist (e.g. racquet sports or using a screwdriver).

Medial epicondylitis is rarer and is due to activity of forced palmar flexion of wrist against resistance.

TABLE 20.4 Abnormalities of the wrist and hand

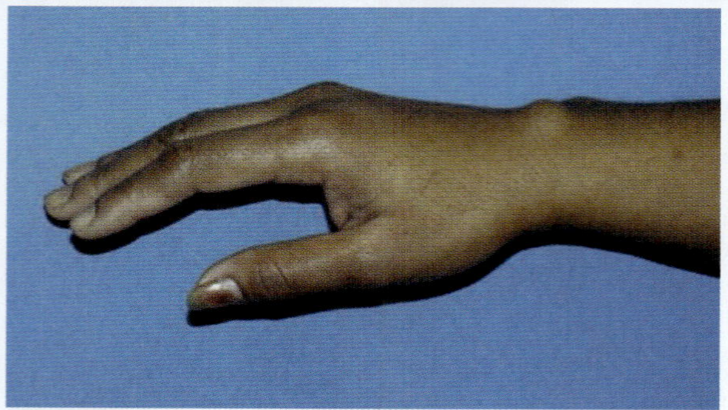

Ganglion cyst

Round, cystic, nontender nodule overlying a tendon sheath or joint capsule, usually on dorsum of wrist. Flexion makes it more prominent. A common benign tumour; it does not become malignant.

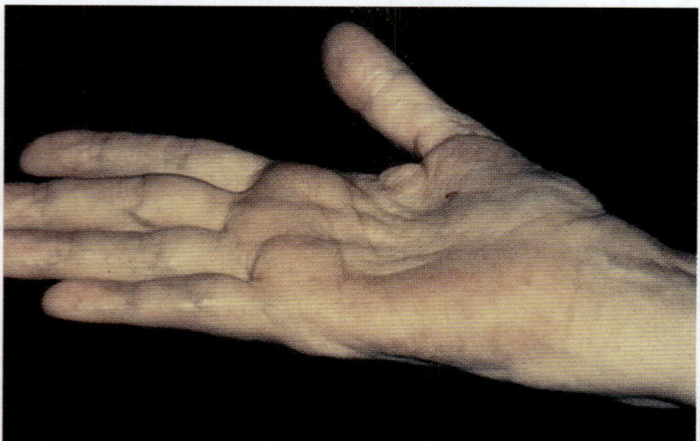

Carpal tunnel syndrome with atrophy of thenar eminence

Atrophy occurs from interference with motor function from compression of the median nerve inside the carpal tunnel. Caused by chronic repetitive motion; occurs between 30 and 60 years of age and is five times more common in women than in men. Symptoms of carpal tunnel syndrome include pain, burning and numbness, positive findings on Phalen's test, positive indication of Tinel's sign and often atrophy of thenar muscles.

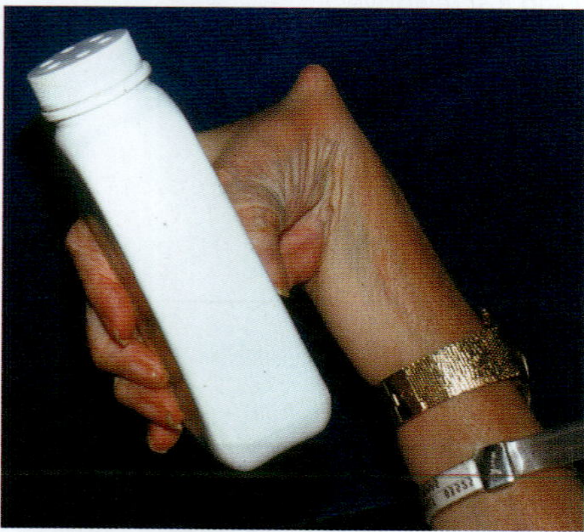

Ankylosis

Wrist in extreme flexion, due to severe rheumatoid arthritis. This is a functionally useless hand because when the wrist is palmar flexed, a good deal of power is lost from the fingers, and the thumb cannot oppose the fingers.

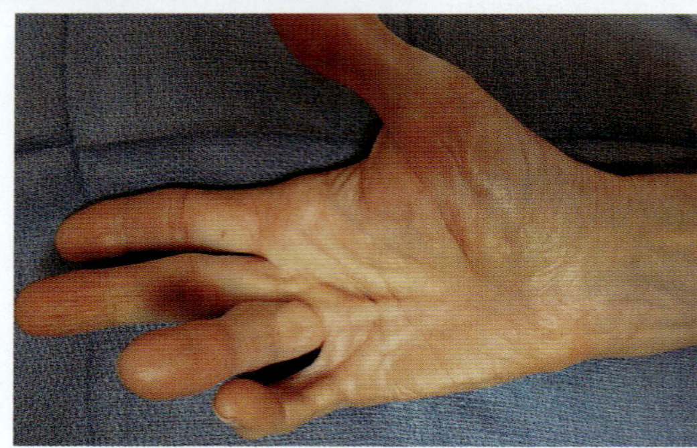

Dupuytren's contracture

Chronic hyperplasia of the palmar fascia causes flexion contractures of the digits, first in the fourth digit, then the fifth digit, and then the third digit. Note the bands that extend from the midpalm to the digits and the puckering of palmar skin. The condition occurs commonly in men past 40 years of age and is usually bilateral. It occurs with diabetes, epilepsy and alcoholic liver disease and as an inherited trait. The contracture is painless but impairs hand function.

CONDITIONS CAUSED BY CHRONIC RHEUMATOID ARTHRITIS

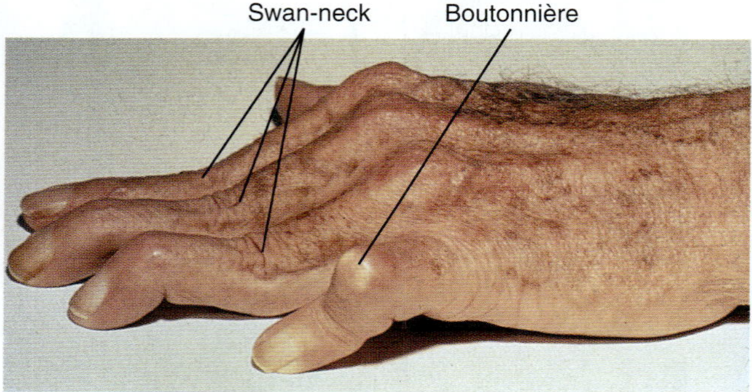

Swan-neck and boutonnière deformity

Flexion contracture resembles curve of a **swan's neck**. Note flexion contracture of metacarpophalangeal joint, then hyperextension of the proximal interphalangeal joint, and flexion of the distal interphalangeal joint. It occurs with chronic rheumatoid arthritis and is often accompanied by ulnar drift of the fingers.

In **boutonnière deformity**, light face the knuckle looks as if it is being pushed through a buttonhole. It is a relatively common deformity and includes flexion of proximal interphalangeal joint with compensatory hyperextension of distal interphalangeal joint.

TABLE 20.4 Abnormalities of the wrist and hand—cont'd

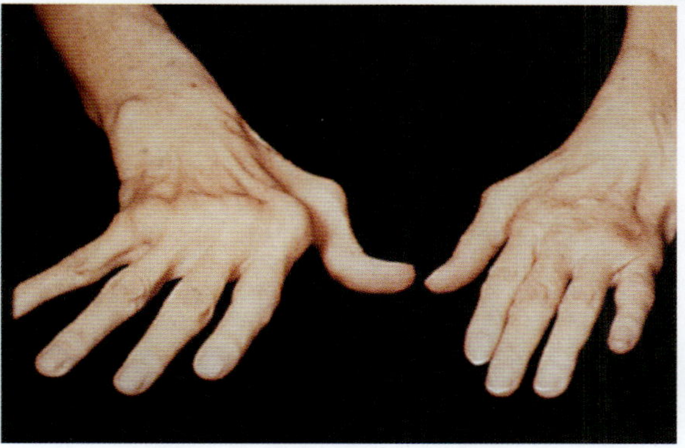

Ulnar deviation or drift

Fingers drift to the ulnar side because of stretching of the articular capsule and muscle imbalance. Also note subluxation and swelling in the joints and muscle atrophy on the dorsa of the hands. This is caused by chronic RA.

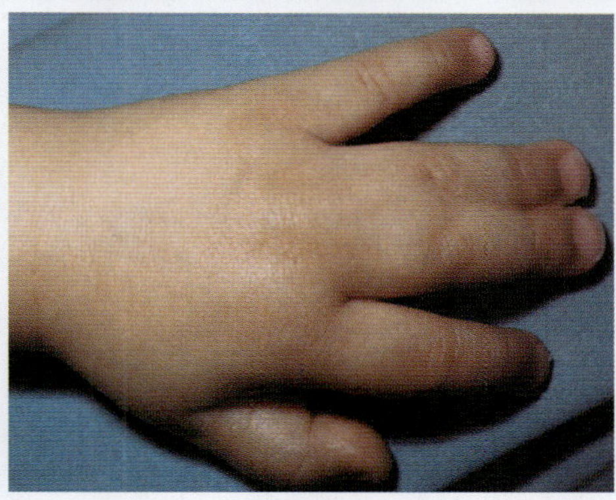

Syndactyly

Webbed fingers are a congenital deformity, usually requiring surgical separation. The metacarpals and phalanges of the webbed fingers are different lengths, and the joints do not line up. To leave the fingers fused would thus limit their flexion and extension.

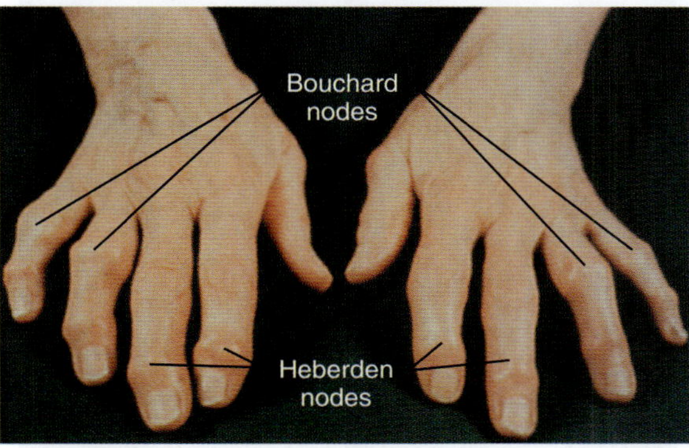

Degenerative joint disease or osteoarthritis

Osteoarthritis is characterised by hard, nontender nodules, 2–3 mm or more. These osteophytes (bony overgrowths) of the distal interphalangeal joints are called Heberden's nodes, and those of the proximal interphalangeal joints are called Bouchard's nodes.

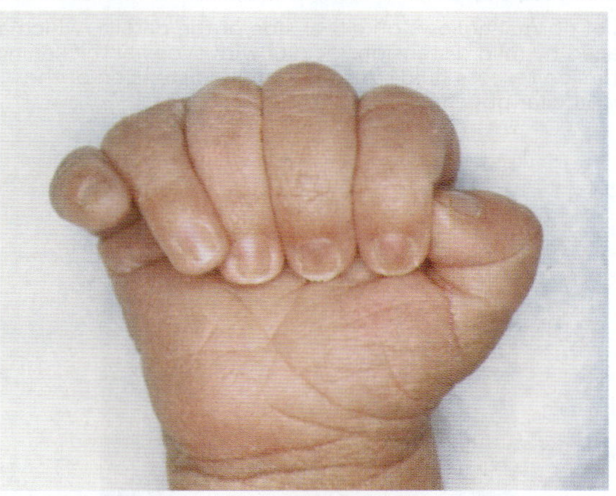

Polydactyly

Extra digits are a congenital deformity, usually occurring at the fifth finger or the thumb. Surgical removal is considered for cosmetic appearance. The sixth finger shown here was not removed because it had full ROM and sensation and a normal appearance.

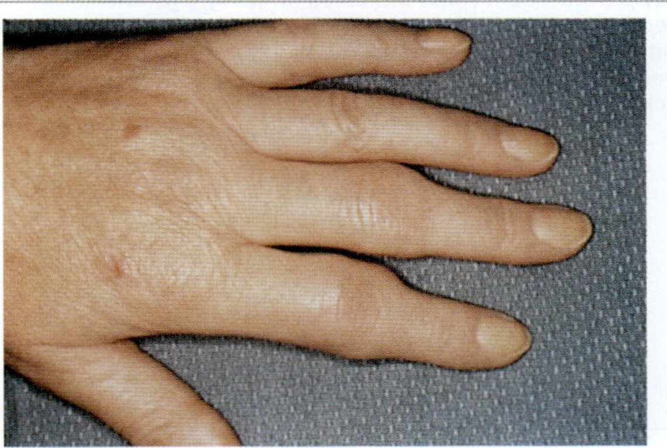

Acute rheumatoid arthritis

Painful swelling and stiffness of joints, with fusiform or spindle-shaped swelling of the soft tissue of proximal interphalangeal joints. Fusiform swelling is usually symmetrical, the hands are warm and the veins are engorged. The inflamed joints have a limited range of motion.

TABLE 20.5 Abnormalities of the knee

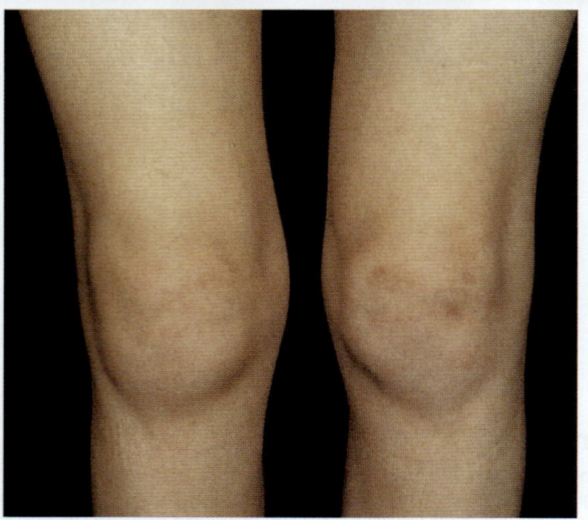

Mild synovitis

Loss of normal hollows on either side of the patella, which are replaced by mild distension. Occurs with synovial thickening or effusion (excess fluid). Also note mild distension of the suprapatellar pouch.

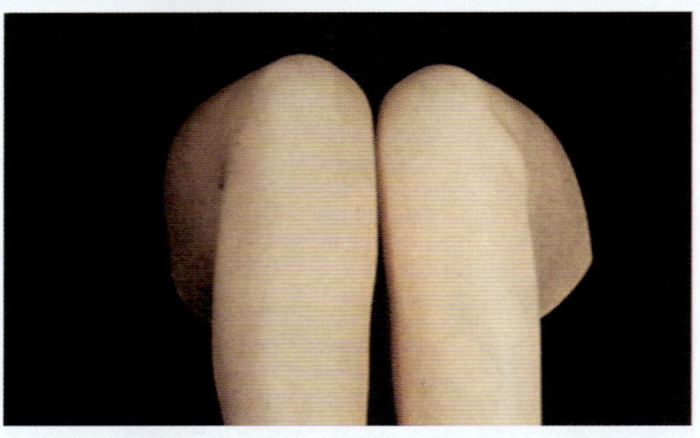

Swelling of menisci

Localised soft swelling from cyst in lateral meniscus shows at the midpoint of the anterolateral joint line. Semiflexion of the knee makes swelling more prominent.

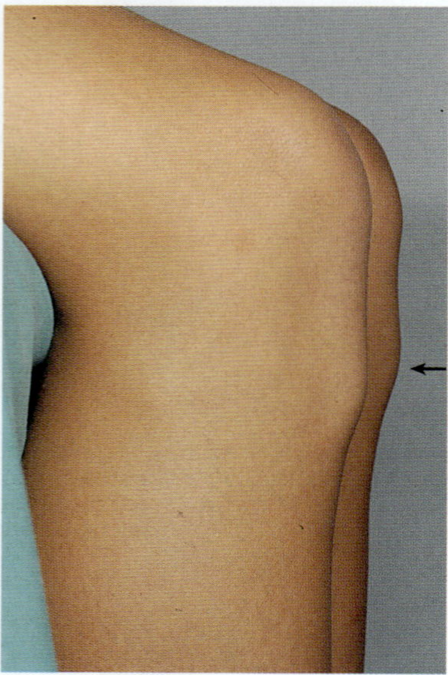

Osgood-Schlatter disease

Painful swelling of the tibial tubercle just below the knee, probably from repeated stress on the patellar tendon. Occurs most in puberty during rapid growth and most often in males. Pain increases with kicking, running, bike riding, stair climbing or kneeling. The condition is usually self-limited, and symptoms resolve with rest.

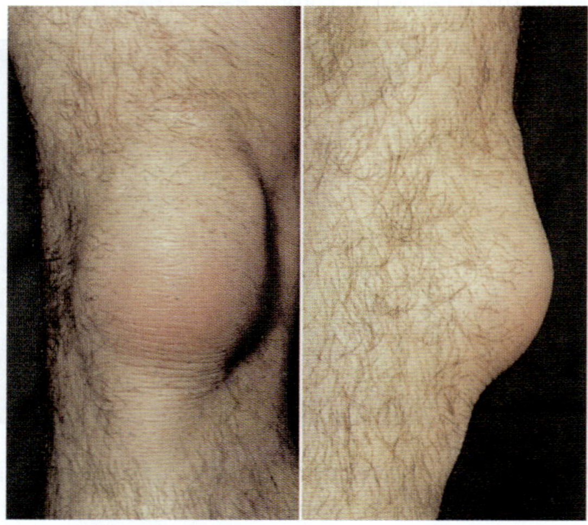

Prepatellar bursitis

Localised swelling on anterior knee between patella and skin. A tender fluctuant mass indicates swelling; in some cases, infection spreads to surrounding soft tissue. The condition is limited to the bursa, and the knee joint itself is not involved. Overlying skin may be red, shiny, atrophic or coarse and thickened.

TABLE 20.6 Abnormalities of the ankle and foot

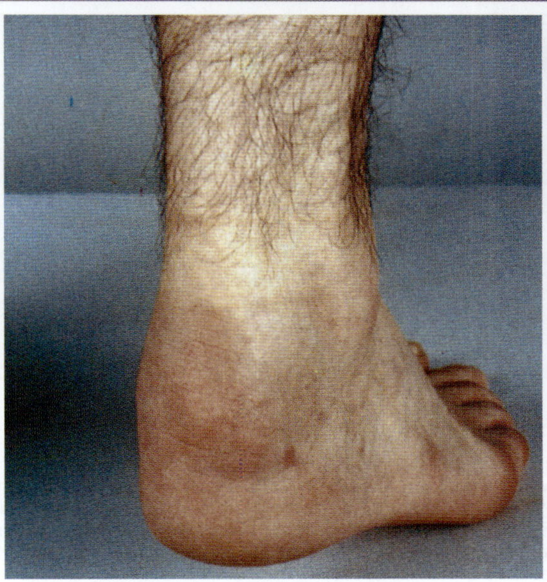

Achilles tenosynovitis

Inflammation of a tendon sheath near the ankle (here, the Achilles tendon) produces a superficial linear swelling and a localised tenderness along the route of the sheath. Movement of the involved tendon usually causes pain.

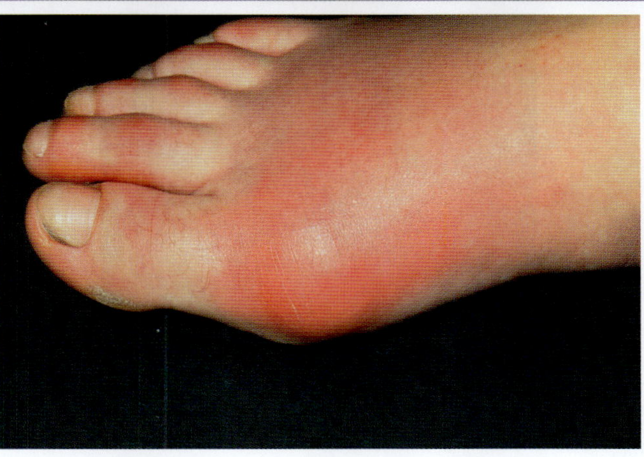

Acute gout

Acute episode of gout usually involves first the metatarso-phalangeal joint. Clinical findings consist of redness, swelling, heat and extreme tenderness. Gout is a metabolic disorder of disturbed purine metabolism, associated with elevated serum uric acid and deposits of urate crystals in the joint space. There is increased risk of gout in obesity, metabolic syndrome, hypertension and hyperlipidaemia. Acute episodes can be triggered by trauma, acute stress and increased alcohol intake.

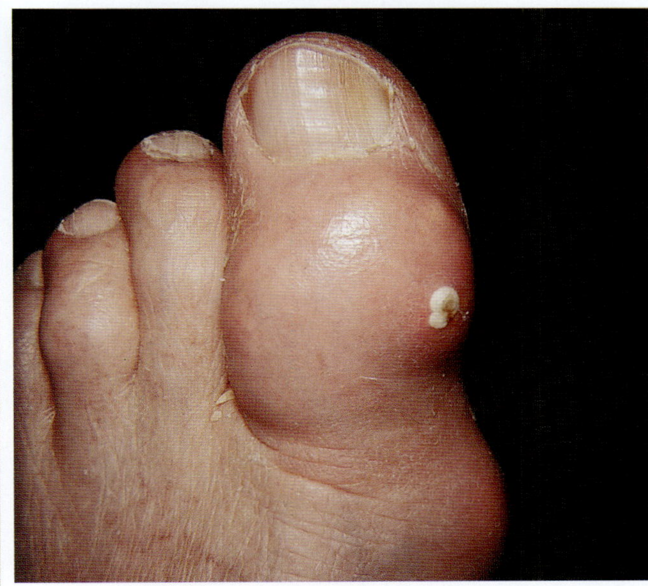

Tophi with chronic gout

Hard, painless nodule (tophi) over metatarsophalangeal joint of first toe. Tophi are collections of sodium urate crystals due to chronic gout in and around the joint that cause extreme swelling and joint deformity. They sometimes burst through the skin with a chalky discharge.

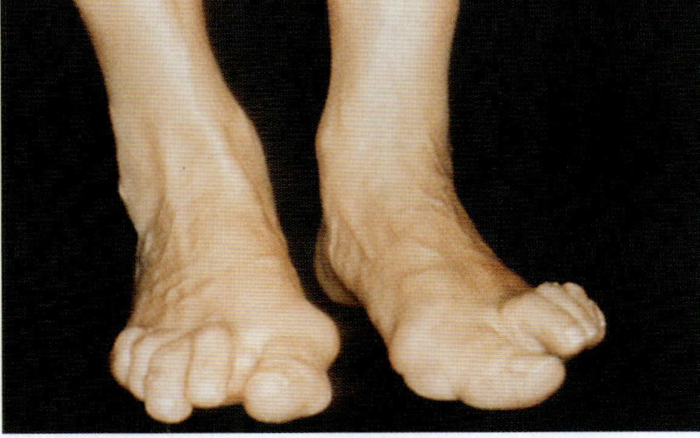

Hallux valgus with bunion and hammertoes

Hallux valgus is a common deformity from rheumatoid arthritis. It is a lateral or outward deviation of the great toe with medial prominence of the head of the first metatarsal. The **bunion** is the inflamed bursa that forms at the pressure point. The great toe loses power to push off while walking; this stresses the second and third metatarsal heads, and they develop calluses and pain. Chronic sequelae include corns, calluses, hammertoes and joint subluxation.

Note the **hammertoe** deformities in the second, third, fourth and fifth toes. Often associated with hallux valgus, hammertoe includes hyperextension of the metatarsophalangeal joint and flexion of the proximal interphalangeal joint.

Corns (thickening of soft tissue) develop on the dorsum over the bony prominence from prolonged pressure from shoes.

(Continued)

TABLE 20.6 Abnormalities of the ankle and foot—cont'd

<table>
<tr><td>
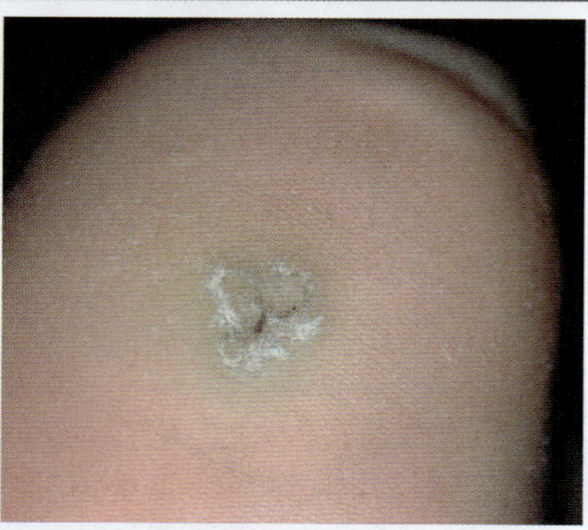

Plantar wart

Vascular papillomatous growth is caused by the *human papillomavirus* and occurs on the sole of the foot, commonly at the ball. The condition is extremely painful when direct pressure is applied (for example when walking).
</td><td>
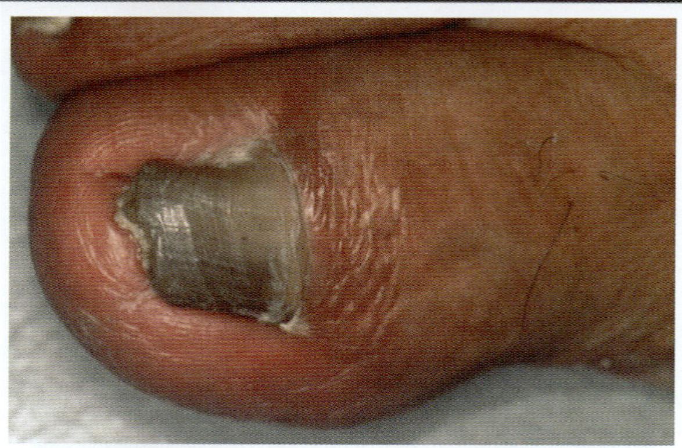

Ingrown toenail

A misnomer; the nail does not grow in, but the soft tissue grows over the nail and obliterates the groove. It occurs almost always on the great toe on the medial or lateral side. It is due to trimming the nail too short or toe-crowding in tight shoes. The area becomes infected when the nail grows and its corner penetrates the soft tissue.
</td></tr>
<tr><td>
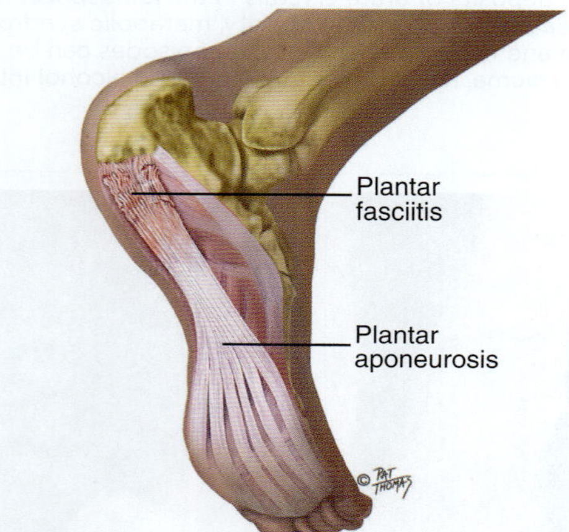

Plantar fasciitis

The plantar fascia is a band of connective tissue that extends lengthwise from the medial tubercle of the heel to the metatarsal heads and the five proximal phalanges of the toes. An inflammatory response to repetitive microtrauma to this fascia is the most frequent cause of heel pain. Risk factors include obesity, high-arched foot, running, standing for long periods on a hard floor, recent injury to lower limbs or change in activity. Pain is unilateral, and described as throbbing, piercing or searing; the pain is worse in the morning or after periods of long rest.
</td><td></td></tr>
</table>

TABLE 20.7 Abnormalities of the spine

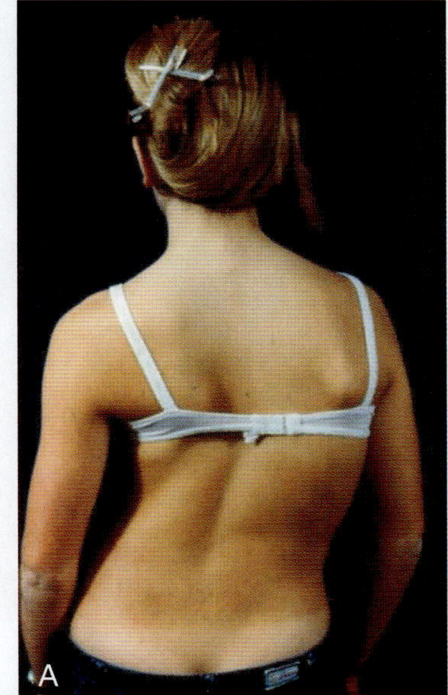

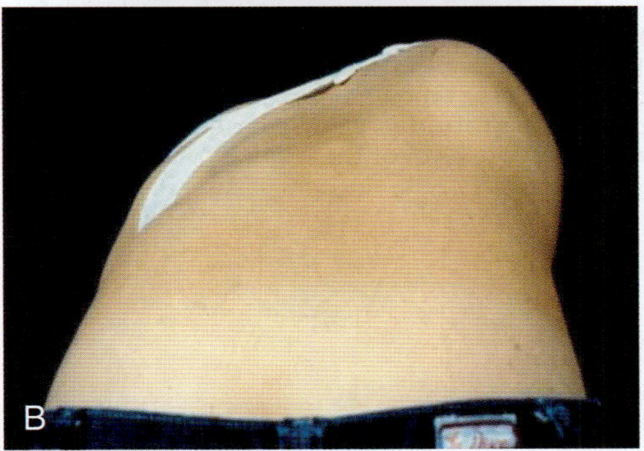

Scoliosis

Lateral curvature of thoracic and lumbar segments of the spine, usually with some rotation of involved vertebral bodies.

Functional scoliosis is flexible; it is apparent with standing and disappears with forward bending. It may be compensatory for other abnormalities such as leg length discrepancy.

Structural scoliosis is fixed; the curvature shows both on standing and on bending forward. Note rib hump with forward flexion. When the person is standing, note unequal shoulder elevation, unequal scapulae, obvious curvature and unequal hip level. At greatest risk are females 10 years of age through adolescence, during the peak of the growth spurt.

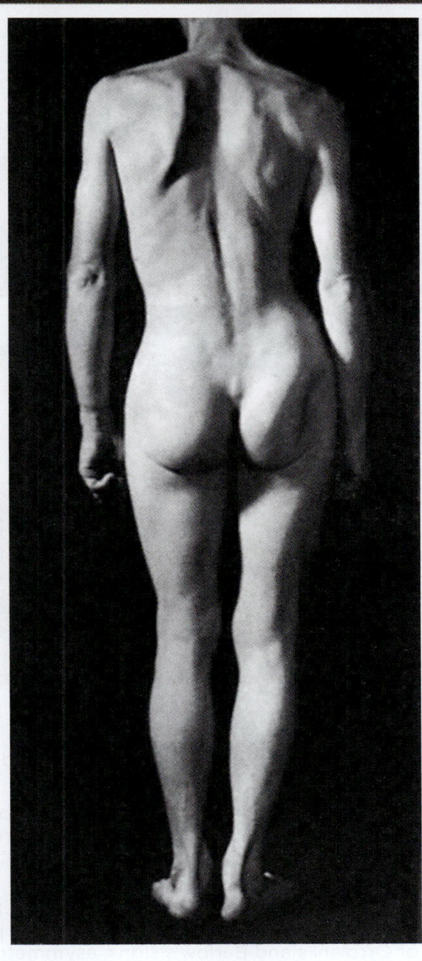

Herniated intervertebral disc

The nucleus pulposus (at the centre of the intervertebral disc) ruptures into the spinal canal and puts pressure on the local spinal nerve root. Usually occurs from stress, such as lifting, twisting, continuous flexion with lifting or fall on buttocks. Occurs mostly in men 20–45 years of age. Lumbar herniations occur mainly in interspaces L4–L5 and L5–S1. Note: sciatic pain, numbness and paraesthesia of involved dermatome; listing away from affected side; decreased mobility; low back tenderness; and decreased motor and sensory function in leg. Straight leg raising tests reproduce sciatic pain.

TABLE 20.8 Common congenital or paediatric abnormalities

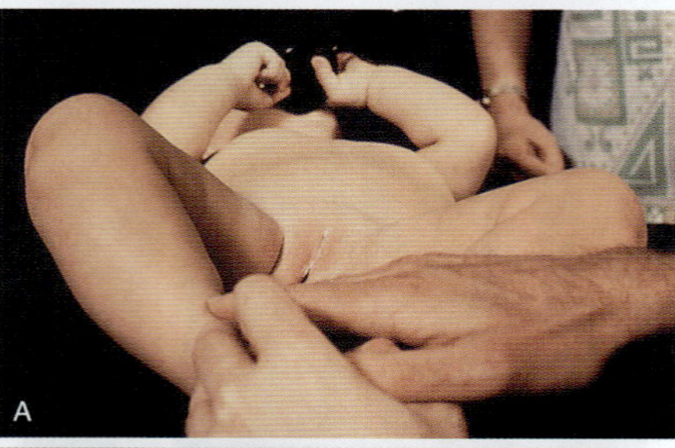

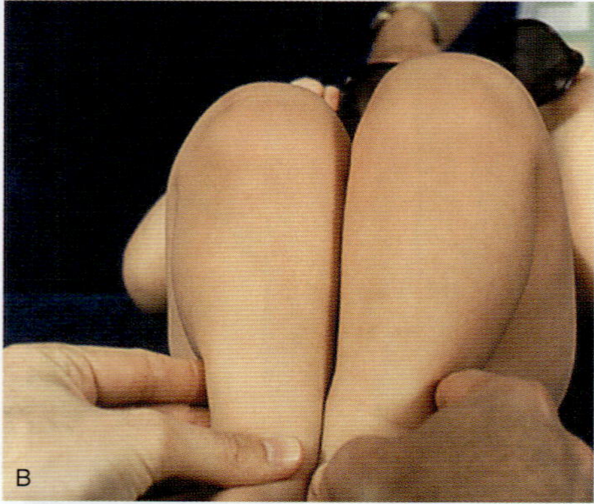

Developmental hip dysplasia

Head of the femur is displaced out of the cup-shaped acetabulum.

The degree of the condition varies; subluxation may occur as stretched ligaments allow partial displacement of femoral head, and acetabular dysplasia may develop because of excessive laxity of hip joint capsule.

Occurrence is 1:500 to 1:1000 births; common in girls by 7:1 ratio. Signs include limited abduction of flexed thigh, positive indications of Ortolani's and Barlow's signs, asymmetrical skin creases or gluteal folds, limb length discrepancy and positive indication of Trendelenburg's sign in older children.

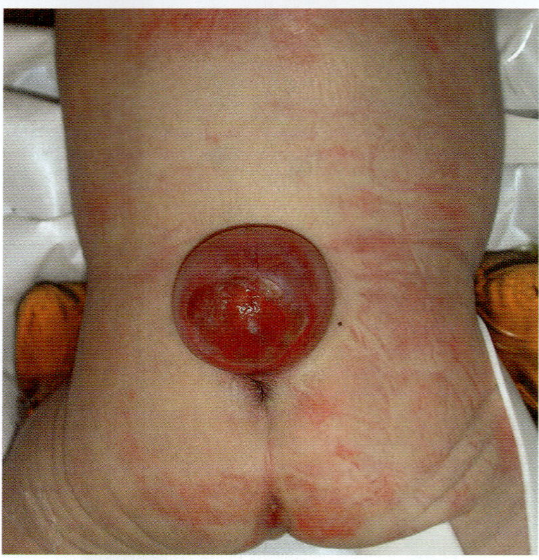

Spina bifida

Incomplete closure of posterior part of vertebrae results in a neural tube defect. Seriousness varies from skin defect along the spine to protrusion of the sac containing meninges, spinal fluid or malformed spinal cord. The most serious type is myelomeningocele (shown here), in which the meninges and neural tissue protrude. In these cases the child is usually paralysed below the level of the lesion.

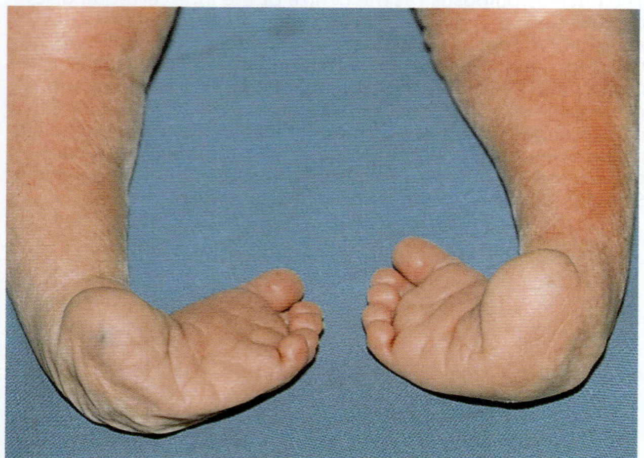

Talipes equinovarus (clubfoot)

Congenital, rigid and fixed malposition of foot, including (1) inversion, (2) forefoot adduction and (3) foot pointing downwards (equinus). A common birth defect, with an incidence of 1:1000 live births. Males are affected twice as frequently as females.

BIBLIOGRAPHY

Australian Commission on Safety and Quality in Health Care. Falls prevention. 2015. Available at: www.safetyandquality.gov.au/our-work/falls-prevention/.

Australian Institute of Health and Welfare (AIHW). Australian burden of disease study: Impact and causes of illness and death in Aboriginal and Torres Strait Islander people 2011. Canberra: AIHW; 2016. Available at: www.aihw.gov.au/reports/burden-of-disease/australian-bod-study-2011-indigenous-australians/contents/table-of-contents.

Australian Institute of Health and Welfare (AIHW). Osteoporosis snapshot. Cat. No. PHE 233. Canberra: AIHW; 2018a. Available at: www.aihw.gov.au/reports/chronic-musculoskeletal-conditions/osteoporosis/contents/what-is-osteoporosis.

Australian Institute of Health and Welfare (AIHW). Trends in hospitalised injury due to falls in older people, 2002–03 to 2014–15. Injury research and statistics series no. 111. Cat. no. INJCAT 191. Canberra: AIHW; 2018b. Available at: www.aihw.gov.au/getmedia/39e62afd-7207-460d-aaa6-4f0c95ae665a/aihw-injcat-191.pdf.aspx?inline=true.

Australian Institute of Health and Welfare (AIHW). Australia's health 2018, Australia's health series no. 16. 2018c. Available at: https://www.aihw.gov.au/reports/australias-health/australias-health-2018/contents/table-of-contents.

Australian Institute of Health and Welfare (AIHW). Aboriginal and Torres Strait Islander health performance framework - Web report. Canberra: Australian Health Ministers' Advisory Council (AHMAC); 2018d. Available at: www.aihw.gov.au/reports/indigenous-health-welfare/health-performance-framework/contents/overview.

Australian Institute of Health and Welfare (AIHW). Chronic musculoskeletal conditions. Canberra: AIHW; 2018e. Available at: www.aihw.gov.au/reports-data/health-conditions-disability-deaths/chronic-musculoskeletal-conditions/overview.

Australian Institute of Health and Welfare (AIHW). Musculoskeletal conditions and comorbidity in Australia. Arthritis series no. 25. Cat. no. PHE 241. Canberra: AIHW; 2019. Available at: www.aihw.gov.au/reports/chronic-musculoskeletal-conditions/musculoskeletal-conditions-comorbidity-australia/contents/table-of-contents.

Christensen L, Vøllestad NK, Veierød MB, et al. The timed up & go test in pregnant women with pelvic girdle pain compared to asymptomatic pregnant and non-pregnant women. Musculoskelet Sci Pract 2019;43:110–16. doi.org/10.1016/j.msksp.2019.03.006

Dacre J. The GALS screen: the rapid rheumatological exam. Med J Aust 2019;210(9):396-7.

de Souto Barreto P, Rolland Y, Vellas B, Maltais M. Association of longterm exercise training with risk of falls, fractures, hospitalizations, and mortality in older adults: a systematic review and meta-analysis. JAMA Intern Med 2019;179(3):394–405.

Department of Health. Pregnancy care guidelines. Canberra: Australian Government Department of Health; 2018. Available at: https://beta.health.gov.au/resources/pregnancy-care-guidelines.

Dhillon RJ, Hasni S. Pathogenesis and management of sarcopenia. Clin Geriatr Med 2017 Feb;33(1):17–26.

Doherty M, Dacre J, Dieppe P, et al. The 'GALS' locomotor screen. Ann Rheum Dis 1992;51:1165-9.

Douglas G, Dova AR, Fairhurst K, editors. MacLeod's clinical examination. 14th ed. Edinburgh: Elsevier; 2018.

Eudy AM, McDaniel G, Clowse MEB. Pregnancy in rheumatoid arthritis: a retrospective study. Clin Rheumatol 2018;37(3):789–94.

Ferrari SL. Pathophysiology of osteoporosis. In Ferrari SL, Roux C, editors. Pocket reference to osteoporosis. Champaign, IL: Springer International Publishing; 2019.

Foster HE, Jandial S. pGALS–paediatric Gait Arms Legs and Spine: a simple examination of the musculoskeletal system. Pediatr Rheumatol 2013;11(1):44.

Gane EM, Brakenridge CL, Smits EJ, et al. The impact of musculoskeletal injuries sustained in road traffic crashes on work-related outcomes: a protocol for a systematic review. Syst Rev 2018;(1):202.

Gutke A, Boissonnault J, Brook G, et al. The severity and impact of pelvic girdle pain and low-back pain in pregnancy: A multi-national study. J Women's Health 2018;27(4):510–17.

Kanis JA. Diagnosis and clinical aspects of osteoporosis. In Ferrari SL, Roux C, editors. Pocket Reference to Osteoporosis. Champaign, IL: Springer International Publishing; 2019

Komaba H. Fragility fractures in hemodialysis patients. Loss of kidney function and system for calcium homeostasis. Clin Calcium 2018;28(8):1057–63.

Krause ML, Makol A. Management of rheumatoid arthritis during pregnancy: challenges and solutions. Open Access Rheumatol 2016;8:23–36.

Kravets I. Paget's disease of bone: diagnosis and treatment. Am J Med 2018;131(11):1298–303.

Lynn M. Management of crush injuries and crush syndrome. In: Lynn M, Lieberman H, Lynn L, et al, editors. Disasters and mass casualty incidents. 2nd ed, Champaign, IL: Springer; 2019. pp. 87–8.

Malacova E, Cheang PR, Dunlop E, et al. Prevalence and predictors of vitamin D deficiency in a nationally representative sample of adults participating in the 2011–2013 Australian Health Survey. Br J Nutr 2019;1–11.

Marieb EM, Keller SM. Essentials of human anatomy & physiology. 12th Global ed. New York: Pearson; 2018.

Marty E, Liu Y, Samuel A, et al. A review of sarcopenia: enhancing awareness of an increasingly prevalent disease. Bone 2017;(105):276–86.

McVeigh JA, Howie EK, Zhu K, et al. Organized sport participation from childhood to adolescence is associated with bone mass in young adults from the Raine study. J Bone Miner Res 2019;34(1):67–74.

Rizzoli R. Diagnosis and clinical aspects of osteoporosis. In: Ferrari SL, Roux C, editors. Pocket reference to osteoporosis. Champaign, IL: Springer International Publishing; 2019. pp. 31–42.

Rouf A, Clayton S, Allman-Farinelli M. The barriers and enablers to achieving adequate calcium intake in young adults: a qualitative study using focus groups. J Hum Nutr Diet 2019;32(4):443–54. doi.org/10.1111/jhn.12653

Royal Australian College of General Practitioners (RACGP). Osteoporosis risk assessment, diagnosis and management. 2017. Available at: https://www.osteoporosis.org.au/sites/default/files/files/RACGP%20Osteoporosis%20Summary%20Guideline%204428%20Nov%202017.pdf.

Royal College of Pathologists of Australia (RCPA). RCPA manual. 2019. Available at: www.rcpa.edu.au/Manuals/RCPA-Manual.

Scoliosis Australia. The national self-detection program for scoliosis. 2019. Available at: www.scoliosis-australia.org/scoliosis/self_detection_prog.html.

Lee S, Oh E, Son Hong G-R. Comparison of factors associated with fear of falling between older adults with and without a fall history. Int J Environ Res Public Health 2018;(5):982.

Studer K, Williams N, Antoniou G, et al. Increase in late diagnosed developmental dysplasia of the hip in South Australia: risk factors, proposed solutions. Med J Aust 2016;204(6):240.

Talley NJ, O'Connor S. Clinical examination: a systematic guide to physical diagnosis. 8th ed. Chatswood, NSW: Elsevier Australia; 2018.

Tatangelo G, Watts J, Lim K, et al. The cost of osteoporosis, osteopenia, and associated fractures in Australia in 2017. J Bone Miner Res 2019;3(5):616–25.

Tiller G, Buckle J, Allen R, et al. Juvenile idiopathic arthritis managed in the new millennium: one-year outcomes of an inception cohort of Australian children. Paediatr Rheumatol 2018;16(1):69.

World Health Organization (WHO). Global status report on road safety 2018: summary. Geneva: (WHO/NMH/NVI/18.20); 2018. Available at: www.who.int/violence_injury_prevention/road_safety_status/2018/en/.

Assessing nutrition and metabolic function

Unit 7

Chapter Twenty-One

Nutritional and metabolic assessment

Written by Joyce K Keithly
Adapted by Trish Burton

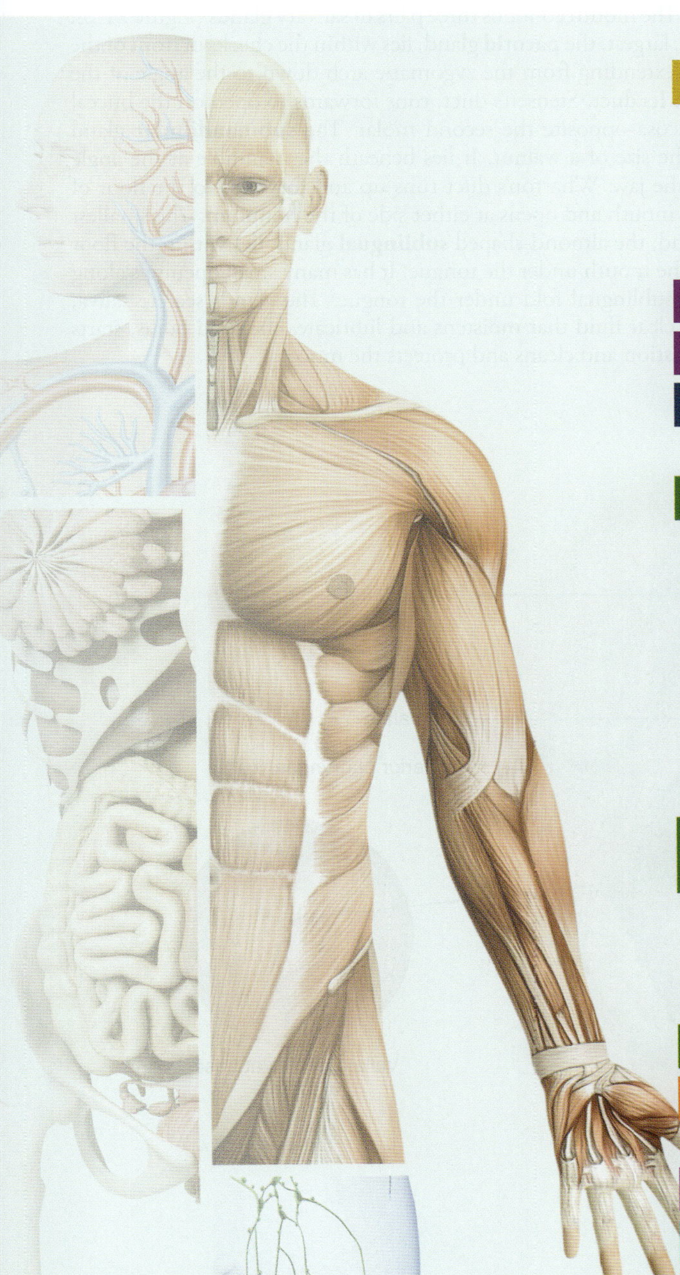

INTRODUCTION

Nutrition plays an essential part in growth, development and general health and wellbeing that every body system needs to be taken into account when considering a person's nutritional status. In terms of relevant anatomy and physiology, you will find relevant information in Chapter 18 as well as in Chapters 23 and 25.

Structure and function

THE MOUTH

The mouth is the first segment of the digestive system and an airway for the respiratory system. The **oral cavity** is a short passage bordered by the lips, palate, cheeks and tongue. It contains the teeth and gums, tongue and salivary glands (Figure 21.1).

The lips are the anterior border of the oral cavity—the transition zone from the outer skin to the inner mucous membrane lining the oral cavity. The arching roof of the mouth is the palate; it is divided into two parts. The anterior **hard palate** is made up of bone and is a whitish colour. Posterior to this is the **soft palate**, an arch of muscle that is pinker in colour and mobile. The **uvula** is the free projection hanging down from the middle of the soft palate. The cheeks are the side walls of the oral cavity.

The floor of the mouth consists of the horseshoe-shaped mandible bone, the tongue and underlying muscles. The **tongue** is a mass of striated muscle arranged in a crosswise pattern so that it can change shape and position. The papillae are the rough, bumpy elevations on its dorsal surface. Note the larger vallate papillae in an inverted **V** shape across the posterior base of the tongue, and do not confuse them with abnormal growths. Underneath, the ventral surface of the tongue is smooth and shiny and has prominent veins. The **frenulum** is a midline fold of tissue that connects the tongue to the floor of the mouth.

The tongue's ability to change shape and position enhances its functions in mastication, swallowing, cleansing the teeth and the formation of speech. The tongue also functions in taste sensation. Microscopic taste buds are in the papillae at the back and along the sides of the tongue and on the soft palate.

The mouth contains three pairs of salivary glands (Figure 21.2). The largest, the **parotid** gland, lies within the cheeks in front of the ear extending from the zygomatic arch down to the angle of the jaw. Its duct, Stensen's duct, runs forwards to open on the buccal mucosa opposite the second molar. The **submandibular** gland is the size of a walnut. It lies beneath the mandible at the angle of the jaw. Wharton's duct runs up and forwards to the floor of the mouth and opens at either side of the frenulum. The smallest gland, the almond-shaped **sublingual** gland, lies within the floor of the mouth under the tongue. It has many small openings along the sublingual fold under the tongue. The glands secrete saliva, the clear fluid that moistens and lubricates the food bolus, starts digestion and cleans and protects the mucosa.

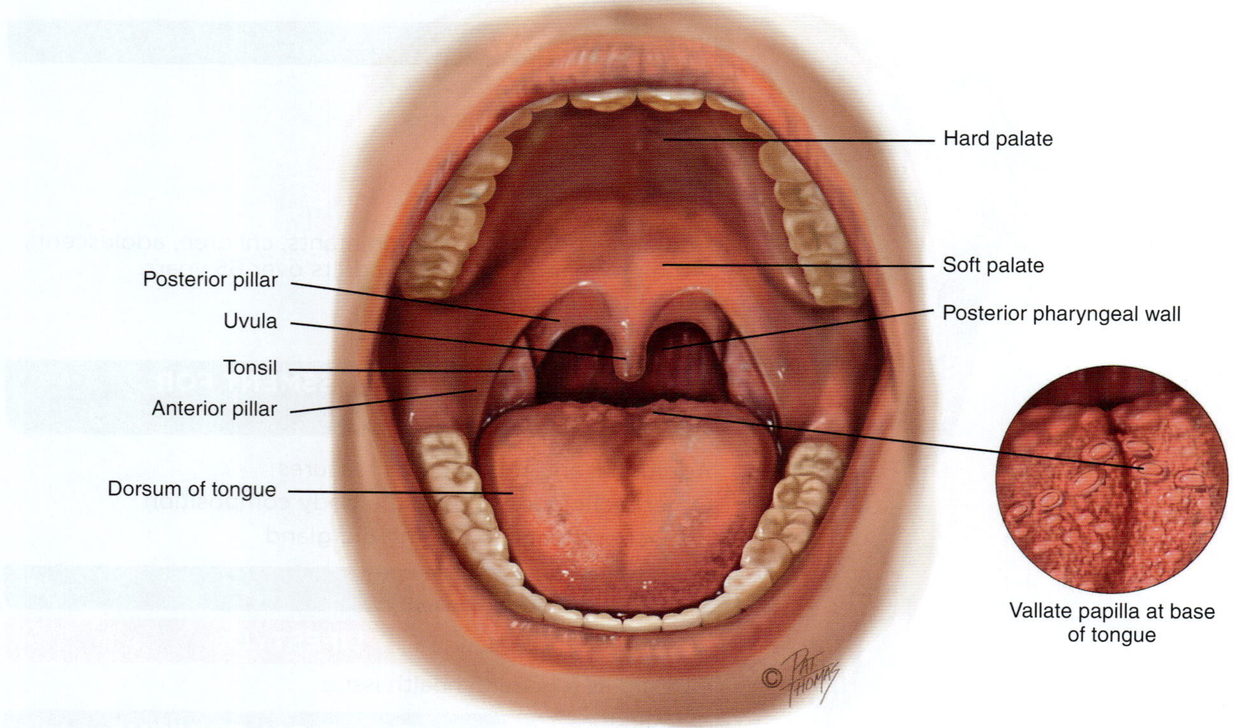

Figure 21.1
Oral cavity. © Pat Thomas, 2010

Adults have 32 **permanent** teeth—16 in each arch. Each tooth has three parts: the crown, the neck and the root (Figure 21.3). The gums (gingivae) collar the teeth. They are thick fibrous tissues covered with mucous membrane. The gums are different from the rest of the oral mucosa because of their pale pink colour and stippled surface. Refer to Chapter 18 for information about the nose, oropharynx and throat.

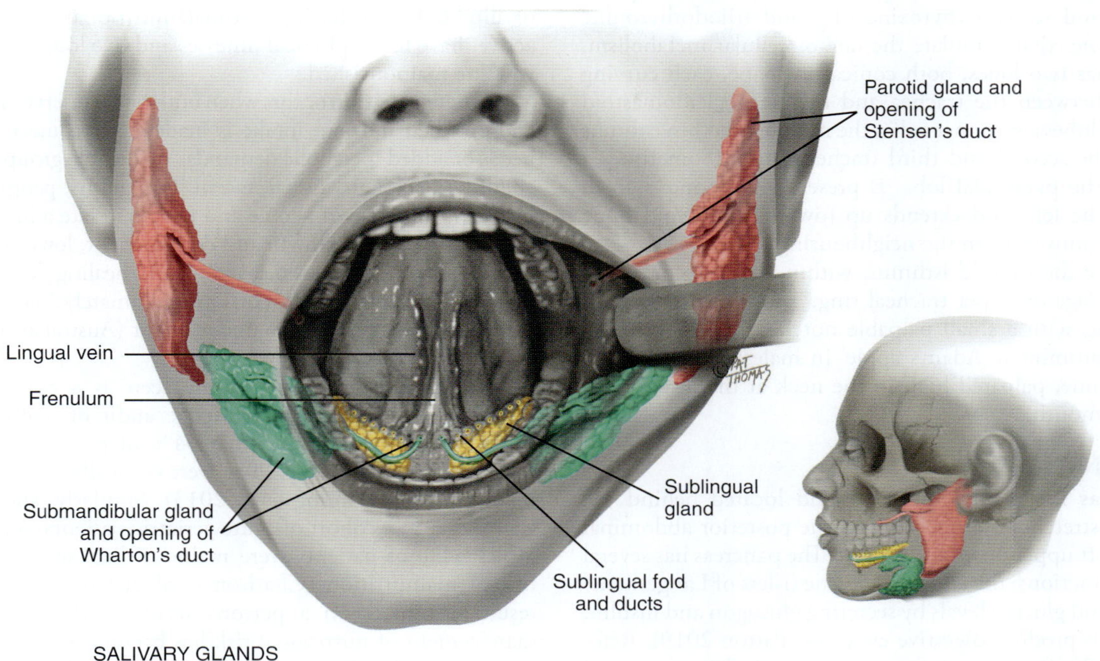

Figure 21.2
Salivary glands.

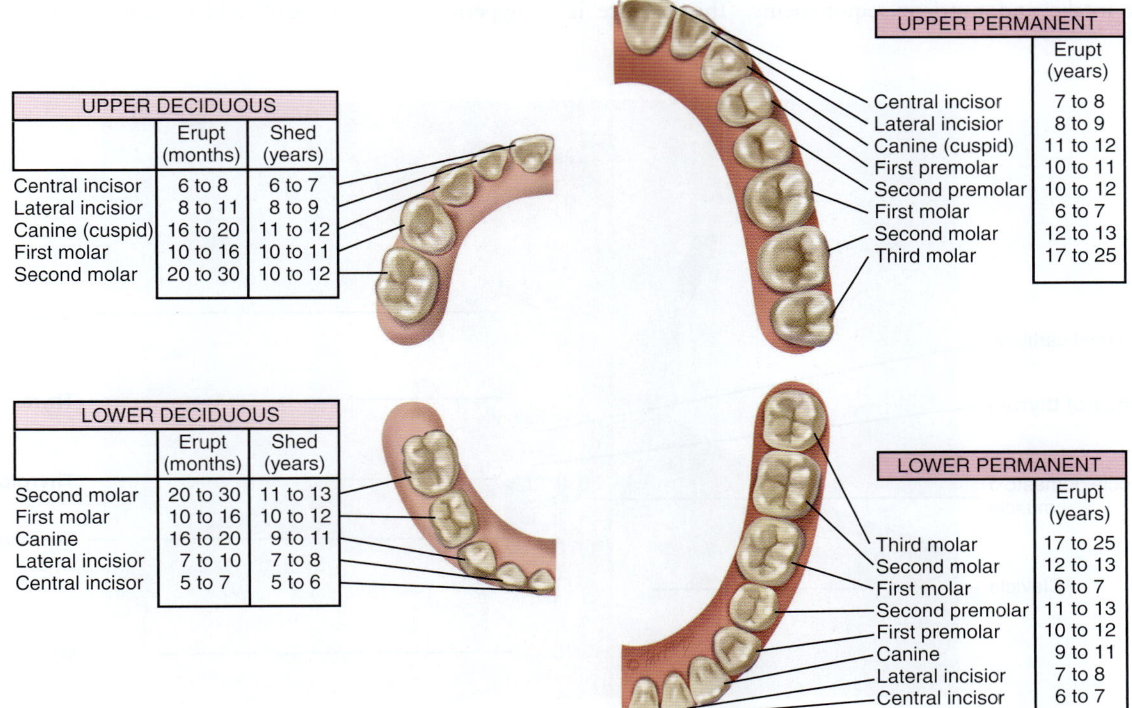

UPPER DECIDUOUS	Erupt (months)	Shed (years)
Central incisor	6 to 8	6 to 7
Lateral incisior	8 to 11	8 to 9
Canine (cuspid)	16 to 20	11 to 12
First molar	10 to 16	10 to 11
Second molar	20 to 30	10 to 12

LOWER DECIDUOUS	Erupt (months)	Shed (years)
Second molar	20 to 30	11 to 13
First molar	10 to 16	10 to 12
Canine	16 to 20	9 to 11
Lateral incisior	7 to 10	7 to 8
Central incisor	5 to 7	5 to 6

UPPER PERMANENT	Erupt (years)
Central incisor	7 to 8
Lateral incisior	8 to 9
Canine (cuspid)	11 to 12
First premolar	10 to 11
Second premolar	10 to 12
First molar	6 to 7
Second molar	12 to 13
Third molar	17 to 25

LOWER PERMANENT	Erupt (years)
Third molar	17 to 25
Second molar	12 to 13
First molar	6 to 7
Second premolar	11 to 13
First premolar	10 to 12
Canine	9 to 11
Lateral incisior	7 to 8
Central incisor	6 to 7

Figure 21.3
Deciduous and permanent teeth. © Pat Thomas, 2006

THE THYROID GLAND

The **thyroid gland** is an important endocrine gland with a rich blood supply. It straddles the trachea in the middle of the neck (Figure 21.4). This highly vascular endocrine gland synthesises and secretes thyroxine (T_4) and triiodothyronine (T_3), hormones that stimulate the rate of cellular metabolism. The gland has two lobes, both conical in shape, each curving posteriorly between the trachea and the sternocleidomastoid muscle. The lobes are connected in the middle by a thin isthmus lying over the second and third tracheal rings. (Sometimes a third lobe, the pyramidal lobe, is present. It is cone shaped, usually on the left, and extends up towards the hyoid bone from the isthmus or from the neighbouring lobe.)

Just above the thyroid isthmus, within about 1 cm, is the **cricoid** cartilage or upper tracheal ring. The **thyroid** cartilage is above that, with a small palpable notch in its upper edge. This is the prominent 'Adam's apple' in males. The highest is the **hyoid** bone, palpated high in the neck at the level of the floor of the mouth.

THE PANCREAS

The **pancreas** is a soft, lobulated gland located behind the stomach. It stretches obliquely across the posterior abdominal wall to the left upper quadrant (LUQ). The pancreas has several important functions; the endocrine tissue (islets of Langerhans) regulates blood glucose levels by secreting glucagon and insulin. Exocrine cells produce digestive enzymes (Patton 2019). Refer to Chapter 23 for more information about the anatomical location of the pancreas in the abdominal cavity.

DEFINING NUTRITIONAL STATUS

Nutritional status refers to the degree of balance between nutrient intake and nutrient requirements. This balance is affected by many factors, including physiological, psychosocial, developmental, cultural and economic.

Optimal nutritional status is achieved when sufficient nutrients are consumed to support day-to-day body needs and any increased metabolic demands due to growth, pregnancy or illness. People having optimal nutritional status are more active, have fewer physical illnesses and live longer than people who are malnourished.

Under-nutrition occurs when nutritional reserves are depleted and/or when nutrient intake is inadequate to meet day-to-day needs or added metabolic demands. Vulnerable groups—infants, children, pregnant women, recent immigrants, people with low incomes, hospitalised people and people in late adulthood—are at risk for impaired growth and development, lowered resistance to infection and disease, delayed wound healing, longer hospital stays and higher healthcare costs. Approximately 2% of Australian adults are considered to be underweight (Australian Institute of Health and Welfare (AIHW) 2014a).

Under-nutrition is commonly seen as a consequence of hospital admission. A retrospective audit of malnutrition in Australian hospitals found that 64% of patients were at risk of malnutrition: of these, 90% were clinically assessed as being malnourished (Boltong et al 2013). Similarly, another study found that in a cohort of acute geriatric patients in New South Wales 34% of patients were malnourished and 55% were at risk of malnutrition (Charlton et al 2013). Considering the resultant impact on a person's recovery, the screening and management of nutritional risk has become a central focus, in particular within the acute and sub-acute setting.

Over-nutrition is caused by the consumption of nutrients—especially kilojoules, sodium and fat—in excess of body needs. A major nutritional problem today, over-nutrition can lead to obesity and is a risk factor for heart disease, type 2 diabetes, hypertension, stroke, gallbladder disease, sleep apnoea, certain

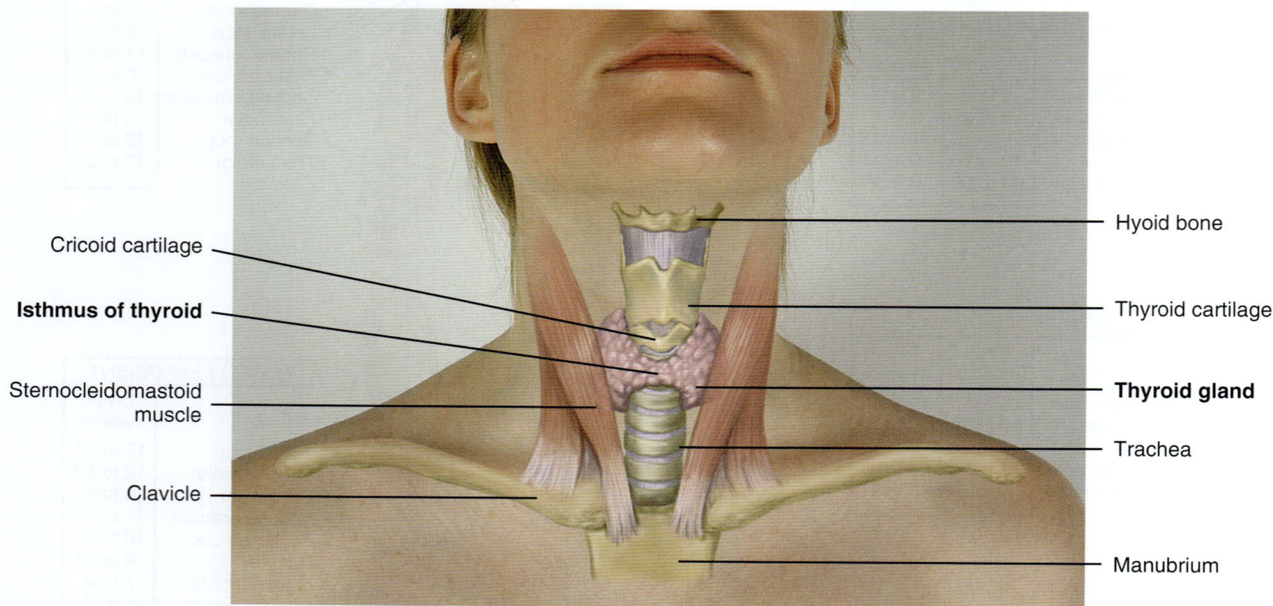

Figure 21.4
Thyroid gland.

cancers and osteoarthritis. More than three in five Australian adults (63%) are considered to be overweight or obese (AIHW 2014a). Twenty-six per cent of children aged 5–17 years are considered to be overweight or obese (AIHW 2014a) and in New Zealand three in 10 adults (31%) of adults and 11% of children were considered to be obese (Ministry of Health 2013). Obesity rates were highest in Pacific adults, where over two-thirds (68%) were obese; one in four Pacific Islander children were obese (27%) and one in five Māori children were obese (19%) (Ministry of Health 2019). For children, overweight is defined as a body mass index (BMI) equal to or greater than the 95th percentile based on age- and gender-specific BMI charts. For adults, overweight is defined as a BMI of 25 or greater, and obesity is defined as a BMI of 30 (AIHW 2014a). Being overweight during childhood and adolescence is associated with increased risk for becoming overweight during adulthood. The incidence of overweight and obesity are more common in people who have a low socioeconomic status (AIHW 2014a, Ministry of Health 2019).

DEVELOPMENTAL CONSIDERATIONS

Infant to school child (birth to 12 years)

The time from birth to 4 months of age is the most rapid period of growth in the life cycle. Although infants lose weight during the first few days of life, birth weight is usually regained by the 7th to 10th day after birth. Thereafter, infants double their birth weight by 4 months and triple it by 1 year of age. Breastfeeding is recommended for full-term infants for the first year of life because breast milk is ideally formulated to promote normal infant growth and development and natural immunity. Although relatively few contraindications to breastfeeding exist, women who are human immunodeficiency virus (HIV) positive should not breastfeed, since HIV can be transmitted through breast milk.

Infants increase their length by 50% during the first year of life and double it by 4 years of age. Brain size also increases very rapidly during infancy and childhood. By age 2 years, the brain has reached 50% of its adult size; by age 4, 75%; and by age 8, 100%. For this reason, infants and children younger than 2 should not drink skim or low-fat milk or be placed on low-fat diets—fat (kilojoules and essential fatty acids) is required for proper growth and central nervous system development.

In the infant, salivation starts at 3 months. The baby will drool periodically for a few months before learning to swallow the saliva. This drooling does not herald the eruption of the first tooth, although many parents think it does.

The teeth, both sets, begin development in utero. Children have 20 **deciduous**, or temporary, teeth. These erupt between 6 months and 24 months of age. All 20 teeth should appear by 2½ years of age. The deciduous teeth are lost beginning at age 6 years through to age 12 years. They are replaced by the permanent teeth, starting with the central incisors. The permanent teeth appear earlier in girls than in boys.

Orofacial clefts describe the incomplete closure of the hard or soft palate of the mouth with or without midline clefting of the upper or lower lip. Clefts are congenital abnormalities arising during development of the oral region. Cleft palate is relatively rare in the Australian population, indicated by rates of around 7.3 per 10,000 live births and even less common in the New Zealand population, at around 5.5 per 10,000 live births (AIHW 2008). The incidence of cleft lip, with or without cleft palate, is somewhat higher in both regions at around 9 per 10,000 births (AIHW 2008). This rate is about 50% higher in Australian Indigenous infants (AIHW 2008).

Adolescent (12 or 13 years to 19 years)

Following a period of slow growth in late childhood, adolescence is characterised by rapid physical growth and endocrine and hormonal changes. Energy and protein requirements increase to meet this demand, and because of bone growth and increasing muscle mass (and, in girls, the onset of menarche), calcium and iron requirements also increase. Typically, these increased requirements cannot be met by three meals per day; therefore, nutritious snacks play an important role in achieving adequate nutrient intake.

In general, boys grow taller and have less body fat than girls. In adolescence, the percentage of body fat increases in females to about 25% and decreases in males (replaced by muscle mass) to about 12%. Typically, girls double their body weight between the ages of 8 and 14; boys double their body weight between the ages of 10 and 17 years.

Adulthood (20 to 64 years)

During adulthood, growth and nutrient needs stabilise. Most adults are in relatively good health. However, lifestyle factors such as cigarette smoking, stress, lack of exercise, excessive alcohol intake and diets high in saturated fat, cholesterol, salt and sugar, and low in fibre can be factors in the development of hypertension, obesity, atherosclerosis, cancer, osteoporosis and diabetes. The adult years, therefore, are an important time for education, to preserve health and to prevent or delay the onset of chronic disease.

Late adulthood (65+ years)

As people age, a number of changes occur that make them prone to under-nutrition or over-nutrition. Poor physical or mental health, social isolation, alcoholism, limited functional ability, poverty and polypharmacy are the major risk factors for malnutrition in older adults (Jaul et al 2018).

Normal physiological changes in late adulthood that directly affect nutritional status include poor dentition, decreased visual acuity, decreased saliva production, slowed gastrointestinal motility, decreased gastrointestinal absorption and diminished olfactory and taste sensitivity. Important nutritional features of the older years are a decrease in energy requirements due to loss of lean body mass, the most metabolically active tissue, and an increase in fat mass.

Socioeconomic conditions frequently have a significant effect on the nutritional status of those in late adulthood. Decline of extended families and increased mobility of families reduce available support systems. Facilities for meal preparation and eating, transportation to grocery stores, physical limitations, income and social isolation are frequent problems and can obviously interfere with the acquisition of a balanced diet. Medications must also be considered, because those in late adulthood frequently take multiple medications that have a potential for interaction with nutrients and with one another.

In the oral cavity, the soft tissues atrophy and the epithelium thins, especially in the cheek and tongue. This results in loss of taste buds, with about an 80% reduction in taste functioning. Further impairments to taste include a decrease in salivary secretion that is needed to dissolve flavouring agents, and the presence of upper dentures that cover secondary taste sites. Atrophic tissues ulcerate easily, which places the older person at risk for infections such as oral moniliasis. An increased risk of malignant oral lesions is also present.

Many dental changes occur with ageing. The tooth surface is abraded. The gums begin to recede and the teeth begin to erode at the gum line. A smooth **V**-shaped cavity forms around the neck of the tooth, exposing the nerve and making the tooth hypersensitive. Some tooth loss may occur from bone resorption (osteoporosis), which decreases the inner tooth structure and its outer support. Natural tooth loss is exacerbated by years of inadequate dental care, decay, poor oral hygiene and cigarette smoking.

If tooth loss occurs, the remaining teeth drift, causing **malocclusion**. The stress of chewing with malocclusing teeth causes further problems: (1) excessive bone resorption with further tooth loss occurs, (2) muscle imbalance results from a mandible and maxilla now out of alignment, which produces muscle spasms, tenderness of muscles of mastication and chronic headaches, and (3) the temporomandibular joint is stressed, leading to osteoarthritis, pain and inability to fully open the mouth.

A diminished sense of taste and smell can decrease the ageing person's interest in food and may contribute to malnutrition. Saliva production decreases; saliva acts as a solvent for food flavours and helps move food around the mouth. Decreased saliva also reduces the mouth's self-cleaning property. The major cause of decreased saliva flow is not the ageing process itself but the use of medications that have anticholinergic effects.

Reduction in or absence of teeth and trouble with mastication encourages older people to eat soft foods (usually high in carbohydrates) and to decrease meat and fresh vegetable intake. This may increase the risk of nutritional deficit for protein, vitamins and minerals.

Pregnancy and lactation

To support the nutritional requirements of the mother and fetus, sufficient kilojoules, protein, vitamins and minerals must be consumed. Weight gain will vary between individuals and can depend on the pre-pregnancy weight and body mass index of the mother. Generally, if a woman's body mass index is between 18.6 and 24.9 (kg/m^2) she is likely to gain 11 to 16 kg. If a woman is underweight (body mass index $<$18.5) she is likely to gain 12.5–18 kg and if she is overweight or obese she is likely to gain 5–11.5 kg. To gain 1 or 2 kg in the first trimester is normal. Women should then gain approximately 400 g per week if in normal weight range, less than 300 g per week if overweight or obese and 500 g per week if underweight. However, the focus should remain on a healthy diet rather than specific weight gain. In addition, dieting during pregnancy is not recommended as this may affect the development of the fetus.

CULTURAL AND SOCIAL CONSIDERATIONS

As foods and eating customs are culturally distinct, each person has a unique cultural heritage that may affect nutritional status. Australia and New Zealand have had a continual influx of immigrants since the time of European settlement. Up until the second half of the 20th century, migrants to Australia and New Zealand were overwhelmingly from the British Isles. They brought with them traditional British and Irish diets. The large-scale arrival of non-British migrants saw new foods enter Australian and New Zealand menus. Migrants from the European continent brought wine, pasta and coffee. The variety of cuisines continued to diversify throughout the latter half of the twentieth century with European, Asian, Middle Eastern and African cuisines commonly found in restaurants and homes, particularly in Australia. Since about 2005, the increased immigration of peoples from Islamic backgrounds, from the African continent in particular, has seen a growing cultural awareness of religious food practices such as halal diets (Table 21.1).

Immigrants commonly maintain traditional eating customs (especially for holidays and observance of religious customs) long after the language and manner of dress of an adopted country have become routine. Occupation, class, religion, gender and health awareness all have a great bearing on eating customs.

Newly arrived immigrants may be at nutritional risk for a variety of reasons. They have frequently emigrated from countries with limited food supplies—caused by poverty, poor sanitation, war or political strife. General under-nutrition, hypertension, diarrhoea, lactose intolerance, osteomalacia (soft bones), scurvy and dental caries are among the more common nutrition-related problems of new immigrants from developing countries. In addition, barriers such as language and cultural differences can further hinder the provision of nutritional information and health promotion among these groups (Lee et al 2013). The best way to learn about the eating patterns of a people is to talk with them, eat with them and ask about their dietary customs.

The cultural factors that must be considered are the cultural definition of food, frequency and number of meals eaten away from home, form and content of ceremonial meals, amount and types of foods eaten and regularity of food consumption.

The 24-hours food history or 3-day food diaries, traditionally used for assessment, may be inadequate when dealing with people from culturally diverse backgrounds. Standard dietary handbooks may fail to provide culture-specific diet information because nutritional content is generally based on Western diets.

Cultural variation in diets can create confusion when completing a health assessment. For example, among Vietnamese migrants, the dietary intake of calcium may appear inadequate, particularly with the low consumption of dairy products common among members of this group. Daily soups prepared by soaking bones in acidified broth or pickled or sweet and sour meats such as pork ribs (vinegar leaches calcium from the bones and makes it available to the body) are, however, commonly consumed, thus providing adequate quantities of calcium to meet daily requirements. Tofu is also a good source of calcium if calcium salts are used to precipitate the curd. In Middle Eastern countries, yoghurt and feta cheese are the major dietary sources of calcium since milk is not commonly consumed by adults. Food itself is only one part of eating. In some cultures, social contacts during meals are restricted to members of the immediate or extended family. For example, in some Middle Eastern cultures, men and women eat meals separately, or women may be permitted to eat with their husbands, but not with other males. Etiquette during meals, the use of hands, type of eating utensils (e.g. chopsticks, special flatware) and protocols

TABLE 21.1 Typical religious dietary practices

RELIGIOUS GROUP	FOOD RESTRICTIONS
Buddhism	All meat
Catholicism	Meat by some denominations on Ash Wednesday, Good Friday and other holy days Alcoholic beverages by some denominations
Hinduism	Beef, pork, and some fowl Alcohol Garlic and onions by some Red-coloured foods (e.g. tomatoes) by some
Islam	All pork and pork products Meat not slaughtered according to ritual Alcoholic beverages and alcohol products (e.g. vanilla extract), coffee and tea Food and beverages before sunset during Ramadan
Mormon	Alcoholic beverages Caffeinated beverages (e.g. coffee, tea, soft drinks) and medicines containing caffeine, stimulants or alcohol (e.g. caffeine-based medications (e.g. NoDoz), some cold and flu medications) Food and beverages on first Sunday of each month
Orthodox Judaism	All pork and pork products Meat not slaughtered according to ritual All shellfish (e.g. crab, lobster, shrimp, oysters) Dairy products and meat at the same meal Leavened bread and cake during Passover Food and beverages on Yom Kippur
Seventh-Day Adventist	All pork and pork products Shellfish Meat, dairy products, and eggs by some Alcoholic beverages, coffee and tea Highly seasoned foods

governing the order in which foods are consumed during a meal all vary cross-culturally.

Australian and New Zealand children generally show good levels of dental health. Australian children particularly appear to have good access to dental care enhancing their good oral health, with two in three Australian and four in five New Zealand children visiting a dentist in each 12-month period (AIHW 2014b, Ministry of Health 2013). The overall incidence of good oral health in children has increased due to factors such as provision of school dental care services, increased access to fluoridated toothpaste and drinking water and improved dental hygiene. However, nearly 50% of children aged 12 years and above have decay in their permanent teeth (AIHW 2014b). Good oral health varies across the population. Children in remote and very rural areas and those from the lowest socioeconomic groups show approximately twice the incidence of decayed, missing or filled teeth of their urban counterparts (AIHW 2014b).

Oral health of adults is also significantly impacted by location and age. Rural residents are twice as likely as city residents to be edentulous which can impact on diet and nutritional status (AIHW 2014b). This percentage significantly increases with age; 5.5% of Australian adults between 45 and 64 years are likely to have no natural teeth, while about 21.1% of adults over 65 have no remaining natural teeth (AIHW 2014b). Compared with Australian adults, New Zealand adults had poorer oral health across a range of clinical oral health indicators, and were also less likely to have visited a dental professional in the previous year (Ministry of Health 2019). The health of teeth and gums is clearly related to access to dental care, with about 49% of city dwellers visiting the dentist regularly compared to 31% of remote area dwellers. This is consistent with the New Zealand experience where poorer oral health and lower dental service attendance rates in adults were found in particular among men, younger adults (aged 25–34 years), Māori, Pacific peoples and people living in areas of higher socioeconomic deprivation (Ministry of Health 2019). Apparent lack of access to regular dental care, together with overall rates of dental decay, seems to impact on levels of *untreated* dental decay. There are several initiatives that have been targeted at improving the oral health of Indigenous Australians, for example the provision of full mouth fluoride varnishes, fissure sealants and clinical services in the Northern Territory (AIHW 2014c).

Overall, however, oral health issues contribute only 0.9 disability-adjusted life years for Australian adults, even though about 600 Australians die each year from oral or oral-related cancers (AIHW 2011). Higher rates of lip and oral cancers are reported in Indigenous people, particularly Indigenous males; often presumed to be associated with higher levels of smoking (AIHW 2011).

Indigenous Australians and Torres Strait Islanders

Prior to European settlement, Indigenous Australians and Torres Strait Islanders lived on traditional diets of native plants and animals which were rich in nutrients and low in fat. Specific diets depended on the area in which the community lived and were affected by seasonal changes. While some groups held permanent settlements, in coastal and river areas, for example, others travelled vast distances seasonally to known food sources. The introduction of high energy and low nutrient modern diets has increased the risk of obesity, cardiovascular disease and diabetes in these and other population groups. Indigenous Australians are six times more likely to have diabetes than the general population, with poor nutrition contributing to morbidity and mortality among Indigenous populations. The persistently poor diet and health status is also attributed to their low socioeconomic status, as food purchases are often restricted to cheap, high energy and nutrient poor foods (Lee et al 2016).

Māori and Pacific Islanders

Like the Indigenous Australian population, the Māori and Pacific peoples existed on a high nutrient, low energy dense diet prior to colonisation. With the settlement of Europeans and urbanisation of New Zealand, the Māori diet and physical activity patterns changed. This led to reduced physical activity and a low nutrient, high energy diet. Māori and Pacific peoples now have a diet higher in fat and lower in vegetables than the general population. Food has a central role in the cultural life of Māori and Pacific peoples and this must be considered when developing approaches to address obesity and nutrition. In addition to the cultural issues, healthy food choices in New Zealand are significantly tied to socioeconomic status. Māori and Pacific peoples are overrepresented in the low socioeconomic groups in New Zealand and this must also be taken into consideration when addressing nutritional issues.

Dietary practices of selected cultural groups

It is necessary to avoid **cultural stereotyping**—the tendency to view individuals of common cultural backgrounds similarly and according to a preconceived notion of how they 'ought' to behave. For example, despite widely held stereotypes, we know that there are Chinese people who do not like rice, Italian people who dislike spaghetti, Irish people who dislike corned beef and cabbage, and so forth. Aggregate dietary preferences among people from certain cultural groups, however, can be described (e.g. characteristic ethnic dishes, methods of food preparation). Cultural food preferences are often interrelated with religious dietary beliefs and practices. Many religions use foods as symbols in celebrations and rituals.

Fasting and other religious observations may limit a person's food or liquid intake during specified times; for example, many Catholics fast and abstain from meat on Ash Wednesday and the Fridays of Lent. Muslims fast from dawn to sunset during the month of Ramadan in the Islamic calendar and eat only twice a day—before dawn and after sunset; Jews observe a 24-hours fast on Yom Kippur.

Knowing the person's religious practices related to food enables you to suggest improvements or modifications that do not conflict with dietary laws. With widespread malnutrition in the hospital or supported care setting, it is imperative that people's cultural food preferences are assessed in order to support optimum nutrition in this unfamiliar environment. Table 21.1 summarises dietary practices for selected religious groups.

PURPOSES AND COMPONENTS OF NUTRITIONAL ASSESSMENT

Nutritional status can be determined by the application of nutritional assessment techniques. In general, these techniques are non-invasive, inexpensive and easy to perform.

The purposes of nutritional assessment are to (1) identify individuals who are malnourished or are at risk of developing malnutrition, (2) provide data for designing a nutrition plan of care that will prevent or minimise the development of malnutrition and (3) establish baseline data for evaluating the efficacy of nutritional care.

Nutrition screening, the first step in assessing nutritional status, may be completed in any setting (e.g. general practice clinic, home, hospital, long-term care). Based on easily obtained data, nutrition screening is a quick and easy way to identify individuals at nutrition risk, such as those with weight loss, inadequate food intake or recent illness. Parameters used for nutrition screening typically include weight and weight history, conditions associated with increased nutritional risk, diet information and routine laboratory data. A variety of valid tools are available for screening different populations. For example, the Malnutrition Universal Screening Tool (MUST) has been validated in many patient groups for use both in the hospital setting as well as in the community (Malnutrition Advisory Group 2013, Morris et al 2018).

Individuals identified at nutritional risk during screening should undergo a **comprehensive nutritional assessment**, which includes dietary history and clinical information, physical examination for clinical signs, anthropometric measures and laboratory tests. The skills needed to collect the clinical and dietary history and to perform the physical examination are described in the Subjective data and Objective data sections that follow.

Various methods for collecting current dietary intake information are available—24-hours food history, food frequency questionnaire and food diary. During hospitalisation, documentation of nutritional intake can best be achieved through a daily food chart which identifies the type as well as the quantity of food consumed.

The easiest and most popular method for obtaining information about dietary intake is the **24-hours food history**. The individual or family member completes a questionnaire or is interviewed and asked to recall everything eaten within the last 24 hours. However, several significant sources of error may occur when this method is used: (1) the individual or family member may not be able to recall the type or amount of food eaten; (2) intake within the last 24 hours may be atypical of usual intake; (3) the individual or family member may alter the truth for a variety of reasons; and (4) snack items and use of gravies, sauces and condiments may be underreported.

To counter some of the difficulties inherent in the 24-hours recall method, a **food frequency questionnaire** may also be completed. With this tool, information is collected on how many times per day, week or month the individual eats particular foods. Drawbacks to the use of the food frequency questionnaire are (1) it does not quantify amount of intake, and (2) like the 24-hours recall, it relies on the individual's or family member's memory for how often a food was eaten.

Food diaries or records require asking the individual or family member to write down everything consumed for a certain period of time. Three days—two weekdays and one weekend day—are customarily used. A food diary is most complete and accurate if the individual is instructed to record information immediately after eating. Potential problems with the food diary include (1) noncompliance, (2) inaccurate recording, (3) atypical intake on the recording days and (4) conscious alteration of diet during the recording period.

Direct observation of the feeding and eating process can lead to detection of problems not readily identified through standard nutrition interviews. For example, observing the typical feeding techniques used by a parent or caregiver and the interaction between the individual and caregiver can be of value when assessing failure to thrive in children or unintentional weight loss in older adults.

The Australian Guide to Healthy Eating and the Summary of Dietary Guidelines for an Adult are examples of guides used to encourage adequate dietary intake (Figure 21.5 and Table 21.2). The Australian and New Zealand Government websites for dietary guidelines are provided to assist the healthcare professional and the client to create individualised nutrition and health plans (see nutrition-related websites below). The plans can be easily adapted to clients with different ages, gender, cultural backgrounds, lifestyles and health problems. For example, the estimated energy requirement for an active 2-year-old boy is 2000 kJ per day compared with 1800 kJ per day for a 2-year-old girl (National Health and Medical Research Council (NHMRC)/Ministry of Health New Zealand 2014).

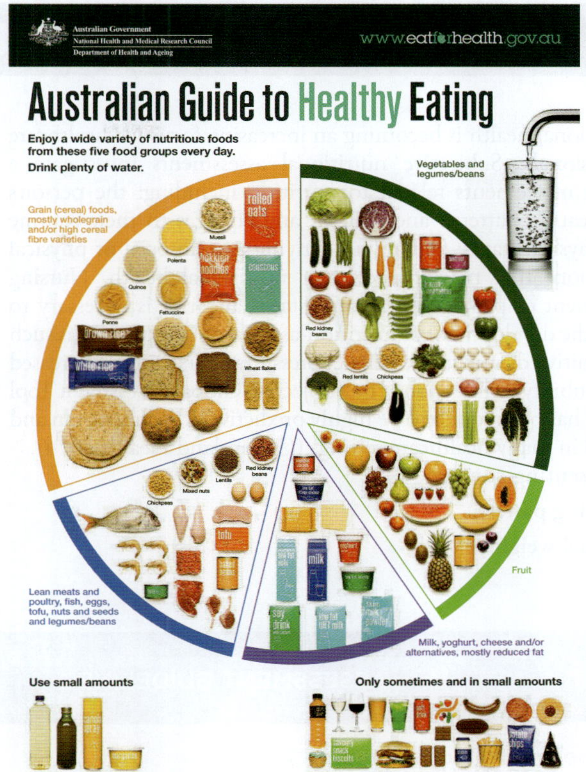

Figure 21.5
Australian Guide to Healthy Eating, National Health and Medical Research Council. ©Commonwealth of Australia 2014, Creative Commons Attribution 3.0 Australia License.

TABLE 21.2 Summary of dietary guidelines for an adult (approximately 8380 kJ per day)
Consume 4 to 7 serves of vegetables each day (e.g. 1 medium potato, 1 cup raw). Choosing a variety of vegetables helps to provide the vitamins, minerals, antioxidants, fibre and carbohydrate that help to keep you healthy.
Consume 2 to 3 serves of fruit each day (e.g. 1 medium piece, 1 cup diced or canned). Choose a variety of fruits.
Consume 4 to 6 serves (e.g. 2 slices of bread, 1 cup rice pasta noodles) of wholegrain products per day. Limit refined carbohydrate (e.g. white bread) to under half of the daily servings.
Consume 2 to 3 serves of low-fat, high calcium milk products (e.g. 1 cup milk, 2 slices of cheese).
Consume 1 to 1.5 serves of meat, fish or eggs (e.g. 65–100 g lean meat, 80–120 g fish, 2 small eggs). Choose meats or other sources of protein that are lean, low-fat or fat-free.
Fats and high sugar foods should be consumed sometimes and in small amounts and limited to 2.5 serves (e.g. 1 tsp butter, 1 can soft drink, ½ small chocolate bar). These foods may be high in fat, salt and sugar. Keep total fat intake to 20% to 35% of energy intake, most from polyunsaturated or monounsaturated fats. Limit intake of saturated fat. Keep *trans* fatty acid consumption as low as possible.
Limit alcohol intake. Men should drink no more than two standard drinks per day and women should aim for no more than one per day (e.g. 1 stubby of beer, 100 mL wine). Alcohol provides little nutrition and adds extra kilojoules.
Consume less than 300 mg/day of cholesterol.
Consume less than 1500 mg (approximately ½ tsp of salt) of sodium per day.
Consume potassium-rich foods, such as fruits and vegetables.
Consume as little added sugar (or other low kJ sweeteners) as possible.
Get at least 30 min of moderate intensity exercise on most days of the week; to lose weight or maintain weight loss, increase to 60–90 min.

Subjective data

Nutritional health is becoming an increasing focus for healthcare professionals. Subjective nutritional assessments investigate a variety of elements related to nutrition including: the person's usual eating patterns and weight; any changes to their routine and physical status; and any underlying psychosocial or physical conditions that may impact their nutritional health. Nursing assessment of people's nutritional status and risk is necessary to avoid the development of nutrition-associated complications such as cognitive dysfunction, fatigue, pressure ulcers and an increased susceptibility to infection. The Subjective Global Assessment Tool (SGA) has been found to be highly predictive of malnutrition and is used in many healthcare settings (Queensland Health 2014).

1. Presenting concern
2. Eating pattern
3. Usual weight
4. Changes in appetite, taste, smell, chewing, swallowing
5. Teeth
6. Recent surgery, burns, trauma, infection
7. Chronic illness
8. Nausea, vomiting, diarrhoea, constipation
9. Food allergies or intolerances
10. Family history
11. Health and lifestyle management

Practice note: Before you commence the assessment, introduce yourself to the person, confirm the person's identity, discuss the purpose and scope of the assessment, clarify any questions the person may have and obtain verbal consent from the person to perform the assessment.

ASSESSMENT GUIDELINES	CLINICAL SIGNIFICANCE AND CLINICAL ALERTS
1. Presenting concern	
Do you feel that you have any problem/s with your nutrition, ability to prepare food and eating? Does this affect your feeling of energy and ability to carry out activities of daily living? It is important to ascertain the person's perception of their nutritional and metabolic function. • If they do perceive a problem—how does this impact on their quality of life?	The person's response to this question will guide areas to focus on in further subjective and objective data collection.
2. Eating patterns	
• Number of meals/snacks per day? • Kind and amount of food eaten? • Fad, special or alternative diets? • Where is food eaten? • Food preferences and dislikes? • Religious or cultural restrictions? • Able to feed self?	Most individuals are knowledgeable about, or interested in, the foods they consume. If misconceptions are present, begin gradual education to enact healthy eating habits. Ethnic/religious beliefs or feeding difficulties may affect intake of certain foods. Alternative diets, if not closely managed, may not be nutritionally adequate.
3. Usual weight	
What is your usual weight? • 20% below or above desirable weight? • Recent weight change? • How much lost or gained? • Over what time period? • Reason for loss or gain?	Persons who have had a recent, unintentional weight loss or who are obese are at nutritional risk. Underweight individuals are vulnerable because their fuel reserves may be depleted. Excess weight is associated with a number of health problems, ranging from hypertension to cancer. Protein and energy needs are often overlooked in acutely ill obese persons.

ASSESSMENT GUIDELINES	CLINICAL SIGNIFICANCE AND CLINICAL ALERTS
4. Changes in appetite, taste, smell, chewing, swallowing	
• Type of change? • When did change occur? • What is current dental and oral health?	**Poor appetite, taste and smell alterations,** as well as chewing and swallowing difficulties, interfere with adequate nutrient intake and increase the likelihood of nutritional risk. **Dysphagia** may occur with cancers in the mouth or oesophagus or neurological conditions such as stroke. **Changes in appetite** associated with weight loss may indicate an increase in metabolic activity such as thyrotoxicosis or diabetes. An increase in appetite with weight gain may indicate the effects of excessive glucocorticoids such as Cushing's syndrome or hypoglycaemia (Talley & O'Connor 2018).
5. Teeth	
• Any toothache? Are your teeth sensitive to heat, cold? Have you lost any teeth?	
6. Recent surgery, trauma, burns, infection	
• When? • Type? • How treated? • Conditions that increase nutrient loss (e.g. draining wounds, effusions, blood loss, dialysis and sepsis)?	Individuals who have had recent surgery, trauma, sepsis or conditions causing nutrient losses may have energy and nutrient needs that are two or three times greater than normal.
7. Chronic illnesses	
• Type? • When diagnosed? • How treated? • Dietary modifications? • Recent cancer chemotherapy or radiation therapy?	Individuals with chronic illnesses that affect nutrient use (e.g. diabetes, pancreatitis, COPD or malabsorption) or those receiving cancer treatment are twice as likely to have nutritional deficits.
8. Nausea, vomiting, diarrhoea, constipation	
• Any problems? • Due to? • How long?	**Gastrointestinal symptoms** such as nausea, vomiting, diarrhoea or constipation may interfere with nutrient intake or absorption. **Diarrhoea** may be associated with hyperactive thyroid function. **Constipation** may be associated with underactive thyroid function (Talley & O'Connor 2018). Any significant changes in bowel function must be further investigated because of the link to bowel cancer. See also Chapter 25.

SUBJECTIVE DATA

ASSESSMENT GUIDELINES	CLINICAL SIGNIFICANCE AND CLINICAL ALERTS
9. Food allergies or intolerances	
• Any problematic foods? • Type of reaction? • How long? • How are food allergies/intolerances managed?	**Food allergies**, especially peanut allergies, are on the rise and a major health concern. Refer to published guidelines for more information on the management of food allergies. **Intolerances** may result in nutrient deficiencies (e.g. diarrhoea after milk ingestion).
10. Family history	
Family or personal history of heart disease, osteoporosis, cancer, gout, GI disorders, obesity, thyroid disorders or diabetes? • Effect of each on eating patterns? • Effect on activity patterns?	**Long-term nutritional deficiencies** or excesses may first become manifest as disease, such as these common examples during the adult years. Early identification of nutritional alterations permits dietary and activity modifications to occur promptly—at a time when the body can recover more fully.
11. Health and lifestyle management	
Meals • Meal preparation facilities? • Transportation for travel to the supermarket? • Adequate income for food purchase? • Who prepares meals and does shopping? • Environment during mealtimes?	Socioeconomic factors may interfere with the ability to purchase a range and amount of food necessary for an adequate diet.
Medications and/or nutritional supplements • Prescription medications? • Nonprescription? • Use over a 24-hours period?	Analgesics, antacids, anticonvulsants, antibiotics, diuretics, laxatives, antineoplastic drugs, steroids and oral contraceptives are among the drugs that can interact with nutrients, impairing their digestion, absorption, metabolism or utilisation.
Type of vitamin/mineral supplement? • Amount? Duration of use? • Herbal and botanical products? Specific type/brand and where obtained? How often used? Who recommended? How does it help you? Any problems?	**Vitamin/mineral supplements** may cause harmful side effects if taken in large amounts. Use of **herbal/botanical supplements** is commonly not reported, so ask about intake and discuss proper use and potential adverse effects. Complementary and alternative medicines can have interactions with other medications; for information refer to National Center for Complementary and Alternative Medicine website (see websites list at end of chapter).

ASSESSMENT GUIDELINES	CLINICAL SIGNIFICANCE AND CLINICAL ALERTS
Smoking, alcohol or non-prescription drug use • When was last drink of alcohol? • Units of alcohol consumed at that time? • Unit of alcohol consumed each day? Each week? • Duration of use? • (Repeat questions for each drug used.) With regard to smoking: • What do you smoke? • How many each day? • How long have you smoked? • Have you ever tried to give up smoking? • How long since you smoked?	These agents are often substituted for nutritious foods and increase requirements for some nutrients. Also, pregnant women who smoke, drink alcohol or use non-prescription drugs give birth to a disproportionate number of infants with low birth weights, failure to thrive and other serious complications. Chronic tobacco use is associated with tooth loss and decay and periodontal disease. Chronic tobacco use combined with heavy alcohol consumption increases risk of oral and pharyngeal cancers.
Exercise and activity patterns • Amount? • Type? • Lethargy or poor exercise tolerance? • Excessive sweating?	**Kilojoule and nutrient needs** increase with increased activity and exercise, especially competitive sports and manual labour. Inactive or sedentary lifestyles often lead to excess weight gain. **Lethargy** is a common symptom of many health problems; for example hypothyroidism, diabetes, anaemia, cardiac or renal failure (Talley & O'Connor 2018). Excessive sweating can indicate a number of metabolic disorders including hypothyroidism and hypoglycaemia (Talley & O'Connor 2018).
Additional subjective data for infants and children (questions for parents or guardians)	
Dietary histories of infants and children are generally obtained from the child's parents, guardian, babysitter or daycare centre. Usually, the person responsible for food preparation is able to provide a fairly accurate dietary history. Having the caregivers keep a thorough daily food diary or asking the caregiver to recall the nutritional intake over the previous 24 hours during clinic visits are the most commonly employed techniques for this population group.	
Gestational nutrition. • Maternal history of alcohol or illegal drug use? • Any diet-related complications during gestation? • Infant's birth weight? • Any evidence of delayed physical or mental growth?	**Low birth weight** (< 2500 g) is a major factor in infant morbidity and mortality. Poor gestational nutrition, low maternal weight gain and maternal alcohol and drug use—all factors in low birth weight—can lead to birth defects and delayed growth and development. Similarly, maternal history of gestational diabetes may affect the infant's blood glucose levels in the early neonatal period.
Infant breastfed or bottle fed. • Type, frequency, amount and duration of feeding? • Any difficulties encountered? • Timing and method of weaning?	Well-nourished infants are more likely to have appropriate physical and social growth and development. Inexperienced mothers may have problems with breastfeeding or bottle-feeding or have questions about whether the infant is receiving adequate amounts of food.

SUBJECTIVE DATA

ASSESSMENT GUIDELINES	CLINICAL SIGNIFICANCE AND CLINICAL ALERTS
Child's willingness to eat what you prepare. • Any special likes or dislikes? • How much will child eat? • How do you control non-nutritious snack foods? • How do you avoid food aspiration?	The preschool period is one of increasing growth and is the period when lifelong food habits form. Use of small portions, finger foods, simple meals and nutritious snacks are strategies to improve dietary intake. Avoid foods likely to be aspirated (e.g. hot dogs, nuts, grapes, round sweets and popcorn).
Teeth. • Did the child's teeth erupt about on time? • Do the teeth seem straight to you? • Is the child using a bottle? How often during the day? Does the child go to sleep with a bottle at night? • Have you noticed any thumb sucking after secondary teeth came in? • Have you noticed the child grinding their teeth?	Delayed eruption may impair nutrition. Prolonged use of the bottle increases risk for tooth decay and middle ear infections. Prolonged thumb sucking (after age 6–7 years) may affect occlusion. Bruxism usually occurs in sleep from dental problems, nervous tension.
Self-care behaviours. • Does the child use a toothbrush regularly? • How often does the child see a dentist? • Is the water fluoridated?	Evaluate child's self-care. Early self-care has best compliance.
Additional subjective data for the adolescent	
Your present weight. • What would you like to weigh? • How do you feel about your present weight? • On any special diet to lose weight? • On other diets to lose weight? If so, were they successful? • Constantly think about 'feeling fat'? • Intentionally vomit or use laxatives or diuretics after eating?	**Obesity**, particularly in girls, may precipitate fad dieting and malnutrition. Because of adolescents' increased body awareness and self-consciousness, they are prone to eating disorders (anorexia nervosa or bulimia), conditions in which the real or perceived body image does not compare favourably to an ideal image found in advertisements or pictures of fashion models.
Use of anabolic steroids or other agents to increase muscle size and physical performance? • When? • How much? • Any problems?	Once confined to male professional athletes, the use of anabolic steroids and other performance-enhancing agents now extends to secondary school and university or TAFE in both males and females. Adverse effects include personality disorders (aggressiveness), liver and other organ damage.
• Use of caffeinated, energy boosting drinks? When? Type? Duration?	Energy boosting drinks like Red Bull, V or XS may contain large amounts of caffeine, other stimulants and/or herbal products. Side effects include dehydration, dangerously high blood pressure and heart rate and sleep problems.
What snacks or fast foods do you like to eat? • When? • How much?	An accurate dietary history may be difficult because of between-meal snacks and meals eaten on the run. These are often omitted or forgotten during the interview or in a food diary.
Age first started menstruating. • What is your menstrual flow like?	Menarche is usually delayed if malnutrition is present. Likewise, amenorrhoea or scant menstrual flow is associated with nutritional deficiency.

ASSESSMENT GUIDELINES	CLINICAL SIGNIFICANCE AND CLINICAL ALERTS
Additional subjective data for the pregnant woman	
How many times have you been pregnant? • When? • Any problems encountered during previous pregnancies? • Problems this pregnancy?	A multiparous mother with pregnancies occurring less than 1 year apart has an increased chance of depleted nutritional reserves. Note previous complications of pregnancy (excessive vomiting, anaemia or gestational diabetes). Slower gastrointestinal motility and pressure from the fetus may cause constipation, haemorrhoids and indigestion. A past history of a low-birth-weight infant suggests past nutritional problems. Giving birth to an infant weighing 4.5 kg or more may signal *latent* diabetes in the mother.
What foods do you prefer when pregnant? • What foods do you avoid? • Crave any particular foods?	The expectant mother is vulnerable to familial, cultural and traditional influences for food choices. Cravings for or aversions to particular foods are common; evaluate for their potential contribution to, or interference with, dietary intake. There are certain foods that should be avoided; for more information, see the Food Standards Australia and New Zealand website in the website list below.
Additional subjective data for middle adulthood (40–64 years)	
Menstrual history, menopausal symptoms Onset of symptoms (irregular period, hot flushes, sleep disturbance, anxiety, etc.)	Normal changes to ovarian function can cause significant symptoms which can affect quality of life. See Chapter 26 for detailed assessment.
Additional subjective data for the adult over 65 years	
How does your diet differ from when you were in your 40s and 50s? • Why? • What factors affect the way you eat?	Note any physiological or psychological changes or socioeconomic changes that affect nutritional status.
Older adults (particularly those over 75 years of age) and adults who have chronic health problems are particularly at risk of malnutrition.	The Nutritional Risk Screening and Monitoring Tool consists of 10 trigger questions for nutrition screening of the older person. This nutrition checklist identifies major risk factors and indicators of poor nutritional status.
Taste, smell and chewing. • Any dryness in the mouth? Are you taking any medications? • Have you had any loss of teeth? Can you chew all types of food? • Are you able to care for your own teeth or dentures? • Have you noticed a change in your sense of taste or smell?	**Xerostomia** (dry mouth) is a side effect of many drugs: antidepressants, anticholinergics, antihypertensives, antipsychotics, bronchodilators. Self-care may be decreased by disabilities such as arthritis, vision impairment, confusion or depression. Some people add extra salt or sugar to enhance food when taste begins to wane. Diminished smell may decrease the person's ability to detect food spoilage, gas leaks or smoke from a fire.

SUBJECTIVE DATA

Objective data

Observation of an individual's appearance—obese, cachectic (fat and muscle wasting) or oedematous—provides an overall indication of a person's nutritional status. In addition, a variety of objective screening tests are used to guide nutritional intervention. Body mass index, the Malnutrition Universal Screening tool and the Subjective Global Assessment are commonly used to screen for nutritional risk. In addition to these tools, specific clinical signs can indicate nutritional deficiencies, most prominently seen in areas in which rapid turnover of epithelial tissue occurs—skin, hair, mouth, lips and eyes. These signs, however, may not be nutritional in origin and consequently laboratory testing can assist in nutritional investigation and diagnosis. Laboratory tests for assessment of nutritional status are reviewed later in this chapter. Refer to Chapter 22 for details of objective assessment of skin, hair and nails.

Equipment needed

Measuring tape
Pen or pencil
Nutritional assessment forms
Hand hygiene solution

PROCEDURES AND NORMAL FINDINGS	ABNORMAL FINDINGS AND CLINICAL ALERTS
General inspection	
During collection of subjective data you will have noticed the condition of the person's skin, lips, hair and mucous membranes, breath odour, ease of breathing, height to weight ratio, body shape, level of hygiene and grooming and general demeanor. All of these factors provide clues to the person's nutrition and metabolic health.	
Anthropometric measures	
Anthropometry is the measurement and evaluation of growth, development and body composition. The most commonly used anthropometric measures for registered nurses are height, weight and waist-to-hip ratio. Measurement of height, weight and head circumference is described in Chapter 10.	
Derived weight measures	
Three derived weight measures are used to depict changes in body weight.	
Body weight as a percentage of ideal body weight is calculated using the following formula:	
$$\text{Percentage ideal body weight} = \frac{\text{Current weight}}{\text{Ideal weight}} \times 100$$	A current weight of 80% to 90% of ideal weight suggests mild malnutrition; 70% to 80%, moderate malnutrition; and <70%, severe malnutrition.
The **per cent usual body weight** is calculated as follows: $$\text{Percentage usual body weight} = \frac{\text{Current weight}}{\text{Ideal weight}} \times 100$$	A current weight of 85% to 95% of usual body weight indicates mild malnutrition; 75% to 84%, moderate malnutrition; and <75%, severe malnutrition.
Recent weight change is calculated using the following formula: $$\frac{\text{Usual weight} - \text{Current weight}}{\text{Usual weight}} \times 100$$	An unintentional loss of >5% of body weight over 1 month, >7.5% of body weight over 3 months or >10% of body weight over 6 months is clinically significant.

PROCEDURES AND NORMAL FINDINGS	ABNORMAL FINDINGS AND CLINICAL ALERTS
Body Mass Index (BMI)	
Body mass index is a practical marker of optimal weight for height and an indicator of obesity or protein–kilojoule malnutrition. It is calculated by: $$\text{Body mass index} = \frac{\text{Weight (in kilograms)}}{\text{Height (in metres)}^2}$$	BMI interpretation for adults (World Health Organization (WHO), 2015a): <18.5 Underweight 18.5–24.99 Normal weight ≥25.0 Overweight ≥30.0 Obesity ≥40 Obesity class III
Waist-to-hip ratio	
The **waist-to-hip ratio** assesses body fat distribution as an indicator of health risk. Obese persons with a greater proportion of fat in the upper body, especially in the abdomen, are described as presenting with android obesity; obese persons with most of their fat in the hips and thighs are described as presenting with gynoid obesity. The equation to calculate waist-to-hip ratio is: $$\text{Waist-to-hip} = \frac{\text{Waist circumference}}{\text{Hip circumference}}$$ where **waist circumference (WC)** is measured in centimetres at the smallest circumference below the rib cage and above the umbilicus (Figure 21.6), and hip circumference is measured in centimetres at the largest circumference of the buttocks. In addition, waist circumference alone can be used to predict greater health risk. 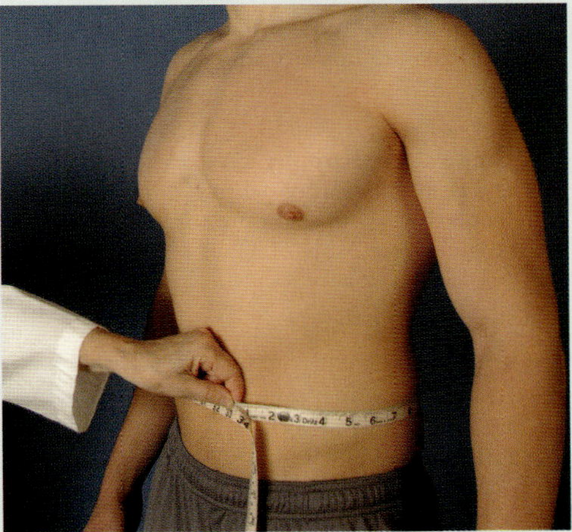 **Figure 21.6** Waist circumference.	A **waist-to-hip ratio** of ≥1.0 in men or ≥0.8 in women is indicative of android (upper body obesity) and increasing risk for obesity-related diseases and early mortality. A WC >88 cm in women and >102 cm in men increases risk of cardiovascular and metabolic diseases. For people of Asian or Aboriginal or Torres Strait Islander descent a WC >80 cm in women and >90 cm in men increases risk of cardiovascular and metabolic diseases (Royal Australian College of General Practitioners and Diabetes Australia 2016).
Inspect the mouth	
Begin with anterior structures and move posteriorly. Use a tongue blade to retract structures and a bright light for optimal visualisation.	
Lips	
Inspect the lips for colour, moisture, cracking or lesions. Retract the lips and note their inner surface as well (Figure 21.7).	**Cherry red lips** may be observed in ketoacidosis. **Cheilitis** (perlèche)—cracking at the corners (see Table 21.6).

OBJECTIVE DATA

PROCEDURES AND NORMAL FINDINGS	ABNORMAL FINDINGS AND CLINICAL ALERTS
Figure 21.7 Lips.	
Teeth and gums	
The condition of the teeth is an index of the person's general health. Your examination should not replace the regular dental examination, but you should note any diseased, absent, loose or abnormally positioned teeth. The teeth normally look white, straight and evenly spaced and clean and free of debris or decay.	Discoloured teeth appear brown with excessive fluoride use, yellow with tobacco use.
Compare the number of teeth with the number expected for the person's age. Ask the person to bite as if chewing something and note alignment of upper and lower jaw. Normal occlusion in the back is the upper teeth resting directly on the lowers; in the front, the upper incisors slightly override the lower incisors.	**Grinding** down of tooth surface. **Plaque**—soft debris. **Caries**—decay. **Malocclusion** (poor biting relationship), protrusion of upper or lower incisors (see Table 21.7).
Normally, the gums look pink or coral with a stippled (dotted) surface. The gum margins at the teeth are tight and well defined. Check for swelling; retraction of gingival margins; and spongy, bleeding or discoloured gums. Dark-skinned people normally may have a dark melanotic line along the gingival margin.	**Gingival hypertrophy**, crevices between teeth and gums, pockets of debris. Gums bleed with slight pressure, indicating gingivitis (see Table 21.7).
Tongue	
Check the tongue for colour, surface characteristics and moisture. The colour is pink and even. The dorsal surface is normally roughened from the papillae. A thin white coating may be present. Ask the person to touch the tongue to the roof of the mouth. Its ventral surface looks smooth, glistening, and shows veins. Saliva is present. If the person is able to move their own tongue ask them to move it so you can visualise the ventral and lateral surfaces. Inspect for any white patches or lesions—normally none are present. If any occur, palpate these lesions for induration.	**Beefy red swollen tongue.** Smooth glossy areas (see Table 21.8). **Enlarged tongue** occurs with mental retardation, hypothyroidism, acromegaly; a small tongue accompanies malnutrition. **Dry mouth** occurs with dehydration, fever; tongue has deep vertical fissures. **Saliva** is decreased while the person is taking anticholinergic and other medication. **Excess saliva** and drooling occur with gingivostomatitis and neurological dysfunction.
If the person is unconscious or otherwise unable to move their tongue on demand, with a gloved hand hold the tongue with a cotton gauze pad for traction and swing the tongue out and to each side (Figure 21.8).	

PROCEDURES AND NORMAL FINDINGS	ABNORMAL FINDINGS AND CLINICAL ALERTS
Figure 21.8 Tongue.	
Inspect carefully the entire **U**-shaped area under the tongue behind the teeth. Oral malignancies are most likely to develop here. Note any white patches, nodules or ulcerations. If lesions are present, or with any person over 50 years old or with a positive history of smoking or alcohol use, use your gloved hand to palpate the area. Place your other hand under the jaw to stabilise the tissue and to 'capture' any abnormality (Figure 21.9). Note any induration. 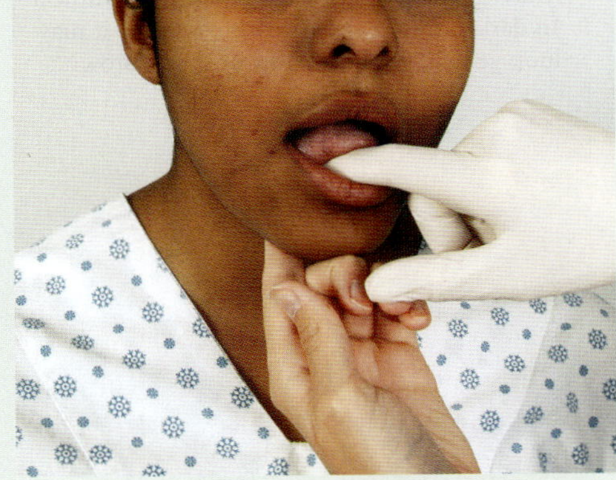 **Figure 21.9** Under tongue.	***Clinical alert:*** Any lesion or ulcer persisting for more than 2 weeks must be investigated. An indurated area may be a mass or lymphadenopathy, and it must be investigated.
Buccal mucosa	
Hold the cheek open with a tongue blade, and check the buccal mucosa for colour, nodules or lesions. It looks pink, smooth and moist, although patchy hyperpigmentation is common and normal in dark-skinned people.	Dappled brown patches are present with Addison's disease (chronic adrenal insufficiency).
An expected finding is **Stensen's duct**, the opening of the parotid salivary gland. It looks like a small dimple opposite the upper second molar. You also may see a raised occlusion line on the buccal mucosa parallel with the level the teeth meet. This is caused by the teeth closing against the cheek.	Orifice of Stensen's duct looks red with mumps. **Koplik's spots**—early prodromal (early warning) sign of measles (see Table 21.9).

PROCEDURES AND NORMAL FINDINGS	ABNORMAL FINDINGS AND CLINICAL ALERTS
A larger patch also may be present along the buccal mucosa. This is **leuco-oedema**, a benign greyish opaque area, more common in dark-skinned people. When it is mild, the patch disappears as you stretch the cheeks. The severity of the condition increases with age, looking greyish white and thickened. The cause of the condition is unknown. Do not mistake leuco-oedema for oral infections such as candidiasis (thrush).	
Fordyce's granules are small, isolated white or yellow papules on the mucosa of cheek, tongue and lips (Figure 21.10). These little sebaceous cysts are painless and not significant. 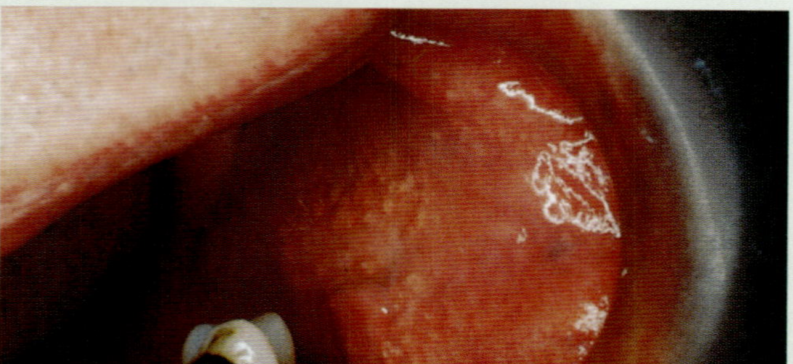 **Figure 21.10** Fordyce's granules.	The chalky white raised patch of **leucoplakia** is abnormal (see Table 21.9).
Palate	
Shine your light up to the roof of the mouth. The more anterior hard palate is white with irregular transverse rugae. The posterior soft palate is pinker, smooth and upwardly movable. A normal variation is a nodular bony ridge down the middle of the hard palate, a **torus palatinus** (Figure 21.11). This benign growth arises after puberty in some people. Figure 21.12 uses a mirror to reflect the image of the torus palatinus, which actually lies in the roof of the mouth. 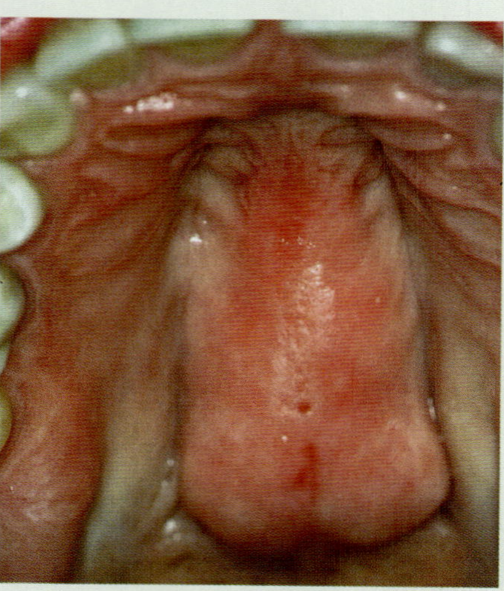 **Figure 21.11** Torus palatinus.	The hard palate appears yellow with jaundice. In dark-skinned people with jaundice, it may look yellow, muddy yellow or green-brown.

OBJECTIVE DATA

PROCEDURES AND NORMAL FINDINGS	ABNORMAL FINDINGS AND CLINICAL ALERTS
Observe the uvula; it normally looks like a fleshy pendant hanging in the midline (Figure 21.12). Ask the person to say 'ahhh' and note the soft palate and uvula rise in the midline. This tests one function of cranial nerve X, the vagus nerve. 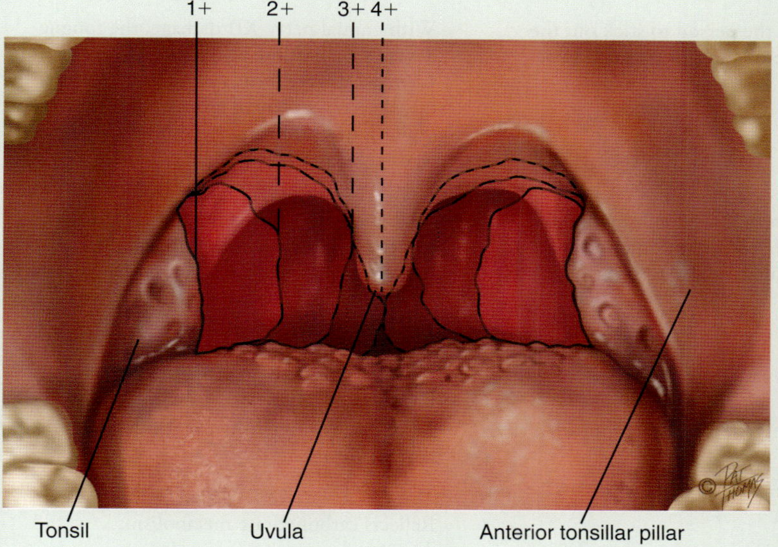 **Figure 21.12** Uvula. © Pat Thomas, 2006	A **bifid** uvula looks like it is split in two (see Table 18.2). Any deviation to the side or absent movement indicates nerve damage, which might occur following a stroke or head injury. ***Clinical alert***: this finding may indicate dysphagia. Further assessment of swallowing ability is required.
Inspect the throat	
Enlarge your view of the posterior pharyngeal wall by depressing the tongue with a tongue blade (Figure 21.13). Push down halfway back on the tongue. Press slightly off centre to avoid eliciting the gag reflex. You can help the person whose gag reflex is easily triggered by offering a tongue blade to depress their own tongue. 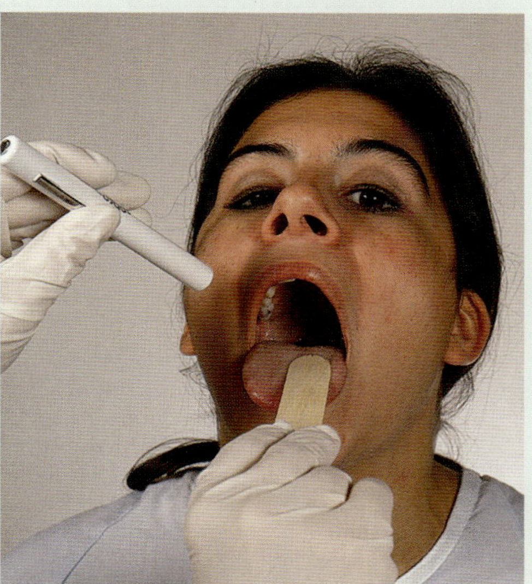 **Figure 21.13** Throat.	Acute tonsillitis may affect appetite and nutritional intake. ***Clinical alert:*** a person who does not have a gag reflex should be nil by mouth to avoid respiratory compromise.

OBJECTIVE DATA

PROCEDURES AND NORMAL FINDINGS	ABNORMAL FINDINGS AND CLINICAL ALERTS
Although usually it is not done in the screening examination, touching the posterior wall with the tongue blade elicits the gag reflex. This tests cranial nerves IX and X, the glossopharyngeal and vagus.	Part of swallowing assessment.
Test cranial nerve XII, the hypoglossal nerve, by asking the person to stick out the tongue. It should protrude in the midline. Note any tremor, loss of movement or deviation to the side.	With cranial nerve XII damage, the tongue deviates *towards* the paralysed side. ***Clinical alert:*** this finding may indicate a raised risk of potential airway compromise and aspiration. Further assessment of swallow and airway patency is required.
During the examination, notice any breath odour, *halitosis*. This is common and usually is due to a local cause, such as poor oral hygiene, consumption of odoriferous foods, alcohol consumption, heavy smoking or dental infection. Occasionally, it may indicate a systemic disease.	**Diabetic ketoacidosis** has a sweet, fruity breath odour; this acetone smell also occurs in children with malnutrition or dehydration. Others are an ammonia breath odour with uraemia; a musty odour with liver disease; a foul, fetid odour with dental or respiratory infections; alcohol odour with alcohol ingestion or chemicals.
Blood glucose monitoring	
Blood glucose levels (BGL) Blood glucose monitoring is a test to identify blood glucose concentration. The test is performed by a finger prick. The blood sample is applied to a disposable test-strip which is inserted into a testing monitor for a calculation of the level of glucose. Because of the wide range of technologies to perform this test, it is important to be familiar with how to use available equipment, including calibration of equipment.	Reflects carbohydrate metabolism. Test may be used: • as a screening measure • to monitor blood glucose levels of people who are at risk of hyper/hypoglycaemia • to monitor the effectiveness of insulin therapy. Normal levels 4.0–6.0 mmol/L before meals 4.0–8.0 mmol/L 2 hours after meals Any random level over 5.5 mmol/L requires further investigation.
Additional objective data for infants, children and adolescents (birth to 19 years)	
Weight. During infancy, childhood and adolescence, height and weight should be measured at regular intervals, because longitudinal growth is one of the best indices of nutritional status over time.	
Body mass index. Determination of body mass index may be useful in evaluating childhood and teenage over- or under-nutrition.	
Mouth and throat. A normal finding in infants is the **sucking tubercle**, a small pad in the middle of the upper lip from friction of breast- or bottle-feeding. Note the number of teeth and whether it is appropriate for the child's age. Also note pattern of eruption, position, condition and hygiene. Use this guide for children under 2 years old; the child's age in months minus the number 6 should equal the expected number of deciduous teeth. Normally, all 20 deciduous teeth are in by 2½ years. Saliva is present after 3 months of age and shows in excess with teething children.	No teeth by age 1 year. Discoloured teeth appear yellow or yellow-brown with infants taking tetracycline or whose mothers took the drug during the last trimester; appear green or black with excessive iron ingestion, although this reverses when the iron is stopped. **Malocclusion:** upper or lower dental arches are out of alignment.
Mobility should allow the tongue to extend at least as far as the alveolar ridge.	**Ankyloglossia**, a short lingual frenulum, can limit protrusion and impair speech development (see Table 21.5).

PROCEDURES AND NORMAL FINDINGS	ABNORMAL FINDINGS AND CLINICAL ALERTS
Note any bruising or laceration on the buccal mucosa or gums of the infant or young child.	Trauma may indicate child abuse from forced feeding of bottle or spoon.
Bednar aphthae are traumatic areas or ulcers on the posterior hard palate on either side of the midline. They result from abrasions while sucking.	
Insert your gloved finger into the baby's mouth and palpate the hard and soft palate as the baby sucks. The sucking reflex can be elicited in infants up to 12 months old.	
Additional objective data for the pregnant woman	
Gum hypertrophy (surface looks smooth and stippling disappears) may occur normally at puberty or during pregnancy (pregnancy gingivitis).	
Weight. Height and weight are measured on the first antenatal visit and BMI calculated. Further weight measurements are offered at subsequent visits. See Chapter 29.	Consider the expectant mother at nutritional risk if her weight is 10% or more below ideal or 20% or more above the norm for her height and age group.
Additional objective data for the adults over 65 years	
In the edentulous person the mouth and lips fold in, giving a 'purse-string' appearance. The teeth may look slightly yellowed, although the colour is uniform. Yellowing results from the dentin visible through worn enamel. The surface of the incisors may show vertical cracks from a lifetime of exposure to extreme temperatures. The teeth may look longer as the gum margins recede.	
The surfaces may look worn down or abraded. Old dental work deteriorates, especially at the gum margins. The teeth loosen with bone resorption and may move with palpation.	
The tongue looks smoother as a result of papillary atrophy. The older adult's buccal mucosa is thinned and may look shinier, as though it was 'varnished'.	
Height. With age, height declines in both men and women very slowly from the early 30s, leading to an average 2.9 cm loss in men and 4.9 cm loss in women. Height measures may not be accurate in individuals confined to a bed or wheelchair or those over 65 years of age (because of osteoporotic changes). Therefore, arm span (see below), which is correlated with height, may be a better measure for older people.	Body mass index and waist-to-hip ratio are better indicators of obesity in this age group.
Laboratory studies	
Routine laboratory tests are objective, can detect preclinical nutritional deficiencies and can be used to confirm subjective findings. Use caution, however, when interpreting test results that may be outside normal ranges, because they do not always reflect a nutritional problem and because standards for persons in late adulthood have not yet been firmly established.	
Haemoglobin. The haemoglobin determination is used to detect iron deficiency anaemia. Normal values are as follows: **infants**, 1 to 3 days—145 to 225 g/L, 2 months—90 to 140 g/L; **children**, 6 to 12 years—115 to 155 g/L; **adults**, males—140 to 180 g/L, females—120 to 160 g/L.	**Increased haemoglobin** levels suggest haemoconcentration due to polycythaemia vera or dehydration. **Decreased haemoglobin** levels may indicate anaemia, recent haemorrhage or haemodilution caused by fluid retention.

OBJECTIVE DATA

PROCEDURES AND NORMAL FINDINGS	ABNORMAL FINDINGS AND CLINICAL ALERTS
Haematocrit. Haematocrit, a measure of cell volume, is also an indicator of iron status. Normal values are as follows: **infants**, 1 to 3 days—44% to 72%, 2 months—28% to 42%; **children**, 6 to 12 years—35% to 45%; **adults**, males—37% to 49%, females—36% to 46%.	A high **haematocrit** can indicate dehydration and subsequent concentration of the blood. A low value indicates insufficient haemoglobin formation, thus haematocrit and haemoglobin values should be interpreted together.
Blood glucose (plasma, serum or whole blood) Laboratory measurement of blood glucose levels is more accurate than finger prick methods. This test may be taken while person is fasting or at random.	**Hypoglycaemia** may indicate imbalance between kilojoule intake, exercise and insulin levels. **Hyperglycaemia** may indicate diabetes. Blood levels: *Fasting*: 3.0–5.4 mmol/L >2 hours after eating (post-prandial) *Random*: 3.0–7.7 mmol/L
Cholesterol. Total cholesterol is measured to evaluate fat metabolism and to assess the risk of cardiovascular disease. Normal cholesterol concentrations vary with age and gender. Normal cholesterol is below 4.0 mmol/L, while the ratio between low density lipoproteins and high density lipoproteins should be less than 4 (i.e. LDL:HDL = <4).	Coronary artery disease risk steadily increases as serum cholesterol rises. **Serum cholesterol** levels of 5.5–6.5 mmol/L (borderline high) are associated with moderate risk and 6.5 mmol/L or more (high) with high risk of coronary artery disease, heart attack, stroke and peripheral vascular disease.
Triglycerides. Serum triglycerides (TGs) are used to screen for hyperlipidaemia and to determine the risk of coronary artery disease. Triglyceride values are age related. Some controversy exists over the most appropriate normal ranges, but the following are fairly widely accepted: **ages 0 to 19**—0.11 to 1.13 mmol/L; **ages 20 to 65**—0.45 to 2.26 mmol/L.	**Serum TG levels** are also associated with coronary artery disease and are categorised as *borderline*, 0.5–1.7 mmol/L, or *high*, more than 1.7 mmol/L.
Vitamin D: essential for bone and muscle health and regulating the immune system and cell activity. Vitamin D is required for effective absorption of calcium. A serum 25-hydroxyvitamin D (25-OHD) level of ≥ 50 nmol/L at the end of winter (10–20 nmol/L higher at the end of summer) (Malacova et al 2019).	**Low vitamin D:** associated with rickets and osteoporosis, bone and muscle pain.
Total lymphocyte count. The most commonly used tests of immune function are total lymphocyte count (TLC) and skin testing, also called delayed cutaneous hypersensitivity testing. TLC is an important indicator of visceral protein status and therefore of cellular immune function.	
The TLC is derived from the white blood cell count (WBC) and the differential count: $$\text{TLC} = \frac{\text{Number of lymphocytes in differential}}{100 \text{ cells}}$$ where TLC is calculated in cells per cubic millimetre. Normal values for all age categories are between 1800 and 3000 cells/mm^3.	Non-nutritional factors that affect TLC include hypoalbuminaemia, metabolic stress (e.g. major surgery, trauma and sepsis), infection, cancer and chronic diseases. **Total lymphocyte** counts of 1500–1800 indicate mild lymphocyte depletion; 900–1500, moderate depletion; and less than 900, severe depletion.
Skin testing. Adequate immunity can also be demonstrated by a positive reaction to multiple skin test antigens. In these tests of immune function, at least six antigens are injected intradermally in the forearm area, and the response (redness and/or induration) is noted at 24 and 48 hours. A 5 mm or greater response to more than one antigen is generally considered to be a positive reaction (i.e. indicative of adequate immunity). Commonly used antigens include *Candida*, tetanus toxoid, diphtheria toxoid, streptococcus, old tuberculin, proteus and trichophyton.	A response of <5 mm indicates anergy or immune-incompetence. Anergy occurs with malnutrition, hepatic failure, infection and immunosuppressive drugs (e.g. chemotherapy agents, steroids). **Lymphocytopenia** and the lack of a positive response to skin test antigens increase the risk of infection and sepsis.

PROCEDURES AND NORMAL FINDINGS	ABNORMAL FINDINGS AND CLINICAL ALERTS
Serum proteins. Serum albumin is another common measurement of visceral protein status. Because of its relatively long half-life (17–20 days) and large body pool (4.0–5.0 g/kg), albumin is not an early indicator of protein malnutrition. Normal serum albumin concentration in infants and children older than 6 months and adults ranges from 35 to 55 g/L.	**Low serum albumin** < levels occur with protein–kilojoule malnutrition, altered hydration status and decreased liver function. A serum albumin level of 28–35 g/L represents moderate visceral protein depletion, and <28 g/L denotes severe depletion (Grodner 2019).
Levels of **serum transferrin**, an iron-transport protein, can be measured directly or by an indirect measurement of total iron-binding capacity. Serum transferrin, with a half-life of 8–10 days, may be a more sensitive indicator of visceral protein status than albumin. The most widely used formula for computing serum transferrin is $\text{Serum transferrin} = (0.8 \times \text{Total iron-binding capacity}) - 43$ The normal values for serum transferrin are 1.7 to 2.5 g/L.	Levels of 1.5 to 1.7 g/L suggest mild protein deficiency; 1.0 to 1.5 g/L, moderate deficiency; and levels less than 1.0 g/L, severe deficiency (Royal Australian College of Pathologists 2019). Because many clinical conditions can alter serum albumin and transferrin levels, consider the person's history in conjunction with these values for accurate interpretation.
Prealbumin, or thyroxin-binding prealbumin, serves as a transport protein for thyroxine (T_4) and retinol-binding protein. With a shorter half-life (48 hours) than either albumin or transferrin, prealbumin is sensitive to acute changes in protein status and sudden demands on protein synthesis. Normal prealbumin levels range from 150 to 250 mg/L.	**Prealbumin levels** are elevated in renal disease and reduced by surgery, trauma, burns and infection. Prealbumin levels of 100–150 mg/L indicate mild depletion; 50–100 mg/L, moderate depletion; and less than 50 mg/L, severe depletion.
C-reactive protein (CRP), a plasma protein marker of inflammatory status produced by the liver, is used to monitor metabolic stress (e.g. trauma, surgery, burns) and as an indicator of when to begin nutritional support in critically ill patients. CRP is generally not detectable in the blood (<6 mg/L) of healthy individuals.	Detectable levels of **CRP** are associated with increased risk of atherosclerosis and may be seen in other inflammatory conditions, such as infections, rheumatoid arthritis or tuberculosis. The use of oral contraceptives and the last 4–5 months of pregnancy may also produce detectable CRP levels.
Nitrogen balance. Nitrogen balance is also used as an index of protein nutritional status. Nitrogen is released with the catabolism of amino acids (proteins) and is excreted in the urine as urea. Nitrogen balance therefore indicates whether the person is anabolic (using the normal energy stores and therefore pooling proteins and nitrogen creating a positive nitrogen balance) or catabolic (breaking down proteins in tissues for energy and therefore excreting nitrogen and creating a negative nitrogen balance within the body).	
Nitrogen balance is estimated by a formula based on urine urea nitrogen (UUN) excreted during the previous 24 hours: $\text{Nitrogen} = \text{Nitrogen intake} - \text{Nitrogen excretion}$ $= \text{Protein intake}/6.25 - (24 \text{ hours UUN} + 4)$ where Nitrogen balance is determined in grams 24 hours UNN = Urinary urea nitrogen, measured in grams 4 = Non-urea nitrogen losses via faeces, skin, sweat and lungs, measured in grams	In response to stress and increased protein demand, the body rapidly mobilises its protein compartments, which results in increased production of urea and excretion of urea in the urine. With infection, an estimated loss of 9–11 g/day of UUN can be expected. In patients with major burns, 12–18 g/day of urea nitrogen may be expected in the urine (Grodner 2019).
Creatinine-height index. The creatinine-height index (CHI) is a method of estimating the amount of skeletal muscle mass. Creatinine is derived from the breakdown of creatine, an energy-containing complex found in muscle. Creatinine is excreted unchanged in the urine at a constant rate in proportion to the amount of body muscle.	

PROCEDURES AND NORMAL FINDINGS	ABNORMAL FINDINGS AND CLINICAL ALERTS
Creatinine height index is calculated by first measuring urinary creatinine using 24-hours urine collection specimen. This value is then compared with ideal urinary creatinine levels from a creatinine-for-height-standard table, by means of the following equation: $$\text{CHI} = \frac{\text{Actual 24-hours urine creatinine}}{\text{Ideal 24-hours urine creatinine for height}} \times 100$$ The person's CHI is then compared with a CHI standard table to determine the degree of skeletal muscle depletion.	The validities of CHI and nitrogen balance studies are dependent on the accuracy of the 24-hours urine collection. Failure to obtain an accurate sample and abnormal renal function result in underestimation of creatinine and nitrogen losses. Assuming an accurate 24-hours urine specimen, a CHI of 60% to 80% of standard indicates a moderate deficit in body mass. A value of <60% indicates a severe deficit of body muscle mass (Royal Australian College of Pathologists 2019). Stress, fever and trauma can increase urinary creatinine excretion.
Developmental considerations in laboratory testing	
In **infancy and childhood**, laboratory tests are performed only when under-nutrition is suspected or if the child has acute or chronic illnesses that affect nutritional status.	
During **adolescence**, unless overt disease is suspected, laboratory evaluation of haemoglobin and haematocrit levels and urinalysis for glucose and protein levels are adequate.	
In **pregnancy**, haemoglobin and haematocrit values can be used to detect deficiencies of protein, folic acid, vitamin B_{12} and iron. Urine is frequently tested for glucose and protein (albumin), which can signal diabetes, pre-eclampsia and renal disease.	
In **late adulthood**, all serum and urine data must be interpreted with an understanding of declining renal efficiency and a tendency for people to be over-hydrated or under-hydrated.	
Serial nuritional assessment	
To monitor nutritional status in malnourished individuals or in individuals at risk for malnutrition, serial measurements of nutritional assessment parameters are made at routine intervals. At a minimum, weight and dietary intake should be evaluated weekly. Because the other nutritional assessment parameters change more slowly, data on these indicators may be collected biweekly or monthly.	Based on the findings of the nutritional assessment, the type of malnutrition can be diagnosed. The four major types of malnutrition are obesity, marasmus, kwashiorkor and marasmus/kwashiorkor mix (Table 21.4). Each type of malnutrition has characteristic clinical and laboratory findings and a distinct cause.

Further objective assessment for advanced practice

The assessments described in the following sections require advanced skill and scope of practice. Nurses working in community settings and specialised clinics may need to develop these skills.

Equipment needed

In addition to the equipment listed previously you will require:
Anthropometer
Skinfold calipers

PROCEDURES AND NORMAL FINDINGS	ABNORMAL FINDINGS AND CLINICAL ALERTS
Additional anthropometric measures	
In addition to measures of height and weight, advanced assessment includes triceps skinfold thickness, ulnar length, elbow breadth and arm circumferences.	

OBJECTIVE DATA

PROCEDURES AND NORMAL FINDINGS	ABNORMAL FINDINGS AND CLINICAL ALERTS
Skinfold thickness	
Skinfold thickness measurements provide an estimate of body fat stores or the extent of obesity or under-nutrition. Although other sites can be used (biceps, subscapular or suprailiac skinfolds), the triceps skinfold (TSF) is most commonly selected because of its easy accessibility and because standards and techniques are most developed for this site. To measure TSF thickness:	
1. Have the ambulatory person stand with arms hanging freely at the sides and back to the examiner. (Non-ambulatory persons should lie on one side. The uppermost arm should be fully extended, with the palm of the hand resting on the thigh.)	
2. Using the thumb and forefinger of your left hand, gently grasp a fold of skin and fat on the posterior aspect of the person's left upper arm, midway between the acromion process of the scapula and the olecranon process (the tip of the elbow). Gently pull the skinfold away from the underlying muscle (Figure 21.14). **Figure 21.14** Skinfold thickness.	
3. While grasping the skinfold, pick up the calipers with your right hand and depress the spring-loaded lever. Apply caliper jaws horizontally to the fat fold. Release the lever of the calipers while holding the skinfold. Wait 3 seconds, then take a reading. Repeat three times and average the three skinfold measurements (Figure 21.15). **Figure 21.15** Caliper method.	**TSF** values 10% below or above standard suggest under-nutrition and over-nutrition, respectively.

OBJECTIVE DATA

PROCEDURES AND NORMAL FINDINGS	ABNORMAL FINDINGS AND CLINICAL ALERTS
4. Record measurements to the nearest 5 mm (0.5 cm) on the nutritional assessment data form. Compare the person's measurements with standards by age, sex and body frame size.	Non-reproducible readings may be due to instrument malfunctions, use of plastic calipers (which are less accurate) or examiner error. Oedema may produce falsely high readings.
Other techniques to measure body composition	
Tests include **bioelectrical impedance analysis (BIA)** and **dual-energy X-ray absorptiometry (DEXA)**. Both BIA and DEXA measure fat and lean body mass; in addition, DEXA measures bone mineral density.	
Arm span or total arm length	
Measurement of arm span is useful for those situations in which height is difficult to measure, such as in children with cerebral palsy or scoliosis or in persons in late adulthood with spinal curvature. Arm span, which is nearly equivalent to height, is sometimes used clinically instead of height (Stewart & Marfell-Jones 2011). Measure the distance from the sternal notch to the tip of the longest finger on one hand and multiply the number by 2.8 (Grodner 2019).	
Inspect and palpate the thyroid gland	
The thyroid gland is difficult to palpate; arrange your setting to maximise your likelihood of success. Position a standing lamp to shine tangentially across the neck to highlight any possible swelling. Supply the person with a glass of water, and first inspect the neck as the person takes a sip and swallows. Thyroid tissue moves up with a swallow.	Look for diffuse enlargement or a nodular lump.
Posterior approach. To palpate, move behind the person (Figure 21.16A). Ask the person to sit up very straight and then to bend the head slightly forwards and to the right. This will relax the neck muscles. Use the fingers of your left hand to push the trachea slightly to the right. **Figure 21.16** Thyroid gland.	
Then curve your right fingers between the trachea and the sternocleidomastoid muscle, retracting it slightly, and ask the person to take a sip of water. The thyroid moves up under your fingers with the trachea and larynx as the person swallows. Reverse the procedure for the left side.	

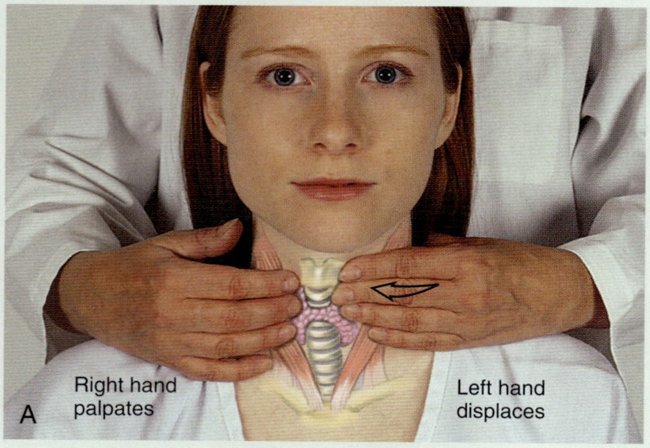

OBJECTIVE DATA

PROCEDURES AND NORMAL FINDINGS	ABNORMAL FINDINGS AND CLINICAL ALERTS
Usually, you cannot palpate the normal adult thyroid. If the person has a long, thin neck, you will sometimes feel the isthmus over the tracheal rings. The lateral lobes are not usually palpable; check them for enlargement, consistency, symmetry and the presence of nodules.	**Abnormalities:** enlarged lobes that are easily palpated before swallowing, or are tender to palpation; or the presence of nodules or lumps (Figure 21.16B). See Table 21.12. 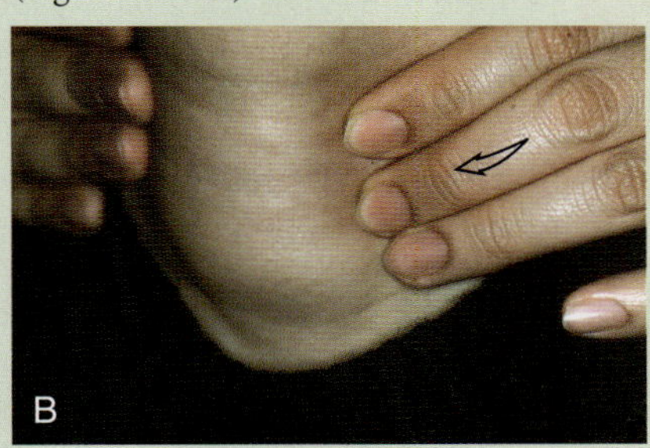
Anterior approach. This is an alternative method of palpating the thyroid, but it is more awkward to perform, especially for a beginning examiner. Stand facing the person. Ask them to tip the head forwards and to the right. Use your right thumb to displace the trachea slightly to the person's right. Hook your left thumb and fingers around the sternocleidomastoid muscle. Feel for lobe enlargement as the person swallows (Figure 21.17). 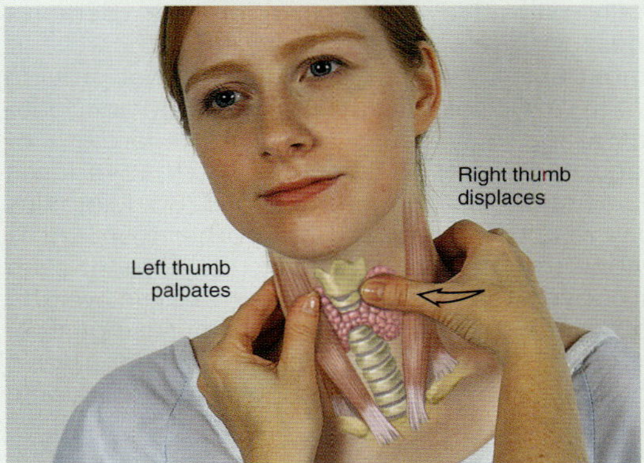 **Figure 21.17** Anterior approach thyroid.	

Summary Checklist

NUTRITIONAL AND METABOLIC ASSESSMENT

Subjective data

1. Presenting concern
2. Eating patterns
3. Usual weight
4. Changes in appetite, taste, smell, chewing, swallowing
5. Teeth
6. Recent surgery, trauma, burns, infection
7. Chronic illnesses
8. Vomiting, diarrhoea, constipation
9. Food allergies or intolerances
10. Family history
11. Health and lifestyle management

Objective data

1. General inspection
2. Anthropometric measures
3. Inspect the mouth
4. Inspect the throat
5. Blood glucose monitoring

OBJECTIVE DATA

PROMOTING A HEALTHY LIFESTYLE

OBJECTIVE DATA

OBESITY AS A GENERATIONAL HEALTH ISSUE

Intergenerational cycle of obesity has been identified as a heath priority in Australia and New Zealand (Gordon et al., 2017).

The statistics for obesity include;

- One in 5 (20%) of 2 to 4 year old children are overweight or obese, with 11% being classified overweight and 8.7% considered obese (AIHW, 2019).
- 1 in 4 (28%) children aged between 5 and 17 years , are overweight or obese, with 20% being overweight and 7.4% classified as obese.
- In relation to gender, similar proportions of boys and girls were obese
- highest prevalence of obesity (8.2%) for boys was at the age 16–17 years, and the age bracket of 5–7 years for girls (12%) (AIHW, 2019).
- in low socioeconomic areas 28% of 2 to 17 year olds were overweight or obese compared to 25% in high socioeconomic areas. The incidence of obesity for lower socioeconomic groups was 10.7% compared to 4.4% in higher socioeconomic groups (AIHW, 2019).

As the Australian population ages the statistics become more prominent;

- with almost two-thirds (63%) of Australians aged 18 and over were classified as being overweight or obese - 36% are overweight, and 28% are obese (AIHW, 2019).
- Male adults having higher rates of being overweight or obese (71%) compared to women (56%). (AIHW, 2019).
- For adults over 18 years of age, from low socioeconomic groups, 72% were overweight or obese compared to 62% in high socioeconomic groups. (AIHW, 2019).

The New Zealand Health Survey 2017/18 found that approximately;

- 1 in 8 children, between the ages of 2 to14 years were obese (12%).
- For Māori children, 17% were identified as obese,
- 30% of Pacific Islander children were obese.
- children living in the most deprived areas were 2.1 times as likely to be obese as children living in the least deprived areas (Ministry of Health New Zealand, 2019).

In the New Zealand adult population,

- 1 in 3 adults (aged 15 years and over) were obese (32%), and within this cohort were Māori adults (47%) and Pacific adults (65%).
- adults living in the most deprived areas were 1.6 times as likely to be obese as adults living in the least deprived areas (Ministry of Health New Zealand, 2019).

Early gestational weight gain has been identified as a predictor for the development of intergenerational obesity. A study conducted in Sydney antenatal clinics found that overweight and obese women and/or women residing in lower socioeconomic areas were at increased risk of excess early gestational weight (Cheney et al., 2017). This impacts on pregnancy outcomes and long-term outcomes for mother and child.

The keys to a healthy diet for adults are (a) eat a variety of foods from all the basic food groups to ensure nutrient adequacy; (b) consume the recommended amounts of fruits/vegetables, whole grains and fat-free or low-fat milk products or equivalents; (c) limit intake of foods high in saturated or trans fats, added sugars, starch, cholesterol, salt and alcohol; (d) match kilojoule intake with kilojoules expended; (e) be physically active for at least 30 minutes each day of the week; and (f) follow food safety guidelines for handling, preparing and storing foods.

Approaches to weight loss for overweight and obesity must be tailored to the individual, be culturally sensitive and consider the person's readiness to lose weight and their healthcare and self-care beliefs. Weight loss programs that provide less than 5020 kilojoules may not provide adequate nutrients and may cause damage. Regardless of macronutrient composition, any diet that reduces kilojoule intake or contains 5860–6280 kilojoules per day results in weight loss. In other words, it is not eating too much of any particular nutrient such as carbohydrate or fat that makes us gain weight, but rather the overall number of kilojoules ingested. The cardinal features of a successful long-term weight loss plan are (a) getting regular physical exercise (i.e. 30 minutes every day).

It has been proposed that to interrupt the cycle of intergenerational obesity, interventions must occur across the lifespan This involves targeted interventions at the preconception stage, prenatal care, paternal roles, birth to 2 years (including physical activity and sleep) and social determinants of health (Haire-Joshu and Tabak, 2016).

Nurses in any setting can focus on;

- Opening the discuss about physical activities, nutrition and long term heath implications of obesity
- Focusing on the interventions with families especially when the child is overweight
- Encouraging breast feeding for at least the first 6 months of life
- Providing readily available nutritional information including authoritive web sources
- Providing support and motivation for change
- Referring to dietician and/or exercise physiologist for specific advice (Braga et al. 2017)

Documentation and critical thinking

FOCUSED ASSESSMENT: CLINICAL CASE STUDY

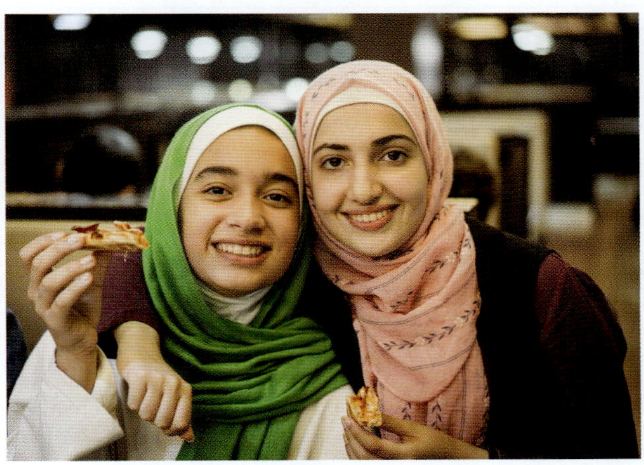

Context

The diabetes education nurse in the general practice setting is an essential member of the healthcare multidisciplinary team that cares for people who have diabetes mellitus (types 1 and 2). Part of the diabetes educator's role is the assessment of the person with diabetes and the subsequent planning of coordinated care.

Subjective

Lisa Alfarsi is a 15-year-old teenager with type 1 diabetes. She has had the condition for the last 2 years and she presents with her mother for the usual 3-monthly check-up. Her mother is concerned that Lisa has not been checking blood glucose levels regularly and administering insulin as prescribed. Lisa states she forgets occasionally and what is the 'big deal' about it?

Objective

General appearance is a well-looking teenager.

Height is 166.4 cm. Current weight is 50.9 kg. BMI: 18.

HbA1c 8% (10.2 mmol) which is slightly elevated.

Collaborative problem

Self-care of type 1 diabetes.

Problem statement/nursing diagnosis

Ineffective health maintenance related to HbA1c levels and management of diabetes.

Abnormal findings

TABLE 21.3 Clinical signs of malnutrition

AREA OF EXAMINATION	NORMAL APPEARANCE	SIGNS ASSOCIATED WITH MALNUTRITION	NUTRIENT DEFICIENCY
Skin	Smooth, no signs of rashes, bruises, flaking	Dry, flaking, scaly	Vitamin A, vitamin B-complex, linoleic acid
		Petechiae/ecchymoses	Vitamins C and K
		Follicular hyperkeratosis (dry, bumpy skin)	Vitamin A, linoleic acid
		Cracks in skin, lesions on the hands, legs, face or neck	Niacin, tryptophan
		Pellagrous dermatosis (hyperpigmentation of skin exposed to sunlight)	Niacin
		Nasolabial seborrhoea	Riboflavin, vitamin B_6
		Acneiform forehead rash	Vitamin B_6
		Eczema	Linoleic acid
		Xanthomas (excessive deposits of cholesterol)	Excessive serum levels of LDLs or VLDLs

(Continued)

ABNORMAL FINDINGS

TABLE 21.3 Clinical signs of malnutrition—cont'd

AREA OF EXAMINATION	NORMAL APPEARANCE	SIGNS ASSOCIATED WITH MALNUTRITION	NUTRIENT DEFICIENCY
Hair	Shiny, firm, does not fall out easily, healthy scalp	Dull, dry, sparse	Protein, zinc, linoleic acid
		Colour changes	Copper or protein
		Corkscrew hair	Copper
Eyes	Corneas are clear, shiny; membranes are pink and moist; no sores at corners of eyelids	Foamy plaques (Bitot's spots)	Vitamin A
		Dryness (xerophthalmia)	Vitamin A
		Softening (keratomalacia)	Vitamin A
		Pale conjunctivae	Iron, vitamins B_6, B_{12}
		Red conjunctivae	Riboflavin
		Blepharitis	B-complex, biotin
Lips	Smooth, not chapped or swollen	Cheilosis (vertical cracks in lips)	Riboflavin, niacin
		Angular stomatitis (red cracks at sides of mouth)	Riboflavin, niacin, iron, vitamin B_6
Tongue	Red in appearance; not swollen or smooth, no lesions	Glossitis (beefy red)	Vitamin B-complex
		Pale	Iron
		Papillary atrophy	Niacin
		Papillary hypertrophy	Multiple nutrients
		Magenta/purplish coloured	Riboflavin
Gums	Reddish-pink, firm, no swelling or bleeding	Bleeding	Vitamin C
Nails	Smooth, pink	Brittle, ridged or spoon shaped (koilonychia)	Iron
		Splinter haemorrhages	Vitamin C
Musculoskeletal	Erect posture, no malformations, good muscle tone, can walk or run without pain	Pain in calves, thighs	Thiamine
		Osteomalacia	Vitamin D, calcium
		Rickets	Vitamin D, calcium
		Joint pain	Vitamin C
		Muscle wasting	Protein, carbohydrate, fat
Neurological	Normal reflexes, appropriate affect	Peripheral neuropathy Hyporeflexia Disorientation or irritability	Thiamine, vitamin B_6 Thiamine Vitamin B_{12}

Detsky AJ, McLaughlin JR, Baker JP et al: What is subjective global assessment of nutritional status? *J Parenter Enteral Nutr*, 11:9, 1987.

TABLE 21.4 Classification of malnutrition

TYPE/AETIOLOGY	CLINICAL FEATURES	ANTHROPOMETRIC MEASURES	LABORATORY FINDINGS
Obesity due to energy excess refers to weights more than 20% above ideal body weight. Persons who are 100% or more above ideal body weight are categorised as morbidly obese. The causes of overweight and obese conditions are complex and multifaceted: genetic, social, cultural, pathological, psychological and physiological factors have all been implicated. Regardless of its cause, the underlying problem is usually an imbalance of kilojoule intake and kilojoule expenditure. In most cases, a small kilojoule surplus over a long period of time results in the extra weight. Although visceral protein levels and immunocompetence are generally normal in the obese individual, anthropometric measures are above normal.	Obese appearance	Weight >120% standard for height Body mass index >30 Triceps skinfold (TSF) >10% standard Waist-to-hip ratio >1.0 (men) or >0.8 (women)	Serum cholesterol <5.5 mmol/L Serum triglycerides <1.7 mmol/L
Marasmus (protein–kilojoule malnutrition) is due to inadequate intake of protein and kilojoules or prolonged starvation. Anorexia, bowel obstruction, cancer cachexia and chronic illness are among the clinical conditions leading to marasmus. Like obesity, marasmus is complex and can result from multifaceted factors; genetic, social, cultural, pathological, psychological and physiological. Marasmus is characterised by decreased anthropometric measures—weight loss and subcutaneous fat and muscle wasting. Visceral protein levels may remain within normal ranges.	Starved appearance	Weight <80% standard for height TSF <90% standard Mid-arm muscle circumference (MAMC) ≥90% standard	Creatinine-height index <80% standard
Kwashiorkor (protein malnutrition) is due to diets that may be high in kilojoules but that contain little or no protein, e.g. low-protein liquid diets, fad diets and long-term use of dextrose-containing intravenous fluids. Individuals with kwashiorkor, in contrast to those with marasmus, have decreased visceral protein levels and depressed immune function, but generally they have adequate anthropometric measures. These individuals may therefore appear well-nourished or even obese.	Well-nourished appearance Oedematous	Weight >100% standard for height TSF >100% standard	Serum albumin <35 g/L Serum transferrin <1.5 g/L Lymphocytes <1500 mm^3 Anergy
Marasmus/kwashiorkor mix is due to prolonged inadequate intake of protein and kilojoules (e.g. severe starvation, severe catabolic states). This mix combines elements of both marasmus and kwashiorkor. Nutritional assessment findings include muscle, fat and visceral protein wasting, along with immune-incompetence. Individuals with marasmus/kwashiorkor mix are usually those who have undergone acute catabolic stress, such as major surgery, trauma or burns in combination with prolonged starvation. Without nutritional support, this type of malnutrition is associated with the highest risk of morbidity and mortality.	Emaciated appearance	Weight <70% standard TSF <80% standard MAMC <60% standard	Serum albumin <28 g/L Serum transferrin <1.0 g/L Lymphocytes <900 mm^3 Anergy Creatinine-height index <60% standard

TABLE 21.5 Abnormalities caused by nutritional deficiencies

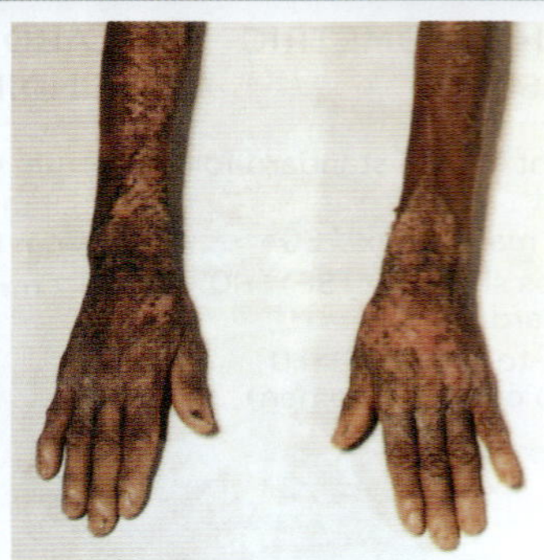

Pellagra

Pigmented keratotic scaling lesions resulting from a deficiency of niacin. These lesions are especially prominent in areas exposed to the sun, such as hands, forearms, neck and legs.

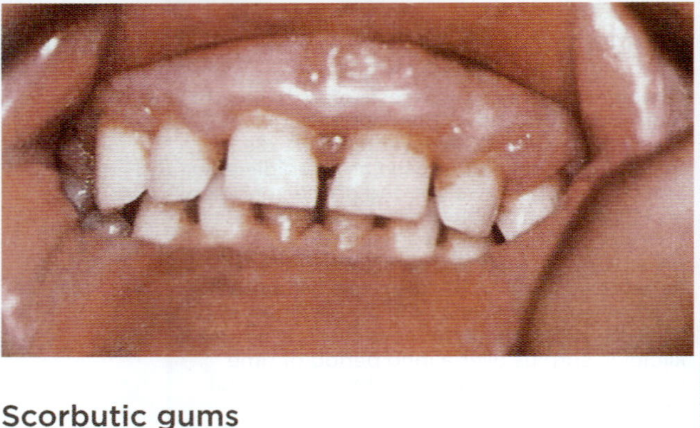

Scorbutic gums

Deficiency of vitamin C. Gums are swollen, ulcerated and bleeding due to vitamin C-induced defects in oral epithelial basement membrane and periodontal collagen fibre synthesis.

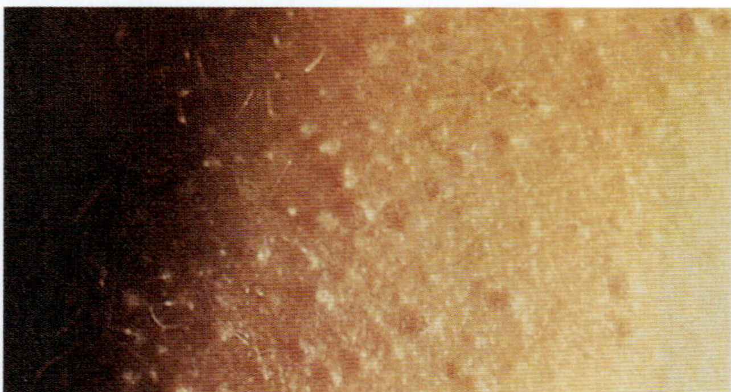

Follicular hyperkeratosis

Dry, bumpy skin associated with vitamin A and/or linoleic acid (essential fatty acid) deficiency. Linoleic acid deficiency may also result in eczematous skin, especially in infants.

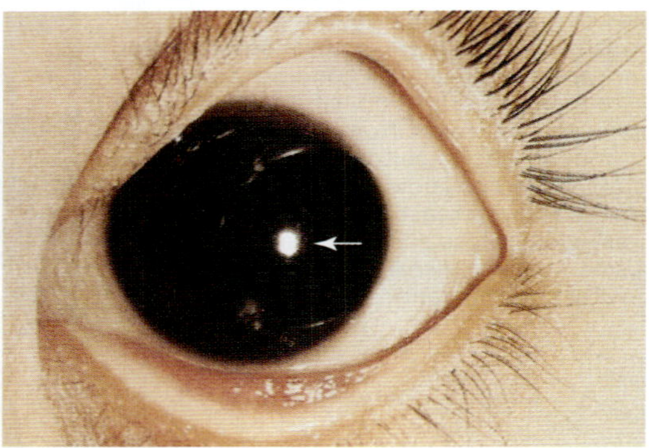

Bitot's spots

Foamy plaques of the cornea that are a sign of vitamin A deficiency. Severe depletion may result in conjunctival xerosis (drying) and progress to corneal ulceration, and finally destruction of the eye (keratomalacia).

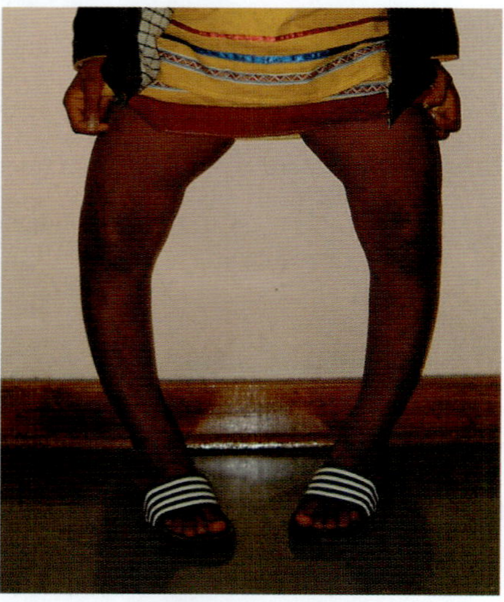

Rickets

Sign of vitamin D and calcium deficiencies in children (disorders of cartilage cell growth, enlargement of epiphyseal growth plates) and adults (osteomalacia).

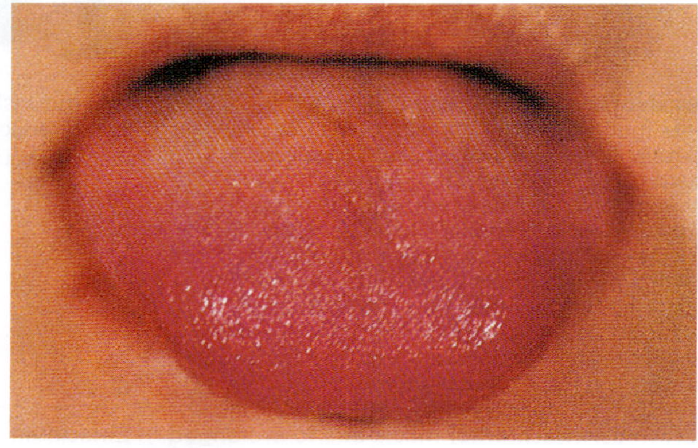

Magenta tongue

'Magenta tongue' is a sign of riboflavin deficiency. In contrast, a pale tongue is probably attributable to iron deficiency; a beefy red-coloured tongue is caused by vitamin B-complex deficiency.

Abnormal findings for advanced practice

TABLE 21.6 Abnormalities of the lips

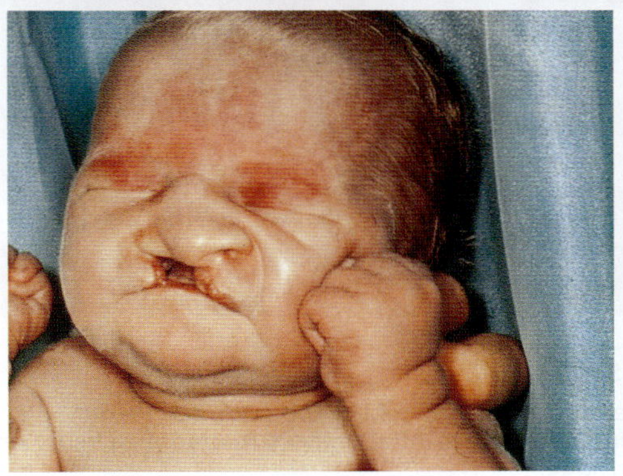

Cleft lip

Orofacial clefts are the most common congenital deformities of the head and neck. The incidence of orofacial clefts in infants born in Australia is 17 per 10,000. The incidence is 50% higher among Indigenous infants (AIHW 2008). Early treatment preserves the functions of speech and language formation and deglutition (swallowing).

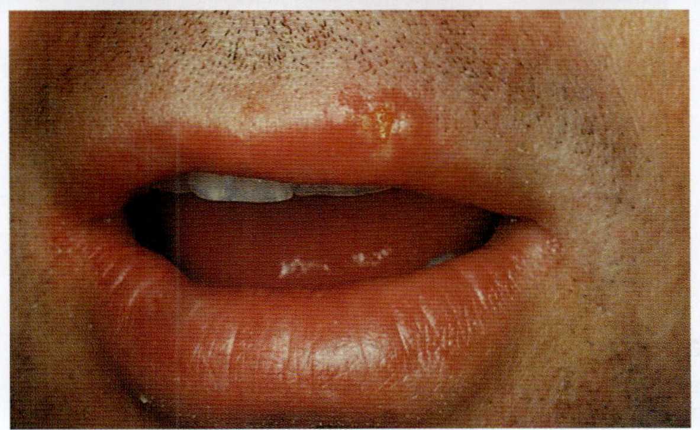

Herpes simplex 1

The cold sores are groups of clear vesicles with a surrounding indurated erythematous base. These evolve into pustules, which rupture, weep and crust, and heal in 4–10 days. The most likely site is the lip-skin junction; infection often recurs in same site. Caused by the herpes simplex virus (HSV-1), the lesion is highly contagious and is spread by direct contact. Recurrent herpes infections may be precipitated by sunlight, fever, colds, allergy. It is a very common lesion, affecting 50% of adults.

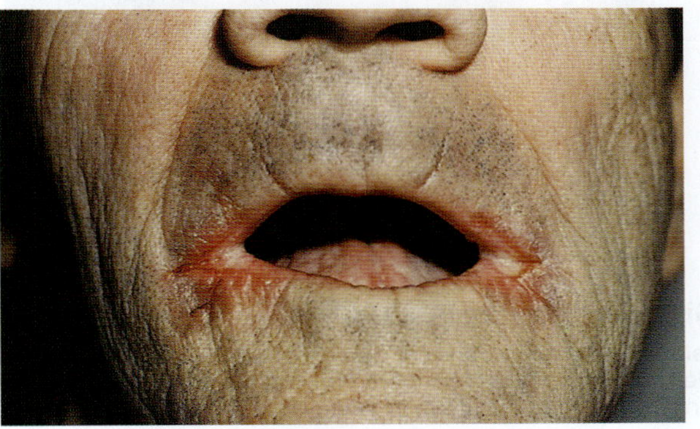

Angular cheilitis (stomatitis, perlèche)

Erythema, scaling, shallow and painful fissures at the corners of the mouth occur with excess salivation and *Candida* infection. It is often seen in edentulous persons and in those with poorly fitting dentures causing folding in of corners of mouth, creating a warm and moist environment favouring growth of yeast.

Retention 'cyst' (mucocoele)

A round, well-defined translucent nodule that may be very small or up to 1 or 2 cm. It is a pocket of mucus that forms when a duct of a minor salivary gland ruptures. The benign lesion also may occur on the buccal mucosa, on the floor of the mouth or under the tip of the tongue.

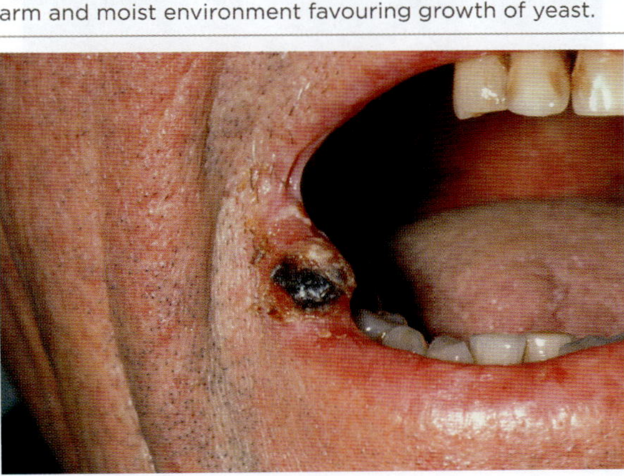

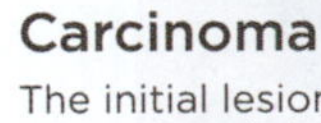

Carcinoma

The initial lesion is round and indurated, then it becomes crusted and ulcerated with an elevated border. The majority occur between the outer and middle thirds of lip. Any lesion that is still unhealed after 2 weeks should be referred.

TABLE 21.7 Abnormalities of the teeth and gums

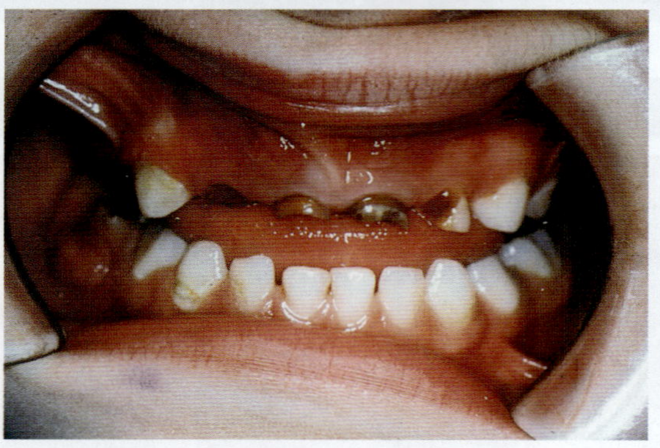

Baby bottle tooth decay

Destruction of numerous deciduous teeth may occur in older infants and toddlers who take a bottle of milk, juice or sweetened drink to bed and prolong bottle feeding past the age of 1 year. Liquid pools around the upper front teeth. Mouth bacteria act on carbohydrates in the liquid, especially sucrose, forming metabolic acids. Acids break down tooth enamel and destroy its protein.

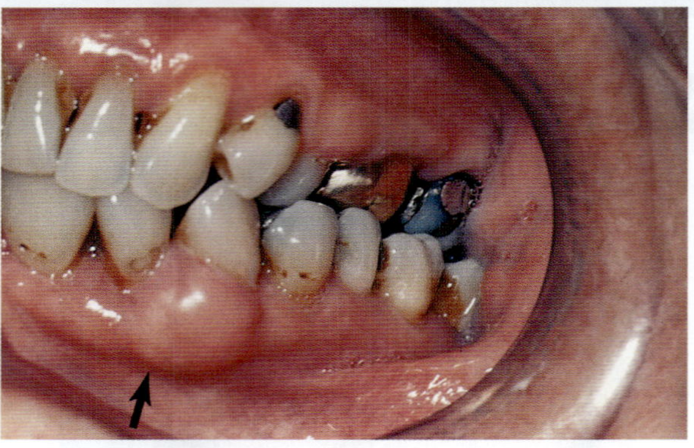

Epulis

A nontender, fibrous nodule of the gum, seen emerging between the teeth; an inflammatory response to injury or haemorrhage.

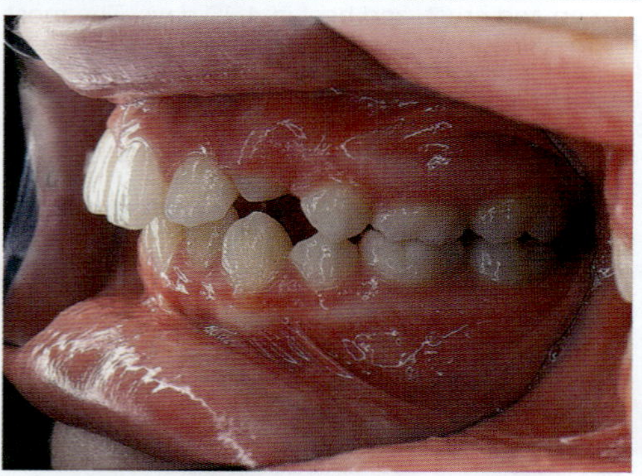

Malocclusion

Upper or lower dental arches are not in alignment and incisors protrude from developmental problem of mandible or maxilla, or incompatibility between jaw size and tooth size. The condition increases risk of facial deformity, negative body image, chewing problems or speech dysfluency.

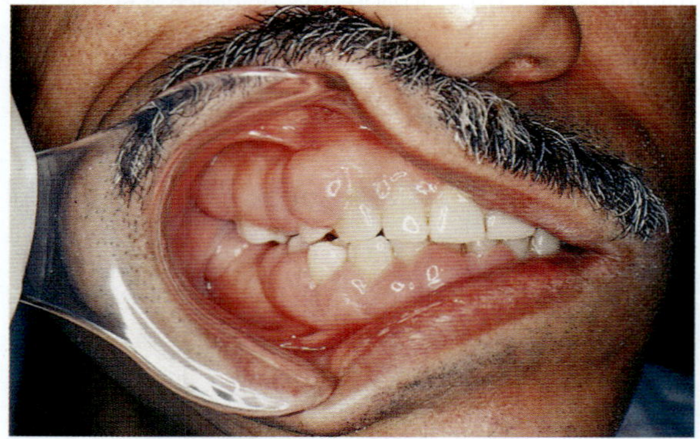

Gingival hyperplasia

Painless enlargement of the gums, sometimes overreaching the teeth. This occurs with puberty, pregnancy, leukaemia and with long-term therapeutic use of phenytoin (Dilantin).

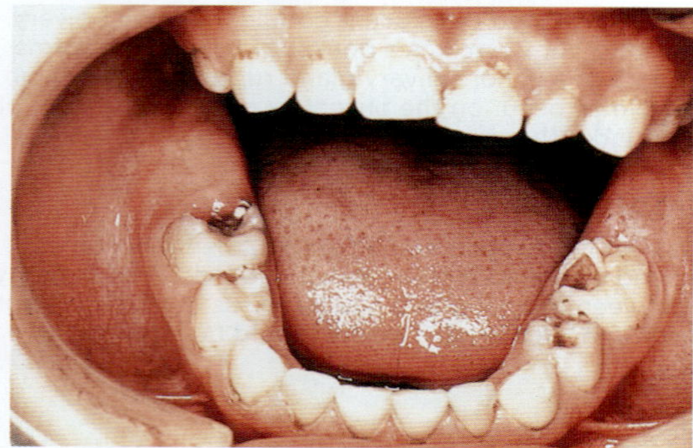

Dental caries

Progressive destruction of tooth. Decay initially looks chalky white. Later, it turns brown or black and forms a cavity. Early decay is apparent only on X-ray study. Susceptible sites are tooth surfaces where food debris, bacterial plaque and saliva collect.

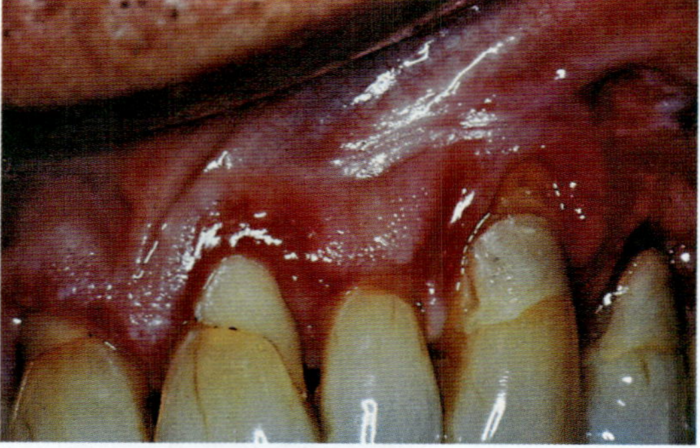

Gingivitis

Gum margins are red, swollen and bleed easily. This case is severe; gingival tissue has desquamated, exposing roots of teeth. Inflammation is usually due to poor dental hygiene or vitamin C deficiency. The condition may occur in pregnancy and puberty because of changing hormonal balance.

TABLE 21.7 Abnormalities of the teeth and gums—cont'd

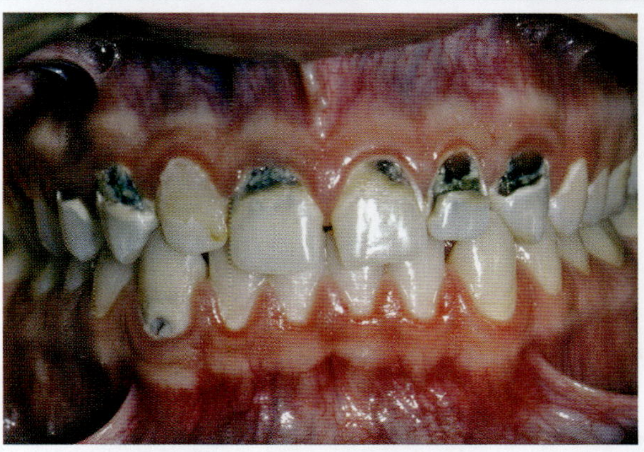

Meth mouth

Illicit methamphetamine abuse (crystal meth, meth ice) leads to extensive dental caries, gingivitis, tooth cracking and edentulism. Methamphetamine causes vasoconstriction and decreased saliva, and its use increases the urge to consume sugars and starches and to give up oral hygiene. Absence of the buffering saliva leads to increased acidity in the mouth, and the increased plaque encourages bacterial growth. These conditions and the presence of carbohydrates set up an oral environment prone to caries, cracking of enamel and the damage seen here.

TABLE 21.8 Abnormalities of the tongue

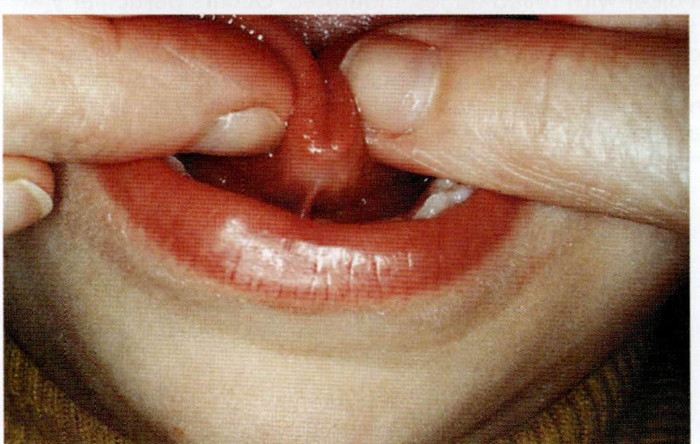

Ankyloglossia

(Tongue-tie.) A short lingual frenulum, here fixing the tongue tip to the floor of the mouth and gums. This limits mobility and will affect speech (pronunciation of a, d, n) if the tongue tip cannot be elevated to the alveolar ridge. A congenital defect.

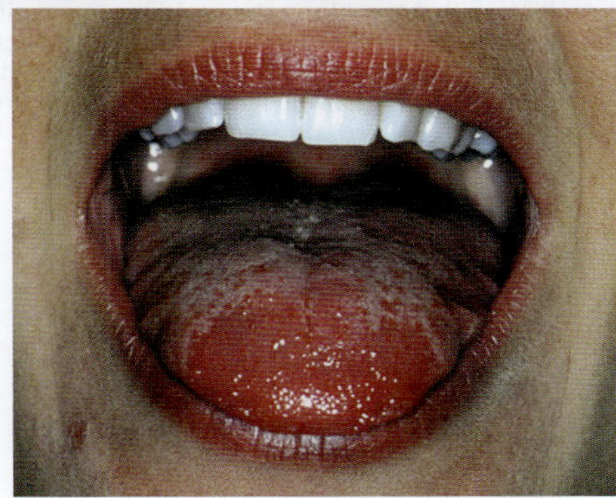

Geographic tongue (migratory glossitis)

Pattern of normal coating interspersed with bright red, shiny, circular bald areas with raised pearly borders. Pattern resembles a map, and changes in a few days. Not significant, and its cause is not known.

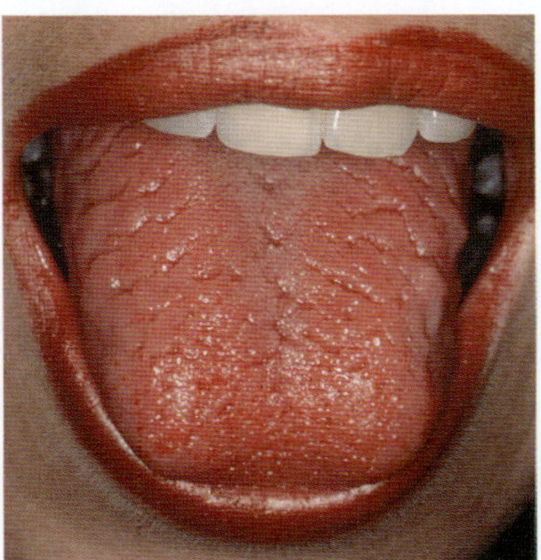

Fissured or scrotal tongue

Deep furrows divide the papillae into small irregular rows. The condition occurs in 5% of the general population and in Down syndrome. The incidence increases with age. (Vertical, or longitudinal, fissures also occur with dehydration because of reduced volume of the tongue.)

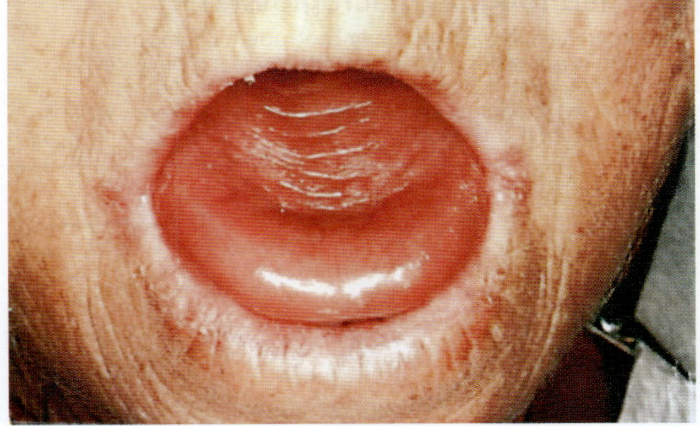

Smooth, glossy tongue (atrophic glossitis)

The surface is slick and shiny; the mucosa thins and looks red from decreased papillae. Accompanied by dryness of tongue and burning. Occurs with vitamin B_{12} deficiency (pernicious anaemia), folic acid deficiency and iron deficiency anaemia. Here, also note angular cheilitis.

(Continued)

TABLE 21.8 Abnormalities of the tongue—cont'd

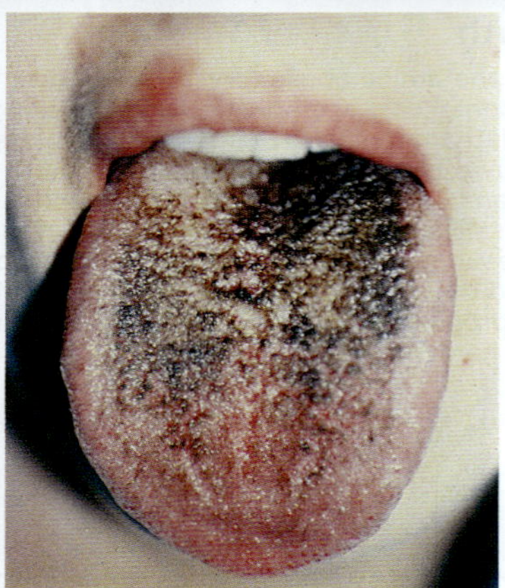

Black hairy tongue

This is not really hair but the elongation of filiform papillae and painless overgrowth of mycelial threads of fungus infection on the tongue. Colour varies from black-brown to yellow. It occurs after use of antibiotics, which inhibit normal bacteria and allow proliferation of fungus.

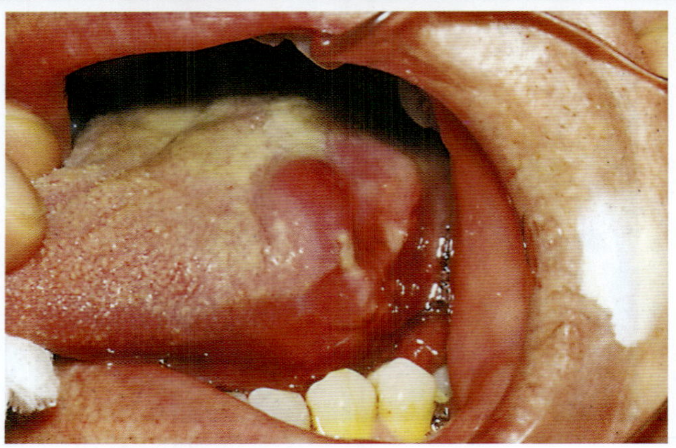

Carcinoma

An ulcer with rolled edges; indurated. Occurs particularly at sides, base and under the tongue. When it is in the floor of mouth, it may cause painful movement or limited movement of tongue. Risk of early metastasis is present because of rich lymphatic drainage. Heavy smoking and heavy alcohol use place persons at greater risk.

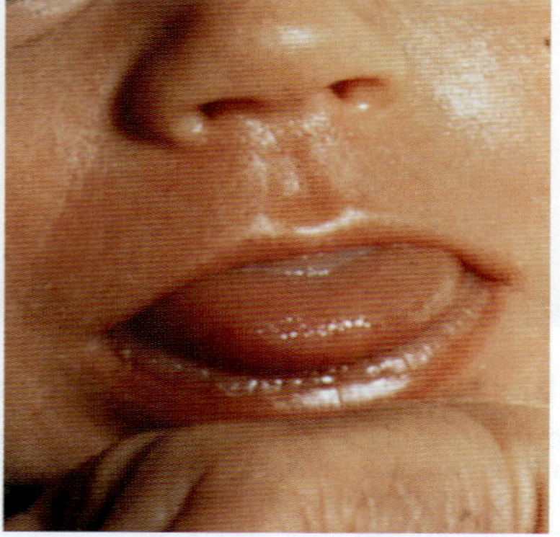

Enlarged tongue (macroglossia)

The tongue is enlarged and may protrude from mouth. The condition is not painful but may impair speech development. Here, it occurs with Down syndrome; it also occurs with cretinism, myxoedema, acromegaly. Also a transient swelling occurs with local infections.

TABLE 21.9 Abnormalities of the buccal mucosa

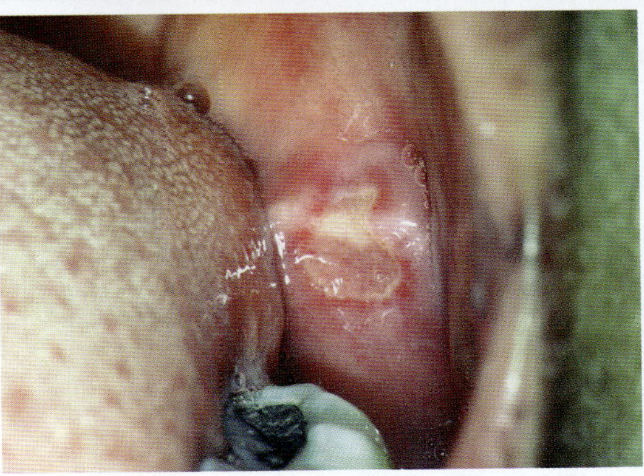

Aphthous ulcers

A 'canker sore' is a vesicle at first, then a small, round, 'punched-out' ulcer with white base surrounded by a red halo. It is quite painful and lasts for 1–2 weeks. The cause is unknown, although it is associated with stress, fatigue and food allergy. It is common, affecting 20% to 60% of the population.

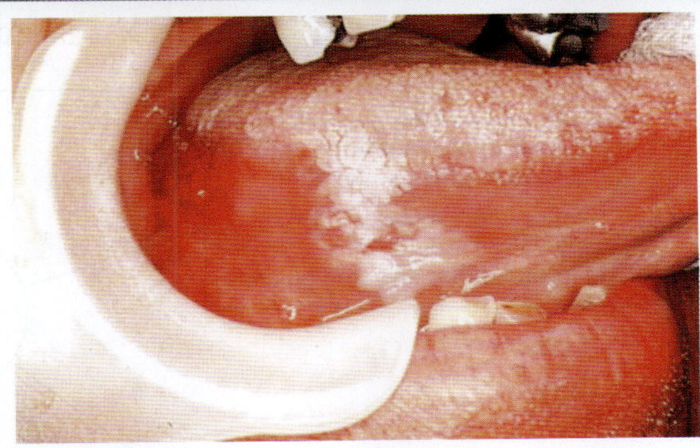

Leucoplakia

Chalky white, thick, raised patch with well-defined borders. The lesion is firmly attached and does not scrape off. It may occur on the lateral edges of tongue. It is due to chronic irritation, and occurs more frequently with heavy smoking and heavy alcohol use. Lesions are precancerous, and the person should be referred. (Here, the lesion is associated with squamous carcinoma.)

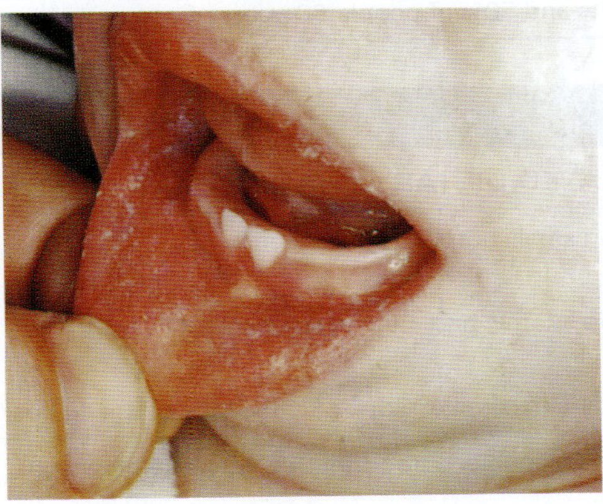

Koplik's spots

Small blue-white spots with irregular red halo scattered over mucosa opposite the molars. An early sign, and pathognomonic, of measles.

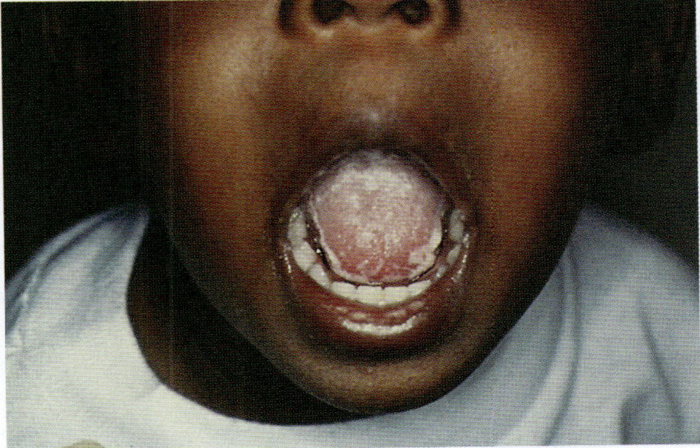

Candidiasis or monilial infection

A white, cheesy, curd-like patch on the buccal mucosa and tongue. It scrapes off, leaving raw, red surface that bleeds easily. Termed 'thrush' in the newborn. It is an opportunistic infection that occurs after the use of antibiotics, corticosteroids and in immunosuppressed persons.

TABLE 21.10 Metabolic syndrome (MetSy)

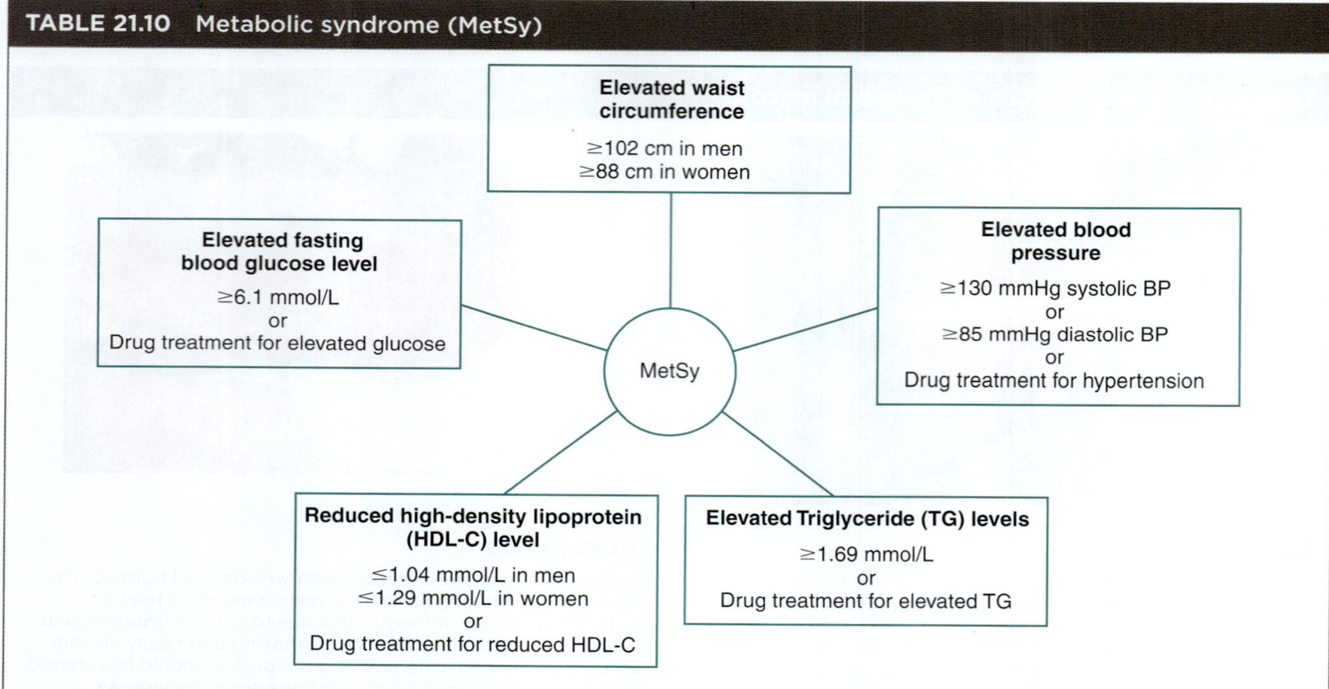

Having 3 of these 5 biomarkers signifies MetS. MetS is associated with increased risk for cardiovascular disease, type 2 diabetes mellitus, and mortality. Its prevalence is estimated to be nearly 35% of adults and 50% of people 60 years of age and older.

TABLE 21.11 Nutritional consequences of bariatric surgery*†

POTENTIAL NUTRITIONAL CONSEQUENCES	RELATED DIETARY CHANGES
Malabsorption of protein and calories caused by decreased absorptive surface and availability of digestive enzymes	Eating small, nutrient-dense meals
Malabsorption of vitamins and minerals caused by achlorhydria or loss of site of absorption	Taking vitamin and mineral supplements
Weight regain	Avoiding excessive intake of calorically dense liquids/foods
Obstruction of bypassed sections or pouch	Avoiding chunks of food that could cause blockage

*Vertical and adjustable gastric banding, Roux-en-Y gastric bypass.

†People who are 100% or more above ideal body weight or have a body mass index (BMI) ≥40 are categorised as morbidly or extremely obese and are possible candidates for bariatric or weight-loss surgery, as are people with BMIs ≥35 and comorbid conditions.

TABLE 21.12 Swellings on the neck

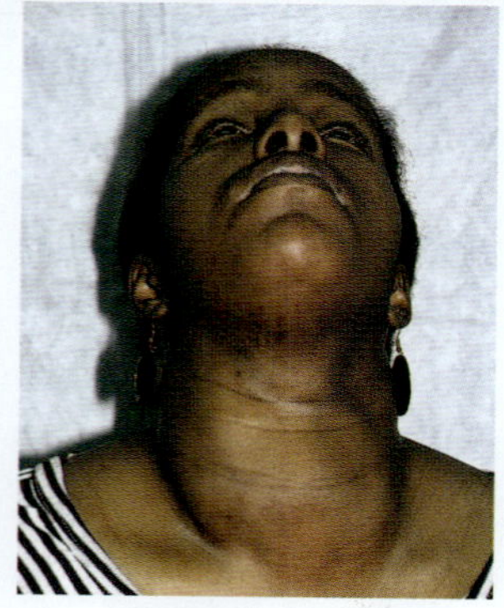

Thyroid—multiple nodules

Multiple nodules usually indicate inflammation or a multinodular goitre rather than a neoplasm. However, suspect any rapidly enlarging or firm nodule.

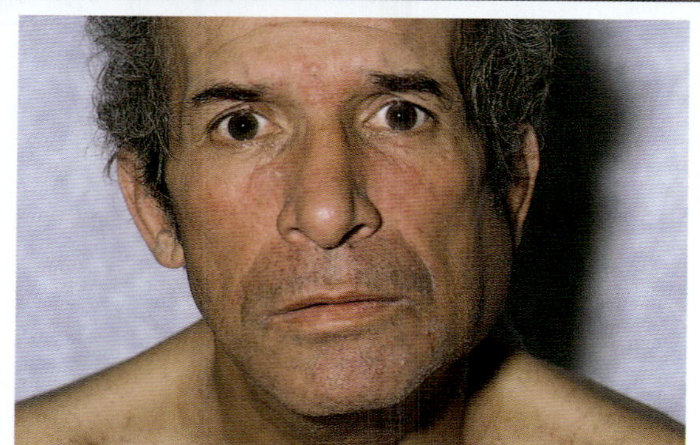

Parotid gland enlargement

Rapid painful inflammation of the parotid occurs with mumps. Parotid swelling also occurs with blockage of a duct, abscess or tumour. Note swelling anterior to lower ear lobe. Stensen's duct obstruction can occur in ageing adults dehydrated from diuretics or anticholinergics.

TABLE 21.13 Paediatric facial abnormalities

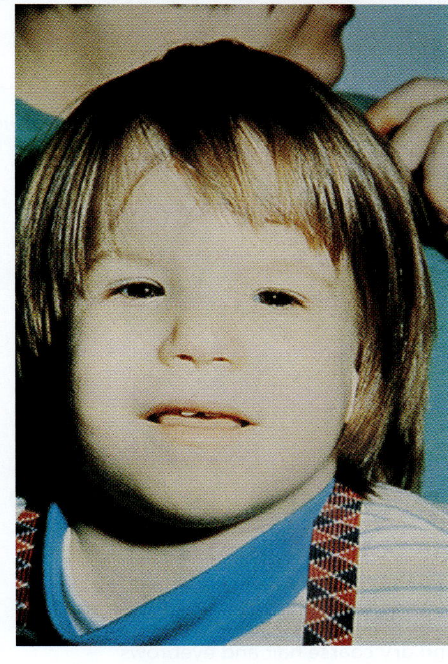

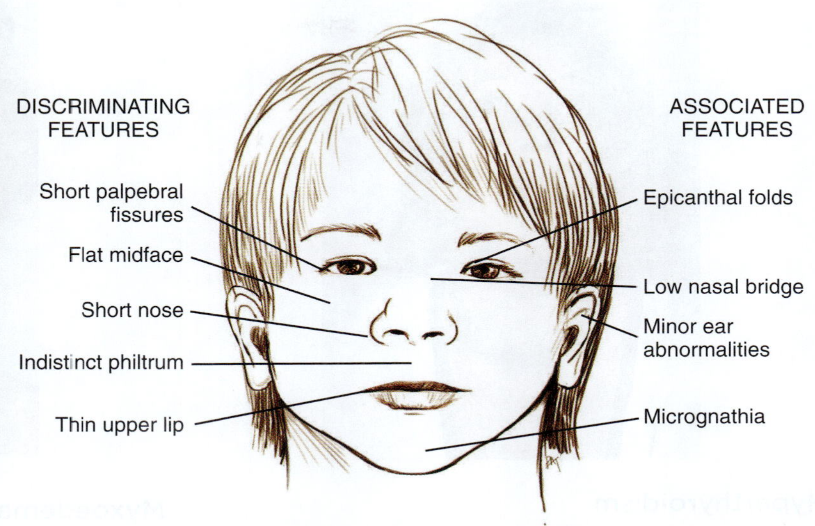

Fetal alcohol syndrome

A pregnant woman who abuses alcohol is at great risk of producing a baby with a wide range of growth and development abnormalities. Facial malformations may be recognisable at birth. Characteristic facies include narrow palpebral fissures, epicanthal folds and midfacial hypoplasia.

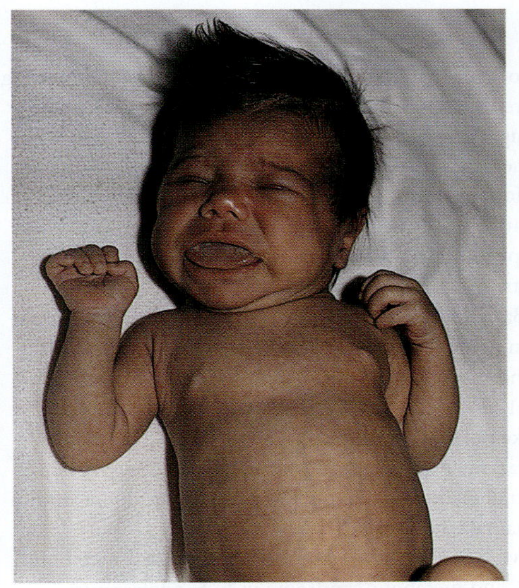

Congenital hypothyroidism

Thyroid deficiency at an early age produces impaired growth and neurological deficit. Without neonatal screening, characteristic facies develop by 3 to 6 months of age: low hairline, hirsute forehead, swollen eyelids, narrow palpebral fissures, widely spaced eyes, depressed nasal bridge, puffy face, thick tongue protruding through an open mouth and a dull expression. Head size is normal but the anterior and posterior fontanels are wide open.

TABLE 21.14 Abnormal facial appearances with chronic illnesses

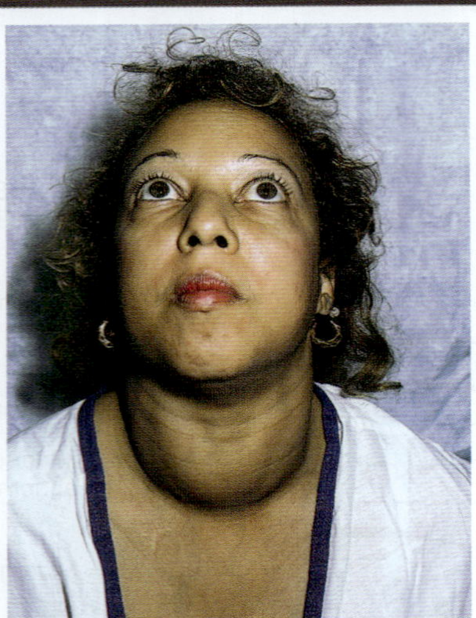

Hyperthyroidism

Goitre is an increase in the size of the thyroid gland and occurs with hyperthyroidism, Hashimoto's thyroiditis and hypothyroidism. Graves' disease (shown here) is the most common cause of hyperthyroidism, manifested by goitre and exophthalmos (bulging eyeballs). Symptoms include nervousness, fatigue, weight loss, muscle cramps and heat intolerance; signs include tachycardia, shortness of breath, excessive sweating, fine muscle tremor, thin silky hair and skin, infrequent blinking and a staring appearance.

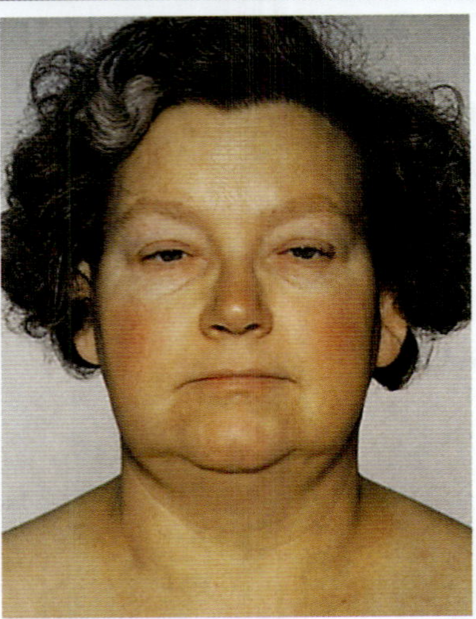

Myxoedema (hypothyroidism)

A deficiency of thyroid hormone, when severe, causes a non-pitting oedema or myxoedema. Note puffy oedematous face, especially around eyes (periorbital oedema), coarse facial features, dry skin and dry coarse hair and eyebrows.

BIBLIOGRAPHY

Australian Institute of Health and Welfare (AIHW). Making progress: the health, development and wellbeing of Australia's children and young people. 2008. Available at: www.aihw.gov.au/publications.

Australian Institute of Health and Welfare (AIHW). Key indicators of progress for chronic disease and associated determinants. 2011. Available at: www.aihw.gov.au/publications.

Australian Institute of Health and Welfare (AIHW). Australia's health 2014. Australia's health series no. 14. Cat. No. AUS 178. Canberra: AIHW; 2014a. Available at: www.aihw.gov.au/publication-detail/?id=60129548265&tab=2.

Australian Institute of Health and Welfare (AIHW). Oral health and dental care in Australia: key facts and figures trends. Cat. no. DEN 228. Canberra: AIHW; 2014b. Available at: www.aihw.gov.au/publication-detail/?id=60129548265&tab=2.

Australian Institute of Health and Welfare (AIHW). Stronger futures in the Northern Territory: oral health services July 2012–December 2013. Cat. no. IHW 144. Canberra: AIHW; 2014c. Available at: www.aihw.gov.au/publication-detail/?id=60129549684.

Australian Institute of Health and Welfare (AIHW). An interactive insight into overweight and obesity in Australia. 2017. Available at: https://www.aihw.gov.au/reports/overweight-obesity/interactive-insight-into-overweight-and-obesity/contents/how-many-people-are-overweight-or-obese.

Australian Institute of Health & Welfare. Overweight & obesity. 2019. Available at: https://www.aihw.gov.au/reports-data/behaviours-risk-factors/overweight-obesity/overview.

Boltong AG, Loeliger JM, Steer BL. Using a public hospital funding model to strengthen a case for improved nutritional care in a cancer setting. Aust Health Rev 2013;37:286–90.

Centers for Disease Control and Prevention (CDC). Growth charts, National Centre for health statistics in collaboration with the National Centre for chronic disease prevention and health promotion. 2012. Available at: www.cdc.gov/growthcharts.

Charlton KE, Batterham MJ, Bowden S, et al. A high prevalence of malnutrition in acute geriatric patients predicts adverse clinical outcomes and mortality within 12 months. e-SPEN Journal 2013;8(3):e120–5.

Cheney K, Berkemeier S, Sim K, et al. Prevalence and predictors of early gestational weight gain associated with obesity risk in a diverse Australian antenatal population: a cross-sectional study. BMC Pregnancy Childbirth 2017;17:296.

Gaston SA, Tulve NS, Ferguson TF. Abdominal obesity, metabolic dysfunction, and metabolic syndrome in U.S. adolescents: National Health and Nutrition Examination Survey 2011–2016. Ann Epidemiol 2019;30:30–6. doi:10.1016/j.annepidem.2018.11.009

Gordon A, Sim K, Lopez-Vargas P, et al. Research priorities in the intergenerational cycle of obesity. J Paediatr Child Health 2017;53(Suppl. 2):37–8.

Grodner M. Nutritional foundations and clinical applications. 7th ed. Chatswood, NSW: Elsevier; 2019.

Haire-Joshu D, Tabak R. Preventing obesity across early life intervention. Annu Rev Public Health 2016;37(1):253–71.

Jaul E, Barron J, Rosenzweig JP, et al. An overview of co-morbidities and the development of pressure ulcers among older adults. BMC Geriatr 2018;18:305–15. doi:10.1186/s12877-018-0997-7.

Lee A, Rainbow S, Tregenza J, et al. Nutrition in remote Aboriginal communities: lessons from Mai Wiru and the Anangu Pitjantjatjara Yankunytjatjara Lands. Aust NZ J Publ Heal 2016;40(Suppl.1):S81–8. doi:10.1111/1753-6405.12419.

Lee SK, Sulaiman-Hill CMR, Thompson SC. Providing health information for culturally and linguistically diverse women: priorities and preferences of new migrants and refugees. Health Promot J Austr 2013;24:98–103.

Malacova E, Cheang PR, Dunlop E, et al. Prevalence and predictors of vitamin D deficiency in a nationally representative sample of adults participating in the 2011–2013 Australian Health Survey. Br J Nutr 2019. doi:10.1017/S0007114519000151.

Malnutrition Advisory Group, British Association for Parenteral and Enteral Nutrition. Malnutrition universal screening tool. 2013. Available at: www.bapen.org.uk/screening-for-malnutrition/must/introducing-must.

Ministry of Health New Zealand. Annual update of key findings 2017/18: New Zealand Health Survey. Wellington: Ministry of Health; 2019. Available at: https://www.health.govt.nz/publication/annual-update-key-results-2017-18-new-zealand-health-survey

Morris NF, Stewart S, Riley MD, et al. A comparison of two malnutrition screening tools in acute medical inpatients and validation of a screening tool among adult Indigenous Australian patients. Asia Pac J Clin Nutr 2018;27(6):1198–206.

National Health and Medical Research Council. Australian dietary guidelines. Canberra: Australian Government, 2013a. Available at: www.nhmrc.gov.au/guidelines/publications/n55.

National Health and Medical Research Council. Clinical practice guidelines for the management of overweight and obesity in adults, adolescents and children in Australia. Canberra: Australian Government; 2013b. Available at: www.nhmrc.gov.au/guidelines/publications/n57.

National Health and Medical Research Council/Ministry of Health New Zealand. Nutrient reference values for Australia and New Zealand. 2014. Available at: www.nrv.gov.au.

National Heart Foundation of Australia and the Cardiac Society of Australia and New Zealand. Reducing risk in heart disease: an expert guide to clinical practice for secondary prevention of coronary heart disease. Melbourne: National Heart Foundation of Australia; 2012. Available at: www.heartfoundation.org.au/SiteCollectionDocuments/Reducing-risk-in-heart-disease.pdf.

Pagana K. Manual of diagnostic and laboratory tests. 6th ed. Chatswood, NSW: Elsevier; 2017.

Patton K. Anatomy and physiology. 10th ed. Chatswood, NSW: Elsevier; 2019.

Queensland Health. Validated nutrition assessment tools: comparison guide. 2014. Available at: www.health.qld.gov.au/nutrition/resources/hphe_asst_tools.pdf.

Royal Australian College of General Practitioners and Diabetes Australia. General practice management of type 2 diabetes—2016–18. Melbourne: Royal Australian College of General Practitioners and Diabetes Australia; 2016. Available at: http://www.racgp.org.au/your-practice/guidelines/diabetes/.

Royal Australian College of Pathologists. RCPA manual. 2019. Available at: https://www.rcpa.edu.au/Manuals/RCPA-Manual.

Stanley SH, Laugharne JD, Chapman C, et al. Kimberley Indigenous mental health: An examination of metabolic syndrome risk factors. Aust J Rural Health 2016;24:300–5. doi:10.1111/ajr.12270.

Stewart A, Marfell-Jones M. International standards for anthropometric assessment. 3rd ed. New Zealand: International Society for the Advancement of Kinanthropometry; 2011.

Talley NJ, O'Connor S. Clinical examination. 8th ed. Chatswood, NSW: Elsevier; 2018.

World Health Organization. BMI classification. 2015a. Available at: http://apps.who.int/bmi/index.jsp?introPage=intro_3.html.

World Health Organization. Growth reference 5–19 years. 2015b. Available at: http://www.who.int/growthref/who2007_bmi_for_age/en/.

Websites

Better Health Channel. Available at: https://www.betterhealth.vic.gov.au/

Dietitians Association of Australia. Available at: www.daa.asn.au/

Food Standards Australia and New Zealand. Available at: www.foodstandards.gov.au/foodstandards/nutritionpanelcalculator/

Heart Foundation of Australia. Available at: https://www.heartfoundation.org.au/healthy-eating

Heart Foundation of New Zealand. Available at: https://www.heartfoundation.org.nz/wellbeing/healthy-eating

National Center for Complementary and Alternative Medicine. Available at: http://nccam.nih.gov/

National Digestive Disease Clearing House. Available at: https://www.niddk.nih.gov/health-information/digestive-diseases

National Health and Medical Research Council—Nutritional guidelines. Available at: https://www.nhmrc.gov.au/about-us/publications/australian-dietary-guidelines

New Zealand Ministry of Health—Food and nutrition guidelines. Available at: https://www.health.govt.nz/our-work/eating-and-activity-guidelines/current-food-and-nutrition-guidelines

Nutrition Australia. Available at: www.nutritionaustralia.org/

Chapter Twenty-Two
Skin, hair and nails assessment

Written by Carolyn Jarvis
Adapted by Trish Burton

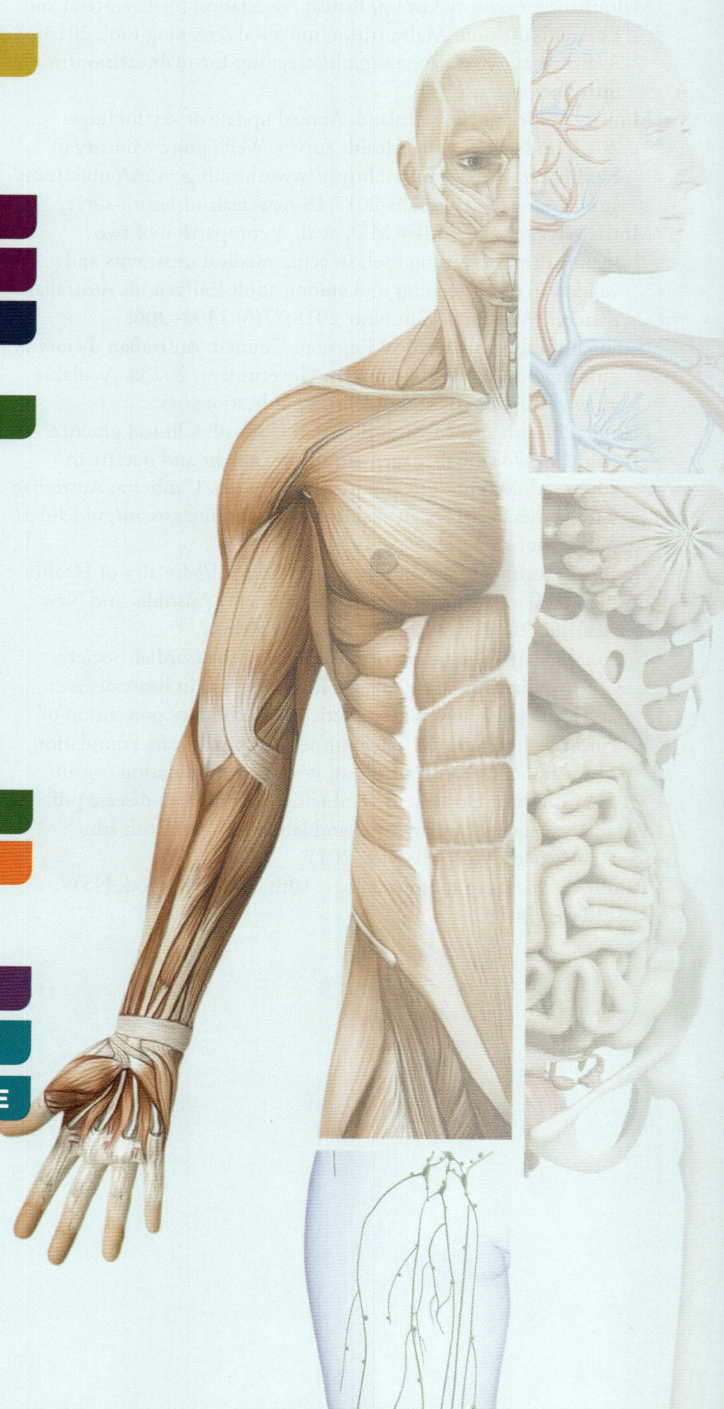

INTRODUCTION

Think of the skin as the body's largest organ system—it covers 6.01 m^2 of surface area in the average adult. The skin is the sentry that guards the body from environmental stresses (e.g. trauma, pathogens, dirt) and adapts it to other environmental influences (e.g. heat, cold). We assess the skin in nearly every area of health assessment. As nutrition is very important to the health of the skin, hair and nails please also refer to Chapter 21.

Structure and function

SKIN

The skin has two layers—the outer highly differentiated *epidermis* and the inner supportive *dermis* (Figure 22.1). Beneath these layers is a third layer, the *subcutaneous* layer of adipose tissue.

Epidermis

The *epidermis* is thin but tough. Its cells are bound tightly together into sheets that form a rugged protective barrier. It is stratified into several zones. The inner **stratum germinativum**, or basal cell layer, forms new skin cells. Their major ingredient is the tough, fibrous protein *keratin*. The melanocytes interspersed along this layer produce the pigment *melanin*, which gives brown tones to the skin and hair. All people have the same number of melanocytes; however, the amount of melanin they produce varies with genetic, hormonal and environmental influences.

From the basal layer, the new cells migrate up and flatten into the **stratum corneum**. This outer horny cell layer consists of dead keratinised cells that are interwoven and closely packed. The cells are constantly being shed, or desquamated, and are replaced with new cells from below. The epidermis is completely replaced every 4 weeks. In fact, each person sheds about ½ kg of skin each year.

The epidermis is uniformly thin except on the surfaces that are exposed to friction, such as the palms and the soles. On these surfaces, skin is thicker because of work and weight bearing. The epidermis is avascular; it is nourished by blood vessels in the dermis below.

Skin colour is derived from three sources: (1) mainly from the brown pigment melanin, (2) also from the yellow-orange tones of the pigment carotene and (3) from the red-purple tones in the underlying vascular bed. All people have skin of varying shades of brown, yellow and red; the relative

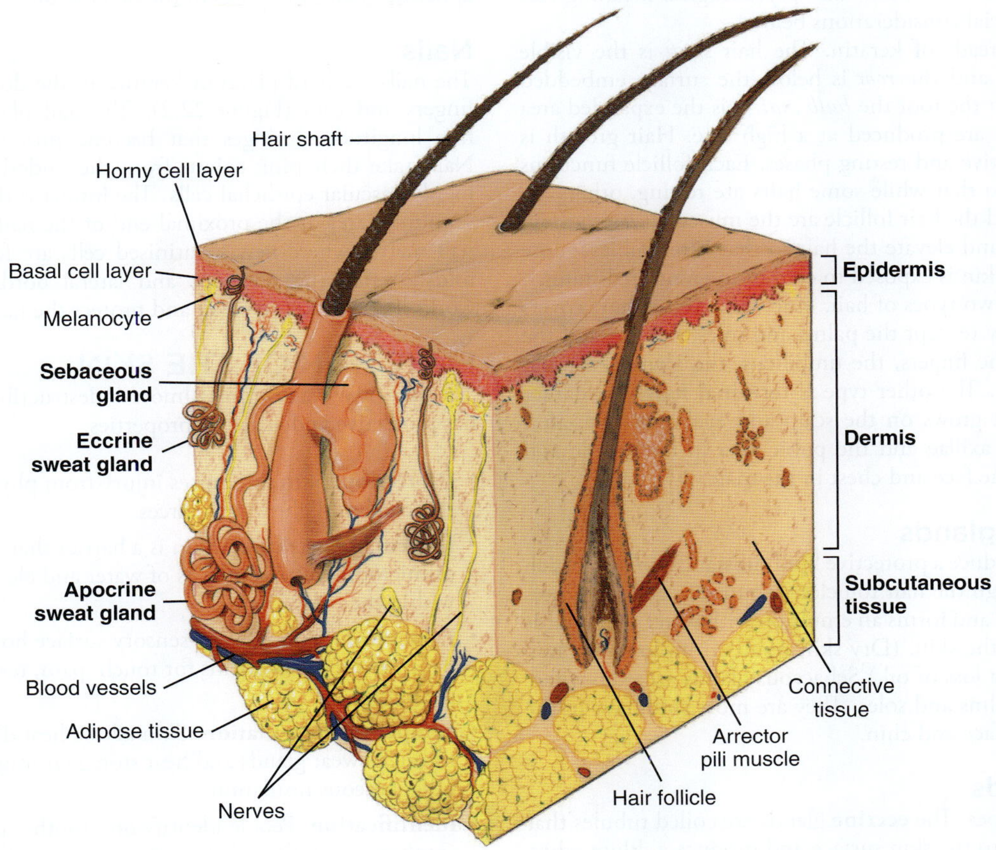

Figure 22.1

proportion of these shades affects the prevailing colour. Skin colour is further modified by the thickness of the skin and by the presence of oedema.

Dermis

The *dermis* is the inner supportive layer consisting mostly of connective tissue, or *collagen*. This is the tough, fibrous protein that enables the skin to resist tearing. The dermis also has resilient elastic tissue that allows the skin to stretch with body movements. The nerves, sensory receptors, blood vessels and lymphatics lie in the dermis. Also, appendages from the epidermis—such as the hair follicles, sebaceous glands and sweat glands—are embedded in the dermis.

Subcutaneous layer

The *subcutaneous layer* is adipose tissue, which is made up of lobules of fat cells. The subcutaneous tissue stores fat for energy, provides insulation for temperature control and aids in protection by its soft cushioning effect. Also, the loose subcutaneous layer gives skin its increased mobility over structures underneath.

EPIDERMAL APPENDAGES

These structures are formed by a tubular invagination of the epidermis down into the underlying dermis.

Hair

Hair is *vestigial* for humans; it is no longer needed for protection from cold or trauma. However, hair is highly significant in most cultures for its cosmetic and psychological meaning (see Cultural and social considerations below).

Hairs are threads of keratin. The hair *shaft* is the visible projecting part, and the *root* is below the surface embedded in the follicle. At the root the *bulb matrix* is the expanded area where new cells are produced at a high rate. Hair growth is cyclical, with active and resting phases. Each follicle functions independently so that while some hairs are resting, others are growing. Around the hair follicle are the muscular *arrector pili*, which contract and elevate the hair so that it resembles 'goose flesh' when the skin is exposed to cold or in emotional states.

People have two types of hair. Fine, faint **vellus hair** covers most of the body (except the palms and soles, the dorsa of the distal parts of the fingers, the umbilicus, the glans penis and inside the labia). The other type is **terminal hair**, the darker thicker hair that grows on the scalp and eyebrows and, after puberty, on the axillae and the pubic area in both male and female and on the face and chest in the male.

Sebaceous glands

These glands produce a protective lipid substance, *sebum*, which is secreted through the hair follicles. Sebum oils and lubricates the skin and hair and forms an emulsion with water that retards water loss from the skin. (Dry skin results from loss of water, not directly from loss of oil.) Sebaceous glands are everywhere except on the palms and soles. They are most abundant in the scalp, forehead, face and chin.

Sweat glands

There are two types. The **eccrine** glands are coiled tubules that open directly onto the skin surface and produce a dilute saline solution called *sweat*. The evaporation of sweat reduces body temperature. Eccrine glands are widely distributed through the body and are mature in the 2-month-old infant.

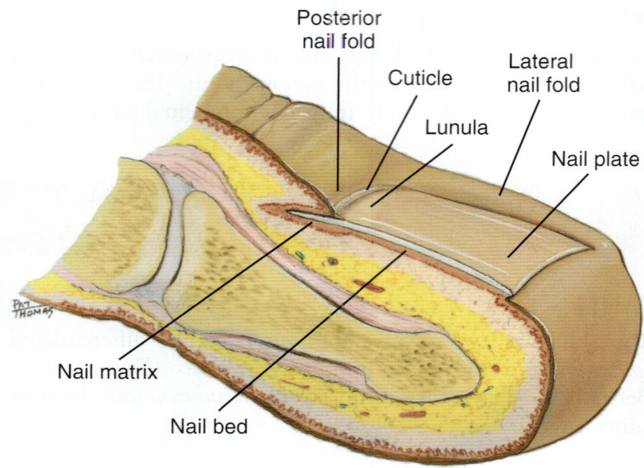

Figure 22.2

The **apocrine** glands produce a thick, milky secretion and open into the hair follicles. They are located mainly in the axillae, anogenital area, nipples and navel and are vestigial in humans. They become active during puberty, and secretion occurs with emotional and sexual stimulation. Bacterial flora residing on the skin surface react with apocrine sweat to produce a characteristic musky body odour. The functioning of apocrine glands decreases in the older adult.

Nails

The nails are hard plates of keratin on the dorsal edges of the fingers and toes (Figure 22.2). The nail plate is clear, with fine longitudinal ridges that become prominent in ageing. Nails take their pink colour from the underlying nail bed of highly vascular epithelial cells. The lunula is the white opaque semilunar area at the proximal end of the nail. It lies over the nail matrix where new keratinised cells are formed. The nail folds overlap the posterior and lateral borders. The cuticle works like a gasket to cover and protect the nail matrix.

FUNCTION OF THE SKIN

The skin is a waterproof, almost indestructible covering that has protective and adaptive properties:

- **Protection.** Skin minimises injury from physical, chemical, thermal and light wave sources.
- **Prevents penetration.** Skin is a barrier that stops invasion of microorganisms and loss of water and electrolytes from within the body.
- **Perception.** Skin is a vast sensory surface holding the neurosensory end-organs for touch, pain, temperature and pressure.
- **Temperature regulation.** Skin allows heat dissipation through sweat glands and heat storage through subcutaneous insulation.
- **Identification.** People identify one another by unique combinations of facial characteristics, hair, skin colour and even fingerprints. Self-image is often enhanced or deterred by the way society's standards of beauty measure up to each person's perceived characteristics.

- **Communication.** Emotions are expressed in the sign language of the face and in the body posture. Vascular mechanisms such as blushing or blanching also signal emotional states.
- **Wound repair.** Skin allows cell replacement of surface wounds.
- **Absorption and excretion.** Skin allows limited excretion of some metabolic wastes, byproducts of cellular decomposition such as minerals, sugars, amino acids, cholesterol, uric acid and urea.
- **Production of vitamin D.** The skin is the surface on which ultraviolet light converts cholesterol into vitamin D.

DEVELOPMENTAL CONSIDERATIONS

Infancy to adolescence (birth to 19 years)

The hair follicles develop in the fetus at 3 months gestation; by midgestation most of the skin is covered with **lanugo**, the fine downy hair of the newborn infant. In the first few months after birth, this is replaced by fine vellus hair. Terminal hair on the scalp, if present at birth, tends to be soft and to suffer a patchy loss, especially at the temples and occiput. Also present at birth is **vernix caseosa**: the thick, cheesy substance made up of sebum and shed epithelial cells.

The newborn's skin is similar in structure to the adult's, but many of its functions are not fully developed. The newborn's skin is thin, smooth and elastic and is relatively more permeable than that of the adult, so the infant is at greater risk for fluid loss. Sebum, which holds water in the skin, is present for the first few weeks of life, producing milia and cradle cap in some babies. Then sebaceous glands decrease in size and production and do not resume functioning until puberty. Temperature regulation is ineffective. Eccrine sweat glands do not secrete in response to heat until the first few months of life and then only minimally throughout childhood. The skin cannot protect much against cold because it cannot contract and shiver and because the subcutaneous layer is inefficient. Also, the pigment system is inefficient at birth.

As the child grows, the epidermis thickens, toughens and darkens and the skin becomes better lubricated. Hair growth accelerates. At puberty, secretion from apocrine sweat glands increases in response to heat and emotional stimuli, producing body odour. Sebaceous glands become more active—the skin looks oily and acne develops. Subcutaneous fat deposits increase, especially in females.

Secondary sex characteristics that appear during adolescence are evident in the integument (i.e. skin). In the female, the diameter of the areola enlarges and darkens, and breast tissue develops. Coarse pubic hair develops in males and females, then axillary hair, then coarse facial hair in males.

The pregnant woman

The change in hormone levels results in increased pigment in the areolae and nipples, vulva and sometimes in the midline of the abdomen **(linea nigra)** or in the face **(chloasma)**. Hyperoestrogenaemia probably also causes the common vascular spiders and palmar erythema. Connective tissue develops increased fragility, resulting in **striae gravidarum**, which may develop in the skin of the abdomen, breasts or thighs. Metabolism is increased in pregnancy; as a way to dissipate heat, the peripheral vasculature dilates, and the sweat and sebaceous glands increase secretion. Fat deposits are laid down, particularly in the buttocks and hips, as maternal reserves for the nursing baby. For further information see Chapter 29.

Late adulthood (65+ years)

The skin is a mirror that reflects ageing changes that proceed in *all* our organ systems; it just happens to be the one organ we can view directly. The ageing process carries a slow atrophy of skin structures. The ageing skin loses its elasticity; it folds and sags. By the 70s to 80s, it looks parchment thin, lax, dry and wrinkled.

The epidermis's outer layer, the *stratum corneum*, thins and flattens. This allows chemicals easier access into the body. Wrinkling occurs because the underlying dermis thins and flattens. A loss of elastin, collagen and subcutaneous fat occurs as well as a reduction in muscle tone. The loss of collagen increases the risk for shearing, tearing injuries.

Sweat glands and sebaceous glands decrease in number and function, leaving dry skin. Decreased response of the sweat glands to thermoregulatory demand also puts the older person at greater risk for heat stroke. The vascularity of the skin diminishes while the vascular fragility increases; a minor trauma may produce dark red discoloured areas, or **senile purpura**.

Sun exposure and, to a somewhat lesser extent, cigarette smoking further accentuate ageing changes in the skin. Coarse wrinkling, decreased elasticity, atrophy, speckled and uneven colouring, more pigment changes and a yellowed, leathery texture occur. Chronic sun damage is even more prominent in pale or light-skinned persons.

An accumulation of factors place the older person at risk for skin disease and breakdown: the thinning of the skin, the decrease in vascularity and nutrients, the loss of protective cushioning of the subcutaneous layer, a lifetime of environmental trauma to skin, the social changes of ageing (e.g. less nutrition, limited financial resources), the increasingly sedentary lifestyle and the chance of immobility. When skin breakdown does occur, subsequent cell replacement is slower, and wound healing is delayed.

In the ageing hair matrix, the number of functioning melanocytes decreases, so the hair looks grey or white and feels thin and fine. A person's genetic script determines the onset of greying and the number of grey hairs. Hair distribution changes. Males may have a symmetrical W-shaped balding in the frontal areas. Some testosterone is present in both males and females; as it decreases with age, axillary and pubic hair decrease. As the female's oestrogen also decreases, testosterone is unopposed and the female may have some bristly facial hairs. Nails grow more slowly. Their surface is lustreless and is characterised by longitudinal ridges resulting from local trauma at the nail matrix.

Because the ageing changes in the skin and hair can be viewed directly, they carry a profound psychological impact. For many people, self-esteem is linked to a youthful appearance. This view is compounded by media advertising in western society. Although sagging and wrinkling skin and greying and thinning hair are usual processes of ageing, they prompt a loss of self-esteem for many adults.

CULTURAL AND SOCIAL CONSIDERATIONS

Awareness of biocultural differences and the ability to recognise the unique clinical manifestations of disease are especially important when dealing with people with dark pigmented skin. As described earlier, melanin is responsible for the various colours and tones of skin observed among people from culturally diverse backgrounds. Melanin protects the skin against harmful ultraviolet rays, a genetic advantage accounting for the lower incidence of skin cancer in people with dark pigmented skin. The incidence of melanoma is higher among Caucasians than among people with dark pigmented skin.

Areas of the skin affected by hormones and, in some cases, differing for culturally diverse people are the sexual skin areas, such as the nipples, areola, scrotum and labia majora. In general, these areas are darker than other parts of the skin in both adults and children.

The apocrine and eccrine sweat glands are important for fluid balance and for thermoregulation. When apocrine gland secretions are contaminated by normal skin flora, odour results. The amount of chloride excreted by sweat glands varies widely.

While the characteristics of hair vary widely between people, hair condition is significant in diagnosing and treating certain disease states. For example, hair texture becomes dry, brittle and lustreless with inadequate nutrition.

Subjective data

Comprehensive assessment of the skin, hair and nails is an important component of health assessment. Skin integrity refers to intact structure and function and relies on adequate perfusion by oxygenated blood and adequate nutrition and hydration. Changes in skin integrity may therefore indicate alterations in perfusion and oxygenation, nutrition and hydration state of the person. Altered skin integrity can also occur as a result of reduced mobility, mechanical or chemical factors, extremes of temperature, bodily excretions or secretions and humidity. Altered skin integrity often results in pain and puts the person at risk of infection.

1. Presenting concern
2. Previous history
3. Changes in pigmentation, moles, moisture
4. Pruritus
5. Excessive bruising
6. Rash or lesion
7. Hair loss
8. Change in nail
9. Environmental or occupational hazards
10. Health and life style management

Practice note: Before you commence the assessment, introduce yourself to the person, confirm the person's identity, discuss the purpose and scope of the assessment, clarify any questions the person may have and obtain verbal consent from the person to perform the assessment.

ASSESSMENT GUIDELINES	CLINICAL SIGNIFICANCE AND CLINICAL ALERTS
1. Presenting concern	
• Do you feel that you have any problem/s with your skin, hair or nails? It is important to ascertain the person's perception of the health of their skin, hair and nails. • If they do perceive a problem—how does this impact on their quality of life?	The person's response to this question will guide areas to focus on in further subjective and objective data collection.
2. Previous history of skin disease	
• Have you had any previous skin disease or problem? How was this treated? Is there any family history of allergies or allergic skin problem?	Some skin disorders have genetic or familial links, e.g. allergies, hay fever, psoriasis, atopic dermatitis (eczema), acne.
• Do you have any allergies to drugs, plants, animals, foods?	Identify offending allergen. Allergic reactions may result in skin symptoms such as redness, swelling and pruritus.
• Do you have any birthmarks, tattoos?	Use of nonsterile equipment to apply tattoos increases risk of hepatitis C.

ASSESSMENT GUIDELINES	CLINICAL SIGNIFICANCE AND CLINICAL ALERTS
3. Change in pigmentation	
• Have you noticed any change in skin colour or pigmentation?	Skin colour will vary from pink to dark brown. Exposed areas are often darker than non-exposed areas. **Hypopigmentation**—loss of pigmentation. **Hyperpigmentation** (increase in colour) such as freckles on the face and arms is common in people with pale skin.
• Is the change in pigmentation generalised (all over), or localised?	Generalised change suggests systemic illness: **Pallor** (pale colour) may be caused by anaemia or vasoconstriction. **Erythema** (red colour). Local redness of skin is indicative of a local inflammation whereas generalised erythema is often related to systemic vasodilation. **Cyanosis** (blue colour). Cyanosis of the oral mucous membranes and lips results from hypoxaemia. Cyanosis of the extremities results from reduced peripheral blood flow. **Jaundice** (yellow colour) is caused by changes in metabolism of bilirubin.
4. Change in mole	
• Have you noticed any **change in a mole**: colour, size, shape, sudden appearance of tenderness, bleeding, itching? • Do you have any 'sores' that do not heal?	Person may be unaware of changes in a mole especially if it is in an area that they cannot see such as on the back, buttocks, soles of feet or between toes. ***Clinical alert:*** any changes in the colour, size or edges, or development of itchiness or bleeding could be signs of malignancy and should be referred to a medical practitioner for further assessment (Ritchie 2017).
5. Excessive dryness or moisture	
• Have you had any change in the feel of your skin: temperature, moisture, texture?	**Seborrhoea**—oily.
• Any excess dryness? Is this seasonal or constant?	**Xerosis**—dry.
6. Pruritus	
• Have you had any skin itching? Is this mild (prickling, tingling) or intense (intolerable)? • Does it awaken you from sleep?	**Pruritus** is the most common of skin symptoms; occurs with dry skin, ageing, drug reactions, allergy, obstructive jaundice, uraemia, lice.
• Where is the itching? When did it start?	Presence or absence of pruritus may be significant for diagnosis. Scratching may cause excoriation of primary lesion.
• Do you have any other skin pain or soreness? Where?	

SUBJECTIVE DATA

SUBJECTIVE DATA

ASSESSMENT GUIDELINES	CLINICAL SIGNIFICANCE AND CLINICAL ALERTS
7. Excessive bruising	
• Do you have any excess bruising? Whereabouts are the bruises? • How did this happen? • How long have you had it?	Multiple cuts and bruises, bruises in various stages of healing, bruises above knees and elbows and illogical explanation—consider the possibility of abuse. Frequent falls may be due to dizziness of neurological or cardiovascular origin. Also, frequent minor trauma may be a side effect of alcoholism or other drug abuse.
8. Rash or lesion	
Have you had a skin rash or lesion? • **Onset.** When did you first notice it?	Rashes are a common reason for seeking healthcare. A careful history is important; it may be an accurate predictor of the type of lesion you will see in the examination and its cause (Thomas et al 2016).
• **Location.** Where did it start?	Identify the primary site—it may give clues as to the cause. Migration pattern, evolution.
• **Character or quality.** Describe the colour. Is it raised or flat? Any crust, odour? Does it feel tender, warm? • **Duration.** How long have you had it?	
• **Setting.** Anyone at home or work with a similar rash? Have you been camping, acquired a new pet, tried a new food, drug? Does the rash seem to come with stress?	Identify new or relevant exposure, any household or social contacts with similar symptoms.
• **Alleviating and aggravating factors.** What home care have you tried? Bath, lotions, heat, cold? Do they help, or make it worse? • **Associated symptoms.** Is it itchy? Have you had a fever?	Myriad over-the-counter remedies are available. Many people try them and seek professional help only when they do not see improvement.
• What do you think the rash/lesion means?	Assess person's perception of cause: fear of cancer, tick-borne illnesses or sexually transmitted diseases.
• How has rash/lesion affected your self-care, hygiene, ability to function at work/home/socially?	Assess effectiveness of coping strategies. Chronic skin diseases may increase risk of loss of self-esteem, social isolation and anxiety.
• Are there any new or increased stressors in your life?	Stress can exacerbate chronic skin illness.
9. Hair loss	
• Have you had any recent hair loss? Was it a gradual or sudden onset? Was the hair loss symmetrical? Was it associated with fever, illness, increased stress?	**Alopecia** is a significant loss of hair. A full head of hair equates with vitality in many cultures. If treated as a trivial problem, the person may seek alternative, unproven methods of treatment.
• Has there been any unusual hair growth? • Has there been a recent change in texture, appearance of your hair?	**Hirsutism** is shaggy or excessive hair.
10. Change in nails	
• Any change in nails? Have there been any changes in the shape, colour or brittleness of your nails? Do you tend to bite or chew nails?	

ASSESSMENT GUIDELINES	CLINICAL SIGNIFICANCE AND CLINICAL ALERTS
11. Environmental or occupational hazards	
• Have you been exposed to any **environmental** or **occupational** hazards?	Majority of skin neoplasms result from occupational or environmental agents.
• Are there any hazard-related problems with your occupation, such as exposure to dyes, toxic chemicals, radiation? • What are your hobbies? Do you perform any household or furniture repair work that involves use of paints or glues?	People at risk include outdoor sports enthusiasts, farmers, sailors, outdoor workers; also creosote workers, tilers, coal workers.
• How much sun exposure do you get from outdoor work, leisure activities, sunbathing?	**Vitamin D** forms in the skin as a result of exposure to sunlight; in particular the ultraviolet B component of sunlight and is important for strong healthy bones. Cancer Council Australia (2018a) recommends exposing the face, arms and hands or the equivalent area of skin to a few minutes of sunlight on either side of the peak UV periods on most days of the week. People at risk of vitamin D deficiency include those who cover their skin, those with naturally very dark skin, elderly people, those who are housebound or are in institutional care and babies of vitamin D-deficient mothers. Overexposure during peak ultraviolet radiation periods (10 am to 3 pm) accelerates ageing of skin and produces lesions. Those at high risk are light-skinned people, those over 40 years old and those regularly in the sun. The Cancer Council Australia (2018b) recommends the use of protection to prevent skin cancer when the UV index is moderate or above (i.e. UV index is 3 or higher). Sun protection includes wearing a hat, using sunscreen and covering skin.
• Have you recently been bitten by an insect: bee, wasp, tick, mosquito, spider?	Identify contactants that produce lesions or contact dermatitis.
• Have you had any recent exposure to plants, animals or been camping?	People with chronic recurrent **urticaria (hives)** can benefit by keeping a diary of meals and environmental contacts to identify precipitating factors.
12. Health and lifestyle management	
• What do you do to care for your skin, hair, nails? What cosmetics, soaps, chemicals do you use? • Do you clip cuticles on nails or use adhesive for false fingernails?	
• If you have known allergies, how do you control your environment to minimise exposure?	
• Do you perform a skin self-examination?	

SUBJECTIVE DATA

SUBJECTIVE DATA

ASSESSMENT GUIDELINES	CLINICAL SIGNIFICANCE AND CLINICAL ALERTS
Medications. What medications do you take? • Prescription and over-the-counter? • Recent change?	Drugs may produce allergic skin eruption: aspirin, antibiotics, barbiturates, some tonics. Drugs may increase sunlight sensitivity and give burn response: sulfonamides, thiazide diuretics, oral hypoglycaemic agents and tetracycline. Drugs can cause hyperpigmentation: antimalarials, antineoplastic agents, hormones, metals, and tetracycline.
• How long have you been taking the medication?	Even after a long time on medication, a person may develop sensitivity.
Additional subjective data for infants and children (questions for parents or guardians)	
• Does the child have any birthmarks?	
• Was there any change in skin colour as a newborn? – Was there any jaundice? On which day after birth did it occur? – Has there been any cyanosis? What were the circumstances?	
• Have you noted any rash or sores? What seems to bring it on? – Have you introduced a new food or formula? When? Does your child eat chocolate, cow's milk or eggs?	Generalised rash—consider allergic reaction to new food. Irritability and general fussiness may indicate the presence of pruritus.
• Does the child have a nappy rash? How do you care for this? Do you use disposable nappies? If not, how do you wash nappies? How often do you change nappies? How do you clean skin?	Infrequent nappy changing may cause rash. Infant may be allergic to a certain detergent or to disposable wipes (Hugill 2017).
• Does the child have any burns or bruises? – Where? – How did it happen?	A careful history is important to distinguish expected childhood bumps and bruises from any lesion that may indicate child abuse or neglect: cigarette burns; excessive bruising, especially above knees or elbows; linear whip marks. With abuse, the history often will not coincide with the physical appearance and location of lesion.
• Has the child had any exposure to contagious skin conditions: scabies, impetigo, lice? Or to communicable diseases: measles, chickenpox, scarlet fever?	
– Are the child's vaccinations up to date?	
• Does the child have any habits or habitual movements, such as nail-biting, twisting hair, rubbing head on mattress?	
• What steps are taken to protect the child from sun exposure? Do you use sunscreen? How do you treat sunburn?	Excessive sun exposure, especially severe or blistering sunburns in childhood, increases risk for melanoma in later life.

ASSESSMENT GUIDELINES	CLINICAL SIGNIFICANCE AND CLINICAL ALERTS
Additional subjective data for the adolescent	
• Have you noticed any skin problems such as pimples, blackheads? – How long have you had them? How do you feel about it? – How do you treat this? Have you sought medical advice? If so what was the advice?	About 70% of teens will have acne, and the psychological effect is often more significant than the physical effect. Self-treatment is common. Many myths surround the cause of acne. Cause is unknown; acne is not caused by poor diet, oily complexion or contagion.
Additional subjective data for the adult over 65 years	
• What changes have you noticed in your skin in the last few years?	Assess impact of ageing on self-concept. Common ageing changes may cause distress. Many changes attributed to ageing are due to chronic sun damage. Most skin cancers appear in older people, although sun damage often begins decades earlier.
• Any delay in wound healing? – Any skin itching?	Pruritus is very common with ageing. Consider side effects of medicine or systemic disease (e.g. liver or kidney disease, cancer, lymphoma), but senile pruritus is usually due to dry skin (xerosis). Exacerbated by too-frequent bathing or use of soap. Scratching with dirty, jagged fingernails produces excoriations.
• Do you have any other skin pain?	Some diseases, such as herpes zoster (shingles), produce more intense sensations of pain, itching in older people. Other diseases (e.g. diabetes) may reduce pain sensation in extremities. Also, some older people tolerate chronic pain as 'part of growing old' and hesitate to 'complain'.
• Have you noticed any changes in your feet or toenails? Do you have any bunions? Are you able to wear shoes?	Some older people cannot reach down to care for their feet/nails.
• Do you experience frequent falls?	Multiple bruises, trauma from falls.
• Do you have a history of diabetes, peripheral vascular disease?	Risk for skin lesions in feet or ankles.
• What do you do to care for your skin?	Application of bland lotions is important to retain moisture in ageing skin. Dermatitis may ensue from certain cosmetics, creams, ointments and dyes applied to achieve a youthful appearance.
	Ageing skin has a delayed inflammatory response when exposed to irritants. If the person is not alerted by warning signs (e.g. pruritus, redness), exposure may continue and dermatitis may ensue.

SUBJECTIVE DATA

Objective data

For most nurses, skin assessment is done in an opportunistic way in which the nurse examines the person's skin when performing other health assessments or nursing care activities; for example, assisting the person with activities of daily living or assisting the person to move and reposition may prompt the need for a more comprehensive assessment of a particular area of the skin. Nurses also assess the colour and moisture level of a person's skin especially the face, lips, nose, ear lobes and periphery every time they interact with the person. Changes in skin colour and moisture along with variations in vital signs and conscious state may indicate clinical deterioration for which immediate further assessment and action is required. On admission to healthcare services, it is expected that nurses will perform a skin assessment to identify risk of or presence of pressure injury. Nurses working in skin cancer clinics adopt a systematic, detailed and comprehensive approach to skin assessment.

To help you focus, pay attention to the person's skin characteristics. The danger is one of omission. You grow so accustomed to seeing the skin that you are likely to ignore it as you assess the organ systems underneath. Yet the skin holds information about the body's circulation, nutritional status and signs of systemic diseases, as well as topical data on the integument itself. Baseline knowledge is important to assess colour or pigment changes. If this is the first time you are examining the person, ask about their usual skin colour and about any self-monitoring practices.

Preparation

When performing a skin assessment, ensure that the room is warm, there is adequate lighting and privacy. Assist the person into a position of comfort and expose only areas of the body being assessed.

Equipment needed

Small centimetre paper ruler
Penlight
Hand hygiene solution
Disposable gloves

PROCEDURES AND NORMAL FINDINGS	ABNORMAL FINDINGS AND CLINICAL ALERTS
General inspection	
During collection of subjective data you will have noticed the colour, smoothness and moisture of the face in particular lips, nose and earlobes, the periphery, height to weight ratio, level of hygiene and grooming and general demeanor. All of these factors provide clues to the condition of the integument.	Condition of skin can be an indicator of a person's general health and wellbeing. Interpretation should be guided by whether the person's skin indicates a health problem or puts the person at risk of a health problem or whether personal choices have been made. ***Clinical alert:*** multiple bruises at different stages of healing and excessive bruising above knees or elbows should raise concern about physical abuse. See Table 22.7. Refer to medical practitioner. Further information on family violence is available in Chapter 5.
Inspect and palpate the skin	
Note the presence of scars, wounds, bruises, piercings, tattoos, enlarged veins and general hygiene and skin condition. Any bruising (ecchymosis) should be consistent with stage of life. For example it is not uncommon for young children to have bruises on their legs as a result of vigorous play activities. For the frail, older person, skin is easily bruised as a result of minor day to day bumps. There are normally no venous dilatations or varicosities.	Varicosities: enlarged or swollen veins. Bruises usually occur as a result of trauma, bleeding disorders or liver dysfunction. ***Clinical alert:*** Multiple bruises at different stages of healing and excessive bruises above knees or elbows should raise concern about physical abuse (see Table 22.7). Refer to Chapter 5.

PROCEDURES AND NORMAL FINDINGS	ABNORMAL FINDINGS AND CLINICAL ALERTS

Colour

General pigmentation. Observe the skin tone. Normally it is consistent with genetic background and varies from pinkish tan to ruddy dark tan or from light to dark brown. People who have dark pigmented skin normally have areas of lighter pigmentation on the palms, nail beds and lips (Figure 22.3A).

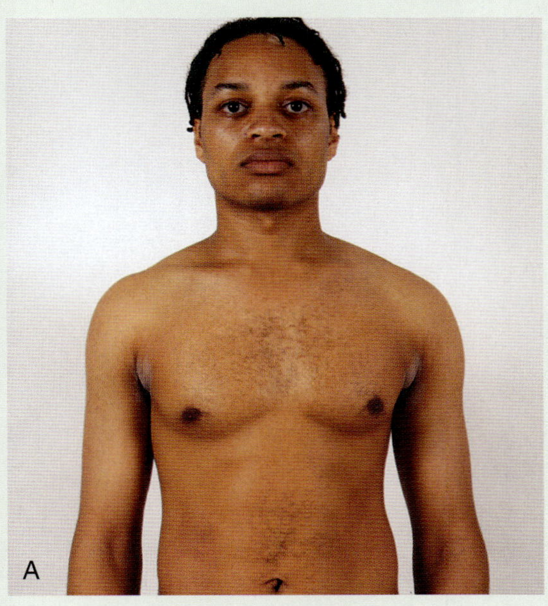

Figure 22.3A

General pigmentation is darker in sun-exposed areas. Common (benign) pigmented areas also occur.

An acquired condition is **vitiligo**, the complete absence of melanin pigment in patchy areas of white or light skin on the face, neck, hands, feet, body folds and around orifices (Figure 22.3B). Vitiligo can occur in any person, although dark-skinned people are more severely affected and potentially suffer a greater threat to their body image.

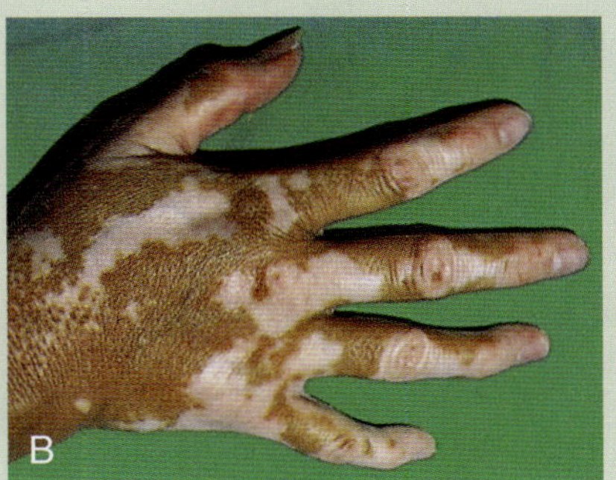

Figure 22.3B
Vitiligo.

TABLE 22.1 External variables influencing skin colour

VARIABLE	CAUSES	MISLEADING OUTCOME
Emotions		
Fear, anger	Peripheral vascconstriction	False pallor
Embarrassment	Flushing in face and neck	False erythema
Environment		
Hot room	Vasodilatation	False erythema
Chilly or air-conditioned room	Vasoconstriction	False pallor, coolness
Cigarette smoking	Vasoconstriction	False pallor
Physical		
Prolonged elevation	Decreased arterial perfusion	Pallor, coolness
Dependent position	Venous pooling	Redness, warmth, distended veins
Immobilisation, prolonged inactivity	Slowed circulation	Pallor, coolness, nail beds pale, prolonged capillary filling time

PROCEDURES AND NORMAL FINDINGS	ABNORMAL FINDINGS AND CLINICAL ALERTS
• **Freckles** (ephelides)—small, flat macules of brown melanin pigment that occur on sun-exposed skin (Figure 22.4A). • **Mole** (naevus)—a proliferation of melanocytes, tan to brown colour, flat or raised. Acquired naevi are characterised by their symmetry, small size (6 mm or less), smooth borders and single uniform pigmentation. The **junctional naevus** (Figure 22.4B) is macular only and occurs in children and adolescents. It progresses to the **compound naevi** in young adults (Figure 22.4C) that are macular and papular. The intradermal naevus (mainly in older age) has naevus cells in the dermis only. • **Birthmarks**—may be red or tan to brown in colour. 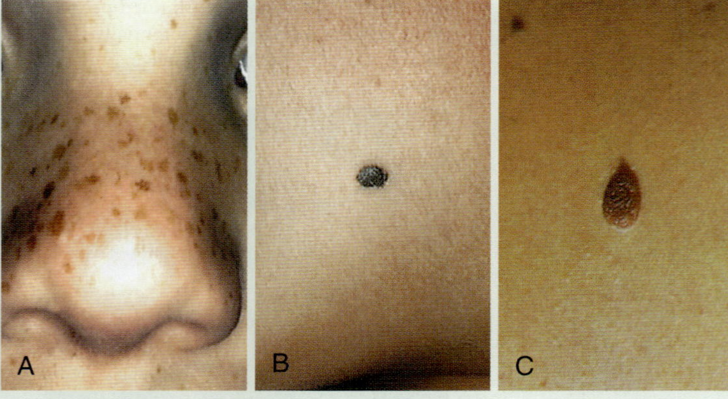 **Figure 22.4** A, Freckles. B, Junctional naevus. C, Compound naevus.	See also Table 22.3.
Widespread colour change. Note any colour change over the entire body skin, such as **pallor** (whitish tone), **erythema** (red), **cyanosis** (blue) and **jaundice** (yellow). Note whether the colour change is transient and expected or if it is due to pathology.	
In people who have dark pigmented skin, the amount of pigment may mask colour changes. Lips and nail beds show some colour change, but they vary with the person's skin colour and may not always be accurate signs. The more reliable sites are those with the least pigmentation, such as under the tongue, the buccal mucosa, the palpebral conjunctiva and the sclera. See Table 22.2 for specific clues to assessment.	Ashen grey colour in a person with dark skin or marked pallor in a person with light coloured skin occurs with anaemia, shock, arterial insufficiency (see Table 22.2).
Look for **pallor** in people with dark skin by the absence of the underlying red tones that normally give brown- or dark-coloured skin its lustre. Generalised pallor can be observed in the mucous membranes, lips and nail beds. The palpebral conjunctiva and nail beds are preferred sites for assessing the pallor of anaemia. When inspecting the conjunctiva, lower the lid sufficiently to visualise the conjunctiva near the *outer* canthus as well as the inner canthus. The colouration is often lighter near the inner canthus.	**Pallor.** When the red-pink tones from the oxygenated haemoglobin in the blood are lost, the skin takes on the colour of connective tissue (collagen), which is mostly white. Pallor is common in acute high-stress states, such as anxiety or fear, because of the powerful peripheral vasoconstriction from sympathetic nervous system stimulation. The skin also looks pale with vasoconstriction from exposure to cold and cigarette smoking and in the presence of oedema.

PROCEDURES AND NORMAL FINDINGS	ABNORMAL FINDINGS AND CLINICAL ALERTS
	Anaemias, particularly chronic iron deficiency anaemia, may show 'spoon' nails, with a concave shape. A lemon yellow tint of the face and slightly yellow sclera accompany pernicious anaemia, also indicated by neurological deficits and a red, painful tongue. Fatigue, exertional dyspnoea, rapid pulse, dizziness and impaired mental function accompany most severe anaemias. ***Clinical alert:*** The pallor of impending shock is accompanied by other subtle manifestations, such as increasing pulse rate, oliguria, apprehension and restlessness. Report changes such as this to medical practitioner immediately.
Erythema. Erythema is an intense redness of the skin from excess blood (hyperaemia) in the dilated superficial capillaries. This sign is *expected* with fever, local inflammation or with emotional reactions such as blushing in vascular flush areas (cheeks, neck and upper chest). When erythema is associated with fever or localised inflammation, it is characterised by increased skin temperature from the increased rate of blood flow through the blood vessels. Because it is more difficult to see inflammation in people with dark skin, it is often necessary to palpate the skin for increased warmth, taut or tightly pulled surfaces that may be indicative of oedema and hardening of deep tissues or blood vessels.	**Erythema** occurs with polycythaemia, venous stasis, carbon monoxide poisoning and the extravascular presence of red blood cells **(petechiae, ecchymoses, haematoma)** (see Tables 22.2 and 22.3).
Cyanosis. This is a bluish mottled colour that signifies that the tissues are not adequately perfused with oxygenated blood (Figure 22.5). Be aware that cyanosis can be a nonspecific sign. A person who is anaemic could have hypoxaemia without ever looking cyanosed because not enough haemoglobin is present (either oxygenated or reduced) to colour the skin. On the other hand, a person with polycythaemia (an increase in the number of red blood cells) looks ruddy blue at all times and may not necessarily be hypoxaemic. This person is just unable to fully oxygenate the massive numbers of red blood cells. 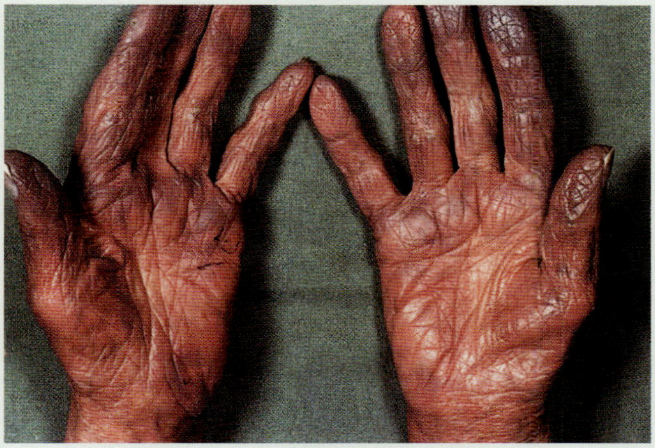 **Figure 22.5**	**Cyanosis** indicates hypoxaemia and occurs with shock, heart failure, chronic bronchitis and congenital heart disease.
Cyanosis is difficult to observe in people with dark skin (see Table 22.2). Given that most conditions causing cyanosis also cause decreased oxygenation of the brain, other clinical signs—such as changes in level of consciousness and signs of respiratory distress—will be evident.	

OBJECTIVE DATA

PROCEDURES AND NORMAL FINDINGS	ABNORMAL FINDINGS AND CLINICAL ALERTS
Jaundice. Jaundice is exhibited by a yellow colour, indicating rising amounts of bilirubin in the blood. Except for physiological jaundice in the newborn (see below), jaundice does not occur normally. Jaundice is *first* noted in the junction of the hard and soft palate in the mouth and in the sclera. But do not confuse scleral jaundice with the normal yellow subconjunctival fatty deposits that are common in the outer sclera of people with dark skin. The scleral yellow of jaundice extends up to the edge of the iris.	**Jaundice** occurs with hepatitis, cirrhosis, sickle-cell disease, transfusion reaction and haemolytic disease of the newborn.
As levels of serum bilirubin rise, jaundice is evident in the skin over the rest of the body. This is best assessed in direct natural daylight. Common calluses on palms and soles often look yellow—do not interpret these as jaundice.	Light or clay-coloured stools and dark golden urine often accompany jaundice.
Temperature	
Note the temperature of your own hands. Then use the backs (dorsa) of your hands to palpate the person bilaterally. The skin should be warm, and the temperature should be equal bilaterally; warmth suggests normal circulatory status. Hands and feet may be slightly cooler in a cool environment.	**Hypothermia.** Generalised coolness may be induced, such as in hypothermia used for surgery or high fever. Localised coolness is expected with an immobilised extremity, as when a limb is in a cast or with an intravenous infusion. **Hyperthermia.** Generalised hyperthermia occurs with an increased metabolic rate, such as in fever or after heavy exercise. A localised area feels hyperthermic with trauma, infection or sunburn.
	General hypothermia accompanies a central circulatory problem such as shock. **Localised hypothermia** occurs in peripheral arterial insufficiency and Raynaud's disease.
	Hyperthyroidism has an increased metabolic rate, causing warm, moist skin.
Moisture	
Perspiration appears normally on the face, hands, axillae and skinfolds in response to activity, a warm environment, fever or anxiety.	**Diaphoresis,** or profuse perspiration, accompanies an increased metabolic rate, such as occurs in heavy activity or fever. Diaphoresis occurs with thyrotoxicosis and with stimulation of the nervous system with anxiety or pain.
Look for dehydration in the oral mucous membranes and the elasticity of the skin. Normally the mucous membranes look smooth and moist and the skin is elastic.	With **dehydration**, mucous membranes look dry and the lips look parched and cracked. With extreme dryness, the skin is fissured, resembling cracks in a dry lake bed and does not recoil quickly when lightly pinched.
Texture	
Normal skin feels smooth and firm, with an even surface.	**Hyperthyroidism**—skin feels smoother and softer, like velvet. **Hypothyroidism**—skin feels rough, dry and flaky.
Thickness	
The epidermis is uniformly thin over most of the body, although thickened callus areas are normal on palms and soles. A callus is a circumscribed overgrowth of epidermis and is an adaptation to excessive pressure from the friction of work and weight bearing.	Very thin, shiny skin (atrophic) occurs with **arterial insufficiency.**

OBJECTIVE DATA

PROCEDURES AND NORMAL FINDINGS	ABNORMAL FINDINGS AND CLINICAL ALERTS
Oedema	
Oedema is fluid accumulating in the intercellular spaces; it is not present normally. To check for oedema, imprint your thumbs firmly against the ankle malleolus or the tibia. Normally, the skin surface stays smooth. If your pressure leaves a dent in the skin, 'pitting' oedema is present. Its presence is graded on a four-point scale: 1+ **Mild pitting,** slight indentation, no perceptible swelling of the leg 2+ **Moderate pitting,** indentation subsides rapidly 3+ **Deep pitting,** indentation remains for a short time, leg looks swollen 4+ **Very deep pitting,** indentation lasts a long time, leg is very swollen This scale is somewhat subjective; outcomes vary among examiners (see further content on grading scale in Chapters 16 and 17). Oedema masks normal skin colour and obscures pathological conditions such as jaundice or cyanosis because the fluid lies between the surface and the pigmented and vascular layers. It makes skin look lighter.	**Oedema** is most evident in dependent parts of the body (feet, ankles and sacral areas), where the skin looks puffy and tight. Oedema makes the hair follicles more prominent, so you note a pigskin or orange-peel look (called *peau d'orange*). **Unilateral oedema**—is usually related to a local or peripheral cause. **Bilateral oedema** or oedema that is generalised over the whole body (*anasarca*)—is usually related to a central problem such as heart failure or kidney failure as a consequence of increased capillary hydrostatic pressure (Todd 2017). **Dependent oedema**
Mobility and turgor	
Pinch up a large fold of skin on the anterior chest under the clavicle (Figure 22.6). Mobility is the skin's ease of rising, and turgor is its ability to return to place promptly when released. This reflects the elasticity of the skin. 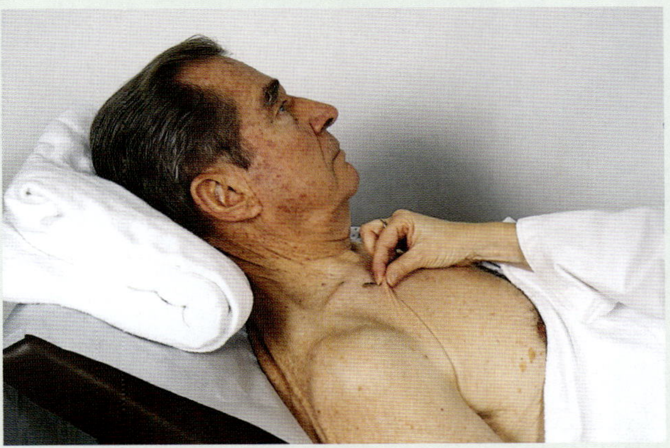 **Figure 22.6**	**Mobility and turgor** is decreased when oedema is present. **Poor turgor** is evident in severe dehydration or extreme weight loss; the pinched skin recedes slowly or 'tents' and stands by itself. **Scleroderma,** literally 'hard skin', is a chronic connective tissue disorder associated with decreased mobility.
Lesions	
If any lesions are present, note the: 1. **Colour** 2. **Elevation:** flat, raised or pedunculated 3. **Pattern or shape:** the grouping or distinctness of each lesion, for example, annular, grouped, confluent, linear. The pattern may be characteristic of a certain disease. 4. **Size,** in centimetres: use a ruler to measure. Avoid household descriptions such as 'pea sized'. 5. **Location and distribution** on body: is it generalised or localised to area of a specific irritant; around jewellery, watchband, around eyes? 6. Any **exudate:** note its colour and any odour.	**Macule:** small pigmented spot on the skin that is neither raised nor depressed **Papule:** a small hard round protuberance on the skin **Naevi:** moles **Danger signs:** abnormal characteristics of pigmented lesions are summarised in the mnemonic **ABCDE:** Asymmetry (not regularly round or oval, two halves of lesion do not look the same) Border irregularity (notching, scalloping, ragged edges or poorly defined margins) Colour variation (areas of brown, tan, black, blue, red, white or combination) Diameter greater than 6 mm (i.e. the size of a pencil eraser), although early melanomas may be diagnosed at a smaller size Elevation and Enlargement

OBJECTIVE DATA

PROCEDURES AND NORMAL FINDINGS	ABNORMAL FINDINGS AND CLINICAL ALERTS
Palpate lesions. Wear a glove if you anticipate contact with blood, mucosa, any body fluid or skin lesion. Roll a nodule between the thumb and index finger to assess depth.	***Clinical alert:*** change in mole's size, a new pigmented lesion and development of itching, burning or bleeding in a mole. Any of these signs should raise suspicion of malignant melanoma and warrant referral to medical practitioner (Ritchie 2017).
Does the lesion blanch with pressure or stretch? Stretching the area of skin between your thumb and index finger decreases (blanches) the normal underlying red tones, thus providing more contrast and brightening the macules. Red macules from dilated blood vessels *will* blanch momentarily, whereas those from extravasated blood (petechiae) do not. Blanching also helps identify a macular rash in people with dark pigmented skin.	
Cherry angiomas are small (1–5 mm), smooth, slightly raised bright red dots that commonly appear on the trunk in all adults over 30 years old (Figure 22.7). They normally increase in size and number with ageing and are not significant. **Figure 22.7** Cherry angioma.	

Assessing for pressure injury

Assessment is an important aspect of the nurse's role in prevention of pressure injury. Risk factors include; • Impaired mobility/reduced activity • Impaired sensory perception • Poor oxygenation • Incontinence • Malnutrition or obesity • Compromised skin integrity • Increasing age and frailty • Compromised or reduced blood supply to pressure points • Severely compromised status of health. • Friction/shear Ensure thorough and regular assessment of bony prominences, skin folds that trap moisture, areas that come in contact with tubing; for example, a patient may require oxygen or tube feeding and the nares or ears are vulnerable to pressure from this equipment. For the Braden scale for predicting pressure injury see: www.bradenscale.com/images/bradenscale.pdf (ACSQHC 2018).	**Pressure injury grading** **Grade 1:** Non-blanchable erythema **Grade 2:** Partial thickness skin loss (damage to epidermis and/or dermis—including abrasion, blisters) **Grade 3:** Full thickness skin loss (damage or necrosis of subcutaneous tissues; does not include underlying fascia or underlying structures) **Grade 4:** Full thickness skin loss with extensive destruction and tissue necrosis extending to underlying bone, tendon or joint capsule. See Table 22.6.

OBJECTIVE DATA

PROCEDURES AND NORMAL FINDINGS	ABNORMAL FINDINGS AND CLINICAL ALERTS
Wound assessment	
Wound assessment is usually taken over time. It is important to use objective measures as described above to monitor healing or deterioration. It is important to note that many healthcare organisations have a specific wound assessment and care chart. Note and describe: • **Anatomical location**— may use a body map. • **Size** (length, width, depth, undermining—wound extends underneath the skin edges). Use a disposable ruler to measure and take a photograph if possible. • **Colour and type of wound tissue** (e.g. granulation, slough, necrotic) • **Exudate or drainage**—amount and type (described at time of dressing change, number of dressing changes required) • **Odour** (offensive, non-offensive) • **Periwound skin condition**—colour and temperature • **Wound margins**—colour and condition of skin • **Pain**—presence or absence and type of pain (Hess 2019).	
Inspect and palpate the hair and scalp	
Colour	
Hair colour comes from melanin production and may vary from pale blonde to total black. Greying begins as early as the third decade of life because of reduced melanin production in the follicles. Genetic factors affect the age of onset of greying.	
Texture	
Scalp hair may be fine or thick and may look straight, curly or kinky. It should look shiny, although this characteristic may be lost with the use of some beauty products such as dyes, rinses or other hair treatments.	Note dull, coarse or brittle scalp hair. Grey, scaly, well-defined areas with broken hairs accompany tinea capitis, a ringworm infection found mostly in school-age children (see Table 22.13).
Distribution	
Fine vellus hair coats the body, whereas coarser terminal hairs grow at the eyebrows, eyelashes and scalp. During puberty, distribution conforms to normal male and female patterns. At first, coarse curly hairs develop in the pubic area, then in the axillae and last in the facial area in boys. In the genital area, the female pattern is an inverted triangle; the male pattern is an upright triangle with pubic hair extending up to the umbilicus. The amount of hair varies from person to person.	Absent or abnormally configured pubic hair suggests endocrine abnormalities. **Hirsutism**—excess body hair. In females, this forms a male pattern of hair distribution on the face and chest and indicates endocrine abnormalities (see Table 22.13).
Lesions	
Separate the hair into sections and lift it, observing the scalp. With a history of itching, inspect the hair behind the ears and in the occipital area as well. All areas should be clean and free of any lesions or pest inhabitants. Many people normally have seborrhoea (dandruff), which is indicated by loose white flakes on the scalp and hair.	Distinguish dandruff from nits (eggs) of lice, which are oval, adhere to hair shaft and cause intense itching (see Table 22.13).
Inspect and palpate the nails	
Shape and contour	
The nail surface is normally slightly curved or flat, and the posterior and lateral nail folds are smooth and rounded. Nail edges are smooth, rounded and clean, suggesting adequate self-care.	Jagged nails, bitten to the quick, or traumatised nail folds from chronic nervous picking suggest nervous habits. Chronically dirty nails suggest poor self-care or some occupations in which it is impossible to keep them clean.

PROCEDURES AND NORMAL FINDINGS	ABNORMAL FINDINGS AND CLINICAL ALERTS
The profile sign. View the index finger at its profile and note the angle of the nail base; it should be about 160 degrees (Figure 22.8). The nail base is firm to palpation. Curved nails are a variation of normal with a convex profile. They may look like clubbed nails, but notice that the angle between nail base and nail is normal (i.e. 160 degrees or less).	**Clubbing** of nails occurs with congenital chronic cyanotic heart disease and with emphysema and chronic bronchitis. In early clubbing, the angle straightens out to 180 degrees and the nail base feels spongy to palpation.

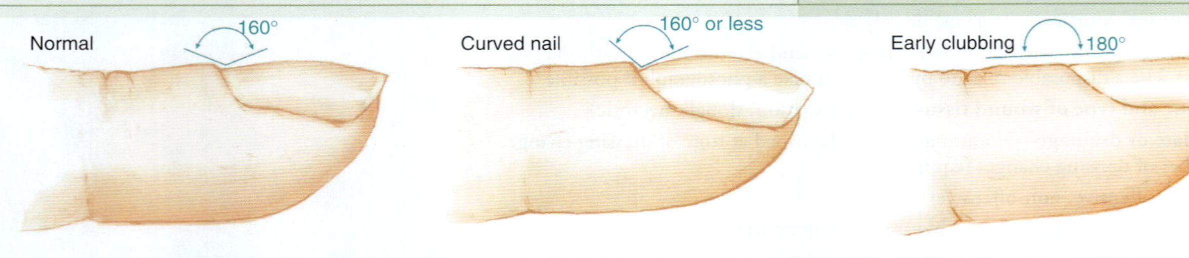

Figure 22.8

Consistency

PROCEDURES AND NORMAL FINDINGS	ABNORMAL FINDINGS AND CLINICAL ALERTS
The surface is smooth and regular, not brittle or splitting.	Pits, transverse grooves or lines may indicate a nutrient deficiency or may accompany acute illness in which nail growth is disturbed (see Table 22.14).
Nail thickness is uniform.	Nails are thickened and ridged with arterial insufficiency.
The nail is firmly adherent to the nail bed, and the nail base is firm to palpation.	A spongy nail base accompanies clubbing.

Colour

PROCEDURES AND NORMAL FINDINGS	ABNORMAL FINDINGS AND CLINICAL ALERTS
The translucent nail plate is a window to the even, pink nail bed underneath. People with dark skin may have brown-black pigmented areas or linear bands or streaks along the nail edge (Figure 22.9). All people may normally have white hairline linear markings from trauma or picking at the cuticle (Figure 22.10). Note any abnormal marking in the nail beds.	**Cyanosis** or marked pallor. **Brown linear streaks** (especially sudden appearance) are abnormal in light-skinned people and may indicate melanoma. **Splinter haemorrhages, transverse ridges or Beau's lines** (see Table 22.14).

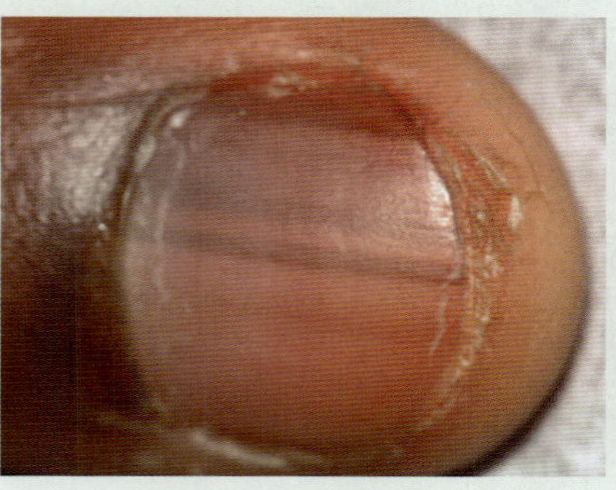

Figure 22.9
Linear pigmentation.

Figure 22.10
Leuconychia pigmentation.

PROCEDURES AND NORMAL FINDINGS	ABNORMAL FINDINGS AND CLINICAL ALERTS
Capillary refill. Depress the nail edge to blanch and then release, noting the return of colour. Normally, colour return is instant, or at least within a few seconds in a cold environment. This indicates the status of the peripheral circulation. A sluggish colour return takes longer than 1 or 2 seconds. Inspect the toenails. Separate the toes and note the smooth skin in between.	**Cyanotic** nail beds or sluggish colour return: consider cardiovascular or respiratory dysfunction.
Additional objective data for infants	
Inspect the skin	
Skin colour—general pigmentation. Light skinned newborns have pink, well perfused intact skin. Dark-skinned newborns initially have lighter-toned skin than their parents because of a pigment function that is not yet in full production. Their full melanotic colour is evident in the nail beds and scrotal folds. The **mongolian spot** is a common variation of hyperpigmentation in infants of South-East Asian, Pacific Island and African descent (Figure 22.11). It is a blue-black to purple macular area at the sacrum or buttocks, but sometimes it occurs on the abdomen, thighs, shoulders or arms. It is due to deep dermal melanocytes. It gradually fades during the first year. By adulthood these spots are lighter but are frequently still visible. 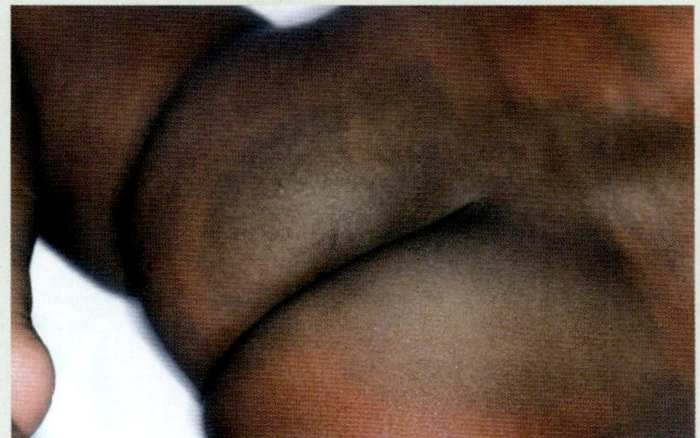 **Figure 22.11** Mongolian spot.	If you are unfamiliar with **mongolian spots**, be careful not to confuse them with bruises. Recognition of this normal variation is particularly important when dealing with children who might be erroneously identified as victims of child abuse. **Bruising** is a common soft tissue injury that follows a rapid, traumatic or breech birth. **Multiple bruises** in various stages of healing, or pattern injury, suggest child abuse (see Table 22.7). ***Clinical alert***: Multiple bruises in various stages of healing,or pattern injury, suggest child abuse. Refer to medical practitioner.
The **café au lait spot** is a large round or oval patch of light-brown pigmentation (hence, the name 'coffee with milk'), which is usually present at birth (Figure 22.12). Most often these patches are normal. 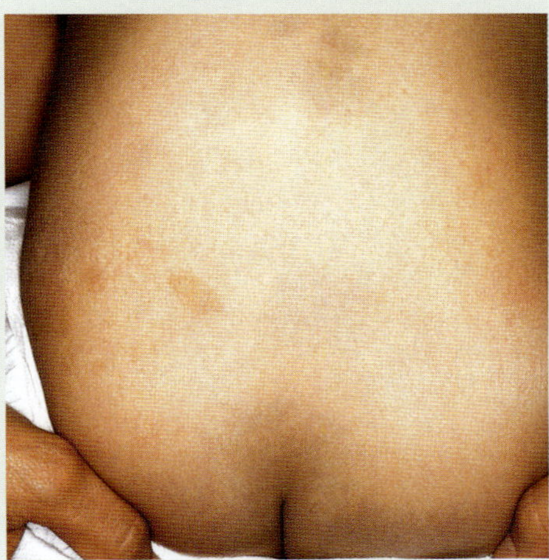 **Figure 22.12** Café au lait.	Six or more café au lait macules, each more than 1.5 cm in diameter, are diagnostic of neurofibromatosis, an inherited neurocutaneous disease.

OBJECTIVE DATA

PROCEDURES AND NORMAL FINDINGS	ABNORMAL FINDINGS AND CLINICAL ALERTS
Moisture. The vernix caseosa is the moist, white, cream cheese-like substance that covers part of the skin in all newborns. Perspiration is present after 1 month of age.	Green-tinged vernix occurs with meconium staining. In children, excessive sweating may accompany hypoglycaemia, heart disease or hyperthyroidism.
Texture. A common variation occurring in the infant is **milia** (Figure 22.15). Milia are tiny white papules on the cheeks, forehead and across the nose and chin caused by sebum that occludes the opening of the follicles. Tell parents not to squeeze the lesions; milia resolve spontaneously within a few weeks.	
Thickness. In the neonate, the epidermis is normally thin, but you will also note well-defined areas of subcutaneous fat. The baby's skin dimples over joints, but there is no break in the skin. Check for any defect or break in the skin, especially over the length of the spine.	Lack of subcutaneous fat occurs in prematurity and malnutrition. A red sacrococcygeal dimple occurs with a pilonidal cyst or sinus (see Table 22.1).
Mobility and turgor. Test mobility and turgor over the abdomen in an infant.	Poor turgor, or 'tenting', indicates dehydration or malnutrition.
Erythematous skin colour changes	
Three erythematous states are common variations in the neonate:	
1. The newborn's skin has a beefy red flush for the first 24 hours because of vasomotor instability; then the colour fades to its normal colour.	
2. Another finding, the **harlequin colour change**, occurs when the baby is in a side-lying position. The lower half of the body turns red and the upper half blanches with a distinct demarcation line down the midline. The cause is unknown, and its occurrence is transient.	
3. Finally, **erythema toxicum** is a common rash that appears in the first 3–4 days of life. Sometimes called the 'flea bite' rash or newborn rash, it consists of tiny, punctate, red macules and papules on the cheeks, trunk, chest, back and buttocks (Figure 22.13). The cause is unknown; no treatment is needed. **Figure 22.13** Erythema toxicum.	
Cyanotic conditions	
A newborn may have **acrocyanosis**, a bluish colour around the lips, hands and fingernails, and feet and toenails. This may last for a few hours and disappear with warming.	Persistent generalised cyanosis indicates distress, such as cyanotic congenital heart disease.

PROCEDURES AND NORMAL FINDINGS	ABNORMAL FINDINGS AND CLINICAL ALERTS
Cutis marmorata is a transient mottling in the trunk and extremities in response to cooler room temperatures (Figure 22.14). It forms a reticulated red or blue pattern over the skin. 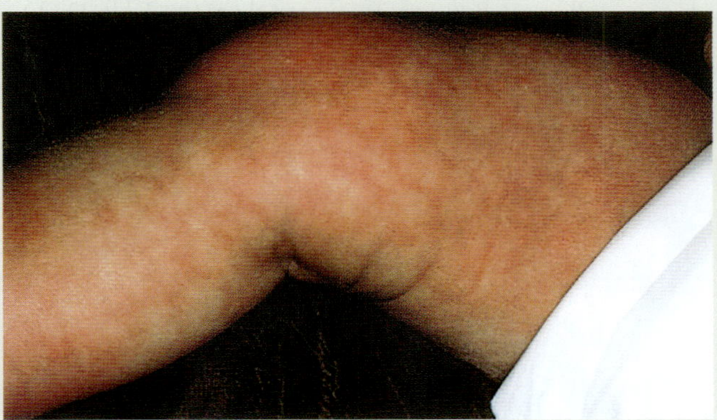 **Figure 22.14** Cutis marmorata.	Persistent or pronounced cutis marmorata occurs with trisomy 21 (Down syndrome) or prematurity. Green-brown discolouration of the skin, nails and cord occurs with passing of meconium in utero, indicating fetal distress.
Other skin colour changes	
Physiological jaundice is a common variation in about half of all newborns. A yellowing of the skin, sclera and mucous membranes develops after the 3rd or 4th day of life because of the increased numbers of red blood cells that haemolyse after birth. The haemoglobin in the red blood cells is metabolised by the liver and spleen; its pigment is converted into bilirubin.	Jaundice on the first day of life may indicate haemolytic disease. Jaundice after 2 weeks of age may indicate biliary tract obstruction.
Carotenaemia also produces a yellow-orange colour in light-skinned persons but no yellowing in the sclera or mucous membranes. It comes from ingesting large amounts of foods containing carotene, a vitamin A precursor. Carotene-rich foods are popular as prepared infant foods, and the absorption of carotene is enhanced by mashing, pureeing and cooking. The colour is best seen on the palms and soles, the forehead, tip of the nose and nasolabial folds, the chin, behind the ears and over the knuckles; it fades to normal colour within 2 to 6 weeks of withdrawing carotene-rich foods from the diet. 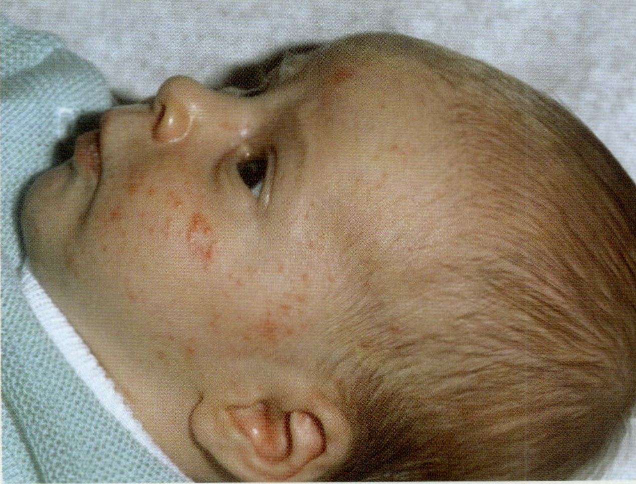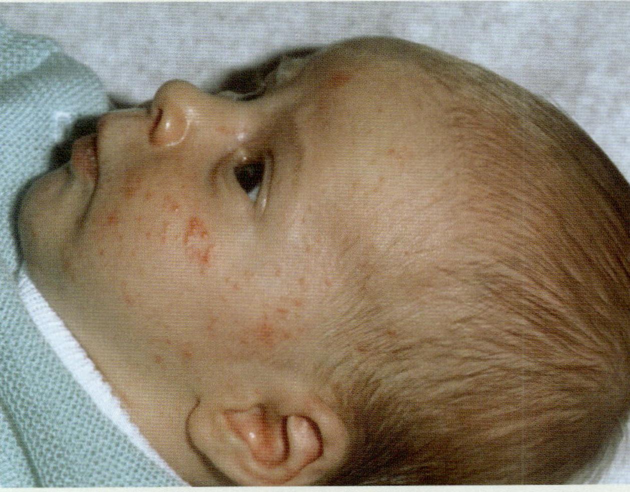 **Figure 22.15** Milia.	

PROCEDURES AND NORMAL FINDINGS	ABNORMAL FINDINGS AND CLINICAL ALERTS
3. Vascularity or bruising. Some vascular markings are common birthmarks in the newborn. A **storkbite** (salmon or strawberry patch) is a flat, irregularly shaped red or pink patch found on the forehead, eyelid or upper lip but most commonly at the back of the neck (nuchal area) (Figure 22.16). It is present at birth and usually fades during the first year. 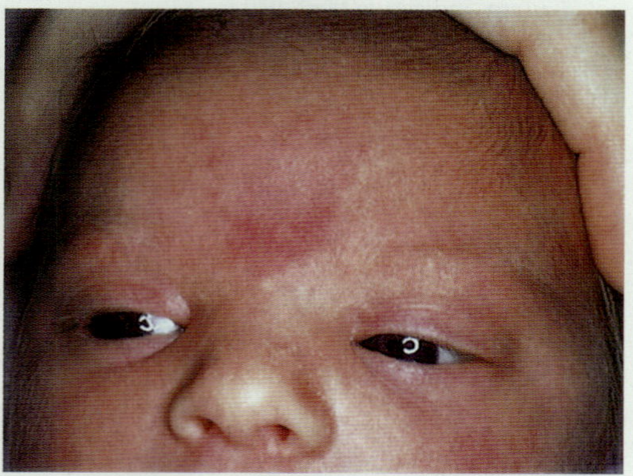 **Figure 22.16** Storkbite.	Port-wine stain, strawberry mark (immature haemangioma), cavernous haemangioma (see Table 22.8). Bruising may suggest abuse (see Table 22.7).
Inspect hair and nails	
Hair. A newborn's skin is covered with fine downy lanugo (Figure 22.17), especially in a preterm infant. Dark-skinned newborns have more lanugo than lighter-skinned newborns. Scalp hair may be lost in the few weeks after birth, especially at the temples and occiput. It grows back slowly. 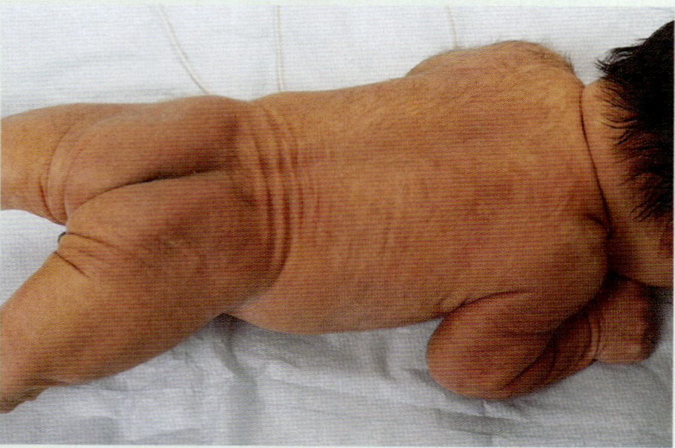 **Figure 22.17** Lanugo.	Scaly crusted scalp occurs with seborrhoeic dermatitis (cradle cap) (see Table 22.13).
Nails. A newborn's nail beds may be blue (cyanotic) for the first few hours of life; then they turn pink.	

PROCEDURES AND NORMAL FINDINGS	ABNORMAL FINDINGS AND CLINICAL ALERTS

Additional objective data for the adolescent

The increase in sebaceous gland activity creates increased oiliness and **acne**. Acne is the most common skin problem of adolescence. Almost all teens have some acne, even if it is the milder form of open comedones (blackheads) (Figure 22.18A) and closed comedones (whiteheads). Severe acne includes papules, pustules and nodules (Figure 22.18B). Acne lesions usually appear on the face and sometimes on the chest, back and shoulders. Acne may appear in children as early as 7–8 years of age; then the lesions increase in number and severity and peak at 14–16 years in girls and at 16–19 years in boys.

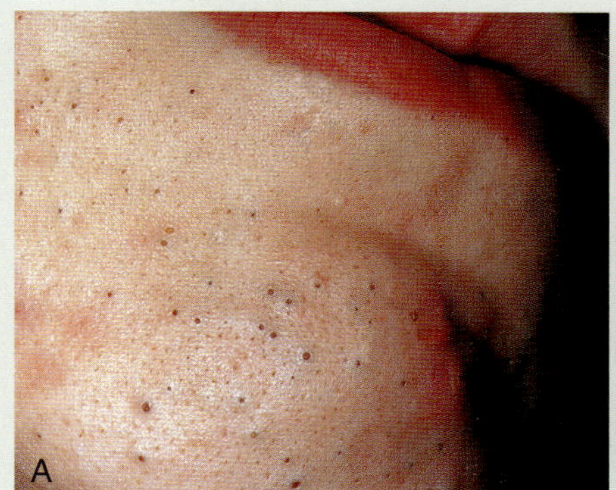

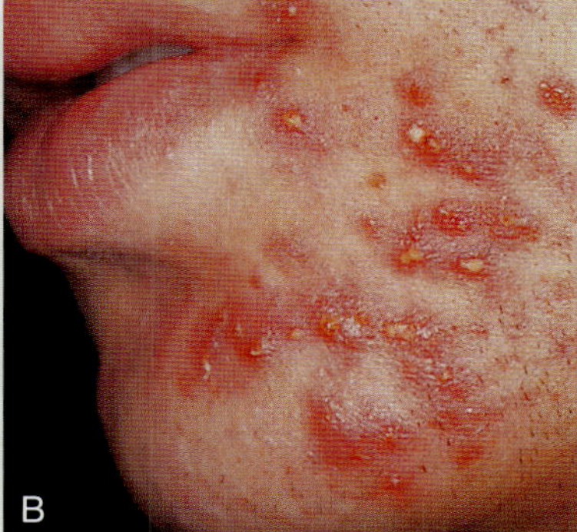

Figure 22.18
A. Open comedones. B. Acne.

Additional objective data for the pregnant woman

Striae are jagged linear 'stretch marks' of silver to pink colour that appear during the second trimester on the abdomen, breasts and sometimes thighs. They occur in half of all pregnancies. They fade after delivery but do not disappear. Another skin change on the abdomen is the linea nigra, a brownish black line down the midline (see Figure 29.3). **Chloasma** is an irregular brown patch of hyperpigmentation on the face. It may occur with pregnancy or in women taking oral contraceptive pills. Chloasma disappears after delivery or stopping the pills. Vascular spiders occur in two-thirds of pregnancies. These lesions have tiny red centres with radiating branches and occur on the face, neck, upper chest and arms.

Additional objective data for the adult over 65 years

Skin colour and pigmentation. Common variations of hyperpigmentation are:

Lentigines. Commonly called liver spots, these are small, flat, brown macules (Figure 22.19). These circumscribed areas are clusters of melanocytes that appear after extensive sun exposure. They appear on the forearms and dorsa of the hands. They are not malignant and require no treatment.

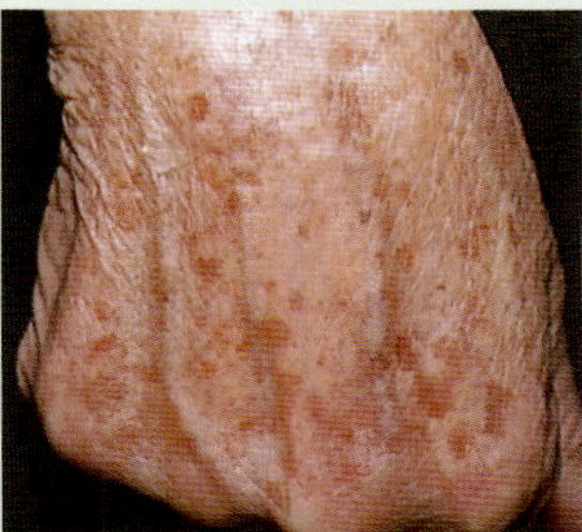

Figure 22.19
Lentigines.

OBJECTIVE DATA

PROCEDURES AND NORMAL FINDINGS	ABNORMAL FINDINGS AND CLINICAL ALERTS
Keratoses. These lesions are raised, thickened areas of pigmentation that look crusted, scaly and warty. One type, **seborrhoeic keratosis**, looks dark, greasy and 'stuck on' (Figure 22.20). They develop mostly on the trunk but also on the face and hands and on unexposed as well as on sun-exposed areas. They do not become cancerous. 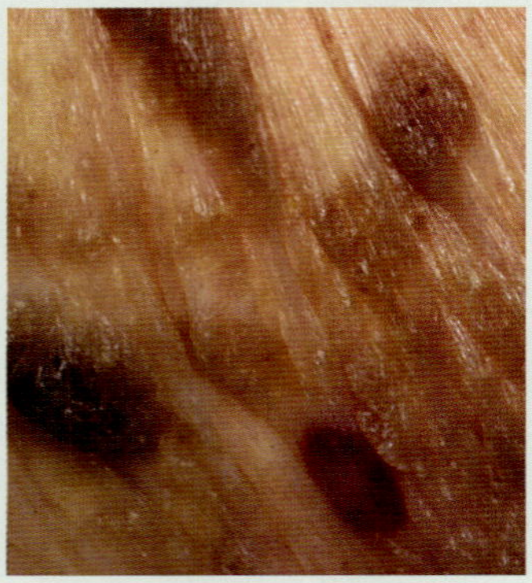 **Figure 22.20** Seborrhoeic keratosis.	
Another type, **actinic (solar) keratosis**, is less common (Figure 22.21). These lesions are red-tan scaly plaques that increase over the years to become raised and roughened. They may have a silvery-white scale adherent to the plaque. They occur on sun-exposed surfaces and are directly related to sun exposure. They are premalignant and may develop into squamous cell carcinoma. 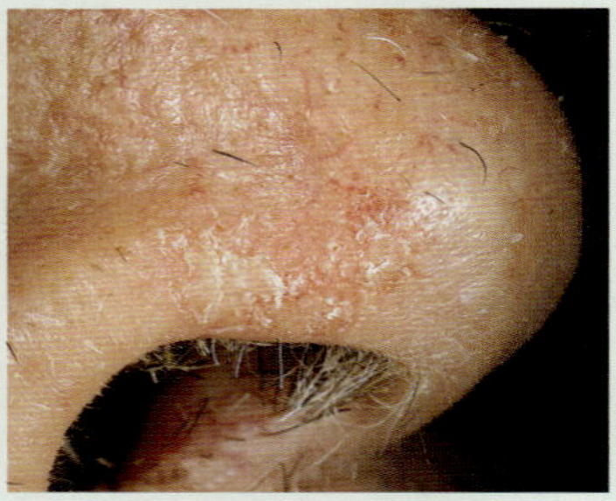 **Figure 22.21** Actinic keratosis.	
Moisture. Dry skin (xerosis) is common in the older person because of a decline in the size, number and output of the sweat glands and sebaceous glands. The skin itches and looks flaky and loose.	
Texture. Common variations occurring in the older adult are **acrochordons**, or 'skin tags', which are overgrowths of normal skin that form a stalk and are polyp-like (Figure 22.22). They occur frequently on eyelids, cheeks and neck and axillae and trunk. 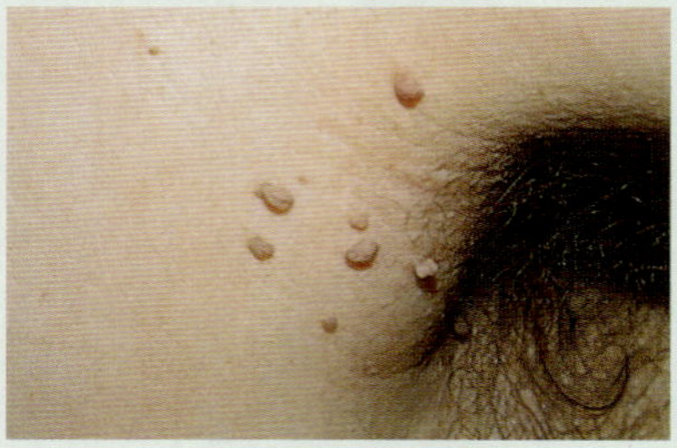 **Figure 22.22** Acrochordons.	

OBJECTIVE DATA

PROCEDURES AND NORMAL FINDINGS	ABNORMAL FINDINGS AND CLINICAL ALERTS
Sebaceous hyperplasia consists of raised yellow papules with a central depression. They are more common in men, occurring over the forehead, nose or cheeks. They have a pebbly look (Figure 22.23). 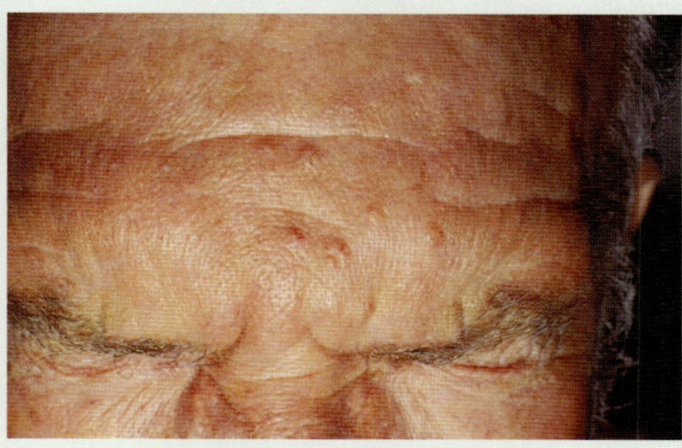 **Figure 22.23** Sebaceous hyperplasia.	
Thickness. With ageing, the skin looks as thin as parchment and the subcutaneous fat diminishes. Thinner skin is evident over the dorsa of the hands, forearms, lower legs, dorsa of feet and over bony prominences. The skin may feel thicker over the abdomen and chest.	
Mobility and turgor. The turgor is decreased (less elasticity), and the skin recedes slowly or 'tents' and stands by itself (Figure 22.24). 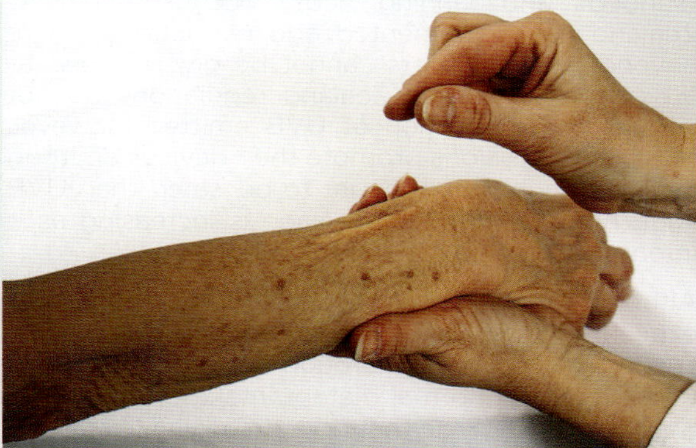 **Figure 22.24**	
Hair. With ageing, the hair growth decreases, and the amount decreases in the axillae and pubic areas. After menopause, some women may develop bristly hairs on the chin or upper lip resulting from unopposed androgens. In men, coarse terminal hairs develop in the ears, nose and eyebrows, although the beard is unchanged. Male-pattern balding, or alopecia, is a genetic trait. It is usually a gradual receding of the anterior hairline in a symmetrical W shape. In men and women, scalp hair gradually turns grey because of the decrease in melanocyte function.	
Nails. With ageing, the nail growth rate decreases, and local injuries in the nail matrix may produce longitudinal ridges. The surface may be brittle or peeling and sometimes yellowed. Toenails are also thickened and may grow misshapen, almost grotesque. The thickening may be a process of ageing or it may be due to chronic peripheral vascular disease.	Fungal infections are common in ageing, with thickened crumbling toenails and erythematous scaling on contiguous skin surfaces (McIntosh 2018).

Summary Checklist

ASSESSING SKIN, HAIR AND NAILS

Subjective data

1. Presenting concern
2. Previous history of skin disease
3. Change in pigmentation
4. Change in mole
5. Excessive dryness or moisture
6. Presence of pruritus
7. Presence of excessive bruising
8. Presence of rash or lesion
9. Hair loss
10. Change in nails
11. Environmental or occupational hazards
12. Health and lifestyle management

Objective data

1. General inspection
2. Inspect and palpate the skin
3. Assessing for pressure injury
4. Wound assessment
5. Inspect and palpate the hair and scalp
6. Inspect and palpate the nails

PROMOTING A HEALTHY LIFESTYLE

ARTIFICIAL TANNING AND SKIN CANCER RISK

The dangers of sun tanning

There are many documented adverse effects of skin tanning whether it is by exposure to UV rays from sunlight or sunbeds/tanning beds. It is well known that prolonged sun exposure can lead to skin cancer. Exposure to UV rays on the skin causes suppression of cutaneous DNA repair and immune functioning, ocular disorders and increased risk of skin cancer, specifically squamous/basal cell carcinoma and melanoma. Further, the amount of UVA light received in a tanning salon may be two to three times more than the UVA light received from the sun and is a known risk factor for melanoma. People who use tanning beds more than once a month are 55% more likely to develop malignant melanoma. In addition, people who use tanning salons are 2.5 times more likely to have squamous cell carcinoma and 1.5 times more likely to have basal cell carcinoma.

Despite public health warnings and increasing evidence of the dangers of artificial UV radiation, indoor tanning salons continue to be popular. While it is illegal to operate commercial solariums (sunbeds and tanning beds) in Australia, New Zealand has implemented age restrictions where anyone under 18 years cannot be given access to a solarium. The New Zealand regulations do not control the proportion of UVB emitted, however. Most tanning salons promote their devices emitting UVA light, which is thought to be 'safer' than UVB light; however, UVB light usage is increasing as it intensifies tanning results.

Although one of the sources of vitamin D is exposure to UV light, an adequate level of vitamin D is typically attained through incidental exposure to the sun and normal dietary intake of vitamin D. Sources of vitamin D that do not carry an increased risk of skin cancer include vitamin D supplements or food sources supplemented with vitamin D.

PROMOTING A HEALTHY LIFESTYLE

TEACH SKIN SELF-EXAMINATION

Nurses are in an ideal position to educate individuals about the dangers of excessive UV exposure. As you examine an individual's skin, take the time to ask about sun exposure, tanning practices and outdoor sun-protective precautions as well.

Teach all adults to examine their skin once a month, using the ABCDE rules (see above) to raise warning signals of any suspicious lesions. Use a well-lit room that has a full-length mirror. It helps to have a small handheld mirror. Ask a friend or relative to search skin areas difficult to see (e.g. behind ears, back of neck, back). Follow the sequence outlined in Figure 22.25 and advise the person to report any suspicious lesions promptly to their general practitioner or nurse.

Cancer Council Australia 2019 Sun Safety. Online. Available: https://www.cancer.org.au/preventing-cancer/sun-protection/

Cancer Council Australia 2018a *How much sun is enough? Getting the balance right—vitamin D and sun protection* (brochure). Online. Available: https://www.cancer.org.au/policy-and-advocacy/position-statements/sun-smart/#jump_3

Ministry of Health New Zealand 2019 Sunbeds. Online. Available: https://www.health.govt.nz/your-health/healthy-living/environmental-health/sunbeds

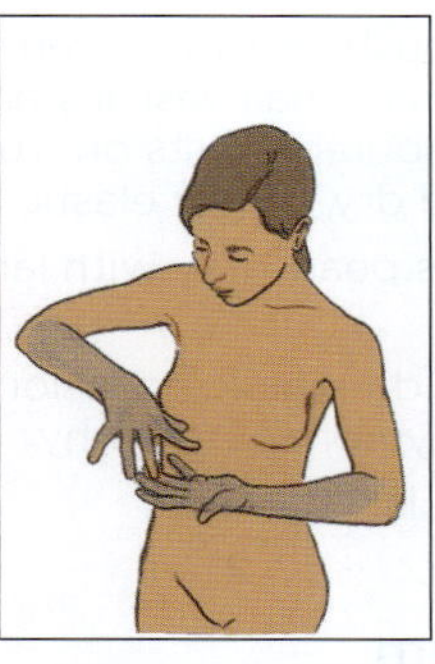

1. Undress completely. Check forearms, palms, space between fingers. Turn over hands and study the backs.

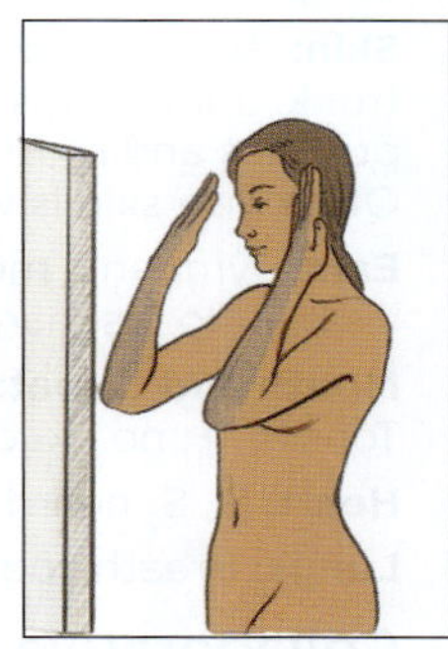

2. Face mirror; bend arms at elbow. Study arms in mirror.

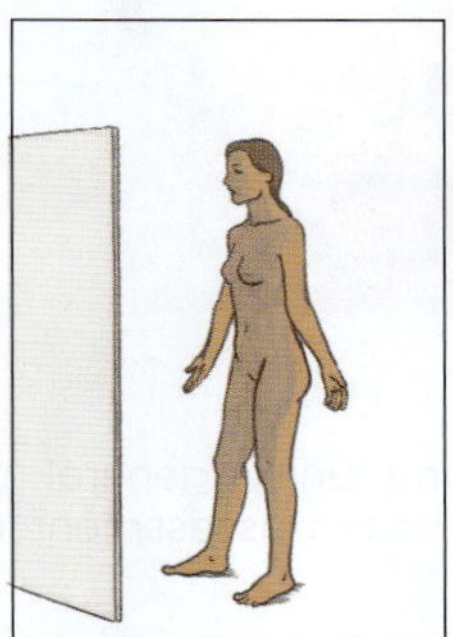

3. Face mirror and study entire front of body. Start at face, neck, torso, working down to lower legs.

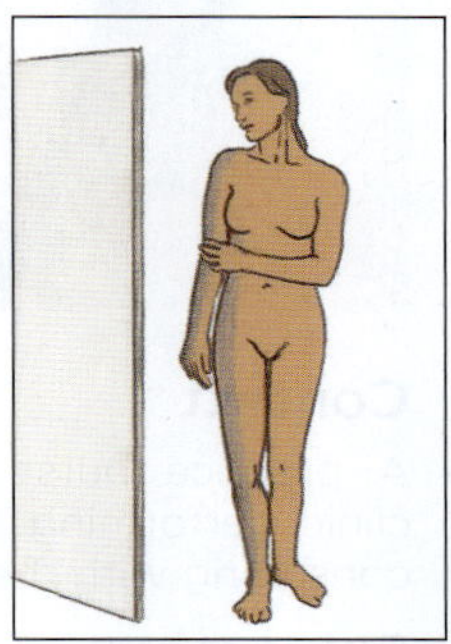

4. Pivot to right side facing mirror. Study sides of upper arms, working down to ankles. Repeat with left side.

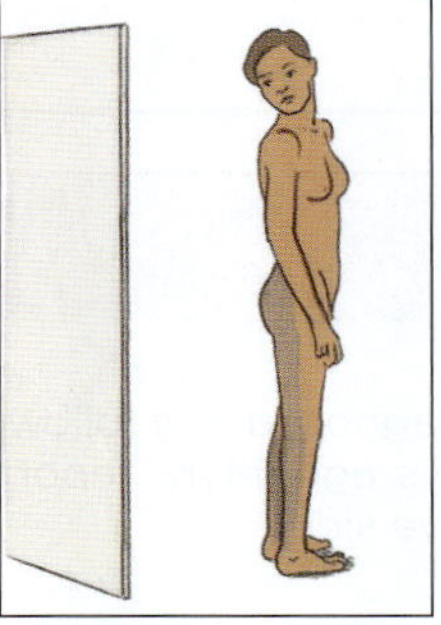

5. With back to mirror, study buttocks, thighs, lower legs.

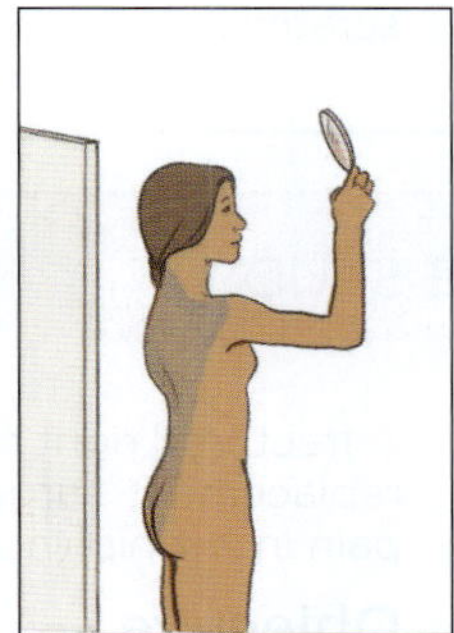

6. Use the handheld mirror to study upper back.

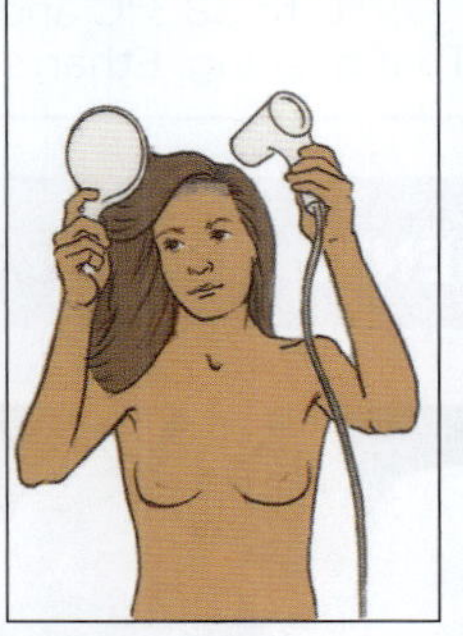

7. Use the handheld mirror to study scalp, lifting the hair. A blow-dryer on a cool setting helps to lift hair.

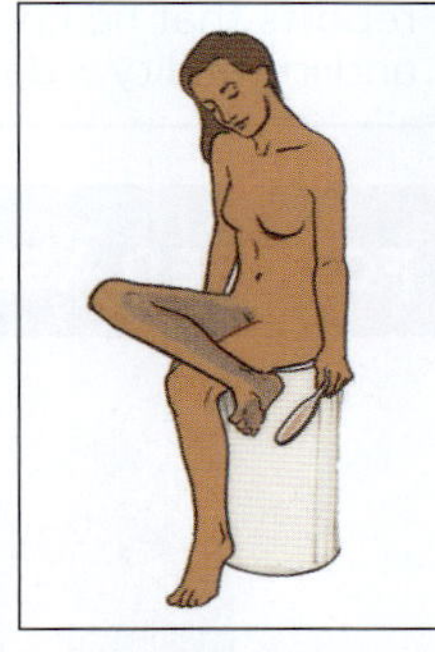

8. Sit on chair or bed. Study insides of each leg and soles of feet. Use the small mirror to help.

Figure 22.25
Skin self-examination.

OBJECTIVE DATA

Documentation and critical thinking

FOCUSED ASSESSMENT: CLINICAL CASE STUDY 1

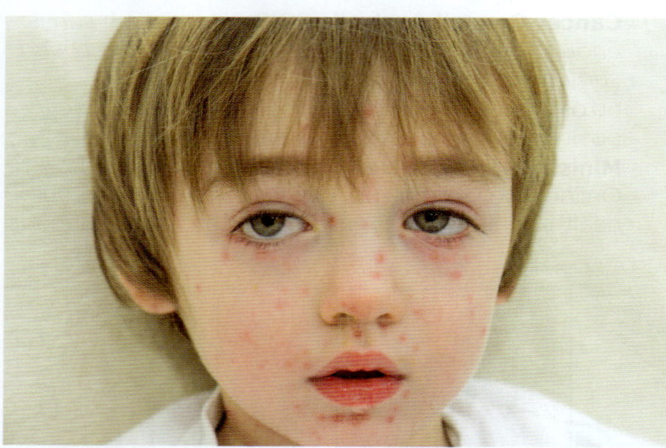

Context

A practice nurse in a community general practice clinic performing an initial health assessment prior to consulting with the GP.

Subjective

Ethan Evans is a 3-year-old male presenting with his mother, who seeks healthcare because of Ethan's fever, fatigue and rash of 3 days' duration. Two weeks ago, Ethan was playing with a child who was subsequently diagnosed as having chickenpox. Ethan's mother reports that he had a fever 37.7°C to 38.3°C and fatigue and irritability 3 days ago. That evening, Ethan's mother noted 'tiny blisters' on his chest and back.

Yesterday, the blisters on Ethan's chest changed to white with a scab on top. New eruptions of blisters on shoulders, thighs, face were noted; they caused intense itching and scratching. Ethan's mother confirms that Ethan has not been immunised against chickenpox.

Objective

Temp: 38.0°C, HR 110, R 24.

Skin: Generalised vesiculopustular rash covering face, trunk, upper arms and thighs. Small vesicles on face, pustules and red-honey-coloured crusts on trunk. Otherwise skin is warm and dry, turgor elastic.

Ears: Tympanic membranes pearl-grey with landmarks visible. No discharge.

Mouth and throat: Mucosa dark pink, no lesions. Tonsils 1+, no exudate. No lymphadenopathy.

Heart: S_1, S_2 heard and regular rhythm.

Lungs: Breath sounds clear.

Collaborative problem

Acute chickenpox (varicella) infection

Problem statement/nursing diagnosis

Impaired skin integrity related to varicella, infection and scratching

FOCUSED ASSESSMENT: CLINICAL CASE STUDY 2

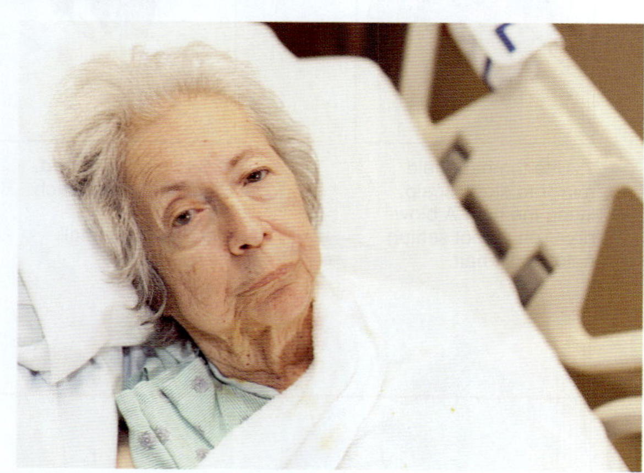

Context

Acute care ward with the registered nurse performing a skin assessment at the beginning of the shift.

Subjective

Myra Gray is a 79-year-old widow and retired academic, in good health up until recent hospitalisation after a fall. A fractured right hip was diagnosed and followed by hip replacement surgery 2 days ago. Myra reports aching pain in left hip (nonoperative side).

Objective

Pressure injury non blanching erythema L ischium 2 × 2 cm (Grade 1 pressure injury). Skin on buttocks, hips and legs generally dry and lacking in moisture. Area over L ischium very warm and tender to touch. Needs assistance with repositioning in bed and transfer to chair.

Collaborative problem

Pressure injury and pain

Problem statement/nursing diagnoses

Impaired skin integrity left hip related to immobility and pressure

Acute pain related to pressure injury

Abnormal findings

TABLE 22.2 Detecting colour changes in light and dark skin

	NOTE APPEARANCE	
AETIOLOGY	**LIGHT SKIN**	**DARK SKIN**
Pallor		
Anaemia—decreased haematocrit Shock—decreased perfusion, vasoconstriction	Generalised pallor	Brown skin appears yellow-brown, dull; dark coloured skin appears ashen grey, dull; skin loses its healthy glow—check areas with least pigmentation, such as conjunctivae, mucous membranes
Local arterial insufficiency	Marked localised pallor (e.g. lower extremities, especially when elevated)	Ashen grey, dull; cool to palpitation
Albinism—total absence of pigment melanin throughout the integument	Whitish pink	Tan, cream, white
Vitiligo—patchy depigmentation from destruction of melanocytes	Patchy milky white spots, often symmetrical bilaterally	Same
Cyanosis		
Increased amount of unoxygenated haemoglobin Central—chronic heart and lung disease cause arterial desaturation	Dusky blue	Dark but dull, lifeless; only severe cyanosis is apparent in skin—check conjunctivae, oral mucosa, nail beds
Peripheral—exposure to cold, anxiety	Nail beds dusky	
Erythema		
Hyperaemia—increased blood flow through engorged arterioles, such as in inflammation, fever, alcohol intake, blushing	Red, bright pink	Purplish tinge, but difficult to see; palpate for increased warmth with inflammation, taut skin and hardening of deep tissues
Polycythaemia—increased red blood cells, capillary stasis	Ruddy blue in face, oral mucosa, conjunctiva, hands and feet	Well-concealed by pigment—check for redness in lips
Carbon monoxide poisoning	Bright cherry red in face and upper torso	Cherry red colour in nail beds, lips and oral mucosa
Venous stasis—decreased blood flow from area, engorged venules	Dusky rubor of dependent extremities; a prelude to necrosis with pressure sore	Easily masked; use palpation for warmth or oedema
Jaundice		
Increased serum bilirubin, more than 2 to 3 mg/100 mL from liver inflammation or haemolytic disease, such as after severe burns, some infections	Yellow in sclera, hard palate, mucous membranes, then over skin	Check sclera for yellow near limbus; do not mistake normal yellowish fatty deposits in the periphery under the eyelids for jaundice—jaundice best noted in junction of hard and soft palate and also palms
Carotenaemia—increased serum carotene from ingestion of large amounts of carotene-rich foods	Yellow-orange in forehead, palms and soles, nasolabial folds, but no yellowing in sclera or mucous membranes	Yellow-orange tinge in palms and soles
Uraemia—renal failure causes retained urochrome pigments in the blood	Orange-green or grey overlying pallor of anaemia; may also have ecchymoses and purpura	Easily masked; rely on laboratory and clinical findings
Brown-tan		
Addison's disease—cortisol deficiency stimulates increased melanin production	Bronzed appearance, an 'eternal tan', most apparent around nipples, perineum, genitalia and pressure points (inner thighs, buttocks, elbow, axillae)	Easily masked; rely on laboratory and clinical findings
Café au lait spots—caused by increased melanin pigment in basal cell layer	Tan to light brown, irregularly shaped, oval patch with well-defined borders	

TABLE 22.3 Common shapes and configurations of lesions

<table>
<tr><td>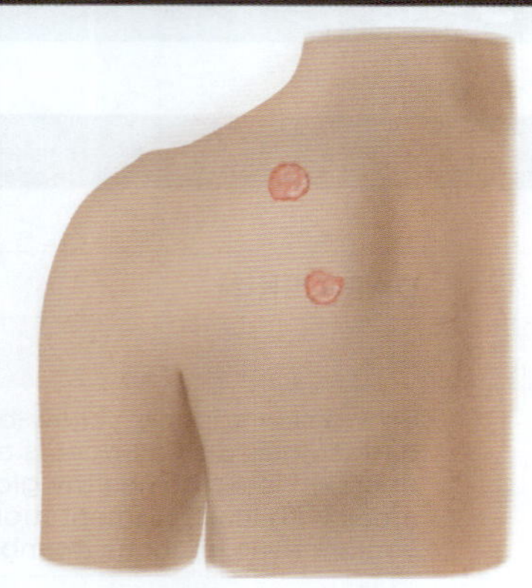
Annular, or circular, begins in centre and spreads to periphery (e.g. tinea corporis or ringworm, tinea versicolour, pityriasis rosea).</td><td>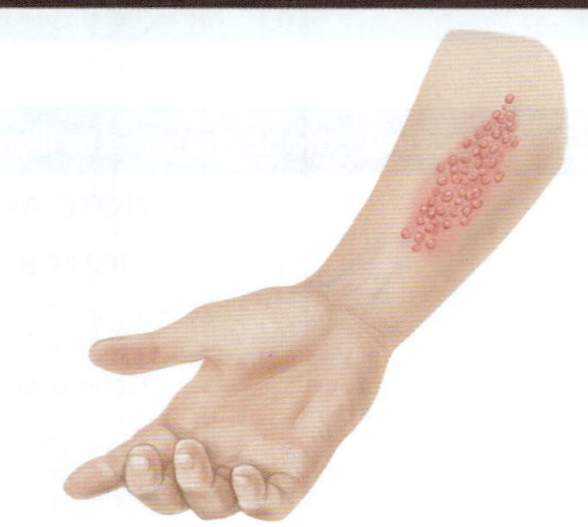
Grouped, clusters of lesions (e.g. vesicles of contact dermatitis).</td></tr>
<tr><td>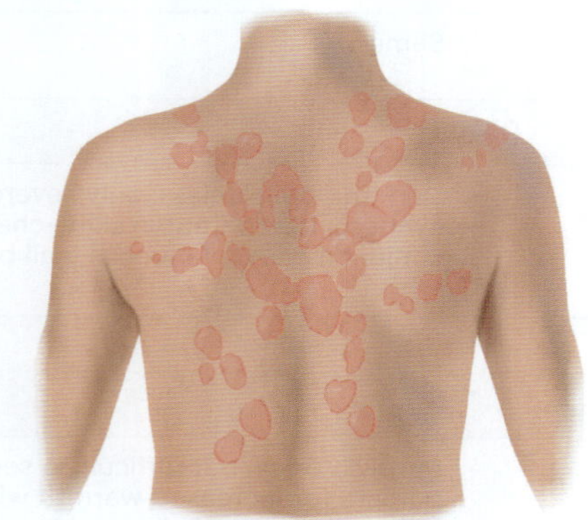
Confluent, lesions run together (e.g. urticaria (hives)).</td><td>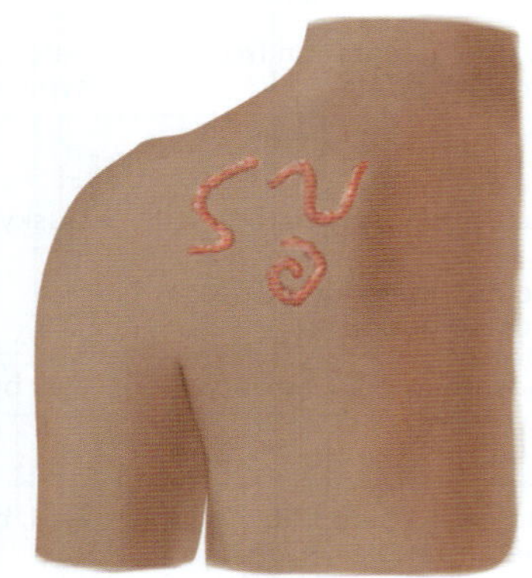
Gyrate, twisted, coiled spiral, snake-like.</td></tr>
<tr><td>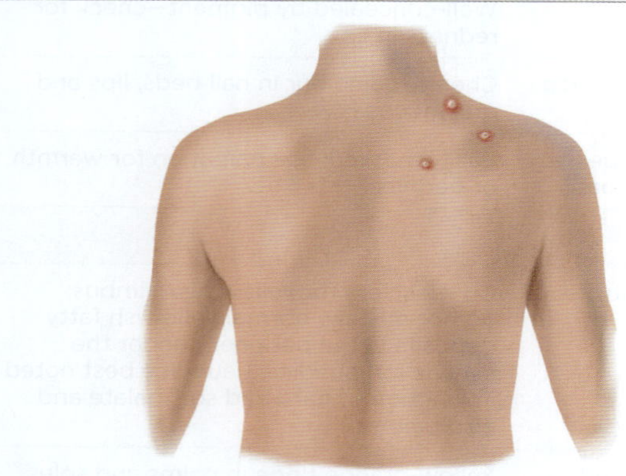
Discrete, distinct, individual lesions that remain separate (e.g. molluscum).</td><td>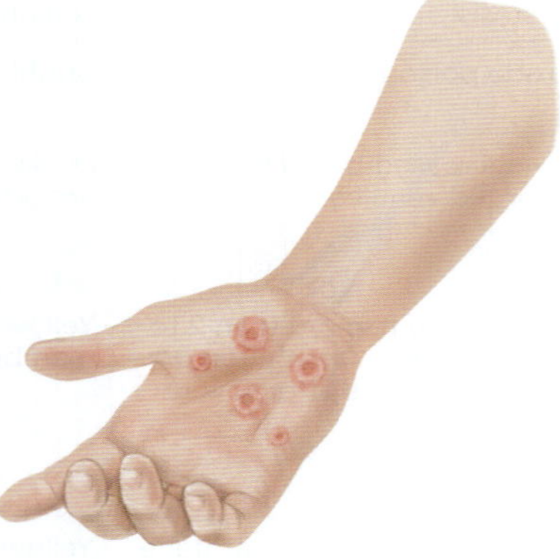
Target, or iris, resembles iris of eye, concentric rings of colour in the lesions (e.g. erythema multiforme).</td></tr>
</table>

TABLE 22.3 Common shapes and configurations of lesions—cont'd

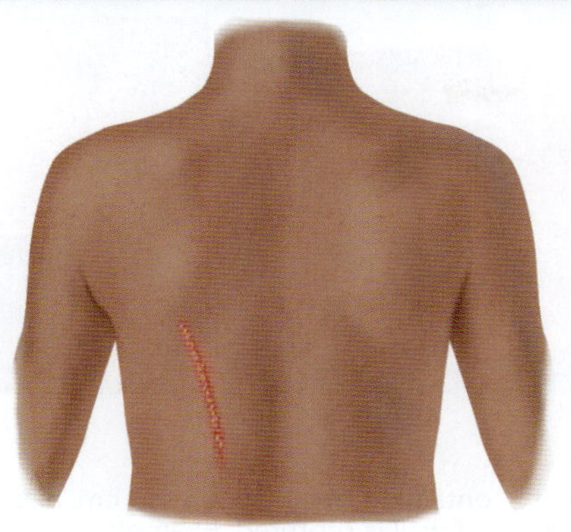

Linear, a scratch, streak, line or stripe.

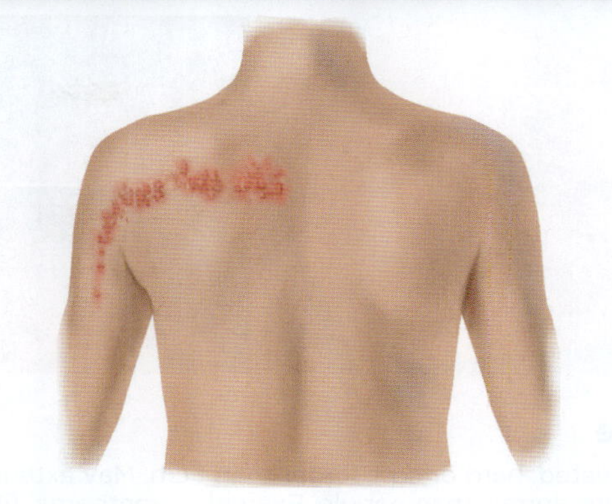

Zosteriform, linear arrangement along a nerve route (e.g. herpes zoster).

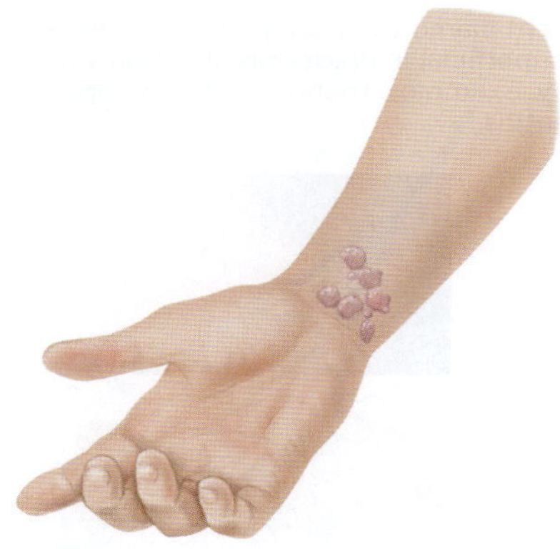

Polycyclic, annular lesions grow together (e.g. lichen planus, psoriasis).

TABLE 22.4 Primary skin lesions*

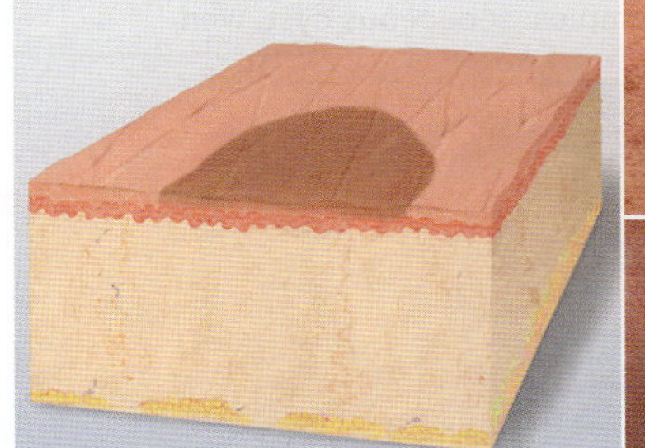

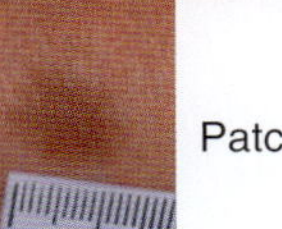

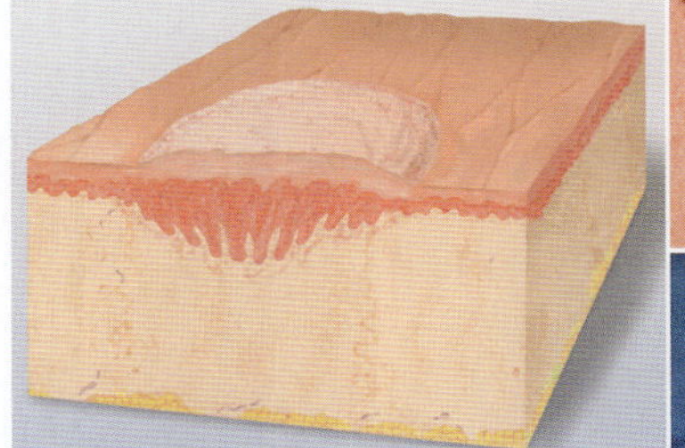

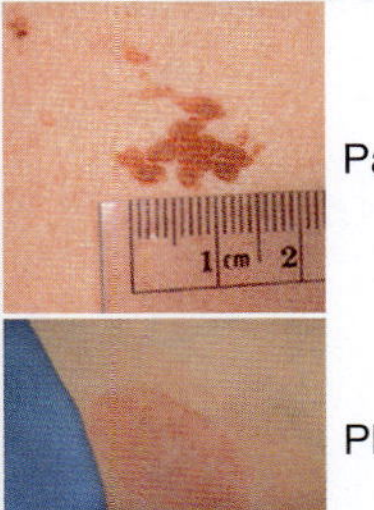

Macule

Solely a colour change, flat and circumscribed, of less than 1 cm. Examples: freckles, flat naevi, hypopigmentation, petechiae, measles, scarlet fever.

Papule

Something you can feel (i.e. solid, elevated, circumscribed, less than 1 cm diameter) caused by superficial thickening in the epidermis. Examples: elevated naevus (mole), lichen planus, molluscum, wart (verruca).

Patch

Macules that are larger than 1 cm. Examples: mongolian spot, vitiligo, café au lait spot, chloasma, measles rash.

Plaque

Papules coalesce to form surface elevation wider than 1 cm. A plateau-like, disc-shaped lesion. Examples: psoriasis, lichen planus.

(Continued)

TABLE 22.4 Primary skin lesions—cont'd

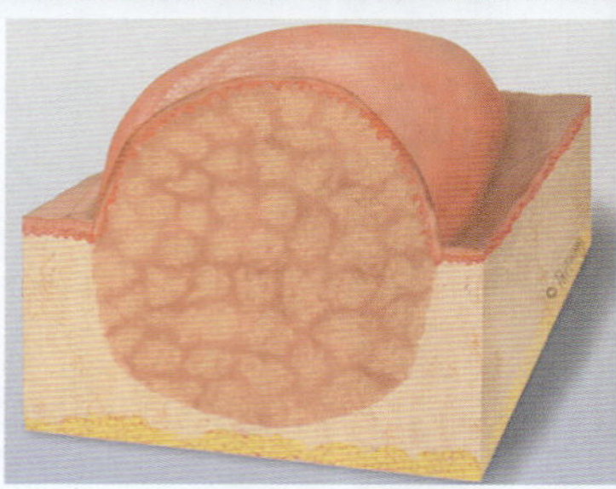
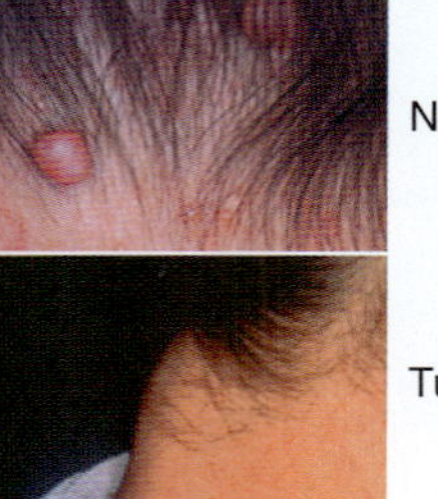

Nodule

Solid, elevated, hard or soft, larger than 1 cm. May extend deeper into dermis than papule. Examples: xanthoma, fibroma, intradermal naevi.

Tumour

Larger than a few centimetres in diameter, firm or soft, deeper into dermis; may be benign or malignant, although 'tumour' implies 'cancer' to most people. Examples: lipoma, haemangioma.

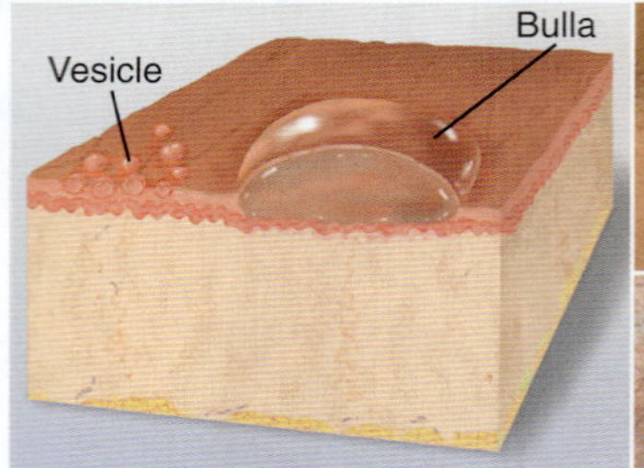

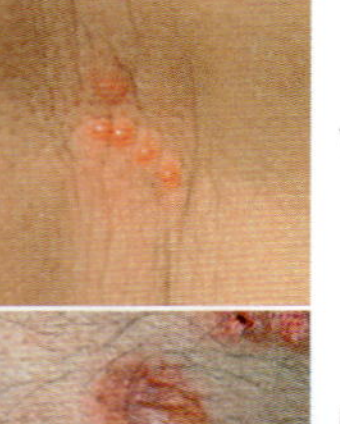

Vesicle

Elevated cavity containing free fluid, up to 1 cm; a 'blister'. Clear serum flows if wall is ruptured. Examples: herpes simplex, early varicella (chickenpox), herpes zoster (shingles), contact dermatitis.

Bulla

Larger than 1 cm diameter; usually single chambered (unilocular); superficial in epidermis; it is thin walled, so it ruptures easily. Examples: friction blister, pemphigus, burns, contact dermatitis.

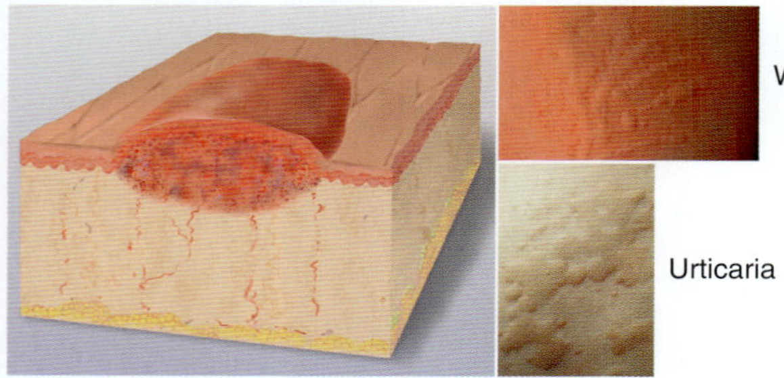

Wheal

Superficial, raised, transient and erythematous; slightly irregular shape due to oedema (fluid held diffusely in the tissues). Examples: mosquito bite, allergic reaction, dermographism.

Urticaria (hives)

Wheals coalesce to form extensive reaction, intensely pruritic.

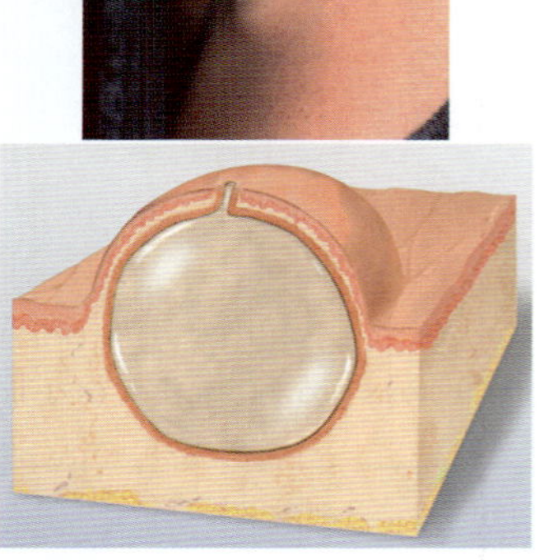

Cyst

Encapsulated fluid-filled cavity in dermis or subcutaneous layer, tensely elevating skin. Examples: sebaceous cyst, wen.

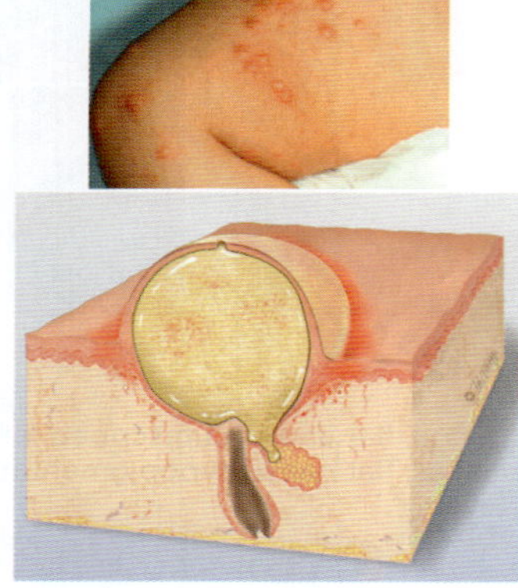

Pustule

Turbid fluid (pus) in the cavity. Circumscribed and elevated. Examples: impetigo, acne.

*The immediate result of a specific causative factor; primary lesions develop on previously unaltered skin.

TABLE 22.5 Secondary skin lesions*

DEBRIS ON SKIN SURFACE

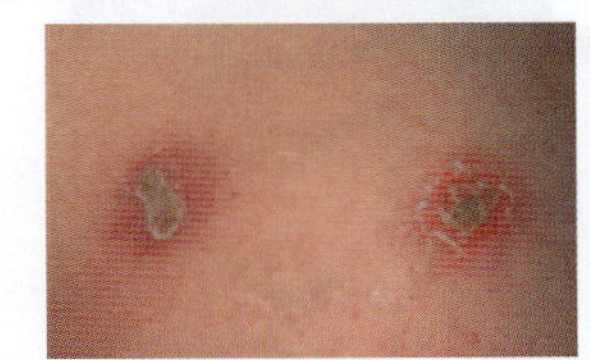
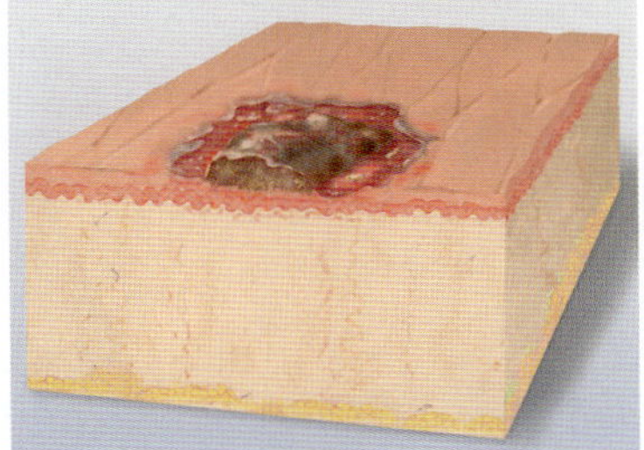

Crust

The thickened, dried-out exudate left when vesicles/pustules burst or dry up. Colour can be red-brown, honey or yellow, depending on the fluid's ingredients (blood, serum, pus). Examples: impetigo (dry, honey coloured), weeping eczematous dermatitis, scab after abrasion.

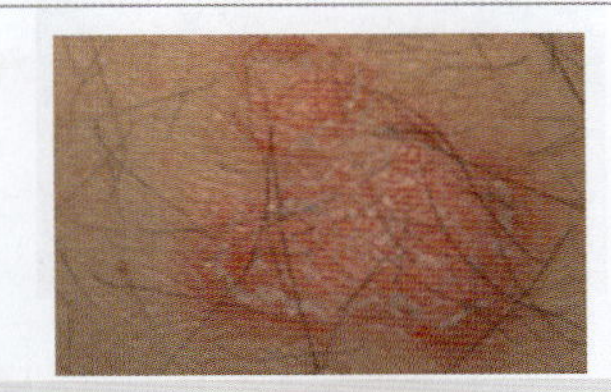
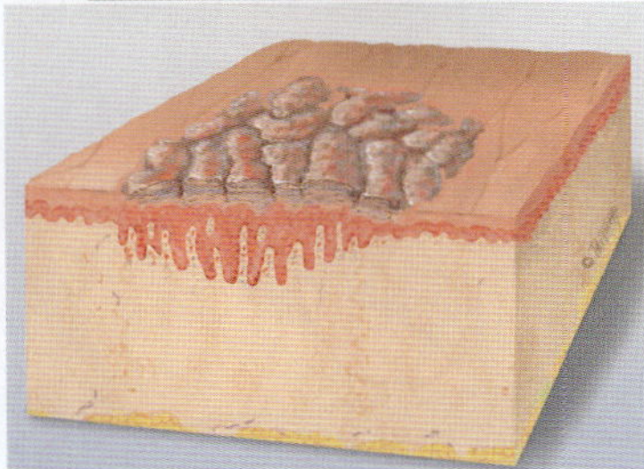

Scale

Compact, desiccated flakes of skin, dry or greasy, silvery or white, from shedding of dead excess keratin cells. Examples: after scarlet fever or drug reaction (laminated sheets), psoriasis (silver, mica-like), seborrhoeic dermatitis (yellow, greasy), eczema, ichthyosis (large, adherent, laminated), dry skin.

BREAK IN CONTINUITY OF SURFACE

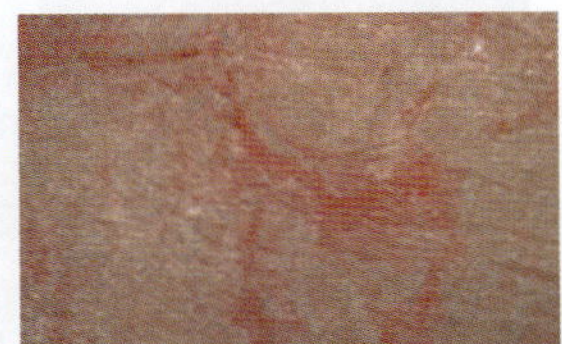
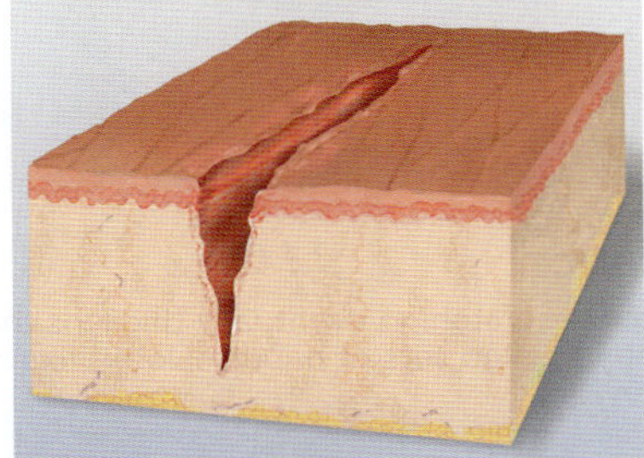

Fissure

Linear crack with abrupt edges, extends into dermis, dry or moist. Examples: cheilosis—at corners of mouth due to excess moisture; athlete's foot.

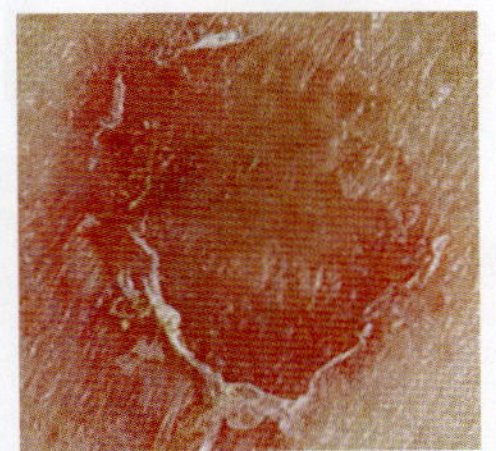
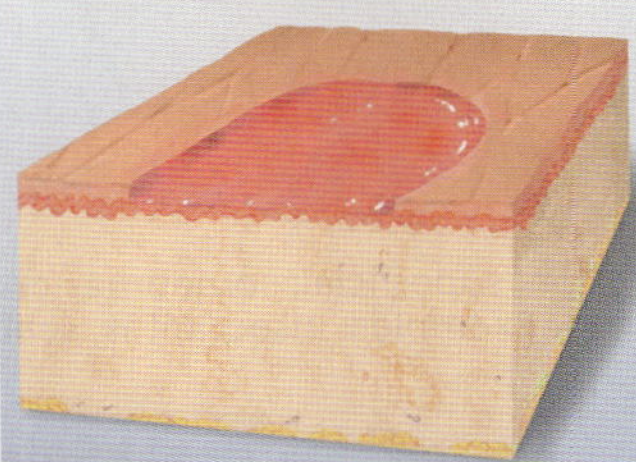

Erosion

Scooped out but shallow depression. Superficial; epidermis lost; moist but no bleeding; heals without scar because erosion does not extend into dermis.

(Continued)

ABNORMAL FINDINGS

TABLE 22.5 Secondary skin lesions—cont'd

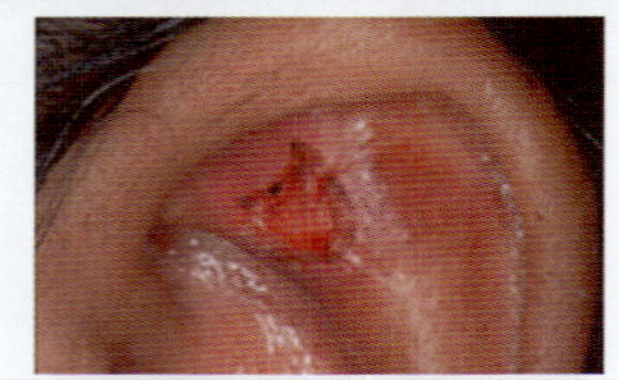 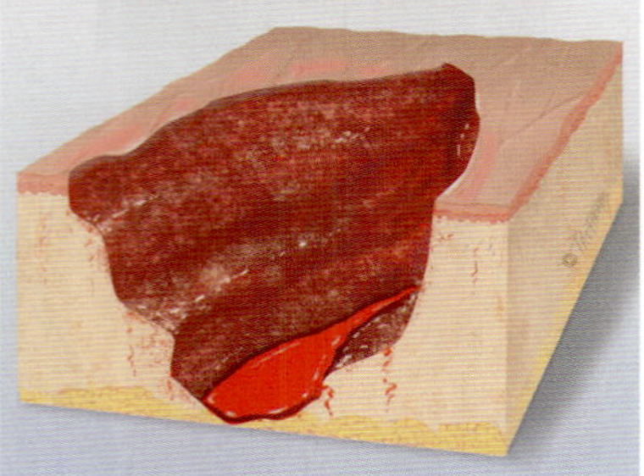 **Ulcer** Deeper depression extending into dermis, irregular shape; may bleed; leaves scar when heals. Examples: stasis ulcer, pressure injury, chancre.	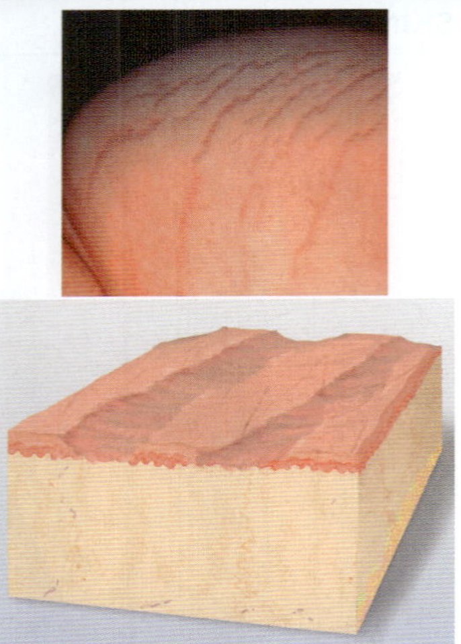 **Atrophic scar** Resulting skin level depressed with loss of tissue; a thinning of the epidermis. Example: striae.
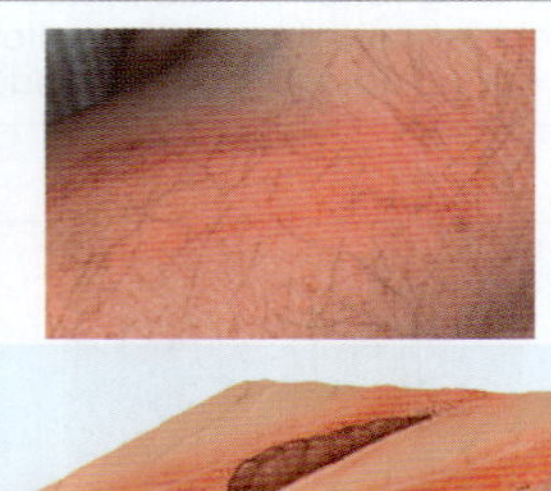 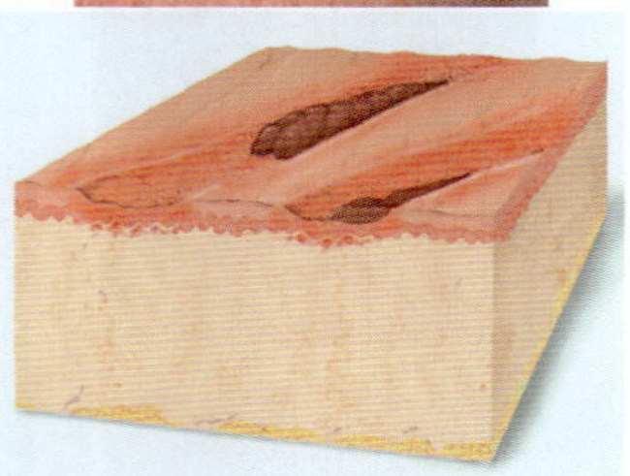 **Excoriation** Self-inflicted abrasion; superficial; sometimes crusted; scratches from intense itching. Examples: insect bites, scabies, dermatitis, varicella.	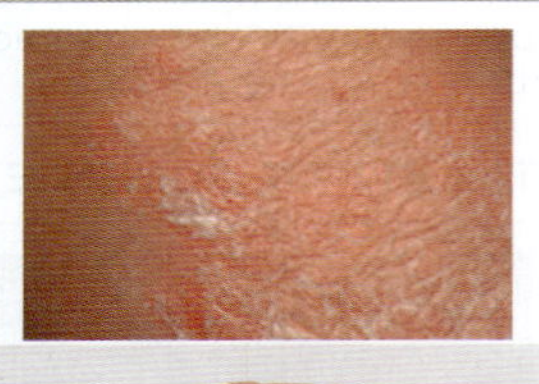 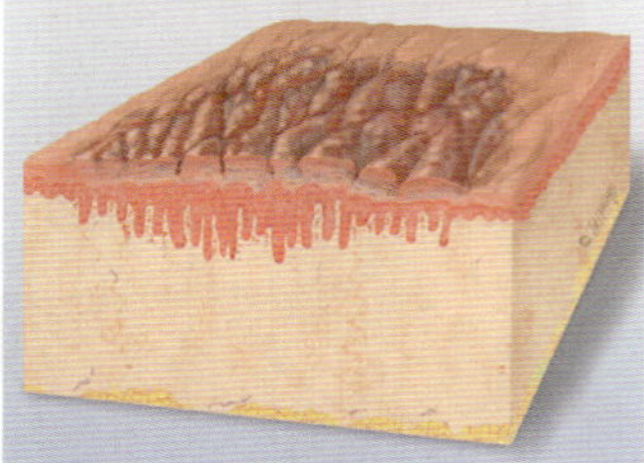 **Lichenification** Prolonged intense scratching eventually thickens the skin and produces tightly packed sets of papules; looks like surface of moss (or lichen).
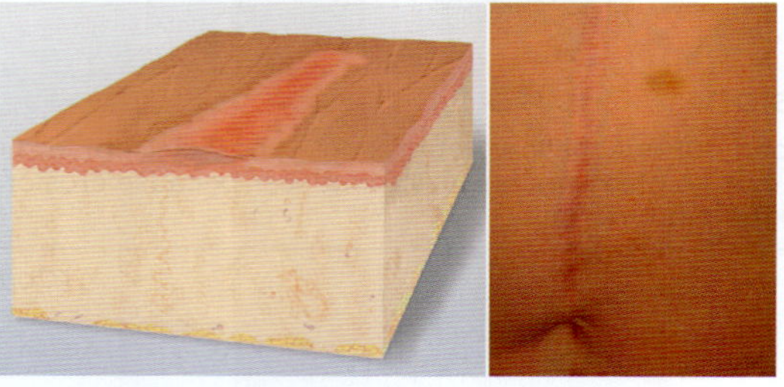 **Scar** After a skin lesion is repaired, normal tissue is lost and replaced with connective tissue (collagen). This is a permanent fibrotic change. Examples: healed area of surgery or injury, acne.	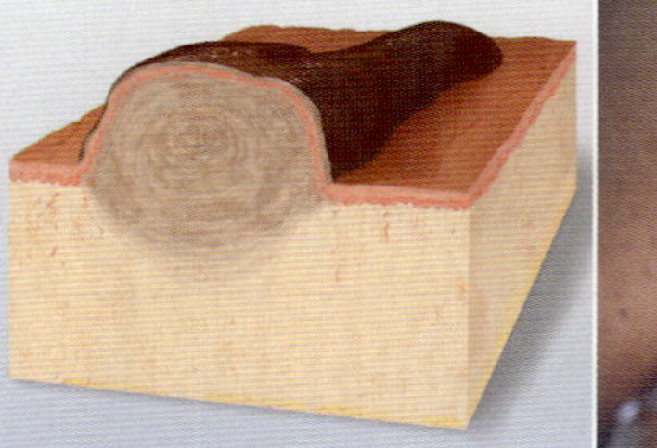 **Keloid** A hypertrophic scar. The resulting skin level is elevated by excess scar tissue, which is invasive beyond the site of original injury. May increase long after healing occurs. Looks smooth, rubbery, 'claw-like', and has a higher incidence among dark-skinned people.

*Resulting from a change in a primary lesion from the passage of time; an evolutionary change.

Note: Combinations of primary and secondary lesions may coexist in the same person. Such combined designations may be termed papulosquamous, maculopapular, vesiculopustular or papulovesicular.

TABLE 22.6 Pressure injury	
Pressure injuries appear on the skin over a bony prominence when circulation is impaired, e.g. when a person is confined to bed or immobilised. Immobilisation impedes delivery of blood carrying oxygen and nutrients to the skin, and it impedes venous drainage carrying metabolic wastes away from the skin. This results in ischaemia and cell death. Common sites for pressure injuries are on the back (heel, ischium, sacrum, elbow, scapula, vertebra, head) or the side (ankle, knee, hip, rib, shoulder, ear). **Risk factors for pressure injuries** include impaired mobility, thin fragile skin of ageing, decreased sensory perception (thus unable to respond to pain accompanying prolonged pressure), impaired level of consciousness (also unable to respond), moisture from urine or stool incontinence, excessive perspiration or wound drainage, shearing injury (being pulled down or across in bed), poor nutrition, infection. Knowledge of risk factors and prevention of pressure injuries is far more easily accomplished than is treatment of existing pressure injuries. However, once pressure injuries occur, they are assessed by stage, depending on the pressure injury depth:	
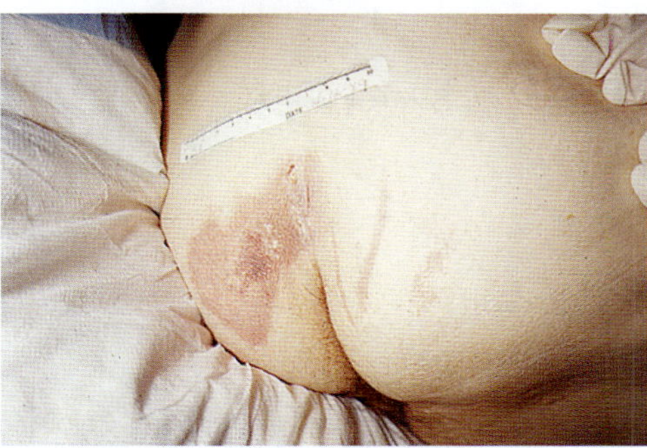 **Stage I** Intact skin appears red but unbroken. Localised redness in lightly pigmented skin does not blanch (turn light with fingertip pressure). Dark skin appears darker but does not blanch.	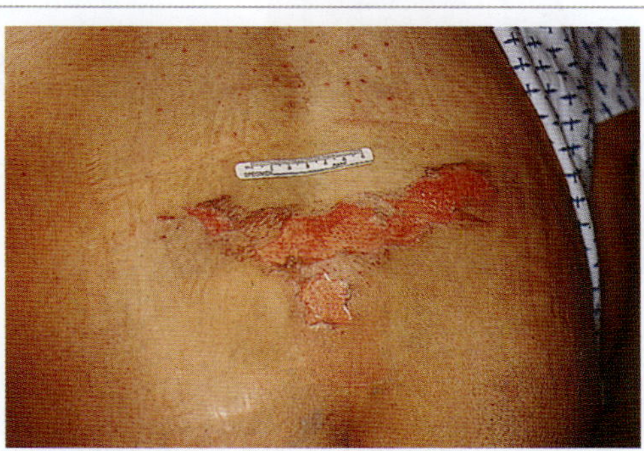 **Stage II** Partial-thickness skin erosion with loss of epidermis or also the dermis. Superficial injury looks shallow, like an abrasion or open blister with a red-pink wound bed.
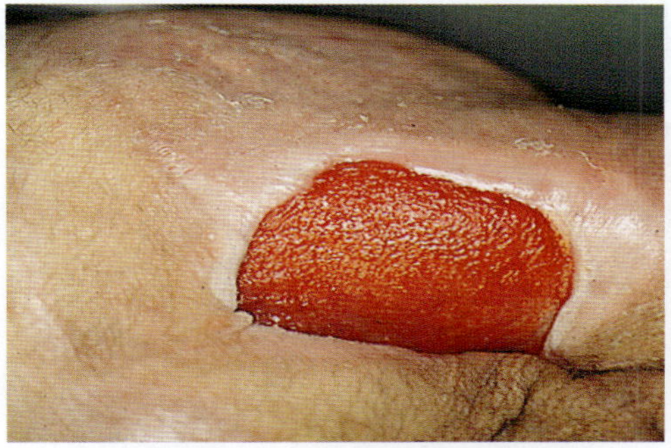 **Stage III** Full-thickness pressure injury extending into the subcutaneous tissue and resembling a crater. May see subcutaneous fat but not muscle, bone or tendon.	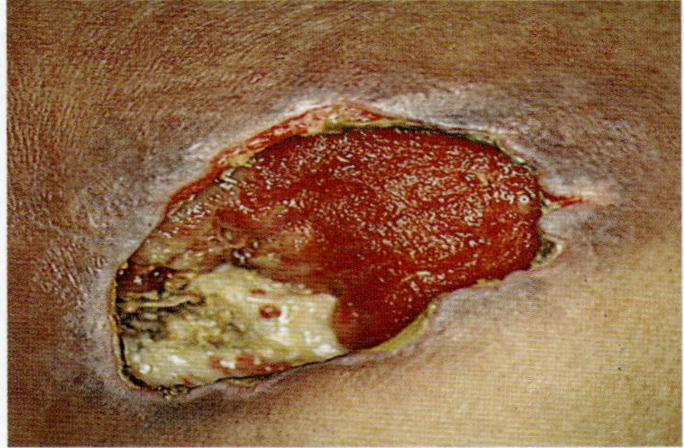 **Stage IV** Full-thickness pressure injury involves all skin layers and extends into supporting tissue. Exposes muscle, tendon or bone, and may show slough (stringy matter attached to wound bed) or eschar (black or brown necrotic tissue).
Once stage III or IV injuries occur, wound size must be measured weekly to provide quantifiable data for wound healing. Use disposable rulers with mm and cm markings, and measure the greatest overall wound length. Then measure the greatest length perpendicular to the first number and multiply.	

TABLE 22.7 Lesions caused by trauma or abuse

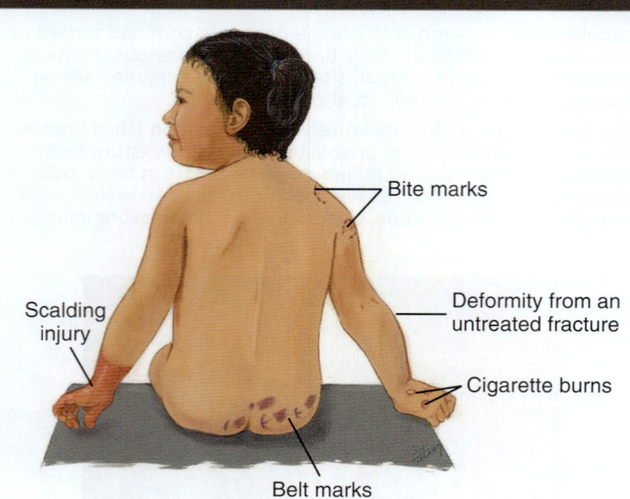

Pattern injury

Pattern injury is a bruise or wound whose shape suggests the instrument or weapon that caused it (e.g. belt buckle, broomstick, burning cigarette, pinch marks, bite marks or scalding hot liquid). Inflicted scalding-water immersion burns usually have a clear border, like a glove or sock, indicating that body part was held under water intentionally. Deformity results from an untreated fracture because the bone heals out of alignment.

These physical signs suggest child abuse, together with a history that does not match the severity or type of injury, and indicates impaired or dysfunctional parent-child relationship.

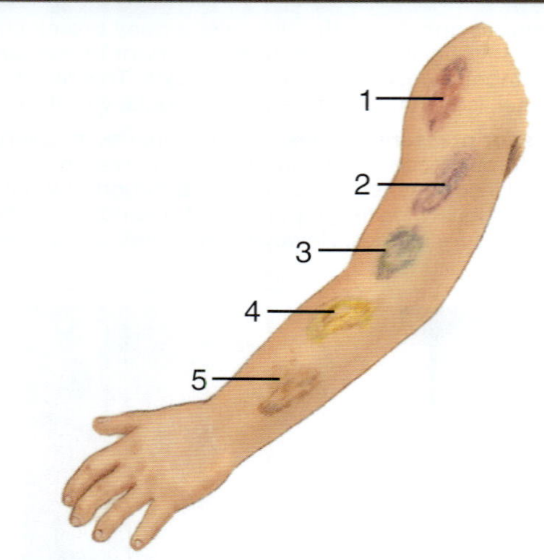

Contusion (bruise)

A large patch of capillary bleeding into tissues. Colour in light-skinned person is usually first 1—red-blue or purple immediately after or within 24 hours of trauma and generally progresses to 2—blue to purple; 3—blue-green; 4—yellow; 5—brown to disappearing. A recent bruise in dark-skinned person is deep, dark purple. Note that it is not possible to date the age of a bruise from its colour.

Pressure on a bruise will not cause it to blanch. A bruise usually occurs from trauma; also from bleeding disorders and liver dysfunction.

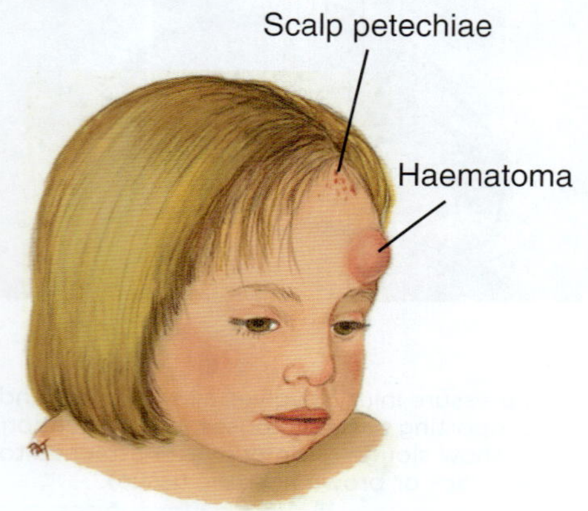

Haematoma

A haematoma is a bruise you can feel. It elevates the skin and is seen as swelling. Multiple petechiae and purpura may occur on the face when prolonged vigorous crying or coughing raises venous pressure.

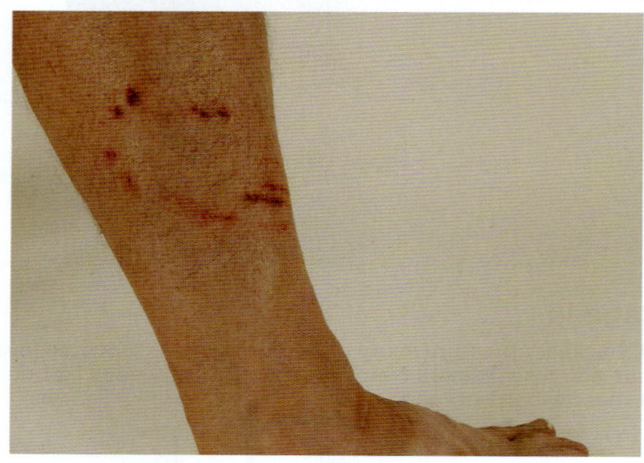

Dog, cat and human bite wounds

Dog bite shown here is a crushing injury with puncture wounds and lacerations. Dog bites on adults occur on arms or legs; on children they are more often on face or scalp. Assess for cosmetic repair and risk of infection. An X-ray image shows bone penetration or tooth fragment left in the wound. Cat bites involve deeply punctured tissue, and over half result in infection. Human bites are even more serious because of abundant microorganisms in human saliva. All are treated with appropriate antibiotics.

Abnormal findings for advanced practice

TABLE 22.8 Vascular lesions

HAEMANGIOMAS

Caused by a benign proliferation of blood vessels in the dermis.

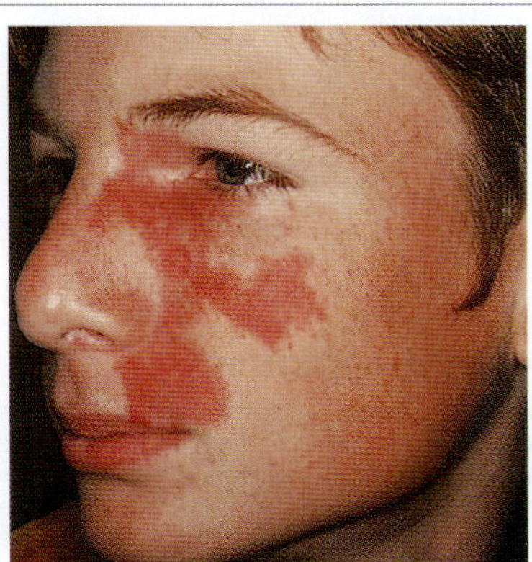

Port-wine stain (naevus flammeus)

A large, flat macular patch covering the scalp or face, frequently along the distribution of cranial nerve V. The colour is dark red, bluish or purplish and intensifies with crying, exertion or exposure to heat or cold. The marking consists of mature capillaries. It is present at birth and usually does not fade. The use of yellow light lasers now makes photoablation of the lesion possible, with minimal adverse effects.

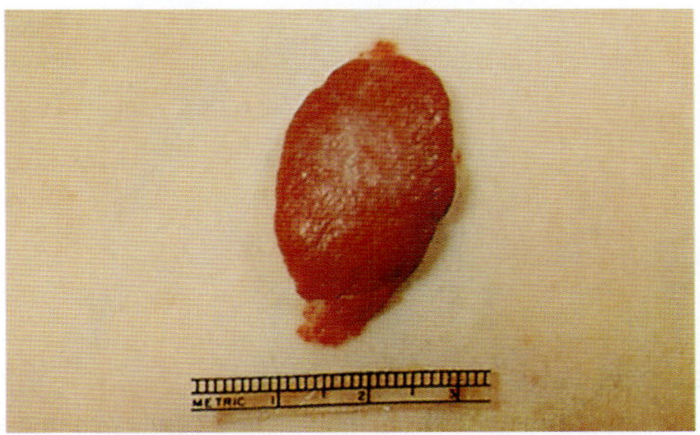

Strawberry mark (immature haemangioma)

A raised bright red area with well-defined borders about 2–3 cm in diameter. It does not blanch with pressure. It consists of immature capillaries, is present at birth or develops in the first few months and usually disappears by age 5–7 years. Requires no treatment, although parental and peer pressure may prompt treatment.

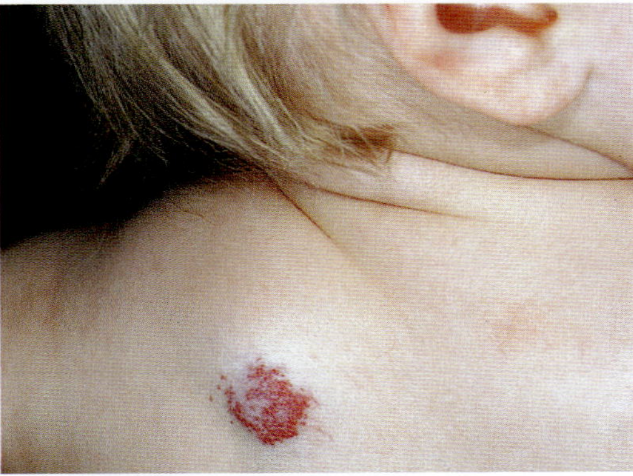

Cavernous haemangioma (mature)

A reddish-blue, irregularly shaped, solid and spongy mass of blood vessels. It may be present at birth, may enlarge during the first 10 to 15 months and will not involute spontaneously.

(Continued)

TABLE 22.8 Vascular lesions—cont'd

TELANGIECTASES

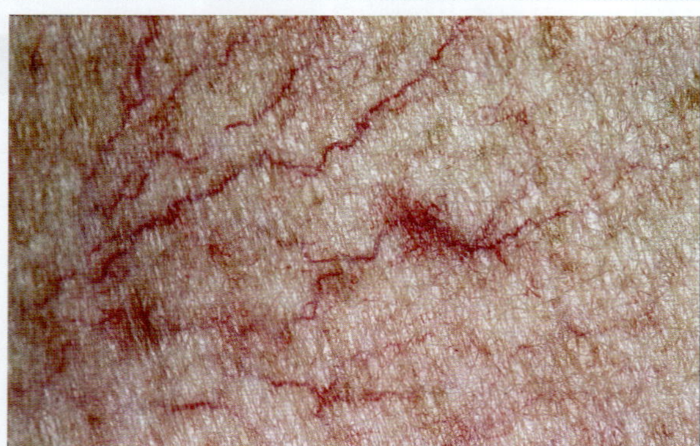

Telangiectasia

Caused by vascular dilatation; permanently enlarged and dilated blood vessels that are visible on the skin surface.

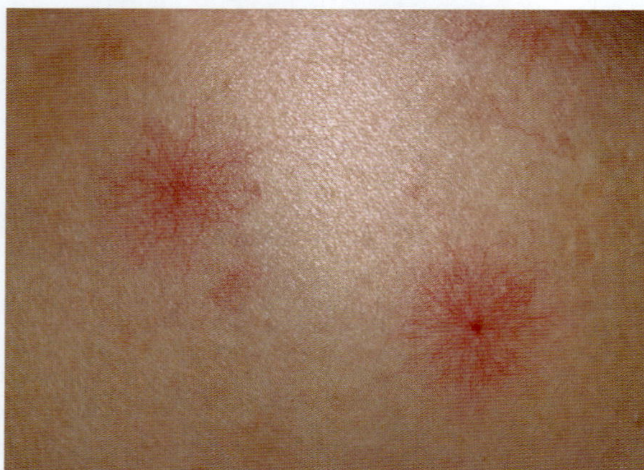

Spider or star angioma

A fiery red, star-shaped marking with a solid circular centre. Capillary radiations extend from the central arterial body. With pressure, note a central pulsating body and blanching of extended legs. Develops on face, neck or chest; may be associated with pregnancy, chronic liver disease or oestrogen therapy or may be normal.

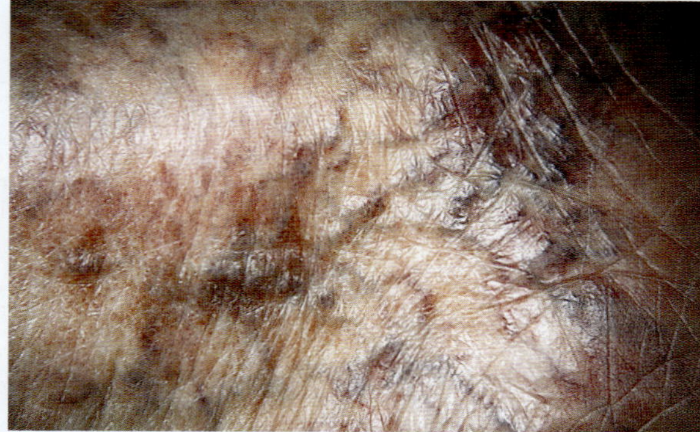

Venous lake

A blue-purple dilatation of venules and capillaries in a star-shaped, linear or flaring pattern. Pressure causes them to empty or disappear. Located on the legs near varicose veins and also on the face, lips, ears and chest.

TABLE 22.8 Vascular lesions—cont'd

PURPURIC LESIONS

Caused by blood flowing out of breaks in the vessels. Red blood cells and blood pigments are deposited in the tissues (extravascular). Difficult to see in dark-skinned people.

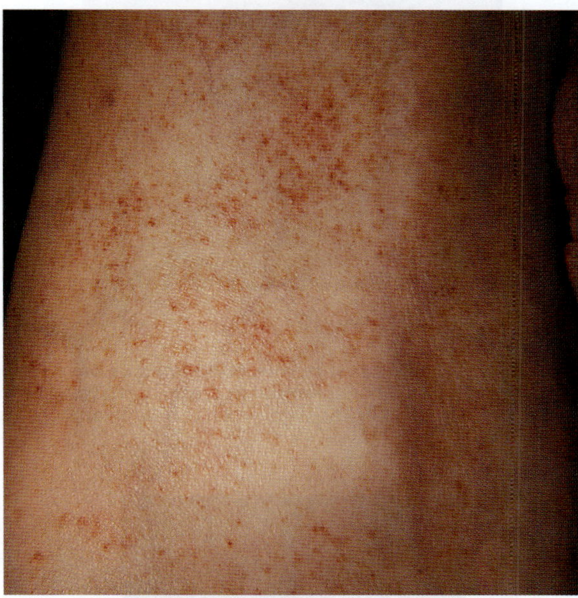

Petechiae

Tiny punctate haemorrhages, 1–3 mm, round and discrete, dark red, purple or brown in colour. Caused by bleeding from superficial capillaries; will not blanch. May indicate abnormal clotting factors. In dark-skinned people, petechiae are best visualised in the areas of lighter melanisation (e.g. the abdomen, buttocks and volar surface of the forearm). When the skin is black or very dark brown, petechiae cannot be seen in the skin.

Most of the diseases that cause bleeding and microembolism formation—such as thrombocytopenia, subacute bacterial endocarditis and other septicaemias—are characterised by petechiae in the mucous membranes as well as on the skin. Thus, you should inspect for petechiae in the mouth, particularly the buccal mucosa, and in the conjunctivae.

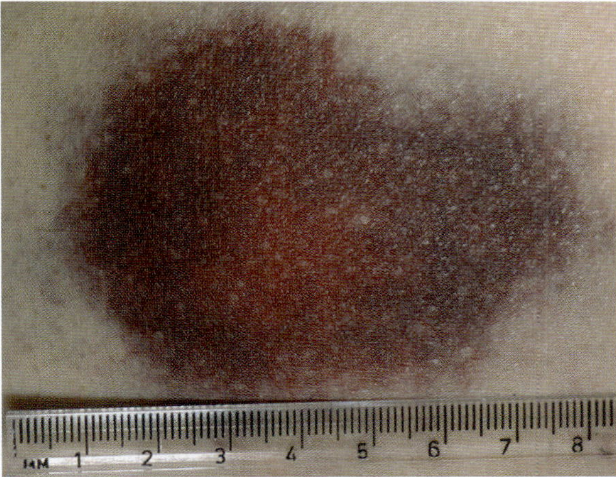

Ecchymosis

A purplish patch resulting from extravasation of blood into the skin, >3 mm in diameter.

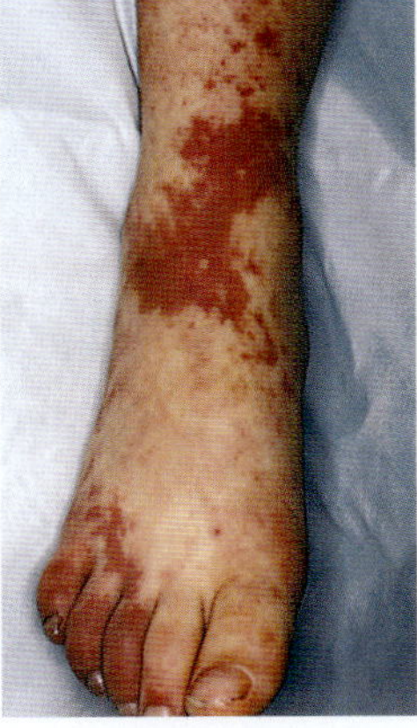

Purpura

Confluent and extensive patch of petechiae and ecchymoses, >3 mm flat, red to purple, macular haemorrhage. Seen in generalised disorders such as thrombocytopenia and scurvy. Also occurs in old age as blood leaks from capillaries in response to minor trauma and diffuses through dermis.

TABLE 22.9 Common skin lesions in children

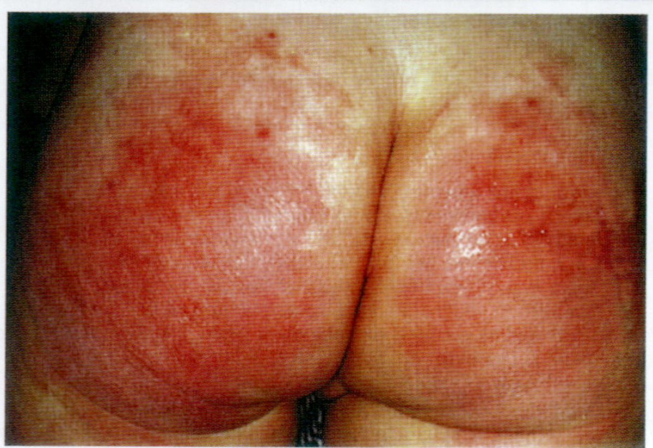

Nappy dermatitis

Red, moist maculopapular patch with poorly defined borders in nappy area, extending along inguinal and gluteal folds. History of infrequent nappy changes or occlusive coverings. Inflammatory disease caused by skin irritation from ammonia, heat, moisture occlusive nappies.

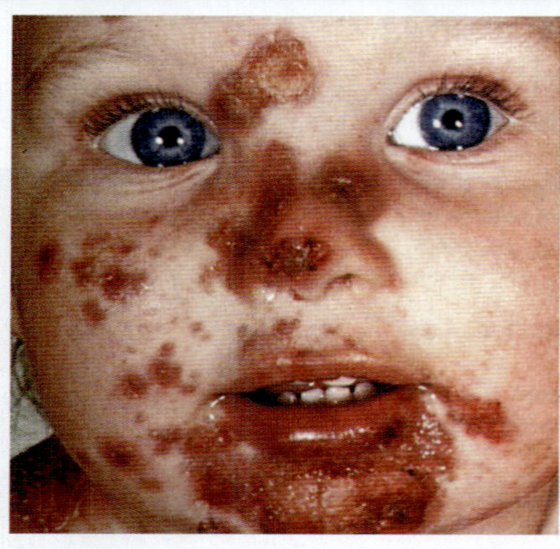

Impetigo

Moist, thin-roofed vesicles with thin, erythematous base. Rupture to form thick, honey-coloured crusts. Contagious bacterial infection of skin; most common in infants and children.

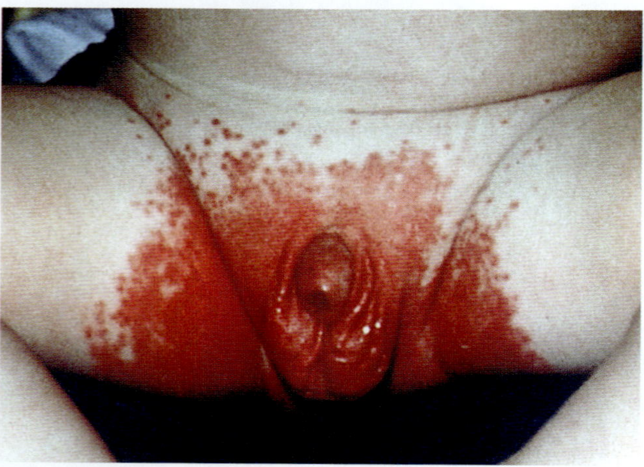

Intertrigo (candidiasis)

Scalding red, moist patches with sharply demarcated borders, some loose scales. Usually in genital area extending along inguinal and gluteal folds. Aggravated by urine, faeces, heat and moisture, the *Candida* fungus infects the superficial skin layers.

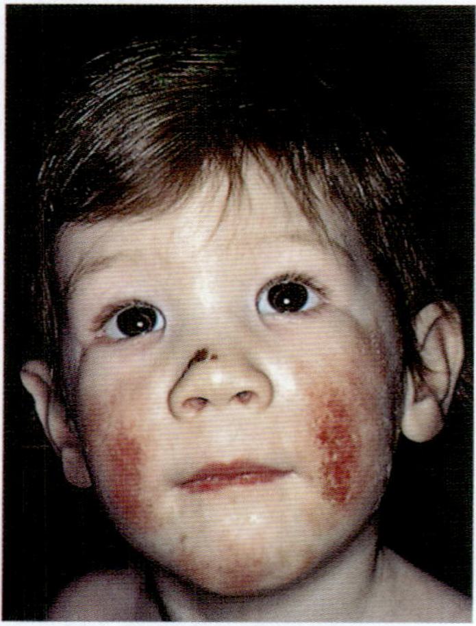

Atopic dermatitis (eczema)

Erythematous papules and vesicles, with weeping, oozing and crusts. Lesions usually on scalp, forehead, cheeks, forearms and wrists, elbows, backs of knees. Paroxysmal and severe pruritus. Family history of allergies.

TABLE 22.9 Common skin lesions in children—cont'd

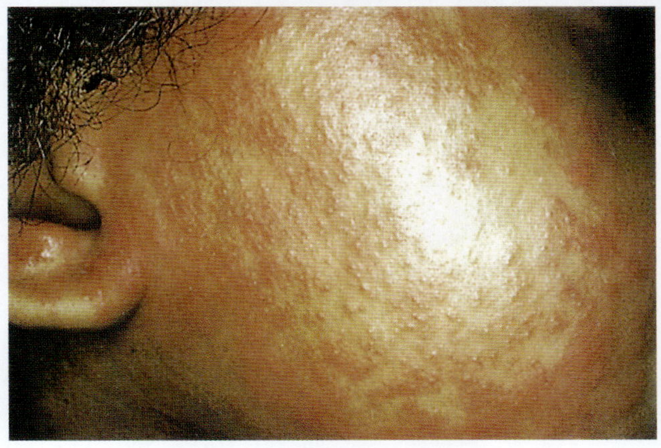

Measles (rubeola) in dark skin

Red-purple maculopapular blotchy rash in dark skin (above) and in light skin (below) appears on third or fourth day of illness. Rash appears first behind ears and spreads over face, then over neck, trunk, arms and legs; looks 'coppery' and does not blanch. Also characterised by Koplik's spots in mouth—bluish white, red-based elevations of 1–3 mm.

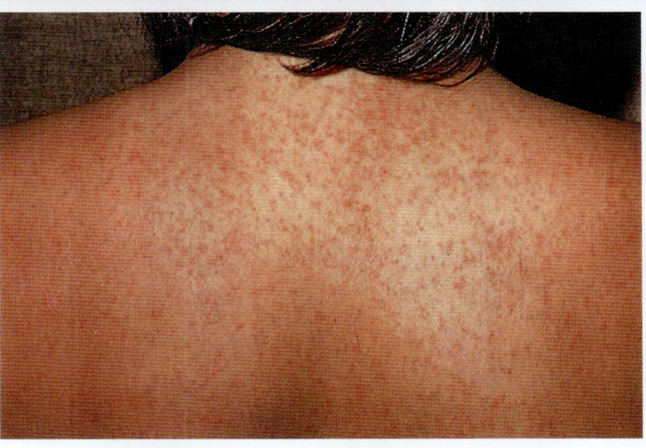

Measles (rubella)

Pink papular rash (similar to rubeola but paler) first appears on face, then spreads. Distinguished from rubeola by presence of neck lymphadenopathy and absence of Koplik's spots.

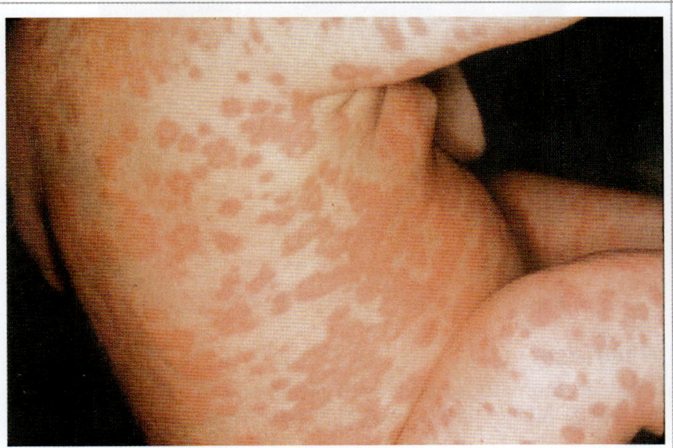

Measles (rubeola) in light skin

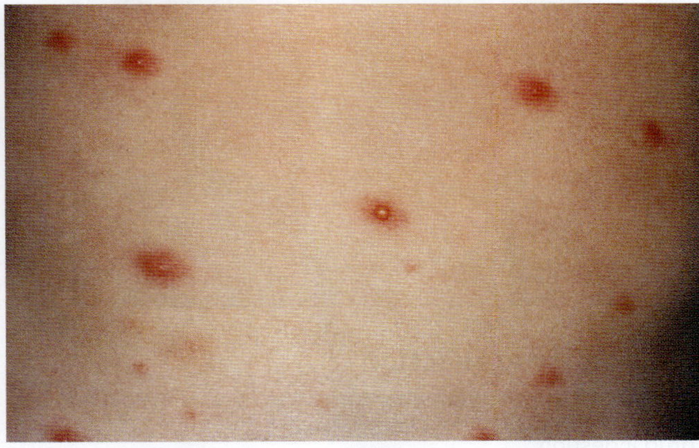

Chickenpox (varicella)

Small tight vesicles first appear on trunk, then spread to face, arms and legs (not palms or soles). Shiny vesicles on an erythematous base are commonly described as the 'dewdrop on a rose petal'. Vesicles erupt in succeeding crops over several days, and then become pustules, then crusts. Intensely pruritic.

TABLE 22.10 Common skin lesions

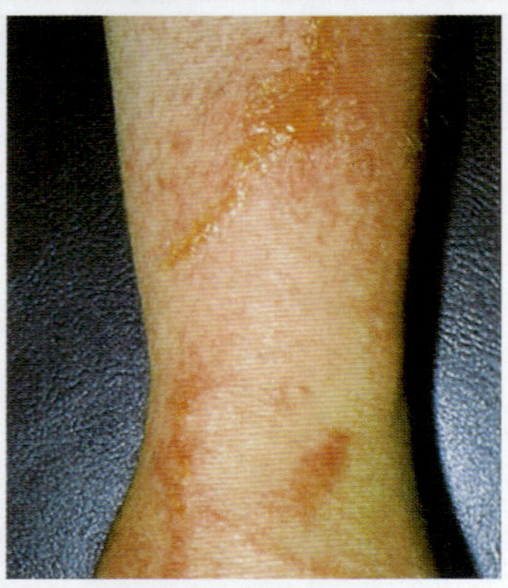

Primary contact dermatitis

Local inflammatory reaction to an irritant in the environment or an allergy. Characteristic location of lesions often gives clue. Often erythema shows first, followed by swelling, wheals (or urticaria) or maculopapular vesicles, scales. Frequently accompanied by intense pruritus.

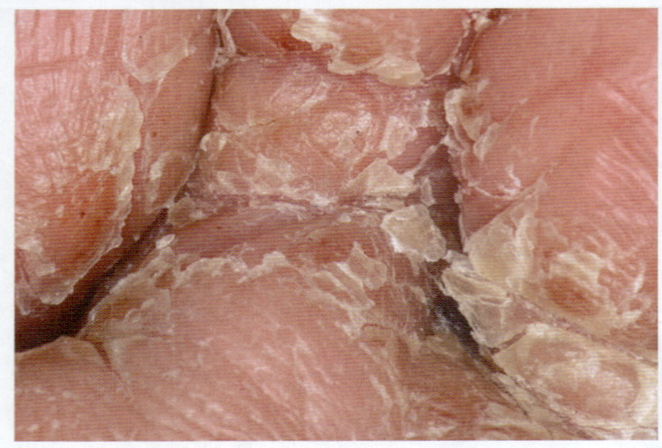

Tinea pedis (ringworm of the foot)

'Athlete's foot', a fungal infection, first appears as small vesicles between toes, sides of feet, soles. Then grows scaly and hard. Found in chronically warm moist feet: children after gymnasium activities, athletes, ageing adults who cannot dry their feet well.

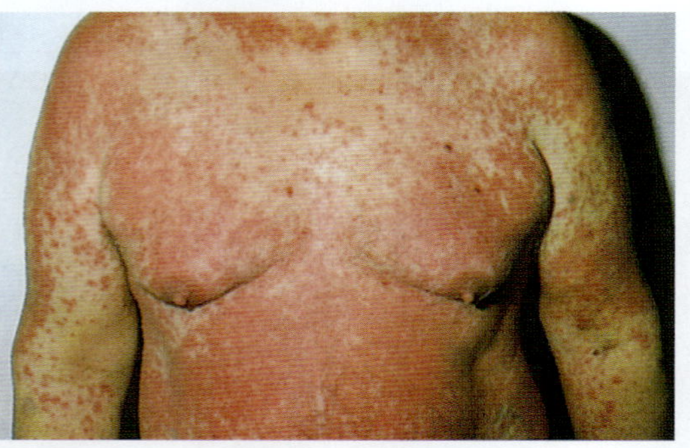

Allergic drug reaction

Erythematous and symmetric rash, usually generalised. Some drugs produce urticarial rash or vesicles and bullae. History of drug ingestion.

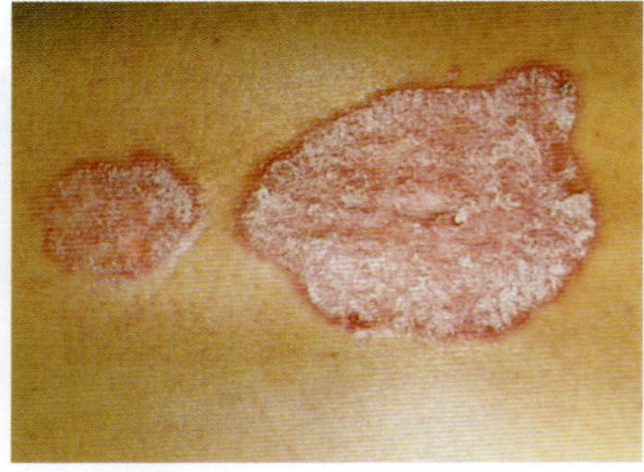

Psoriasis

Scaly erythematous patch, with silvery scales on top. Usually on scalp, outside of elbows and knees, low back and anogenital area.

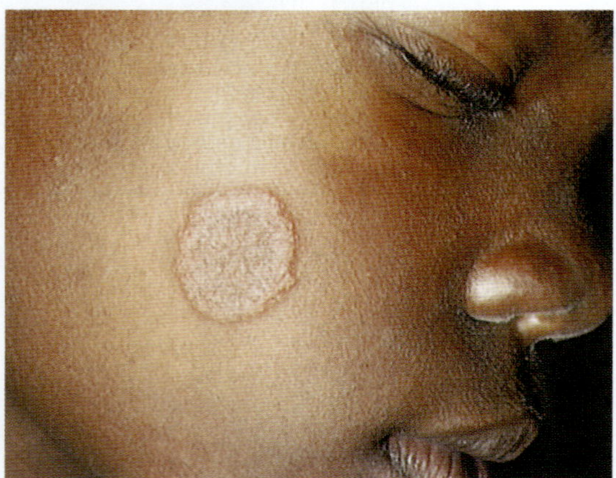

Tinea corporis (ringworm of the body)

Scales—hyperpigmented in whites, depigmented in dark-skinned persons—on chest, abdomen, back of arms forming multiple circular lesions with clear centres.

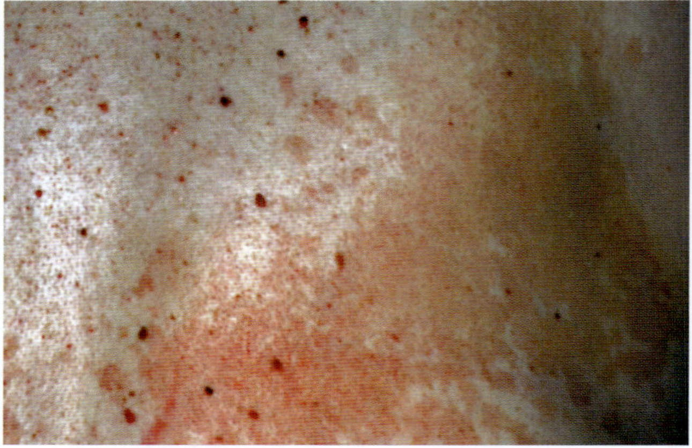

Tinea versicolour

Fine, scaling, round patches of pink, tan or white that (hence the name) do not tan in sunlight, caused by a superficial fungal infection. Usual distribution is on neck, trunk and upper arms—a short-sleeved turtleneck sweater area. Most common in otherwise healthy young adults.

TABLE 22.10 Common skin lesions—cont'd

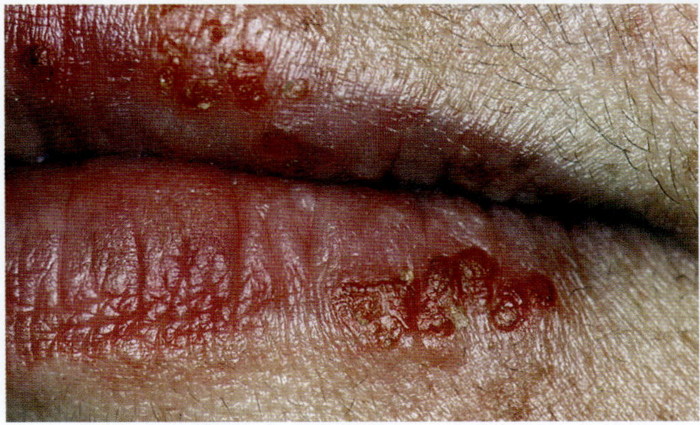

Herpes simplex (cold sores)

Herpes simplex virus (HSV) infection has a prodrome of skin tingling and sensitivity. Lesion then erupts with tight vesicles followed by pustules and then produces acute gingivostomatitis with many shallow, painful ulcers. Common location is upper lip, also in oral mucosa and tongue.

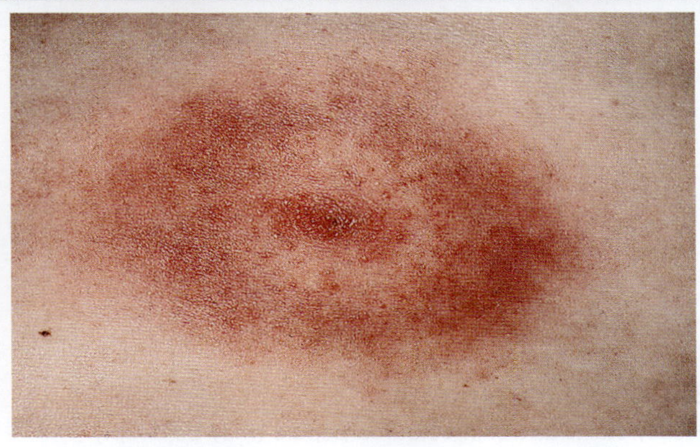

Lyme disease

Lyme disease (LD) is not fatal but may have serious arthritic, cardiac or neurological sequelae. It is caused by a spirochaete bacterium carried by ticks.

The first stage (early localised LD) has the distinctive bull's eye, red macular or papular rash (shown above) in 50% of cases. The rash radiates from the site of the tick bite (5 cm or larger) with some central clearing; it is usually located in axillae, midriff, inguinal region or behind knees, with regional lymphadenopathy. Rash fades in 4 weeks; untreated individual may then have disseminated disease with fatigue, anorexia, fever, chills or joint or muscle aches. Antibiotic treatment shortens symptoms and decreases risk for sequelae (Graves & Stenos 2017).

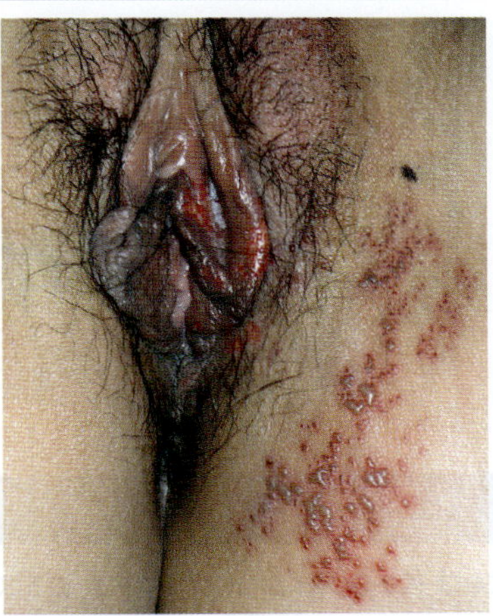

Herpes zoster (shingles)

Small grouped vesicles emerge along route of cutaneous sensory nerve, then pustules, then crusts. Caused by the varicella zoster virus (VZV), a reactivation of the dormant virus of chickenpox. Acute appearance, unilateral, does not cross midline. Commonly on trunk; can be anywhere. If on ophthalmic branch of cranial nerve V, it poses risk to eye. Most common in adults older than 50 years old. Pain is often severe and long-lasting in ageing adults; called *postherpetic neuralgia*.

NOTE: Be observant! The photo above is not genital herpes. This is herpes zoster with a linear lesion on only one side.

TABLE 22.11 Malignant skin lesions

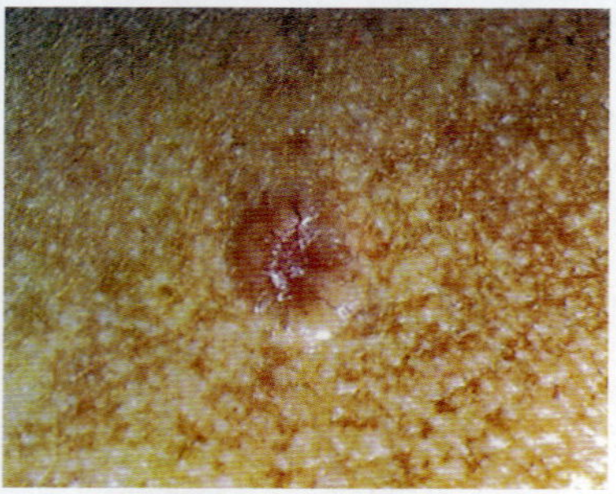

Basal cell carcinoma

Usually starts as a skin-coloured papule (may be deeply pigmented) with a translucent top and overlying telangiectasia. Then develops rounded pearly borders with central red ulcer, or looks like large open pore with central yellowing. Most common form of skin cancer; slow but inexorable growth.

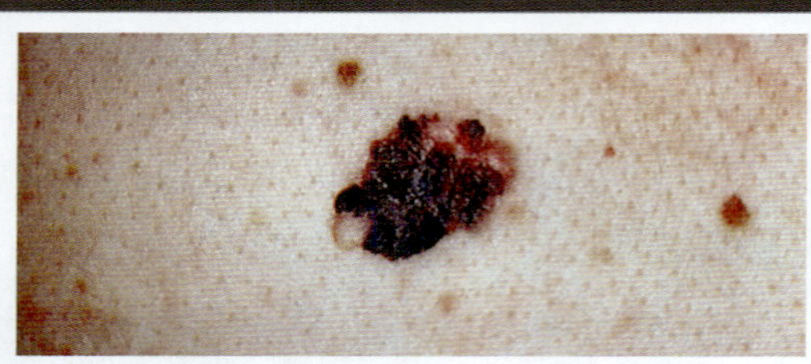

Malignant melanoma

Half 'of the occurrences of these' (to eliminate ambiguity: 'half the size' or 'half the occurrences') lesions arise from preexisting naevi. Usually brown; can be tan, black, pink-red, purple or mixed pigmentation. Often irregular or notched borders. May have scaling, flaking, oozing texture. Common locations are on the trunk and back in men and women, on the legs in women and on the palms, soles of feet and the nails in dark-skinned people.

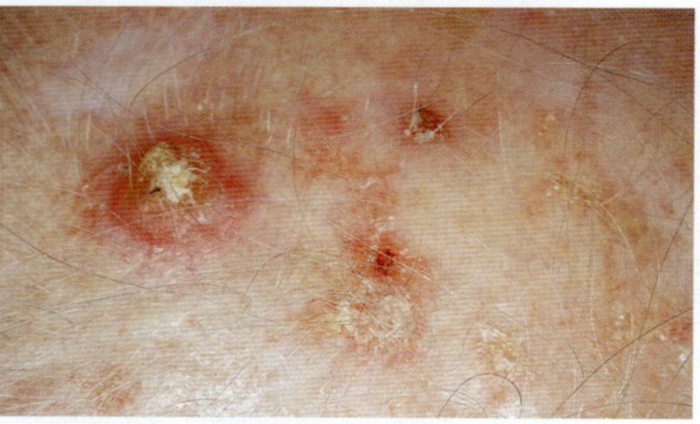

Squamous cell carcinoma

Erythematous scaly patch with sharp margins, 1 cm or more. Develops central ulcer and surrounding erythema. Usually on hands or head, areas exposed to solar radiation. Less common than basal cell carcinoma but grows rapidly.

TABLE 22.12 Skin lesions associated with AIDS

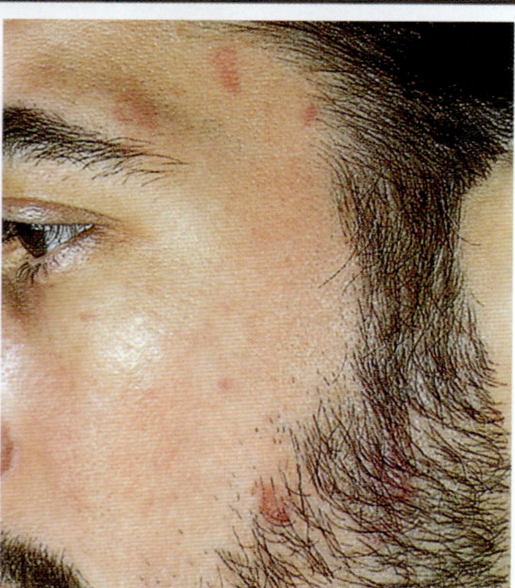

AIDS related Kaposi's sarcoma: patch stage

An aggressive form of Kaposi's sarcoma is one of the diseases that may occur with the acquired immune deficiency disorder (AIDS). Here, multiple patch-stage early lesions are faint pink on the temple and beard area. They could easily be mistaken for bruises or naevi and be ignored.

TABLE 22.13 Abnormal conditions of hair

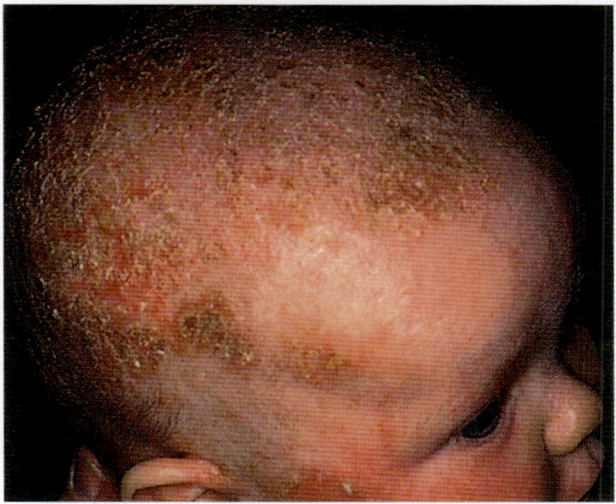

Seborrhoeic dermatitis (cradle cap)

Thick, yellow to white, greasy, adherent scales with mild erythema on scalp and forehead; very common in early infancy. Resembles eczema lesions except cradle cap is distinguished by absence of pruritus, 'greasy' yellow-pink lesions and negative family history of allergy.

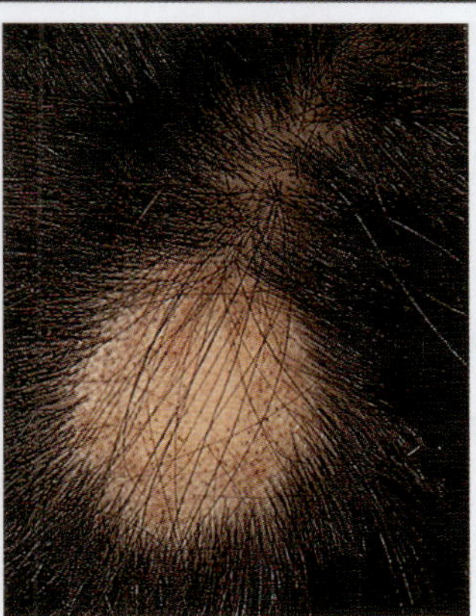

Alopecia areata

Sudden appearance of a sharply circumscribed, round or oval balding patch, usually with smooth, soft, hairless skin underneath. Unknown cause; when limited to a few patches, person usually has complete regrowth.

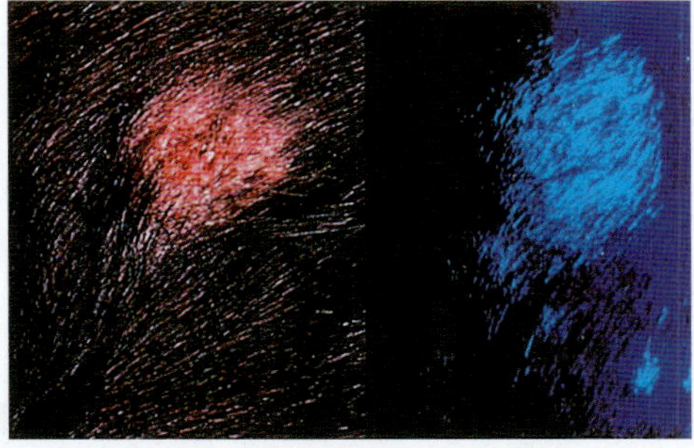

Tinea capitis (scalp ringworm)

Rounded patchy hair loss on scalp, leaving broken-off hairs, pustules and scales on skin. Caused by fungal infection; lesions may fluoresce blue-green under Wood's light. Usually seen in children and farmers; highly contagious, may be transmitted by another person, by domestic animals or from soil.

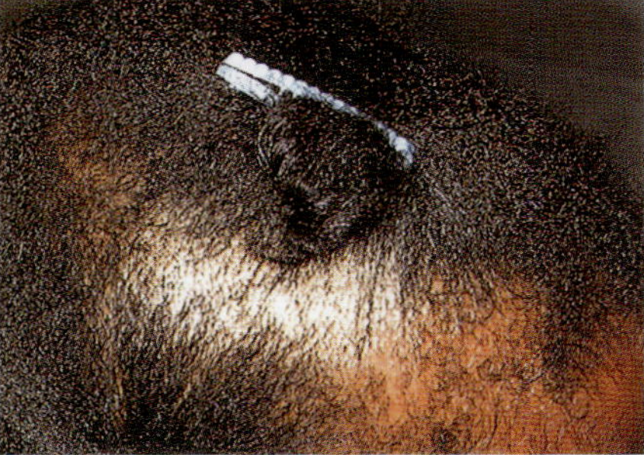

Traumatic alopecia: traction alopecia

Linear or oval patch of hair loss along hair line, a part or scattered distribution; caused by trauma from hair rollers, tight braiding, tight ponytail, hair clips.

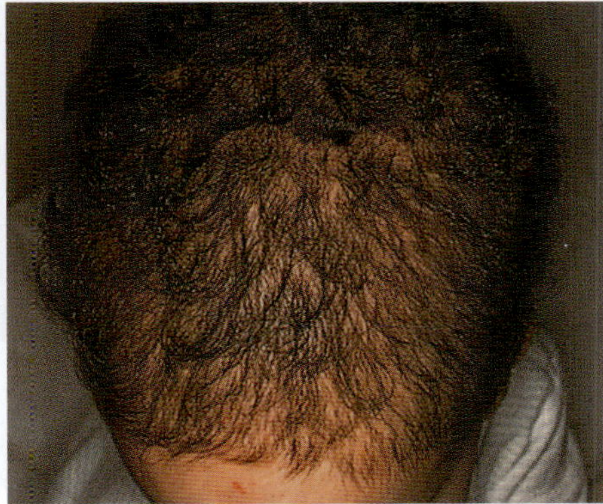

Toxic alopecia

Patchy, asymmetric balding that accompanies severe illness or use of chemotherapy where growing hairs are lost and resting hairs are spared. Regrowth occurs after illness or discontinuation of toxin.

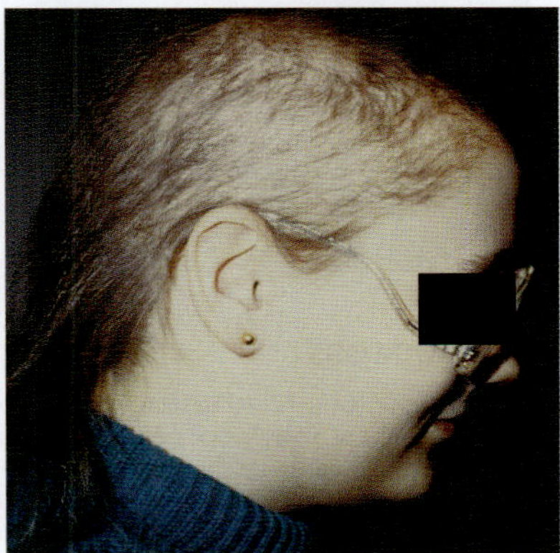

Trichotillomania

Traumatic self-induced hair loss usually the result of compulsive twisting or plucking. Forms irregularly shaped patch, with broken-off, stub-like hairs of varying lengths; person is never completely bald. Occurs as child rubs or twists area absently while falling asleep, reading or watching television. In adults, it can be a serious problem and is usually a sign of a personality disorder.

(Continued)

TABLE 22.13 Abnormal conditions of hair—cont'd

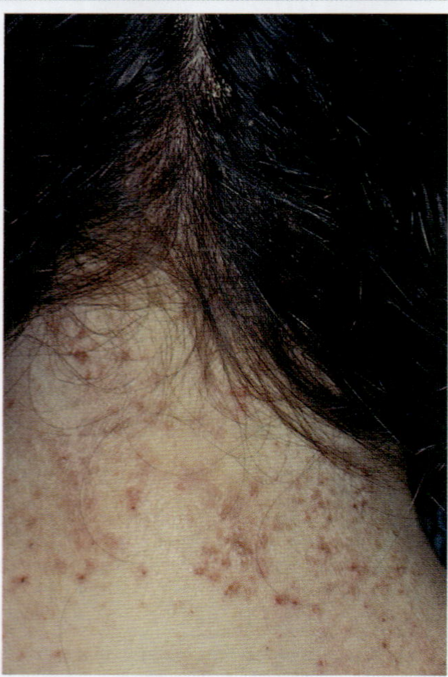

Pediculosis capitis (head lice)

History includes intense itching of the scalp, especially the occiput. The nits (eggs) of lice are easier to see in the occipital area and around the ears, appearing as 2- to 3-mm oval translucent bodies, adherent to the hair shafts. Common among school-age children. Over-the-counter pediculicide shampoos are available; however, nit removal by daily combing of wet hair with a fine-tooth metal comb is especially important.

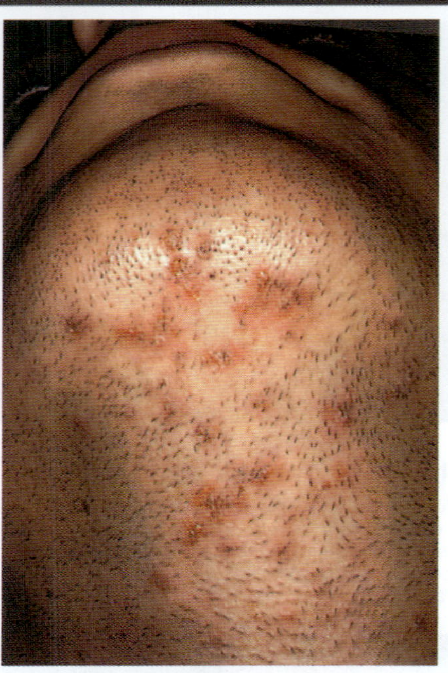

Folliculitis (razor bumps)

Superficial infection of hair follicles. Multiple pustules, 'whiteheads', with hair visible at centre and erythematous base. Usually on arms, legs, face and buttocks.

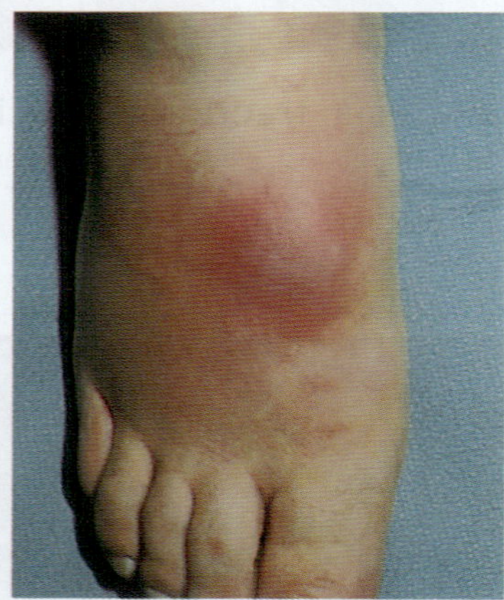

Furuncle and abscess

Red, swollen, hard, tender, pus-filled lesion caused by acute localised bacterial (usually staphylococcal) infection; usually on back of neck, buttocks, occasionally on wrists or ankles. Furuncles are due to infected hair follicles, whereas abscesses are due to traumatic introduction of bacteria into the skin. Abscesses are usually larger and deeper than furuncles.

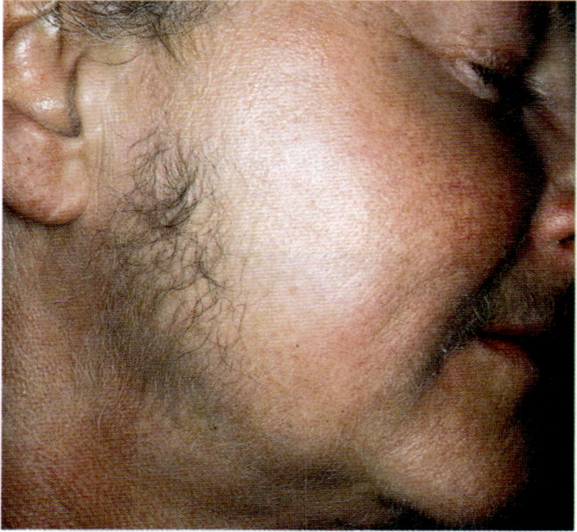

Hirsutism

Excess body hair in females forming a male sexual pattern (upper lip, face, chest, abdomen, arms, legs); caused by endocrine or metabolic dysfunction, or occasionally is idiopathic.

TABLE 22.14 Abnormal conditions of nails and hands	
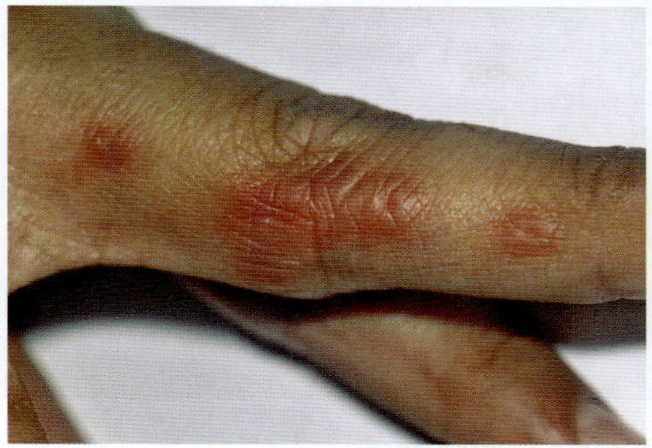 **Scabies** An intensely pruritic contagion caused by the scabies mite. Mites form a linear or curved elevated burrow on the fingers, web spaces of hands, and wrists. Other family members are usually infected. The patient cannot stop scratching.	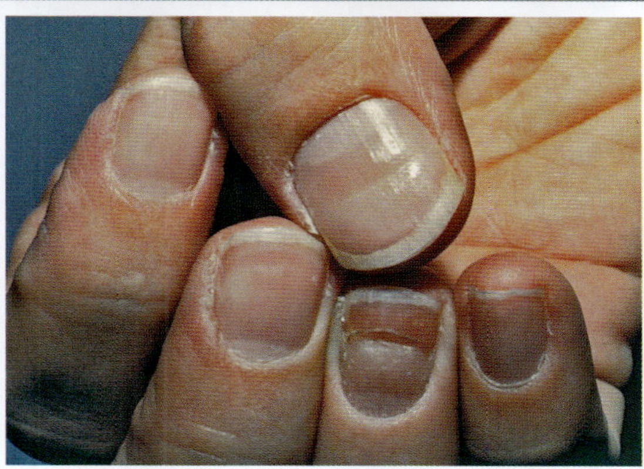 **Beau's line** Transverse furrow or groove. A depression across the nail that extends down to the nail bed. Occurs with any trauma that temporarily impairs nail formation, such as acute illness, toxic reaction or local trauma. Dent appears first at the cuticle and moves forward as nail grows.
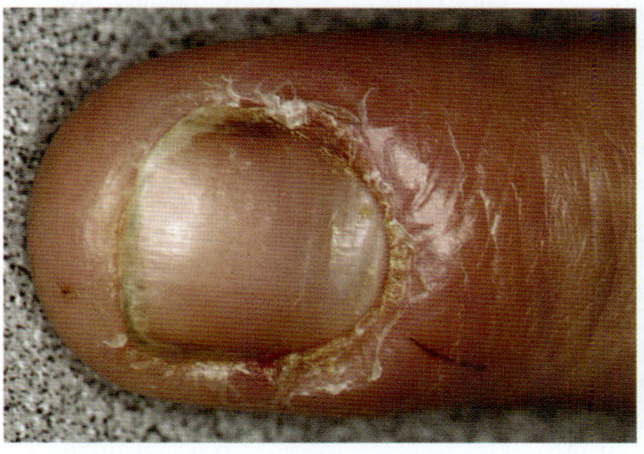 **Paronychia** Red, swollen, tender inflammation of the nail folds. Acute paronychia is usually a bacterial infection; chronic paronychia is most often a fungal infection from a break in the cuticle in those who perform 'wet' work.	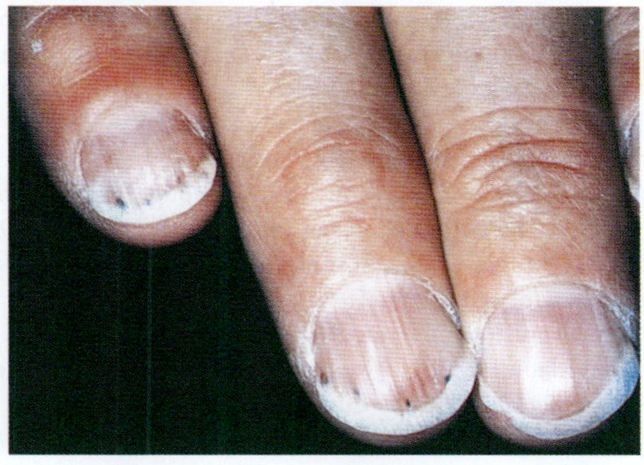 **Splinter haemorrhages** Red-brown linear streaks, embolic lesions, occur with subacute bacterial endocarditis; may also occur with minor trauma.
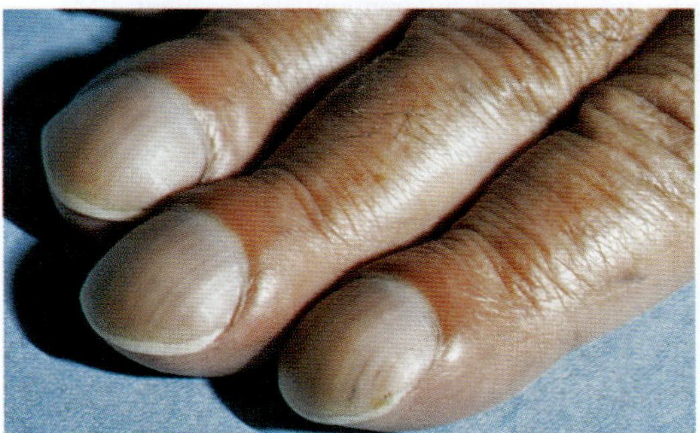 **Late clubbing** Proximal edge of nail elevates; angle is greater than 180 degrees. Distal phalanx looks rounder and wider. Seen with chronic obstructive pulmonary disease and congenital heart disease with cyanosis. Occurs first in thumb and index finger.	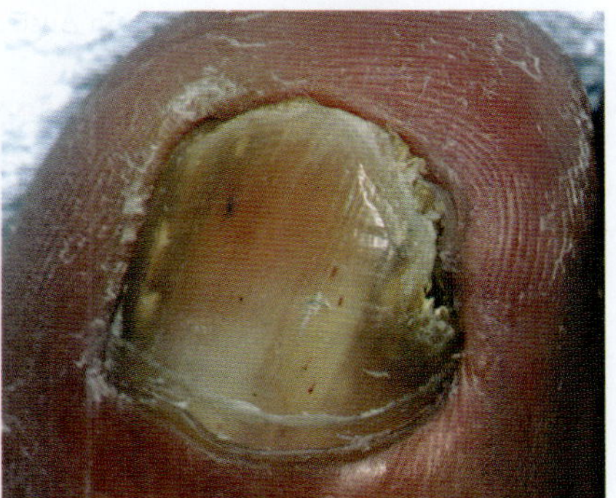 **Onycholysis** This is a slow, persistent fungal infection of fingernails and, more often, toenails, common in older adults. Fungus causes change in colour (green where nail plate separated from bed), texture, thickness, with nail crumbling or breaking, and loosening of the nail plate, usually beginning at the distal edge and progressing proximally.

(Continued)

TABLE 22.14 Abnormal conditions of nails and hands—cont'd

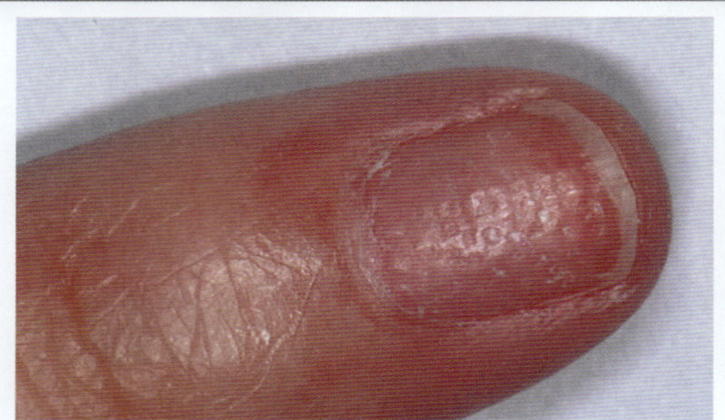

Pitting

Sharply defined pitting and crumbling of the nails with distal detachment often occurs with psoriasis.

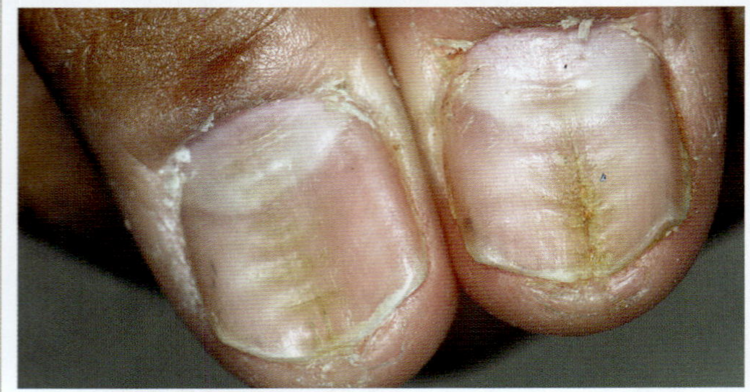

Habit-tic dystrophy

Depression down middle of nail or multiple horizontal ridges, caused by continuous picking of cuticle by another finger of same hand, which causes injury to nail base and nail matrix.

BIBLIOGRAPHY

Australasian College of Dermatologists. 2019. Information for Skin, Hair and Nail Conditions. Available at: www.dermcoll.edu.au.

Australian Institute of Health and Welfare. Cancer. 2019. Available at: https://www.aihw.gov.au/reports-data/health-conditions-disability-deaths/cancer/overview.

Cancer Council Australia. How much sun is enough? Getting the balance right—vitamin D and sun protection (brochure). 2018a. Available at: https://www.cancer.org.au/policy-and-advocacy/position-statements/sun-smart/#jump_3.

Cancer Council Australia. National Cancer Prevention Policy 9. 2018b. Available at: https://www.aihw.gov.au/reports-data/health-conditions-disability-deaths/cancer/overview.

Cancer Council Australia. Sun safety. 2019. Available at: https://www.cancer.org.au/preventing-cancer/sun-protection/.

Campbell K, Baronoski S, Gloeckner M, Holloway S, Idensohn P, Langemo D, et al. Skin tears: prediction, prevention, assessment and management. Nurse Prescr 2018;16(12):600-7.

Cohen J, Powderly W, Opal S. Infectious diseases. 4th ed. Chatswood, NSW: Elsevier; 2016.

Graves S, Stenos J. Tick-borne Infectious diseases in Australia. Med J Aust 2017;206(7):320–24.

Hess CT. Comprehensive patient and wound assessments. Adv Skin Wound Care 2019;32(6):287–8.

Hugill K. Revisiting nappy dermatitis: causes and preventative care. Br J Midwifery 2017;25(3):150–4.

Lebwohl M, Heymann W, Berth-Jones J, Coulson I. Treatment of skin disease. 5th ed. Chatswood, NSW: Elsevier; 2017.

McIntosh I. Nail disorders and their significance. Nail Disord 2018;75(1):6–7.

Ministry of Health, New Zealand. Sunbeds. 2019. Available at: https://www.health.govt.nz/your-health/healthy-living/environmental-health/sunbeds.

Pagana K. Manual of diagnostic and laboratory tests. 6th ed. Chatswood, NSW: Elsevier; 2017.

Patton K. Anatomy and physiology. 10th ed. Chatswood, NSW: Elsevier; 2019.

Ritchie S. Distinguishing benign and malignant skin lesions. Nurs Pract 2017;(95):26–9.

Royal College of Pathologists of Australian. RCPA manual. 2019. Available at: https://www.rcpa.edu.au/Manuals/RCPA-Manual.

Stokholm J, Sevelsted A, Anderson U, Bisgaard H. Preeclampsia associates with asthma, allergy, and eczema in childhood. Am J Respir Crit Care Med 2017;195(5):614-21. doi:10.1164/rccm.201604-0806OC.

Thomas A, Baird S, Anderson J. Purpuric and petechial rashes in adults and children: initial assessment. BMJ 2016;352(8050):1285–87.

Todd M. Lymphoedema and chronic oedema. Nurse Prescr 2017;15(6):276–80.

Urinary and bowel function

Unit 8

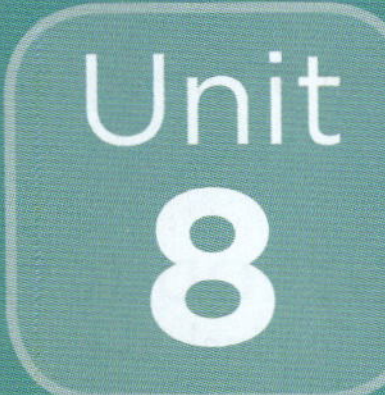

Chapter Twenty-Three

Abdominal assessment

Written by Carolyn Jarvis
Adapted by Elizabeth Watt

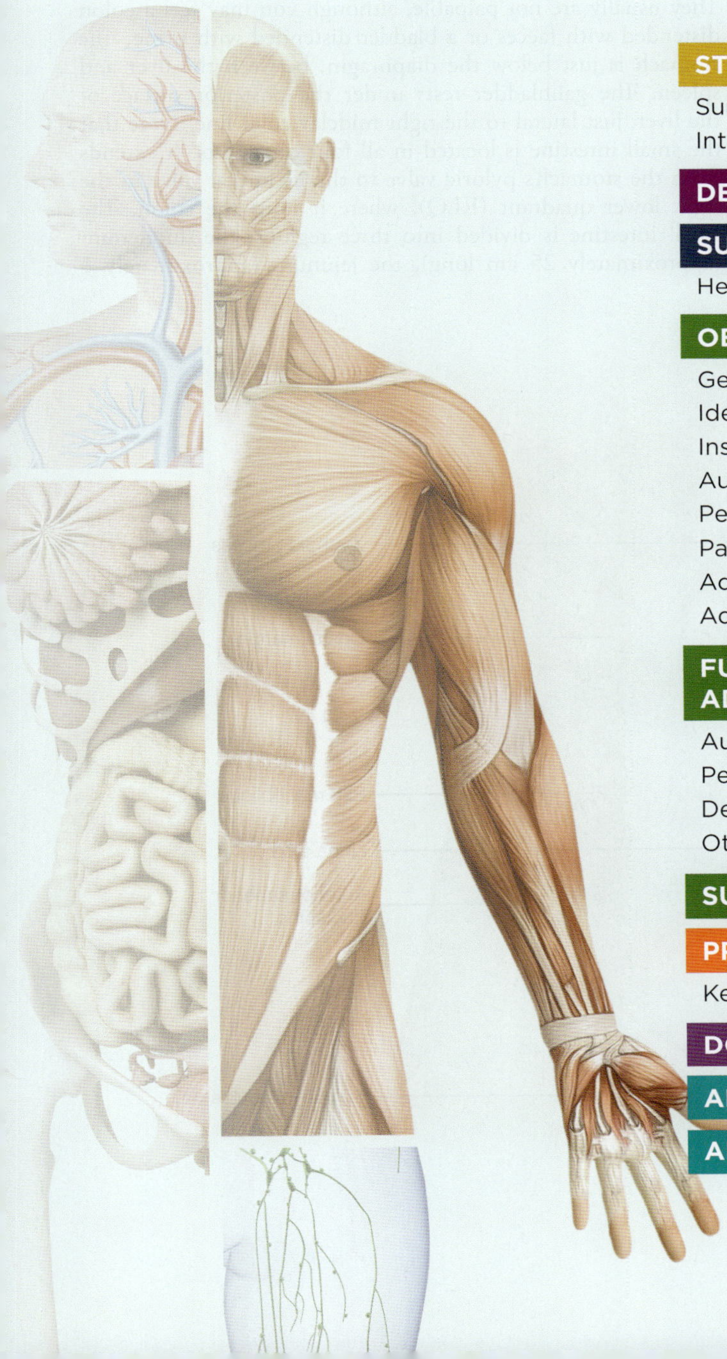

STRUCTURE AND FUNCTION

Surface landmarks
Internal anatomy

DEVELOPMENTAL CONSIDERATIONS

SUBJECTIVE DATA

Health history questions

OBJECTIVE DATA

General inspection
Identify abdominal landmarks
Inspection
Auscultation—bowel sounds
Percussion—general tympany
Palpation—surface and light
Additional objective data for infants and children
Additional objective data for adults over 65 years

FURTHER OBJECTIVE ASSESSMENT FOR ADVANCED PRACTICE

Auscultate vascular sounds
Percuss general tympany, liver span and splenic dullness
Deep palpation
Other procedures for advanced practice

SUMMARY CHECKLIST

PROMOTING A HEALTHY LIFESTYLE

Keeping your liver healthy

DOCUMENTATION AND CRITICAL THINKING

ABNORMAL FINDINGS

ABNORMAL FINDINGS FOR ADVANCED PRACTICE

INTRODUCTION

Abdominal assessment is frequently performed in nursing. It forms part of an assessment of nutrition and metabolic function, urinary and bowel function and assessment during pregnancy. Structures relevant to abdominal assessment include all of the abdominal organs and the abdominal wall. You will find other relevant anatomy and physiology in Chapters 24 and 25. Information relevant to abdominal examination in pregnancy is detailed in Chapter 29.

Structure and function

SURFACE LANDMARKS

The **abdomen** is a large oval cavity extending from the diaphragm down to the brim of the pelvis. It is bordered at its back by the vertebral column and paravertebral muscles and at the sides and front by the lower rib cage and abdominal muscles (Figure 23.1). Four layers of large, flat muscles form the ventral (anterior) abdominal wall. These are joined at the midline by a tendinous seam, the **linea alba**. One set, the **rectus abdominis**, forms a strip extending the length of the midline, and its edge is often palpable.

INTERNAL ANATOMY

Inside the abdominal cavity, all the internal organs are called the viscera (Figure 23.2). You must be able to visualise each organ as you listen to or palpate through the abdominal wall.

The **solid viscera** are those that maintain a characteristic shape (liver, pancreas, spleen, adrenal glands, kidneys, ovaries and uterus). The liver fills most of the right upper quadrant (RUQ) and extends over to the left midclavicular line. The lower edge of the liver and the right kidney may normally be palpable. The ovaries normally are palpable only on bimanual examination during the pelvic examination.

The shapes of the **hollow viscera** (stomach, gallbladder, small intestine, colon and bladder) depend on the contents. They usually are not palpable, although you may feel a colon distended with faeces or a bladder distended with urine. The stomach is just below the diaphragm, between the liver and spleen. The gallbladder rests under the posterior surface of the liver, just lateral to the right midclavicular line. Note that the small intestine is located in all four quadrants. It extends from the stomach's pyloric valve to the ileocaecal valve in the right lower quadrant (RLQ), where it joins the colon. The small intestine is divided into three regions, the duodenum (approximately 25 cm long), the jejunum (approximately 1

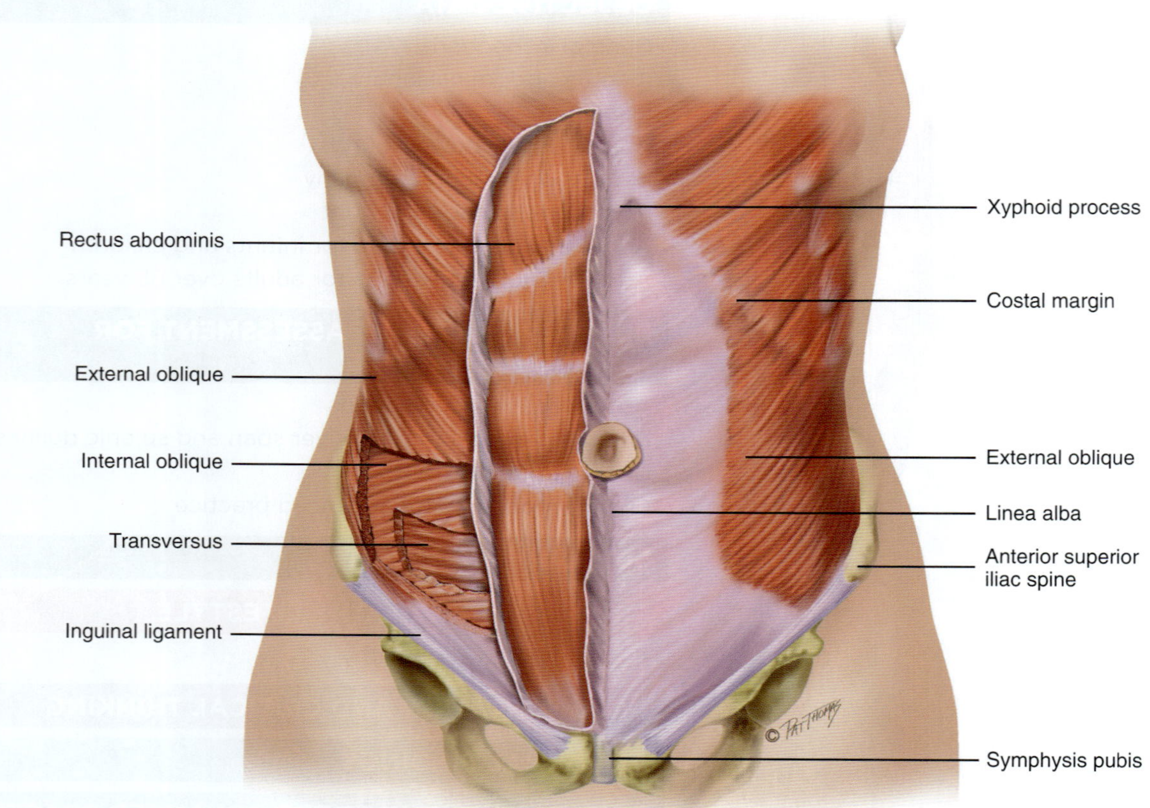

Figure 23.1
© Pat Thomas, 2006.

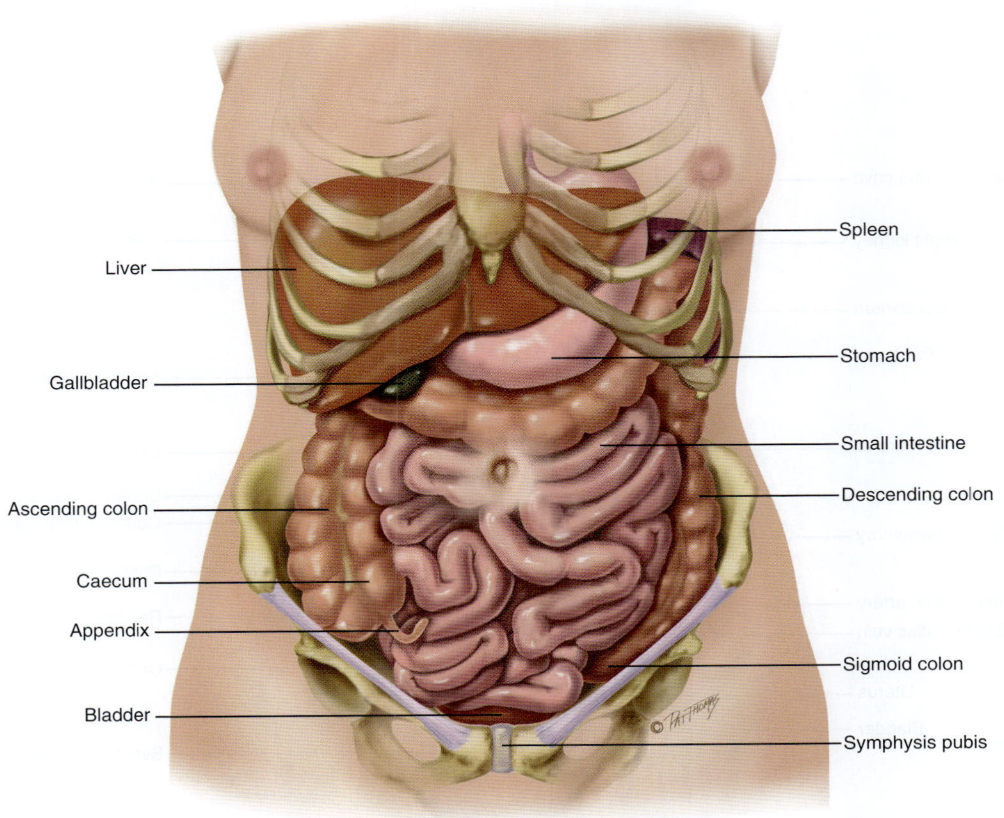

Figure 23.2
© Pat Thomas, 2006.

m long) and the ileum (approximately 2 m long). The small intestine joins the large intestine at the ileocaecal valve. The large intestine is approximately 1.5 m long and extends from the ileum to the anus. It is divided into four major areas; the caecum, colon, rectum and anal canal. The colon is divided according to its position in the abdomen; the ascending colon, the transverse colon, the descending colon and the sigmoid colon. See Chapter 25 for detail about the anatomy of the anus and rectum.

The **spleen** is a soft mass of lymphatic tissue on the posterolateral wall of the abdominal cavity, immediately under the diaphragm (Figure 23.3). It lies obliquely with its long axis behind and parallel to the tenth rib, lateral to the midaxillary line. Its width extends from the ninth to the eleventh rib, about

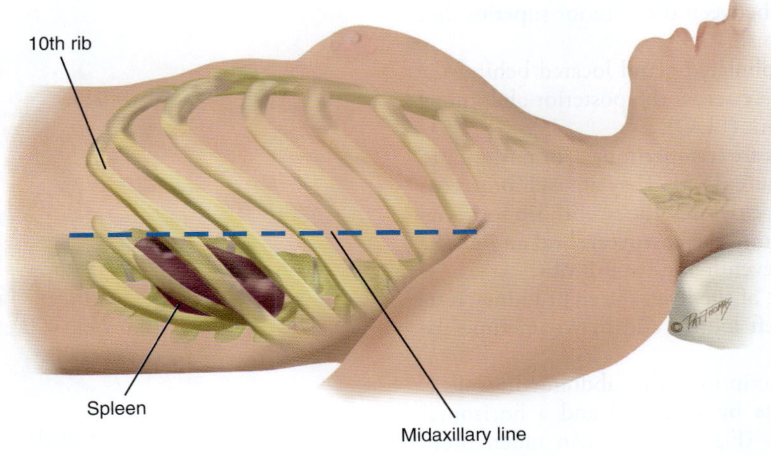

Figure 23.3
© Pat Thomas, 2006.

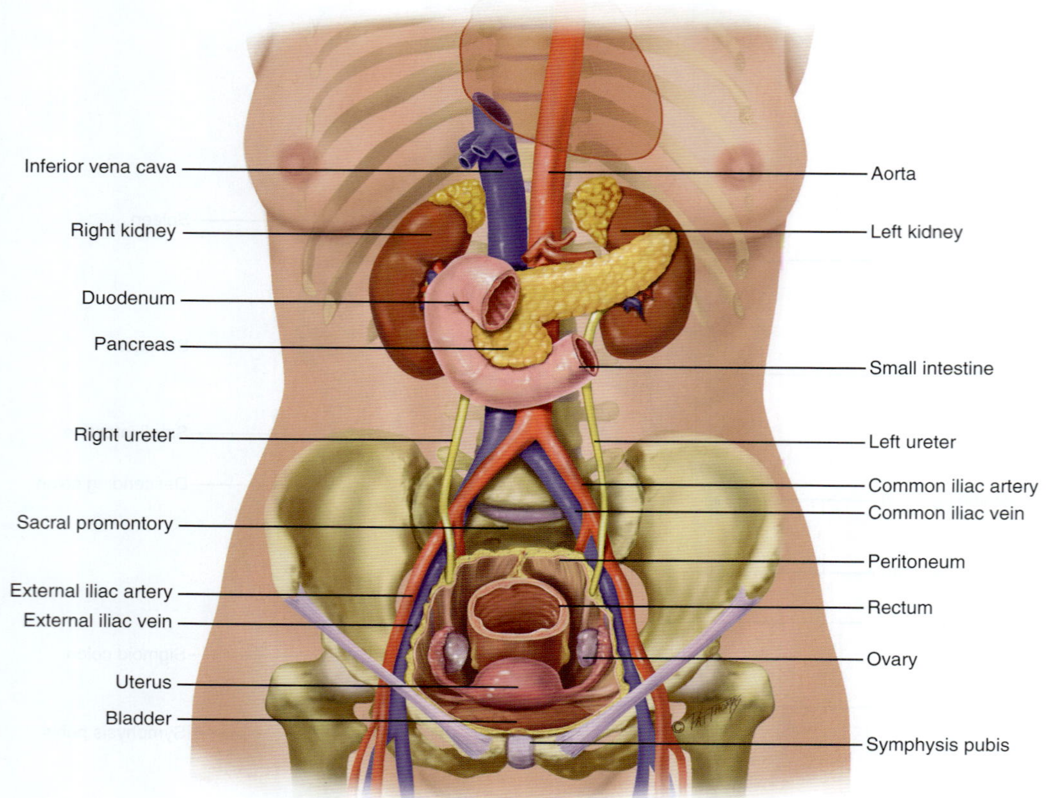

Figure 23.4
© Pat Thomas, 2006.

7 cm. It is not palpable. If it becomes enlarged, its lower pole moves downwards and towards the midline.

The **aorta** is just to the left of midline in the upper part of the abdomen (Figure 23.4). It descends behind the peritoneum and, at 2 cm below the umbilicus, it bifurcates into the right and left common iliac arteries opposite the fourth lumbar vertebra. You can palpate the aortic pulsations in the upper anterior abdominal wall. The right and left iliac arteries become the femoral arteries in the groin area. Their pulsations are easily palpated at a point halfway between the anterior superior iliac spine and the symphysis pubis.

The **pancreas** is a soft, lobulated gland located behind the stomach. It stretches obliquely across the posterior abdominal wall to the left upper quadrant (LUQ).

The bean-shaped **kidneys** are retroperitoneal, or posterior to the abdominal contents (Figure 23.5). They are well protected by the posterior ribs and musculature. The twelfth rib forms an angle with the vertebral column, the **costovertebral angle**. The left kidney lies here at the eleventh and twelfth ribs.

Because of the placement of the liver, the right kidney rests 1 to 2 cm lower than the left kidney and may sometimes be palpable.

For convenience in description, the abdominal wall is divided into **four quadrants** by a vertical and a horizontal line bisecting the umbilicus (Figure 23.6). (An older, more complicated scheme divided the abdomen into nine regions. Although the old system generally is not used, some regional

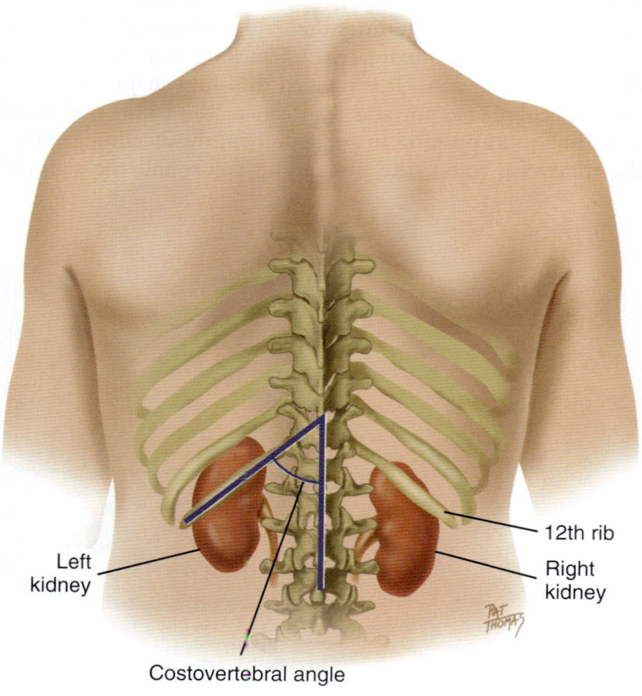

Figure 23.5

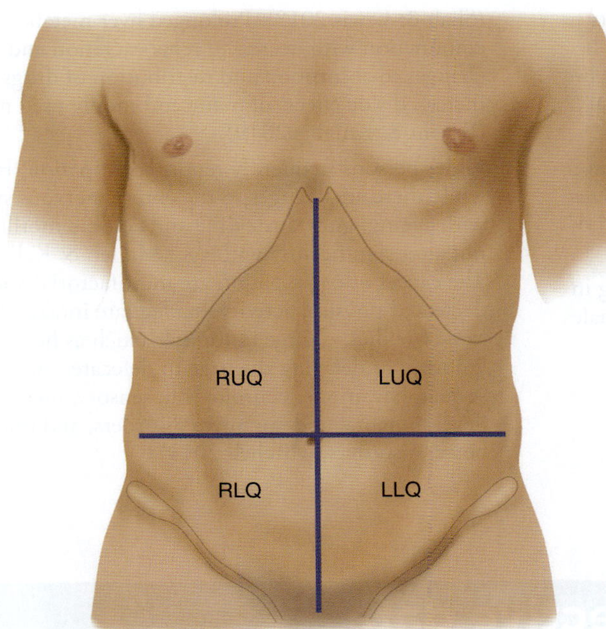

Four quadrants

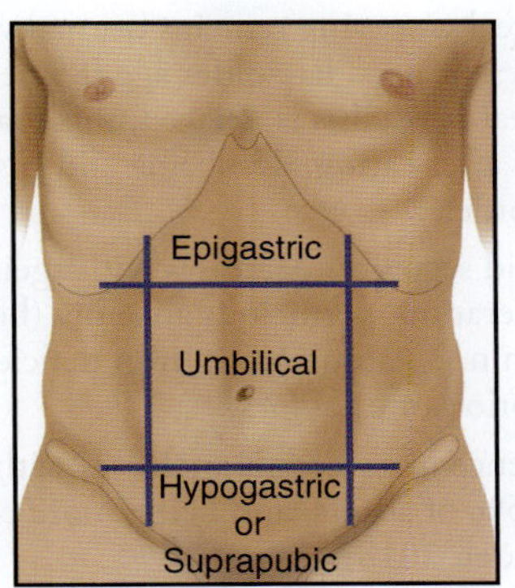

Figure 23.6

names persist, such as **epigastric** for the area between the costal margins, **umbilical** for the area around the umbilicus and **hypogastric** or **suprapubic** for the area above the pubic bone.)

The anatomical location of the organ by quadrants is:

Right upper quadrant (RUQ)
Liver
Gallbladder
Duodenum
Head of pancreas
Right kidney and adrenal
Hepatic flexure of colon
Part of ascending and transverse colon

Left upper quadrant (LUQ)
Stomach
Spleen
Left lobe of liver
Body of pancreas
Left kidney and adrenal
Splenic flexure of colon
Part of transverse colon and descending colon

Right lower quadrant (RLQ)
Caecum
Appendix
Right ovary and tube
Right ureter
Right spermatic cord

Left lower quadrant (LLQ)
Part of descending colon
Sigmoid colon
Left ovary and tube
Left ureter
Left spermatic cord

Midline
Aorta
Uterus (if enlarged)
Bladder (if distended)

DEVELOPMENTAL CONSIDERATIONS

Infants and children

In the newborn, the umbilical cord shows prominently on the abdomen. It contains two arteries and one vein. The liver takes up proportionately more space in the abdomen at birth than in later life. In healthy term neonates, the lower edge may be palpated 0.5 to 2.5 cm below the right costal margin. Age-related values of expected liver span are listed in the objective data section of the chapter. The urinary bladder is located higher in the abdomen than in the adult. It lies between the symphysis pubis and the umbilicus. Also, during early childhood, the abdominal wall is less muscular, so the appearance is rounded and the organs may be easier to palpate.

The pregnant woman

Nausea and vomiting, or 'morning sickness', is an early sign of pregnancy for many pregnant women, starting between the first and second missed menstrual periods. The cause is unknown but may be due to hormone changes such as the production of human chorionic gonadotrophin (hCG). Another symptom is 'acid indigestion' or heartburn (pyrosis) caused by oesophageal reflux. Gastrointestinal motility decreases, which prolongs gastric emptying time. The decreased motility causes more water to be reabsorbed from the colon, which may lead to constipation. Persistent straining to eliminate hard stool, as well as increased venous pressure in the lower pelvis, may lead to haemorrhoids.

The enlarging uterus displaces the intestines upwards and posteriorly and therefore bowel sounds are diminished. The appendix is displaced upwards and to the right. Skin changes on the abdomen, such as striae and the linea nigra, are discussed later in this chapter and in Chapter 29.

Late adulthood (65+ years)

Ageing alters the appearance of the abdominal wall. With further ageing, adipose tissue is redistributed away from the face and extremities to the abdomen and hips; the abdominal musculature may reduce in tone. Changes of ageing occur in the gastrointestinal system but do not significantly affect function when no disease is present.

- Salivation may decrease, causing a dry mouth and a decreased sense of taste. Further changes are discussed in Chapter 21.

- Oesophageal emptying remains normal when there is no disease present until late older age (85 years and older). If oesophageal peristalsis is delayed, this may result in a feeling of fullness after eating, dysphagia and gastro-oesophageal reflux disorder.
- Gastric acid secretion decreases with ageing. This may cause gastric ulceration, pernicious anaemia (because it interferes with vitamin B_{12} absorption), iron deficiency anaemia and malabsorption of calcium.
- The incidence of gallstones increases with age, occurring in 10% to 15% of adults, and being more common in females (Shabanzadeh 2018).
- Liver size and hepatic blood flow decrease with age, particularly after 80 years, although most liver function remains normal. However, liver metabolism that is responsible for the enzymatic oxidation, reduction and hydrolysis of drugs is substantially decreased with age (Shah & Lewis 2018). Prolonged liver metabolism, in conjunction with decreased renal excretion and aged related changes to absorption and distribution of drugs, can cause increased side effects of many commonly used medications (Bryant & Knights 2019).
- Older persons frequently report constipation. However, while there are changes to the enteric nervous system with ageing, gut transit time and colonic motility do not alter significantly with age (Marieb & Keller 2018). The causes of constipation are multifactorial and include decreased physical activity, inadequate intake of water, a low-fibre diet, change in lifestyle (such as hospitalisation), ignoring or delaying the urge to defecate, the side effect of some medications, neurological, sensory, mental health, developmental and cognitive disorders, and underlying bowel disorders (Mitchell 2019).

Subjective data

Abdominal assessment is commonly performed in conjunction with assessment of bowel and bladder function and/or nutritional and oral assessment. Therefore, the focus of the abdominal assessment outlined below is primarily related to investigation of abdominal pain. You will need to adjust the questioning to fit the purpose of the examination. For example, if the focus of the assessment is about bowel function you would include the questions related to bowel function; however, if the abdominal assessment is related to nutrition you would focus on the questions related to that area and expand the questions to include those related to eating, appetite, etc.

1. Presenting concern
2. Food intolerance
3. Abdominal pain
4. Nausea/vomiting
5. Bowel function
6. Past abdominal history
7. Health and lifestyle management

Practice note: Before you commence the assessment, introduce yourself to the person, confirm the person's identity, discuss the purpose and scope of the assessment, clarify any questions the person may have and obtain verbal consent from the person to perform the assessment.

ASSESSMENT GUIDELINES	CLINICAL SIGNIFICANCE AND CLINICAL ALERTS
1. Presenting concern	
• It is important to ascertain the person's perception of their presenting health concern. Do you feel that you have any abdominal problems? • If they do perceive a problem—how does this impact on their quality of life?	
2. Food intolerance	
• Are there any foods you cannot eat? What happens if you do eat them: allergic reaction, heartburn, belching, abdominal pain, bloating, indigestion, diarrhoea? • Have you sought any assistance from a health professional (GP, registered nurse, dietitian, natural therapist) for these symptoms? • Do you use antacids or any other medication or therapy for these symptoms? Which substance? How often?	**Food intolerance** (e.g. lactase deficiency resulting in bloating or excessive gas after taking milk products).

ASSESSMENT GUIDELINES	CLINICAL SIGNIFICANCE AND CLINICAL ALERTS
3. Abdominal pain	
Review pain assessment strategies and tools from Chapter 13. Use a pain assessment tool as appropriate to the person's age, context and capacity to communicate. In general, you need to ask the person to describe: • **Character:** How would you describe the pain you are experiencing: cramping (colic type), burning in pit of stomach, dull, stabbing, aching? • **Onset:** duration, variation. How did it start? How long have you had it? • **Location:** Where is the pain? Please point to it (you could use a body diagram to report these findings). Is the pain in one spot or does it move around? • **Duration:** Is the pain constant or does it come and go? Does it occur before or after meals? Does it peak? When? • **Severity:** How intense is the pain, rated from 1–10? • **Pattern:** What makes the pain worse: e.g. food, position, stress, medication, activity? What have you tried to relieve pain: rest, heating pad, change in position, medication? • **Associated factors:** Is the pain associated with any other symptoms? For example, menstrual period or irregularities, stress, dietary indiscretion, fatigue, nausea and vomiting, gas, fever, rectal bleeding, frequent urination, vaginal or penile discharge?	Abdominal pain may be visceral from an internal organ (dull, general, poorly localised), parietal from inflammation of overlying peritoneum (sharp, precisely localised, aggravated by movement) or referred from a disorder in another site (see Table 23.3).
4. Nausea/vomiting	
• Do you have any **nausea** or **vomiting**? How often? How much comes up? What is the colour? Is there an odour?	Nausea/vomiting is a common side effect of many medications, with gastrointestinal disease, early pregnancy.
• Is it bloodstained?	This could be bright red or dark brown coloured (digested blood commonly termed 'coffee-ground'). **Haematemesis** occurs with stomach or duodenal ulcers and oesophageal varices.
• Is the nausea and vomiting associated with any other symptoms such as colicky pain, diarrhoea, fever, chills?	
• What foods did you eat in the last 24 hours? Where? At home, school, restaurant? Is there anyone else in the family with same symptoms in last 24 hours?	Consider food poisoning.
5. Bowel function	
• How often do you have a **bowel movement**? • What is the colour? Consistency? (use Bristol stool chart described in Chapter 25) • Any **diarrhoea** or **constipation?** How long? • Any recent change in bowel habits?	Detailed assessment of bowel function is covered in Chapter 25. Black stools may be tarry due to occult blood **(melaena)** from gastrointestinal bleeding or non-tarry from iron medications. Grey stools occur with **hepatitis**. Red blood in stools occurs with gastrointestinal bleeding or localised bleeding around the anus.
6. Past history	
• Have you had any **history** of gastrointestinal problems: gastric ulcer or ***Helicobacter pylori*** infection, gallbladder disease, hepatitis/jaundice, appendicitis, colitis, diverticulitis, **Crohn's disease**, constipation, hernia? If so, describe. • Do you have any history of urinary tract infections, kidney problems, ovarian or menstrual problems? If so, describe.	
• Have you ever had any surgery in the abdomen? Please describe.	Past surgery to the abdomen can predispose the person to **abdominal adhesions** which can cause bowel obstruction (see Table 23.2).
• Have you any problems after surgery?	

ASSESSMENT GUIDELINES	CLINICAL SIGNIFICANCE AND CLINICAL ALERTS
7. Health and lifestyle management	
• What prescribed **medications** are you currently taking? • Are you taking any **over-the-counter, complementary or natural therapies**? • How about **alcohol**—how much would you say you drink (estimate in mL or standard drinks) each day? Each week? What type? When was your last alcoholic drink? • How about **cigarettes**—do you smoke? How many packs per day? For how long?	**Gastric ulcer disease** can occur with frequent use of non-steroidal anti-inflammatory drugs (NSAIDs), alcohol, smoking and *Helicobacter pylori* infection.
Additional subjective data for infants and children (questions for parents or guardian)	
• **Does the child have abdominal pain?** Please describe what you have noticed and when it started. If the child is able to respond address the question to them: Do you have any pain? Point to where the pain is. Use a paediatric pain chart to assess the significance of the pain to the child (refer to Chapter 13 for details). • Refer also to nutritional assessment, and assessment of urinary and bowel function (Chapters 21, 24 and 25).	This symptom is hard to assess with young children. Many conditions of unrelated organ systems are associated with vague abdominal pain (e.g. otitis media). Children cannot articulate specific symptoms and often focus on 'the tummy'. Abdominal pain accompanies inflammation of the bowel, constipation, urinary tract infection and anxiety.

OBJECTIVE DATA

Objective data

Conduct the examination using the following sequence; inspection, auscultation, percussion and palpation. Note that this is a different sequence to other assessments.

Preparation

Adequate lighting is essential. Expose the abdomen so that it is fully visible. Drape (using a clean towel, small sheet or light blanket) below the suprapubic area and female breasts. Make sure belts are loosened and clothing is moved above the costal margin and below the symphysis pubis.

The following measures will enhance abdominal wall relaxation:

- The person should have emptied the bladder, saving a urine specimen if needed.
- The room should be warm to avoid chilling and tensing of muscles.
- Position the person supine, with the head on a pillow, the knees bent or on a pillow and the arms at the sides or across the chest. (Note: Discourage the person from placing their arms over the head because this tenses abdominal musculature.)
- Warm the stethoscope endpiece and your hands to avoid abdominal tensing. Your fingernails must be short.
- Inquire about any painful areas. Examine these areas last to avoid any muscle guarding.
- Finally, learn to use distraction: enhance muscle relaxation. For example, encourage slow breathing; use emotive imagery; use a low, soothing voice; and ask the person to relate their abdominal history while you palpate.

Equipment needed

Secondary light source if needed
Stethoscope
Disinfectant wipes (to clean stethoscope endpiece)
One pillow under the person's head
Hand hygiene solution

PROCEDURES AND NORMAL FINDINGS	CLINICAL SIGNIFICANCE AND CLINICAL ALERTS
General inspection	
During collection of subjective data you will have noticed the colour and moisture of the person's skin and mucous membranes, ease of movement, presence of pain or nausea, hygiene and grooming and height/weight ratio. All of these factors provide clues to gastrointestinal function and the potential for abdominal health issues. A comfortable person is relaxed quietly on the bed or examining table and has a relaxed facial expression and slow, even respirations.	Restlessness and constant turning to find comfort occur with the colicky pain of gastroenteritis or bowel obstruction. Absolute stillness, resisting any movement, occurs with the pain of peritonitis. Knees flexed up, facial grimacing and shallow rapid, uneven respirations also indicate pain.

PROCEDURES AND NORMAL FINDINGS	CLINICAL SIGNIFICANCE AND CLINICAL ALERTS
Identify abdominal landmarks	
Identify the following abdominal landmarks: costal margins, symphasis pubis, xiphoid process, inferior-superior illiac spines, umbilicus. Draw an imaginary line with your finger to identify the four abdominal quadrants: right upper quadrant, right lower quadrant, left upper quadrant, left lower quadrant. These quadrants will provide a structure for you to document your findings accurately.	Refer to Figures 23.1, 23.2, 23.4 and 23.6 for underlying anatomy.
Inspect the abdomen	
Umbilicus	
Normally, the umbilicus is midline and inverted, with no sign of discolouration, inflammation or hernia. It becomes everted and pushed upwards with pregnancy. The umbilicus is a common site for skin piercings. The site should not be red or crusted.	Everted with ascites, or underlying mass (see Table 23.1). Deeply sunken with obesity. Enlarged and everted with umbilical hernia. Bluish periumbilical colour occurs with intraabdominal bleeding (Cullen's sign).
Contour	
Stand on the person's side and look down on the abdomen. Then stoop or sit to gaze across the abdomen. Your head should be slightly higher than the abdomen. Determine the profile from the rib margin to the pubic bone. The contour is related to the nutritional and fitness state of the person and normally ranges from flat to rounded (Figure 23.7). A rounded abdomen is a normal finding in a woman who has been pregnant.	Scaphoid abdomen, protuberant abdomen, abdominal distension (see also Table 23.1).

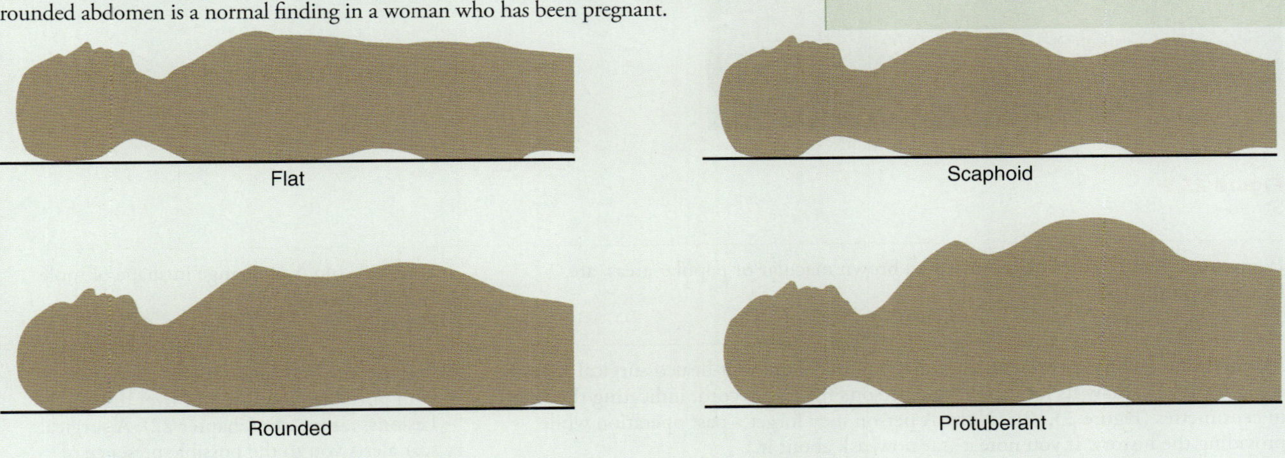

Figure 23.7

PROCEDURES AND NORMAL FINDINGS	CLINICAL SIGNIFICANCE AND CLINICAL ALERTS
Symmetry	
The abdomen should be symmetrical bilaterally (Figure 23.8). Note any localised bulging, visible mass or asymmetric shape. Even small bulges will be highlighted by shadow.	Bulges, **masses**. **Hernia**—protrusion of abdominal viscera through abnormal opening in muscle wall (see Table 23.4).

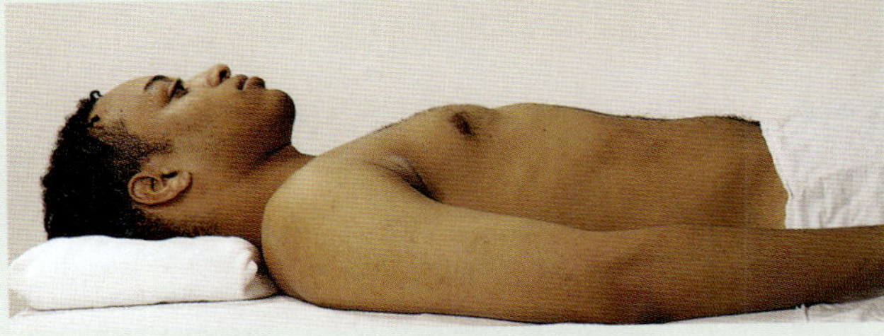

Figure 23.8

PROCEDURES AND NORMAL FINDINGS	CLINICAL SIGNIFICANCE AND CLINICAL ALERTS
Move to the end of the bed and inspect the person's exposed abdomen for symmetry. Ask the person to take a deep breath to further highlight any change. Ask the person to place their chin on their chest and raise their head off the pillow. The abdomen should stay smooth and symmetrical.	Note any localised bulging. Hernia, enlarged liver or spleen may show.
Skin	
The surface is smooth and even, with homogeneous colour. This is a good area to judge skin colour because it is often protected from sun.	Redness with localised inflammation. **Jaundice** (shows best in natural daylight). Skin glistening and taut occurs with **ascites**.
One common pigment change is **striae** (lineae albicantes), silvery white, linear, jagged marks about 1–6 cm long (Figure 23.9). They occur when elastic fibres in the reticular layer of the skin are broken after rapid or prolonged stretching, as in pregnancy or excessive weight gain. Recent striae are pink or blue; then they turn silvery white. **Figure 23.9** Striae.	
Pigmented naevi (moles), circumscribed brown macular or papular areas, are common on the abdomen.	Unusual colour or change in shape of mole (see Chapter 22). **Petechiae.**
Normally, no lesions are present, although you may note well-healed surgical scars. If a scar is present, draw its location in the person's medical record, indicating the length in centimetres (Figure 23.10). (**Note:** A person may forget a past operation while providing the history. If you note a scar now, ask about it.) 6 cm 11 cm **Figure 23.10**	**Cutaneous angiomas** (spider naevi) occur with portal hypertension or liver disease. Lesions, rashes (see Chapter 22). A surgical scar alerts you to the possible presence of underlying adhesions and excess fibrous tissue.

OBJECTIVE DATA

PROCEDURES AND NORMAL FINDINGS	CLINICAL SIGNIFICANCE AND CLINICAL ALERTS
Veins are not usually seen, but a fine venous network may be visible in thin people.	Prominent, dilated veins occur with **portal hypertension, cirrhosis,** ascites or vena caval obstruction. Veins are more visible with malnutrition as a result of thinned adipose tissue.
Good skin turgor reflects healthy nutrition and hydration. Gently pinch up a fold of skin; then release. Note how long it takes the skin to return to original position.	Slow return to the original position, referred to as 'poor turgor', occurs with dehydration, which often accompanies gastrointestinal disease.
Pulsation or movement	
Normally, you may see the pulsations from the aorta beneath the skin in the epigastric area, particularly in thin people. Respiratory movement also shows in the abdomen, particularly in males. Finally, waves of peristalsis may be visible in very thin people. These ripple slowly and obliquely across the abdomen.	Marked pulsation of aorta occurs with widened pulse pressure (e.g. hypertension, aortic insufficiency, thyrotoxicosis) and with aortic aneurysm. Marked visible peristalsis, together with a distended abdomen, indicates **intestinal obstruction** (see Table 23.2).
Auscultate bowel sounds	
Depart from the usual examination sequence and auscultate the abdomen next. This is done because percussion and palpation can increase peristalsis, which would give a false interpretation of bowel sounds. Use the diaphragm endpiece because bowel sounds are relatively high pitched. Hold the stethoscope lightly against the skin; pushing too hard may stimulate more bowel sounds (Figure 23.11). It is usual practice to begin in the RLQ at the ileocaecal valve area because bowel sounds are normally always present here. If bowel sounds are heard in one area it is likely that they will be present throughout the abdomen (Talley & O'Connor 2018). 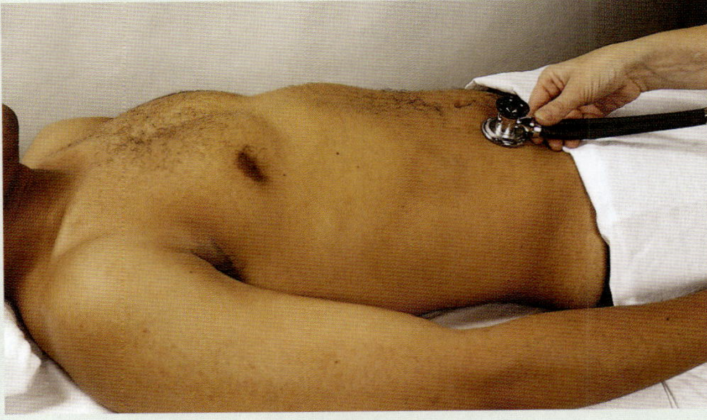 Figure 23.11	

OBJECTIVE DATA

PROCEDURES AND NORMAL FINDINGS	CLINICAL SIGNIFICANCE AND CLINICAL ALERTS
Bowel sounds—present or absent	
There is no accepted time that you should listen for bowel sounds—just listen until you hear them. Bowel sounds originate from the movement of air and fluid through the small intestine. Depending on the time elapsed since eating, a wide range of normal sounds can occur (Talley & O'Connor 2018). Bowel sounds are normally high pitched, gurgling, cascading sounds, occurring irregularly anywhere from 5 to 30 times per min. Do not bother to count them. Record if they are present or absent. A perfectly 'silent abdomen' is uncommon. Listen for at least 4 min if bowel sounds are not heard initially (Talley & O'Connor 2018).	Two distinct patterns of abnormal bowel sounds may occur: 1. **Hyperactive sounds** are loud, high-pitched, rushing, tinkling sounds that signal increased motility. 2. **Hypoactive or absent sounds** follow abdominal surgery or with inflammation of the peritoneum (see Table 23.5). ***Clinical alert:*** The finding of absent bowel sounds may indicate the development of a paralytic ileus and the person should be referred to a medical practitioner for further assessment if this is a new finding or the person has other symptoms such as abdominal pain, abdominal distension, nausea and vomiting.
Percussion	
Percussion can be used to identify the presence and extent of faecal loading or a distended bladder, especially if there is no access to a bladder ultrasound machine. Percussion is a skill that takes time to master and takes experience to interpret the various sounds. Percussion is rarely used by registered nurses to assess the relative density of abdominal contents, to locate organs or to screen for abnormal fluid or masses (see section titled 'Further assessment for advanced practice').	
First, percuss lightly in all four quadrants to determine the prevailing amount of tympany and dullness (Figure 23.12). Move clockwise. **Tympany** should predominate because air in the intestines rises to the surface when the person is supine. 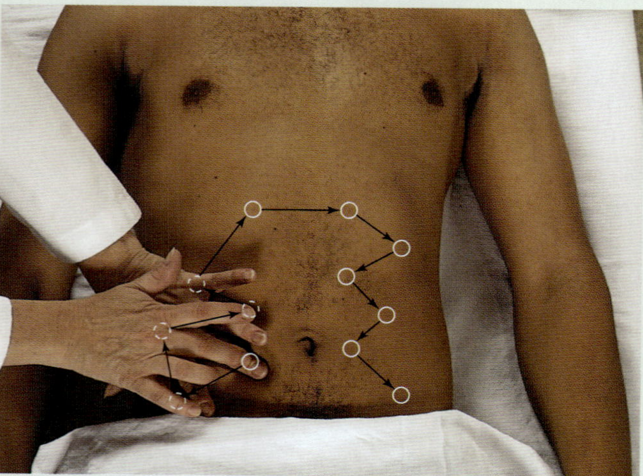 **Figure 23.12**	**Dullness** occurs over a distended bladder, faecal loading, adipose tissue, fluid or a mass. **Hyperresonance** is present with gaseous distension.

OBJECTIVE DATA

PROCEDURES AND NORMAL FINDINGS	CLINICAL SIGNIFICANCE AND CLINICAL ALERTS
Palpation	
Perform palpation to judge the size, location and consistency of an **abnormal mass or tenderness**. Review comfort measures at the beginning of this section. Because most people are naturally inclined to protect the abdomen, you need to use additional measures to enhance complete muscle relaxation.	
1. Ask the person to bend their knees.	
2. Hold your palpating hand low and parallel to the abdomen. Use the finger pads, not the tips.	Holding the hand high and pointing down could make the person tense up.
3. Instruct the person to breathe slowly (in through the nose, and out through the mouth).	
4. Keep your own voice low and soothing. Conversation may relax the person.	
5. Try 'emotive imagery'. For example, you might say, 'Now I want you to imagine you are dozing on the beach, with the sun warming your muscles and the sound of the waves lulling you to sleep. Let yourself relax.'	
Surface palpation	
Begin with **surface palpation**. With the first four fingers close together, depress the skin about 1 cm (Figure 23.13). Make a gentle rotary motion, sliding the fingers and skin together. Then lift the fingers (do not drag them) and move clockwise to the next location around the abdomen. The objective here is not to search for masses but to form an overall impression of the skin surface and superficial musculature. Save the examination of any identified tender areas until last. This method avoids pain and the resulting muscle rigidity that would obscure deeper palpation later in the examination. **Figure 23.13**	**Muscle guarding.** **Rigidity.** Large masses. Tenderness.
As you circle the abdomen, discriminate between voluntary muscle guarding and involuntary rigidity. **Voluntary guarding** occurs when the person is cold, tense or ticklish. It is bilateral, and you will feel the muscles relax slightly during exhalation. Use the relaxation measures to try to eliminate this type of guarding, or it will interfere with deep palpation. If the rigidity persists, it is probably involuntary.	**Involuntary rigidity** is a constant board-like hardness of the muscles. It is a protective mechanism accompanying acute inflammation of the peritoneum. It may be unilateral, and the same area usually becomes painful when the person increases intraabdominal pressure by attempting a sit-up.

OBJECTIVE DATA

PROCEDURES AND NORMAL FINDINGS	CLINICAL SIGNIFICANCE AND CLINICAL ALERTS
Light palpation	
Now perform **light palpation** using the technique described in surface palpation but push down about 5–8 cm depending on the amount of abdominal fat (Figure 23.14). Moving clockwise, explore the entire abdomen. The objective of light palpation is to identify masses (location, shape and size). 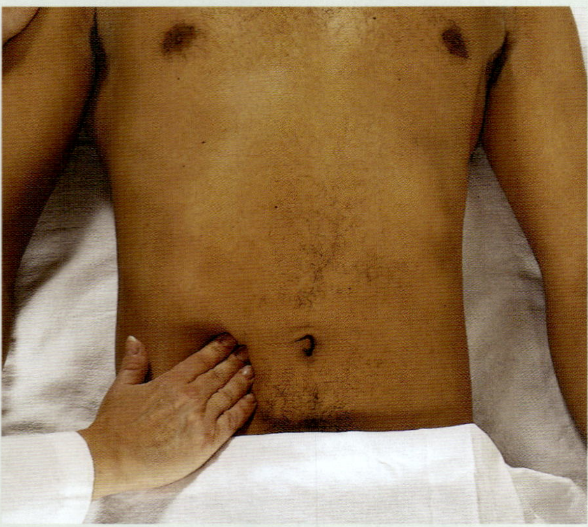 Figure 23.14	
To overcome the resistance of a very large or obese abdomen, you may need to use a two-handed technique. Place your two hands on top of each other (Figure 23.15). The top hand does the pushing; the bottom hand is relaxed and can be free to focus on the sense of palpation. 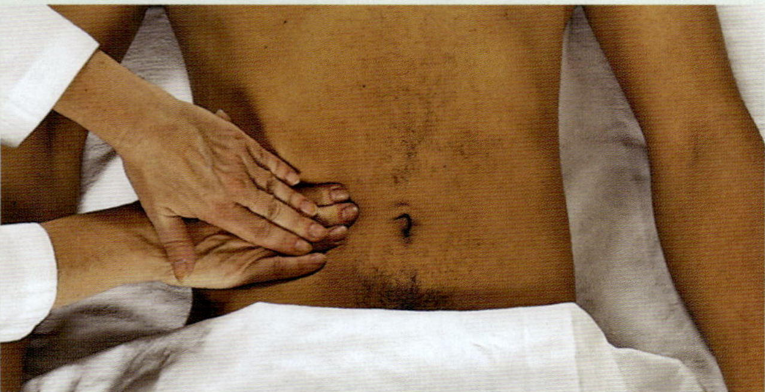 Figure 23.15	
With either technique, note the **location, size, consistency and mobility** of masses. Making sense of what you are feeling is more difficult than it looks. It helps to memorise the anatomy and visualise what is under each quadrant as you palpate. Refer to Figures 23.2 and 23.4.	

OBJECTIVE DATA

PROCEDURES AND NORMAL FINDINGS	CLINICAL SIGNIFICANCE AND CLINICAL ALERTS
Mild tenderness is normally present when palpating the sigmoid colon. Any other tenderness should be investigated.	Tenderness occurs with local inflammation, with inflammation of the peritoneum or underlying organ and with an enlarged organ whose capsule is stretched. **Rebound tenderness** is present when the person experiences a sudden sharp pain on removal of the palpating hand from the abdominal surface (Talley & O'Connor 2018). ***Clinical alert:*** If the person experiences any significant abdominal tenderness, stop the examination and refer the person to a medical practitioner for further assessment.
If you identify a mass note the following: **1.** Location (quadrant) **2.** Size (measured) and shape **4.** Consistency (soft, firm, hard) **5.** Surface (smooth, nodular) **6.** Mobility (including movement with respirations) **7.** Pulsatility (you can feel a pulse in the mass) **8.** Tenderness	***Clinical alert:*** If you palpate a pulsatile mass, especially if there is also abdominal tenderness, stop the examination and refer the person to a medical practitioner for further assessment. A pulsatile abdominal mass may indicate the presence of an abdominal aortic aneurysm.
Additional objective data for infants	
Inspection. The contour of the abdomen is **protuberant** because of the immature abdominal musculature. The skin contains a fine, superficial venous pattern. This may be visible in lightly pigmented children up to the age of puberty.	A scaphoid shape occurs with dehydration. Dilated veins may indicate underlying abdominal pathology such as liver enlargement.
Inspect the umbilical cord throughout the neonatal period. At birth, it is white and contains two umbilical arteries and one vein surrounded by mucoid connective tissue, called Wharton's jelly. The umbilical stump dries within a week, hardens and falls off by 10–14 days. Skin covers the area by 3–4 weeks.	The presence of only one artery signals the risk of congenital defects. Inflammation. Discharge after cord falls off.
The abdomen should be symmetrical, although two bulges are common. You may note an **umbilical hernia**. It appears at 2–3 weeks and is especially prominent when the infant cries. The hernia reaches maximum size at 1 month (up to 2.5 cm) and usually disappears by 1 year. Another common variation is **diastasis recti**, a separation of the rectus muscles with a visible bulge along the midline.	Refer any umbilical hernia larger than 2.5 cm (see Table 23.4) continuing to grow after 1 month.
The abdomen shows respiratory movement. The only other abdominal movement you should note is occasional peristalsis, which may be visible because of the thin musculature.	Marked peristalsis suggests pyloric stenosis (see Table 23.5).
Auscultation. Auscultation for the presence or absence of bowel sounds.	
Percussion. Percussion elicits tympany over the stomach (the infant swallows some air with feeding). Percussing the spleen is not done. The abdomen sounds tympanitic, although it is normal to percuss dullness over the bladder. This dullness may extend up to the umbilicus.	
Palpation. Aid palpation by flexing the baby's knees with one hand while palpating with the other (Figure 23.16). Alternatively, you may hold the upper back and flex the neck slightly with one hand.	

PROCEDURES AND NORMAL FINDINGS	CLINICAL SIGNIFICANCE AND CLINICAL ALERTS
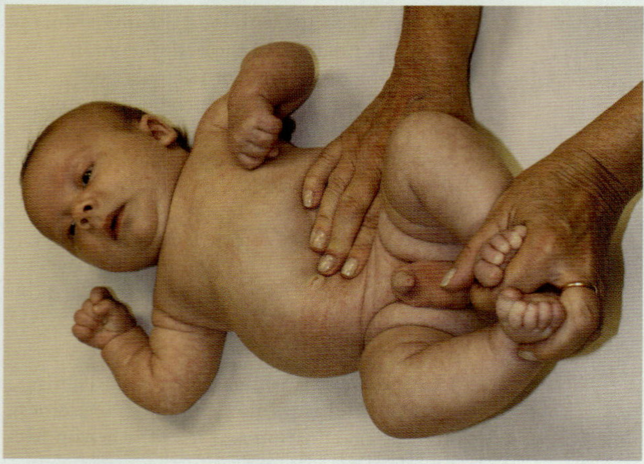 Figure 23.16	
Additional objective data for children	
Under age 4 years, the abdomen looks protuberant when the child is both supine and standing. After age 4 years, the potbelly remains when standing because of lumbar lordosis, but the abdomen looks flat when supine. Normal movement on the abdomen includes respirations, which remain abdominal until 7 years of age.	A scaphoid abdomen is associated with dehydration or malnutrition. Under 7 years of age, the absence of abdominal respirations occurs with inflammation of the peritoneum.
To **palpate the abdomen,** position the young child on the parent's lap as you sit knee-to-knee with the parent (Figure 23.17). Flex the child's knees up and elevate the head slightly. Hold your entire palm flat on the abdominal surface for a moment before starting palpation. This accustoms the child to being touched. If the child is very ticklish, hold their hand under your own as you palpate or apply the stethoscope and palpate around it. 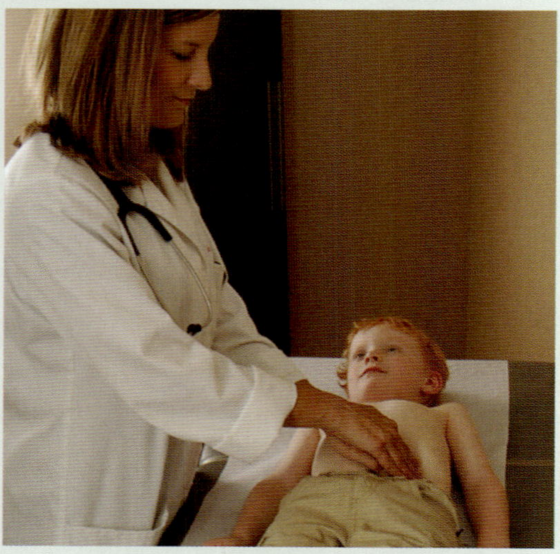 Figure 23.17	

PROCEDURES AND NORMAL FINDINGS	CLINICAL SIGNIFICANCE AND CLINICAL ALERTS
Additional objective data for the adult over 65 years	
As a person ages, on inspection, you may note increased deposits of subcutaneous fat on the abdomen and hips because it is redistributed away from the extremities. The abdominal musculature is often thinner and has less tone than that of the younger adult, so in the absence of obesity you may note peristalsis.	
Because of the thinner, softer abdominal wall, the organs may be easier to palpate (in the absence of obesity).	Abdominal rigidity with acute abdominal conditions is less common in the older person. With an acute abdomen, the older person often complains of less pain than a younger person would.

Further objective assessment for advanced practice

The assessments that are described in the following sections require advanced skill and scope of practice. Nurses working in specialist settings and some community nurses would need to develop these skills.

Preparation

Same preparation as previously described.

Equipment needed

Small centimetre ruler
Skin-marking pen
Hand hygiene solution

PROCEDURES AND NORMAL FINDINGS	CLINICAL SIGNIFICANCE AND CLINICAL ALERTS
Auscultate vascular sounds	
As you listen to the abdomen for bowel sounds, note the presence of any **vascular sounds** or **bruits**. Using firmer pressure, listen over the aorta, renal arteries, iliac and femoral arteries, especially in people with hypertension (Figure 23.18). Note location, pitch and timing of a vascular sound. There should be no bruits present. 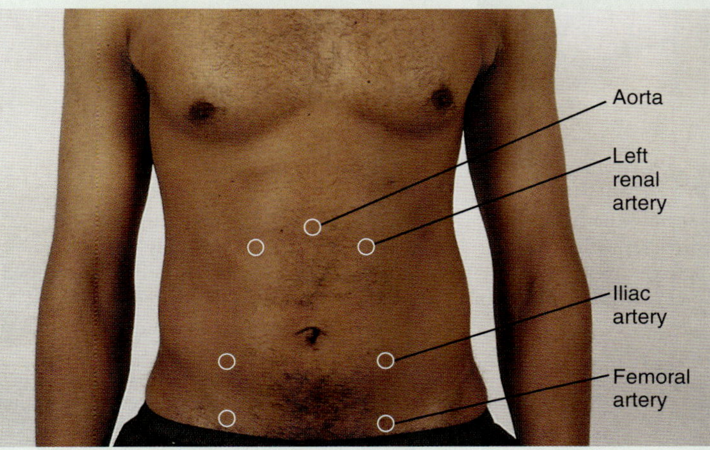 Figure 23.18	A **systolic bruit** is a pulsatile blowing sound and occurs with stenosis or occlusion of an artery. **Venous hum and peritoneal friction rub** are rare (see Table 23.6).

OBJECTIVE DATA

PROCEDURES AND NORMAL FINDINGS	CLINICAL SIGNIFICANCE AND CLINICAL ALERTS
Percussion	
Percuss to assess the relative density of abdominal contents, to locate organs and to screen for abnormal fluid or masses.	
General tympany	
First, percuss lightly in all four quadrants to determine the prevailing amount of tympany and dullness (see Figure 23.12). Move clockwise. Tympany should predominate because air in the intestines rises to the surface when the person is supine.	**Dullness** occurs over a distended bladder, faecal loading, adipose tissue, fluid or a mass. **Hyperresonance** is present with gaseous distension.
Liver span	
Next, percuss to map out the boundaries of certain organs. Measure the height of the liver in the right midclavicular line. (For a consistent placement of the midclavicular line landmark, remember to palpate the acromioclavicular and the sternoclavicular joints and judge the line at a point midway between the two.)	
Begin in the area of lung resonance and percuss down the midclavicular line and the interspaces of the ribs until the sound changes to a dull quality (Figure 23.19). Mark the spot, usually in the fifth intercostal space. Then find abdominal tympany and percuss up the midclavicular line. Mark where the sound changes from tympany to a dull sound, normally at the right costal margin. Figure 23.19	
Measure the distance between the two marks; the normal liver span in the adult ranges from 6 to 12 cm (Figure 23.20). The height of the liver span correlates with the height of the person; taller people have longer livers. Also males have a larger liver span than females of the same height. Overall, the mean liver span is 10.5 cm for males and 7 cm for females.	An enlarged liver span indicates liver enlargement or **hepatomegaly**. Accurate detection of liver borders is confused by dullness above the fifth intercostal space, which occurs with lung disease (e.g. pleural effusion or lung consolidation). Accurate detection at the lower border is confused when dullness is pushed up with ascites or pregnancy or with gas distension in the colon, which obscures lower border.

PROCEDURES AND NORMAL FINDINGS	CLINICAL SIGNIFICANCE AND CLINICAL ALERTS
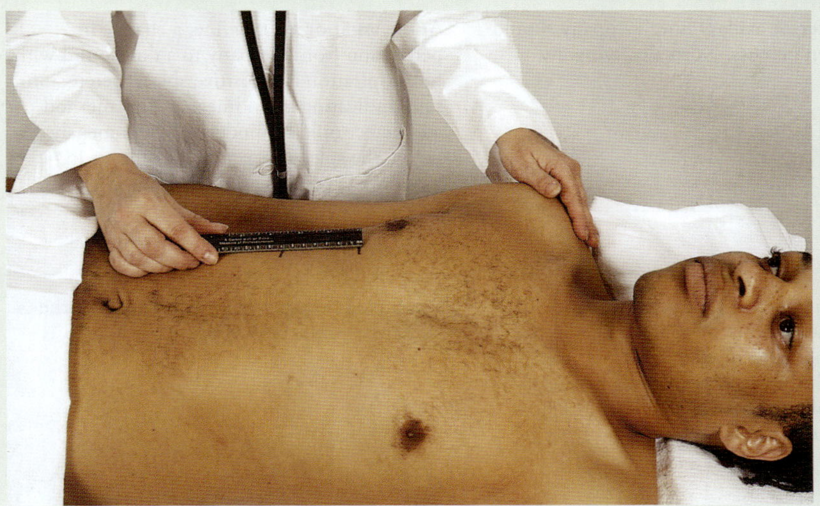 Figure 23.20	
One variation occurs in people with chronic emphysema, in which the liver is displaced downwards by the hyperinflated lungs. Although you hear a dull percussion note well below the right costal margin, the overall span is still within normal limits.	
Clinical estimation of liver span is important to screen for hepatomegaly and to monitor changes in liver size. However, this measurement is a gross estimate; the liver span may be underestimated because of inaccurate detection of the upper border and/ or the lower border is too high.	
Spleen	
Often the spleen is obscured by stomach contents, but you may locate it by percussing for a dull note from the ninth to 11th intercostal space just behind the left midaxillary line (Figure 23.21). The area of **splenic dullness** is normally not wider than 7 cm in the adult and should not encroach on the normal tympany over the gastric air bubble. 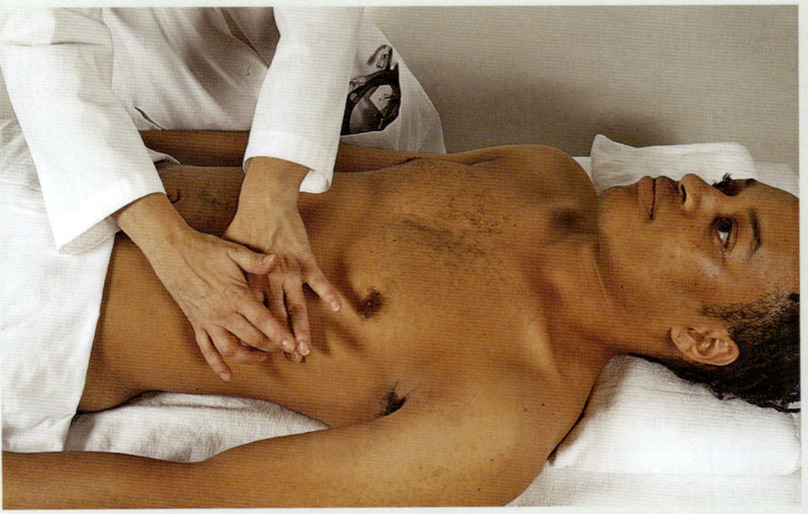 Figure 23.21	A dull note forward of the midaxillary line indicates enlargement of the spleen, as occurs with mononucleosis, trauma and infection.

OBJECTIVE DATA

PROCEDURES AND NORMAL FINDINGS	CLINICAL SIGNIFICANCE AND CLINICAL ALERTS
Now percuss in the lowest interspace in the left **anterior** axillary line. Tympany should result. Ask the person to take a deep breath and then percuss. Normally, tympany remains through full inspiration.	At the anterior axillary line, a change in percussion from tympany to a dull sound with full inspiration is a positive spleen percussion sign, indicating splenomegaly. This method will detect mild to moderate splenomegaly before the spleen becomes palpable, as in mononucleosis, malaria or hepatic cirrhosis.
Costovertebral angle tenderness	
Indirect fist percussion causes the tissues to vibrate instead of producing a sound. To assess the kidney, place one hand over the 12th rib at the costovertebral angle on the back (Figure 23.22). Thump that hand with the ulnar edge of your other fist. The person normally feels a thud but no pain. (Although this step is explained here with percussion techniques, its usual sequence in a complete examination is with thoracic assessment, when the person is sitting up and you are standing behind.) 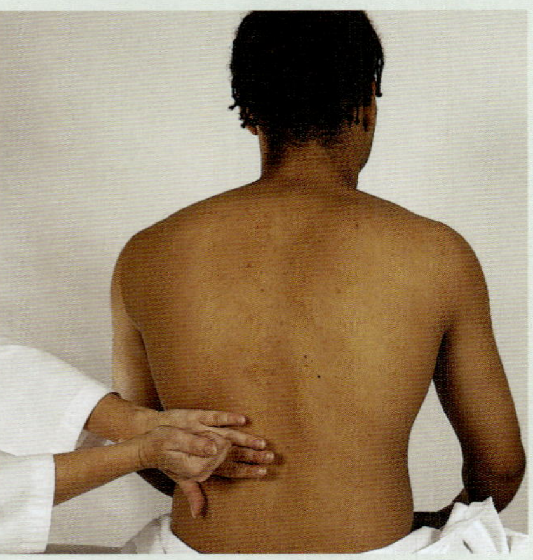 **Figure 23.22**	Sharp pain occurs with inflammation of the kidney or paranephric area.
Palpation of deeper abdominal areas	
Perform palpation to judge the size, location and consistency of certain organs and to screen for an abnormal mass or tenderness. Review comfort measures at beginning of this section. Because most people are naturally inclined to protect the abdomen, you need to use additional measures to enhance complete muscle relaxation. Use the techniques described above to perform surface and light palpation.	***Clinical alert:*** If the person experiences any significant abdominal tenderness stop the examination and refer the person to a medical practitioner for further assessment.
Liver	
Next, palpate for specific organs, beginning with the liver in the RUQ (Figure 23.23). Place your left hand under the person's back parallel to the 11th and 12th ribs and lift up to support the abdominal contents. Place your right hand on the RUQ, with fingers parallel to the midline. Push deeply down and under the right costal margin. Ask the person to take a deep breath. It is normal to feel the edge of the liver bump your fingertips as the diaphragm pushes it down during inhalation. It feels like a firm regular ridge. Often, the liver is not palpable and you feel nothing firm.	Except with a depressed diaphragm, a liver palpated more than 1–2 cm below the right costal margin is enlarged. Record the number of centimetres it descends and note its consistency (hard, nodular) and tenderness (see Table 23.7).

PROCEDURES AND NORMAL FINDINGS	CLINICAL SIGNIFICANCE AND CLINICAL ALERTS
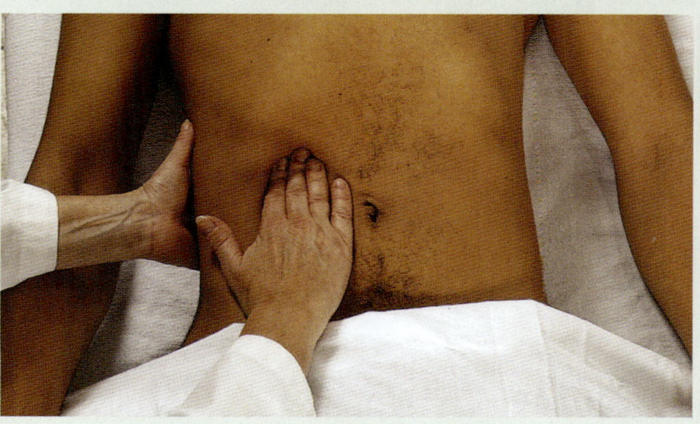 Figure 23.23	
Hooking technique. An alternative method of palpating the liver is to stand up at the person's shoulder and swivel your body to the right so that you face the person's feet (Figure 23.24). Hook your fingers over the costal margin from above. Ask the person to take a deep breath. Try to feel the liver edge bump your fingertips. 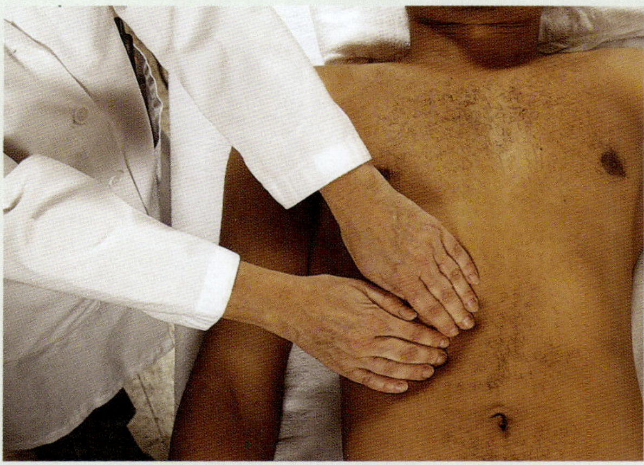 Figure 23.24	
Spleen	
The spleen is not normally palpable and must be enlarged three times its normal size to be felt. If you feel an enlarged spleen refer the person to a medical practitioner; do not proceed with the palpation. To search for it, reach your left hand over the abdomen and behind the left side at the 11th and 12th ribs (Figure 23.25A). Lift up for support. Place your right hand obliquely on the LUQ with the fingers pointing towards the left axilla and just inferior to the rib margin. Push your hand deeply down and under the left costal margin and ask the person to take a deep breath. You should feel nothing firm.	The spleen enlarges with mononucleosis and trauma (see Table 23.7). An enlarged spleen is friable and can rupture easily with overpalpation. Describe the number of centimetres it extends below the left costal margin.

OBJECTIVE DATA

PROCEDURES AND NORMAL FINDINGS	CLINICAL SIGNIFICANCE AND CLINICAL ALERTS
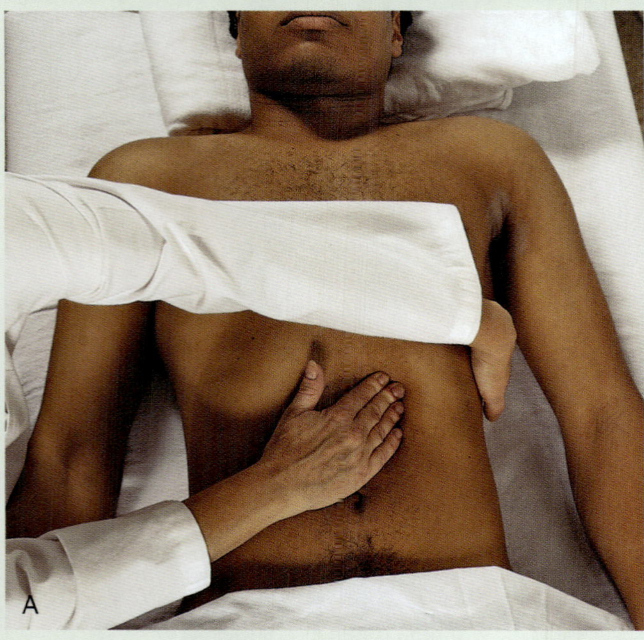 Figure 23.25A	
When enlarged, the spleen slides out and bumps your fingertips. It can grow so large that it extends into the lower quadrants. When this condition is suspected, start low so you will not miss it. An alternative position is to roll the person onto their right side to displace the spleen more forwards and downwards (Figure 23.25B). Then palpate as described earlier. 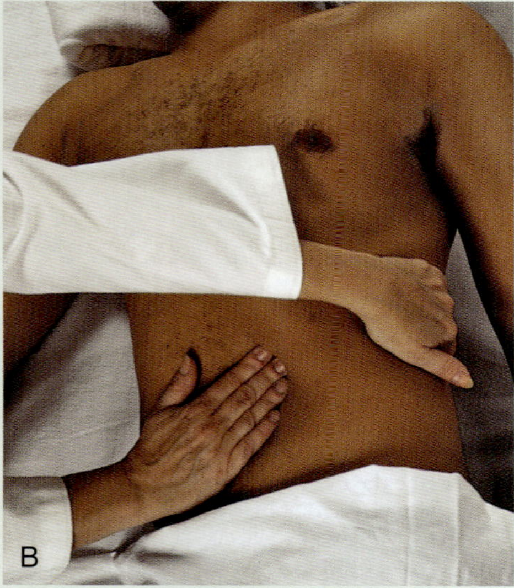 Figure 23.25B	

PROCEDURES AND NORMAL FINDINGS	CLINICAL SIGNIFICANCE AND CLINICAL ALERTS
Kidneys	
Search for the right kidney by placing your hands together in a 'duck-bill' position at the person's right flank (Figure 23.26A). Press your two hands together firmly (you need deeper palpation than that used with the liver or spleen) and ask the person to take a deep breath. In most people, you will feel no change. Occasionally, you may feel the lower pole of the right kidney as a round, smooth mass slide between your fingers. Either condition is normal. 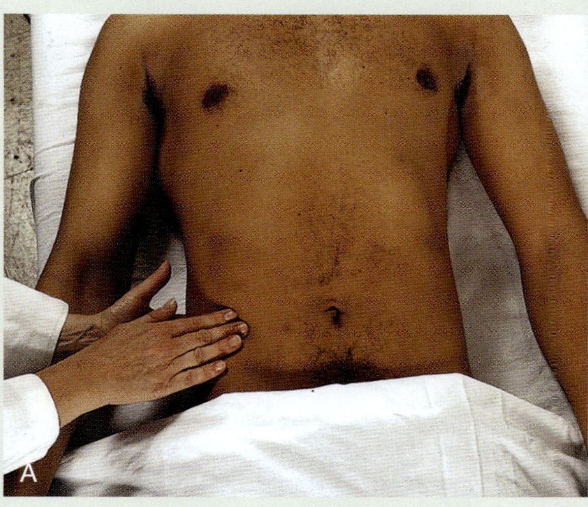 Figure 23.26A	Enlarged kidney. Kidney mass.
The left kidney sits 1 cm higher than the right kidney and is not palpable normally. Search for it by reaching your left hand across the abdomen and behind the left flank for support (Fig. 23.26B). Push your right hand deep into the abdomen and ask the person to breathe deeply. You should feel no change with the inhalation. 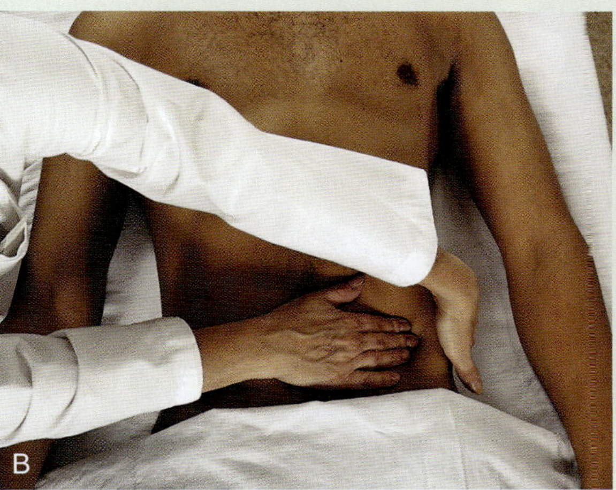 Figure 23.26B	

PROCEDURES AND NORMAL FINDINGS	CLINICAL SIGNIFICANCE AND CLINICAL ALERTS
Aorta	
Using your opposing thumb and fingers, palpate the aortic pulsation in the upper abdomen slightly to the left of midline (Figure 23.27). Normally, it is 2.5–4 cm wide in the adult and pulsates in an anterior direction. 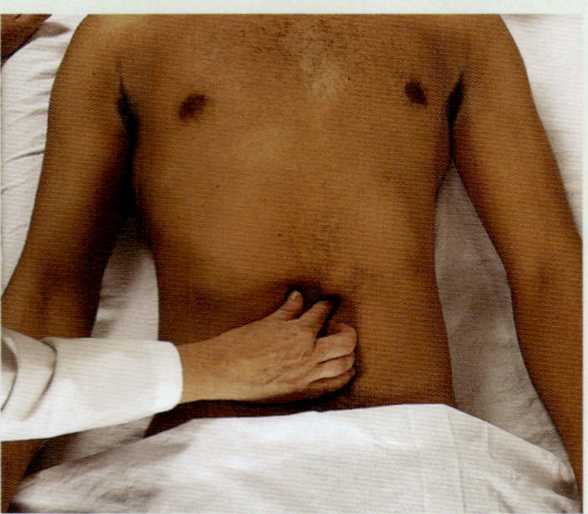 Figure 23.27	Widened with **aneurysm** (see Tables 23.6 and 23.7). Prominent lateral pulsation with aortic aneurysm.
Other procedures for advanced practice nurses	
Rebound tenderness (Blumberg's sign). Assess rebound tenderness when the person reports abdominal pain or when you elicit tenderness during palpation. Choose a site away from the painful area. Hold your hand at 90 degrees, or perpendicular, to the abdomen. Push down slowly and deeply; then lift up *quickly* (Figures 23.28A and 23.28B). This makes structures that are indented by palpation rebound suddenly. A normal, or negative, response is no pain on release of pressure. Perform this test at the end of the examination, because it can cause severe pain and muscle rigidity. 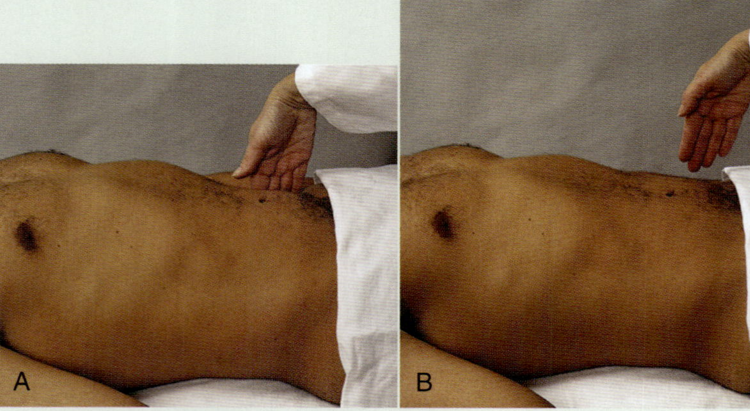 Figure 23.28 Rebound tenderness.	Pain on release of pressure confirms rebound tenderness, which is a reliable sign of peritoneal inflammation. **Peritoneal inflammation** accompanies appendicitis.
Inspiratory arrest (Murphy's sign). Normally, palpating the liver causes no pain. In a person with inflammation of the gallbladder, or cholecystitis, pain occurs. Hold your fingers under the liver border. Ask the person to take a deep breath. A normal response is to complete the deep breath without pain.	When the test is positive, as the descending liver pushes the inflamed gallbladder onto the examining hand, the person feels sharp pain and abruptly stops inspiration midway.

PROCEDURES AND NORMAL FINDINGS	CLINICAL SIGNIFICANCE AND CLINICAL ALERTS
Iliopsoas muscle test. Perform the iliopsoas muscle test when the acute abdominal pain of appendicitis is suspected. With the person supine, lift the right leg straight up, flexing at the hip (Figure 23.29); then push down over the lower part of the right thigh as the person tries to hold the leg up. When the test is negative, the person feels no change. 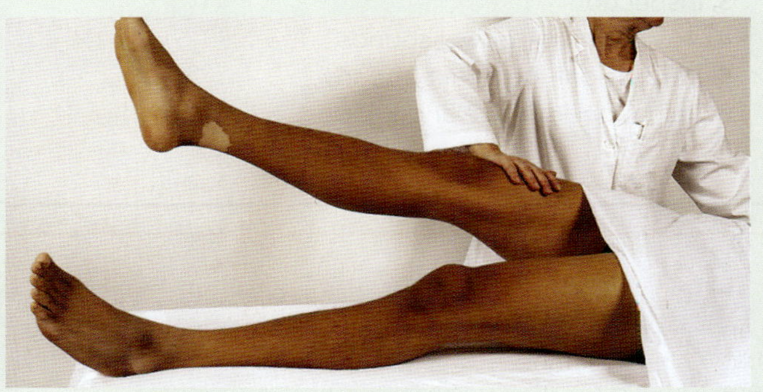 **Figure 23.29** Iliopsoas muscle test.	When the iliopsoas muscle is inflamed (which occurs with an inflamed or perforated appendix), pain is felt in the right lower quadrant.
Additional objective data for infants	
The liver fills the RUQ. It is normal to feel the liver edge at the right costal margin or 1–2 cm below. Normally, you may palpate the spleen tip and both kidneys and the bladder. Also easily palpated are the caecum in the RLQ, and the sigmoid colon, which feels like a sausage in the left inguinal area.	
Make note of the newborn's first stool, a sticky, greenish-black meconium stool within 24 hours of birth. By the fourth day, stools of breast-fed babies are golden-yellow, pasty and smell like sour milk, whereas those of formula-fed babies are brown-yellow, firmer and more faecal smelling.	
Additional objective data for children	
The liver remains easily palpable 1–2 cm below the right costal margin (this is not a sign of hepatomegaly). The edge is soft and sharp and moves easily. On the left, the spleen is also easily palpable with a soft, sharp, movable edge. Usually you can feel 1–2 cm of the right kidney and the tip of the left kidney. Percussion of the liver span measures about 3.5 cm at age 2 years, 5 cm at age 6 years and 6–7 cm during adolescence.	
In assessing abdominal tenderness, remember that the young child often answers this question affirmatively no matter how the abdomen actually feels. Use objective signs to aid assessment, such as a cry changing in pitch as you palpate, facial grimacing, moving away from you and guarding.	***Clinical alert:*** If the child experiences any significant abdominal tenderness, stop the examination and refer the child to a medical practitioner for further assessment.
The school-age child has a slim abdominal shape as they lose the potbelly. This slimming trend continues into adolescence. The adolescent may be embarrassed with exposure of the abdomen, and adequate draping is necessary. The physical findings are the same as those listed for the adult.	

OBJECTIVE DATA

Summary Checklist

ABDOMINAL ASSESSMENT

Subjective data

1. Presenting concern
2. Food intolerance
3. Abdominal pain
4. Nausea/vomiting
5. Bowel function
6. Past abdominal history
7. Health and lifestyle management

Objective data

1. General inspection
2. Identify abdominal landmarks
3. Inspection
4. Auscultation—bowel sounds
5. Percussion—general tympany
6. Palpation—surface and light

PROMOTING A HEALTHY LIFESTYLE

KEEPING YOUR LIVER HEALTHY

The liver is the largest organ in the body. It has an immense capacity to heal and regenerate, but that capacity is not infinite. Unfortunately, signs of severe liver damage or disease usually do not become apparent until the liver has been significantly harmed. The best protection for the liver is prevention!

There are many things an individual can do to protect the liver:

- **Watch your diet and weight.** Obesity can cause a condition called nonalcoholic fatty liver disease, which may include cirrhosis (Pedersen & Bendtsen 2019).
- **Drink alcohol in moderation.** The current Australian Guidelines to Reduce Health Risks from Drinking Alcohol (National Health and Medical Research Council 2019) recommend that healthy men and women drink no more than two standard drinks on any day to reduce the lifetime risk of harm from alcohol-related disease or injury.
- **Use medications wisely.** Use prescription and over-the-counter medications only when needed. Be sure to take only the recommended doses. Several commonly used medications such as amoxicillin/clavulanate can induce drug-induced liver injury in some people (Shung & Lim 2019). Certain medications, including complementary therapies and illicit drugs, can form toxic compounds that can cause liver damage. Make sure that all medications, including over-the-counter, complementary therapies and illicit drugs, are reviewed as part of any health history.
- **Get vaccinated.** A vaccine is available for both hepatitis A and hepatitis B.
- **Be aware of your risk for hepatitis.** The three leading causes of hepatitis are hepatitis A, hepatitis B and hepatitis C infection.

  Hepatitis A is primarily spread through food or water contaminated by faeces from an infected person. In Australia and New Zealand hepatitis A is more common among specific groups of people including:
  - Children in daycare centres and pre-schools
  - Men who have sex with men
  - Injecting drug users
  - Residents in care facilities for the intellectually disabled
  - Travellers to regions where hepatitis A is common (e.g. Asia, Africa, the South Pacific and Central and South America).

  Hepatitis B is a potentially life-threatening health problem and one of the most common infectious diseases in the world. It is primarily spread through contact with infected blood or body fluids (including saliva, semen, vaginal secretions and breast milk). Chronic hepatitis B infection can lead to liver cancer. The most common ways that hepatitis is spread include:
  - Having unprotected sex
  - Sharing and re-use of needles or other injecting equipment
  - Needlestick injury in the healthcare setting
  - Mother-to-child transmission at birth
  - Child-to-child transmission through contact such as biting or scratching
  - Sharing personal items such as razors and toothbrushes
  - During medical, surgical or dental procedures or tattooing.

  Hepatitis C can be acute or chronic and can range from a mild short-term illness to a serious life-long illness. A significant number of people who have chronic infection will develop liver cancer and cirrhosis (WHO 2018). It is primarily spread through contact with infected blood by injecting drug users. Other ways in which hepatitis C can be spread include:
  - Unsterile medical procedures
  - Needlestick injury in the healthcare setting
  - Unscreened blood and blood products.

You can get more information about liver health and hepatitis from the following websites:

The Liver Foundation: www.liver.org.au

Hepatitis Australia: www.hepatitisaustralia.com

Hepatitis Foundation of New Zealand: www.hepatitisfoundation.org.nz

World Health Organization: www.who.int/hepatitis/en/

Documentation and critical thinking

FOCUSED ASSESSMENT: CLINICAL CASE STUDY

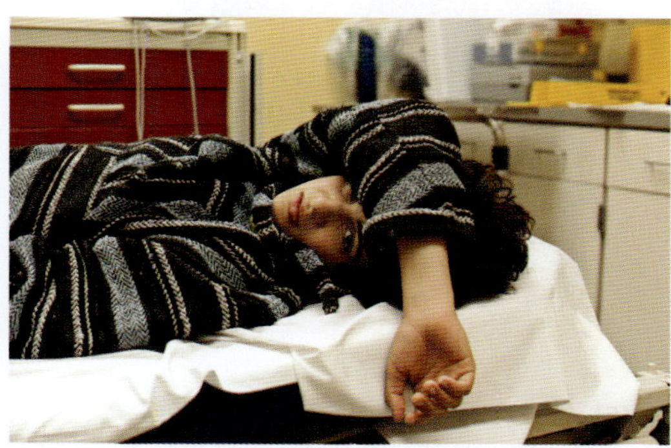

Context

The registered nurse is working in triage at an emergency department of a public hospital. The initial assessment is conducted to assess the urgency of the person's need for medical care.

Subjective

Dan Groves is a 17-year-old male high school student who presents at the emergency department with abdominal pain. He is accompanied by his parents (Jo and Peter Groves).

Two days ago, Dan noted general abdominal pain in umbilical region. Now the pain is sharp and severe, and Dan points to location in right lower quadrant. Pain score 9/10 at rest. No bowel movement for 2 days. Nausea and vomiting off and on for 1 day. He says that no one else in his household has these symptoms and that he has only eaten home prepared meals in the last few days.

Objective

BP 112/70, temp. 38°C, HR 116, RR 18.

Lying on side with knees drawn up under chin. Resists any movement. Face tight and occasionally grimacing. Cries out with any sudden movement.

No bowel sounds present on auscultation.

On palpation, abdominal wall is rigid and board-like. Extreme tenderness to light palpation in RLQ—no further assessment undertaken until medical consultation.

Collaborative problem

Acute abdominal pain in RLQ (? appendicitis)—requires urgent medical assessment

Problem statements/nursing diagnoses

Nausea related to possible acute appendicitis

Abdominal pain related to possible acute appendicitis

Potential for anxiety related to uncertain diagnosis and need for further assessment

Abnormal findings

TABLE 23.1 Abdominal distension*

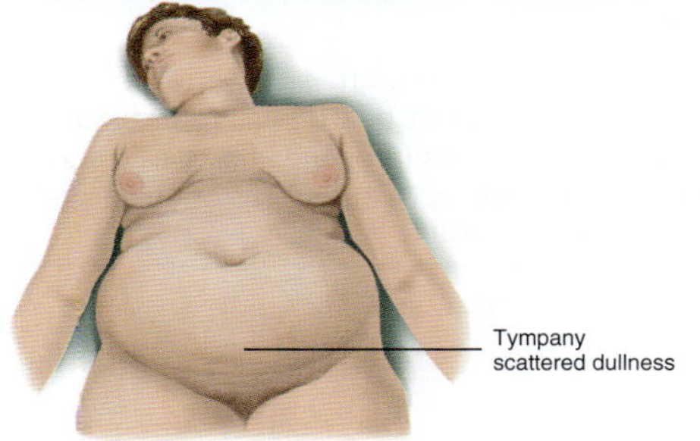	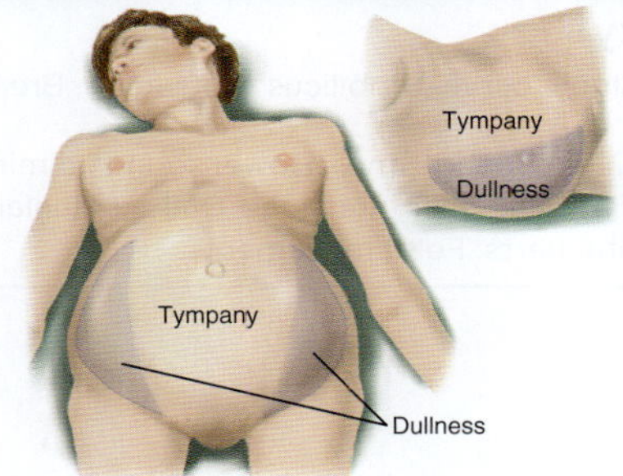
Obesity **Inspection.** Uniformly rounded. Umbilicus sunken (it adheres to peritoneum, and layers of fat are superficial to it). **Auscultation.** Bowel sounds heard in all four quadrants. **Percussion.** Tympany. Scattered dullness over adipose tissue. **Palpation.** Soft. May be hard to palpate through thick abdominal wall.	**Ascites** **Inspection.** Single curve. Everted umbilicus. Bulging flanks when supine. Taut glistening skin, recent weight gain, increase in abdominal girth. **Auscultation.** Bowel sounds heard in all four quadrants. Diminished over ascitic fluid. **Percussion.** Tympany at top where intestines float. Dull over fluid. Produces fluid wave and shifting dullness. **Palpation.** Taut skin and increased intraabdominal pressure limit palpation.

(Continued)

TABLE 23.1 Abdominal distension—cont'd

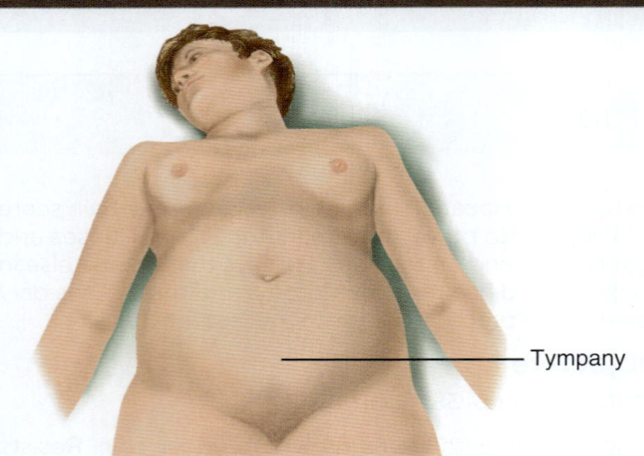

Air or gas

Inspection. Single round curve.
Auscultation. Depends on cause of gas (e.g. decreased or absent bowel sounds with ileus); hyperactive with early intestinal obstruction.
Percussion. Tympany over large area.
Palpation. May have muscle spasm of abdominal wall.

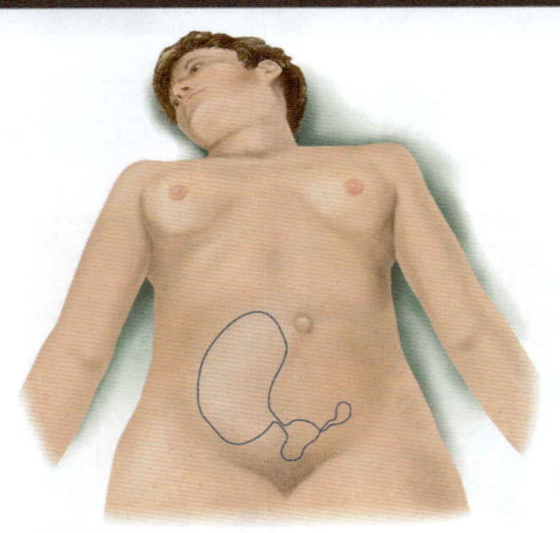

Ovarian cyst (large)

Inspection. Curve in lower half of abdomen, midline. Everted umbilicus.
Auscultation. Bowel sounds heard in all four quadrants.
Percussion. Top dull over fluid. Intestines pushed superiorly. Large cyst produces fluid wave and shifting dullness.
Palpation. Transmits aortic pulsation while ascites does not.

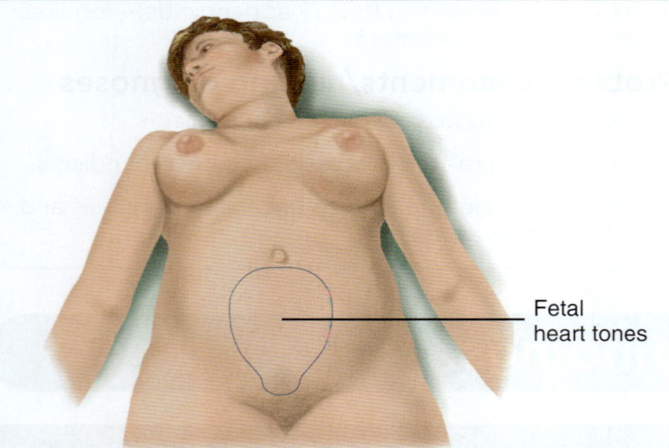

Pregnancy†

Inspection. Single curve. Umbilicus protruding. Breasts engorged.
Auscultation. Fetal heart tones. Bowel sounds diminished.
Percussion. Tympany over intestines. Dull over enlarging uterus.
Palpation. Fetal parts. Fetal movements.

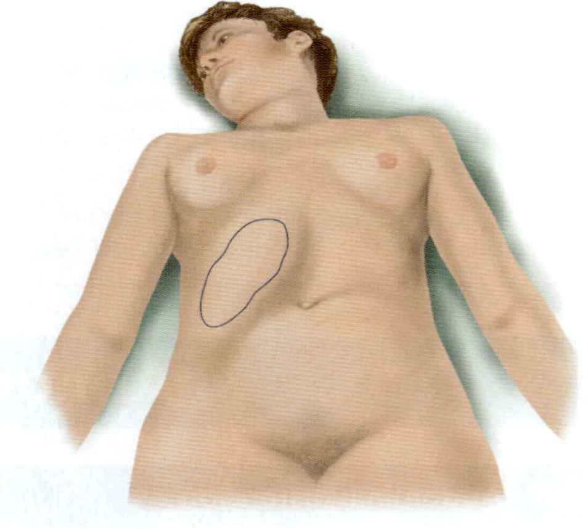

Tumour

Inspection. Localised distension.
Auscultation. Bowel sounds heard in all four quadrants.
Percussion. Dull over mass if reaches up to skin surface.
Palpation. Define borders. Distinguish from enlarged organ or normally palpable structure.

TABLE 23.1 Abdominal distension—cont'd

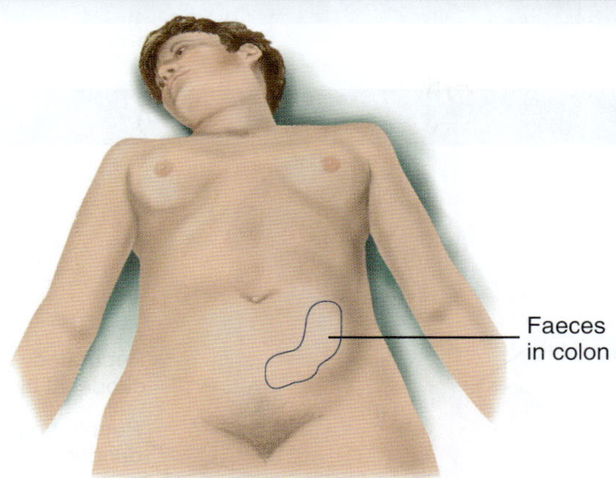

Faeces

Inspection. Localised distension.

Auscultation. Bowel sounds heard in all four quadrants.

Percussion. Tympany predominates. Scattered dullness over faecal mass.

Palpation. Firm rope-like mass with faeces in intestines (likely to be in descending colon and sometimes transverse colon).

*A mnemonic device to recall the common causes of abdominal distension is the seven Fs: fat, flatus, fluid, fetus, faeces, fetal growth and fibroid.

†Obviously a normal finding, pregnancy is included for comparison of conditions causing abdominal distension.

TABLE 23.2 Clinical portrait of intestinal obstruction

SUBJECTIVE DATA:

History of previous abdominal surgery with adhesions

Vomiting, nausea

Colicky pain from strong peristalsis above the obstruction

Absence of stool or passage of flatus

OBJECTIVE DATA:

Restless, ill-appearing person

Distended abdomen

Hyperactive bowel sounds in early obstruction; hypoactive or silent in late obstruction

Tenderness on palpation

Hypovolaemic shock due to dehydration and sepsis may occur (increased pulse, decreased BP, cool skin, dry mucous membranes)

DIAGNOSTIC TESTS

Laboratory: Evidence of dehydration, loss of electrolytes and possibly sepsis

Radiology: accumulation of fluid and gas in bowel proximal (above) to obstruction

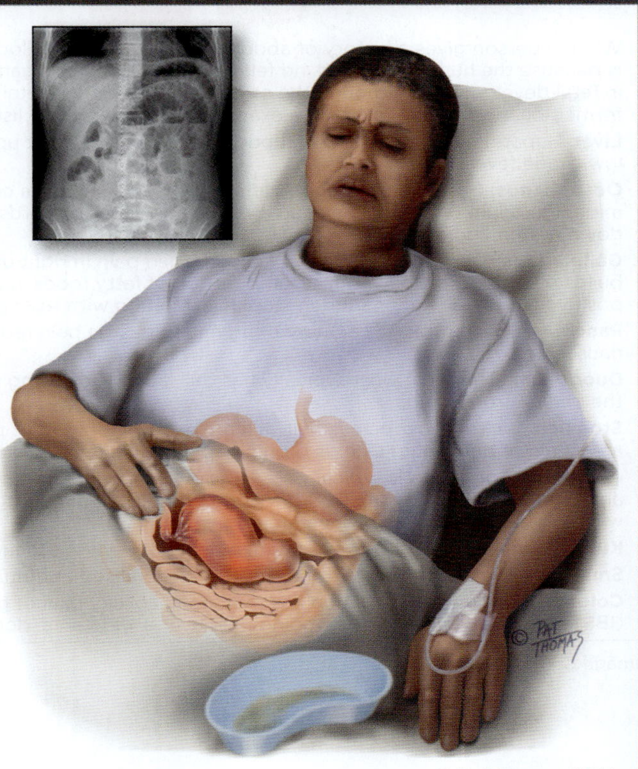

© Pat Thomas, 2014.

Abnormal findings for advanced practice

TABLE 23.3 Common sites of referred abdominal pain

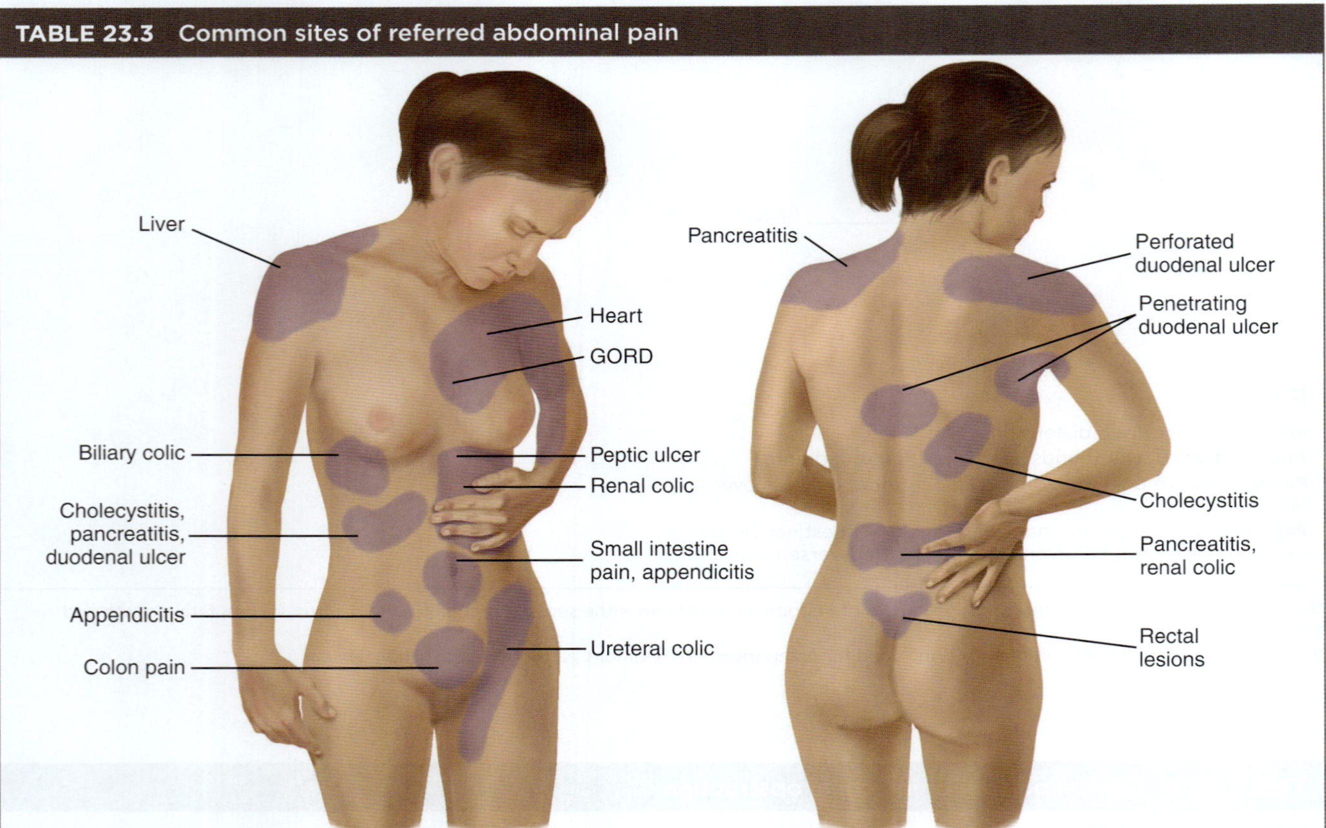

When a person gives a history of abdominal pain, the pain's location may not necessarily be directly over the involved organ. That is because the human brain has no felt image for internal organs. Rather, pain is referred to a site where the organ was located in fetal development. Although the organ migrates during fetal development, its nerves persist in referring sensations from the former location. The following are examples, not a complete list.

Liver. Hepatitis may have mild to moderate, dull pain in right upper quadrant or epigastrium, along with anorexia, nausea, malaise, low-grade fever.

Oesophagus. Gastro-oesophageal reflux disease (GORD) is a complex of symptoms of oesophagitis, including burning pain in midepigastrium or behind lower sternum that radiates upwards, or 'heartburn'. Occurs 30–60 min after eating; aggravated by lying down or bending over.

Gallbladder. Cholecystitis is biliary colic, sudden pain in right upper quadrant that may radiate to right or left scapula, and which builds over time, lasting 2–4 h, after ingestion of fatty foods, alcohol or caffeine. Associated with nausea and vomiting, and positive Murphy's sign or sudden stop in inspiration with RUQ palpation.

Pancreas. Pancreatitis has acute, boring midepigastric pain radiating to the back and sometimes to the left scapula or flank, severe nausea and vomiting.

Duodenum. Duodenal ulcer typically has dull, aching, gnawing pain, does not radiate, may be relieved by food and may awaken the person from sleep.

Stomach. Gastric ulcer pain is dull, aching, gnawing epigastric pain, usually brought on by food, radiates to back or substernal area. Pain of perforated ulcer is burning epigastric pain of sudden onset that refers to one or both shoulders.

Appendix. Appendicitis typically starts as dull, diffuse pain in periumbilical region that later shifts to severe, sharp, persistent pain and tenderness localised in RLQ (McBurney's point). Pain is aggravated by movement, coughing and deep breathing; associated with anorexia, then nausea and vomiting, fever.

Kidney. Kidney stones prompt a sudden onset of severe, colicky flank or lower abdominal pain.

Small intestine. Gastroenteritis has diffuse, generalised abdominal pain, with nausea, diarrhoea.

Colon. Large bowel obstruction has moderate, colicky pain of gradual onset in lower abdomen, bloating. Irritable bowel syndrome (IBS) has sharp or burning, cramping pain over a wide area; does not radiate. Brought on by meals, relieved by bowel movement.

TABLE 23.4 Abnormalities on inspection

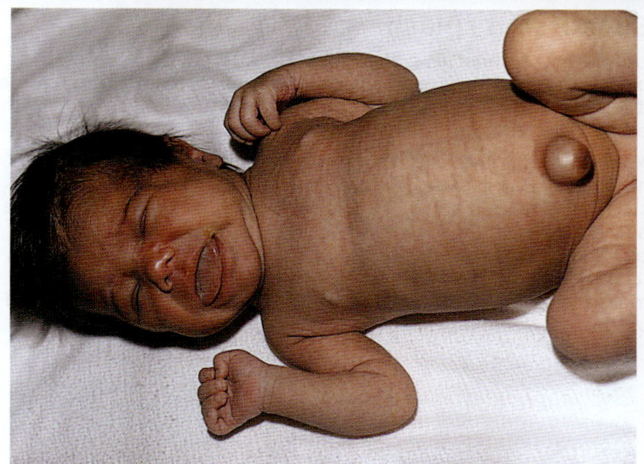

Umbilical hernia

Umbilical hernia is a soft, skin-covered mass, which is the protrusion of the omentum or intestine through a weakness or incomplete closure in the umbilical ring. It is accentuated by increased intraabdominal pressure as with crying, coughing, vomiting or straining, but the bowel rarely incarcerates or strangulates. Most umbilical hernias resolve spontaneously by 1 year; parents should avoid affixing a belt or coin at the hernia because this will not help closure and may cause contact dermatitis.

In an adult, it occurs with pregnancy, chronic ascites or from chronic intrathoracic pressure (e.g. asthma, chronic bronchitis).

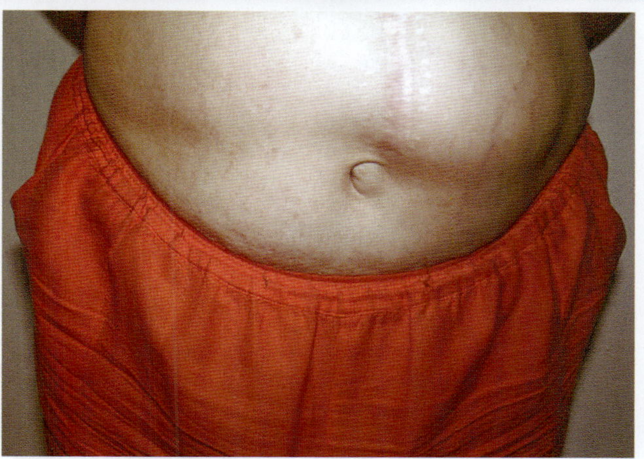

Incisional hernia

A bulge near an old operative scar that may not show when person is supine but is apparent when the person increases intraabdominal pressure by a sit-up, stand or Valsalva manoeuvre.

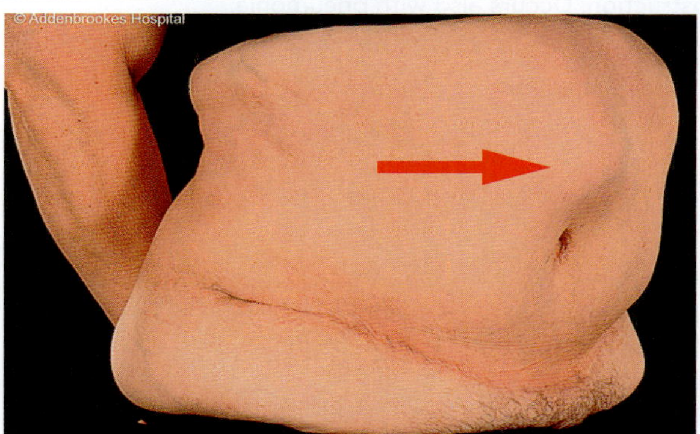

Epigastric hernia

A small, fatty nodule at epigastrium in midline, through the linea alba. Usually one can feel it rather than observe it. May be palpable only when standing.

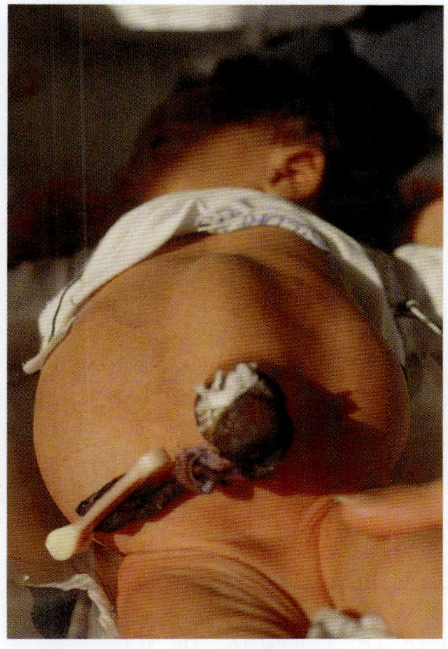

Diastasis recti

Diastasis recti, or a midline longitudinal ridge, is a separation of the abdominal rectus muscles. Ridge is revealed when intra-abdominal pressure is increased by raising head while supine. Occurs congenitally and as a result of pregnancy or marked obesity in which prolonged distension or a decrease in muscle tone has occurred. It is not clinically significant.

TABLE 23.5 Abnormal bowel sounds

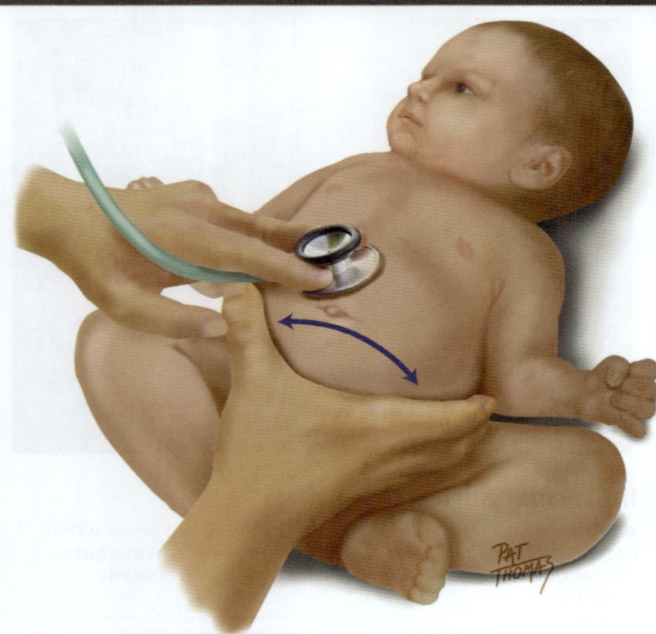

Succussion splash

Unrelated to peristalsis, this is a very loud splash auscultated over the upper abdomen when the infant is rocked side to side. It indicates increased air and fluid in the stomach, as seen with pyloric obstruction or large hiatus hernia.

Marked peristalsis, together with projectile vomiting in the newborn, suggests pyloric stenosis, an obstruction of the stomach's pyloric valve. Pyloric stenosis is a congenital defect and appears in the second or third week. After feeding, pronounced peristaltic waves cross from left to right, leading to projectile vomiting. Then one can palpate an olive-sized mass in the RUQ midway between the right costal margin and umbilicus. Refer promptly because of the risk of weight loss.

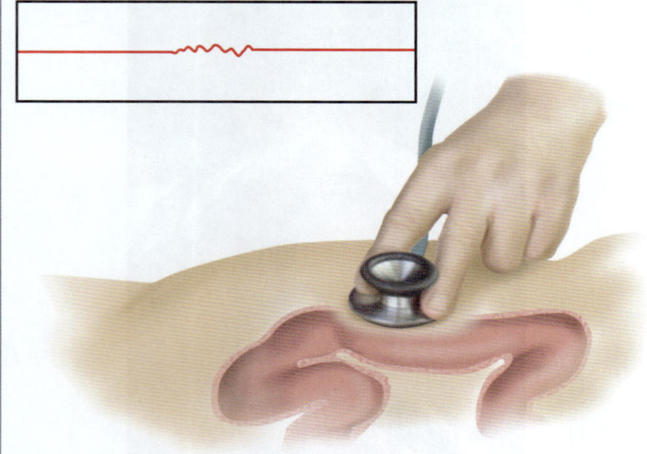

Hypoactive bowel sounds

Diminished or absent bowel sounds signal decreased motility as a result of inflammation as seen with peritonitis, from paralytic ileus following abdominal surgery or from late bowel obstruction. Occurs also with pneumonia.

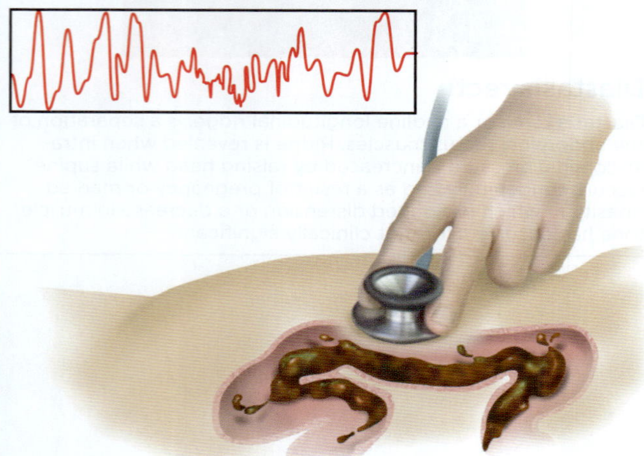

Hyperactive bowel sounds

Loud, gurgling sounds, 'borborygmi', signal increased motility. They occur with early mechanical bowel obstruction (high pitched), gastroenteritis, brisk diarrhoea, laxative use and subsiding paralytic ileus.

TABLE 23.6 Abdominal friction rubs and vascular sounds

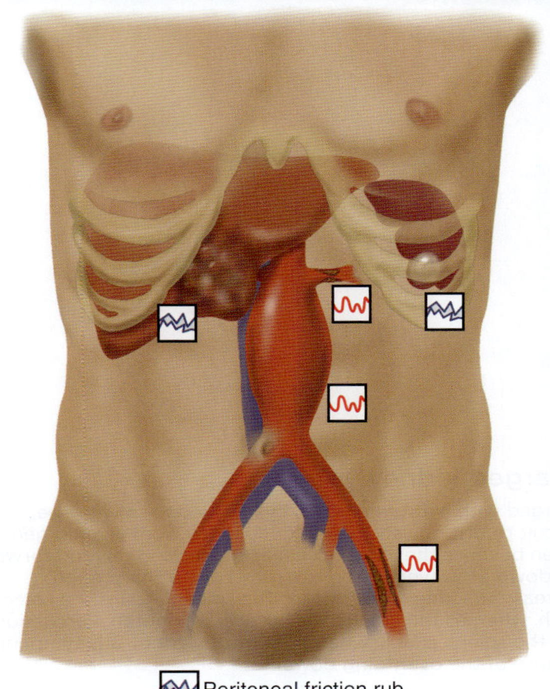

Peritoneal friction rub

A rough, grating sound, like two pieces of leather rubbed together, indicates peritoneal inflammation. Occurs rarely. Usually occurs over organs with a large surface area in contact with the peritoneum.

Liver—friction rub over lower right rib cage, from abscess or metastatic tumour.

Spleen—friction rub over lower left rib cage in left anterior axillary line, from abscess, infection or tumour.

Vascular sounds

Arterial—a **bruit** indicates turbulent blood flow, as found in constricted, abnormally dilated or tortuous vessels. Listen with the bell. Occurs with the following three conditions:

Aortic aneurysm—murmur is harsh, systolic or continuous and accentuated with systole. Note in person with hypertension.

Renal artery stenosis—murmur is midline or towards flank, soft, low-to-medium pitch.

Partial occlusion of femoral arteries

Venous hum—occurs rarely. Heard in periumbilical region. Originates from inferior vena cava. Medium pitch, continuous sound, pressure on bell may obliterate it. May have palpable thrill. Occurs with portal hypertension and cirrhotic liver.

TABLE 23.7 Abnormalities on palpation of enlarged organs

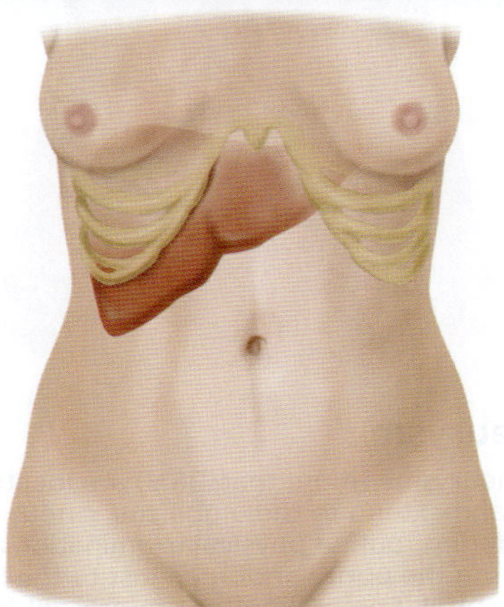

Enlarged liver

An enlarged, smooth and nontender liver occurs with fatty infiltration, portal obstruction or cirrhosis, high obstruction of inferior vena cava and lymphocytic leukaemia.

The liver feels enlarged and smooth but is tender to palpation with early heart failure, acute hepatitis or hepatic abscess.

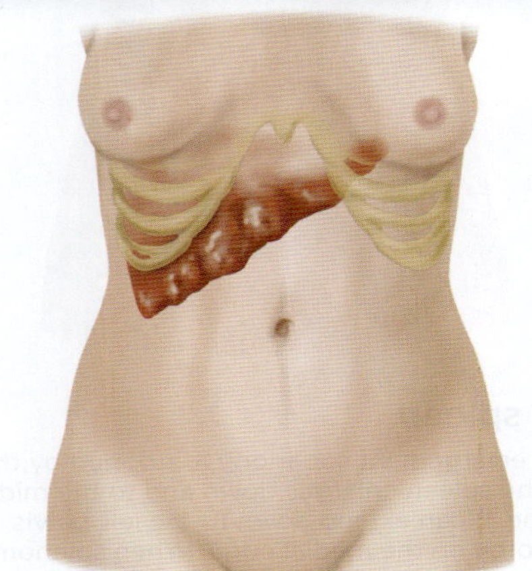

Enlarged nodular liver

An enlarged and nodular liver occurs with late portal cirrhosis, metastatic cancer or tertiary syphilis.

TABLE 23.7 Abnormalities on palpation of enlarged organs—cont'd

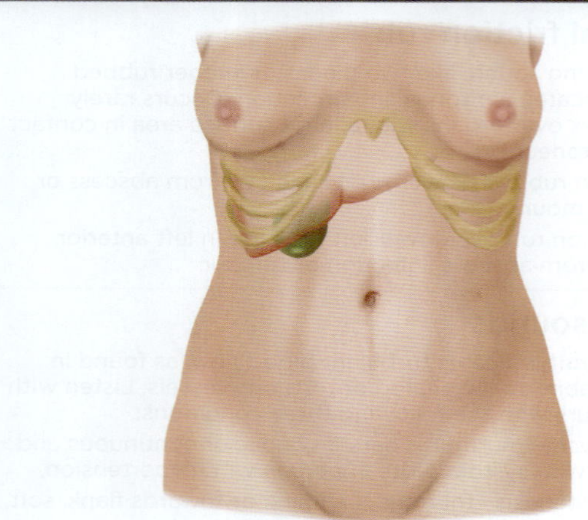

Enlarged gallbladder

An enlarged, tender gallbladder suggests acute cholecystitis. Feel it behind the liver border as a smooth and firm mass like a sausage, although it may be difficult to palpate because of involuntary rigidity of abdominal muscles. The area is exquisitely painful to fist percussion, and inspiratory arrest (Murphy's sign) is present.

An enlarged, nontender gallbladder also feels like a smooth, sausage-like mass. It occurs when the gallbladder is filled with stones, as with common bile duct obstruction.

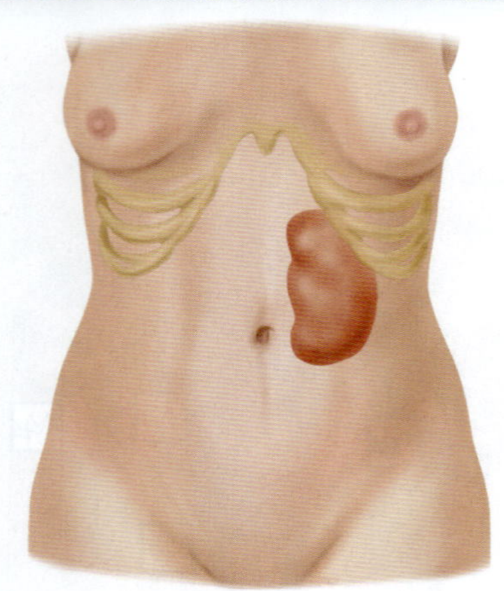

Enlarged kidney

Enlarged with hydronephrosis, cyst or neoplasm. May be difficult to distinguish an enlarged kidney from an enlarged spleen because they have a similar shape. Both extend forwards and down. However, the spleen may have a sharp edge, whereas the kidney never does. The spleen retains the splenic notch, whereas the kidney has no palpable notch. Percussion over the spleen is dull, whereas over the kidney it is tympanitic because of the overriding bowel.

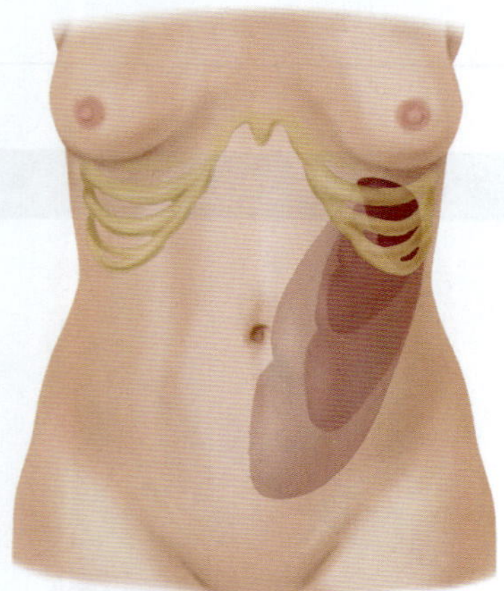

Enlarged spleen

Because any enlargement superiorly is stopped by the diaphragm, the spleen enlarges down and to the midline. When extreme, it can extend down to the left pelvis. It retains the splenic notch on the medial edge. When splenomegaly occurs with acute infections (mononucleosis), it is moderately enlarged and soft, with rounded edges. When the result of a chronic cause, the enlargement is firm or hard, with sharp edges. An enlarged spleen is usually not tender to palpation; it is tender only if the peritoneum is also inflamed.

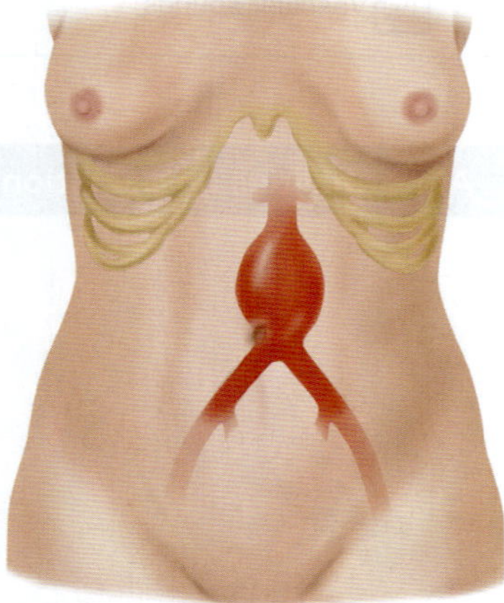

Aortic aneurysm

Most aortic aneurysms (more than 95%) are located below the renal arteries and extend to the umbilicus. About 80% of these are palpable during routine physical examination and feel like a pulsating mass in the upper abdomen just to the left of midline. You will hear a bruit. Femoral pulses are present but decreased.

Additional information on abdominal aneurysm is illustrated in Table 23.6.

BIBLIOGRAPHY

Bryant B, Knights K. Pharmacology for health professionals. 5th ed. Chatswood, NSW: Elsevier; 2019.

Chen J, Brady P. Gastroesophageal reflux disease: pathophysiology, diagnosis, and treatment. Gastroenterol Nurs 2019;42(1):20–8.

de Burlet KJ, Ing AJ, Larsen PD, Dennett ER. Systematic review of diagnostic pathways for patients presenting with acute abdominal pain. Int J Qual Health Care 2018;30(9):678–83.

Di Costanzo M, Canani RB. Lactose intolerance: common misunderstandings. Ann Nutr Metab 2018;73(4):30–7.

Kelly D, Sharif K, Hartley J, editors. Atlas of pediatric hepatology. Cham: Springer; 2019.

Marieb EM, Keller SM. Essentials of human anatomy & physiology. 12th Global ed. New York: Pearson; 2018.

Mitchell A. Carrying out a holistic assessment of a patient with constipation. Br J Nurs 2019;28(4):230–2.

Miwa H, Oshima T, Tomita T, et al. Recent understanding of the pathophysiology of functional dyspepsia: role of the duodenum as the pathogenic center. J Gastroenterol 2019;54(4):305–11.

National Health and Medical Research Council: Draft. Australian guidelines to reduce health risks from drinking alcohol. Canberra: Commonwealth of Australia; 2019. Available at: https://www.nhmrc.gov.au/health-advice/alcohol.

Pedersen JS, Bendtsen F. Adult Non-alcoholic Fatty Liver Disease (NAFLD). In: Krag A, Hansen T, editors. The human gut-liver-axis in health and disease. Champaign, IL: Springer; 2019. pp. 23–46.

Reddy SR, Cappell MS. A systematic review of the clinical presentation, diagnosis, and treatment of small bowel obstruction. Curr Gastroenterol Rep 2017;19(6):28.

Shabanzadeh DM. Incidence of gallstone disease and complications. Curr Opin Gastroenterol. 2018;34(2):81–9. doi: 10.1097/MOG.0000000000000418.

Shah S, Lewis MC. Renal, metabolic, and endocrine aging. In: Reves J, Barnett S, McSwain J, editors. Geriatric anesthesiology. Cham: Springer; 2018. p. 197–202.

Shung DL, Lim JK. Drug-induced liver injury. In: Cohen S, Davitkov P, editors. Liver disease. Champaign, IL: Springer; 2019. pp. 1–10.

Sturm A, White L, editors. Inflammatory bowel disease nursing manual. Cham: Springer; 2019.

Talley NJ, O'Connor S. Clinical examination: a systematic guide to physical diagnosis. 8th ed. Chatswood: Elsevier; 2018.

Tortora GJ. Principles of anatomy and physiology, 2nd Asia-Pacific ed. Melbourne: Wiley; 2018.

World Health Organization (WHO). Hepatitis C key facts. 2018. Available at: www.who.int/news-room/fact-sheets/detail/hepatitis-c.

Chapter Twenty-Four

Assessment of urinary function

Written by Carolyn Jarvis
Adapted by Elizabeth Watt

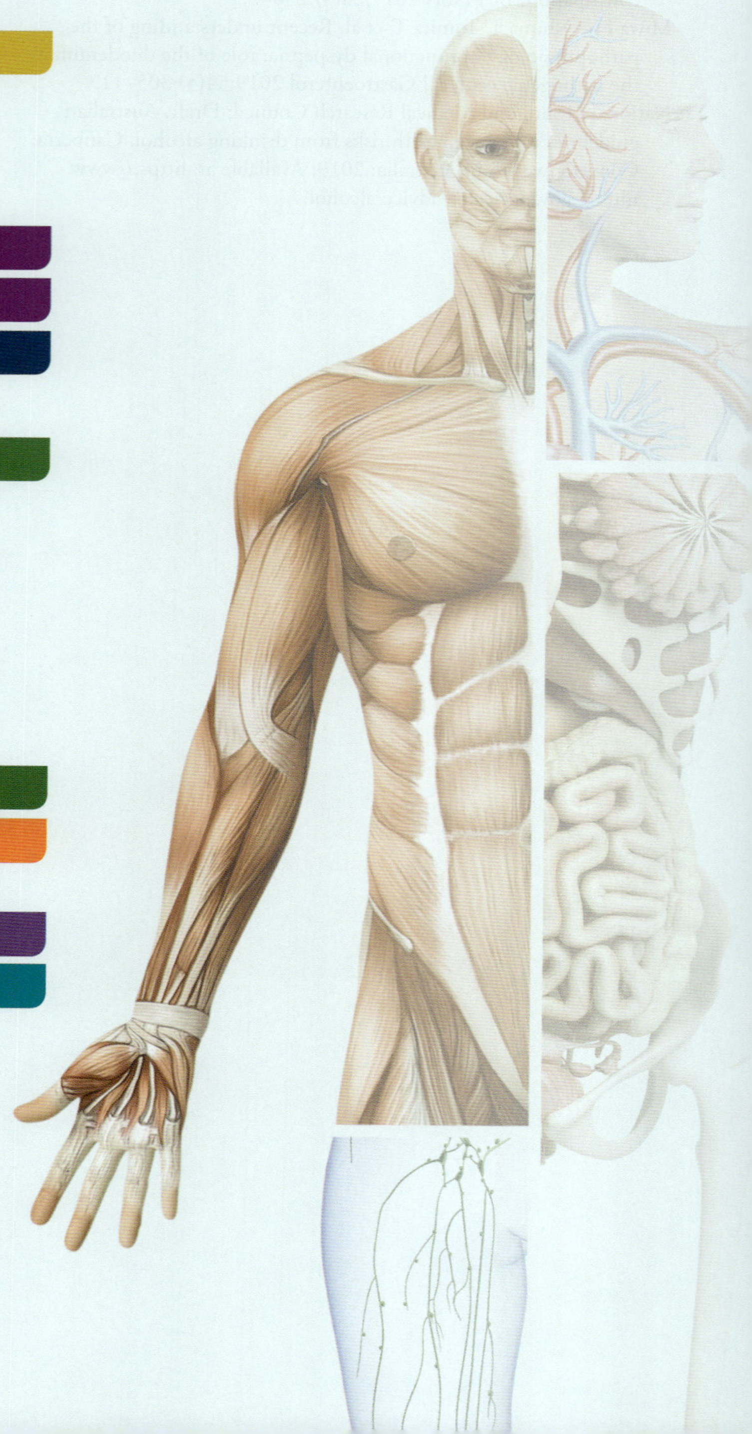

INTRODUCTION

Structures relevant to assessment of urinary tract function include the kidneys, ureters, bladder and urethra. The upper urinary tract consists of the kidneys and ureters. The lower urinary tract consists of the bladder and urethra. The male prostate gland, while not related to the urinary tract in terms of urine production, drainage of urine, storage and voiding, is an important structure to consider in this chapter as any enlargement of the prostate can lead to obstructed urine flow through the urethra. The structure and function of the prostate gland is described in Chapter 27. Likewise, the pelvic floor muscles play an important role in the maintenance of continence (see Chapter 26).

Structure and function

The urinary system has several important functions including the regulation of blood volume and composition; assisting in the regulation of blood pressure; production of hormones (calcitriol and erythropoietin); regulation of blood glucose levels; excretion of wastes in the urine; passing urine from the kidney to the bladder via the ureters; storage of urine in the bladder; emptying the stored urine from the bladder via the urethra (Tortora 2018).

KIDNEYS

The bean-shaped **kidneys** are retroperitoneal, or posterior to the abdominal contents (Figure 24.1). They are well protected by the posterior ribs and musculature. The twelfth rib forms an angle with the vertebral column, the **costovertebral angle** (Figure 24.2). The left kidney lies here at the eleventh and twelfth ribs. An average-sized adult kidney is approximately 10–12 cm long and 5–7 cm wide and weighs approximately 130–150 g (Tortora 2018). Each kidney is covered by three layers of tissue: the renal capsule, adipose capsule and renal fascia which all help to maintain the position of the kidney and protect it from trauma. Near the centre of each kidney is a narrowing (the renal hilum) through which the ureter, renal artery and renal vein, lymphatic vessels and nerves enter and exit. A longitudinal section through the kidney (Figure 24.3) reveals two distinct regions; the outer layer (renal cortex) and the inner layer (the medulla). The medulla consists of a number

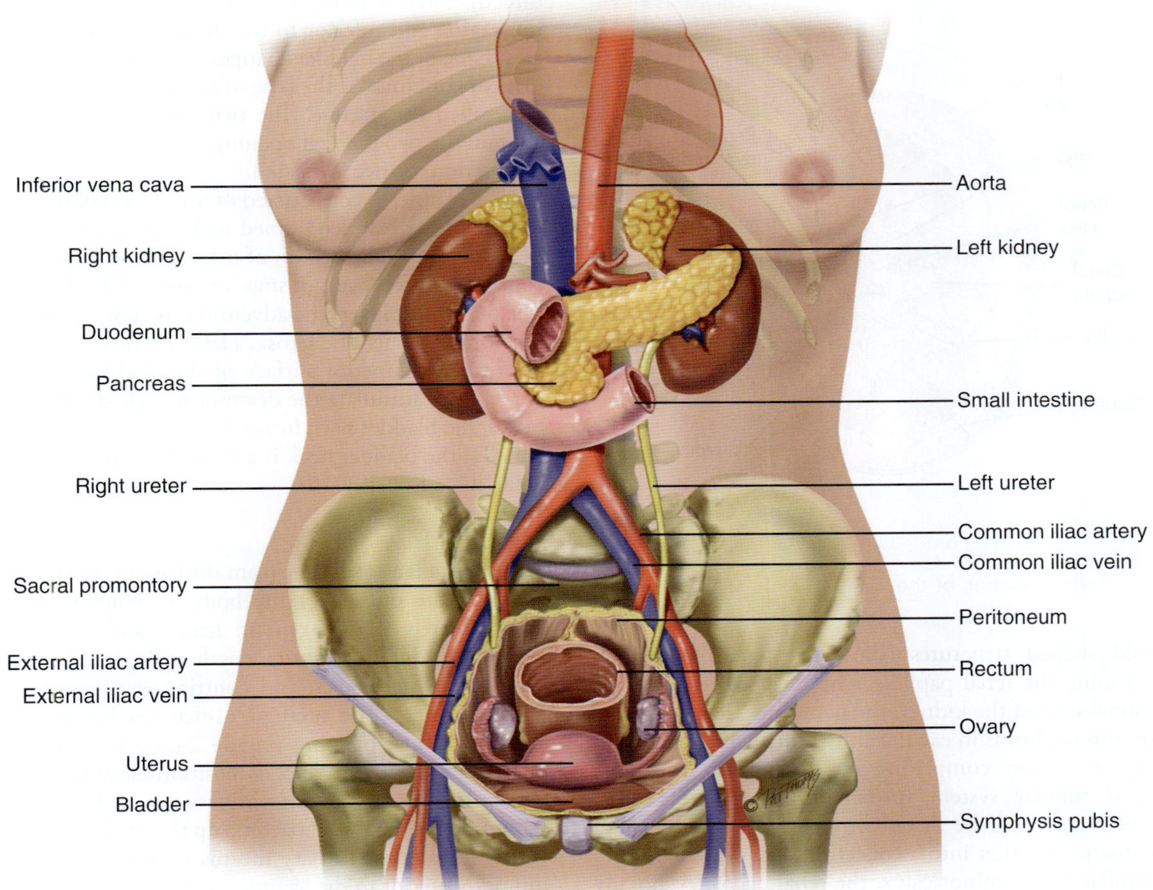

Figure 24.1
© Pat Thomas, 2006.

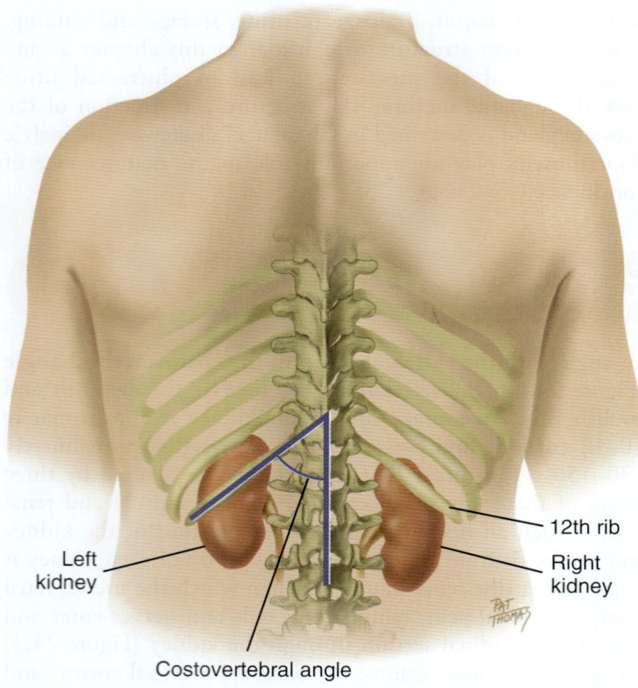

Figure 24.2

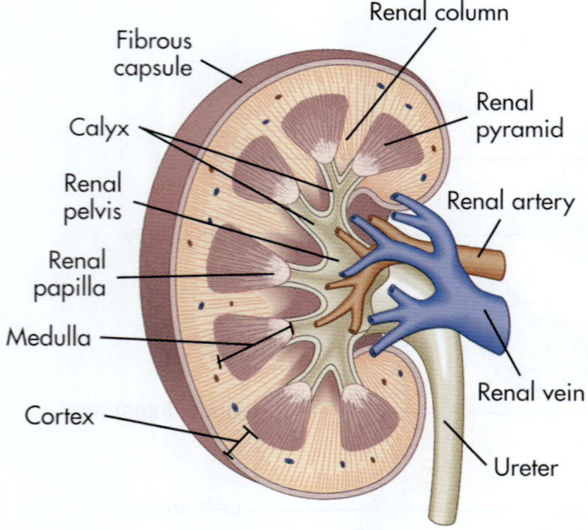

Figure 24.3
Longitudinal section of the kidney.

of pyramid shaped structures (the renal pyramids) which narrow, forming the renal papillae. The renal cortex contains the functional unit of the kidney, the nephron. There are more than 1 million nephrons in each healthy kidney. Each nephron is a complex system comprising a glomerulus, Bowman's capsule and tubular system (proximal convoluted tubule, the loop of Henle and the distal convoluted tubule). Several nephrons merge together into a collecting duct which empties via the papillae to the minor calyx, the renal pelvis, eventually draining into the ureters. The two kidneys receive 25% of the resting cardiac output into the renal arteries. In adults, renal blood flow is approximately 1200 mL per min. The amount of filtrate formed in the renal corpuscle (a Bowman's capsule and a glomerulus) of both kidneys each minute is known as the glomerular filtration rate (GFR). The urine output does depend on intake of fluids; however the normal adult output of urine is approximately 1500–1600 mL/24 hours.

URETERS

The two ureters extend in a continuous tube from the renal pelvis (pelvoureteric junction) to the trigone of the bladder (vesicoureteric junction) and carry urine from the kidney. Peristaltic contractions of the muscle walls of the ureters help move urine down each ureter into the bladder. Each ureter is 25–30 cm long and has a diameter of approximately 3–4 mm (Marieb & Keller 2018). Three layers of muscle form the ureters (the mucosa, the lamina propria and the muscularis). The inner layer (the mucosa) is composed of transitional epithelium which is able to stretch to accommodate a varying volume of fluid. The distal end of the ureter enters the bladder on an angle at the vesicoureteric junction. The muscle of bladder and ureter in combination with the angle of entry of the ureter into the bladder acts as a valve-like mechanism to prevent reflux of urine back up into the ureter from the bladder during micturition.

BLADDER

The urinary bladder is a hollow, distensible, muscular organ designed to store and expel urine. It lies in the pelvic cavity posterior to the symphysis pubis. In men, the bladder lies directly anterior to the rectum and in women it is anterior to the vagina and inferior to the uterus (Tortora 2018). The size and shape of the bladder changes to comply with the amount of urine it contains. At the base of the bladder there is a triangular area called the trigone. The two upper corners of the trigone contain the two ureteral openings and the lower corner is where the urethral orifice is located.

The bladder is constructed of four layers of tissue. The inner surface of the bladder is lined with transitional cell epithelium that prevents reabsorption of urine. The muscle of the bladder consists of three layers of smooth muscle (the detrusor muscle). The outermost layer (the adventitia) is composed of fibroelastic connective tissue. The serosa, a layer of the visceral peritoneum, lies over the superior surface of the bladder. Parasympathetic nerve fibres stimulate the detrusor muscle during urination. In males, the bladder neck forms the internal urinary sphincter. In females, the bladder neck is a far weaker structure than in men (Marieb & Keller 2018).

URETHRA

The urethra is a small tube from the base of the bladder (bladder neck) to the outside of the body. In women, the urethra is approximately 3.5–5.5 cm in length and leaves the bladder neck at an angle. The entire length of the female urethra acts as a sphincter mechanism and contributes to continence during bladder filling. The urethral orifice lies between the clitoris and the vaginal opening (Figure 24.4). The relative shortness of the female urethra and its position close to the vagina and anus predisposes women to urinary tract infection (UTI) from ascending movement of bacteria up the urethra into the bladder. In the female, the urinary meatus is located between the labia minora, anterior to the vagina and posterior to the clitoris.

In males, the urethra is approximately 18–23 cm long and is divided into three sections: the prostatic urethra, the membranous urethra and the spongy (or penile) urethra (Tortora 2018) (Figure 24.5). The prostatic urethra originates

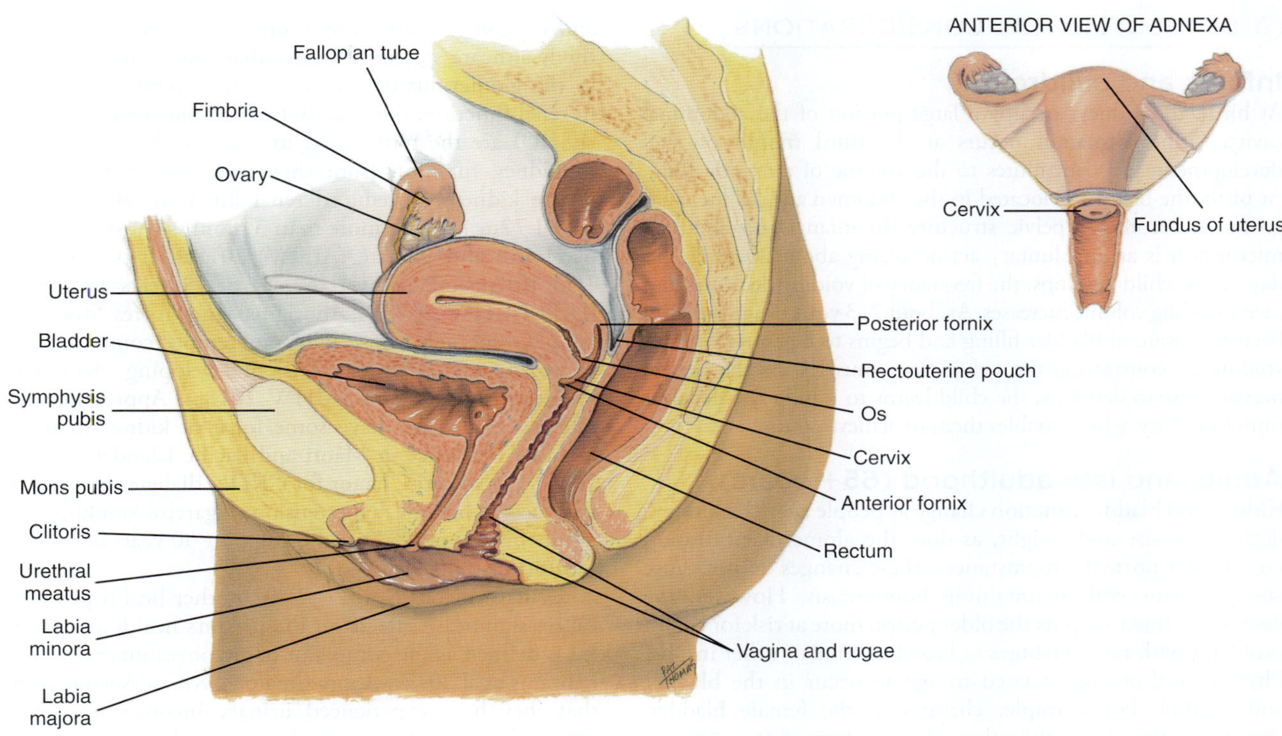

Figure 24.4

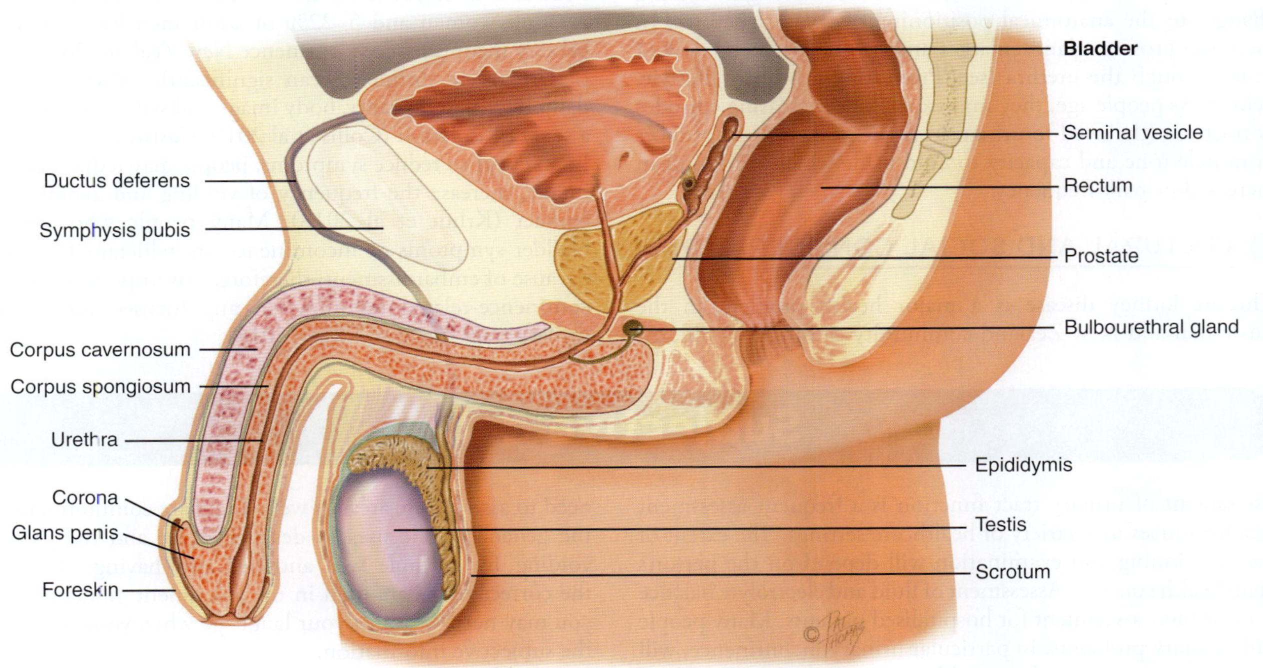

Figure 24.5

at the bladder neck and travels through the prostate gland. The prostate gland encircles the male urethra at the base of the bladder. The membranous urethra passes through the deep muscle of the perineum. These two sections form the sphincter mechanism in males. The spongy urethra consists of four parts: the bulbous urethra, pendulous urethra, fossa navicularis and the meatus. The male urethra transverses the corpus spongiosum, and its meatus forms a slit at the glans tip. The urethra consists of a mucosa and muscularis with circular smooth muscle fibres continuous with the wall of the bladder.

 DEVELOPMENTAL CONSIDERATIONS

Infants and children

At birth, the kidneys occupy a large portion of the abdominal cavity. Urine formation occurs at the third month of fetal development and contributes to the volume of amniotic fluid. At birth, the bladder is located in the abdomen and, as the child grows, it becomes a pelvic structure. In infants and children, micturition is an involuntary act occurring about 20 times per day. As the child develops, the frequency of voiding decreases and mean voiding volume increases. At about 2–3 years of age the child becomes aware of bladder filling and begins to be able to inhibit voiding by contracting the pelvic floor muscles. As the central nervous system develops, the child learns to inhibit the detrusor muscle activity, which enables them to achieve continence.

Adults and late adulthood (65+ years)

Kidney and bladder function change as people age. The kidneys decrease in size and weight, as does the glomerular filtration rate. Under normal circumstances, these changes do not cause any problems with maintaining homeostasis. However, the decrease in function puts the older person more at risk for health problems with rapid changes to blood volume or other insults. Physiological changes related to ageing occur in the bladder and urethra. For example, changes to the female bladder, urethra, vagina and pelvic floor due to decreasing oestrogen following menopause can cause these structures to become less vascular, thinner and less elastic. The muscles that surround the urethra and support the bladder can lose strength, causing changes to the anatomical positioning of these structures. In men, the prostate gland enlarges and can obstruct the flow of urine through the urethra (see 'Promoting a healthy lifestyle' below). As people age, they may experience increasing episodes of nocturia (the need to urinate at night). The bladder reduces in muscle tone and capacity to hold urine which can result in increased urinary frequency.

CULTURAL AND SOCIAL CONSIDERATIONS

Chronic kidney disease is a major health problem in the Australian and New Zealand community causing a significant and on-going health burden on the person, their family and the healthcare system. Diseases that cause irreversible damage to the glomerulus or tubules result in permanent alterations in renal function. Chronic (CKD) or end-stage kidney disease (ESKD) are the terms used to describe the resulting decline in kidney function from these processes. CKD is damage to the kidneys or reduced renal function (eGFR <60 mL/min/1.72m^2) lasting more than 3 months (Australian Institute of Health and Welfare (AIHW) 2018a). It is estimated that 1 in 10 Australians over the age of 18 years are living with CKD (AIHW 2018a). Aboriginal and Torres Strait Islander people, especially those living in remote communities, have approximately 2.1 times the risk of developing CKD than non-indigenous Australians (AIHW 2018a). Approximately 12% of New Zealanders have some form of kidney damage, and a higher incidence in Māori and Pacific Islanders (Lloyd et al 2019). A major risk factor for CKD is diabetes mellitus. Other risk factors include hypertension, cigarette smoking, obesity, family history of CKD and being over 50 years of age (Kidney Health Australia 2019).

Urinary incontinence (UI) is another health problem that causes significant effects on the person's health and wellbeing. UI is defined as the complaint of any involuntary loss of urine (Abrams et al 2017). Approximately 38% of Australians report that they have experienced urinary incontinence and 10% report that they frequently lose control of their bladder or bowel. The majority (74%) are women and half of those with incontinence are aged from 40–59 years of age (Continence Foundation of Australia 2019). In New Zealand, 25–34% of adult women and 5–22% of adult men have experienced urinary incontinence (Continence New Zealand 2019).

Urinary incontinence can significantly affect the person's daily activities, sexuality, body image and self-esteem and create a sense of isolation (Collis et al 2019, Castro Diaz et al 2017). In an effort to reduce symptoms, people may reduce their fluid intake, increase the frequency of voiding and avoiding social contact (Krhut et al 2018). Many people who experience bladder symptoms or incontinence are reluctant to seek help because of embarrassment; therefore, it is important to include continence-related questions in any focused assessment of urinary tract function (Wagg 2018).

Subjective data

Assessment of urinary tract function is a frequent assessment area for nurses in a variety of healthcare settings. The extent of the questioning and examination will depend on the person's main health concern. Assessment of fluid and electrolyte balance is a common assessment for hospitalised patients. Many people with urinary problems, in particular urinary incontinence, will be reluctant to discuss their problem so you need to pose these questions with tact and empathy. You need to keep in mind the intimate and private nature of many aspects of this assessment. Therefore, it is important to ensure the privacy and comfort of the environment, and be mindful of the need for some people to have a health professional of the same gender performing the assessment. You also need to keep in mind that bladder problems often coincide with bowel problems, especially constipation and, in men, erectile dysfunction, so you may need to assess these areas as well. There are common terms that the general public uses to describe urine and the process of voiding, for example 'wee' and 'pee' and 'having a leak'; while the correct terms are used in the assessment guidelines below, you may need to adjust your language when you are collecting the subjective information.

There are many tools available to assist in the collection of subjective data, specifically in relation to the presence and severity of urinary symptoms, including incontinence, and the impact of these symptoms on the quality of life. These validated tools are used in clinical practice and research. The following are some—not all—of the most commonly used tools:

- Assessment of incontinence and LUTS in men (ICIQ—MLUTS Male LUT symptoms questionnaire)

- Assessment of lower urinary tract symptoms in men (I-PPS—International Prostate Symptom Score).
- Assessment of quality of life in prostate cancer (UCLA—Prostate Cancer Index or EPIC—Expanded Prostate Cancer Index).
- Assessment of sexual function in men (IEEF—International index of erectile function) and women (SQoL-F).
- Impact of incontinence on quality of life (ICIQ—UI Short Form).

1. Presenting concern
2. Usual urinary pattern
3. Fluid intake (type and amount)
4. History of change or disturbance to urinary tract function
5. Pain
6. Lower urinary tract symptoms (LUTS)
7. Other symptoms (including fever, weight gain/loss, fatigue)
8. Past history (including obstetric history)
9. Health and lifestyle management
10. Environmental issues related to bladder function

Practice note: Before you commence the assessment, introduce yourself to the person, confirm the person's identity, discuss the purpose and scope of the assessment, clarify any questions the person may have and obtain verbal consent from the person to perform the assessment.

ASSESSMENT GUIDELINES	CLINICAL SIGNIFICANCE AND CLINICAL ALERTS
1. Presenting concern	
• Do you feel that you have any problem with kidney or bladder function? It is important to ascertain the person's perception of their urinary tract function. • If they do perceive a problem—how does this impact on their quality of life?	
2. Usual urinary pattern	
• How often do you empty your bladder (void) during the day? • How often do you get up to empty your bladder (void) overnight?	There is a usual pattern to voiding over a 24-hour period although there is variation between individuals. It is considered normal for an adult to void 3–5 hourly during the daytime and not need to void overnight. The adult bladder capacity is approximately 500 mL (Marieb & Keller 2018). **Oliguria**—diminished quantity, <400 mL/24 hours. **Polyuria**—excessive quantity.
3. Characteristics of the urine	
What colour is your urine? Does it have an unpleasant odour? (If so, describe.) Is the urine clear, cloudy, blood stained, does it contain mucus?	Urine should normally be clear, light yellow coloured and have a non-offensive odour. **Cloudy**—urinary tract infection. **Haematuria**—for example, can indicate urinary tract infection, bladder or renal cancer, urinary calculi and chronic inflammation of the bladder. Can be **microscopic or macroscopic**. Some colour changes are temporary or harmless. However, when there is blood in urine, or a colour change lasting >1 day, the person should seek medical advice. For a complete description, see Table 24.1.

SUBJECTIVE DATA

ASSESSMENT GUIDELINES	CLINICAL SIGNIFICANCE AND CLINICAL ALERTS
4. Fluid intake (type and amount)	
• Assessment of 'fluid balance' is often conducted for hospitalised patients using a fluid balance chart to record intake and output over a 24-hour period. • It is often difficult for people to accurately estimate the amount of fluid they consume in a day. In community and clinic settings accurate assessment of fluid intake and output is also important for those people with renal and urinary tract health problems (and others, for example with heart failure). The person (or their carer) should be asked to keep a written record usually over three 24-hours periods. See further information in the voiding diary section below.	It is important to ascertain the types of fluids consumed over the day and night because some types of fluids are known to irritate the bladder in certain individuals; e.g. caffeine-containing fluids such as coffee and cola drinks. Alcohol is a diuretic and can cause exacerbation of urinary symptoms, especially frequency and urgency.
5. History of change or disturbance to urinary tract function	
• Have you noticed any change in your usual urinary tract function—bladder or kidneys? Can you describe this change for me? How long has this been happening? What have you been doing about this?	Changes in urinary tract function can be a symptom of underlying significant health problems such as malignancy and require further assessment. You need to fully investigate and document the details of the typical symptoms that the person is experiencing.
6. Pain	
• Review pain assessment strategies and tools from Chapter 13. Use a pain assessment tool as appropriate to the person's age, context and capacity to communicate. In general you need to ask the person to describe: **Character:** How would you describe the pain you are experiencing: dull, stabbing, aching, burning? **Onset:** duration, variation: How did it start? How long have you had it? **Location:** Where is the pain? Please point to it (you could use a body diagram to report these findings). Is the pain in one spot or does it move around? **Duration:** Is the pain constant or does it come and go? Does it peak (for example, when urinating, after urinating)? **Severity:** How intense is the pain—rate from 1–10. **Pattern:** What makes the pain worse: e.g. voiding or having bowels opened, sexual intercourse? • **What** have you tried to relieve pain: rest, heating pad, fluids, medication etc? Associated factors: Is the pain associated with any other symptoms? E.g. menstrual period or irregularities, stress, fatigue, nausea and vomiting, frequent urination (see also point 6, lower urinary tract symptoms, below), vaginal or penile discharge?	There are several sites for pain associated with upper and/or lower urinary tract dysfunction. Keep in mind that pain may be referred from another organ or site and may be associated with general symptoms such as fever or nausea. **Flank pain** (costovertebral angle) is usually associated with a disorder of the renal pelvis or kidney, especially when it is unilateral. A continuous dull ache is associated with chronic obstruction or infection. An acute pain in the flank region may be the result of acute obstruction of the renal pelvis or proximal (upper) ureter and is commonly termed 'renal colic'. Pain may also radiate to upper lateral aspect of the abdomen. It is often described as moderate to severe in intensity and will cause the person to seek help. The pain tends to occur in waves during which the pain intensifies for periods of time as the pressure in the ureter and renal pelvis increases in response to the peristaltic waves. If the obstruction is in the lower ureter the pain may also radiate to the inguinal area and/or groin and upper thigh. The person with this type of pain should also be questioned about haematuria, fever and other urinary tract symptoms that might indicate infection (e.g. cloudy, foul-smelling urine, dysuria, frequency) (Talley & O'Connor 2018). See also Table 24.2. Lower urinary tract and pelvic pain—most commonly caused by urinary tract infection (including prostatitis in the male). **Dysuria** (painful urination) is a common symptom related to urinary tract dysfunction. Typically, the person complains of burning on urination which is associated with lower urinary tract infection and, less commonly, prostatitis in men. ***Clinical alert:*** People with pain indicating renal colic and signs and symptoms of infection need urgent medical referral for further assessment and intervention to prevent septicaemia.

ASSESSMENT GUIDELINES	CLINICAL SIGNIFICANCE AND CLINICAL ALERTS
7. Lower urinary tract symptoms (LUTS)	
Storage symptoms: • *Daytime voiding frequency* (see questions related to usual urinary pattern above).	**Increased daytime frequency**—voiding more than 8 times per day. It is important to take into account the volume of urine per void and fluid intake when assessing urinary frequency. The increased urinary frequency could be the result of an unusually high fluid intake or an underlying problem with renal function.
• *Urgency* Do you feel that you are able to delay going to the toilet?	**Urgency**—inability to defer voiding after feeling the desire to void. Can lead to urge urinary incontinence if the person is unable to quickly respond to the desire to void. Urgency can be a debilitating urinary symptom that significantly affects activities of daily living and decreases a person's quality of life (Caruso et al 2017). Urgency often accompanies urinary frequency.
• *Nocturia* Do you need to get up at night to pass urine? How often? How long has this been occurring? Has it increased over this time?	**Nocturia** is defined as waking up to void during the main sleep period, more than once (Hashim et al 2019). It is commonly associated with benign prostatic enlargement in men over the age of 50 years and can be severe. Some men have to void more than six times per night; this results in sleep disturbance, relationship tensions and a general decrease in health and wellbeing (Everaert et al 2018). Other causes are heart failure, urinary tract infection, hyperglycaemia and diuretic medication.
• *Urinary incontinence* Do you ever leak urine when you don't want to? Keep in mind that people will frequently underestimate their urinary symptoms, especially if they have urinary incontinence. Often, if asked directly about urinary incontinence, they will answer 'no'. However, if you ask about whether they use pads so their clothes don't get wet they may answer 'yes'. This happens because people are embarrassed; and some may have had the problem for a long time and now consider it 'normal'. When does the leakage occur (changing position, coughing, sneezing, laughing or no provocation)? How much urine is lost (estimate in terms of dampness to clothing)? How often does this happen?	**Urinary incontinence** is any involuntary loss of urine which is sufficient to be a social or hygienic problem (Abrams et al 2017). A comprehensive assessment of urinary incontinence takes time and expertise to determine the exact type of urinary incontinence. The person may need referral to a continence nurse specialist for further assessment and advice. The International Continence Society classifies the varying types of urinary incontinence according to the typical symptoms (Abrams et al 2017, pp. 2551): **Stress urinary incontinence**—involuntary leakage of urine on effort or exertion, such as coughing, sneezing or running. This type of incontinence is often caused by weakness of the pelvic floor muscles. Usually small amounts of urine are leaked.

SUBJECTIVE DATA

ASSESSMENT GUIDELINES	CLINICAL SIGNIFICANCE AND CLINICAL ALERTS
Do you ever lose urine because you are unable to get to the toilet in time?	**Overactive bladder** is the term used to describe the symptoms of bothersome urgency, frequency, nocturia and sometimes urine leakage. **Urgency urinary incontinence** is the involuntary leakage of urine accompanied by or immediately preceded by a sense of urgency. The person may not be able to inhibit the urge and this can result in the entire bladder contents being leaked. Urge incontinence can be caused by a number of factors including neurological conditions such as stroke and multiple sclerosis, and local causes such as urinary tract infection, faecal impaction or prostatic enlargement (Salvatore et al 2017). **Mixed urinary incontinence**—a combination of stress and urge symptoms.
Do you ever lose urine at night when you are asleep?	**Nocturnal enuresis**—any involuntary loss of urine occurring during sleep. Most commonly occurs in children but can also occur in adults. Loss of urine at night can also occur in people who have acute or chronic urinary retention (see below).
Does urine leak regardless of what you are doing? Do you feel that you completely empty your bladder after you have been to the toilet?	**Continuous urinary leakage**—can be a sign of anatomical abnormality; for example, a fistula formation from bladder to vagina, or continuous overflow of urine where there is an acute or chronic obstruction causing retention with some overflow of urine. The most common cause of retention of urine is enlargement of the prostate gland in men.
Do you have trouble getting to the toilet—e.g. walking, transferring from chair to standing, standing to toilet? Are you able to undress/redress for toileting unassisted? See also below on environmental factors.	**Functional incontinence**—urinary leakage that is associated with impairment of the person's mobility, dexterity or cognitive function. This type of incontinence is a significant problem for frail older people and those people with a disability. The person's or their carer's answers to these questions may lead to the need for a more in-depth assessment of the home environment and referral to an occupational therapist.
Voiding symptoms: • *Urinary stream* Do you feel that the force at which you pass urine has decreased? For men—do you ever find that you need to stand closer to the toilet or urinal? If so, how long has this been happening? Do you find it difficult to start passing urine?	**Slow urinary stream**—perception that the urinary stream has slowed. If the person has a severe slowing of the urinary stream they may describe it as a dribble or trickle. Sometimes described as a weak stream. See also Table 24.2. **Intermittent/interrupted stream**—starting and stopping voiding. **Hesitancy**—a delay in the starting of a urinary stream despite the desire to urinate. All of these symptoms can be associated with poor detrusor (bladder) contraction and bladder outlet obstruction.

ASSESSMENT GUIDELINES	CLINICAL SIGNIFICANCE AND CLINICAL ALERTS
• *Straining* Do you ever have to strain (bear down) to start or continue urinating? Do you ever have to strain to completely empty your bladder?	**Straining**—using muscular effort to initiate, maintain or improve the urinary stream. This is abnormal and may indicate an underlying dysfunction of the detrusor or bladder outlet obstruction.
• *Post micturition symptoms* Do you ever dribble urine after going to the toilet? How often does this happen? Does the leakage stop after a small loss of urine? Do you feel that you empty your bladder completely when you have gone to the toilet? If no, how long have you had this feeling?	**Post-micturition dribble**—a symptom most commonly affecting men where there is a small loss if urine after urination is completed, happening even when the man is redressing. **Feeling of incomplete emptying**—the perception that the bladder is not fully emptied following voiding. This may or may not indicate that the person has a raised post void residual volume (ICS 2019).
• *Difficulty or complete inability to void* In this situation ask: Do you feel that you need to pass urine but can't?	The two most likely causes of significant difficulty with voiding are urinary retention (acute or chronic) and oliguria or anuria. People experiencing severe pain or who have undergone surgery (especially with epidural anaesthesia) can experience transient difficulty in voiding and may require urinary catheterisation until their general health improves. Acute and chronic retention is most often associated with enlargement of the prostate in men (Serlin et al 2018). Acute retention can cause significant lower abdominal pain and restlessness. Chronic urinary retention can result in renal damage due to increased pressures and/or infection in the urinary tract.
• *Lack of sensation of the need to void* In this situation ask: Do you have any sensation to pass urine? Do you lose urine but have no sensation of this happening?	Lack of sensation to void is associated with neurogenic dysfunction of the bladder which can be caused by disease or injury of the central or peripheral nervous system (e.g. multiple sclerosis, spinal cord injury, spina bifida, diabetes mellitus). For some people the bladder contracts without the sensation of the need to void, causing urinary incontinence. For others, the bladder may fail to contract (atonic bladder) resulting in retention of urine (Serlin et al 2018). The bladder can retain large amounts of urine which can cause further damage to the detrusor muscle and increased pressures in the urinary tract resulting in renal damage.
8. Other symptoms (including fever, weight gain/loss, fatigue)	
• **Fever**—Have you experienced fever now or recently? • **Nausea and vomiting**—Have you experienced nausea and/or vomiting now or recently? Anorexia? • **Weight gain/loss and peripheral oedema**—Have you had a weight increase/loss now or recently? Do you have any swelling in your lower legs? Are you experiencing excessive thirst? • **Fatigue/lethargy**—Have you experienced fatigue now or recently? • **For men**—Erectile dysfunction (see Chapter 27). • **Any other symptoms** (e.g. headache, itching skin)?	Fever is associated with infection of the urinary tract and may be accompanied by other symptoms. The presence of a high body temperature with other symptoms such as flank pain, nausea and chills usually indicates the need for urgent referral to a medical practitioner. Nausea and vomiting can accompany pain and fever or can be a sign of increased creatinine levels indicating renal failure. Weight gain/loss in the person with a renal disorder is an indicator of general fluid balance. Fatigue and lethargy can be associated with chronic urinary tract disorders including renal failure.

SUBJECTIVE DATA

ASSESSMENT GUIDELINES	CLINICAL SIGNIFICANCE AND CLINICAL ALERTS
9. Past history (including obstetric history)	
• Do you or your family have any past history of renal or urinary tract health problems (infection, urinary stones, cancer)? • Do you or your family have any past history of neurological disorders? Are you diabetic? For how long? Current treatment? • Have you had any problem with your bowel function, including constipation? • History of mental health problems? • For men—any history of prostate cancer in your family? • For women—obstetric history: How many births? Were forceps used for any of these? Did you have an episiotomy? What were the babies' birth weights? Did you have any bladder control issues after the births? Menopausal symptoms? • Surgical history—including gynaecological, spinal, bowel surgery? • Obesity? • General health—including cognitive function?	Diabetes mellitus is a major risk factor for renal failure and bladder dysfunction. Constipation is a risk factor for urinary incontinence and voiding dysfunction. There is a higher incidence of prostate cancer in men who have a first degree relative with the disease. Pregnancy and childbirth are risk factors for the development of urinary incontinence. Obesity is a risk factor for the development of urinary incontinence. Older people may experience acute confusion rather than the more typical symptoms of urinary tract infection (such as frequency, urgency and dysuria).
10. Health and lifestyle management	
• **Activity and exercise**—What regular exercise do you take? Are you able to manage your personal hygiene and toileting? • **Smoking**<—How much? For how long? • **Continence aids and appliances**—Do you use any continence aids to assist you with toileting or incontinence (e.g. commodes, urinals, toilet seats, grab bars and rails)? If so, which ones? For how long? How effective are they? • Do you use any continence products to assist you with bladder leakage (e.g. pads, pants, condom (sheath) drainage catheters (sometimes referred to as external catheters))? If so which ones? For how long? How effective are they? • **Medications**—What medications are you currently taking (both over-the-counter and prescribed)? • **Screening** (for men over 50 years)—Do you discuss prostate cancer screening with your general practitioner? (See 'Promoting a healthy lifestyle' below.)	Some exercise activities can contribute to bladder symptoms and pelvic floor dysfunction, especially high impact activities or those which cause increased intraabdominal pressure. Smoking is a known risk factor for bladder and renal cancer and can contribute to urinary dysfunction. It is common for the person with urinary incontinence to self-manage their problem. You may need to assess the effectiveness of these aids and appliances and the person's knowledge of matters such as skin care, fluid intake, voiding position. They may need referral to a continence nurse specialist for further assessment and advice. Many medications affect bladder function, in particular anticholinergics, antidepressants and sedatives. Polypharmacy is a major contributor to the risk of incontinence in older people.
11. Environmental issues related to bladder function	
• **Mobility and dexterity issues**—Any mobility and dexterity issues related to getting to and from the toilet and/or dressing/undressing? Do you have any vision problems? • **Home environment**—location and access to the toilet? • **Work environment**—location and access to the toilet, work restrictions related to fluid intake and/or going to the toilet?	All of these factors may contribute to urinary incontinence or other voiding dysfunction and can significantly affect the person's ability to cope with the problem.
Additional subjective data for infants and children (questions for parents or guardian)	
• Does your child have any problem urinating?	
– Any pain with urinating, crying or holding the genitals? Any other symptoms or signs—for example, not feeding normally?	

ASSESSMENT GUIDELINES	CLINICAL SIGNIFICANCE AND CLINICAL ALERTS
– Do you think that your child urinary tract infection?	
• **Toilet training:** (if child older than 2 to 2½ years of age.) Has toilet training started? How is it progressing?	
• **Bed wetting:** (if child 5 years or older.) Does the child wet the bed at night? How often—nightly? Is this a problem for child or for you (parents)? What have you done about this? How does the child feel about it? Any day time wetting?	**Nocturnal enuresis**—involuntary passing of urine that occurs at night during the main sleep period (ICS 2019).

Objective data

Objective data collection focuses on further explanation related to the symptoms experienced by the person which have been revealed in the history taking. Some of the areas for objective assessment required for the assessment of urinary tract function are described in other chapters and will only be mentioned briefly below. Other relevant areas for assessment could include bowel function, skin, genitals (including digital rectal palpation of the prostate in men and vaginal examination and pelvic muscle function in women), mobility and cognitive examination. Refer to the relevant chapters for details.

Preparation

The positioning of the person is dependent on the area being assessed.

Equipment needed

You may need:
Urine jug or jar to collect a clean specimen
Urine testing equipment (dipsticks)
Non-sterile gloves
Portable bladder scanner and ultrasound transmission gel
Paper towel or tissues to remove ultrasound gel
Disinfectant wipes (to clean ultrasound transducer)
Hand hygiene solution (use before and after the physical examination)

OBJECTIVE DATA

PROCEDURES AND NORMAL FINDINGS	ABNORMAL FINDINGS AND CLINICAL ALERTS
General inspection	
During collection of subjective data you will have noticed the person's height to weight ratio, body shape, ability to move around with ease, presence of persistent cough, level of hygiene and grooming, any obvious body odour and the person's general demeanor. All of these factors provide clues to the person's urinary tract function and potential risk factors for dysfunction.	
Vital signs	
Temperature and BP—see Chapter 10.	It is important to assess presence of fever which may be related to infection and could indicate the need for urgent assessment by a medical practitioner. One of the consequences of renal impairment or renal failure is hypertension.
Abdominal examination	
Inspection, percussion and palpation of the lower abdomen to determine bladder distension (see Chapter 23). Normally the bladder would not be palpable above the symphysis pubis after voiding.	Lower abdominal pain on palpation may accompany **urinary retention** or **urinary tract infection.**

PROCEDURES AND NORMAL FINDINGS	ABNORMAL FINDINGS AND CLINICAL ALERTS
Inspection of the genitalia (if indicated)	
For urethral discharge, excoriation. Refer to Chapters 26 and 27 for details.	Urethral discharge is abnormal. See Table 24.2 for image of urethral discharge.
Post-void residual bladder volume	
The portable bladder scanner is commonly used by nurses in hospitals and in the community to assess post-void residual urine volume. The use of this specialised piece of equipment has reduced the need for intermittent urethral catheterisation to assess residual volume. There are various scanning devices available. Most will have an integrated digital screen, a transducer which is placed on the lower abdomen and a printer for displaying the bladder volume measurements. You need to read the instructions for the scanner that you are using; however, the following are general guidelines: • Explain the procedure to the person. • Have the person void into the collection jug or jar as usual—the volume of this void should be measured. Save the sample for dipstick testing after the scan is completed. (The scan should be performed as soon as possible after the person has voided to obtain accurate results.) • Ask the person to lie down (use one pillow if tolerated) and remove clothing on the lower abdomen down to the level of the symphysis pubis. • Have the scanning device placed on a trolley beside the person. • Wipe the transducer head with an disposable disinfectant wipe and allow to dry. • Turn the device on—male or female setting (male setting for a woman who has had a hysterectomy). • Apply transmission gel to the transducer head. • Place the transducer head onto the abdomen approximately 2.5 cm above the symphysis pubis and pointing down towards the bladder. Move the transducer head around until you have the bladder positioned centrally on the scanner screen, then avoid moving the transducer during scanning process. • The scanning device will signal when the scanning is complete. • Remove the transducer head from the abdomen and clean. Offer the person tissues to wipe their abdomen and assist them, if necessary, to redress.	An increased **post-void residual volume (PVR)** is not necessarily a clinical problem; however in situations where there is high pressure in the bladder, an increased PVR can lead to infection, hydronephrosis and renal insufficiency (Castro Diaz et al 2017). Multiple ultrasounds may be needed to identify a trend. In a healthy person the PVR should normally be no more than 50 mL. Over 200 mL is considered to be inadequate emptying (Castro Diaz et al 2017). However, an acceptable PVR is very patient-specific and you should always check with the attending medical officer as to what is considered acceptable for a particular person. Keep in mind that the amount of PVR must be interpreted in light of the volume of urine the person had in their bladder in the first place. For example, if the person voided 100 mL and had a PVR of 100 mL, the finding is significant.
• Label the printed results with the date and time, the volume voided prior to the bladder scan and the person's name and date of birth. The printed results should be fixed into the person's medical history/progress notes. (Note: some scanners use thermal printing that fades over time. In this case photocopy the results.)	
In the normal bladder there should be less than 50 mL of urine left in the bladder after voiding (Castro Diaz et al 2017).	
Examination of urine	
Collect a clean specimen of urine • You should always collect a clean specimen for urinalysis. It should never be taken from a urine drainage bag. • Ask the person to void into a clean container (urinal, bed pan or clean urine measuring jug). • The specimen should be tested as soon as possible after collection. • For the person who has a urethral or suprapubic catheter, the drainage bag tubing should be positioned so that there are loops at the level of the bladder (so that the urine collects in the tubing rather than dripping into the urine drainage bag). When the urine has collected in the tubing, draw approximately 10 mL of the urine from the access port in the tubing. (Never disconnect the tubing from the catheter to take a urine specimen: this breaks the closed system and increases the risk of urinary tract infection.)	

PROCEDURES AND NORMAL FINDINGS	ABNORMAL FINDINGS AND CLINICAL ALERTS
Characteristics	
• Volume of void, colour, clarity and odour. • Urine should normally be clear, light yellow coloured and have a non-offensive odour.	See Table 24.1 for interpretation of urine colour.
Urinalysis	
• Urinalysis can produce quick and useful information on the person's health status, and bladder and kidney function. It may indicate the need for further investigations such as midstream urine (MSU) for microscopy and culture. There are various brands of reagent strips available which test for a variety of urine characteristics and abnormalities. These need to be stored and used in accordance with the manufacturer's instructions. The following are general guidelines: – Don non-sterile gloves. – Open the reagent strip container and remove a reagent strip. Avoid touching the reagent test pads on the stick. – Dip the stick into the urine specimen making sure that all of the reagent test pads are moistened. Remove the stick, making sure that you don't flick the stick causing spray. Start timing the test. Let the stick drain above the urine container to reduce dripping of urine. – Some test pads can be read immediately, others require a specific time for the result to be finalised. Follow the instructions on the container regarding the time requirements. – After the required time frame, compare the colour of the reagent test pad to the chart for the specific test located on the reagent strip container. Avoid touching the urine-soaked reagent strip on the container chart. Discard the test strip and then your gloves into the waste bin. – Perform hand hygiene. – Record the results.	
• Normal urine dip stick (reagent strip) test results: – pH—4.5–8.0 (average 5.0–6.0) – Bilirubin—none or trace – Urobilinogen—none or trace – Protein—none – Blood—none – Glucose—none – Ketones—none – Specific gravity—1.005–1.030 – Leucocyte esterase—none – Nitrite—none	***Clinical alert:*** A person should be referred to a medical or nurse practitioner where there is a positive finding for blood, protein, nitrates or leukocytes.

OBJECTIVE DATA

PROCEDURES AND NORMAL FINDINGS	ABNORMAL FINDINGS AND CLINICAL ALERTS
Fluid balance chart/voiding diary	
In hospitalised people, a **'fluid balance'** chart is commonly issued to record intake and output as well as type and amount of fluid intake and any accompanying voiding symptoms. In situations where estimation of fluid balance is vital to the overall health of the person, urinary catheterisation may be required so that accurate, frequent urine volumes may be obtained. **A voiding diary** (sometimes called a bladder chart, bladder diary or frequency/volume chart) can be used to record a person's voiding and incontinence pattern over a period of time. The form used will depend on the information to be elicited, e.g. information on intake and types of fluids, volume voided, accompanying symptoms such as urgency, dysuria, incontinence and precipitating factors, use of continence pads. This data is sometimes combined with a bowel chart/diary. It is common practice to collect at least 3 full (24-hour) days of charting to establish if a voiding pattern exists. During this time the person or their carer should make no attempt to alter their usual patterns, as the purpose of the chart is to establish the person's usual voiding patterns. You need to review the following data: **Pattern of urinary elimination** • Voiding frequency during the daytime • Presence and severity of nocturia (each void is preceded by sleep) • Proportion of urine formed overnight (voided volume after going to bed to sleep including the first void of the morning) • 24-hours frequency • Maximum voided volume • Average voided volume (sum of volumes voided divided by the number of voids) • 24-hour total voided volume	Output should be roughly similar to intake. In an adult the amount of urine produced per hour is 0.5 mL/kg/hr or 30–40 mL per hour in an average sized adult. Proportion of urine voided overnight. Up to one-third of daily urine production overnight is considered normal
Patterns of urinary leakage • Frequency of incontinence episodes and relationship to voiding and precipitating events (e.g. coughing, sneezing) • Volume of leakage **Fluid consumption** • Intake compared with output • Patterns of intake • Types of fluids • Relationship of intake and voiding or incontinence (Castro Diaz et al 2017, Nelles 2016)	
Additional objective data for infants and children	
It may be difficult to obtain an accurate measurement of urine volume in infants and young children. Observation of the number of wet nappies and the colour and concentration of urine can give an indication of urine output. In sick children, urinary catheterisation may be required to accurately measure urine output.	The expected urine output for infants and young children is 1 mL/kg/h.

OBJECTIVE DATA

Summary Checklist

URINARY TRACT FUNCTION ASSESSMENT

Subjective data

1. Presenting concern
2. Usual urinary pattern
3. Characteristics of the urine
4. Fluid intake
5. History of change or disturbance to urinary tract function.
6. Pain
7. Lower urinary tract symptoms
8. Other symptoms
9. Past history
10. Health and lifestyle management
11. Environmental issues related to bladder function

Objective data

1. General inspection
2. Vital signs
3. Abdominal examination
4. Inspection of genitalia
5. Post void residual urine volume
6. Examination of urine
7. Fluid balance chart/voiding diary

PROMOTING A HEALTHY LIFESTYLE

UNDERSTANDING PROSTATE CHANGES

The discussion of prostate health and the examination of the prostate gland is a unique aspect of male health assessment. Men should be offered the opportunity to discuss changes in their urinary elimination patterns and sexual concerns. These discussions often give rise to the early signs and symptoms of prostatic changes that may indicate the need for further studies and workup.

Through much of a man's life, the prostate gland is typically the size of a walnut. However, by the time a man is 40, it may grow slightly larger. Although this varies between individuals, this gradual enlargement is considered to be a normal part of ageing. This enlargement is termed benign prostatic hypertrophy (BPH). It does not raise an individual's risk for prostate cancer. However, benign enlargement of the prostate can cause significant and bothersome lower urinary tract symptoms including urinary urgency, frequency, poor stream, hesitancy, post micturition dribble and acute or chronic urinary retention. Treatment can include ongoing monitoring of symptoms, medications, and surgical interventions (typically transurethral resection of the prostate—TURP) (Jiwrajka et al 2018).

Prostate cancer is the most common cancer that occurs in men. The risk of developing prostate cancer to age 75 years is 1 in 23 and to age 85 is 1 in 9 for Australian men (AIHW 2018b). In New Zealand males, the incidence of prostate cancer is estimated to be 1 in 13 to age 75 (Prostate Cancer Foundation of New Zealand 2019). Prostate cancer is essentially a disease of older men with 63% diagnosed after 65 years of age (Cancer Council of Australia 2019). The five-year survival rate for prostate cancer is 95% (AIHW 2019).

Part of the concern for men and for healthcare workers is the non-specific nature of the typical presenting signs and symptoms associated with prostate cancer. In the early stages, they are likely to be asymptomatic. Prostate cancer is typically detected by testing the blood for prostate-specific antigen (PSA) and/or on digital rectal exam (DRE). Differential diagnosis involves a health assessment and will include a prostatic-specific antigen (PSA) test, digital rectal examination (DRE), multiparametric MRI and biopsy (PCFA & CCA 2019). PSA is a substance made by the normal prostate gland. When prostate cancer develops, the PSA level increases. However, benign or non-cancerous enlargement of the prostate (BPH), age and prostatitis can also cause the PSA to increase. Treatment options for prostate cancer include active surveillance, surgery (radical prostatectomy), androgen deprivation therapy, radiation therapy, chemotherapy and immunotherapy.

Documentation and critical thinking

FOCUSED ASSESSMENT: CLINICAL CASE STUDY

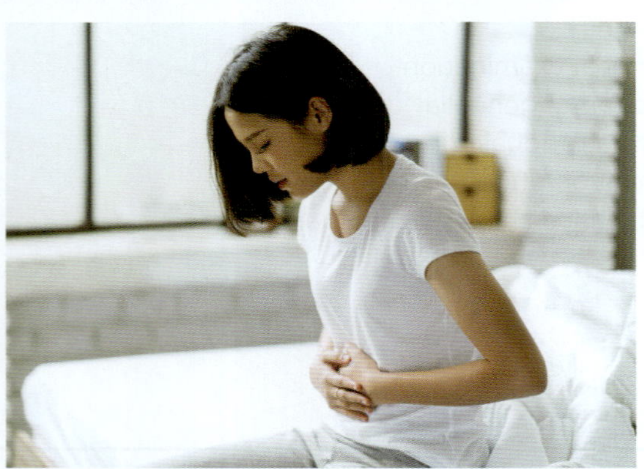

Context

The registered nurse works as a practice nurse in a busy community multidisciplinary health clinic. The role includes screening assessments for people who have not attended the clinic previously.

Subjective

Ms Wan Ching Chee is a 26-year-old woman attending a general practice clinic following sudden onset today of dysuria, urinary frequency and urgency. She has no fever, nausea or flank pain but is complaining of suprapubic pain and discomfort. She has never had a urinary tract infection and has no past medical health problems or surgery. She has recently started a sexual relationship with her boyfriend of 3 months. She takes the oral contraceptive pill but no other medications. Last sexual health check and Pap smear was 1 year ago.

Objective

Vital signs: temp 37°C. HR 72/min. RR 14/min. BP 110/70.

Suprapubic tenderness on palpation. No other areas of tenderness noted. Urine—cloudy and foul smelling. Dipstick test: pH 7.0, protein nil, leucocytes +++, nitrites +++, blood (microscopic) +.

Collaborative problem

Probable lower urinary tract infection.

Problem statements/nursing diagnoses

Pain—dysuria related to probable UTI.

Knowledge deficit about UTI prevention and management (including antibiotic therapy and follow up).

Abnormal findings

TABLE 24.1 Urine colour and discolourations

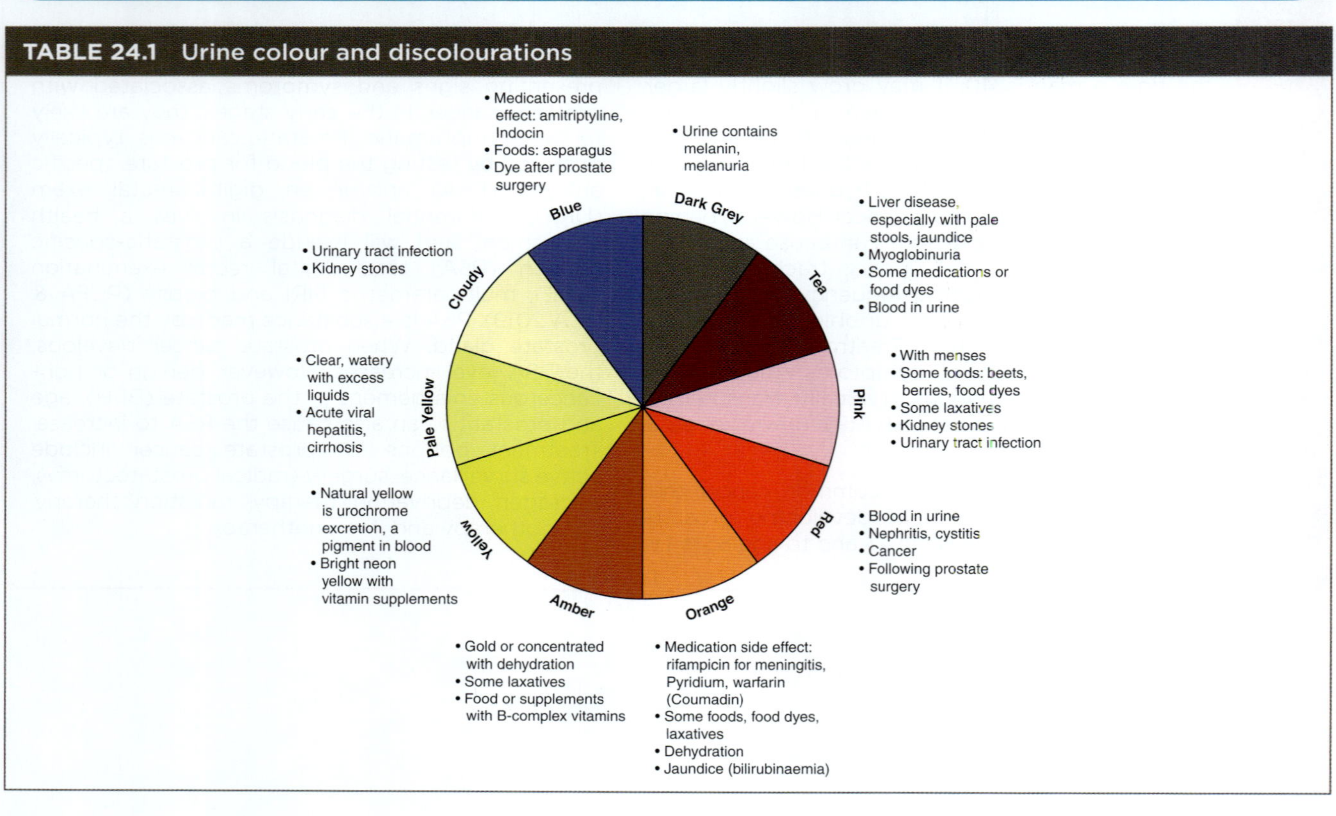

TABLE 24.2 Urinary problems

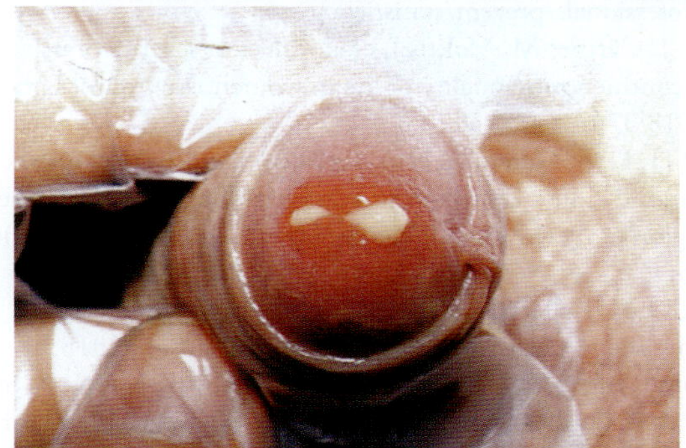

Urethritis (Urethral Discharge and Dysuria)

Infection of urethra causes painful, burning urination or pruritus. Meatus edges are reddened, everted and swollen with purulent discharge. Urine is cloudy with discharge and mucus shreds. Cause determined by urine screen: (1) gonococcal urethritis has thick, profuse, yellow or grey-brown discharge; (2) nongonococcal urethritis (NGU) may have similar discharge but often has scanty, mucoid discharge. Of these, about 40% are caused by chlamydia infection. Guidelines are to treat for both infections if either are found.

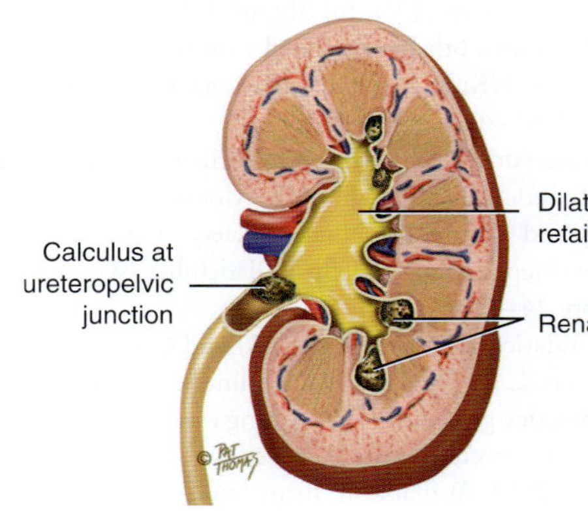

Renal Calculi

Renal stones (crystals of calcium oxalate or uric acid) form in kidney tubules and then migrate and become urgent when they pass into ureter, become lodged and obstruct urine flow, causing hydronephrosis. Cause abrupt severe flank pain with radiation to the groin or abdomen, nausea and vomiting, restlessness, gross or microscopic haematuria.

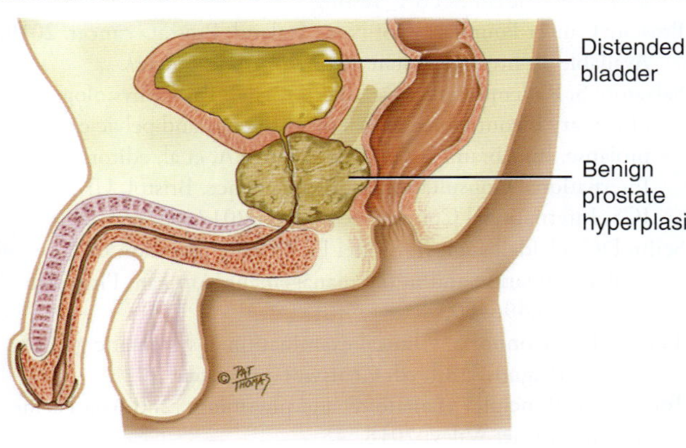

Acute Urinary Retention and Urinary Tract Infection

Inability to pass urine with bladder distension and lower abdominal pain. Common in older men due to bladder outlet obstruction of BPH (see Chapter 26). This can cause UTI, owing to stasis and turbulent flow. UTI incidence increase among men ages ≥60 years and presents with dysuria, frequency, urgency, nocturia, suprapubic pain, occasionally gross haematuria, possibly fever. Treat with antibiotics and address underlying problem.

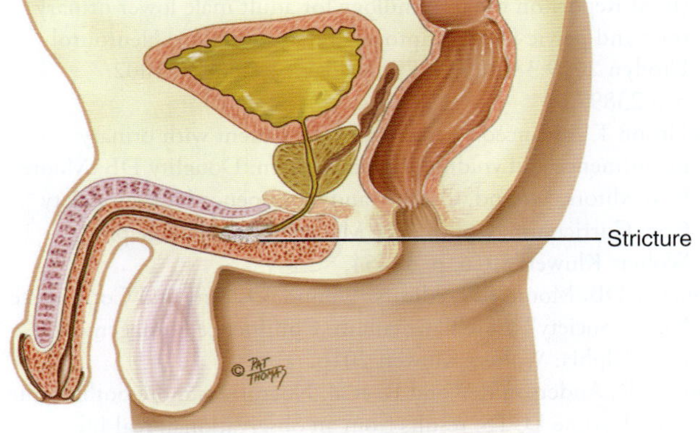

Urethral Stricture

Pinpoint, constricted opening at meatus or inside along urethra. Occurs congenitally or secondary to urethral injury. Gradual decrease in force and calibre of urine stream is most common symptom. Shaft feels indurated along ventral aspect at site of stricture.

BIBLIOGRAPHY

Abrams P, Cardozo P, Wagg A, et al, editors. Incontinence - 6th international consultation on incontinence. 6th ed. Bristol, UK: ICI-ICS, International Continence Society; 2017.

Australian Institute of Health and Welfare (AIHW). Australia's Health 2018. Australia's health, series no. 16. AUS 221. Canberra: AIHW; 2018a. Available at: www.aihw.gov.au/reports/australias-health/australias-health-2018/contents/table-of-contents.

Australian Institute of Health and Welfare (AIHW). Cancer data in Australia – web report. Cat. no: CAN 122. Canberra: AIHW; 2018b. Available at: www.aihw.gov.au/reports/cancer/cancer-in-australia-2019/contents/table-of-contents.

Australian Institute of Health and Welfare (AIHW). Cancer in Australia: In brief 2019. Cancer series no. 122. Cat no. CAN 126. Canberra: AIHW; 2019. Available at: www.aihw.gov.au/publication-detail/?id=60129550047.

Bower W, Everaert K, Ong T, Ervin C, Norgaard J, Whishaw M. Questions to ask a patient with nocturia. Aust J Gen Pract 2018;47:465–9.

Cancer Council of Australia. Cancer types: prostate cancer. 2019. Available at: www.cancer.org.au/about-cancer/types-of-cancer/prostate-cancer.html.

Caruso S, Brescia R, Matarazzo MG, et al. Effects of urinary incontinence subtypes on women's sexual function and quality of life. Urology 2017;108:59–64.

Castro Diaz D, Robinson D, Bosch R, et al. Initial assessment of incontinence in adult male and female patients. In: Abrams P, Cardozo P, Wagg A, et al, editors. 6th International consultation on incontinence. 6th ed. Bristol, UK: ICI-ICS, International Continence Society; 2017. p. 515–56.

Collis D, Kennedy-Behr A, Kearney L. The impact of bowel and bladder problems on children's quality of life and their parents: a scoping review. Child Care Health Dev 2019;45(1):1–14.

Continence Foundation of Australia. Continence in Australia: a snapshot. Melbourne: Continence Foundation of Australia; 2019. Available at: https://continence.org.au/data/files/Reports/Continence_in_Australia_Snapshot.pdf.

Continence New Zealand. Epidemiology—statistics. 2019. Available at: https://www.continence.org.nz/pages/Epidemiology-Statistics/102/.

D'Ancona C, Haylen B, Oelke M, Abranches-Monteiro L, Arnold E, Goldman H, et al. The International Continence Society (ICS) Report on the terminology for adult male lower urinary tract and pelvic floor symptoms and dysfunction. Neurourol Urodyn 2019;38(2):433–77. Available at: doi:10.1002/nau.23897.

Dickinson T. Advanced assessment of the patient with urinary incontinence and voiding dysfunction. In: Doughty DB, Moore KN, editors. Wound, Ostomy and Continence Nurses Society™ Core Curriculum: Continence Management. Philadelphia: Wolters Kluwer; 2016. p. 42–54.

Doughty DB, Moore KN, editors. Wound, Ostomy and Continence Nurses Society™ Core Curriculum: Continence Management. Philadelphia: Wolters Kluwer; 2016.

Everaert K, Anderson P, Wood R, et al. Nocturia is more bothersome than daytime LUTS: results from an observational, real-life practice database including 8659 European and American LUTS patients. Int J Clin Pract 2018;72(6):e13091.

Gammie A, Drake MJ. The fundamentals of uroflowmetry practice, based on International Continence Society good urodynamic practices recommendations. Neurourol Urodyn 2018;37(S6):S44–9. Available at: https://onlinelibrary.wiley.com/doi/abs/10.1002/nau.23777.

Hashim H, Blanker MH, Drake MJ, et al. International Continence Society (ICS) report on the terminology for nocturia and nocturnal lower urinary tract function. Neurourol Urodyn 2019;38(2):499–508.

International Continence Society. Glossary. 2019. Available at: https://www.ics.org/glossary/symptom/feelingofincompletebladderemptying?q=incomplete%20emptying.

Jiwrajka M, Yaxley W, Perera M, et al. Review and update of benign prostatic hyperplasia in general practice. Aust J Gen Pract 2018;47(7):471–5.

Kidney Health Australia. Statistics – Chronic kidney disease in Australia. 2019. Available at: https://kidney.org.au/health-professionals/prevent/statistics.

Krhut J, Gärtner M, Mokris J, et al. Effect of severity of urinary incontinence on quality of life in women. Neurourol Urodyn 2018;37(6):1925–30.

Lloyd H, Li G, Tomlin A, et al. Prevalence and risk factors for chronic kidney disease in primary health care in the southern region of New Zealand. Nephrology (Carlton) 2019;24(3):308–15.

Marieb EM, Keller SM. Essentials of human anatomy and physiology. 12th Global ed. New York: Pearson; 2018.

Milsom I, Altman D, Cartwright R, Lapitan MC, Nelson R, Sjöström S, et al. Epidemiology of urinary incontinence (UI) and other lower urinary tract symptoms (LUTS), pelvic organ prolapse (POP) and anal incontinence (AI). In: Abrams P, Cardozo P, Wagg A, Wein A, editors. 6th International Consultation on Incontinence. Bristol, UK; ICI-ICS, International Continence Society; 2017. p. 2303–426.

Nelles KK. Primary assessment of patients with urinary incontinence and voiding dysfunction. In: Doughty DB, Moore KN, editors. Wound, Ostomy and Continence Nurses Society™ Core Curriculum: Continence Management. Philadelphia: Wolters Kluwer; 2016. pp. 24–43.

Prostate Cancer Foundation of Australia (PCFA) and Cancer Council Australia (CCA). PSA testing guidelines expert advisory panel. Clinical practice guidelines PSA testing and early management of test-detected prostate cancer. Sydney: Cancer Council Australia; 2019. Available at: https:/wiki.cancer.org.au/australia/Guidelines:PSA_Testing.

Prostate Cancer Foundation of New Zealand. Prostate cancer. 2019. Available at: https://prostate.org.nz/prostate-cancer/.

Salvatore S, Rademakers K, DeLancey J, et al. Pathophysiology of urinary incontiennce, faecal incontinence and pelvic organ prolapse. In: Abrams P, Cardozo P, Wagg A, et al, editors. 6th International Consultation on Incontinence. Bristol, UK: ICI-ICS, International Continence Society; 2017. pp. 361–496.

Serlin DC, Heidelbaugh JJ, Stoffel JT. Urinary retention in adults: evaluation and initial management. Am Fam Physician 2018;98(8):496–503.

Talley NJ, O'Connor S. Clinical examination: a systematic guide to physical diagnosis. 8th ed. Chatswood: Elsevier; 2018.

Tortora GJ. Principles of anatomy and physiology. 2nd Asia-Pacific ed. Melbourne: Wiley; 2018.

Wagg A. Why incontinence gets no respect: An international and multidisciplinary perspective. Aust N Z Continence J 2018;24(1):4–6.

Yates A. Understanding incontinence in the older person in community settings. Br J Community Nurs 2019;24(2):72–6.

Websites

Continence Foundation of Australia: www.continence.org.au
International Continence Society: www.ics.org
Kidney Health Australia: www.kidney.org.au
Kidney Health New Zealand: www.kidneys.co.nz
New Zealand Continence Association: www.continence.org.nz
Prostate Cancer Foundation of Australia: www.prostate.org.au
Prostate Cancer Foundation of New Zealand: www.prostate.org.nz

Chapter Twenty-Five

Assessment of bowel function

Written by Carolyn Jarvis
Adapted by Elizabeth Watt

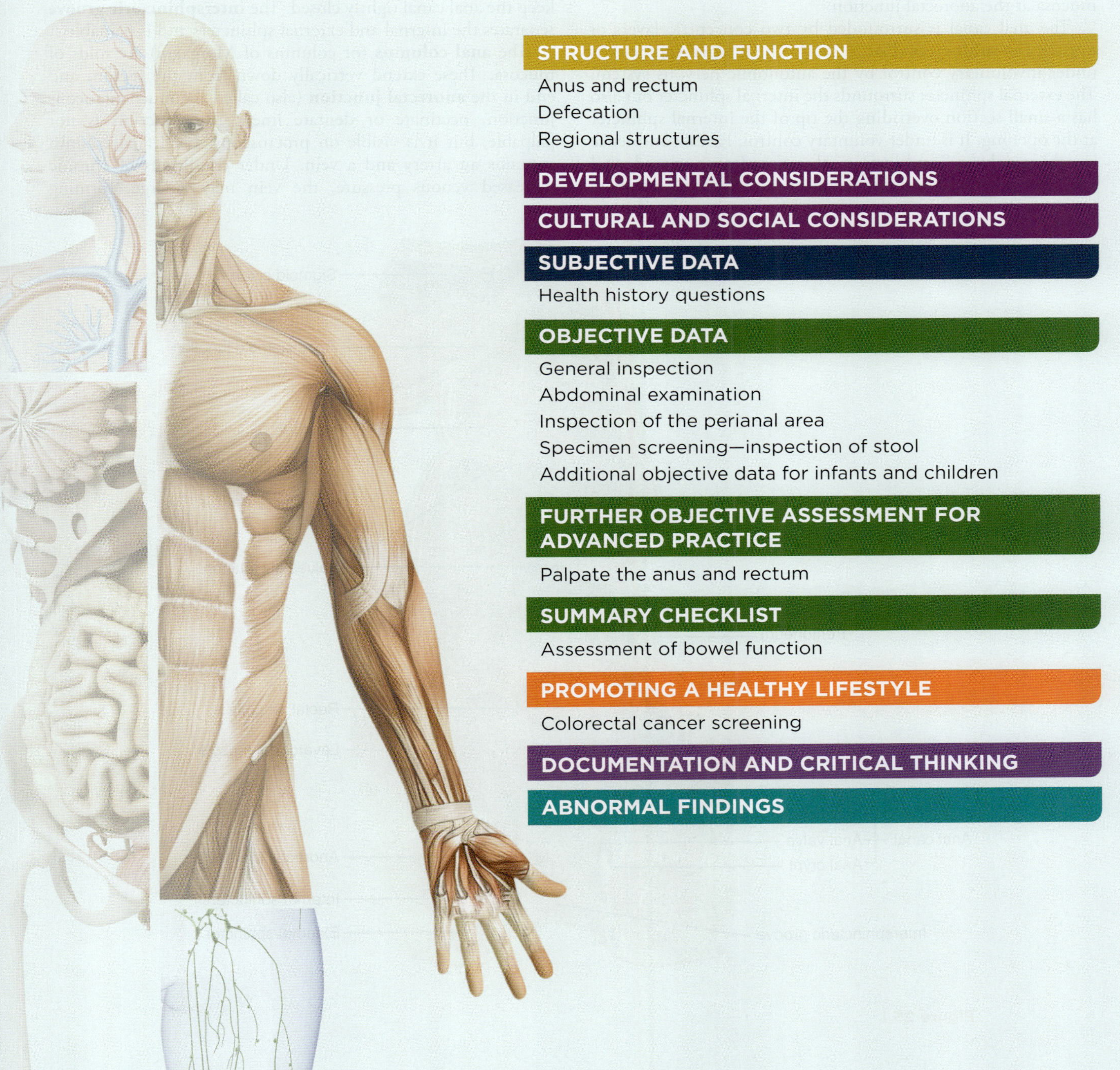

INTRODUCTION

Bowel function assessment is a frequent focus for nurses. Many people have a primary problem concerned with bowel elimination or can develop a bowel health issue secondary to illness, hospitalisation, medical treatments or change of lifestyle. Because so many body systems are involved, as you progress through this chapter you also need to take into account the structure and function related to eating (mouth, teeth and throat) and nutrition (Chapter 21) and the small and large bowel (Chapter 23), as well as the anus and rectum described in this chapter.

Structure and function

ANUS AND RECTUM

The **anal canal** is the outlet of the gastrointestinal tract and is about 3.8 cm long in the adult. It is lined with modified skin (having no hair or sebaceous glands) that merges with rectal mucosa at the anorectal junction.

The anal canal is surrounded by two concentric layers of muscle, the **sphincters** (Figure 25.1). The internal sphincter is under involuntary control by the autonomic nervous system. The external sphincter surrounds the internal sphincter but also has a small section overriding the tip of the internal sphincter at the opening. It is under voluntary control. Faecal continence is achieved by a combination of a competent, closed anal sphincter, normal anorectal sensation and reflexes, adequate rectal capacity and compliance, conscious control, as well as other factors such as stool consistency (Salvatore et al 2017). The pelvic floor also plays an important role in the maintenance of faecal continence and successful defecation (Marieb & Keller 2018). Except for the passing of faeces and gas, the sphincters keep the anal canal tightly closed. The **intersphincteric groove** separates the internal and external sphincters and is palpable.

The **anal columns** (or columns of Morgagni) are folds of mucosa. These extend vertically down from the rectum and end in the **anorectal junction** (also called the mucocutaneous junction, pectinate or dentate line). This junction is not palpable, but it is visible on proctoscopy. Each anal column contains an artery and a vein. Under conditions of chronic increased venous pressure, the vein may enlarge, forming

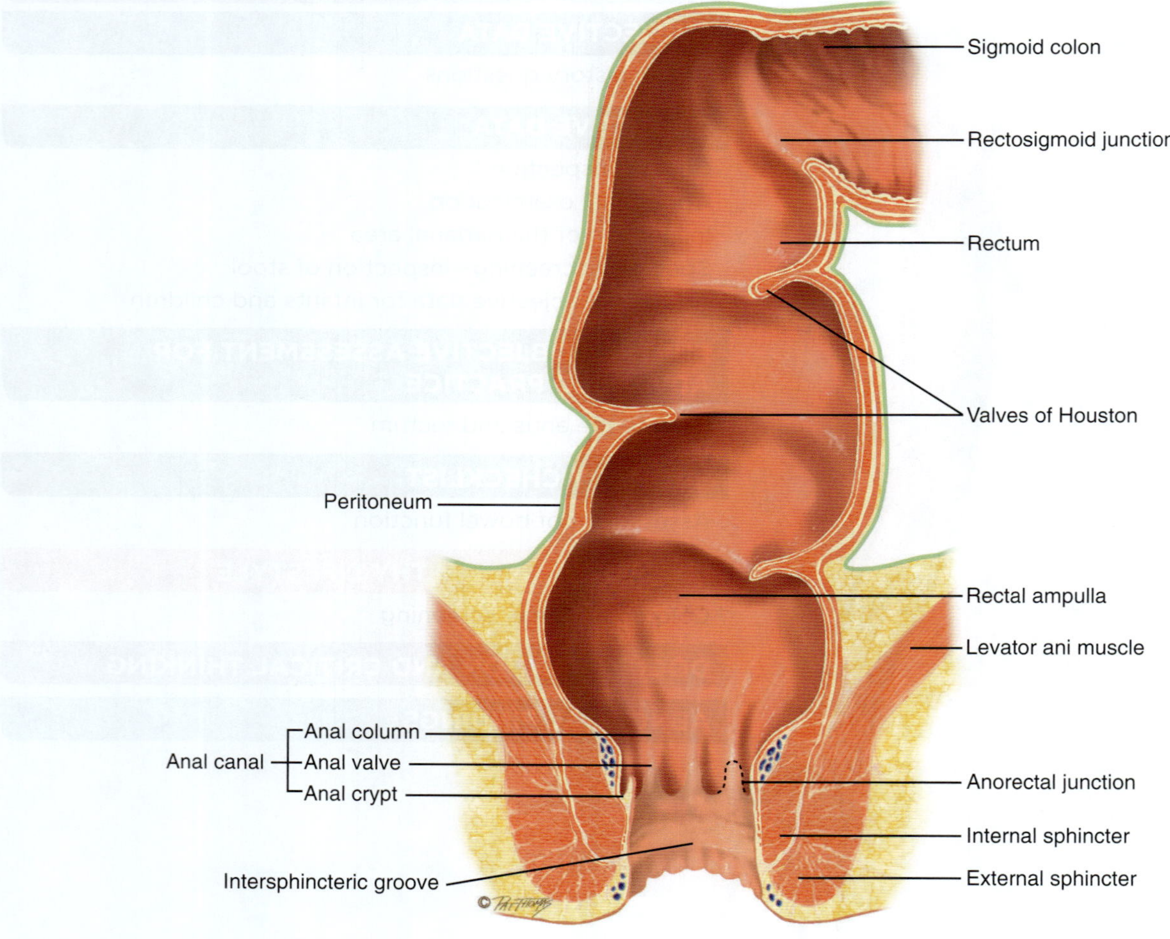

Figure 25.1

a haemorrhoid. At the lower end of each column is a small crescent fold of mucous membrane, the **anal valve**. The space above the anal valve (between the columns) is a small recess, the **anal crypt**.

The canal slants forwards towards the umbilicus, forming a distinct right angle with the rectum, which rests back in the hollow of the sacrum. Although the rectum contains only autonomic nerves, numerous somatic sensory nerves are present in the anal canal and external skin, so a person feels sharp pain from any trauma to the anal area.

The **rectum**, which is approximately 12 cm long, is the distal portion of the large intestine. It extends from the sigmoid colon, at the level of the third sacral vertebra, and ends at the anal canal. Just above the anal canal, the rectum dilates and turns posteriorly, forming the rectal ampulla. The rectal interior has three semilunar transverse folds called the **valves of Houston**. These folds cover half the circumference of the rectal lumen. Their function is unclear, but they may serve to hold faeces as the flatus passes. The lowest is within reach of palpation, usually on the person's left side, and must not be mistaken for an intrarectal mass.

Peritoneal reflection. The peritoneum covers only the upper two-thirds of the rectum. In the male, the anterior part of the peritoneum reflects down to within 7.5 cm of the anal opening, forming the **rectovesical pouch** (Figure 25.2) then covers the bladder. In the female, this is termed the **recto-uterine pouch** and extends down to within 5.5 cm of the anal opening.

DEFECATION

Faecal continence is achieved by a combination of a competent, closed anal sphincter, normal anorectal sensation and reflexes, adequate rectal capacity and compliance, conscious control as well as other factors such as stool consistency (Salvatore et al 2017). The pelvic floor also plays an important role in the maintenance of faecal continence and successful defecation (Marieb & Keller 2018).

Peristaltic movements push faeces from the sigmoid colon into the rectum. As the rectal walls distend, the defecation reflex is stimulated via nerve impulses and the sacral spinal cord, resulting in contraction of the rectal muscles, an increase in pressure within the rectum and relaxation of the **internal anal sphincter** (Tortora 2018). The internal sphincter is a smooth muscle innervated by the autonomic nervous system. As the rectum distends, more faeces enter the rectum. At the same time, impulses travel to the brain to create conscious awareness of the need to defecate. The **external sphincter** is voluntarily controlled. Voluntary constriction of the levator ani muscles will close the anus and defecation can be delayed for a period of time. At the time of defecation, the external sphincter relaxes (Marieb & Keller 2018). A voluntary contraction of abdominal muscles during forced expiration with a closed glottis (Valsalva manoeuvre) causes a rise in intraabdominal pressure to be exerted to assist in expelling faeces.

REGIONAL STRUCTURES

In the female, the uterine cervix lies in front of the anterior rectal wall and may be palpated through it (see Chapter 26). In the male, the prostate gland lies in front of the anterior wall and 2 cm behind the symphysis pubis (see Chapter 27).

The combined length of the anal canal and the rectum is about 16 cm in the adult. The average length of the examining finger is from 6 cm to 10 cm, bringing many rectal structures within reach.

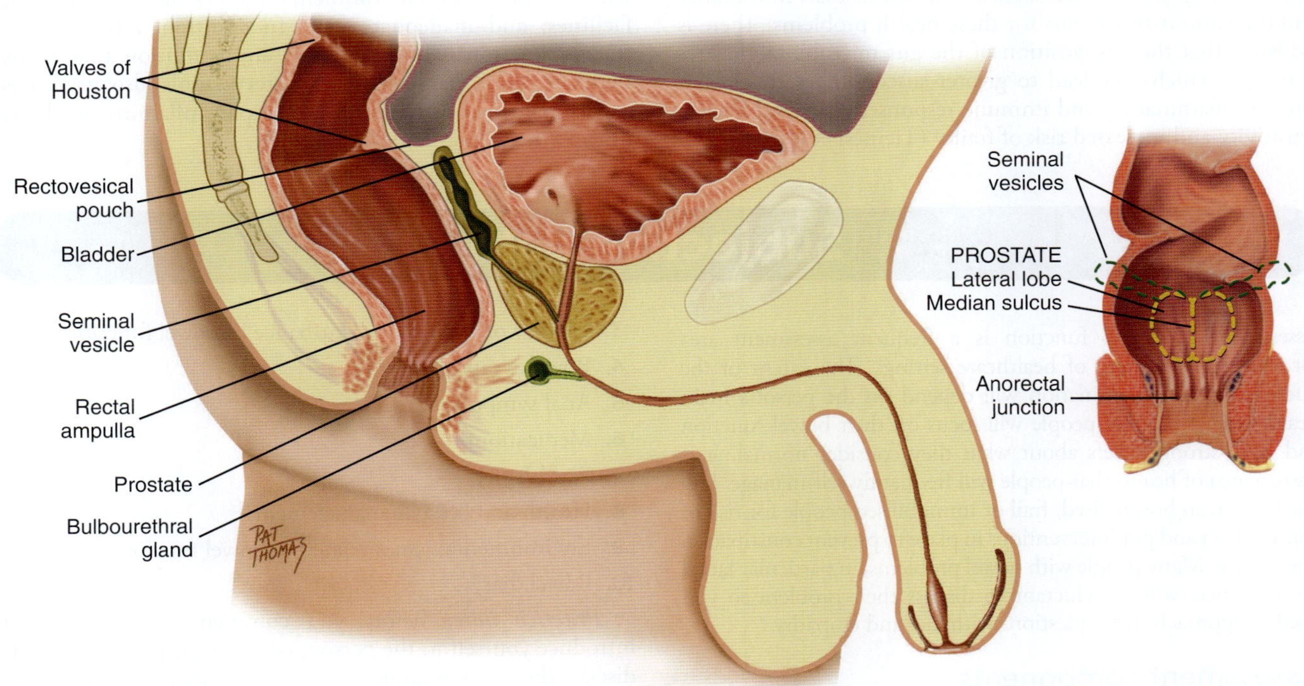

Figure 25.2

The sigmoid colon is named from its **S**-shaped course in the pelvic cavity. It extends from the iliac flexure of the descending colon and ends at the rectum. It is 40 cm long and is accessible to examination only through the colonoscope. The flexible fibreoptic endoscope in current use provides a view of the entire mucosal surface of the sigmoid, as well as the colon.

DEVELOPMENTAL CONSIDERATIONS

Infants

The first stool passed by the newborn is dark green meconium and occurs within 24 to 48 hours of birth, indicating anal patency. From that time on, the infant usually has a stool after each feeding. This response to eating is a wave of peristalsis called the gastrocolic reflex which continues throughout life, although children and adults usually produce no more than one or two stools per day.

The infant passes stools by reflex. Voluntary control of the external anal sphincter cannot occur until the nerves supplying the area have become fully myelinated, usually around 1½ to 2 years of age. Toilet training usually starts after age 2 years.

Late adulthood (65+ years)

There is a widely accepted belief that people are more likely to develop health problems related to bowel function as they age. While there is degeneration of the enteric nervous system with age, gut transit time and colonic motility tend to be consistent throughout life (Marieb & Keller 2018), and most older people maintain the same frequency of bowel movements that they had in their younger years. Known changes that occur with ageing which can affect defecation include a decrease in the resting anal sphincter pressure and impaired rectal sensation (Feldstein et al 2017). However, bowel function is more likely to be influenced by other factors such as chronic disease, immobility and the various treatments for these health problems. There is evidence that the composition of the gut microbiota changes with age, which may lead to greater susceptibility to disease, altered inflammatory and immune response, decreased insulin sensitivity and increased risk of frailty (Ticinesi et al 2019).

CULTURAL AND SOCIAL CONSIDERATIONS

Colorectal cancer is the second most common cancer in Australian men and women (AIHW 2019). There is an increase in the incidence of colorectal cancer with ageing, rising sharply after the age of 50 years. The lifetime risk of developing colorectal cancer for Australians to age 85 years is 1 in 12 men and 1 in 17 women (AIHW 2019). In non-indigenous Australians, there is a 69.5% five-year survival rate for men and a 70.4% five-year survival rate for women (AIHW 2019). New Zealand has similar incidence and survival rates for colorectal cancer in non-indigenous people (Ministry of Health New Zealand 2018). The survival rate from colorectal cancer in Māori people is lower than non-Māori in New Zealand due to disparities in access to cancer screening and treatment and follow-up when a cancer diagnosis is made (Sharples et al 2018). There are also higher colorectal cancer mortality rates for Indigenous Australians (AIHW 2018a). For more information about colorectal cancer and screening programs see 'Promoting a healthy lifestyle' below.

Like urinary incontinence, faecal incontinence has a significant impact on the person. Faecal incontinence is defined as the complaint of involuntary loss of faeces (may be solid and/or liquid) (ICS 2020). It is estimated that faecal incontinence affects approximately 8–15% of adults (Milsom et al 2017) and up to 42% in people living in residential care (de Moraes Lopes et al 2018). Risk factors for faecal or anal incontinence include: acute trauma to the organs, tissues, muscles or nerves involved in defecation; abnormal anal sphincter or pelvic floor function; chronic neurological impairment; congenital anorectal malformations; secondary to degenerative neurological disease; obstruction and impaction with overflow; and environmental factors such as poor toilet facilities; and inadequate care. In addition, advanced age, frailty, functional limitation and any condition that creates frequent, loose, large-volume, watery stools also predispose a person to incontinence; for example, inflammatory bowel disease (de Moraes Lopes et al 2018).

Subjective data

Assessment of bowel function is a frequent assessment area for nurses in a variety of healthcare settings. The extent of the questioning and examination will depend on the person's main health concern. Some people will focus on their bowel function and have strong beliefs about what they consider normal. It is also an area of health that people will frequently self-manage. You need to screen hospitalised, frail or immobilised people for risk of constipation and put interventions in place to prevent constipation developing. Many people with bowel problems, in particular faecal incontinence, will be reluctant to discuss their problem so you need to approach these questions with tact and empathy.

Assessment components

1. Presenting concern
2. Usual bowel pattern
3. History of change or disturbance in bowel function
4. Bowel symptoms
5. Anal symptoms
6. Medications
7. Past history
8. Health and lifestyle management
9. Environmental issues related to bowel function
10. Bowel diary

Practice note: Before you commence the assessment, introduce yourself to the person, confirm the person's identity, discuss the purpose and scope of the assessment, clarify any questions the person may have and obtain verbal consent from the person to perform the assessment.

ASSESSMENT GUIDELINES	CLINICAL SIGNIFICANCE AND CLINICAL ALERTS
1. Presenting concern	
• Do you feel that you have any **problem with bowel function**? • It is important to ascertain the person's perception of their bowel function. • If they do perceive that they have a bowel problem, how does this impact on their quality of life?	
2. Usual bowel pattern	
• Do you have a regular bowel movement? • How often? • Do you have any pain while passing a bowel movement? • Is this relieved when you have finished?	The frequency of bowel movements varies from person to person. Appearance and consistency of the stool is more relevant than frequency of bowel movements. Pain may be due to a local condition (haemorrhoid, fissure), constipation or pathology within the colon.
3. History of change or disturbance in bowel pattern	
• Any **change** in usual **bowel habits**? Can you describe this change for me? • Loose stools or diarrhoea? When did this start? • Is the diarrhoea associated with nausea and vomiting, abdominal pain, something you ate recently?	***Clinical alert:*** Any recent change in bowel pattern could indicate an underlying disease or malignancy; therefore the person should be referred to a medical practitioner for further assessment. **Diarrhoea** can occur with **gastroenteritis, ulcerative colitis, Crohn's disease** and **irritable bowel syndrome**.
• Have you eaten take away food or at a restaurant recently? Does anyone else in your group or family have the same symptoms?	Consider food poisoning.
• Have you travelled overseas or to a remote or rural area during the last 6 months? • Do you live with a pet or farm animals? If so, are they up to date with their immunisations and/or worming treatments?	Consider parasitic infection.
• Have you noticed that it is difficult to have a bowel movement? Do your stools have a hard consistency? Do you have to strain to have a bowel movement? When did this start? • Do you feel that you have completely emptied your bowel when you have been to the toilet?	Consider **constipation**.
4. Bowel symptoms	
• **Rectal bleeding,** blood in the stool: have you ever had black or bloody stools? • When did you first notice blood in the stools? • What is the colour, bright red or dark red-black? • How much blood: spotting on the toilet paper or outright passing of blood with the stool? • Do the bloody stools have a particular smell?	Black stools may be tarry due to occult blood (**melaena**) from gastrointestinal bleeding, or non-tarry from ingestion of iron medications. ***Clinical alert:*** Red blood in stools occurs with gastrointestinal bleeding or localised bleeding around the anus, and also with colon and rectal cancer. The person should be referred to a medical practitioner for further assessment.
• Have you ever had **clay-coloured stools**?	**Clay** colour indicates absent bile pigment.
• **Frothy stool?**	**Steatorrhoea** is excessive fat in the stool as in malabsorption of fat.

SUBJECTIVE DATA

ASSESSMENT GUIDELINES	CLINICAL SIGNIFICANCE AND CLINICAL ALERTS
• **Flatus:** Can you control wind? Passage of flatus is a normal finding. Do you feel that you have excessive wind? Are you able to distinguish between flatus and stool?	The amount of flatus can be affected by diet and underlying intestinal pathology such as food sensitivities. Inability to control the passage of flatus can indicate anal sphincter dysfunction.
• **Urgency:** Do you have any difficulty making it to the toilet in time? How often? What happens? How long can you hang on? • With normal bowel control the person can usually defer for a long period of time after the first urge to defecate.	Consider faecal incontinence. If the person is unable to defer defecation even when the stool consistency is normal they are likely to have poor external anal sphincter function. In this situation the person should be referred to a nurse continence nurse specialist or medical practitioner for further assessment.
• **Passive soiling:** Do you ever experience any leakage from the bowel? Were you aware of this happening? Was it liquid or solid stool? How often does this happen? Does it happen only after you have used your bowels?	Any weakness of the anal sphincter can result in the sphincter not keeping the anal canal closed. Passive soiling is associated with weakness or damage to the anal sphincter.
• **Description of stool:** Ask the person to describe their bowel movement using the Bristol stool chart (Figure 25.3). The Bristol stool chart is a validated tool for describing stool appearance. It is a 7-point scale. Types 3 and 4 are considered to be the most usual or 'normal' consistency.	

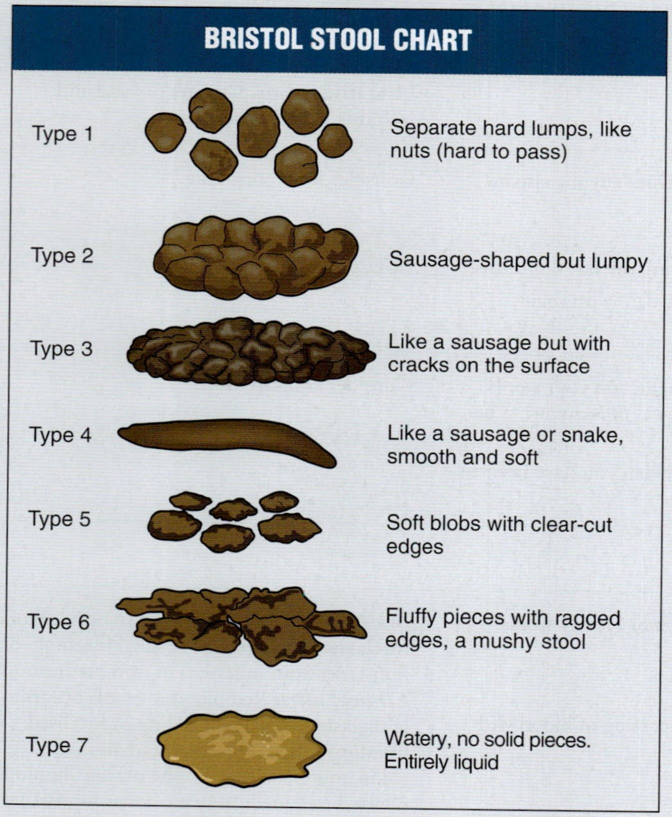

BRISTOL STOOL CHART

Type 1	Separate hard lumps, like nuts (hard to pass)
Type 2	Sausage-shaped but lumpy
Type 3	Like a sausage but with cracks on the surface
Type 4	Like a sausage or snake, smooth and soft
Type 5	Soft blobs with clear-cut edges
Type 6	Fluffy pieces with ragged edges, a mushy stool
Type 7	Watery, no solid pieces. Entirely liquid

Figure 25.3
Bristol stool chart.

ASSESSMENT GUIDELINES	CLINICAL SIGNIFICANCE AND CLINICAL ALERTS
5. Anal symptoms	
• Any problems in anal area: itching, pain or burning, haemorrhoids? How do you treat these? • Any haemorrhoid preparations? • Ever had a fissure, or fistula? How was this treated?	**Pruritus.**
6. Medications	
• What **medications** do you take—prescription, over-the-counter, traditional and complementary therapies? • Laxatives or stool softeners? Which ones? How often? • Iron pills? • Do you ever use suppositories or enemas to move your bowels? How often?	Many prescription medications can cause bowel problems (e.g. narcotic medications). It is important to note what laxatives a person takes on a regular basis. If these are stopped abruptly for any reason this could result in sudden and severe constipation, especially if the laxatives have been taken over many years.
7. Past history	
• Any **family history**: polyps or cancer in colon or rectum, inflammatory bowel disease, prostate cancer? • Any surgery or medical condition which may have contributed to disturbed bowel function? (e.g. gynaecological surgery, abdominal surgery, neurological disease) • For women—obstetric history: How many births? Were forceps used for any of these? Did you have an episiotomy? What were the babies' birth weights? • Did you have any bowel control issues after the births?	Risk factors for colorectal cancer. Labour and delivery, especially prolonged labour and instrumental delivery, can damage the anal sphincter which can predispose the woman to faecal incontinence (Salvatore et al 2017).
8. Health and lifestyle management	
• Diet and fluids: What is the usual amount of **high-fibre foods** in your daily diet: cereals, apples or other fruits, vegetables, wholegrain breads? Spicy foods? How many glasses of water do you drink each day?	High-fibre foods of the soluble type (beans, prunes, barley, carrots, broccoli, cabbage) have been shown to lower cholesterol, while insoluble fibre foods (cereals, wheatgerm) reduce the risk of constipation and colon cancer. Also, fibre foods fight obesity, stabilise blood sugar and help certain gastrointestinal disorders. Inadequate fluid intake is significantly related to the development of constipation. If you find significant risk factors in this area you may need to complete a more detailed nutritional assessment—see Chapter 21.
• **Activity and exercise:** What regular exercise do you undertake? Describe your usual day in terms of exercise and activity. If the person has a very sedentary lifestyle, what do they feel is stopping them being more active?	Lack of activity and exercise are significantly related to the development of constipation. Lack of activity may be related to another health problem; e.g. chronic obstructive pulmonary disease which can cause significant breathlessness on exertion.
• **Smoking:** How much? How long?	Smoking can affect bowel function and is a risk factor for colorectal cancer.
• **Screening:** If 50 years or over—date of last: bowel cancer screening or colonoscopy.	Early detection for cancer. See 'Promoting a healthy lifestyle' below.
• **Pads or pants:** When people disclose bowel control issues ask them if they ever need to wear a pad to protect their clothes from leakage from their bowel. This may give you an indication of the severity of the problem.	

ASSESSMENT GUIDELINES	CLINICAL SIGNIFICANCE AND CLINICAL ALERTS
9. Environmental issues related to bowel function	
You need to make a judgement about whether the following questions are relevant to the individual's situation: • Do you need assistance to get to the toilet? Get the person to describe the level of assistance required. • Do you need assistance with toileting (e.g. undressing, getting onto the toilet)? Get the person to describe the level of assistance required. • Do you find it difficult to get to the toilet (e.g. stairs, distance from living area or bedroom)? Get the person to describe the difficulty. • Do you use toileting aids (e.g. commode chairs, raised toilet seats, support rails)?	Some people will have difficulties getting to the toilet or with activities associated with toileting that may cause them to be incontinent. These need to be investigated so that appropriate interventions can be put in place to improve the situation.
10. Bowel diary	
If the person is experiencing bowel dysfunction it is often necessary to ask them to complete a bowel diary. A bowel diary is used to collect information about the frequency, amount and consistency of bowel movements over a period of time, preferably at least one week. The person is asked to complete a simple chart which details the date and time, description (using the Bristol stool chart, Figure 25.3) and notes about bowel-related symptoms. The data from the chart provides useful information about the severity of symptoms (including incontinence episodes) and the person's actual bowel elimination patterns.	
Additional subjective data for infants and children (questions for parents or guardian)	
• Have you ever noticed any irritation in your child's anal area: redness, raised skin, frequent itching?	In children, pinworms are a common cause of intense itching and irritated anal skin.
• How are your child's bowel movements? Frequency? Any problems? Any pain or straining with bowel movements?	Assess usual elimination pattern. Constipation is a decrease in BM frequency, with difficult passing of very hard, dry stools. **Encopresis** is persistent passing of stools into clothing in a child older than age 4 years, at which age continence would be expected. Can be primary—the child has never attained bowel continence; or secondary—when the soiling occurs after a period of continence (Jinbo 2016).

Objective data

People who have bowel problems frequently have skin excoriation and/or anal abnormalities. The focus in objective assessment is on inspection of the skin and perianal area and inspection of stool. These findings of subjective data collection will guide in deciding if this examination is required. Many people who have bowel problems may also have urinary problems, immobility or nutritional issues. See Chapters 21, 23 and 24 for details of these assessments.

Preparation

The person needs to remove pants/trousers/shorts, as well as underwear and/or stockings.

Ask the person to move into the left (or right) lateral position on a bed or examination couch. Use a sheet, blanket or towel to cover the person.

Make sure that the room is warm and that privacy is maintained.

Equipment needed

Penlight
Non-sterile gloves
Hand hygiene solution

PROCEDURES AND NORMAL FINDINGS	ABNORMAL FINDINGS AND CLINICAL ALERTS
General inspection	
During collection of subjective data you will have noticed the person's height to weight ratio, body shape, ability to move around with ease, level of hygiene and grooming, any obvious body odour and the persons general demeanor. All of these factors provide clues to the person's bowel function and risk factors for dysfunction.	
Abdominal examination	
An abdominal examination should be conducted to identify any factors that can indicate bowel dysfunction. See Chapter 23 for details.	Bloated or rigid abdomen Absence of bowel sounds, or hyperactive bowel sounds Dullness on percussion, especially over the left lower quadrant—may indicate faecal mass Tenderness or mass on palpation
Inspect the perianal area	
• Don non-sterile gloves. • Spread the buttocks wide apart and observe the perianal region. The anus normally looks moist and hairless, with coarse folded skin that is more pigmented than the perianal skin. The anal opening is tightly closed. No lesions are present. Skin is clean.	Inflammation. Lesions or scars. Linear split—**fissure**. Flabby skin sac—haemorrhoid. Shiny blue skin sac—thrombosed haemorrhoid. Small round opening in anal area—**fistula** (see Table 25.1). Perineal soiling may indicate loss of anal sphincter tone and/or poor hygiene practices.
• Inspect the sacrococcygeal area. Normally, it appears smooth and even.	Inflammation or tenderness, swelling, tuft of hair or dimple at tip of coccyx may indicate pilonidal cyst (see Table 25.1).
• Instruct the person to breathe in, hold the breath and bear down by performing a **Valsalva manoeuvre**. No break in skin integrity or protrusion through the anal opening should be present. Describe any abnormality in clock-face terms, with 12:00 as the anterior point towards the symphysis pubis and 6:00 towards the coccyx.	Appearance of fissure, or **haemorrhoids**. Circular red doughnut of tissue—rectal prolapse.
Specimen screening—Inspection of stool	
• Inspect the faecal specimen. Normally, the colour is brown and the consistency is soft. • Use the Bristol stool chart (Figure 25.3) to determine consistency. • Estimate amount of faeces in cups. • See 'Promoting a healthy lifestyle' below for information about the National Bowel Screening Program.	Jelly-like mucus shreds mixed in stool indicate inflammation. Bright red blood on stool surface indicates rectal bleeding. Bright red blood mixed with faeces indicates possible colonic bleeding.
	Black tarry stool with distinct malodour indicates upper gastrointestinal bleeding with blood partially digested. (Must lose more than 50 mL from upper gastrointestinal tract to be considered melaena.) **Black stool**—also occurs with ingesting iron or bismuth preparations. **Grey, tan stool**—absent bile pigment, e.g. obstructive jaundice. **Pale yellow, greasy stool**—increased fat content (steatorrhoea), as occurs with malabsorption syndrome. **Occult bleeding** may indicate pathology within the colon.

PROCEDURES AND NORMAL FINDINGS	ABNORMAL FINDINGS AND CLINICAL ALERTS
Additional objective data for infants and children	
For the newborn, hold the feet with one hand and flex the knees up onto the abdomen. Note the presence of the anus. Confirm a patent rectum and anus by noting the first meconium stool passed within 24 to 48 hours of birth. To assess sphincter tone, check the **anal reflex**. Gently stroke the anal area and note a quick contraction of the sphincter.	**Imperforate anus.**
• Note that the buttocks are firm and rounded with no masses or lesions. Recall that the **mongolian spot** is a common variation of hyperpigmentation in newborns (see Chapter 22).	Flattened buttocks in cystic fibrosis or coeliac syndrome. Coccygeal mass. **Meningocele** (sac containing meninges that protrude through a defect in the bony spine). Tuft of hair or **pilonidal dimple**.
• The **perianal skin** is free of lesions. However, nappy rash is common in children younger than 1 year of age and is exhibited as a generalised reddened area with papules or vesicles.	Pustules indicate secondary infection of nappy rash. Signs of physical or sexual abuse, e.g. anal abrasions, perianal tears. Fissure—common cause of constipation or rectal bleeding in child. (Painful, so the child does not defecate.)
• Inspect the **perianal region** of the school-age child and adolescent during examination of the genitalia.	

OBJECTIVE DATA

Further objective assessment for advanced practice

Nurses working in the acute care setting rarely perform a screening rectal examination; however, they may need to perform a rectal examination as part of a comprehensive assessment of a person with severe constipation, prior to deciding on the most appropriate treatment. You need to make a clinical judgement about the need to perform a rectal examination. Nurse continence specialists may perform this assessment as part of a comprehensive assessment of constipation and faecal incontinence.

You need to fully explain the procedure to be performed and get the person's consent. Make sure that the room is warm and privacy is maintained.

Preparation

The person needs to remove pants/trousers/shorts, as well as underwear and/or stockings.

Ask the person to move into the left (or right) lateral position on a bed or examination couch. Use a sheet, blanket or towel to cover the person.

Make sure that the room is warm and that privacy is maintained.

Equipment needed

Lubricating jelly
Non-sterile gloves
Hand hygiene solution

PROCEDURES AND NORMAL FINDINGS	ABNORMAL FINDINGS AND CLINICAL ALERTS
Palpate the anus and rectum	
Drop lubricating jelly onto your gloved index finger. Instruct the person that palpation is not painful but may feel like needing to move the bowels. Place the pad of your index finger gently against the anal verge (Figure 25.4). You will feel the sphincter tighten, then relax. As it relaxes, flex the tip of your finger and slowly insert it into the anal canal in a direction towards the umbilicus. *Never* approach the anus at right angles with your index finger extended. Such a jabbing motion does not promote sphincter relaxation and is painful.	

PROCEDURES AND NORMAL FINDINGS	ABNORMAL FINDINGS AND CLINICAL ALERTS
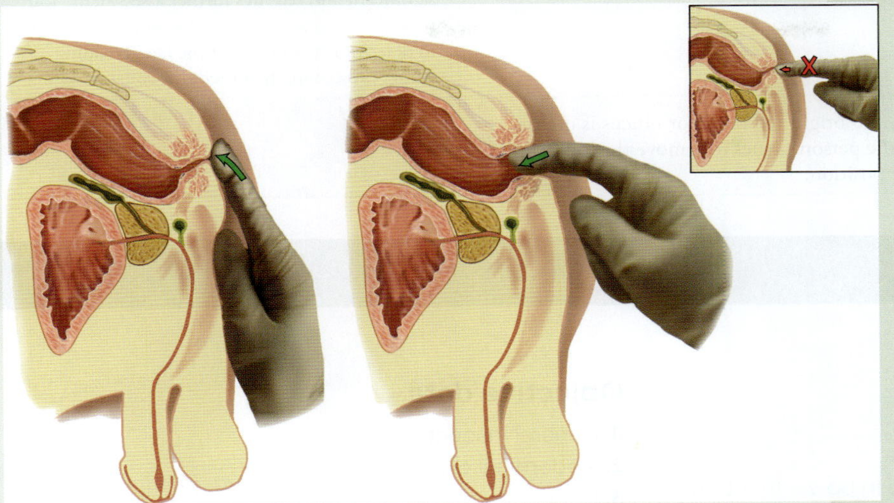 Figure 25.4	
Rotate your examining finger to palpate the entire muscular ring. The canal should feel smooth and even. Note the intersphincteric groove circling the canal wall. To assess tone, ask the person to tighten the muscle. The sphincter should tighten evenly around your finger with no pain to the person. Use a bidigital palpation with your thumb against the perianal tissue (Figure 25.5). Press your examining finger towards it. This manoeuvre highlights any swelling or tenderness and helps assess the bulbourethral glands. 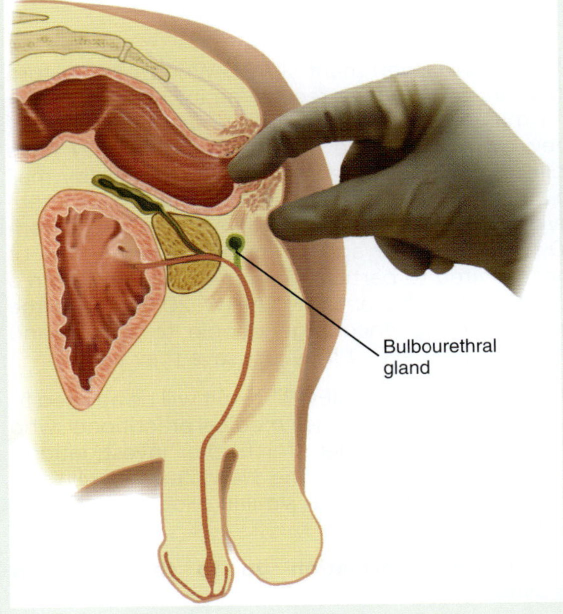 Figure 25.5	Decreased tone. Increased tone occurs with inflammation and anxiety. Tenderness.
Above the anal canal, the rectum turns posteriorly, following the curve of the coccyx and sacrum. Insert your finger further and explore all around the rectal wall. It normally feels smooth with no nodularity. Promptly report any mass you discover for further examination.	Internal haemorrhoid above anorectal junction is not palpable unless thrombosed. A soft, slightly movable mass may be a polyp. A firm or hard mass with irregular shape or rolled edges may signify carcinoma (see Table 25.2).

PROCEDURES AND NORMAL FINDINGS	ABNORMAL FINDINGS AND CLINICAL ALERTS
Palpate any stool in the rectum and assess consistency. Stool should be soft.	Presence of hard stool in the rectum in addition to a history that indicates constipation is significant and requires further assessment. You may also need to perform an abdominal palpation to determine the extent of the faecal loading before prescribing treatment for constipation.
Withdraw your examining finger; normally, no bright red blood or mucus is on the glove. To complete the examination, offer the person tissues to remove the lubricant and help the person to a more comfortable position.	

Summary Checklist

BOWEL ELIMINATION

Subjective data

1. Presenting concern
2. Usual bowel pattern
3. History of change or disturbance in bowel function
4. Bowel symptoms
5. Anal symptoms
6. Medications
7. Past history
8. Health and lifestyle management
9. Environmental issues related to bowel function
10. Bowel diary

Objective data

1. General inspection
2. Abdominal examination
3. Inspection of the perianal area
4. Specimen screening—inspection of stool

PROMOTING A HEALTHY LIFESTYLE

COLORECTAL CANCER SCREENING

National Bowel Cancer Screening Program

Colorectal (bowel) cancer is the second most common cancer in Australian men and women (AIHW 2019). There is an increase in the incidence of colorectal cancer with ageing, rising sharply after the age of 50 years. The lifetime risk of developing colorectal cancer for Australians to age 85 years is 1 in 12 men and 1 in 17 women (AIHW 2019). New Zealand has similar incidence and survival rates for colorectal cancer (Ministry of Health New Zealand 2018). In addition to the risk factors of advancing age and positive family history of colorectal cancer, several signs and symptoms have been associated with colorectal cancer; for example: unexplained weight loss, rectal bleeding, persistent change in bowel habits, and unexplained anaemia (Adelstein et al 2018).

Colorectal cancer screening with an immunochemical faecal occult blood test (iFOBT) has been shown to significantly reduce the morbidity and mortality from bowel cancer (AIHW 2018b). Screening aims to detect colorectal cancer before any obvious signs and symptoms, improving longterm survival. People with a family history of bowel cancer or other risk factors need more intensive screening with regular colonoscopy and other diagnostic tests.

In Australia, the Federal Government funds the National Bowel Cancer Screening Program (Australian Government 2019). When people turn 50 years of age, they receive an invitation through the mail to complete an iFOBT in the privacy of their own home, free of charge. When they have collected the specimens, they return them by mail to a pathology laboratory for analysis. The program invites people for screening every two years from 50 to 74 years of age. Unfortunately, only 41% of those invited to participate in the program return a completed kit for analysis (AIHW 2018c). Take the opportunity to encourage people to collect and return their iFOBT—it may just save their life!

People with a positive iFOBT result will be advised to discuss the result with their medical practitioner, who will generally refer them for further investigations, usually a colonoscopy. The New Zealand Ministry of Health has funded a similar pilot program for New Zealanders.

For further information go to the following websites:

National (Australian) Bowel Cancer Screening Program: www.cancerscreening.gov.au/internet/screening/publishing.nsf/Content/bowel-screening-1

Ministry of Health (New Zealand) National Bowel Cancer Programme: www.health.govt.nz/our-work/preventative-health-wellness/screening/national-bowel-screening-programme

Documentation and critical thinking

FOCUSED ASSESSMENT: CLINICAL CASE STUDY

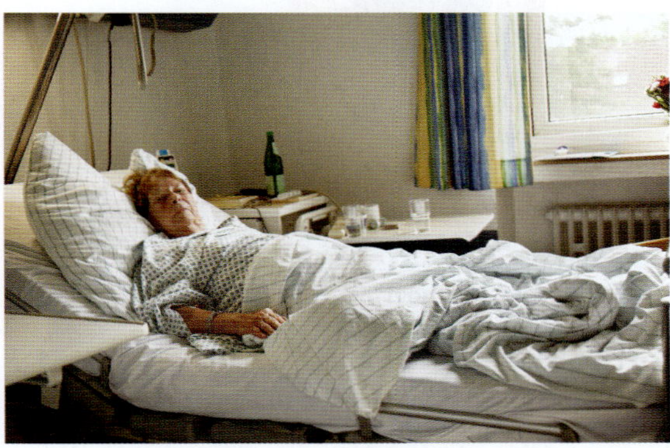

Context

The registered nurse is working on the orthopaedic surgical ward of a large hospital. Mrs Wishart is a 78-year-old woman who had a left total knee replacement 2 days ago. She was previously well with no major health problems other than severe osteoarthritis in the left knee and milder osteoarthritis in the right knee. The surgical procedure went well with no complications. The assessment was performed as part of a general survey on meeting Mrs Wishart at the start of a shift.

Subjective

Mrs Wishart expressed concern that she had not had her bowels opened for 3 days. Normally she has a bowel movement every day and has a soft formed stool which she estimates is Bristol score 3–4 using the Bristol stool chart. She says she now feels bloated and uncomfortable.

She has been eating small amounts of food but feels that her appetite is not good. She normally makes her own breakfast muesli which contains raw oats and oat bran as well as dried fruit and nuts. While in hospital she has been eating buttered toast for breakfast with a cup a tea. She normally eats several pieces of fresh fruit per day but has not been ordering fruit from the menu.

She is drinking tea when offered but not drinking much water as she says it tastes bad.

She took Panadol Osteo for joint pain relief prior to surgery.

Objective

Sitting out of bed for most of the day and walking a short distance several times per shift with gutter frame and assistance. Requiring regular pain medication—oxycodone and paracetamol which has good effect.

Slightly rounded abdomen. Bowel sounds present on auscultation. Abdomen soft on palpation, firm mass in left lower quadrant with mild tenderness—consistent with a faecal mass.

Rectal examination not performed.

Collaborative problem/s

Constipation related to recent surgery, narcotic pain medication, reduced mobility and change of diet.

Problem statement/nursing diagnoses

Constipation related to decreased bowel motility secondary to recent surgery, narcotic pain medication, reduced mobility and change of diet.

Abnormal findings

TABLE 25.1 Abnormalities of the anus and perianal region

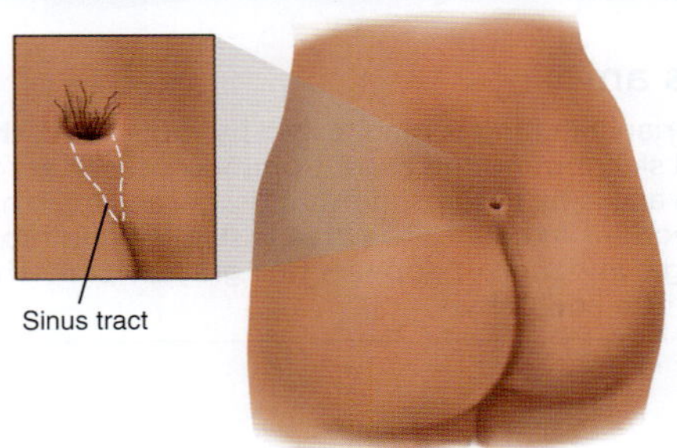

Pilonidal cyst or sinus

A hair-containing cyst or sinus located in the midline over the coccyx or lower sacrum. Often opens as a dimple with visible tuft of hair and, possibly, an erythematous halo. Or, may appear as a palpable cyst. When advanced, has a palpable sinus tract. Although it is a congenital disorder, the lesion is first diagnosed between the ages of 15 and 30 years.

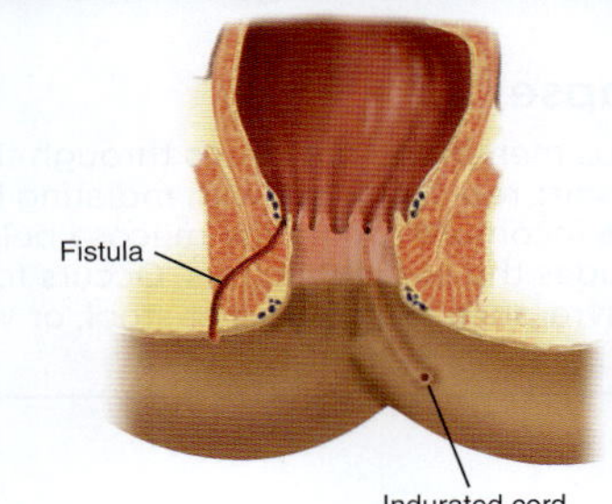

Anorectal fistula

A chronically inflamed gastrointestinal tract creates an abnormal passage from inner anus or rectum out to skin surrounding anus. May result from a local abscess. The red, raised tract opening may drain serosanguinous or purulent matter when pressure is applied. Bidigital palpation may reveal an indurated cord.

(Continued)

TABLE 25.1 Abnormalities of the anus and perianal region—cont'd

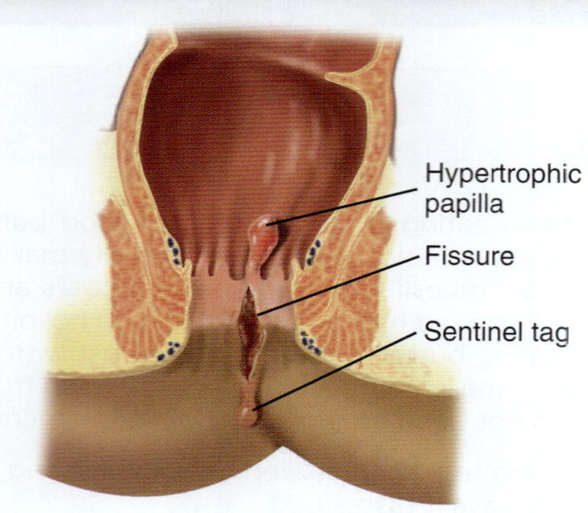

Fissure

A painful longitudinal tear in the superficial mucosa at the anal margin. Most fissures (>90%) occur in the posterior midline area. They are frequently accompanied by a papule of hyperplastic skin, called a sentinel tag, on the anal margin below. Fissures often result from trauma, e.g. passing a large, hard stool or from irritant diarrhoeal stools. The person has itching, bright bleeding (may be noticed on the toilet paper or on stool) and significant pain on defecation. As resulting spasm in the sphincters makes the area painful to examine, local anaesthesia may be indicated.

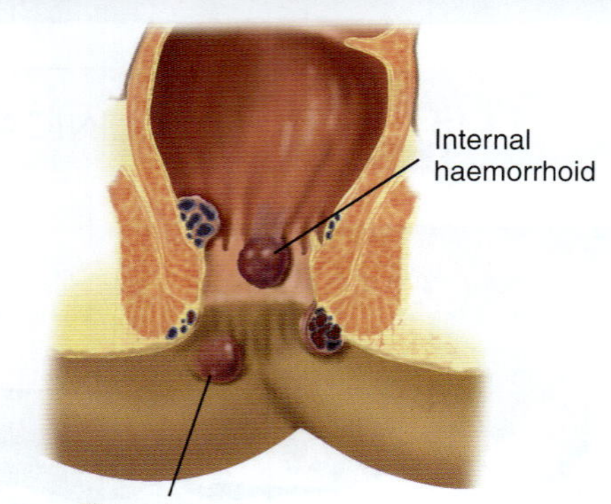

Haemorrhoids

These painless, flabby papules are due to a varicose vein of the haemorrhoidal plexus. An external haemorrhoid originates below the anorectal junction and is covered by anal skin. When thrombosed, it contains clotted blood and becomes a painful, swollen, shiny blue mass that itches and bleeds with defecation. When it resolves, it leaves a painless, flabby skin sac around the anal orifice. An internal haemorrhoid originates above the anorectal junction and is covered by mucous membrane. When the person performs a Valsalva manoeuvre, it may appear as a red mucosal mass. It is not palpable. All haemorrhoids result from increased portal venous pressure, as occurs with straining at stool, chronic constipation, pregnancy, obesity, chronic liver disease or the low-fibre diet common in western society.

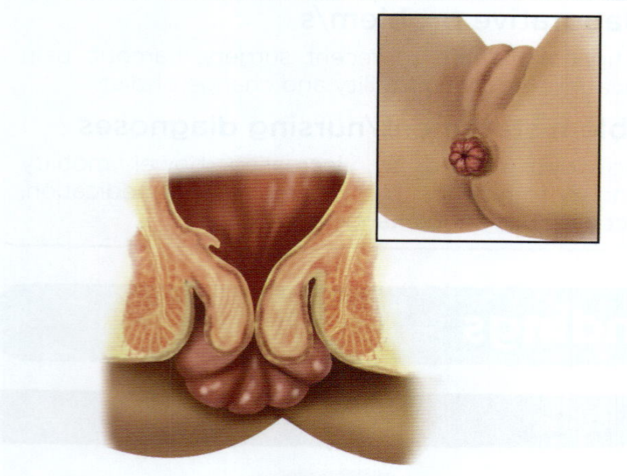

Rectal prolapse

The rectal mucous membrane protrudes through the anus, appearing as a moist red doughnut with radiating lines. When prolapse is incomplete, only the mucosa bulges. When complete, it includes the anal sphincters. Occurs following a Valsalva manoeuvre, such as straining at stool, or with exercise.

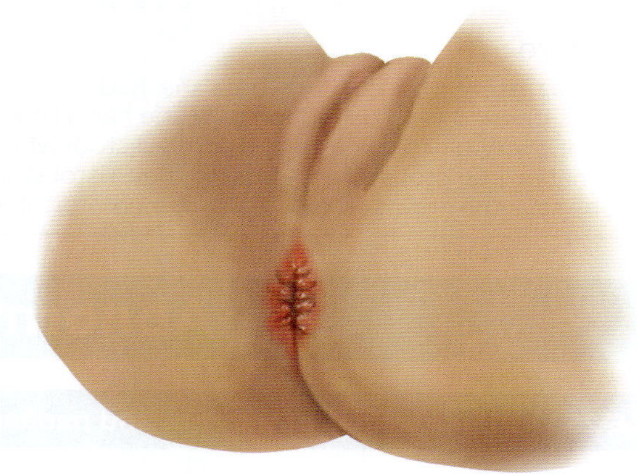

Pruritus ani

Intense perianal itching is manifested by red, raised, thickened, excoriated skin around the anus. Common causes are pinworms in children and anal fissures, dermatitis, chronic diarrhoea, fungal infections in adults. The area is swollen and moist, and with a fungal infection, it appears dull greyish-pink. The skin is dry and brittle and itchy.

TABLE 25.2 Abnormalities of the rectum

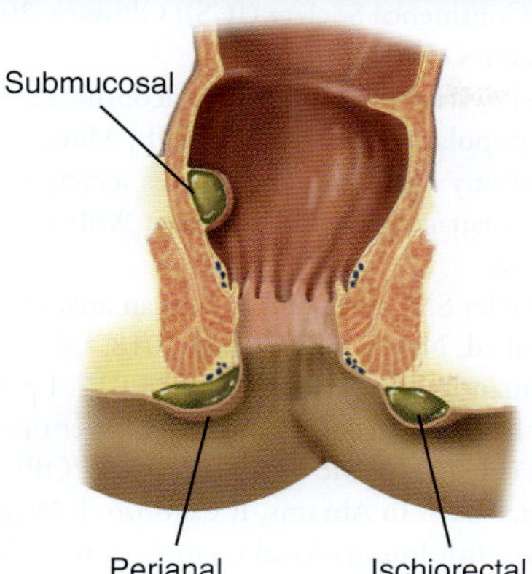

Abscess

A localised cavity of pus from infection in a pararectal space. Infection usually extends from an anal crypt. Characterised by persistent throbbing rectal pain. Termed by the space it occupies, e.g. a perianal abscess is superficial around the anal skin, and appears red, hot, swollen, indurated and tender. An ischiorectal abscess is deep and tender to bidigital palpation. It occurs laterally between the anus and ischial tuberosity and is uncommon.

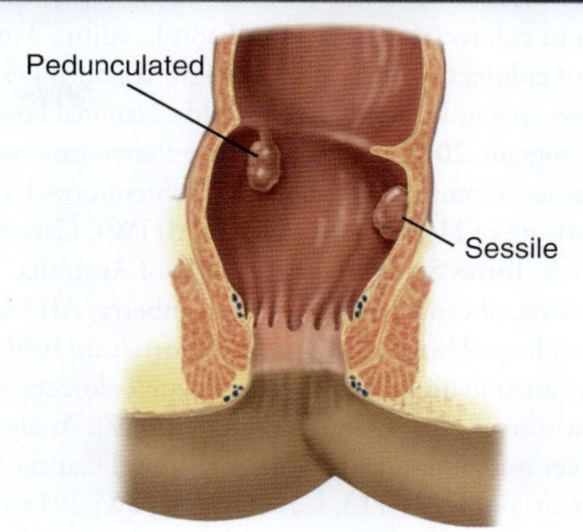

Rectal polyp

A protruding growth from the rectal mucous membrane that is fairly common. The polyp may be *pedunculated* (on a stalk) or *sessile* (a mound on the surface, close to the mucosal wall). The soft nodule is difficult to palpate. Proctoscopy is needed as well as biopsy to screen for a malignant growth.

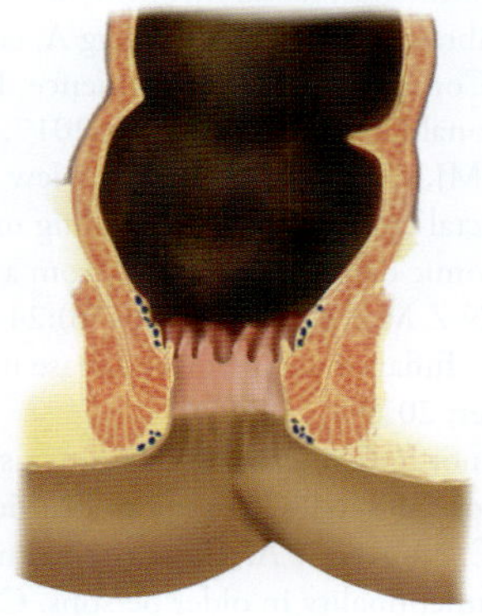

Faecal impaction

A collection of hard, desiccated, immovable faeces in the rectum. The obstruction often results from decreased bowel motility, in which more water is reabsorbed from the stool. For example, in people who have spinal cord injuries, poor diet, lack of exercise, opiate use, cognitive impairment. The person may complain of constipation or of diarrhoea and/or faecal incontinence as a faecal stream passes around the impaction.

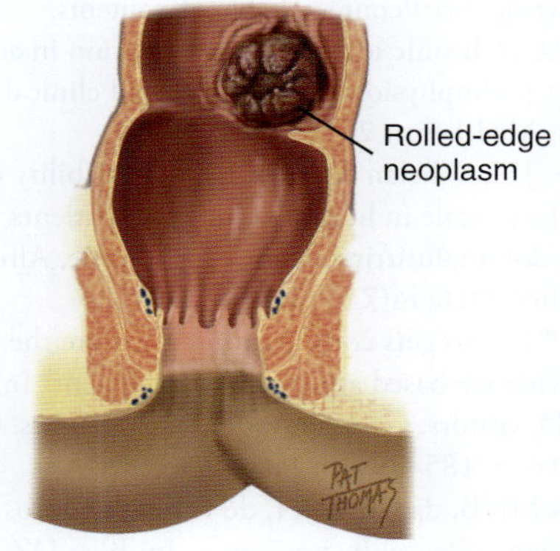

Carcinoma

A malignant neoplasm in the rectum is asymptomatic, thus the importance of routine bowel cancer screening. An early lesion may be a single firm nodule which may bleed. As the lesion grows, it has an irregular cauliflower shape and is fixed and stone hard.

BIBLIOGRAPHY

Adelstein BA, Macaskill P, Katelaris PH, et al. Bowel symptoms in relation to colorectal cancer. In: Olsson L, editor. Timely diagnosis of colorectal cancer. Champaign, IL: Springer; 2018.

Australian Government, Department of Health. National bowel screening program. 2019. Available at: http://www.cancerscreening.gov.au/internet/screening/publishing.nsf/Content/bowel-screening-1.

Australian Institute of Health and Welfare (AIHW). Cancer in Aboriginal & Torres Strait Islander people of Australia. Web report. Colorectal cancer (C18–C20). Canberra: AIHW; 2018a. Available at: https://www.aihw.gov.au/reports/can/109/cancer-in-indigenous-australians/contents/cancer-type/colorectal-cancer.

Australian Institute of Health and Welfare (AIHW). Analysis of bowel cancer outcomes for the National Bowel Cancer Screening Program, Cat. no. CAN 113. Canberra: AIHW; 2018b. Available at: https://www.aihw.gov.au/reports/cancer-screening/analysis-of-bowel-cancer-outcomes-nbcsp-2018/contents/summary.

Australian Institute of Health and Welfare (AIHW). National Bowel Cancer Screening Program: monitoring report 2018. Cat. no. CAN 112. Canberra: AIHW; 2018c. Available at: https://www.aihw.gov.au/reports/cancer-screening/national-bowel-cancer-screening-program-2018/contents/summary.

Australian Institute of Health and Welfare (AIHW). Cancer in Australia 2019. Cancer series no.119. Cat. no. CAN 123. Canberra: AIHW; 2019. Available at: https://www.aihw.gov.au/reports/cancer/cancer-in-australia-2019/contents/table-of-contents.

Black CJ, Ford AC. Chronic idiopathic constipation in adults: epidemiology, pathophysiology, diagnosis and clinical management. Med J Aust 2018;209(2):86-91.

Blake MR, Raker JM, Whelan K. Validity and reliability of the Bristol stool form scale in healthy adults and patients with diarrhoea-predominant irritable bowel syndrome. Aliment Pharmacol Ther 2016;44(7):693-703.

Caffrey J, Pensa G. Who gets constipation? What are the causes? What is an evidence-based approach management? In: Graham A, Carlberg D, editors. Gastrointestinal emergencies. Cham: Springer; 2019. p. 185–7.

de Moraes Lopes MHB, da Costa JN, de Gouveia Santos VLC, et al. Epidemiology of faecal incontinence. In: Bliss DZ, editor. Management of faecal incontinence for the advanced practice nurse. Champaign, IL: Springer; 2018. p. 49–62.

Feldstein RC, Beyda DJ, Katz S. Ageing and the gastrointestinal system. In: Fillit HM, Rockwood K, Young J, editors. Brocklehurst's textbook of geriatric medicine and gerontology. 8th ed. Philadelphia: Elsevier; 2017. pp. 127–32.

International Continence Society (ICS). Glossary. 2020. Available at: https://www.ics.org/glossary.

Jinbo A. Bowel dysfunction and faecal incontinence in the paediatric population. In: Doughty DB, Moore KN, editors. Wound, ostomy and continence nurses society core curriculum: continence management. Philadelphia: Wolters Kluwer; 2016. pp. 238–356.

Marieb EM, Keller SM. Essentials of human anatomy and physiology. 12th Global ed. New York: Pearson; 2018.

Milsom I, Altman D, Cartwright R, et al. 2017. Epidemiology of urinary incontinence (UI) and other lower urinary tract symptoms (LUTS), pelvic organ prolapse (POP) and anal incontinence (AI). In Abrams, P, Cardozo, P, Wagg, A, et al, editors. 6th International Consultation on Incontinence. International Continence Society, Bristol, UK.: ICI-ICS, pp. 2303–2426.

Ministry of Health New Zealand. New cancer registrations. Wellington: Ministry of Health; 2018. Available at: https://www.health.govt.nz/nz-health-statistics/health-statistics-and-data-sets/cancer-new-registrations-and-deaths-series.

Mitchell A. Carrying out a holistic assessment of a patient with constipation. Br J Nurs 2019;28(4):230-2.

Salvatore S, Rademakers K, DeLancey J, et al. Pathophysiology of urinary incontinence, faecal incontinence and pelvic organ prolapse. In: Abrams P, Cardozo P, Wagg A, et al, editors. 6th International Consultation on Incontinence. Bristol, UK: ICI-ICS, International Continence Society; 2017. pp. 361–496.

Sharples KJ, Firth MJ, Hinder VA, et al. The New Zealand PIPER Project: colorectal cancer survival according to rurality, ethnicity and socioeconomic deprivation-results from a retrospective cohort study. N Z Med J 2018;131(1476):24–39.

Sturm A, White L. Inflammatory bowel disease nursing manual. Cham: Springer; 2019.

Talley NJ, O'Connor S. Clinical examination: a systematic guide to physical diagnosis. 8th ed. Chatswood: Elsevier; 2018.

Ticinesi A, Tana C, Nouvenne A. The intestinal microbiome and its relevance for functionality in older persons. Curr Opin Clin Nutr Metab Care 2019;22(1):4–12.

Tortora GJ. Principles of anatomy and physiology. 2nd Asia-Pacific ed. Melbourne: Wiley; 2018.

Assessing sexuality and reproductive function

Unit 9

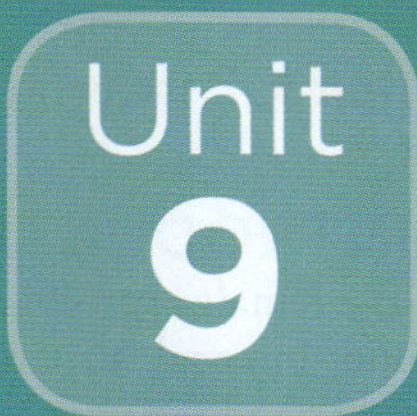

Chapter Twenty-Six

Female sexual and reproductive assessment

Written by Carolyn Jarvis
Adapted by David Lee

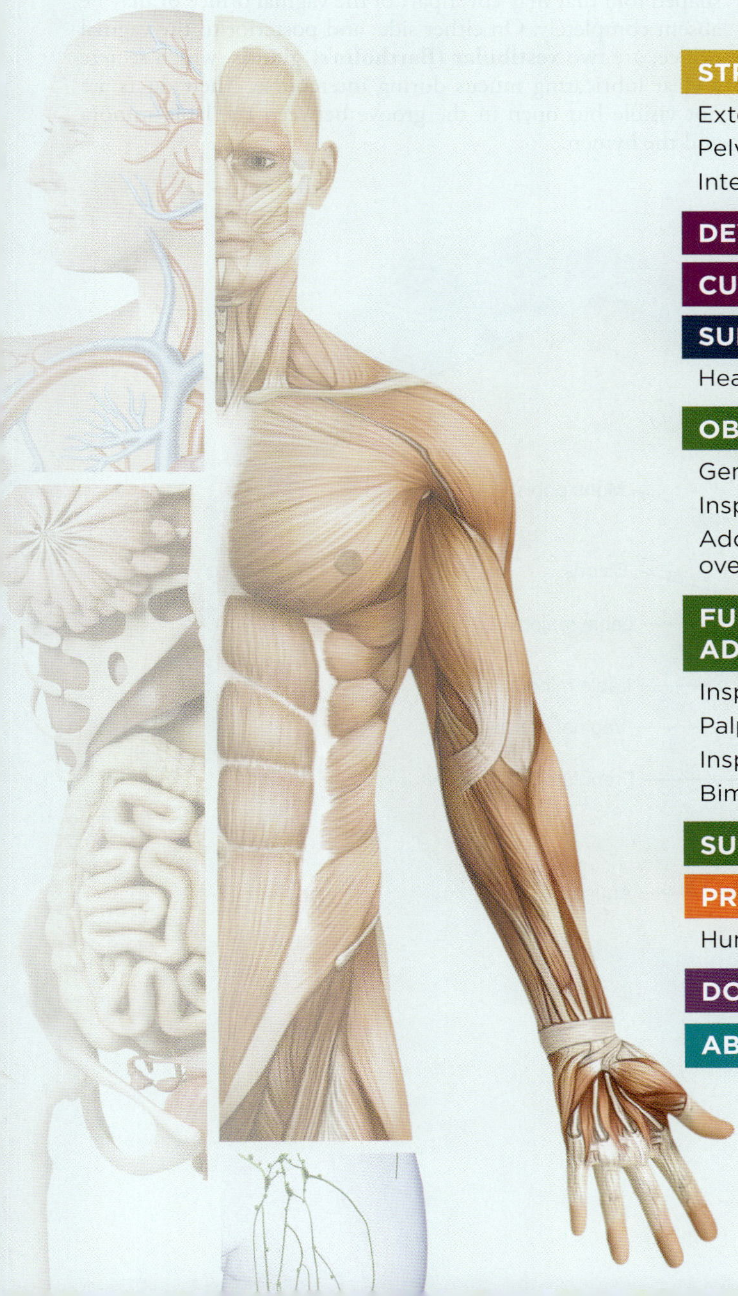

INTRODUCTION

The female reproductive structures include the external genitalia and internal structures: the vagina, cervix, uterus, fallopian tubes and ovaries. The pelvic floor muscles, ligaments and fascia form an important support structure for the internal organs of the lower pelvis. As the organs and muscles of the abdomen, urinary tract and bowel are also relevant to female sexual and reproductive function (refer to Chapters 23, 24 and 25).

Structure and function

EXTERNAL GENITALIA

The external genitalia are called the **vulva**, or pudendum (Figure 26.1). The **mons pubis** is a round, firm pad of adipose tissue covering the symphysis pubis. After puberty, it is covered with hair in the pattern of an inverted triangle. The **labia majora** are two rounded folds of adipose tissue extending from the mons pubis down and around to the perineum. After puberty, hair covers the outer surfaces of the labia, whereas the inner folds are smooth and moist and contain sebaceous follicles.

Inside the labia majora are two smaller, darker folds of skin, the **labia minora**. These are joined anteriorly at the clitoris where they form a hood, or prepuce. The labia minora are joined posteriorly by a transverse fold, the **frenulum** or fourchette. The **clitoris** is a small, pea-shaped erectile body, homologous with the male penis and highly sensitive to tactile stimulation.

The labial structures encircle a boat-shaped space, or cleft, termed the **vestibule**. Within it are numerous openings. The **urethral meatus** appears as a dimple 2.5 cm posterior to the clitoris. Surrounding the urethral meatus are the tiny, multiple **paraurethral (Skene's) glands**. Their ducts are not visible but open posterior to the urethra at the 5 and 7 o'clock positions.

The **vaginal orifice** is posterior to the urethral meatus. It appears either as a thin median slit or as a large opening with irregular edges, depending on the presentation of the membranous **hymen**. The hymen is a thin, circular or crescent-shaped fold that may cover part of the vaginal orifice or may be absent completely. On either side, and posterior to the vaginal orifice, are two **vestibular (Bartholin's) glands**, which secrete a clear lubricating mucus during intercourse. Their ducts are not visible but open in the groove between the labia minora and the hymen.

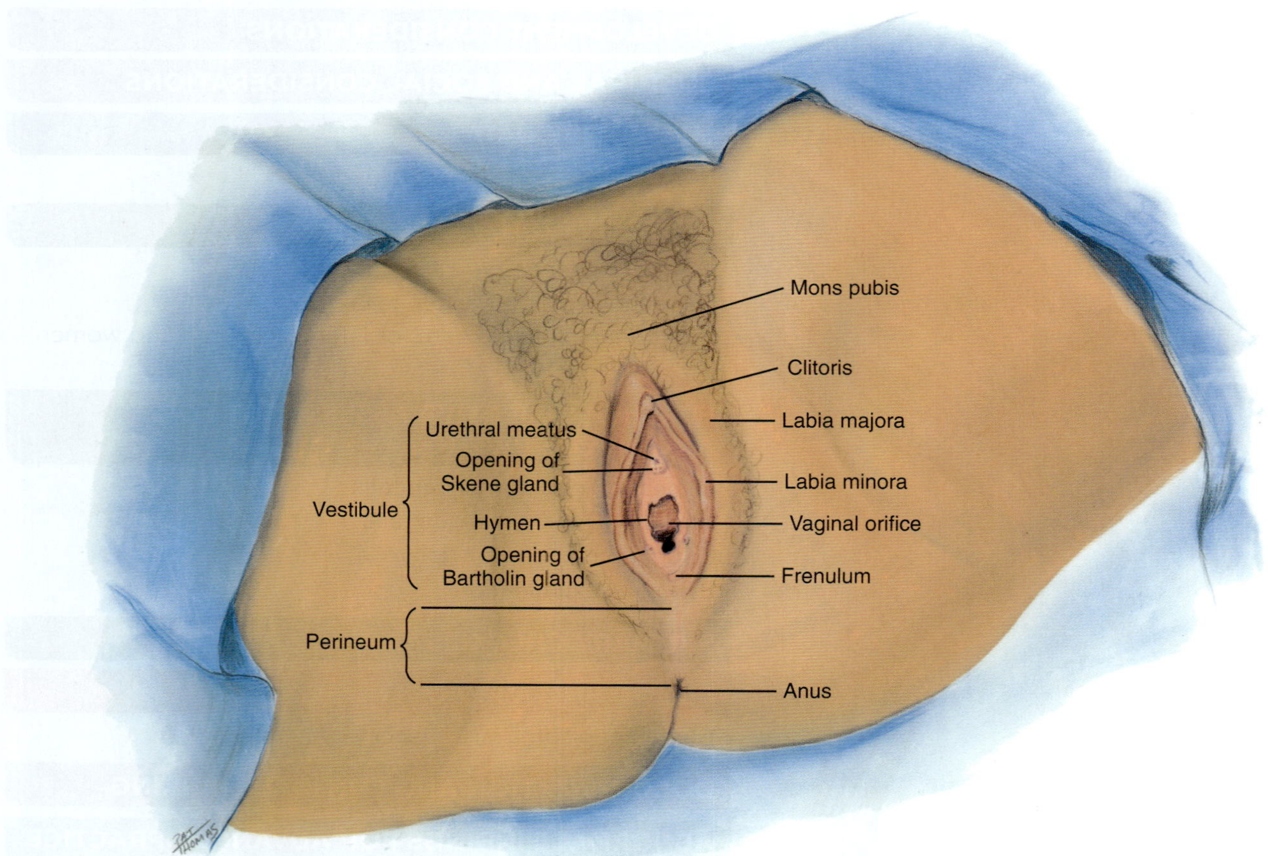

Figure 26.1

PELVIC FLOOR MUSCLES AND PERINEUM

The bony pelvis forms the solid structure for the muscles and ligaments of the anterior, posterior and lateral pelvic walls and pelvic floor which play such an important role in supporting the position of the pelvic organs. The pelvic floor muscles include the coccygeus muscle and the levator ani and are referred to as the pelvic diaphragm, which stretches from the pubic bone anteriorly to the coccyx posteriorly and from the right and left lateral pelvic walls. The anal canal, urethra and vagina pass through the pelvic diaphragm. The levator ani muscles support the pelvic organs and functions as a sphincter for the anal canal and urethra (Tortora et al 2019).

The perineum is located inferior to the pelvic diaphragm. The perineum extends from the symphysis pubis anteriorly to the coccyx posteriorly and the ischial tuberosities laterally. The muscles of the perineum are in two layers, superficial and deep. The superficial layer includes the superficial transverse perineal, bulbospongiosus and the ischiocavernosus muscles which help to maintain erection of the clitoris. The deep layer of the perineum includes the deep transverse perineal muscle, the external urethral sphincter and external anal sphincter which assist in maintaining urinary and faecal continence (Tortora et al 2019).

INTERNAL GENITALIA

The internal genitalia include the **vagina**, a flattened, tubular canal extending from the orifice up and backwards into the pelvis (Figure 26.2). It is 9 cm long and sits between the rectum posteriorly and the bladder and urethra anteriorly. Its walls are in thick transverse folds, or **rugae**, enabling the vagina to dilate widely during childbirth.

At the end of the canal, the uterine **cervix** projects into the vagina. In the nulliparous female, the cervix appears as a smooth doughnut-shaped area with a small circular hole, or **os**. After childbirth, the os is slightly enlarged and irregular. The cervical epithelium is of two distinct types. The vagina and cervix are covered with smooth, pink, stratified squamous epithelium. Inside the os, the endocervical canal is lined with columnar epithelium that looks red and rough. The point where these two tissues meet is the **squamocolumnar junction** and is not visible.

A continuous recess is present around the cervix, termed the **anterior fornix** in front and the **posterior fornix** at the back. Behind the posterior fornix, another deep recess is formed by the peritoneum. It dips down between the rectum and cervix to form the **rectouterine pouch**, or **cul-de-sac of Douglas**.

The **uterus** is a pear-shaped, thick-walled, muscular organ. It is flattened anteroposteriorly, measuring 5.5 to 8 cm long by 3.5 to 4 cm wide and 2 to 2.5 cm thick. It is freely movable, not fixed, and usually tilts forwards and superior to the bladder (a position labelled as anteverted and anteflexed; see Figure 26.21 below).

The **fallopian tubes** are two pliable, trumpet-shaped tubes, 10 cm in length, extending from the uterine fundus laterally to the brim of the pelvis. There they curve posteriorly, their fimbriated ends located near the **ovaries**. The two ovaries are located one on each side of the uterus at the level of the anterior superior iliac spine. Each is oval shaped, 3 cm long by 2 cm wide by 1 cm thick and serves to develop ova (eggs) and the female hormones.

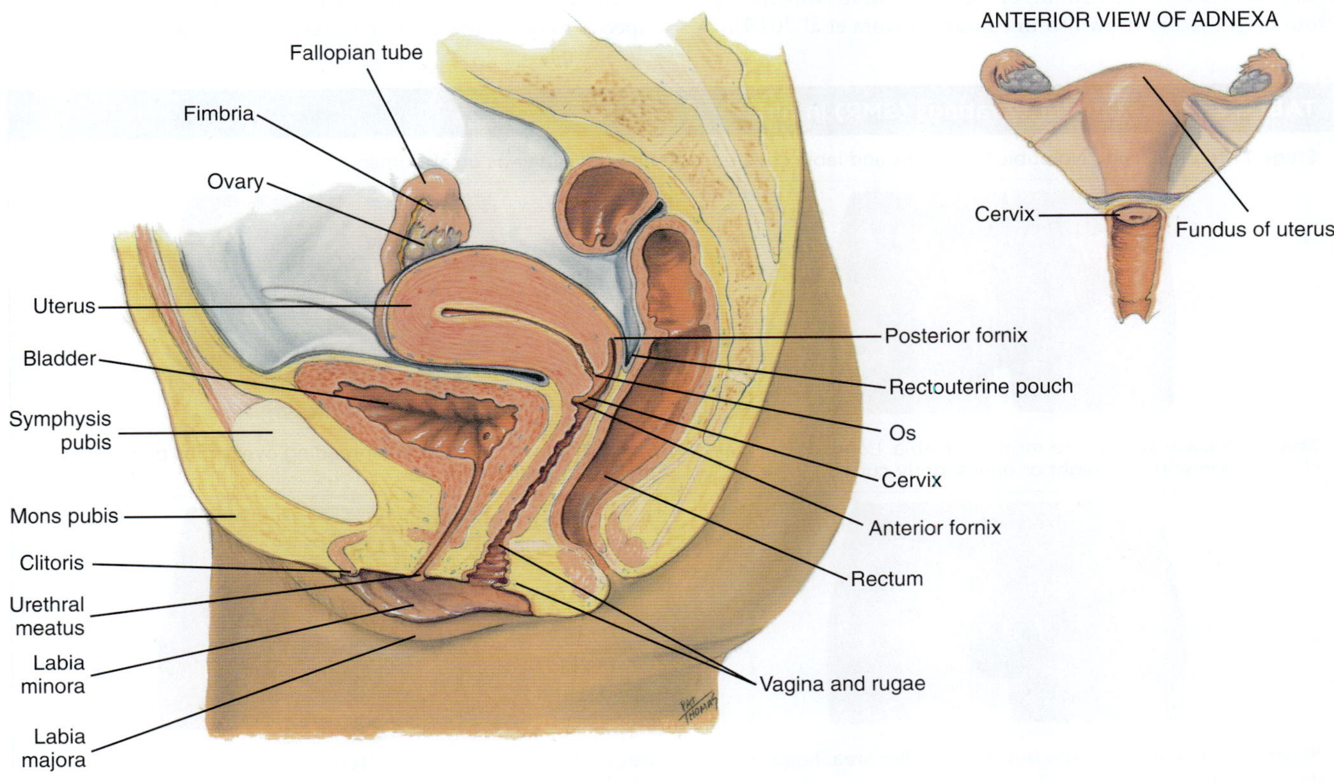

Figure 26.2

DEVELOPMENTAL CONSIDERATIONS

Infants and adolescents

At birth, the external genitalia are engorged because of the presence of maternal oestrogen. The structures recede in a few weeks, remaining small until puberty. The ovaries are located in the abdomen during childhood. The uterus is small with a straight axis and no anteflexion.

At puberty, oestrogens stimulate the growth of cells in the reproductive tract and the development of secondary sex characteristics. The first signs of puberty are breast and pubic hair development, beginning between the ages of 8½ and 13 years. Menarche occurs during the latter half of this sequence, just after the peak of growth velocity. Irregularity of the menstrual cycle is common during adolescence because of the girl's occasional failure to ovulate. With menarche, the uterine body flexes on the cervix. The ovaries are now in the pelvic cavity.

Tanner's table on the five stages of pubic hair development (sex maturity ratings) is helpful in teaching girls the expected sequence of sexual development (see Table 26.1). These data may not necessarily generalise to all people as there are wide individual variations in development.

The adult woman

A woman will experience an average of 450 to 500 menstrual bleeding (or a period) throughout her lifetime. The menstrual cycle start is counted from the first day of a bleed (period) and ends on the first day of bleeding of the next cycle. The menstrual cycle varies for each individual and averages between 21 to 42 days. Periods (bleeding) tends to last between 4 and 8 days and loses 40 to 150 mL of menstrual fluid, which ranges from bright red to brownish in colour (Tortora et al 2019).

The ovulatory phase of the period (mid-cycle) occurs before Day 14 (of a 28 day cycle) when there is a surge of luteinising hormone (LH) which stimulates mature follicles in an ovary to release an egg (ovulation) and this is the time when fertility is high, and pregnancy is most likely to occur (Tortora et al 2019). Some women may experience this phase of their cycle when she experiences 'period pain' (mittelschmerz) unilaterally localised on either side of the abdomen and may be described as 'a twinge' to 'severe abdominal pain' lasting a few minutes to a few hours (Tortora et al 2019).

The menstrual cycle is a conjoint of hormonal hypothalmus control and hormonal release from the ovaries and it aims to prepare the body for pregnancy. The resultant of a non-pregnant state will result in a period. This complex hormonal relationship ends up with ovulation (release of eggs from the ovaries) and thickens the lining of the endometrium (proliferative phase) (Figure 26.3). Further to preparing the woman for pregnancy, the menstrual cycle has no other known physiological features.

The vaginal microbiome (or environment) has an important role in sexual and reproductive health and provides a protective physical and immunological barrier to invasive organisms. The vaginal microbiome protects pathogens from bypassing the cervix through metabolism of glycogen, which produces lactic acid and acidifies the vaginal environment. The optimal vaginal microbiota is dominated by beneficial *Lactobacillus* species (for example *L. crispatus*, *L. iners*). The healthy vaginal pH is typically < 4.5, in which *Lactobacillus* can survive but is too acidic for several other types of bacteria (Champer et al 2018). Changes in the microbiome may be caused hormonally, neurologically, physiologically or by medical treatments such as antibiotic use. These factors can cause a change in the pH towards a less acidic environment and enable other vaginal bacteria or *Candida* species to overgrow, causing infection (Champer et al 2018).

TABLE 26.1 Sex maturity ratings (SMR) in girls

Stage 1 Preadolescent. No pubic hair. Mons and labia covered with fine vellus hair as on abdomen.	
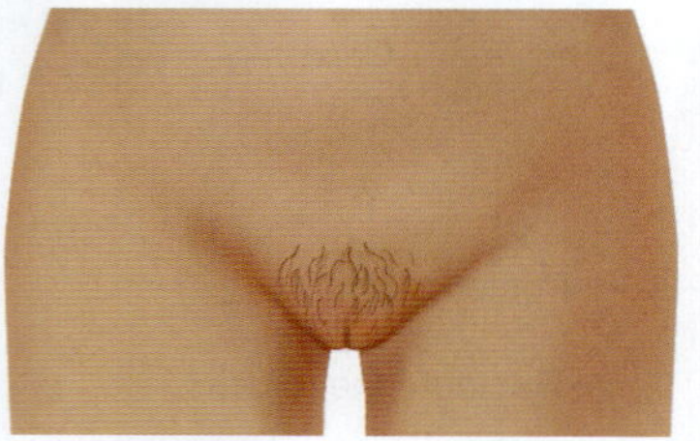 **Stage 2** Growth sparse and mostly on labia. Long, downy hair, slightly pigmented, straight or only slightly curly.	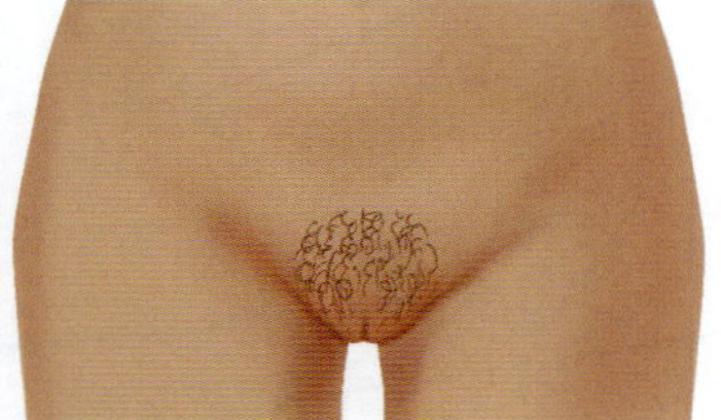 **Stage 3** Growth sparse and spreading over mons pubis. Hair is darker, coarser and curlier.
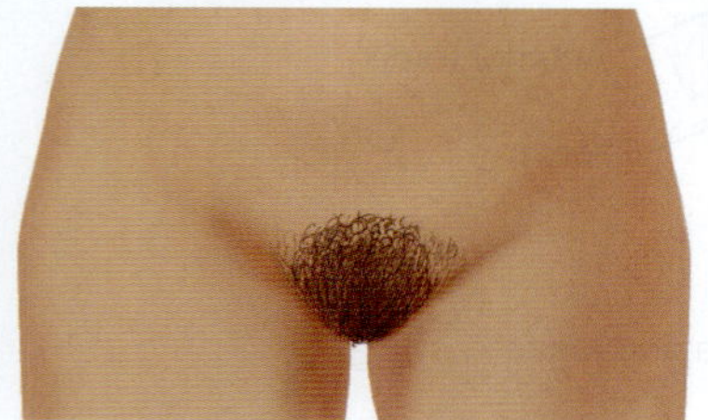 **Stage 4** Hair is adult in type but over smaller area; none on medial thigh.	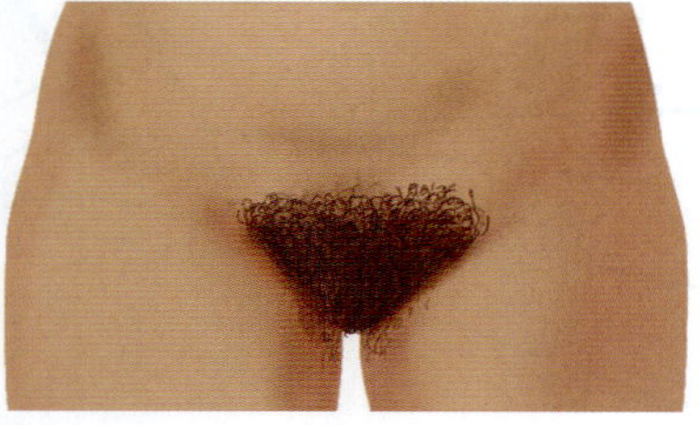 **Stage 5** Adult in type and pattern; inverse triangle. Also on medial thigh surface.

Adapted from Tanner JM: *Growth at adolescence*. Oxford, 1962, Blackwell Scientific.

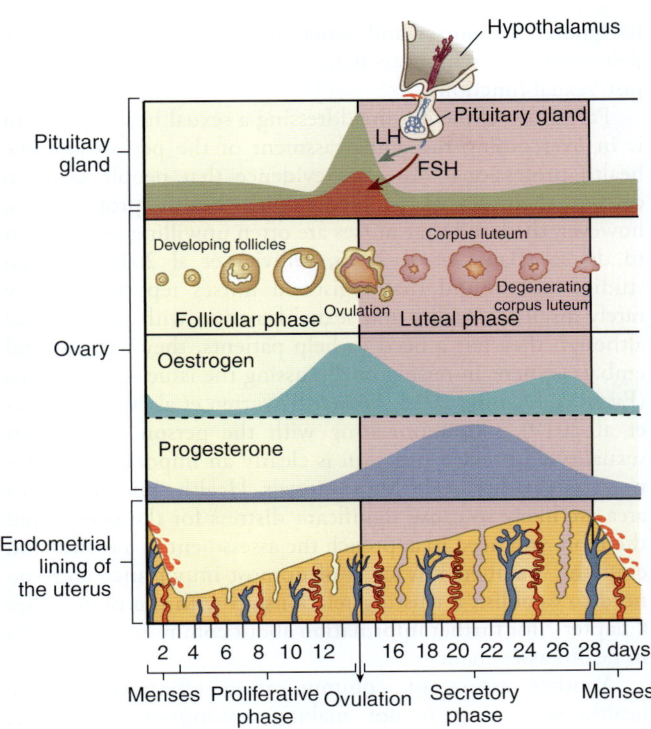

Figure 26.3
Events of the menstrual cycle.

Fertility, infertility and pregnancy choices

Society places demands, and perhaps high expectations and pressure, on women to be fertile. Perhaps one of the most important scientific breakthroughs has been the oral contraceptive pill, and more recently long-acting reversible contraception (LARC), which has provided women with a choice of planning their personal life journey. Women who choose not to go down the medical contraceptive pathway also have a choice in accessing post-coital intervention (PCI) or the morning-after pill as soon as possible after unprotected sex (can be taken up to 4 or 5 days after unprotected sex depending on the type of drug) (Family Planning Victoria 2018). The morning-after pill is available 'over-the-counter' from local pharmacies, without the need for a medical prescription.

Unplanned pregnancies remain an issue in Australia although there are no accurate data on the rates of unintended pregnancies. A survey has shown that in a 10-year period, 25% of women reported an unplanned pregnancy (Taft et al 2018). It is estimated that 25–33% of women who had an unintended pregnancy chose to terminate the pregnancy (TOP). There are safe and effective options for women who choose a termination as this can be a medical choice (using Mifepristone and Misoprostol) or a surgical termination. Surgical TOP is done only after 6 weeks' gestation and medical TOP may not be suitable after 9 weeks gestation (Family Planning Victoria 2019). The cost of these procedures may not be fully covered by the Australian public health insurance Medicare (there may be a 'gap cost' in addition to the Medicare rebate). In New Zealand, termination of pregnancy is covered for residents and requires two consultant medical practitioners to 'certify' that continuation of the pregnancy would result in serious mental or physical health to either the woman or the baby (Family Planning New Zealand 2019).

The shift of women planning pregnancy past 30 years of age has increased since the 1970s. Unfortunately, this also means an increase in 'infertility' as the fertile period appears to decline in women after 30 years of age. Assisted reproductive techniques, such as in-vitro fertilisation, has improved vastly since the 1980s and has successfully assisted many women towards healthy family planning.

The pregnant woman

A complete discussion of the pregnant female is presented in Chapter 29. In summary, shortly after the first missed menstrual period, the genitalia show signs of the growing fetus. The cervix softens (*Goodell's sign*) at 4 to 6 weeks, and the vaginal mucosa and cervix look cyanotic (*Chadwick's sign*) at 8 to 12 weeks. These changes occur because of increased vascularity and oedema of the cervix and hypertrophy and hyperplasia of the cervical glands. The isthmus of the uterus softens (*Hegar's sign*) at 6 to 8 weeks.

The greatest change is in the uterus itself. It increases in capacity by 500 to 1000 times its nonpregnant state, at first because of hormone stimulation and then because of the increasing size of its contents (Marieb & Keller 2018). The nonpregnant uterus has a flattened pear shape. Its early growth encroaches on the space occupied by the bladder, producing the symptom of urinary frequency. By 10 to 12 weeks' gestation, the uterus becomes globular in shape and is too large to stay in the pelvis. At 20 to 24 weeks, the uterus has an oval shape. It rises almost to the liver, displacing the intestines superiorly and laterally.

The female over 65 years

In contrast to the slowly declining hormones in the ageing male, the female's hormonal milieu decreases rapidly. *Menopause* is cessation of the menses. Usually this occurs around 48 to 53 years, although a wide variation of ages from 35 to 60 years exists. The stage of menopause includes the preceding 1 to 2 years of decline in ovarian function, shown by irregular menses that gradually become further apart and produce a lighter flow. Ovaries stop producing progesterone and oestrogen. Because cells in the reproductive tract are oestrogen dependent, decreased oestrogen levels during menopause bring dramatic physical changes.

The uterus reduces in size because of decreased myometrium. The ovaries atrophy to 1 to 2 cm and are not palpable after menopause. Ovulation still may occur sporadically after menopause. The sacral ligaments relax and the pelvic musculature weakens, predisposing the woman to pelvic organ prolapse, particularly in women who have had vaginal births. The cervix decreases in size and looks paler with a thick, glistening epithelium.

The vagina becomes shorter, narrower and less elastic because of increased connective tissue. The vaginal epithelium atrophies, becoming thinner and drier. This results in a fragile mucosal surface that is at risk for bleeding and vaginitis. Decreased vaginal secretions leave the vagina dry and at risk for irritation and pain with intercourse (dyspareunia). The vaginal pH becomes more alkaline, and decreased glycogen content occurs from the decreased oestrogen. These factors also increase the risk of vaginitis because they create a suitable medium for pathogens.

In late older age, externally, the mons pubis looks smaller because the fat pad atrophies. The labia and clitoris gradually decrease in size. Pubic hair becomes thin and sparse. Sexual desire and sexuality do not diminish with age.

CULTURAL AND SOCIAL CONSIDERATIONS

There are varying cultural requirements about the examination of sexual and reproductive function in women, including for some woman the requirement to be examined only by a female healthcare practitioner. You need to ascertain the woman's requirements before the examination commences.

Family relationship and violence

Family can be narrowly defined as individuals that share a common lineage through marriage, birth, ancestry or 'blood line'. Family or 'kin' is also legally defined in terms of marriage, birth parents, power of attorney, property and inheritance. However, such a narrow definition defies many contemporary 'families', where genetics and lineage are not factors that are common that binds individuals together. A broader definition of family exists in many forms and in as many families as there are. De-facto heterosexual couples, once socially frowned upon, are now commonplace, with perhaps siblings of different ancestral lineage. Same sex couples who opt for fertility consider their partnership and offspring to be part of a nuclear family, who may or may not have contact with the 'sperm or egg donor' or the 'surrogate Mum'. Children who are adopted or who are brought up by grandparents might be part of a nuclear family, but also have a broader definition of family.

Nurses and legislated health professionals have a duty of care in mandatory reporting of family violence. Domestic violence includes socio-cultural issues such as female-genital mutilation (FGM), forced marriage and arranged child-marriage from birth. Questions about domestic violence in history taking should then be offered routinely and questions asked with respect, courteously and in a manner that values ethical principles of autonomy, beneficence, non-maleficence, justice and informed consent in a safe and private environment. (Please refer to Chapter 5 for more on family violence and abuse).

Communicating effectively with people about sexuality and sexual function

Many health issues and their treatments can have an adverse effect on a person's sexuality and sexual functioning. Our perceptions of our sexuality affect the way we view ourselves as humans. The World Health Organisation (WHO 2006) has a definition of human sexuality that is useful to consider:

> [Sexuality is]... a central aspect of being human throughout life and encompasses sex, gender identities and roles, sexual orientation, eroticism, pleasure, intimacy and reproduction. Sexuality is experienced and expressed in thoughts, fantasies, desires, beliefs, attitudes, values, behaviours, practices, roles and relationships. While sexuality can include all of these dimensions, not all of them are always experienced or expressed. Sexuality is influenced by the interaction of biological, psychological, social, economic, political, cultural, ethical, legal, historical, religious and spiritual factors.

It is clear to see from this definition that sexuality is an important aspect of human existence and therefore should not be ignored by nurses and other healthcare clinicians. These definitions also remind us that sexuality is much broader than just 'sexual function'.

Part of the difficulty in addressing a sexual health problem is in overcoming the embarrassment of the person and the health professional. There is evidence that people want to discuss their sexual problems with health professionals; however, they find that nurses are often unwilling or reluctant to do so (Bauer et al 2016, Ollivier et al 2019). Several studies have found that registered nurses report that they rarely discuss sexuality and sexual function with patients and although they felt a need to help patients, they felt fear and embarrassment in raising or discussing the issue with patients (Evcili & Demirel 2018, Leonardi-Warren et al 2016, Ollivier et al 2019). Communicating with the person about their sexuality and sexual function is clearly an important skill for nurses and other health professionals. Health concerns in this area are likely to cause significant distress for the person and therefore you need to approach the assessment in a tactful and empathic manner. Privacy is of upmost importance and you need to establish a trusting relationship with the person. See Chapter 7 for further information about communication skills in health assessment.

Another aspect of communicating effectively in the healthcare context is not making assumptions. This was discussed in Chapter 4: Cultural safety. In the context of sexuality and sexual health, this includes not making assumptions about a person's sexual orientation and gender identity. Specifically, this means not making the assumption that the person identifies as heterosexual, lesbian, gay, bisexual or a particular gender. Language is important in conveying acceptance of the person and respect of the person's self-worth and inherent dignity (Australian Human Rights Commission 2018); therefore, it is important to understand commonly used terminology related to gender identity and sexuality. The following terms are a general guide; each LGBTI person has their own preferred language describing their sexuality and terms evolve and change over time (adapted from Australian Human Rights Commission 2018, Queensland Government 2017, Telfer et al 2018):

- **Biological sex** *(What sex were you assigned at birth?)*—an anatomical descriptor of the person's genitals, chromosomes, hormones and other physical and reproductive traits.
- **Gender or gender identity** (*What is your current gender identity?*)—the deeply held internal and individual feeling of gender (male, female or other identity). The gender identity of the person may be reflected in the pronouns they use to describe themselves (for example, he/him/she/her/they/their). *What pronouns would you prefer I refer you as?*
- **Cisgender**—people who identify their gender in the same way that was legally assigned to them at birth.
- **Sexual orientation**—sexual and personal attraction towards another person; including (but not confined to heterosexual, gay, lesbian, bisexual, asexual or same-sex attracted).
- **LGBTI/LGBTIQ+**—acronym for Lesbian, Gay, Bisexual, Transgender, Intersex and Queer people collectively. Sometimes referred to as GLBT+.
- **Lesbian**—refers to women whose long-term sexual, romantic and personal attraction is exclusively towards other women.

- **Gay**—a person whose primary sexual, romantic and personal attraction is to people of the same sex. The term is most commonly used to refer to men, although some women use it.
- **Men who have sex with men**—(or males who have sex with males)—males who have sex with members of the same sex regardless of how they identify themselves (can be gay, heterosexual, bisexual, etc., or not identify with a specific orientation).
- **Bisexual**—a person who is sexually, romantically or emotionally attracted to people of the same sex or gender as well as people of other sexes or genders.
- **Non-binary**—A term to describe someone who does not identify exclusively as male or female.
- **Queer**—used as an umbrella term including a range of sexual orientations and gender identities. Some LGBTIQ+ people may still perceive 'queer' to be an insult.
- **Gender dysphoria**—is defined in DSM-5 (American Psychiatric Association (APA) 2013) as the 'distress caused and experiences as a result of the sex and gender they were assigned at birth'. The removal of the word 'disorder' from previous DSM editions sought to de-stigmatise and reduce societal discrimination against gender-diverse peoples. These clinical criteria are used to access gender affirmation treatments hormonally or surgically.
- **Transgender**—or transgender diverse are terms for people whose gender identity is different than that legally assigned to them at birth. These people may also refer to themselves as 'trans', 'transsexual' or 'transgender'. Being transgender is not related to the person's sexual orientation; the transgender person may be heterosexual, gay, lesbian, bisexual or other sexual orientation. A transgender person may or may not choose to have surgery or hormonal treatments to live as their preferred gender (transition) and they should be referred to as their preferred gender regardless of whether sex-reassignment surgery has been performed. Transition may involve social, medical, surgical and/or legal processes to affirm a person's gender identity.
- **Social transition**—the process by which a person changes their gender expression to better match their gender identity.
- **Medical transition**—the process by which a person changes their physical sex characteristics via hormonal intervention and/or surgery to more closely align with their gender identity.
- **Intersex**—refers to people who are born with physical, hormonal or genetic characteristics that do not conform to medical norms for male or female bodies. Intersex people have a diversity of bodies and identities.
- **Brotherboy** —A culturally specific term to describe Aboriginal and Torres Strait Islander transgender men.
- **Sistergirl** —A culturally specific term to describe Aboriginal and Torres Strait Islander transgender women.
- **Takatāpui** —A Māori term, which is often used to roughly mean 'rainbow person' or 'rainbow community'. It is culturally specific and not easily translated into English. Māori and Pacific Islander peoples have their own terms for gender identity (see Rainbow Youth NZ for more information).

Be cautious about recording information about sexual orientation, gender identity or intersex condition in a person's medical or health record. You should seek consent from the person and inform them about why the information is needed and to whom it will be made available (Victoria Government 2018). There are many excellent resources available to health professionals to assist them in communicating and engaging with people from diverse backgrounds, and some of these are referred to in the bibliography at the end of this chapter.

Subjective data

Assessment in the area of female reproductive function is closely linked to assessment of bladder and bowel function and breast health. Detailed questions and physical examination techniques related to urinary and bowel functions are covered in Chapters 23, 24 and 25. The person's responses to the opening questions below will guide the sequence of the rest of the health interview; the list below is a guide only. You need to be flexible with the structure of this part of the health assessment to ensure that you follow up with the issues that are important to the person first, and then complete the other relevant areas.

1. Presenting concern
2. General health history
3. Sexual health history
4. Reproductive health history
5. Health and lifestyle management

Preparation

As you approach the health assessment interview it is important that you:

- Don't make assumptions about the person's gender identity and sexual orientation based on appearance.
- Use open and inclusive questions that are gender neutral and inclusive.
- Make sure that in your approach to the sexual health history the person is encouraged to discuss their sexual orientation, gender identity, relationship status and that heterosexuality is not assumed.
- A person may choose not to disclose their sexual or gender identity; their choice should be respected.
- Respond positively when the person is prepared to be open about their sexual orientation, gender identity or intersex condition.
- If you are unsure of how to address the person, ask them how they would like to be addressed.
- Begin with open-ended question to assess individual needs.

Practice note: Before you commence the assessment, introduce yourself to the person, confirm the person's identity, discuss the purpose and scope of the assessment, clarify any questions the person may have and obtain verbal consent from the person to perform the assessment.

SUBJECTIVE DATA

ASSESSMENT GUIDELINES	CLINICAL SIGNIFICANCE AND CLINICAL ALERTS
1. Presenting concern	
It is important to ascertain the person's perception of their sexual and/or reproductive health. From the presenting concern, the person would be able to provide you with some insight into their symptoms and perhaps other health issues. If they do perceive a problem—*how does this impact on their quality of life?* The responses to these questions will guide the sequence of the rest of the subjective data collection. Take the cues from the person. If the person is unable to articulate their health concern, use questions below to assist them to verbalise their health situation. A suggested approach: • I would like to ask you some questions to find out more about how I can help you today. Some of the questions might appear intrusive and personal but will assist me in identifying your healthcare needs. Is it OK with you if I ask these questions? • What brings you here today? What concerns do you have about your sexual and reproductive health?	
2. General health history	
Recent illness • Have you experienced any recent illness?	
Personal health history • Any surgery? • Any medical conditions? • Any allergies? • Any health difficulties (mobility, pain, disability)?	
Family history • Any significant family history of diabetes, epilepsy, clotting disorders, hypertension or cardiovascular disease, reproductive cancer, etc.?	
Current and past cigarette smoking • How many for how long?	**Oral contraceptives**, together with cigarette smoking, increase the risk of cardiovascular health issues.
Current and past alcohol and illicit substance use • How much alcohol, how often and for how long. • Which drugs, how much and how often (including injecting drug use)?	Personal health risks as well as putting the person at risk of unsafe sex or sexual violence.
Current medication • Are you taking any prescribed medications, complementary and traditional therapies and over-the-counter medications.	Oral contraceptives increase glycogen content of vaginal epithelium, providing fertile medium for some organisms which cause **vaginitis**. Broad-spectrum antibiotics alter balance of normal flora which can predispose to **candida vaginal infection**.
Psychosocial history (see also Chapter 8: The health history and Chapter 11: Mental health assessment). • What is your highest educational achievement? High school, TAFE or university? • Living arrangements? • Contact and support from family members? Friends? • Hobbies and activities?	

ASSESSMENT GUIDELINES	CLINICAL SIGNIFICANCE AND CLINICAL ALERTS
3. Sexual health history	
A general statement such as, 'When I conduct a health assessment, I ask people about their sexual health. Is it alright with you if I ask questions about your sexual health?' may help you open up the discussion with the person. Only ask the questions that are relevant to the particular situation.	
Genital signs and symptoms If a woman presents with symptoms, then concentrate on a symptom history—length of time, precipitating factors, pain, improvement and past experience. • Ask about current or past symptoms related to urethral, vaginal or anal discharge (amount, odour, colour and character). Questions may include: • Have you experienced any abnormal vaginal or rectal bleeding, genital rashes, lumps or sores? If present, ask the person to describe the sign or symptom: • When it started? • What have they done about it, and did this reduce the symptom? Normal vaginal discharge is small, clear or cloudy, and always nonirritating.	Abnormal vaginal discharge may be described as white, yellow-green, grey, curd-like, foul smelling. Suggests **vaginal infection**; character of discharge often suggests causative organism (see Table 26.5). May be acute or chronic.
• If the person has an abnormal vaginal discharge, is this associated with vaginal itching, rash, pain with intercourse?	Occurs as a result of irritation from discharge. **Dyspareunia** (pain with sexual intercourse) occurs with **vaginitis** of any cause.
• Do you ever experience a feeling of fullness or dragging in the vagina, perineum or rectum? If yes, ask the person to describe the sign or symptom: • When it started? • What have they done about it, and did this reduce the symptom?	These symptoms (and sometimes urinary and/or bowel symptoms) may indicate **pelvic organ prolapse. Cystocele**—anterior vaginal wall defect causing the bladder to prolapse posteriorly into the vagina. **Rectocele**—posterior vaginal wall defect causing the rectum to prolapse anteriorly into the vagina. These symptoms require further assessment by a medical or nurse practitioner.
Urinary or bowel symptoms/lower abdominal pain. • Have you experienced any problem with your bladder or bowel or experienced any abdominal pain (urinary symptoms such as urgency, slow stream, feeling of incomplete emptying or incontinence; typical bowel symptoms such as constipation, difficulty in defecation or feeling of incomplete emptying)? If yes, ask the person to describe the sign or symptom: • When it started? • What have they done about it, and did this reduce the symptom?	**Urinary or faecal incontinence** or bothersome lower urinary tract symptoms can significantly affect a person's sexuality and sexual function and requires further assessment. For details about assessment of urinary function see Chapter 24; bowel function, see Chapter 25; and assessment of abdominal pain, see Chapter 23.
Breast symptoms. • Have you experienced any pain or other abnormal symptoms in your breasts? If yes, ask the person to describe the sign or symptom: • When it started? • What have they done about it, and did this reduce the symptom?	Breast symptoms are often associated with hormonal changes. Any unusual change in the breast should be further assessed and/or referred to a medical practitioner. For details about breast assessment see Chapter 28.

SUBJECTIVE DATA

ASSESSMENT GUIDELINES	CLINICAL SIGNIFICANCE AND CLINICAL ALERTS
Sexual activity (if relevant). • Are you currently sexually active? • Age at first sexual contact? • When was the last time that you had sex? • Do you have a regular or casual sexual partner? How long have you been with this person? • Type of sexual contact (oral, vaginal, anal)? • How many sexual partners have you had in the last 12 months? • Have you had sex that you can't remember because of alcohol or substance use? • Any history with a partner/s from overseas?	Determining the person's sexual practices will enable you to identify areas for health education or the need for further questioning to identify risk factors for sexually transmitted infections, personal safety and/or the need for specific physical examination and other investigations.
Contraception (if relevant). • Are you currently using contraception to avoid pregnancy? What specifically? – If on the combined oral contraceptive pill (COC), ask about adherence—have you missed any pills in the last two packs? – If on the progestogen only pill (POP), ask about adherence—have you taken the pill at the same time daily in the past two packets? – If using long active reversible contraception (LARC), some women will have amenorrhoea and others will have a 'break-through bleed'. – If using intrauterine device (IUD) such as a Mirena, have you had any side-effects? – Use of condoms? – Use of morning after pill? When? Side effects?	
• Assess knowledge of effects, precautions and side effects of contraceptive. – Are you happy with this form of contraception? – Have you experienced any side effects? If so what? How have you managed this?	This information will give direction to possible areas for further discussion and health information or the need for referral to family planning services.
History of sexually transmitted infection (STI). • Do you have any symptoms today—such as an abnormal vaginal discharge, pain passing urine or any abnormal bleeding? • Have you or your partner ever been diagnosed with a STI (such as chlamydia)? • If so, what symptoms did you experience? How long ago? How was it treated? • Have you ever had a test for HIV or hepatitis B or C? • Screen for knowledge of prevention of STIs—use of condoms.	An **STI** includes all conditions that can be transmitted during intercourse or intimate sexual contact with an infected partner.
Sexual function and satisfaction (if relevant). • Are you satisfied with the sexual relationship you have with your partner/s? • Are you satisfied with the way that you and your partner communicate about sex? • Are you satisfied with your ability to respond sexually?	There are validated sexual health/satisfaction assessment tools available (e.g. the female sexual function questionnaire (FSFI).
• Have you experienced any sexual difficulties or dysfunction? – Low sexual desire or sexual arousal – Vaginal dryness (lack of lubrication, 'wetness', on arousal or during sexual activity) – Difficulty in achieving an orgasm, lack of sexual satisfaction – Pain during intercourse – Any other sexual issue? – If you are experiencing any difficulties, how much does this bother you (scale of 1–5; 1 is not bothered at all/5 is extremely bothered)?	**Dyspareunia**—pain with sexual intercourse which can be deep or superficial. **Vaginismus**—an involuntary spasm or contraction of the pelvic floor muscles making penetration painful or impossible causing person/oral and relationship distress. Women who are concerned about their sexual health should be referred to a medical or nurse practitioner/sexual health clinic for further assessment.

ASSESSMENT GUIDELINES	CLINICAL SIGNIFICANCE AND CLINICAL ALERTS
Family violence, sexual abuse, assault or unwanted sexual experiences (if relevant). • See questions and approach to assessment described in Chapter 5 for detail on assessment related to screening for family violence and abuse.	May prompt need for follow-up and referral for follow-up and counselling. See Chapter 5.
4. Reproductive health history	
Menstrual history	
• What was the date of your last normal menstrual period?	**LMP**—last menstrual period.
• At what age did you have your first period?	**Menarche**—mean age at onset at 12–13 years; delayed onset suggests endocrine or underweight problem. **Primary amenorrhoea**—failure to start menstruating by 17 years of age (Talley & O'Connor 2018).
• How often are your periods? Cycle—normally every 18 to 45 days	**Amenorrhoea**—absent menses. **Secondary amenorrhoea**—cessation of menstruation for 6 months or more (Talley & O'Connor 2018).
• How many days does your period last? Duration—average 3 to 7 days.	
• Usual amount of flow: light, medium, heavy? How many pads or tampons do you use each day or hour?	**Menorrhagia**—heavy menses.
• Any clotting?	Clotting indicates heavy flow or vaginal pooling.
• Do you experience any pain or cramps before or during period? How do you treat it? Does it interfere with your day-to-day activities? • Do you experience any other associated symptoms: bloating, breast tenderness, moodiness? • Do you have any spotting between periods?	**Dysmenorrhoea.**
• Do you experience any abnormal vaginal bleeding (post-coital, bleeding between periods)? If so, what have you done about it? • Do you take medication to regulate your menstrual cycle (contraceptive pill or other hormonal medication)?	Bleeding between periods can be an indication of hormonal imbalance or side effect of hormonal contraception. Abnormal vaginal bleeding can also be present with infection, or changes in the cervix and uterus that require further assessment by a medical practitioner.
Menopause • Have your periods slowed down or stopped?	**Menopause**—cessation of menstruation, usually considered to be after 12 months of cessation of menstruation.
• Do you experience any associated symptoms of menopause (e.g. hot flushes, numbness and tingling, headache, palpitations, drenching sweats, mood swings, vaginal dryness, itching)? What have you done about these symptoms if any?	**Perimenopausal period** from 40 to 55 years has hormone shifts, resulting in vasomotor instability.
• If using menopausal hormone therapy (MHT), what is the dose? How effective is the medication in reducing the menopausal side effects? Any unwanted effects of the medication? How long have you been using hormone replacement therapy?	Side effects of **menopausal hormone therapy** include fluid retention, breast pain or enlargement and vaginal bleeding.
• Are you using any other therapies to help relieve menopausal symptoms? For example, herbs and other complementary therapies, exercise, yoga?	

SUBJECTIVE DATA

SUBJECTIVE DATA

ASSESSMENT GUIDELINES	CLINICAL SIGNIFICANCE AND CLINICAL ALERTS
• Has menopause affected your quality of life and sense of wellbeing? If yes, in what ways?	Although this is a normal life stage, reaction varies from acceptance to feelings of loss.
Obstetric history • Have you ever been pregnant?	
• How many occasions have you been pregnant?	**Gravida**—number of pregnancies.
• How many births have you had?	**Para**—number of births (over 20 weeks gestation—live or stillborn).
• Have you had any miscarriages (spontaneous abortion) or a termination of pregnancy (induced abortion)? The woman may not want to share this information. Be aware that partners and other family members may not be aware of this history, therefore it is important to try to consult with a woman by herself in the first instance.	**Abortion**—interrupted pregnancy, including elective termination of pregnancy (medical or surgical) and spontaneous miscarriage.
• For each pregnancy describe: duration, any complication, labour and birth, baby's sex, birth weight, condition.	
• Are you planning a pregnancy? Do you think you may be pregnant now? What symptoms have you noticed?	
• Have you ever had any problems becoming pregnant?	**Infertility** is considered after 1 year of engaging in unprotected sexual intercourse without becoming pregnant.
5. Health and lifestyle management	
Cervical screening test • Have you had a cervical screening test (CST), or what was previously known as the Pap test? • When was your last CST? • Have you had any previously abnormal CST (or Pap test) result? Take the opportunity to reinforce the need for regular CST.	**Cervical screening tests** (CSTs) are recommended for women from 25 years old. See the section titled 'Promoting a healthy lifestyle' later in the chapter for more information about CSTs.
Immunisation • Have you been immunised against human papillomavirus (HPV)? For more information about HPV vaccination see 'Promoting a healthy lifestyle' section of this chapter.	**HPV** can cause cancers of the penis, anus, cervix, vulva, vagina and throat. The virus causes genital warts. Warts that are visible are caused by a sub-type of HPV that is benign and is self-limiting. Warts cause a lot of angst but are self-limiting as they will resolve spontaneously with time. Treatments of genital warts are cosmetic. For further information about HPV vaccination, see the section titled 'Promoting a healthy lifestyle' later in the chapter.
• Have you been immunised against hepatitis B? Hepatitis B vaccination is part of the Australian Immunisation schedule in Australia and New Zealand. Most Australians under the age of 30 would have been given the vaccine and the herd immunity is high >80% but there are sub-populations that may not have been vaccinated. These include migrants, those whose parents are vaccine conscientious objectors and those who missed out at school.	**Hepatitis B** is a sexually transmissible infection and vertical transmission from mother to baby continues to be the main way of acquiring hepatitis B with long term sequelae that includes hepatocellular carcinoma.
• Have you been immunised against Measles, Mumps and Rubella (MMR)? While this is not sexually transmitted, the unvaccinated pregnant woman may vertically transmit the infections to their unborn baby and cause significant morbidity and mortality. It is thus important to ascertain that women of child-bearing age have had the MMR vaccine before they start family planning.	

ASSESSMENT GUIDELINES	CLINICAL SIGNIFICANCE AND CLINICAL ALERTS
Breast health Ask questions about breast health awareness. • Have you ever had a mammogram or breast ultrasound?	For more information on assessment of breast health see Chapter 28.
Safer sex practices See points in sexual health history above.	
Activity and exercise • Ask about usual activity and exercise patterns.	Part of a general health history. May provide an opportunity to provide more information about the importance of exercise to general health and wellbeing.
Additional subjective data for infants and children (questions for parent or guardian)	
• Does your child have any problem urinating? • Have you noticed any evidence of pain with urinating such as crying, holding genitals? • Has your child had a previous urinary tract infection?	For more information on assessment of urinary function see Chapter 24.
• Has your child experienced any problems with genital area: itching, rash, vaginal or anal discharge?	Occurs with poor perineal hygiene or insertion of foreign body in vagina/rectum.
• Questions related to suspected child abuse. Please read the important information about the Australian legal requirements about mandatory reporting of suspected child abuse. See Chapter 5 for details and specific approach to screening.	For more information about signs and symptoms related to child abuse refer to Chapter 5.
Additional subjective data for preadolescents and adolescents	
Use the following questions, as appropriate, to assess sexual growth and development and sexual behaviour. Use the same principles as discussed at the beginning of the health history section related to the approach to gender identity and sexual orientation outlined in the sexual health history.	
Ask questions that seem appropriate for girl's age but be aware that norms vary widely.	
• Around age 9 or 10, girls start to develop breasts and pubic hair. Have you ever seen charts and pictures of normal growth patterns for girls? Let us go over these now.	
• Have your periods started? How did you feel? Were you prepared or surprised?	Assess attitude of girl and parents. Note inadequate preparation or attitude of distaste.
• Who in your family do you talk to about your body changes and about sex information? How do these talks go? Do you think you get enough information? • What about sex education classes at school? Is there a teacher, a nurse, doctor or counsellor to whom you can talk?	
• Often girls your age have questions about having sex. Do you have questions? If appropriate in the situation, ask further questions about sexual activity (use similar questions to that of the adult outlined in the previous section including questions regarding STI protection and prevention of unplanned pregnancy if relevant).	Determining the young person's sexual practices will enable you to identify areas for health education or the need for further questioning to identify risk factors for sexually transmitted infections and/or the need for specific physical examination and other investigations.
• Questions related to suspected child abuse. Please read the important information about the Australian legal requirements about mandatory reporting of suspected child abuse. See Chapter 5 for details and specific approach to screening.	For more information about signs and symptoms related to child abuse refer to Chapter 5.

ASSESSMENT GUIDELINES	CLINICAL SIGNIFICANCE AND CLINICAL ALERTS
Additional subjective data for the woman over 65 years	
• Have you experienced any vaginal itching, discharge, pain with sexual activity?	Associated with **atrophic vaginitis**—inflammation, thinning and dryness of the vaginal tissue and labia due to a reduction in oestrogen following menopause. Can also cause urinary symptoms such as urgency, dysuria and incontinence.

Objective data

The techniques and extent of the objective data collection in this area will depend on the presenting signs and symptoms. Nurses working in sexual health clinics and some urological settings may need to develop skill in a more comprehensive assessment of female sexual and reproductive function. For most nurses asking questions about the woman's reproductive health will be sufficient for a nursing assessment. **Physical examination, including inspection of the genitalia, is only performed when there is a valid reason to do so.**

In the case of a child or adolescent, the parent or guardian normally provides legal informed consent for assessment and treatment. Young people have the legal right to confidential healthcare unless they cannot be considered a mature minor and/or there is a significant concern or risk, for example, harm to self, physical or sexual abuse. It is generally accepted that most young people over the age of 16 years are capable of giving informed consent. Those under 16 years may sometimes be considered mature minors. In some cases, such as adolescents under 16 years, it is legally permissible for a mature adolescent to consent to assessment and treatment (Royal Children's Hospital 2019). The mature minor (Gillick principle) is confirmed in Australian common law that those under 18 years may be able to give informed consent if they have sufficient understanding and intelligence to understand proposed assessment and/or treatment (Australian Law Reform Commission 2010). However, it is always advisable to obtain verbal consent from a child or adolescent before an examination and this should be documented in the health history.

Preparation

Before you start, explain what you are going to assess and why; answer any questions the woman may have; and gain the woman's consent to be examined.

- Ask her if she would like a partner, family member or friend to be present.
- Ask her to empty her bladder before the examination.
- Allow the woman to undress in privacy.
- Explain each step in the examination before you do it.
- Assure the woman that she can stop the examination at any point should she feel any discomfort.
- Communicate throughout the examination. Maintain a dialogue to share information.

For the examination of the external genitalia, the woman should be assisted to lie down in the supine position with one or two pillows under her head. Ensure privacy before exposing the genital area and cover as much bare skin as possible. Have the woman place her ankles together and let her knees drop to the side exposing the perineal area. If the woman has a partner, friend or family member present, ask them to stand at the top (head) of the bed or examination couch to support the woman.

Equipment needed

Non-sterile gloves
Appropriate lighting (examination light)
Hand hygiene solution

PROCEDURES AND NORMAL FINDINGS	ABNORMAL FINDINGS AND CLINICAL ALERTS
General inspection	
During collection of subjective data you will have noticed the condition of the person's skin, hair, posture, height to weight ratio, body shape, level of hygiene and grooming and general demeanor. All of these factors provide clues to the woman's sexual and reproductive health.	
Inspection of external genitalia	
• **Skin colour** (Figure 26.4).	

PROCEDURES AND NORMAL FINDINGS	ABNORMAL FINDINGS AND CLINICAL ALERTS
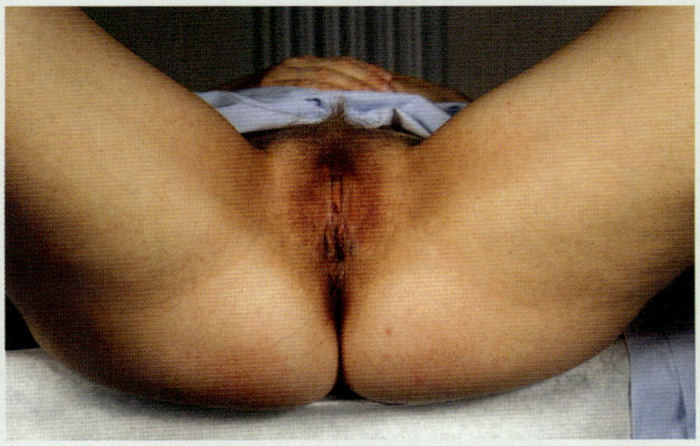 Figure 26.4	
• **Hair distribution** is in the usual female pattern of inverted triangle, although it normally may trail up the abdomen towards the umbilicus. However, it is not uncommon for women to remove some or all of the pubic hair.	Consider delayed puberty if no pubic hair or breast development has occurred by age 13 years. Nits or lice at the base of pubic hair.
• **Labia majora** normally are symmetrical, plump and well formed. In the nulliparous (woman who has never had a baby) woman, labia meet in the midline; after a vaginal birth, the labia are usually gaping and slightly shrivelled.	Swelling.
• No lesions should be present, except for occasional sebaceous cysts. These are yellowish, 1-cm nodules that are firm, non-tender and often multiple.	Be aware that not all lesions are abnormal. There are normal anatomical variants, however. ***Clinical alert:*** If any suspicious lesion is identified, the woman should be referred to a medical or nurse practitioner for further assessment.
With your gloved hand, separate the labia majora to inspect (see Figure 26.5):	
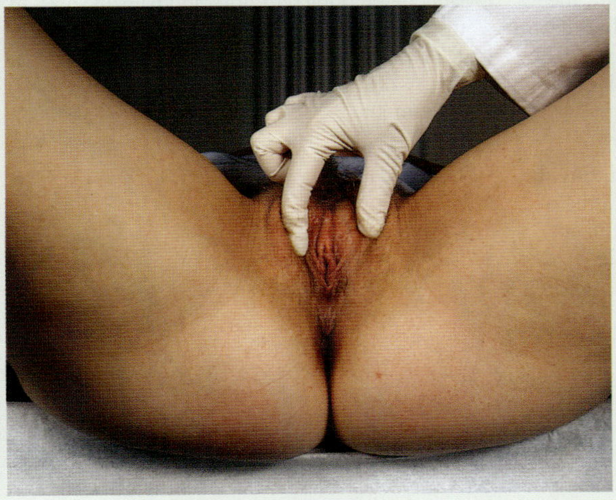 Figure 26.5	Excoriation, nodules, rash or lesions (see Table 26.2).

OBJECTIVE DATA

PROCEDURES AND NORMAL FINDINGS	ABNORMAL FINDINGS AND CLINICAL ALERTS
• **Clitoris.**	
• **Labia minora** are dark pink and moist, usually symmetrical.	**Inflammation** or lesions.
• **Urethral opening** appears stellate or slit-like and is midline.	**Polyp.**
• **Vaginal opening**, or introitus, may appear as a narrow vertical slit or as a larger opening.	Foul-smelling, irritating **discharge**.
• **Perineum** is smooth. A well-healed episiotomy scar, midline or mediolateral, may be present after a vaginal birth.	
• **Anus** has coarse skin of increased pigmentation (see Chapter 25).	
Additional objective data for infants and children	
Preparation A parent or guardian should be present.	
• Infant—place on examination table.	
• Toddler/preschooler—place on parent's lap.	
Frog-leg position—hips flexed, soles of feet together and up to bottom.	
No drapes—the young girl wants to see what you are doing.	
• School-age child—place on examination table, frog-leg position, no drapes.	
During childhood, a routine screening is limited to inspection of the external genitalia to determine that (1) the structures are intact, (2) the vagina is present and (3) the hymen is patent.	
The newborn's genitalia are somewhat engorged. The labia majora are swollen, the labia minora are prominent and protrude beyond the labia majora, the clitoris looks relatively large and the hymen appears thick. Because of transient engorgement, the vaginal opening is more difficult to see now than it will be later. Place your thumbs on the labia majora. Push laterally while pushing the perineum down and try to note the vaginal opening above the hymenal ring. Do not palpate the clitoris because it is very sensitive.	**Ambiguous genitalia** are rare but are suggested by a markedly enlarged clitoris, fusion of the labia (resembling scrotum), and palpable mass in fused labia (resembling testes) (see Table 26.8). ***Clinical alert:*** Any abnormalities should be referred to a medical practitioner for further assessment.
A sanguineous vaginal discharge or leucorrhoea (mucoid discharge) is normal during the first few weeks because of the maternal oestrogen effect. (This also may cause transient breast engorgement and secretion.) During the early weeks, the genital engorgement resolves, and the labia minora atrophy and remain small until puberty (Figure 26.6).	**Lesions, rash.**

PROCEDURES AND NORMAL FINDINGS	ABNORMAL FINDINGS AND CLINICAL ALERTS
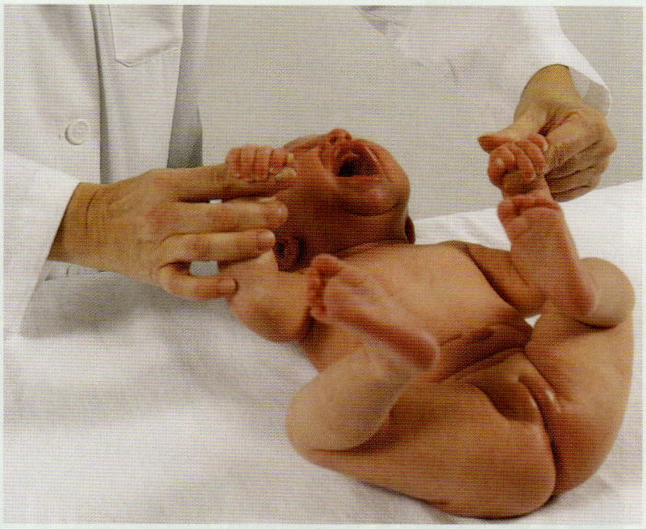 Figure 26.6	
Between the ages of 2 months and 7 years, the labia majora are flat, the labia minora are thin, the clitoris is relatively small, and the hymen is tissue-paper thin. Normally, no irritation or foul-smelling discharge is present.	Poor perineal hygiene. **Excoriations.** During and after toddler age, foul-smelling discharge occurs with lodging of foreign body, pinworms or infection.
In the young school-age girl (7 to 10 years), the mons pubis thickens, the labia majora thicken and the labia minora become slightly rounded. Pubic hair appears beginning around age 11 years, although sparse pubic hair may occur as early as age 8 years. Normally, the hymen is perforate.	Absence of pubic hair by 13 years indicates delayed puberty. **Amenorrhoea** in adolescent, together with bluish and bulging hymen, indicates imperforate hymen and warrants referral.
Almost always in these age groups, an external examination will suffice. If needed, an internal pelvic examination is best performed by a paediatric gynaecologist using specialised instruments.	
Additional objective data for the woman over 65 years	
Natural vaginal lubrication is decreased; to avoid a painful examination, take care to lubricate the examining hand adequately.	
Menopause and the resulting decrease in oestrogen production cause numerous physical changes. Pubic hair gradually decreases, becoming thin and sparse in later years. The skin is thinner and fat deposits decrease, leaving the mons pubis smaller and the labia flatter. Clitoris size also decreases after age 60 years.	

Further objective assessment for advanced practice

The assessments that are described in the following sections require advanced skill and scope of practice. Nurses working in specialist women's health and sexual health settings and urological and continence nurses need to develop these skills. Advanced assessment for infants and children would be performed by specialist neonatal and paediatric nurses, some midwives and maternal and child health nurses. **Physical examination, including vaginal inspection and palpation, are intimate invasive assessments and are only performed when there is a valid reason to do so.** It is critical that clear communication with the person is maintained throughout the procedure to ensure that the person fully understands the purpose, nature and extent of the assessment. You will have to make a professional judgement about the need for another health professional (a chaperone) to be present during the examination.

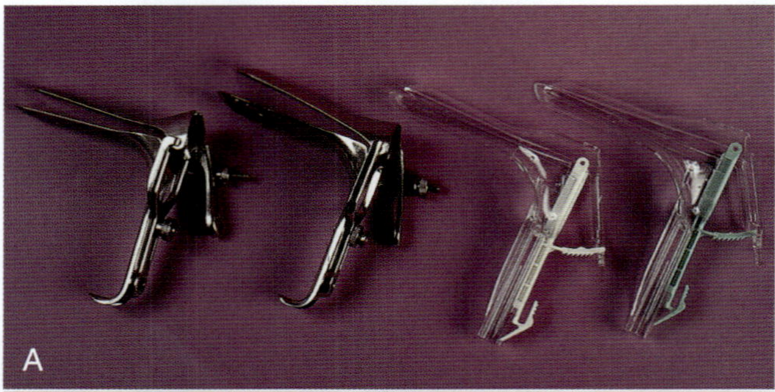

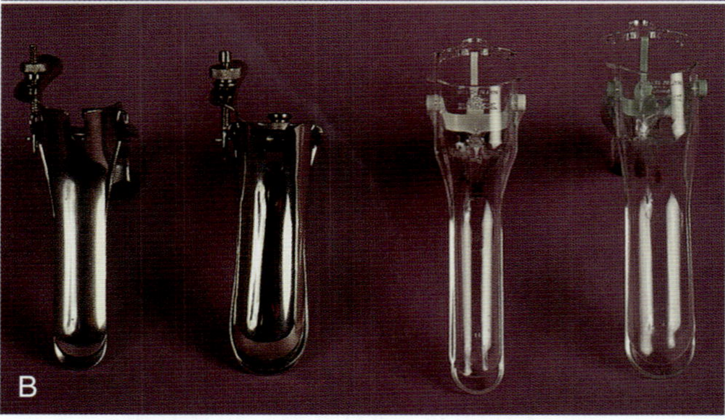

Figure 26.7

Preparation

See previous comments about positioning of the woman. Internal examination usually follows examination of external structures. Take time to reconfirm consent to be examined internally. Familiarise yourself with the vaginal speculum before the examination. Practise opening and closing the blades, locking them into position and releasing them. Try both metal and plastic types. Note that the plastic speculum locks and unlocks with a resounding click that can be alarming to the uninformed woman.

Equipment needed

In addition to the equipment listed previously you will require:

Vaginal speculum of appropriate size (Figure 26.7)
Materials for cytological study—this is dependent on the preference of the laboratory. Make yourself familiar with the equipment and how to collect, prepare and transport the specimen.
Specimen containers for specific STI cultures if needed
Warm water (to lubricate vaginal speculum)
Non-sterile gloves
Water-based lubricant (depending on the purpose and extent of the examination)

PROCEDURES AND NORMAL FINDINGS	ABNORMAL FINDINGS AND CLINICAL ALERTS
Inspection	
In addition to the detailed inspection described previously, you may need to assess for pelvic organ prolapse and stress incontinence. While observing the perineum, ask the woman to cough and note any loss of urine when coughing. Observe for any sign of bulging of the vaginal walls at the introitus and bulging of the urethral meatus. There should be no prolapse of the vaginal walls and no urine loss during coughing.	Loss of urine when coughing is an indicator of **stress incontinence**. Bulging of the anterior vaginal wall is termed a **cystocele** where the pelvic musculature fails to support the bladder and it falls posteriorly into the vagina. This can cause voiding dysfunction and incontinence. Similarly, a bulge in the posterior vaginal wall is termed a **rectocele**. A rectocele can cause defecatory dysfunction and can contribute to constipation. ***Clinical alert:*** Any degree of pelvic organ prolapse should be referred to a medical practitioner for further assessment.

PROCEDURES AND NORMAL FINDINGS	ABNORMAL FINDINGS AND CLINICAL ALERTS
Palpation	
Assess the urethra and Skene's glands	
Dip your gloved finger in a bowl of warm water to lubricate. Then insert your index finger into the vagina, and gently milk the urethra by applying pressure up and out. This procedure should produce no pain. If any discharge appears, culture it. See Figure 26.8. 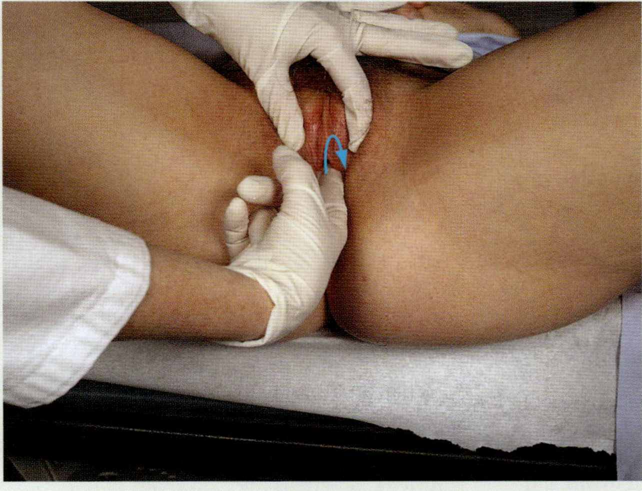 Figure 26.8	**Tenderness.** **Induration** along urethra. **Urethral discharge.**
Assess Bartholin's glands	
Palpate the posterior parts of the labia majora with your index finger in the vagina and your thumb outside (Figure 26.9). Normally, the labia feel soft and homogeneous. 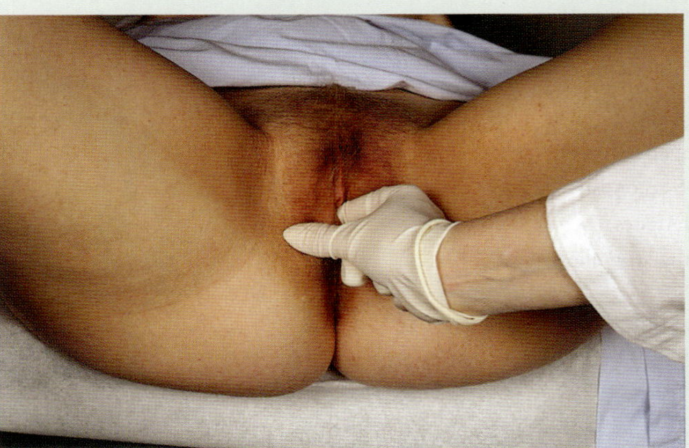 Figure 26.9	Swelling (see Table 26.2). Induration. **Pain** with palpation. **Erythema** around or discharge from duct opening.
Palpate the perineum	
Normally, it feels thick, smooth and muscular in the nulliparous woman, and may be thinner and more rigid in the multiparous woman.	Tenderness. Paper-thin perineum.

OBJECTIVE DATA

PROCEDURES AND NORMAL FINDINGS	ABNORMAL FINDINGS AND CLINICAL ALERTS
Palpate the vagina	
Insert a gloved finger into the vagina and assess for tenderness, descent of the cervix, anterior and posterior vaginal wall. If no specimens are being collected, a water-based lubricant can be applied to your gloved fingers.	Tenderness. Descent of cervix into vagina. **Anterior or posterior prolapse.**
Assessment of pelvic muscle strength	
This is performed to: • Establish a baseline of neuromuscular function and contractility of the pelvic floor muscles; • Assess the woman's ability to identify, isolate, contract and relax the pelvic floor muscles (Castro Diaz et al 2017). Good pelvic muscle function is important in maintaining the position of pelvic organs and structures and in maintaining urinary and faecal continence.	Digital palpation of pelvic floor muscle assessment is subjective and hard to quantify reliably; however, it does offer a clinically useful way to determine pelvic floor muscle function (Guevara 2018).
• Should be performed in the supine position with hips and knees flexed and relaxed. Depending on the purpose of the assessment (and the findings from the assessment in the supine position), it can be repeated in the standing position. • Begin by inserting one gloved finger (index finger) into the woman's vagina (approx. 4 cm). If you cannot feel the vaginal walls tightly around one examining finger you may need to use two fingers (index and middle fingers). • If using one finger, ask the woman to 'lift and squeeze' or 'pull up and tighten' the pelvic floor muscles around your finger. If using two examining fingers, spread the fingers laterally in the anterior–posterior position and ask the woman to 'lift and squeeze' or 'pull up and tighten' the pelvic floor muscles around your fingers.	Absent or decreased contraction—little sensation of pressure on the examiner's fingers. Inability to maintain the contraction (< 3 seconds). Women with poor pelvic floor muscle strength are likely to experience urinary incontinence and should be referred to a nurse continence specialist or continence physiotherapist for further assessment and development of an individualised pelvic floor muscle-strengthening program.
You should feel a brisk contraction of the muscles firmly and evenly around your fingers. The **modified Oxford grading system** is used to quantify pelvic floor muscle strength: 0/5 = nil/none (no discernible peri-vaginal muscle contraction) 1/5 = flicker (fluttering or quivering of the peri-vaginal muscle contraction) 2/5 = weak (weak contraction of the peri-vaginal muscles with or without elevation/lifting) 3/5 = moderate (compressing the examiner's fingers with or without elevation/lifting of the finger/s) 4/5 = good (a firm contraction with good compression of the examiner's fingers causing elevation/lifting of the examiner's finger/s) 5/5 = strong (strong contraction of the of the peri-vaginal muscles on the examiner's finger/s and strong elevation/lifting of the examiner's finger/s • **Assess the duration of the contraction** (in seconds)—normally 3–6 seconds. • **Number of contractions** that can be performed before the muscle fatigues. • **Assess how fast the woman can contract the muscles**. Make sure that you allow the woman to rest the muscles for a few seconds between contractions. • **Assess extent of muscle movement**. Normally the contraction should lift the examiner's fingers upwards. Note the evenness of the contraction (anterior–posterior, circumferential). (Castro Diaz et al 2017, Newman & Laycock 2008, Nelles 2016).	
Inspection of internal genitalia	
Select the proper-sized speculum. Warm and lubricate the speculum under warm running water.	

OBJECTIVE DATA

PROCEDURES AND NORMAL FINDINGS	ABNORMAL FINDINGS AND CLINICAL ALERTS
A good technique is to dedicate one hand to the person and the other hand to picking up equipment in the room. For example, hold the speculum in your left hand (the equipment hand), with the index and the middle fingers surrounding the blades and your thumb under the thumbscrew. This prevents the blades from opening painfully during insertion. With your right index and middle fingers (the patient hand), push the introitus down and open to relax the pubococcygeal muscle (Figure 26.10). Tilt the width of the blades obliquely and insert the speculum past your right fingers, applying any pressure *downwards*. This avoids pressure on the sensitive urethra above it. 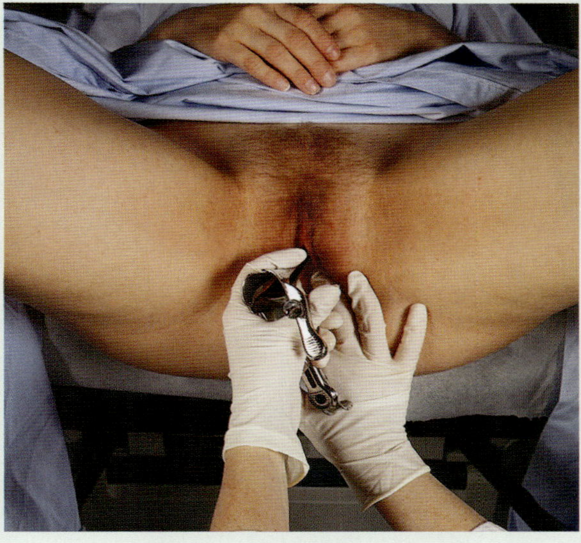 **Figure 26.10**	
Ease insertion by informing the woman of what you are doing. Tell her you are placing the speculum externally. This method relaxes the perineal muscles and opens the introitus. (With experience, you can combine speculum insertion with assessing the support of the vaginal muscles.) As the blades pass your right fingers, withdraw your fingers. Now change the hand holding the speculum to your right hand and turn the width of the blades horizontally. Continue to insert in a 45-degree angle *downwards* towards the small of the woman's back (Figure 26.11). This matches the natural slope of the vagina. 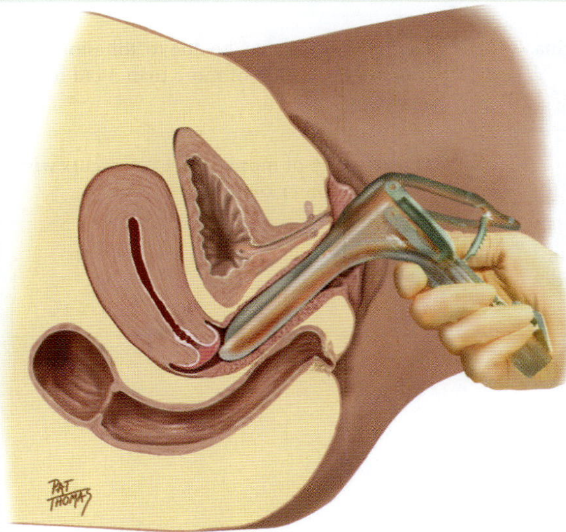 **Figure 26.11**	

OBJECTIVE DATA

PROCEDURES AND NORMAL FINDINGS	ABNORMAL FINDINGS AND CLINICAL ALERTS
After the blades are fully inserted, open them by squeezing the handles together (Figure 26.12). The cervix should be in full view. Sometimes this does not occur (especially with beginning examiners) because the blades are angled above the location of the cervix. Try closing the blades, withdrawing about halfway and reinserting in a more *downwards* plane. Then slowly sweep upwards. Once you have the cervix in full view, lock the blades open by tightening the thumbscrew. 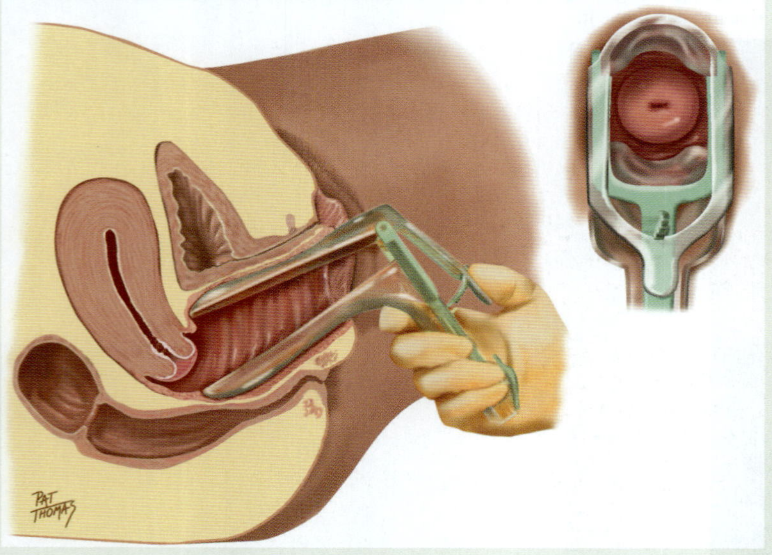 Figure 26.12	
Inspect the cervix and its os	
Note: • **Colour.** Normally the cervical mucosa is pink and even. During the 2nd month of pregnancy it looks blue (Chadwick's sign) and after menopause it is pale.	Redness, inflammation. Pallor with anaemia. Cyanotic other than with pregnancy (see Table 26.4).
• **Position.** Midline, either anterior or posterior. Projects 1–3 cm into the vagina.	Lateral position may be due to adhesion or tumour. Projection of more than 3 cm may be a prolapse.
• **Size.** Diameter is 2.5 cm.	Hypertrophy of more than 4 cm occurs with inflammation or tumour.
• **Os.** This is small and round in the nulliparous woman. In the parous woman, it is a horizontal irregular slit and also may show healed lacerations on the sides (Figure 26.13).	

OBJECTIVE DATA

PROCEDURES AND NORMAL FINDINGS	ABNORMAL FINDINGS AND CLINICAL ALERTS

NORMAL VARIATIONS OF THE CERVIX

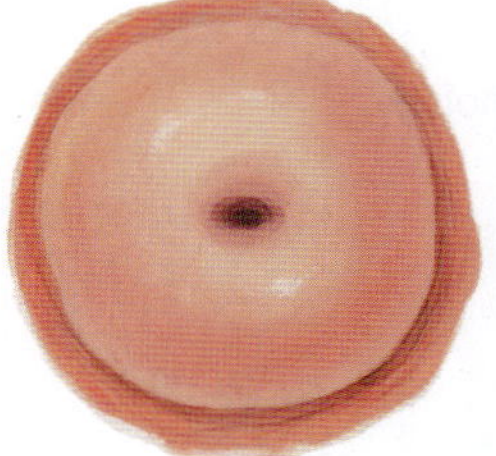
Nulliparous

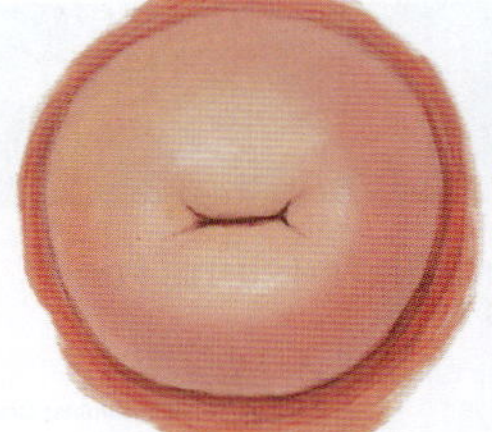
Parous (after childbirth)

LACERATIONS

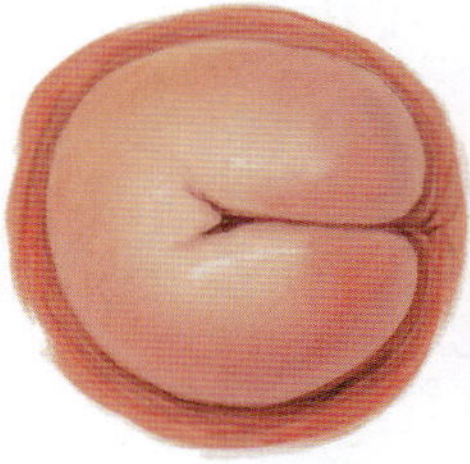
Unilateral transverse

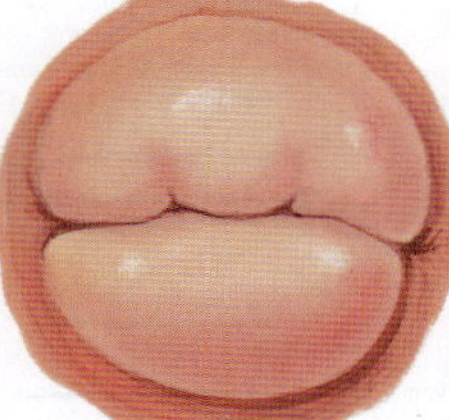
Bilateral transverse

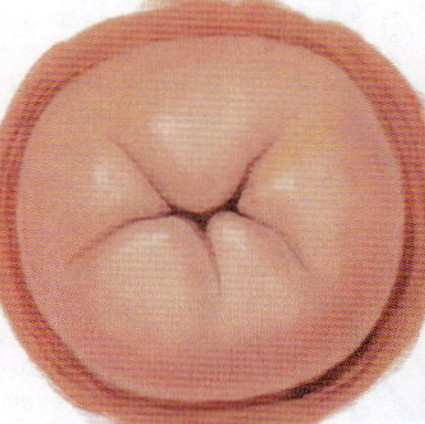
Stellate

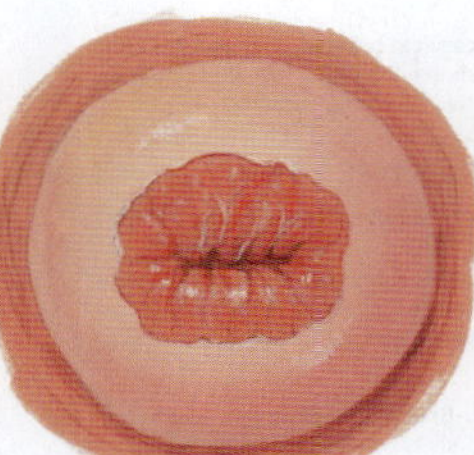
Cervical eversion

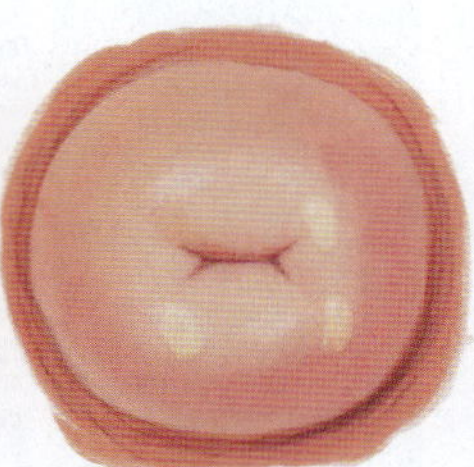
Nabothian cysts

Figure 26.13

PROCEDURES AND NORMAL FINDINGS	ABNORMAL FINDINGS AND CLINICAL ALERTS
• **Surface.** This is normally smooth, but **cervical eversion**, or ectropion, may occur normally after vaginal deliveries. The endocervical canal is everted or 'rolled out'. It looks like a red, beefy halo inside the pink cervix surrounding the os. It is difficult to distinguish this normal variation from an abnormal condition (e.g. erosion or carcinoma) and biopsy may be needed.	Surface reddened, granular and asymmetrical, particularly around os. Friable, bleeds easily. Any lesions: white patch on cervix; strawberry spot. Refer any suspicious red, white or pigmented lesion for biopsy (see erosion, ulceration and carcinoma, Table 26.4).
• **Nabothian cysts** are benign growths that commonly appear on the cervix after childbirth. They are small, smooth, yellow nodules that may be single or multiple. Less than 1 cm, they are retention cysts caused by obstruction of cervical glands.	Cervical polyp—bright red growth protruding from the os (see Table 26.4).
Note the cervical secretions. Depending on the day of the menstrual cycle, secretions may be clear and thin, or thick, opaque and stringy. Always they are odourless and non-irritating.	Foul-smelling, irritating, with yellow, green, white or grey discharge (see Table 26.5).
If secretions are copious, swab the area with a thick-tipped swab. This method sponges away secretions and you have a better view of the structures.	
Obtain cervical smears and cultures	
The Cervical Screening Test (CST) screens for HPV sub-types that are precursors to cervical cancers. Do not obtain during the woman's menses or if a heavy infectious discharge is present. Instruct the woman not to douche, have intercourse or put anything into the vagina within 24 hours before collecting the specimens. Obtain the CST before other specimens so you will not disrupt or remove cells. Laboratories may vary in method of collection of the CST (see Figure 26.14 for an example of ThinPrep technique); however, the test usually consists of three specimens:	

OBJECTIVE DATA

PROCEDURES AND NORMAL FINDINGS | ABNORMAL FINDINGS AND CLINICAL ALERTS

NATIONAL CERVICAL SCREENING PROGRAM GUIDELINES

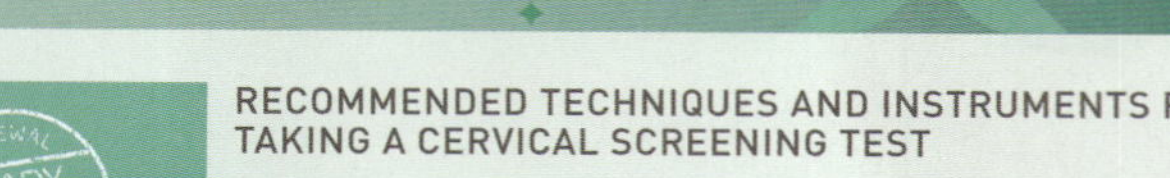

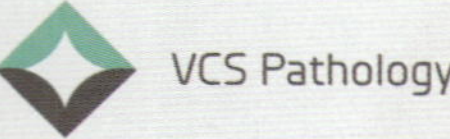

RENEWAL READY SET GO! 2017

A GUIDE TO TAKING A HIGH-QUALITY CERVICAL SCREENING TEST

If you would like to watch a video demonstrating the correct technique for taking a high-quality Cervical Screening Test (CST) visit www.vcspathology.org.au/practitioners/resources1.

For more information about CST technique, the new National Cervical Screening Program, and testing for HPV, contact VCS Pathology on 03 9250 0300 and ask to speak to a Liaison Physician or email On-CallP@vcs.org.au

RECOMMENDED TECHNIQUES AND INSTRUMENTS FOR TAKING A CERVICAL SCREENING TEST

FOR PRE-MENOPAUSAL WOMEN

Cervical sampler broom: rotate 3-5 times

or

Cervex-Brush® Combi: insert central part of the brush into os and rotate clockwise twice

or

Spatula: rotate once or twice, taking care to keep contact with the ecto-cervix

plus

Endocervical brush: insert ensuring that you can see the lower row of the bristles and make a quarter rotation

FOR PERI AND POST-MENOPAUSAL WOMEN

Cervical sampler broom: rotate 3-5 times

plus

Endocervical brush: insert ensuring that you can see the lower row of the bristles and make a quarter rotation

or

Cervix-Brush® Combi: insert central part of the brush into os and rotate clockwise twice

or

Spatula: rotate once or twice, taking care to keep contact with the ecto-cervix

plus

Endocervical brush: insert ensuring that you can see the lower row of the bristles and make a quarter rotation.

FOR THINPREP

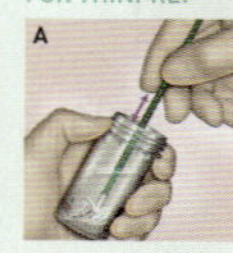

A. Cervical sampler Broom / Cervex-Brush® Combi: rinse the broom/brush as quickly as possible into the vial by pushing the broom into the bottom of the vial 10 times, forcing the bristles apart. As a final step, swirl the broom vigorously to further release material. Discard the collection device.

B. Spatula (Plastic): Rinse the spatula as quickly as possible into the vial by swirling the spatula vigorously in the vial 10 times. Discard the spatula.

C. Endocervical Brush: Rinse the brush as quickly as possible in the solution by rotating the device in the solution 10 times while pushing against the vial wall. Swirl the brush vigorously to release material. Discard the brush.

D. Tighten the cap so that the black line on the cap passes the black line on the vial.

Images supplied by Hologic (Australia) Pty Ltd

RECORDING PATIENT DETAILS

Record the woman's surname and date of birth on the vial.

OR

Apply sticker with details.

Record the woman's information and medical history on the request form.

VCS IS ABLE TO PROCESS THINPREP AND SUREPATH

ThinPrep

- Do not leave any part of the sampling device in the fluid.

SurePath

- Instruments should be broken off and left in the fluid

Sampling instrumments

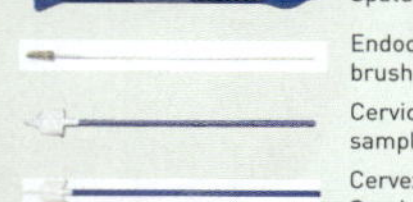

SPECIAL NOTES

Eversion: take care to sample the squamo-columnar junction. This is the junction where the columnar epithelium of the endocervical canal meets the squamous epithelium of the vagina. It is the area where changes occur.

Pregnancy: do not use the endocervical brush or Cervex-Brush® Combi.

www.vcspathology.org.au

NATIONAL CERVICAL SCREENING PROGRAM GUIDELINES

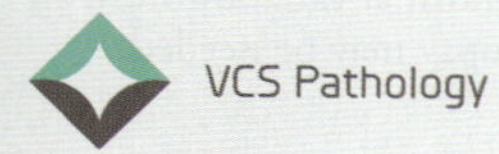

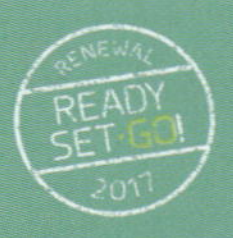

This resource is a guide for practitioners to assist them in identifying visual cervical appearances.

The images shown here are some examples of cervices you may see when taking a cervical sample.

Visual cervical abnormality may need further investigation even if screening tests are negative.

If you are uncertain about the appearance of the cervix, we recommend you seek a second opinion.

Further investigation not required in asymptomatic women

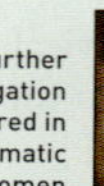
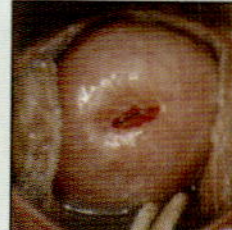
Nulliparous[1]

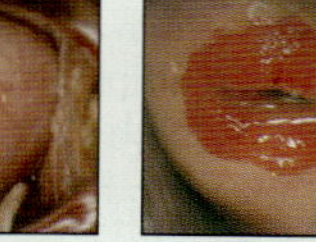
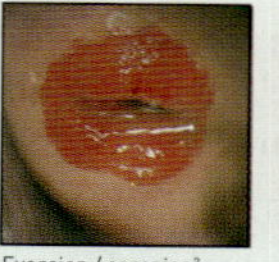
Eversion / ecropion[2]

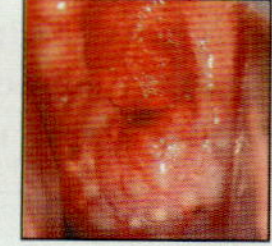
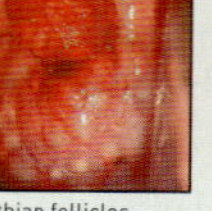
Nabothian follicles

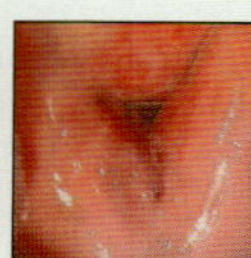
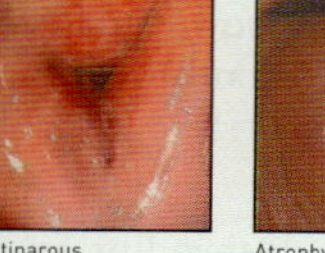
Multiparous

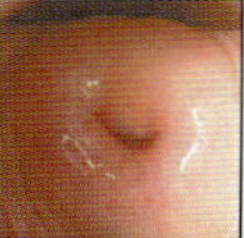
Atrophy

Consider further investigation

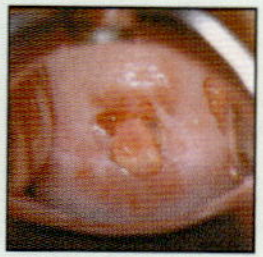
Polyp

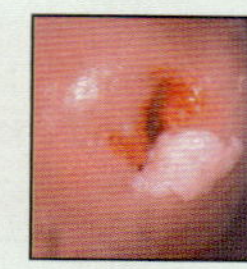
Cervical wart

Should be investigated

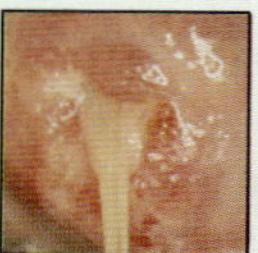
Mucopurulent discharge[3]

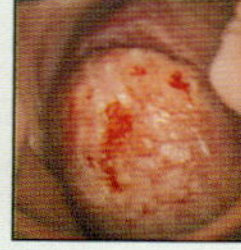
Cancer[2]

Post-intervention - further investigation not required in asymptomatic women

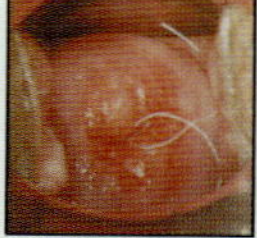
Intra Uterine Device (IUD)

Stenosis

Post treatment[2]

Reproduced with permission from:
1 Wolfendale, Margaret, 1995. Taking Cervical Smears. British Society for Clinical Cytology: page 12.
2 Burghardt, Erich, 1984. Colposcopy Cervical Pathology Textbook and Atlas. Georg Thiem Verlag. Germany: pages 162 & 174.
3 Cartier, René, 1984. Practical Colposcopy. Laboratoire Cartier. Switzerland: page 168.

www.vcspathology.org.au

Corp-Mkt-Pub-11 V6

Figure 26.14
Cervical screening card.

OBJECTIVE DATA

PROCEDURES AND NORMAL FINDINGS	ABNORMAL FINDINGS AND CLINICAL ALERTS
Vaginal pool. Gently rub the blunt end of an Ayre spatula (or cervical brush depending on the equipment required by the particular laboratory) over the vaginal wall under and lateral to the cervix (Figure 26.15). 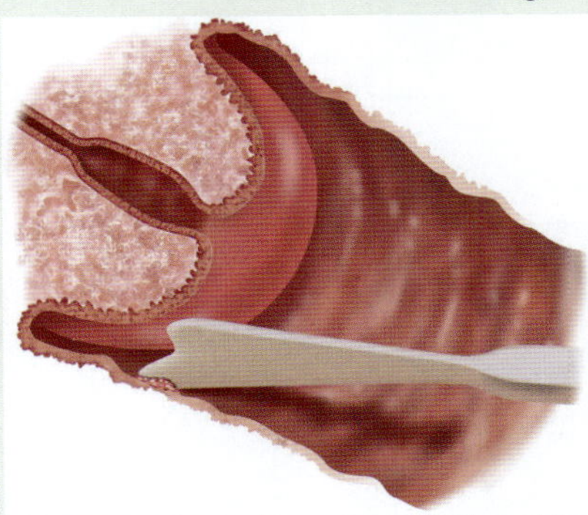 **Figure 26.15**	
Collection of a cervical specimen (Figure 26.16). Insert the bifid end of the Ayre spatula into the vagina with the more pointed bump into the cervical os. Rotate it 360 to 720 degrees, using firm pressure. The rounded cervix fits snugly into the spatula's groove. The spatula scrapes the surface of the squamocolumnar junction (SCJ) and cervix as you turn the instrument. It is important not to screen adolescents and women under 25 years old whose endocervical cells have not yet migrated into the endocervical canal. 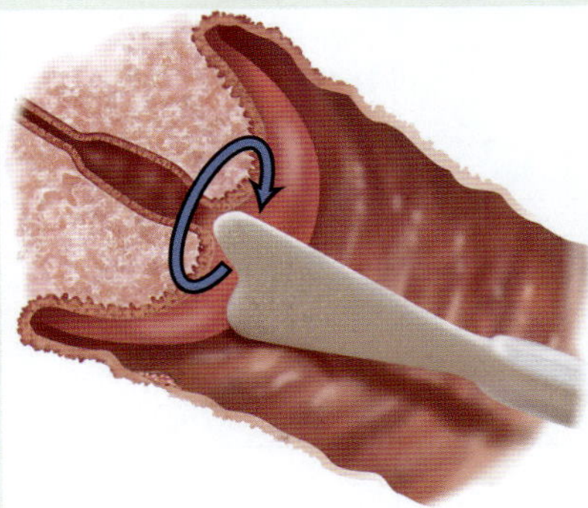 **Figure 26.16**	
Endocervical specimen (Figure 26.17). Insert a cervical brush (instead of a cotton applicator) into the os. The woman may feel a slight pinch with the brush and scant bleeding may occur. 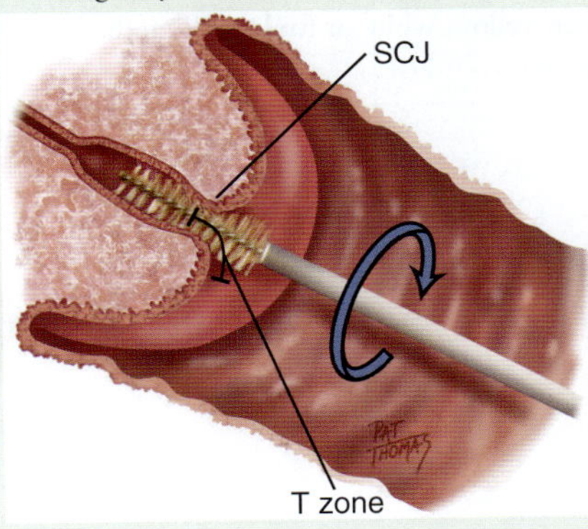 **Figure 26.17**	

OBJECTIVE DATA

PROCEDURES AND NORMAL FINDINGS	ABNORMAL FINDINGS AND CLINICAL ALERTS
Rotate the brush 720 degrees in ONE direction in the endocervical canal, either clockwise or counterclockwise. Then rotate the brush gently on a slide to deposit all the cells. Rotate in the opposite direction from the one in which you obtained the specimen. Avoid leaving a thick specimen that would be hard to read under the microscope. Immediately (within 2 seconds) spray the slide with fixative to avoid drying.	
For the woman after hysterectomy whose cervix has been removed, collect a scrape from the end of the vagina and a vaginal pool.	
Immediately spray the slides with fixative. The frosted ends of the slides should be labelled with the woman's name. Send these to the laboratory with the following necessary data: • Date of specimen • Woman's date of birth • Date of last menstrual period • Any hormone medication • If pregnant, with estimated date of birth • Known infections • Prior surgery or radiation • Prior abnormal cytology • Abnormal findings on physical examination	
These data are important for accurate interpretation; for example, a specimen may be interpreted as positive unless the laboratory technicians know the woman has had prior radiation treatment. Newer methods of cervical screening use a liquid-based thin-layer preparation. Instead of transferring the cervical sample onto a slide, the swab with the sample is deposited into a transportation fluid. The thin uniform layer of suspended cervical cells has improved sensitivity and a lower false–positive rate.	
To screen for STIs, and if you note any abnormal vaginal discharge, obtain a specimen of the discharge. Insert a sterile cotton applicator into the os, rotate it 360 degrees and leave it in place 10–20 seconds for complete saturation. Insert into labelled specimen container. Follow laboratory guidelines for collection, preparation and transport of specimens for possible STIs.	
Inspect the vaginal wall	
Loosen the thumbscrew but continue to hold the speculum blades open. Slowly withdraw the speculum, rotating it as you go, to fully inspect the vaginal wall. Normally, the wall looks pink, deeply rugated, moist and smooth and is free of inflammation or lesions. Normal discharge is thin and clear, or opaque and stringy, but always odourless.	Inflammation or lesions. Leucoplakia: appears as spot of dried white paint. Vaginal discharge: thick, white and curd-like with candidiasis; profuse, watery, grey-green and frothy with trichomoniasis; or any grey, green-yellow, white or foul-smelling discharge (see Table 26.5).
When the blade ends near the vaginal opening, let them close, but be careful not to pinch the mucosa or catch any hairs. Turn the blades obliquely to avoid stretching the opening. Place the metal speculum in a basin to be cleaned later and soaked in a sterilising and disinfecting solution; discard the plastic variety. Discard your gloves and wash hands.	

PROCEDURES AND NORMAL FINDINGS	ABNORMAL FINDINGS AND CLINICAL ALERTS
Bimanual examination	
Drop lubricant onto the index and middle fingers of your gloved hand (Figure 26.18). With the index and middle fingers extended, the last two flexed onto the palm and the thumb abducted; gently insert your fingers into the vagina, with any pressure directed posteriorly. Wait until the vaginal walls relax, then insert your fingers fully. 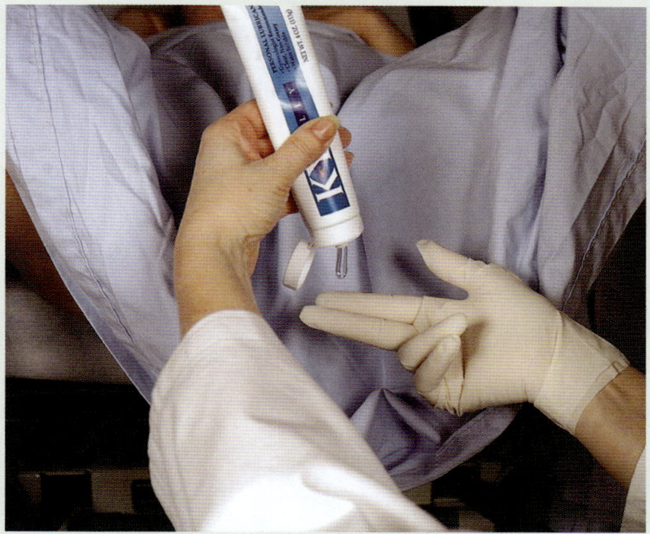 **Figure 26.18**	
You will use both hands to palpate the internal genitalia to assess their location, size and mobility and to screen for any tenderness or mass. One hand is on the abdomen while the other (often the dominant, more sensitive hand) inserts two fingers into the vagina (Figure 26.19). It does not matter which you choose as the intravaginal hand; try each way, and settle on the more comfortable method for you. 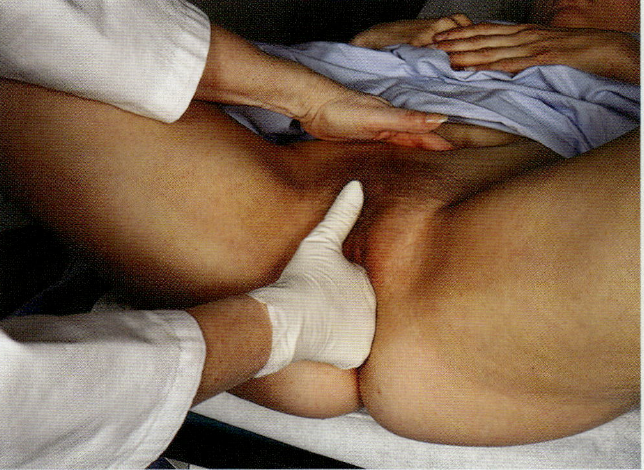 **Figure 26.19**	
Palpate the vaginal wall. Normally, it feels smooth and has no area of induration or tenderness.	Nodule. Tenderness.

PROCEDURES AND NORMAL FINDINGS	ABNORMAL FINDINGS AND CLINICAL ALERTS
Cervix. Locate the cervix in the midline, often near the anterior vaginal wall. The cervix points in the opposite direction of the fundus of the uterus. Palpate using the palmar surface of the fingers. Note these characteristics of a normal cervix:	
• **Consistency**—feels smooth and firm, has the consistency of the tip of the nose. It softens and feels velvety at 5 to 6 weeks of pregnancy (Goodell's sign).	Hard with malignancy. Nodular.
• **Contour**—evenly rounded.	Irregular.
• **Mobility**—With a finger on either side, move the cervix gently from side to side. Normally, this produces no pain (Figure 26.20). 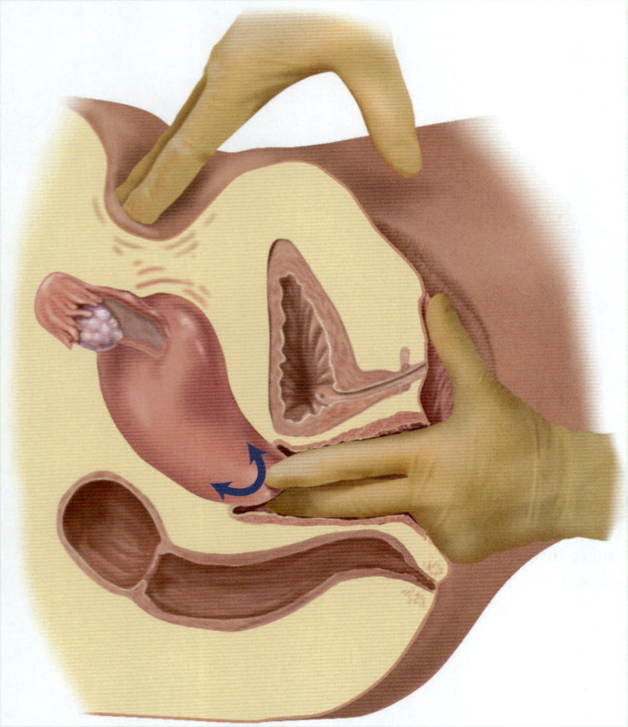 **Figure 26.20**	Immobile with malignancy.
Palpate all around the fornices; the wall should feel smooth.	Painful with inflammation or ectopic pregnancy.
Next, use your abdominal hand to push the pelvic organs closer for your intravaginal fingers to palpate. Place your hand midway between the umbilicus and the symphysis; push down in a slow, firm manner, fingers together and slightly flexed. Brace the elbow of your pelvic arm against your hip, and keep it horizontal. The woman must be relaxed.	
Uterus. With your intravaginal fingers in the anterior fornix, assess the uterus. Determine the position, or *version*, of the uterus (Figure 26.21). This compares the long axis of the uterus with the long axis of the body. In many women, the uterus is anteverted; you palpate it at the level of the pubis with the cervix pointing posteriorly. Two other positions occur normally (midposition and retroverted), as well as two aspects of flexion, where the long axis of the uterus is not straight but is flexed.	

PROCEDURES AND NORMAL FINDINGS	ABNORMAL FINDINGS AND CLINICAL ALERTS

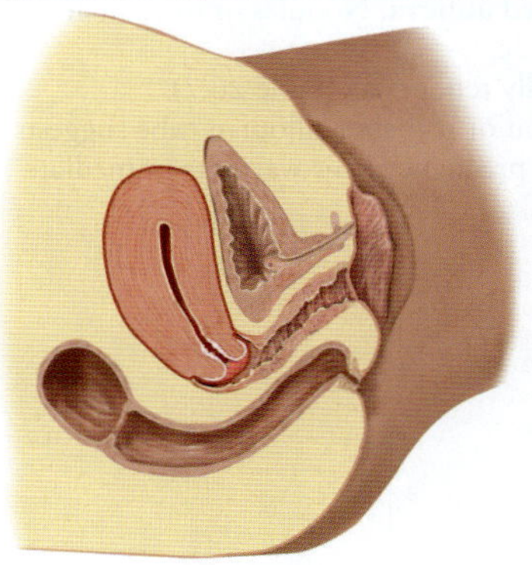

Anteverted

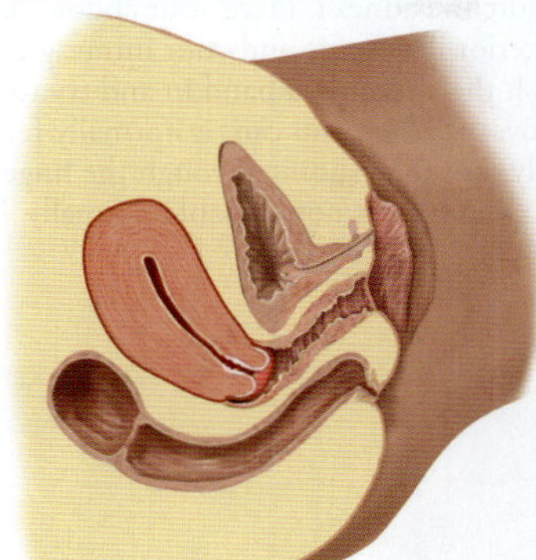

Midposition

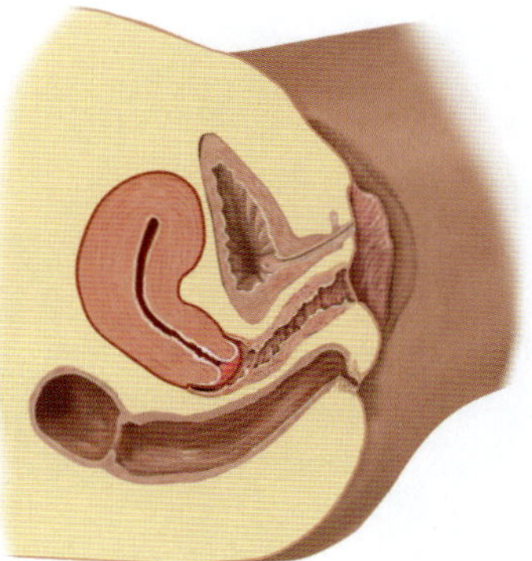

Anteflexed

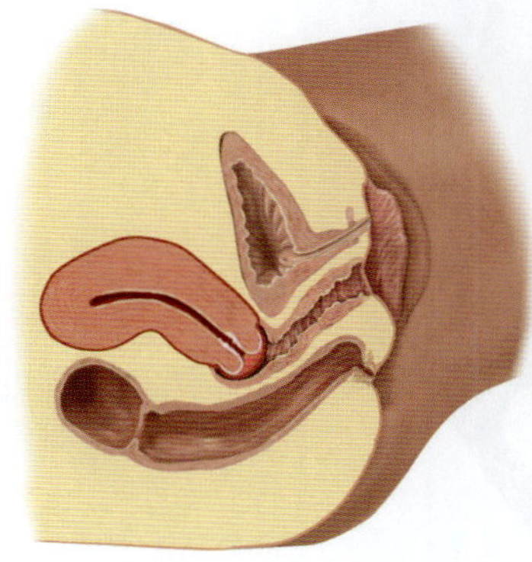

Retroflexed

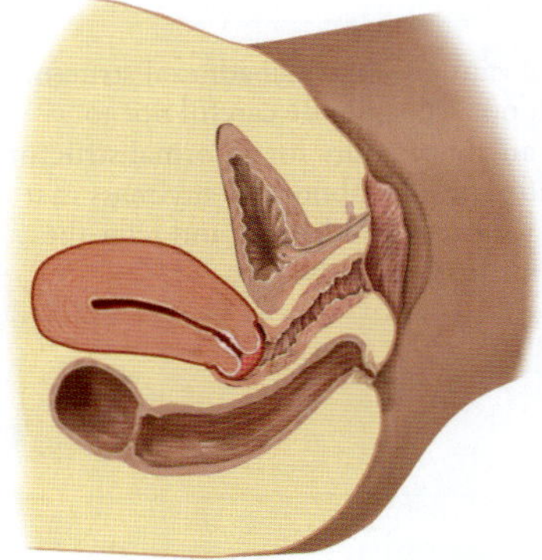

Retroverted

Figure 26.21

Palpate the uterine wall with your fingers in the fornices. Normally, it feels firm and smooth, with the contour of the fundus rounded. It softens during pregnancy. Bounce the uterus gently between your abdominal and intravaginal hand. It should be freely movable and nontender.	Enlarged uterus (see Table 26.6). Lateral displacement. Nodular mass. Irregular, asymmetrical uterus. Fixed and immobile. Tenderness.

OBJECTIVE DATA

PROCEDURES AND NORMAL FINDINGS	ABNORMAL FINDINGS AND CLINICAL ALERTS
Adnexa. Move both hands to the right to explore the adnexa. Place your abdominal hand on the lower quadrant just inside the anterior iliac spine and your intravaginal fingers in the lateral fornix (Figure 26.22). Push the abdominal hand in and try to capture the ovary. Often, you cannot feel the ovary. When you can, it normally feels smooth, firm and almond shaped, and is highly movable, sliding through the fingers. It is slightly sensitive but not painful. The fallopian tube is not palpable normally. No other mass or pulsation should be felt. 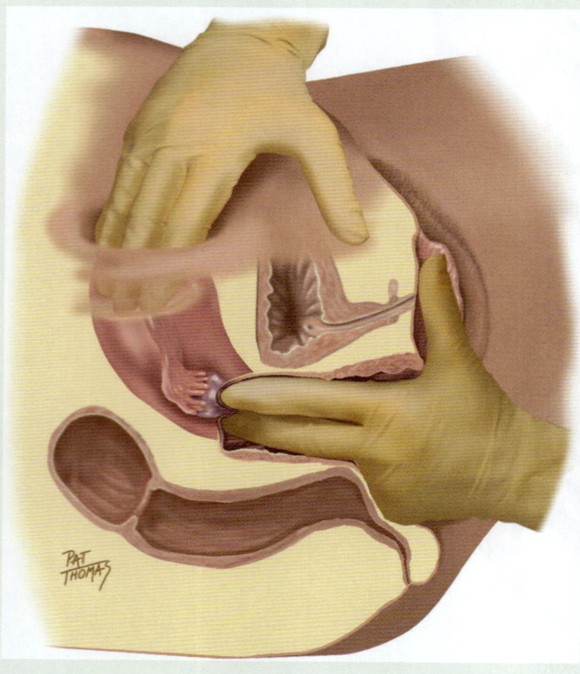 Figure 26.22	**Enlarged adnexa.** Nodules or mass in adnexa. Immobile. Markedly tender (see Table 26.7). Pulsation or palpable fallopian tube suggests ectopic pregnancy; this warrants immediate referral.
	A note of caution—normal adnexal structures are often not palpable. Be careful not to mistake an abnormality for a normal structure. To be safe, consider abnormal any mass that you cannot *positively* identify, and refer the woman for further study.
Move to the left to palpate the other side. Then, withdraw your hand and check secretions on the fingers before discarding the glove. Normal secretions are clear or cloudy and odourless.	
Following the examination make sure that you give the woman some tissues to clean herself and allow time for her to redress before completing the assessment.	
Addition objective data for the adolescent	
The adolescent girl has special needs during the genitalia examination. Examine her alone, without the parent present. Assure her of privacy and confidentiality. Allow plenty of time for health education and discussion of pubertal progress. Assess her growth velocity and menstrual history, and use the SMR charts to teach breast and pubic hair development. Assure her that increased vaginal fluid (physiological **leucorrhoea**) is normal because of the oestrogen effect.	

PROCEDURES AND NORMAL FINDINGS	ABNORMAL FINDINGS AND CLINICAL ALERTS
Perform pelvic examination when contraception is desired, when the girl's sexual activity includes intercourse. Start periodic Pap smears when intercourse begins. Although the techniques of the examination are listed in the adult section, you will need to provide additional time and psychological support for the adolescent having her first pelvic examination.	
The experience of the first pelvic examination determines how the adolescent will approach future care. Your accepting attitude and gentle, unhurried approach are important. You have a unique teaching opportunity here. Take the time to teach, using the girl's own body as illustration. Your frank discussion of anatomy and sexual behaviour communicates that these topics are acceptable to discuss and not taboo with healthcare providers. This affirms the girl's self-concept.	
During the bimanual examination, note that the adnexa are not palpable in the adolescent.	Pelvic or adnexal mass.
Additional objective data for the pregnant woman	
Depending on the week of gestation of the pregnancy, inspection shows the enlarging abdomen. The height of the fundus ascends gradually as the fetus grows. At 16 weeks, the fundus is palpable halfway between the symphysis and umbilicus; at 20 weeks, at the lower edge of the umbilicus; at 28 weeks, halfway between the umbilicus and the xiphoid; and at 34 to 36 weeks, almost to the xiphoid. Then, close to term, the fundus drops as the fetal head engages in the pelvis. See Chapter 29.	***Clinical alert:*** Any serious abdominal pain in a woman who could be or is pregnant should be referred to a medical practitioner urgently for further assessment. Serious abdominal pain in very early pregnancy could be an ectopic pregnancy which can be life-threatening (see Table 26.7).
The external genitalia show hyperaemia of the perineum and vulva because of increased vascularity. Varicose veins may be visible in the labia or legs. Haemorrhoids may show around the anus. Both are caused by interruption in venous return from the pressure of the fetus.	
Routine vaginal examination is not recommended during pregnancy (Department of Health 2019). See Chapter 29 for further details of assessment during pregnancy.	
Additional objective data for the woman over 65 years	
Natural lubrication is decreased; to avoid a painful examination, take care to lubricate instruments and the examining hand adequately. Use the Pedersen speculum (rather than the Graves) because its narrower, flatter blades are more comfortable in women with vaginal stenosis or dryness.	
Internally, the rugae of the vaginal walls decrease, and the walls look pale pink because of the thinned epithelium. The cervix shrinks and looks pale and glistening. It may retract, appearing to be flush with the vaginal wall. In some, it is hard to distinguish the cervix from the surrounding vaginal mucosa. Alternatively, the cervix may protrude into the vagina if the uterus has prolapsed.	Refer any suspicious red, white or pigmented lesion for biopsy. Vaginal atrophy increases the risk of infection and trauma.
With the bimanual examination, you may need to insert only one gloved finger if vaginal stenosis exists. The uterus feels smaller and firmer, and the ovaries are not palpable normally.	Refer any mass for prompt evaluation.
Prior surgery for hysterectomy does not preclude the need for routine gynaecological care, including cervical screening. Cervical screening can help detect gynaecological malignancies even when the cervix has been removed. Be aware that older women may have special needs and will appreciate the following plans of care: for those with arthritis, taking a mild analgesic or anti-inflammatory before the appointment may ease joint pain in positioning; schedule appointment times when joint pain or stiffness is at its least; allow extra time for positioning and 'unpositioning' after the examination; and be careful to maintain dignity and privacy.	

Summary Checklist

FEMALE SEXUALITY AND REPRODUCTIVE FUNCTION ASSESSMENT

Subjective data

1. Presenting concern
2. General health history
3. Sexual health history
4. Reproductive health history
5. Health and lifestyle management

Objective data

1. General inspection
2. Inspection of external genitalia

PROMOTING A HEALTHY LIFESTYLE

HUMAN PAPILLOMA VIRUS VACCINE

Vaccine to prevent cervical cancer—a breakthrough in cancer prevention

In Australia and New Zealand vaccination to prevent human papillomavirus (HPV) infection is part of the National Immunisation Program Schedule. HPV consists of a group of viruses that can cause skin and genital warts and some cancers, including cervical cancer. The vaccine targets HPV, the virus responsible for most cases of cervical cancer. It is recommended for girls and boys (usually 12–13 years of age) *before* they become sexually active because it is not effective if the individual is already infected with HPV. The vaccine (Gardasil®) is given in two separate injections over a 6-month period (or three doses if over 15 years).

HPV is a very common sexually transmitted virus. Most people who have had sex, both men and women, have been infected at some point in their lives. Most people never even know they have HPV because the virus usually does not cause any symptoms. However, sometimes the virus lingers in a woman's cervix and can cause changes that may eventually lead to cervical cancer. Other than the vaccine, the only way to prevent HPV is to abstain from all sexual activity. With the introduction of HPV immunisation, it is estimated that, in Australia, the age-standardised annual incidence of cervical cancer will decrease to fewer than six new cases per 100,000 women by 2020 and be considered a rare cancer (Hall et al 2019).

However, it is important to remind women that being immunised against HPV does not mean that women can forget about routine cervical screening tests. The vaccine will protect against the major types of HPV that cause cervical cancer, but not all types. Cervical screening tests (CST) are recommended for women from 25 years old. In Australia, this diagnostic test screens for HPV subtypes through Nucleic Acid Amplification Test (DNA) testing. Women are advised to screen every five years if normal until the age of 74 years old (Australian Government Department of Health 2019). Abnormal CST has a robust follow up algorithm, so reassure the woman that she will be contacted if there is an abnormal result.

In New Zealand, the CST will change from the traditional 'Pap smear' to the HPV primary screening in 2021. At present, screening is recommended for women 25 years of age and older every two years (National Screening Unit, NZ 2019).

For more information:

Australian HPV Vaccination program: https://www.health.gov.au/resources/collections/hpv-campaign

National (Australian) Cervical Cancer Screening Program: http://www.cancerscreening.gov.au/internet/screening/publishing.nsf/Content/cervical-screening-1

New Zealand Government National Cervical Screening Program: https://www.timetoscreen.nz/cervical-screening/

New Zealand Ministry of Health HPV Program: https://www.health.govt.nz/your-health/healthy-living/immunisation/immunisation-older-children/human-papillomavirus-hpv

Documentation and critical thinking

FOCUSED ASSESSMENT: CLINICAL CASE STUDY

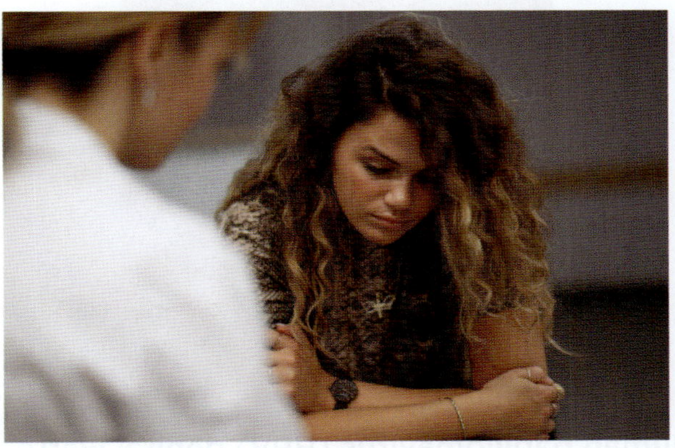

Context

Jacinta Knight, a 27-year-old woman, presents at a women's health clinic with 'urinary burning, vaginal itching and discharge (4 days)'.

Subjective

3 weeks ago: Jacinta was treated at GP clinic for bronchitis with erythromycin, following a respiratory tract virus which progressed to a bacterial infection. No history of asthma, generally healthy but has been very busy at work, working long hours. She says she was very tired before becoming ill. Non-smoker. She says the chest infection improved within 5 days after commencing antibiotics and taking 3 days off work.

She is married to Paul and has never been pregnant. 4 to 5 days ago: noted burning on urination, intense vaginal itching, thick white discharge. Says that Paul has no symptoms.

No previous history of vaginal infection, urinary tract infection or pelvic surgery.

Monogamous sexual relationship. Has used combined oral contraceptive pill for 7 years with no side effects.

Objective

On inspection, vulva and vagina erythematous and oedematous. Thick, white, curd-like discharge clinging to vaginal walls and labia.

Collaborative problem

Likely *Candida* vaginitis following antibiotic use and illness.

Problem statements/nursing diagnoses

Pain and discomfort related to inflammation and itch.

Knowledge deficit related to prevention and treatment of candida (thrush) infection.

Abnormal findings for advanced practice

TABLE 26.2 Abnormalities of the external genitalia

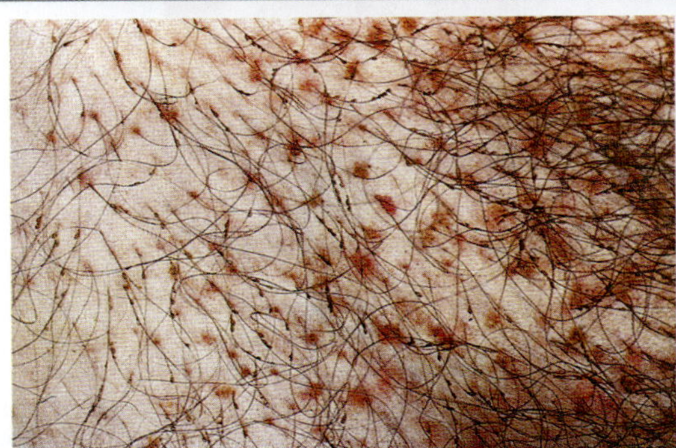 **Pediculosis pubis (crab lice)** The person will complain of severe perineal itching. Appears as excoriations and erythematous areas. May see little dark spots (lice are small), nits (eggs) adherent to pubic hair near roots. Usually localised in pubic hair, occasionally in eyebrows or eyelashes.	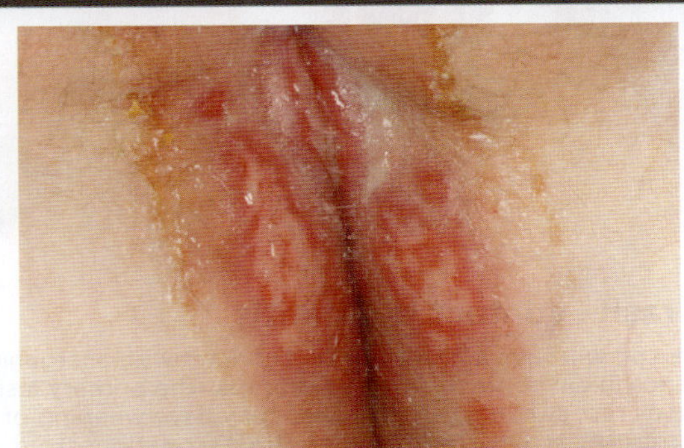 **Herpes simplex virus—type 2 (herpes genitalis)** The person will complain of episodes of local pain, dysuria, and fever. Appears as clusters of small, shallow vesicles with surrounding erythema; erupt on genital areas and inner thigh. Also, inguinal adenopathy, oedema. Vesicles on labia rupture in 1–3 days, leaving painful ulcers. Initial infection lasts 7–10 days. Virus remains dormant indefinitely; recurrent infections last 3–10 days with milder symptoms.

(Continued)

TABLE 26.2 Abnormalities of the external genitalia—cont'd

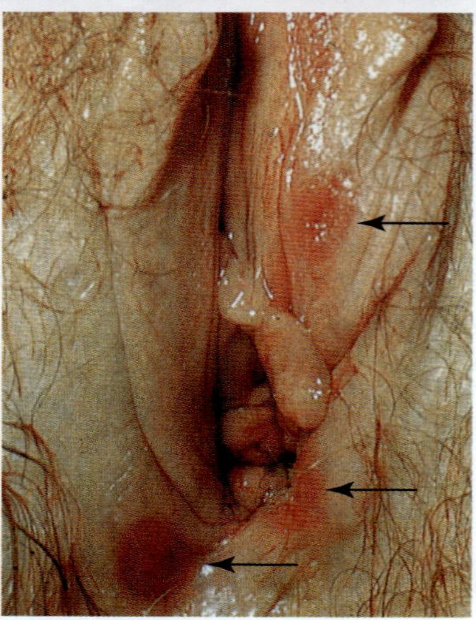

Syphilitic chancre

Begins as a small, solitary silvery papule that erodes to a red, round or oval, superficial ulcer with a yellowish serous discharge. Palpation—nontender indurated base; can be lifted like a button between thumb and finger. Nontender inguinal lymphadenopathy.

Reprinted from *Colour Atlas of Infectious Diseases*, 3rd edn. Emond, p. 173, 1995, by permission of the publisher Mosby.

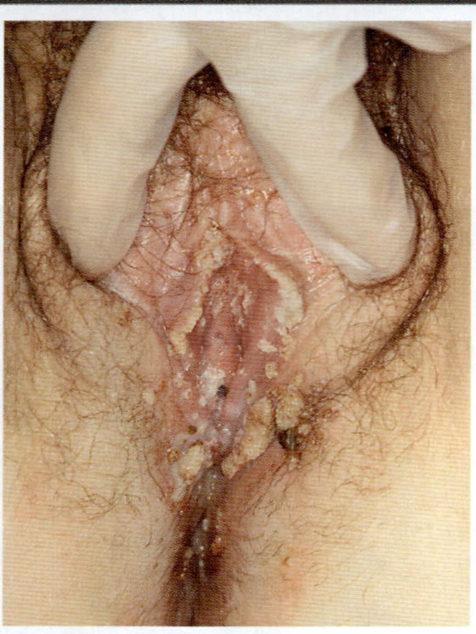

Human papillomavirus (HPV) genital warts

The painless warty growths may be unnoticed by woman (this image shows an advanced case).

The lesions appear as pink or flesh-coloured, soft, pointed, moist, warty papules. Single or multiple in a cauliflower-like patch. Occur around vulva, introitus, anus, vagina and cervix.

HPV infection is common among sexually active women, especially adolescents, regardless of ethnicity or socioeconomic status. Risk factors include early age at menarche and multiple sexual partners. The long incubation period (6 weeks to 8 months) makes it difficult to establish history of exposure. A strong association of HPV infection and abnormal cervical cytology exists. See also 'Promoting a healthy lifestyle' section for information on HPV immunisation.

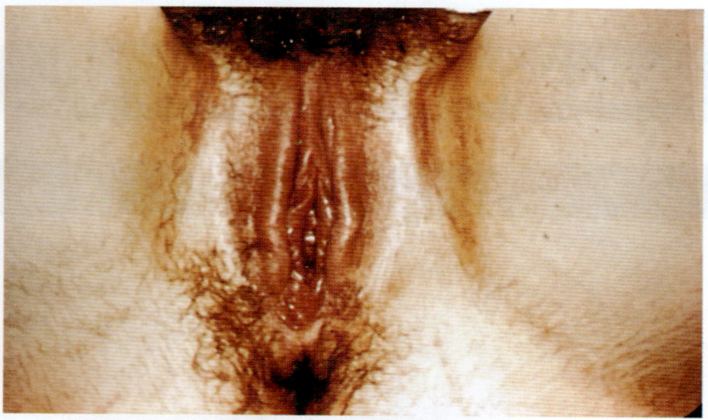

Red rash—contact dermatitis

The person will have a history of skin contact with allergenic substance in environment, intense pruritus. The primary lesions appear as red, swollen, vesicles. Then may have weeping of lesions, crusts, scales, thickening of skin, excoriations from scratching. May result from reaction to feminine hygiene spray or synthetic underclothing.

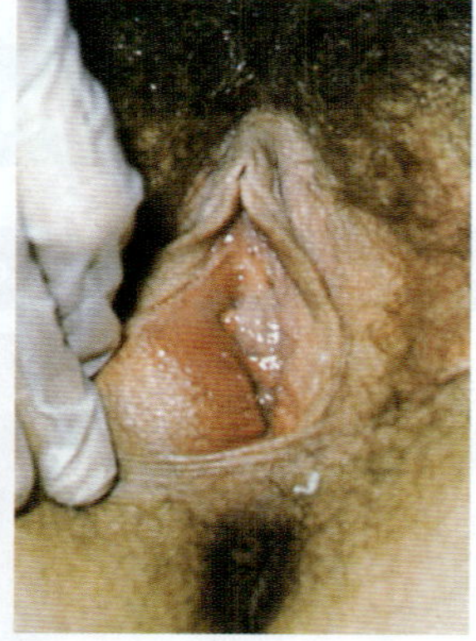

Abscess of Bartholin's gland

The person complains of local pain, which can be severe.

On inspection, the overlying skin red and hot. Posterior part of labia swollen; palpable fluctuant mass and tenderness. Mucosa shows red spot at site of duct opening; can express purulent discharge.

Reprinted from *Colour Atlas of Infectious Diseases*, 3rd edition. Emond, p. 161, 1995, by permission of the publisher Mosby.

TABLE 26.2 Abnormalities of the external genitalia—cont'd

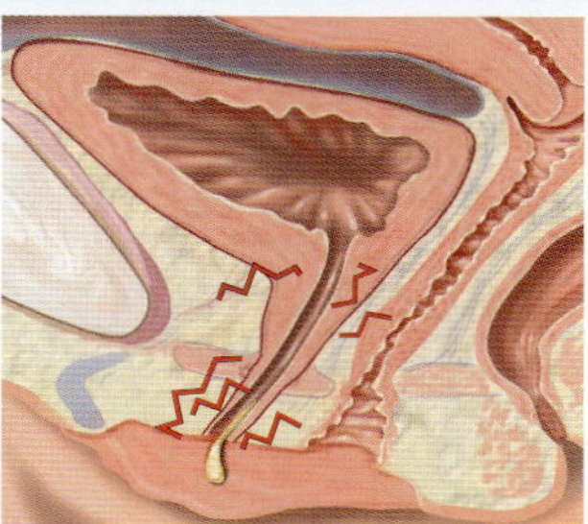
Urethritis

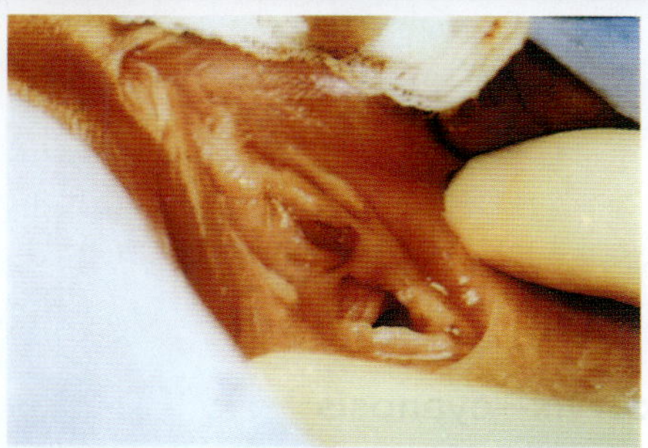

Urethritis

The person complains of dysuria and a burning sensation.

Palpation of anterior vaginal wall shows erythema, tenderness, induration along urethra, purulent discharge from meatus. May be caused by *Neisseria gonorrhoeae*, *Chlamydia* or *Staphylococcus* infection.

Urethral caruncle

The person complains of tenderness, painful urination, urinary frequency, haematuria, dyspareunia or may be asymptomatic.

The lesion appears as a small, deep red mass protruding from meatus; usually secondary to urethritis or skenitis; lesion may bleed on contact.

TABLE 26.3 Abnormalities of the pelvic musculature—pelvic organ prolapse

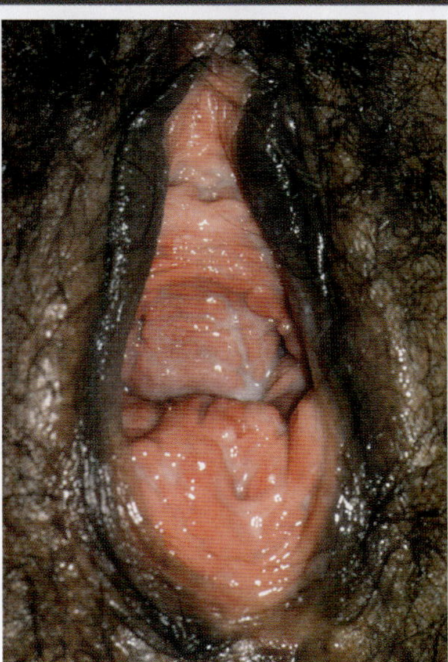

Cystocele

The woman may complain of a feeling of pressure in vagina, stress incontinence.

With straining or standing, note introitus widening and the presence of a soft, round anterior bulge. The bladder, covered by vaginal mucosa, prolapses into vagina.

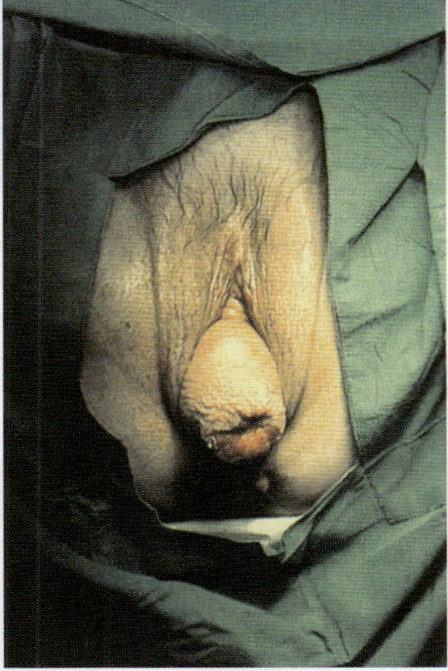

Uterine prolapse

With straining or standing, the uterus protrudes into vagina. Prolapse is graded: 1st degree, cervix appears at introitus with straining; 2nd degree, cervix bulges outside introitus with straining; 3rd degree (in this case), whole uterus protrudes even without straining—essentially, uterus is inside out.

TABLE 26.4 Abnormalities of the cervix

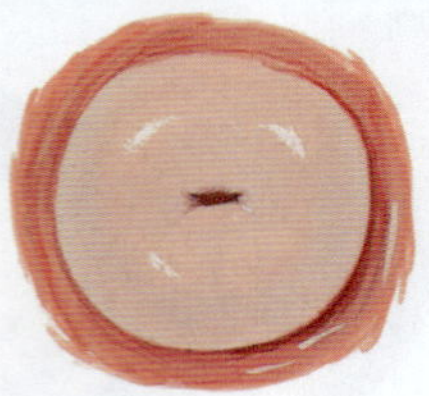

Bluish cervix—cyanosis

Bluish discolouration of the mucosa occurs normally in pregnancy (Chadwick's sign at 6 to 8 weeks' gestation) and with any other condition causing hypoxia or venous congestion (e.g. heart failure, pelvic tumour).

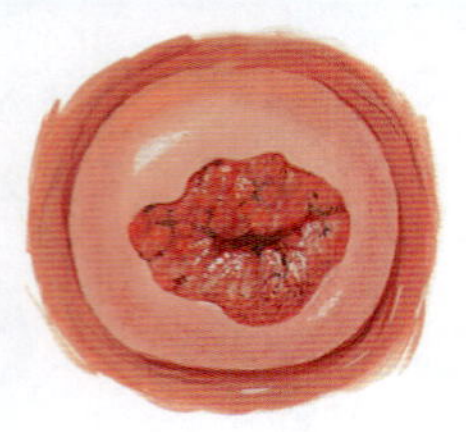

Erosion

Cervical lips inflamed and eroded. Reddened granular surface is superficial inflammation, with no ulceration (loss of tissue). Usually secondary to purulent or mucopurulent cervical discharge. Biopsy needed to distinguish erosion from carcinoma; cannot rely on inspection.

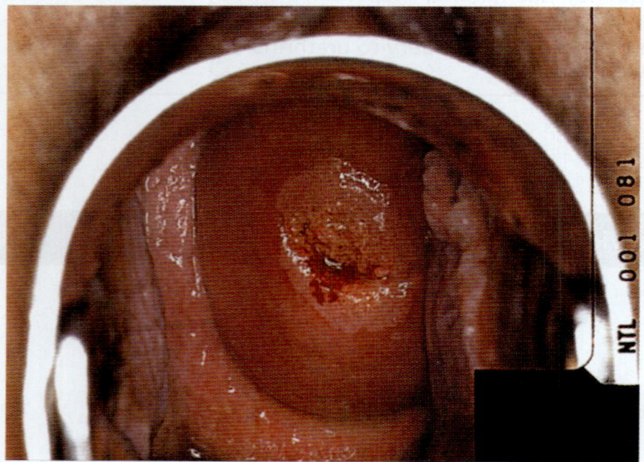

Human papillomavirus (HPV, condylomata)

The virus can appear in various forms when affecting cervical epithelium. Here, warty growth appears as abnormal thickened white epithelium. Visibility of lesion is enhanced by acetic acid (vinegar) wash, which dissolves mucus and temporarily causes intracellular dehydration and coagulation of protein. This must be treated as it can progress to cervical cancer.

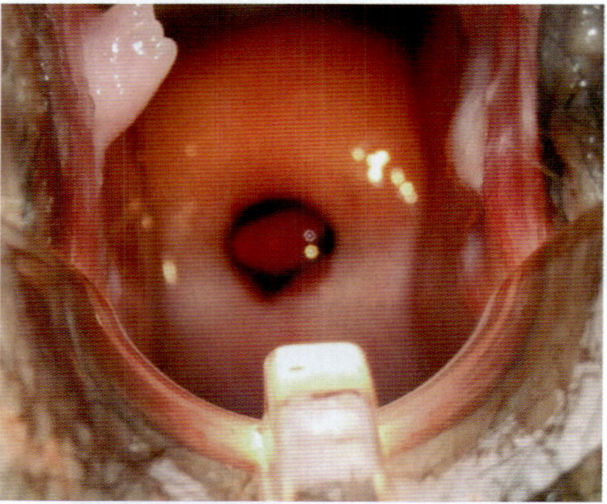

Polyp

The person may have mucoid discharge or bleeding.

The polyp will appear as a bright red, soft, pedunculated growth emerging from os. It is a benign lesion, but this must be determined by biopsy. May be lined with squamous or columnar epithelium.

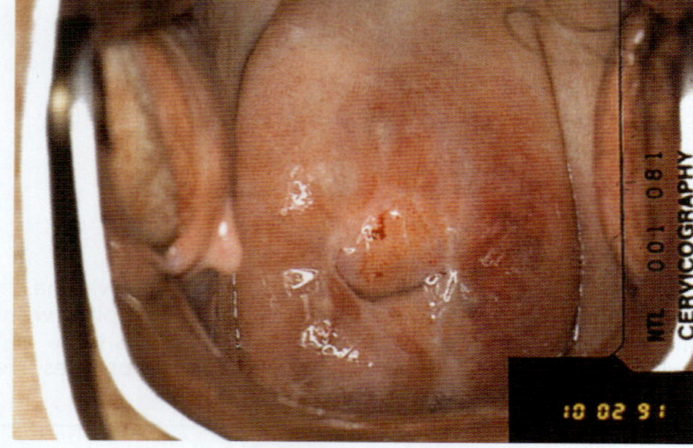

Cervical cancer

The person may complain of bleeding between menstrual periods or after menopause, unusual vaginal discharge.

Chronic ulcer and induration are early signs of carcinoma, although the lesion may or may not show on the exocervix. (Here, lesion is mostly around the external os.) Diagnosed by Pap smear and biopsy. Risk factors for cervical cancer are HPV infection (most common cause), early age at first intercourse, multiple sex partners, cigarette smoking, certain sexually transmitted diseases.

TABLE 26.5 Vulvovaginal infections

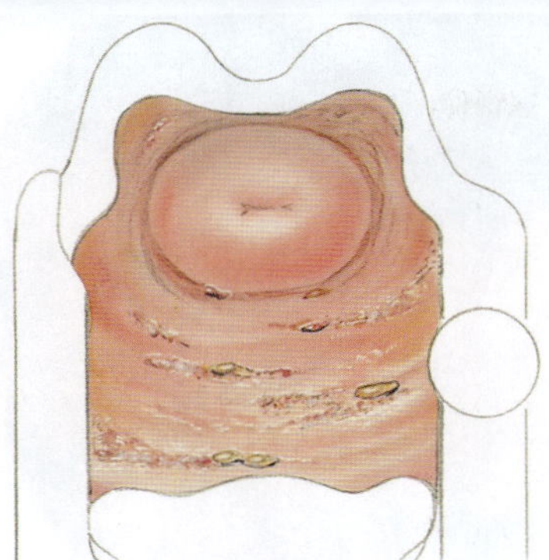

Atrophic vaginitis

Postmenopausal vaginal itching, dryness, burning sensation, dyspareunia, mucoid discharge (may be flecked with blood).

Pale mucosa with abraded areas that bleed easily; may have bloody discharge. Labial mucosa may appear to be thin and fragile, bleeding easily on touch.

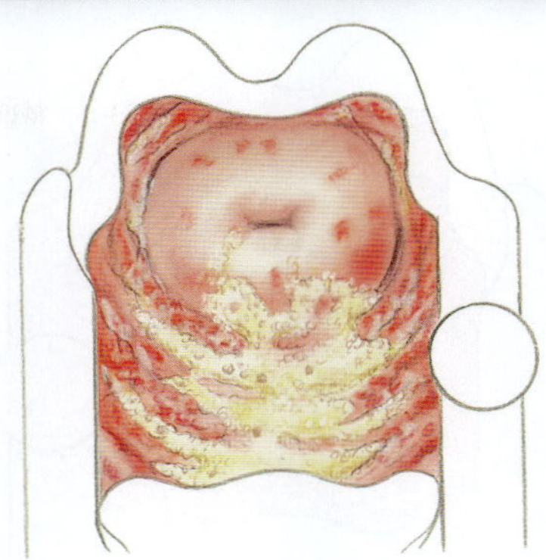

Trichomoniasis

Pruritus, watery and often malodorous vaginal discharge, urinary frequency, terminal dysuria. Symptoms are worse during menstruation when the pH becomes optimal for the organism's growth.

Vulva may be erythematous. Vagina diffusely red, granular, occasionally with red raised papules and petechiae ('strawberry' appearance). Frothy, yellow-green, foul-smelling discharge. Microscopic examination of saline wet mount specimen shows characteristic flagellated cells.

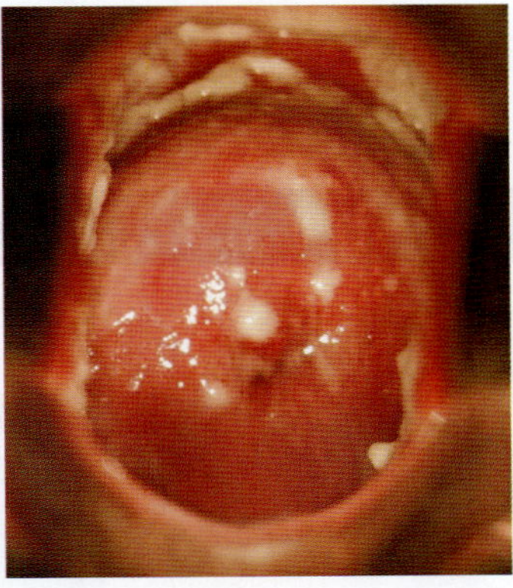

Candidiasis (moniliasis)

Intense pruritus, thick whitish discharge.

Vulva and vagina are erythematous and oedematous. Discharge is usually thick, white, and curdy, 'like cottage cheese'. Diagnose by microscopic examination of discharge on potassium hydroxide wet mount.

Predisposing causes—recent use of antibiotics or some oral contraceptives, more alkaline vaginal pH (as with menstrual periods, postpartum, menopause), also pregnancy from increased glycogen and diabetes types 1 and 2.

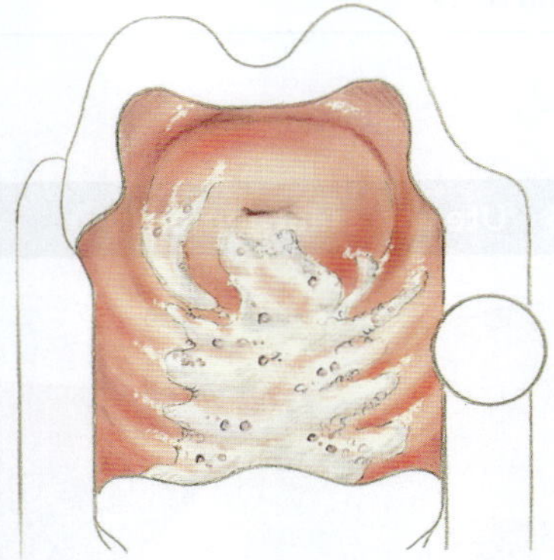

Bacterial vaginosis (*Gardnerella vaginalis, Haemophilus vaginalis* or nonspecific vaginitis)

Profuse discharge, 'constant wetness' with 'foul, fishy, rotten' odour.

Thin, creamy, grey-white, malodorous discharge. No inflammation on vaginal wall or cervix because this is a surface parasite. Microscopic view of saline wet mount specimen shows typical 'clue cells'.

(Continued)

TABLE 26.5 Vulvovaginal infections—cont'd

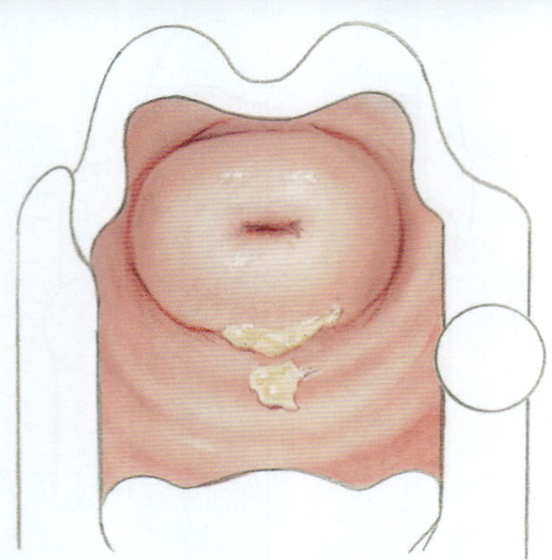

Chlamydia

Minimal symptoms. May have urinary frequency, dysuria or vaginal discharge, postcoital bleeding.

May have yellow or green mucopurulent discharge, friable cervix or cervical motion tenderness. Signs are subtle, easily mistaken for gonorrhoea. The two are important to distinguish because antibiotic treatment is different; if the wrong drug is given or if the condition is untreated, chlamydia can ascend the reproductive tract to cause pelvic inflammatory disease (PID), and result in infertility.

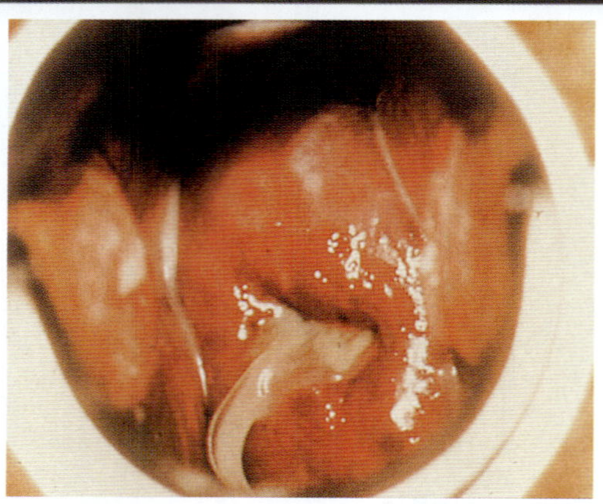

Gonorrhoea

Variable symptoms: vaginal discharge, dysuria, abnormal uterine bleeding, abscess in Bartholin's or Skene's glands; the majority of cases are asymptomatic.

Often no signs are apparent. May have purulent vaginal discharge. Diagnose by positive culture of organism. If the condition is untreated, it may progress to acute salpingitis, pelvic inflammatory disease (PID).

TABLE 26.6 Uterine enlargement

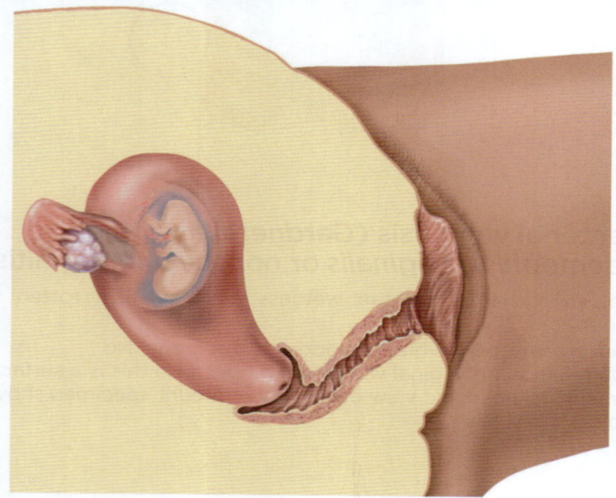

Pregnancy

Obviously a normal condition, pregnancy is included here for comparison.

Amenorrhoea, fatigue, breast engorgement, nausea, changes in food tolerance, weight gain.

Early signs: cyanosis of vaginal mucosa and cervix (Chadwick's sign). Palpation—soft consistency of cervix, enlarging uterus with compressible fundus and isthmus (Hegar's sign at 10 to 12 weeks).

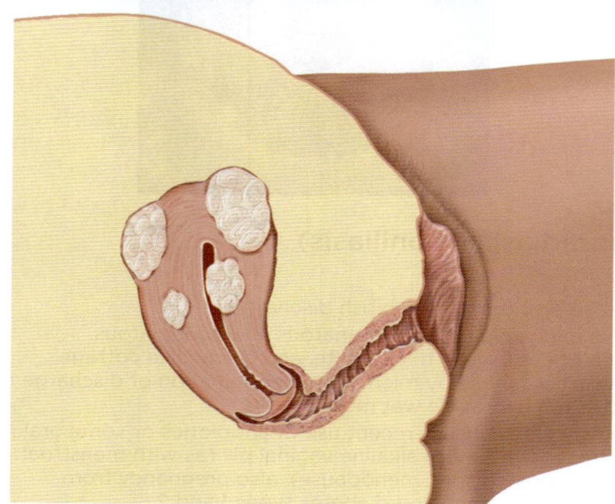

Myomas (leiomyomas, uterine fibroids)

Symptoms vary, depending on size and location. Often no symptoms. When symptoms do occur, include vague discomfort, bloating, heaviness, pelvic pressure, dyspareunia, urinary frequency, backache or hypermenorrhoea if myoma disturbs endometrium. Heavy bleeding produces anaemia.

Uterus irregularly enlarged, firm, mobile and nodular with hard, painless nodules in the uterine wall.

They are usually benign. Highest incidence between the ages of 30 and 45 years and in African-Americans. Myomas are oestrogen dependent; after menopause, the lesions usually regress but do not disappear. Surgery may be indicated.

TABLE 26.6 Uterine enlargement—cont'd

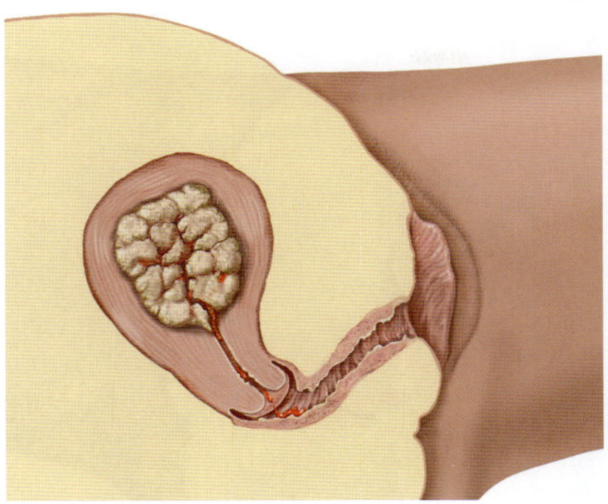

Carcinoma of the endometrium

Abnormal and intermenstrual bleeding before menopause; postmenopausal bleeding or mucosanguineous discharge. Pain and weight loss occur late in the disease.

Uterus may be enlarged.

The Pap smear is rarely effective in detecting endometrial cancer. Women with abnormal vaginal bleeding or at high risk should have an endometrial tissue sample. Risk factors for endometrial cancer are early menarche, late menopause, history of infertility, failure to ovulate, tamoxifen, unopposed oestrogen therapy (which continually stimulates the endometrium, causing hyperplasia) and obesity (which increases endogenous oestrogen).

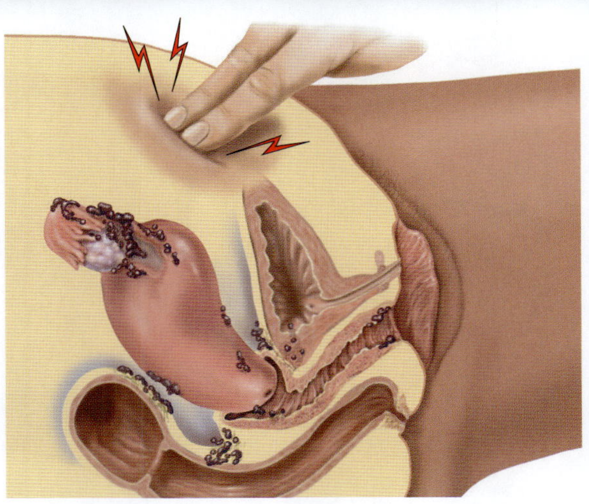

Endometriosis

Symptoms include cyclic or chronic pelvic pain, occurring as dysmenorrhoea or dyspareunia, low backache. Also may have irregular uterine bleeding or hypermenorrhoea or may be asymptomatic.

Uterus fixed, tender to movement. Small, firm nodular masses tender to palpation on posterior aspect of fundus, uterosacral ligaments, ovaries, sigmoid colon. Ovaries often enlarged.

Masses are aberrant growths of endometrial tissue scattered throughout pelvis as a result of transplantation of tissue by retrograde menstruation. Ectopic tissue responds to hormone stimulation; builds up between periods, sloughs during menstruation. May cause infertility from pelvic adhesions, tubal obstruction, decreased ovarian function.

TABLE 26.7 Adnexal enlargement

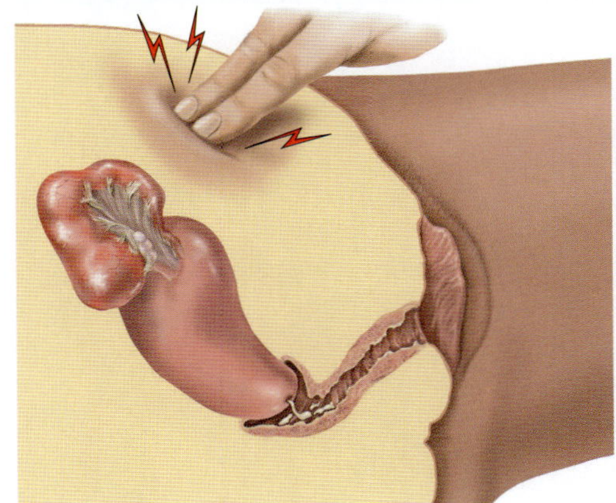

Fallopian tube mass—acute salpingitis (pelvic inflammatory disease (PID))

Sudden fever >38°C, suprapubic pain and tenderness.

Acute—rigid board-like lower abdominal musculature. May have purulent discharge from cervix. Movement of uterus and cervix causes intense pain. Pain in lateral fornices and adnexa. Bilateral adnexal masses difficult to palpate because of pain and muscle spasm. Chronic—bilateral, tender, fixed adnexal masses.

Complications include ectopic pregnancy, infertility and reinfection. PID usually caused by *Neisseria gonorrhoeae* and *Chlamydia trachomatis*.

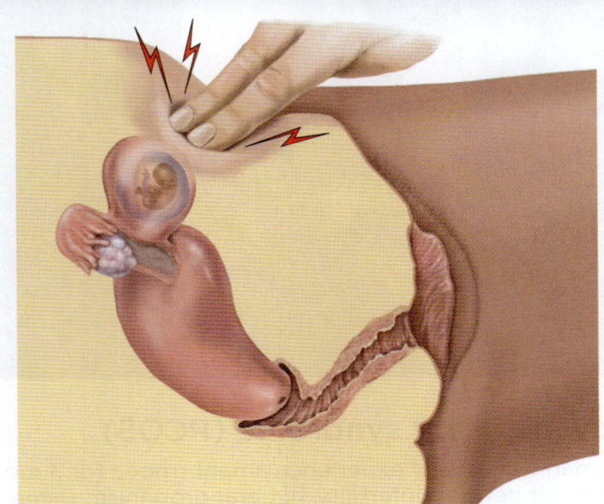

Fallopian tube mass—ectopic pregnancy

Amenorrhoea or irregular vaginal bleeding, pelvic pain.

Softening of cervix and fundus; movement of cervix and uterus causes pain; palpable tender pelvic mass, which is solid, mobile, unilateral. Late signs may indicate rupture: decreased BP, tachycardia, diaphoresis, shock. This is a medical emergency and requires urgent medical referral.

(Continued)

TABLE 26.7 Adnexal enlargement—cont'd

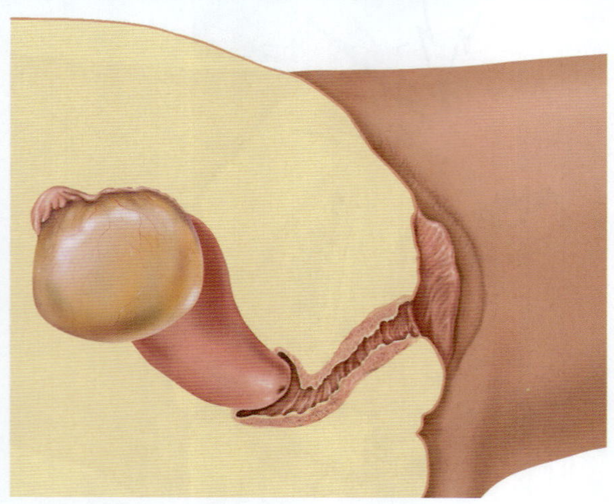

Fluctuant ovarian mass—ovarian cyst

Usually asymptomatic.

Smooth, round, fluctuant, mobile, nontender mass on ovary. Some cysts resolve spontaneously within 60 days but must be followed closely.

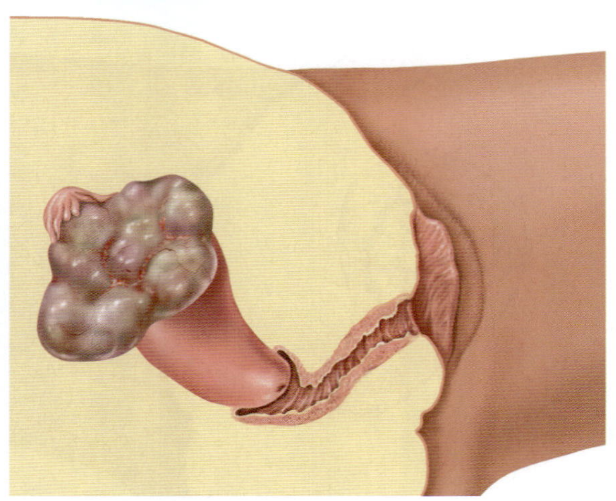

Solid ovarian mass—ovarian cancer

Usually asymptomatic. May have abdominal enlargement from fluid accumulation.

May or may not be able to palpate a solid tumour on the ovary. Heavy, solid, fixed, poorly defined mass suggests malignancy; benign mass may feel mobile and solid.

Biopsy necessary to distinguish the two types of masses. The Pap test does not detect ovarian cancer.

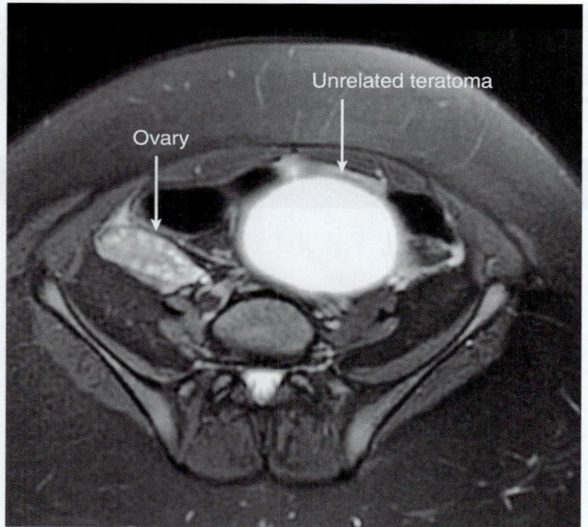

Polycystic ovary syndrome (PCOS)

The woman will usually experience amenorrhoea for 3 months or infrequent periods, infertility, hyperandrogenism (acne, facial hirsutism, hair loss), weight gain. May also have insulin resistance and diabetes.

This MRI image shows a right ovary with multiple cysts.

TABLE 26.8 Abnormalities in paediatric genitalia

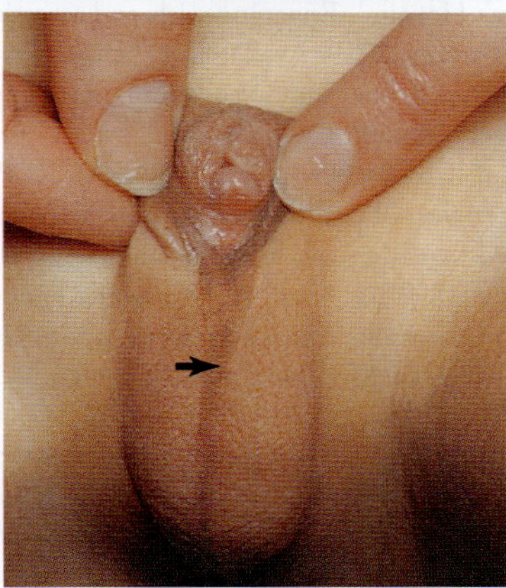

Ambiguous genitalia

Female pseudohermaphroditism is a congenital anomaly resulting from hyperplasia of the adrenal glands, which exposes the female fetus to excess amounts of androgens. This causes masculinised external genitalia, here shown as enlargement of the clitoris and fusion of the labia. Ambiguous means the enlarged clitoris here may look like a small penis with hypospadias, and the fused labia look like an incompletely formed scrotum with absent testes. Other forms of intersexual conditions occur, and the family must be referred for diagnostic evaluation.

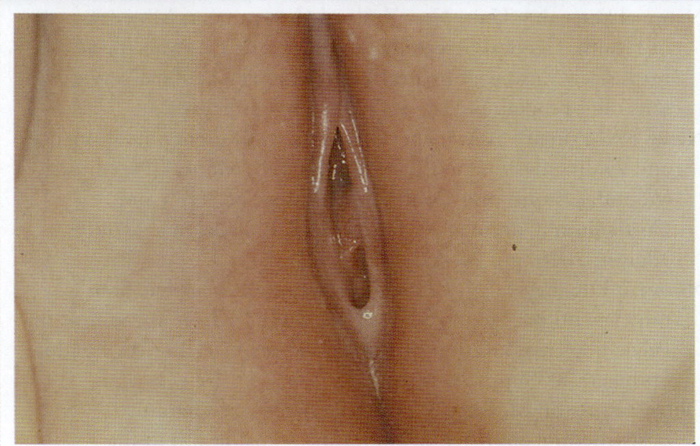

Vulvovaginitis in a child

This is an acute, nonspecific vulvovaginitis in a child. Symptoms include pruritus and burning when urine touches excoriated area. Examination shows red and shiny vulva and surrounding area.

Common causes of vulvovaginitis in the prepubertal child include infection from a respiratory or bowel pathogen, *Candida albicans* infection, sexually transmitted infection or presence of a foreign body.

BIBLIOGRAPHY

American Psychiatric Association (APA). Diagnostic and statistical manual of mental disorders. 5th ed. Arlington, VA: American Psychiatric Association; 2013.

Australian Government Department of Health. National cervical screening program. 2019. Available at: http://www.cancerscreening.gov.au/internet/screening/publishing.nsf/Content/healthcare-providers.

Australian Human Rights Commission. LGBTI Terminology. 2018. Available at: https://www.humanrights.gov.au/our-work/lgbti/terminology.

Australian Law Reform Commission, Australian Government. Capacity and health information. 2010. Available at: https://www.alrc.gov.au/publication/for-your-information-australian-privacy-law-and-practice-alrc-report-108/68-decision-making-by-and-for-individuals-under-the-age-of-18/capacity-and-health-information.

Bauer M, Heasler E, Fetherstonhaugh D. Let's talk about sex: Older people's views on the recognition of sexuality and sexual health in the health-care setting. Health Expect 2016;19(6):1237–50.

Cardozo L, Staskin D. Textbook of female urology and urogynaecology, 3rd ed. Abingdon: Informa Healthcare; 2010.

Cardozo L, Staskin D. Textbook of female urology and urogynecology, two-volume set. Boca Raton, FL: CRC Press; 2017.

Castro Diaz D, Robinson D, Bosch R, et al. Initial assessment of incontinence in adult male and female patients. In Abrams P, Cardozo P, Wagg A. et al., editors. 6th International Consultation on Incontinence. Bristol: ICI-ICS, International Continence Society; 2017. pp. 515–56.

Champer M, Wong AM, Champer J, et al. The role of the vaginal microbiome in gynaecological cancer. BJOG 2018;125(3):309–15.

Department of Health. Clinical practice guidelines: pregnancy care. Canberra: Australian Government Department of Health; 2019. Available at: https://www.health.gov.au/resources/pregnancy-care-guidelines.

Evcili F, Demirel G. Patient's sexual health and nursing: a neglected area. Int J Caring Sci 2018;11(2):1282–8.

Family Planning New Zealand. The Law around Abortion. 2019. Available at: https://www.familyplanning.org.nz/advice/abortion/the-law-around-abortion.

Family Planning Victoria. Medical termination of pregnancy—Medical consultant checklist. 2019. Available at: https://www.fpv.org.au/professional-learning-support/clinical-support.

Family Planning Victoria. Morning after pill—Emergency contraception. 2018. Available at: https://www.fpv.org.au/for-you/contraception/emergency-contraception/morning-after-pill-emergency-contraception.

Guevara GV, editor. Digital palpation of the pelvic floor muscles. International Continence Society; 2018. Available at: https://www.ics.org/committees/standardisation/terminologydiscussions/digitalpalpationofthepelvicfloormuscles

Hall MT, Simms KT, Lew JB, et al. The projected timeframe until cervical cancer elimination in Australia: a modelling study. Lancet Public Health 2019;4(1):e19–27.

Leonardi-Warren K, Neff I, Mancuso M, et al. Sexual health: exploring patient needs and healthcare provider comfort and knowledge. Clin J Oncol Nurs 2016;20(6):E162–7.

Marieb EM, Keller SM. Essentials of human anatomy and physiology. 12th Global ed. New York: Pearson; 2018.

National Screening Unit, New Zealand Government, Ministry of Health. Cervical Screening Guidelines. 2019. Available at: https://www.nsu.govt.nz/health-professionals/national-cervical-screening-programme/cervical-screening-guidelines.

Nelles KK. Primary assessment of patients with urinary incontinence and voiding dysfunction. In: Doughty DB, Moore KN, editors. Wound, Ostomy and Continence Nurses Society™ Core Curriculum: Continence Management. Philadelphia: Wolters Kluwer; 2016. pp. 24–43.

Newman DK, Laycock J. Clinical evaluation of the pelvic floor muscles. In: Baessler K, Schüssler B, Burgio KL, et al., editors. Pelvic floor re-education principles and practice. 2nd ed. London: Springer; 2008. pp. 91–104.

Ollivier R, Aston M, Price S. Let's talk about sex: a feminist poststructural approach to addressing sexual health in the healthcare setting. J Clin Nurs 2019;28(3-4):695–702.

Queensland Government. Queensland public sector LGBTIQ+ inclusion strategy: a strategy for sexual orientation, gender diversity and intersex inclusion 2017-2022. Brisbane: State of Queensland (Public Service Commission); 2017. Available at: https://www.forgov.qld.gov.au/sites/default/files/lgbtiq-inclusion-strategy.pdf?v=1491458841.

Rogers RG, Pauls RN, Thakar R, Morin M, Kuhn A, Petri E, et al. An International Urogynecological Association (IUGA)/ International Continence Society (ICS) joint report on the terminology for the assessment of sexual health of women with pelvic floor dysfunction. Int Urogynecol J 2018;29(5):647-66.

Rosen R, Brown C, Heiman J, Leiblum S, Meston C, Shabsigh R, et al. The Female Sexual Function Index (FSFI): a multidimensional self-report instrument for the assessment of female sexual function. J Sex Marital Ther 2000;26:191-208. Available at: www.fsfiquestionnaire.com.

Royal Children's Hospital. Engaging with and assessing the adolescent patient. 2019. Available at: https://www.rch.org.au/clinicalguide/guideline_index/Engaging_with_and_assessing_the_adolescent_patient/.

Royal College of Pathologists Australia (RCPA). RCPA manual of use and interpretation of pathology tests. 2019. Available at: https://www.rcpa.edu.au/Manuals/RCPA-Manual.

Taft AJ, Shankar M, Black KI, et al. Unintended and unwanted pregnancy in Australia: a cross-sectional, national random telephone survey of prevalence and outcomes. Med J Aust 2018;209(9):407–8.

Talley NJ, O'Connor S. Clinical examination: a systematic guide to physical diagnosis. 8th ed. Chatswood, NSW: Elsevier; 2018.

Telfer MM, Tollit MA, Pace CC, et al. Australian standards of care and treatment guidelines for transgender and gender diverse children and adolescents. Med J Aust 2018;209(3):132–6.

Tortora GJ, Derrickson B, Burkett B, et al. Principles of anatomy and physiology. 2nd Asia-Pacific ed. Melbourne: Wiley; 2019.

Victoria Government—VicHealth. Actions for inclusive practice. 2018. Available at: https://www2.health.vic.gov.au/about/populations/lgbti-health/rainbow-equality/best-practice-examples/actions-for-inclusive-practice.

World Health Organization. Defining sexual health. Report of a technical consultation on sexual health. 28–31 January 2002, Geneva. Geneva: WHO; 2006.

Websites

Jean Hailes for Women's Health: http://jeanhailes.org.au
New Zealand Sexual Health Society (Inc.): www.nzshs.org
Rainbow Network (Australia): https://www.rainbownetwork.com.au
Rainbow Youth (New Zealand): https://www.ry.org.nz

Chapter Twenty-Seven

Male sexual and reproductive assessment

Written by Carolyn Jarvis
Adapted by David Lee

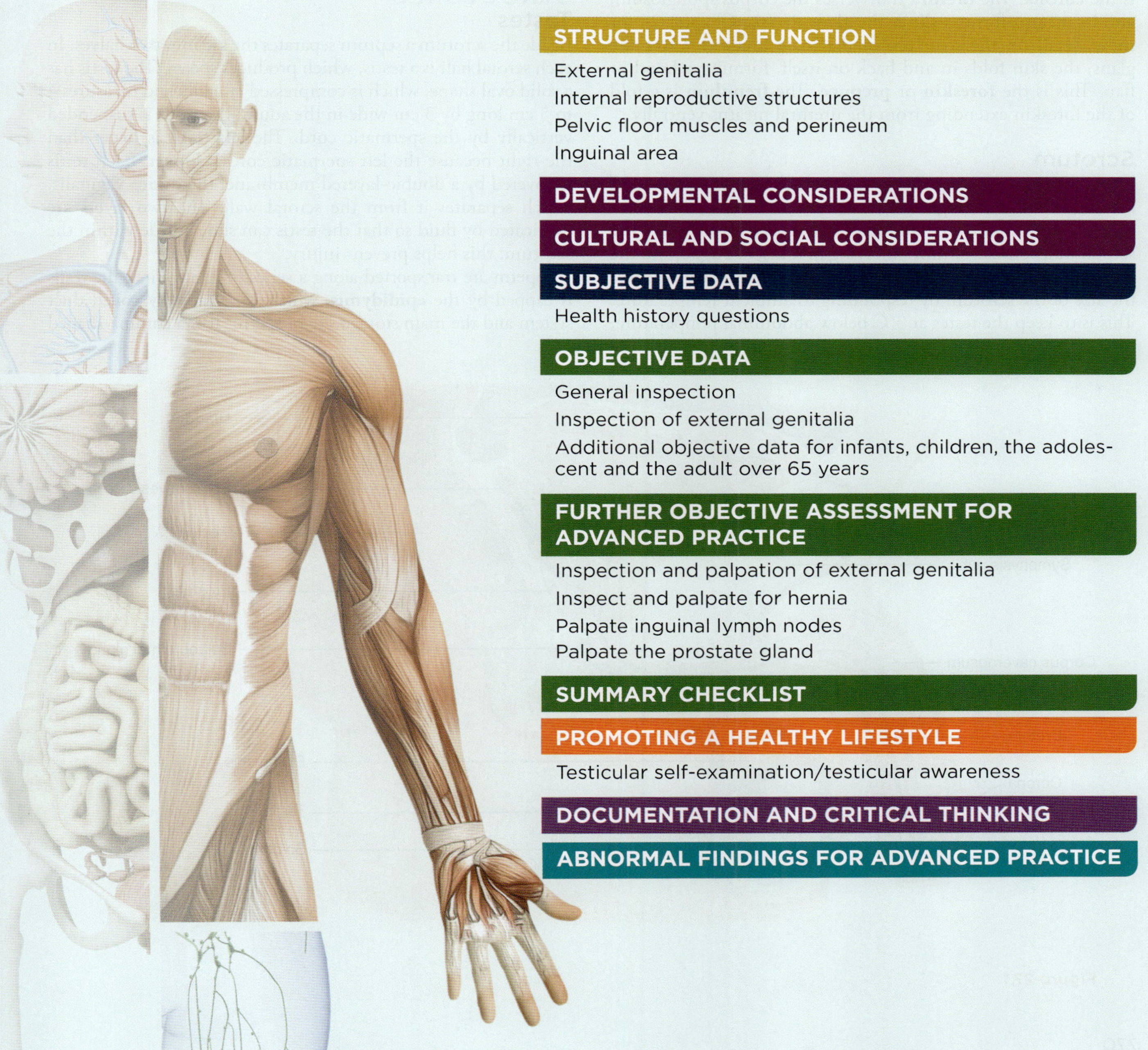

INTRODUCTION

The male reproductive structures include the penis and scrotum externally and the testis, epididymis and ductus deferens internally. They also include glandular structures accessory to the genital organs (the prostate, seminal vesicles and bulbourethral glands). As the organs, muscles and structures of the urinary tract, abdomen and bowel are relevant to male sexual and reproductive function you should also revise Chapters 23, 24 and 25.

Structure and function

EXTERNAL GENITALIA

Penis

The **penis** is composed of three cylindrical columns of erectile tissue: the two corpora cavernosa on the dorsal side and the corpus spongiosum ventrally (Figure 27.1). At the distal end of the shaft, the corpus spongiosum expands into a cone of erectile tissue, the **glans**. The shoulder where the glans joins the shaft is the **corona**. The **urethra** transverses the corpus spongiosum, and its meatus forms a slit at the glans tip (see Chapter 24 for more detail on the structure of the male urethra). Over the glans, the skin folds in and back on itself, forming a hood or flap. This is the **foreskin** or **prepuce**. The **frenulum** is a fold of the foreskin extending from the urethral meatus ventrally.

Scrotum

The **scrotum** is a loose protective sac, which is a continuation of the abdominal wall (Figure 27.2). After adolescence, the scrotal skin is deeply pigmented and has large sebaceous follicles. The scrotal wall consists of thin skin lying in folds, or **rugae**, and the underlying cremaster muscle. The **cremaster muscle** controls the size of the scrotum by responding to ambient temperature. This is to keep the testes at 3°C below abdominal temperature, the best temperature for producing sperm. When it is cold, the muscle contracts, raising the sac and bringing the testes closer to the body to absorb heat necessary for sperm viability. As a result, the scrotal skin looks corrugated. When it is warmer, the muscle relaxes, the scrotum lowers and the skin looks smoother.

INTERNAL REPRODUCTIVE STRUCTURES

Testes

Inside the scrotum a septum separates the sac into two halves. In each scrotal half is a testis, which produces sperm. The testis has a solid oval shape, which is compressed laterally and measures 4 to 5 cm long by 3 cm wide in the adult. The testis is suspended vertically by the spermatic cord. The left testis is lower than the right because the left spermatic cord is longer. Each testis is covered by a double-layered membrane, the tunica vaginalis, which separates it from the scrotal wall. The two layers are lubricated by fluid so that the testis can slide a little within the scrotum; this helps prevent injury.

Sperm are transported along a series of ducts. First, the testis is capped by the **epididymis**, which is a markedly coiled duct system and the main storage site of sperm. It is a comma-shaped

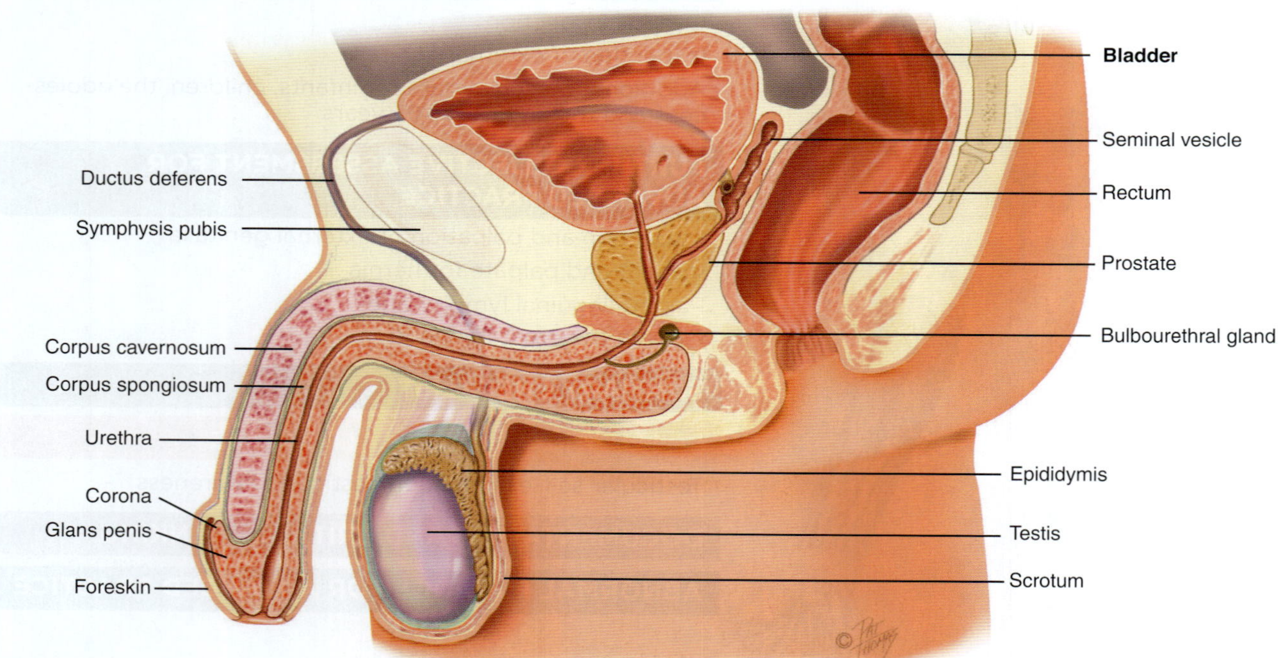

Figure 27.1

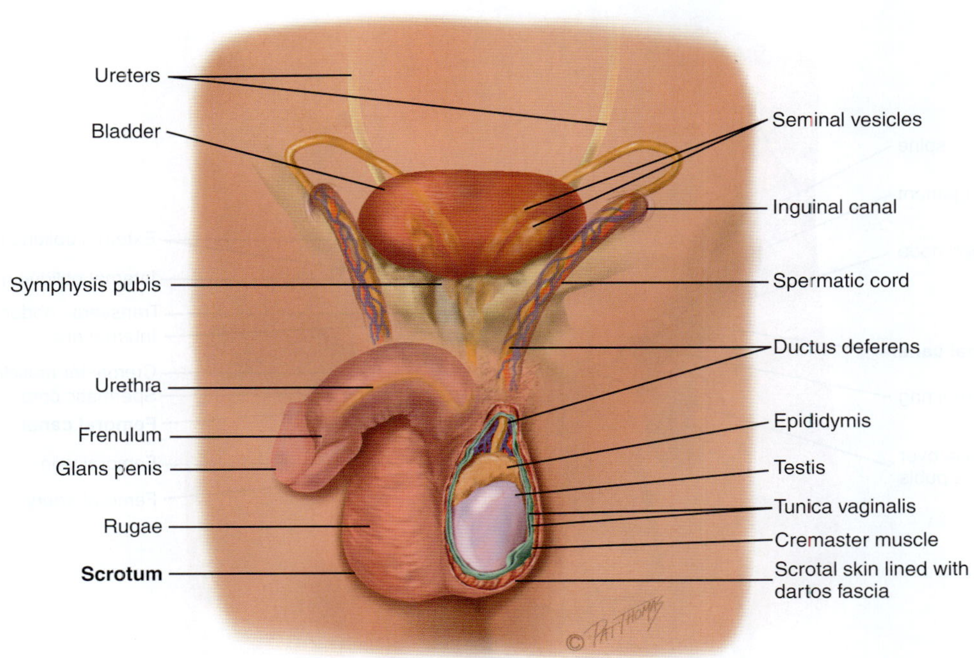

Figure 27.2

structure, curved over the top and the posterior surface of the testis. Occasionally (in 6–7% of males), the epididymis is anterior to the testis.

The lower part of the epididymis is continuous with a muscular duct, the **ductus deferens**. This duct approximates with other vessels (arteries and veins, lymphatics, nerves) to form the **spermatic cord**. The spermatic cord ascends along the posterior border of the testis and runs through the tunnel of the inguinal canal into the abdomen. Here, the ductus deferens continues back and down behind the bladder, where it joins the duct of the seminal vesicle to form the **ejaculatory duct**. This duct empties into the urethra.

The **lymphatics** of the penis and scrotal surface drain into the inguinal lymph nodes, whereas those of the testes drain into the abdomen. Abdominal lymph nodes are not accessible to clinical examination.

Prostate

In the male, the **prostate gland** lies in front of the anterior wall of the rectum and 2 cm behind the symphysis pubis. It surrounds the bladder neck and the urethra and has 15 to 30 ducts that open into the urethra. The prostate secretes a thin, milky alkaline fluid that helps sperm viability. It is a bilobed structure with a round or heart shape. It measures 2.5 cm long and 4 cm in diameter. The two lateral lobes are separated by a shallow groove called the **median sulcus**.

The two **seminal vesicles** project like rabbit ears above the prostate. The seminal vesicles secrete a fluid that is rich in fructose, which nourishes the sperm, and contains prostaglandins. The two **bulbourethral** (Cowper's) **glands** are each the size of a pea and are located inferior to the prostate on either side of the urethra. They secrete a clear, viscid mucus.

PELVIC FLOOR MUSCLES AND PERINEUM

The bony pelvis forms the solid structure for the muscles and ligaments of the anterior, posterior and lateral pelvic walls and pelvic floor which play such an important role in supporting the position of the pelvic organs. The pelvic floor muscles include the coccygeus muscle and the levator ani and are referred to as the pelvic diaphragm, which stretches from the pubic bone anteriorly to the coccyx posteriorly and from the right and left lateral pelvic walls. The anal canal and urethra pass through the pelvic diaphragm. The levator ani muscles support the pelvic organs and functions as a sphincter for the anal canal and urethra (Tortora et al 2019).

The perineum is located inferior to the pelvic diaphragm. The perineum extends from the symphysis pubis anteriorly to the coccyx posteriorly and the ischial tuberosities laterally. The muscles of the perineum are in two layers, superficial and deep. The superficial layer includes the superficial transverse perineal, bulbospongiosus and the ischiocavernosus muscles which help to maintain erection of the penis and facilitate ejaculation. The deep layer of the perineum includes the deep transverse perineal muscle, the external urethral sphincter and external anal sphincter which assist in maintaining urinary and faecal continence as well as ejaculation (Tortora et al 2019).

INGUINAL AREA

The **inguinal area**, or groin, is the juncture of the lower abdominal wall and the thigh (Figure 27.3). Its diagonal borders are the anterior superior iliac spine and the symphysis pubis. Between these landmarks lies the **inguinal ligament** (Poupart's ligament). Superior to the ligament lies the **inguinal canal**, a narrow tunnel passing obliquely between layers of abdominal muscle. It is 4 to 6 cm long in the adult. Its openings are an

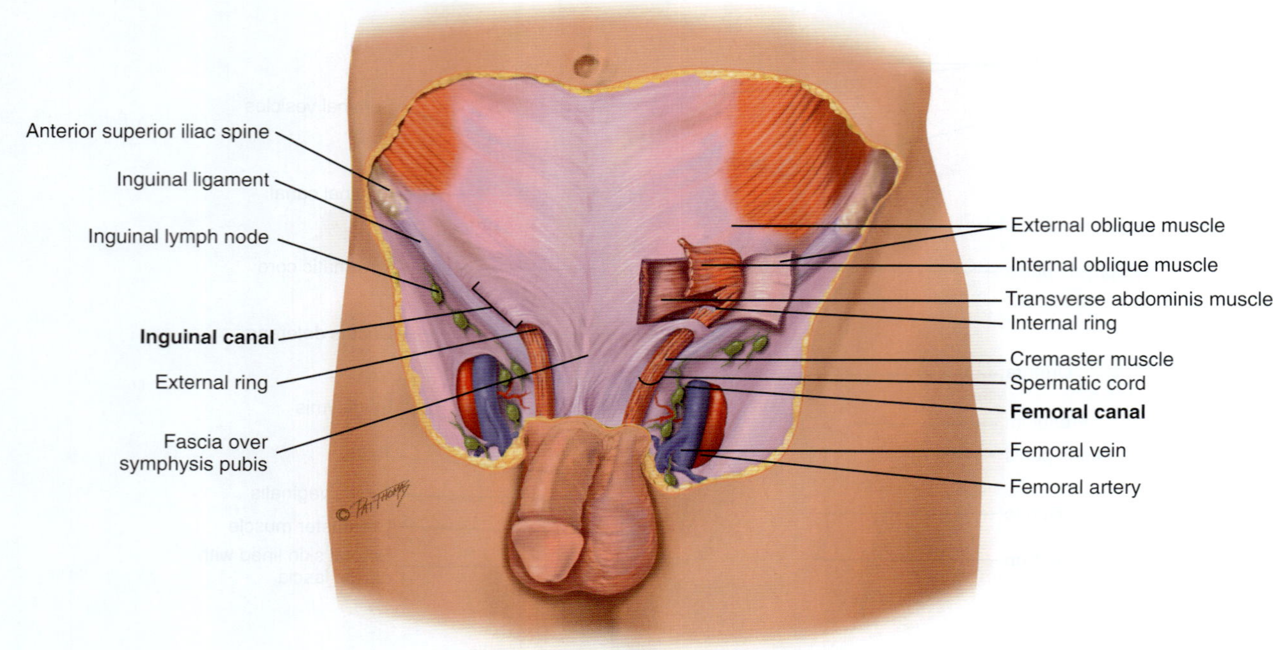

Figure 27.3
©Pat Thomas

internal ring, located 1 to 2 cm above the midpoint of the inguinal ligament, and an external ring, located just above and lateral to the pubis.

Inferior to the inguinal ligament is the **femoral canal**. It is a potential space located 3 cm medial to and parallel with the femoral artery. You can use the artery as a landmark to find this space. There are superficial and deep lymph nodes around the inguinal canal located in the femoral triangle of Scarpa. Lymph nodes are glands that function to maintain blood fluid balance, filter waste and are a protective defence system from pathogens. These lymph nodes may be palpable in thinner men and are smooth, mobile in consistency and non-tender when palpated. The inguinal lymph nodes can become painful and enlarged (lymphadenitis) when there is localised infection. Knowledge of these anatomical areas in the groin is useful because they are potential sites for a hernia, which is a loop of bowel protruding through a weak spot in the musculature.

DEVELOPMENTAL CONSIDERATIONS

Infants

Prenatally, the testes develop in the abdominal cavity near the kidneys. During the later months of gestation the testes migrate, pushing the abdominal wall in front of them and dragging the ductus deferens, the blood vessels and nerves behind. The testes descend along the inguinal canal into the scrotum before birth. At birth, each testis measures 1½ to 2 cm long and 1 cm wide. Only a slight increase in size occurs during the prepubertal years.

Adolescents

Puberty begins sometime between the ages of 9½ and 13. The first sign is enlargement of the testes. Next, pubic hair appears then penis size increases. The stages of development are documented in Tanner's sexual maturity ratings (SMR) (Table 27.1). The complete change in development from a preadolescent to an adult takes about 3 years, although the normal range is 2 to 5 years.

The level of sexual development at the end of puberty remains constant through young and middle adulthood, with no further genital growth and no change in circulating sex hormone. The male does not experience a definite end to fertility as the female does. Around age 40 years, the production of sperm begins to decrease, although it continues into the 80s and 90s.

Testosterone (or androgen) and oestrogen are important hormones in both men and women. When blood levels are depleted or elevated, physiological, physical, emotional and psychological concerns may arise. Men have higher levels of testosterone than women and lower levels of oestrogen. Testosterone maintains sex drive, production of sperm, muscle strength and bone mass and plays a role in overall wellbeing and energy levels. Low levels of testosterone (hypogonadism) may lead to mood changes, poor concentration, lethargy, low libido or sex drive, hot flushes and sweats, reduced body hair growth, reduced muscle strength and breast enlargement (gynaecomastia) (Healthy Male 2019). The misuse of steroids and other appearance and performance enhancing drugs (APEDs) have significant and detrimental impact on physiology, neurological function and mental health (Alcohol and Drug Foundation 2019).

Adults, men over 65 years

At male puberty, the prostate gland undergoes a very rapid increase to more than twice its prepubertal size. During young adulthood its size remains fairly constant. The prostate gland commonly starts to enlarge during the middle adult years. This

TABLE 27.1 Sex maturity ratings (SMR) in boys

DEVELOPMENTAL STAGE	PUBIC HAIR	PENIS	SCROTUM
1	No pubic hair. Fine body hair on abdomen (vellus hair) continues over pubic area	Preadolescent, size and proportion the same as during childhood	Preadolescent, size and proportion the same as during childhood
2	Few straight slightly darker hairs at base of penis. Hair is long and downy	Little or no enlargement	Testes and scrotum begin to enlarge. Scrotal skin reddens and changes in texture
3	Sparse growth over entire pubis. Hair darker, coarser and curly	Penis begins to enlarge, especially in length	Further enlarged
4	Thick growth over pubic area but not on thighs. Hair coarse and curly as in adult	Penis grows in length and diameter, with development of glans	Testes almost fully grown, scrotum darker
5	Growth spread over medial thighs, although not yet up towards umbilicus. After puberty, pubic hair growth continues until the mid-20s, extending up the abdomen towards the umbilicus	Adult size and shape	Adult size and shape

benign prostatic hypertrophy (BPH) is a common condition affecting more than 20% of men by 60 years of age and 40% of men over 70 years of age (Patel & Bariol 2019). It is thought that hypertrophy is caused by hormonal imbalance that leads to the proliferation of benign adenomas. These gradually impede voiding because they obstruct the urethra.

Prostate cancer is the most common cancer that occurs in men and the second leading cause of cancer deaths in men. The risk of developing prostate cancer to age 75 years is 1 in 23 and to age 85 is 1 in 9 for Australian men (AIHW 2019). In New Zealand males the incidence of prostate cancer is estimated to be 1 in 13 to age 75 (Prostate Cancer Foundation of New Zealand 2019). Prostate cancer is essentially a disease of older men with 63% diagnosed after 65 years of age; it is rare before the age of 40 and its incidence rises rapidly after age 60 (Cancer Council of Australia 2019). The cause of prostate cancer is unknown. Apart from advancing age and being male, the strongest established risk factor is a family history of the disease; the risk depends on the number of relatives affected. In the early stages of prostate cancer, the man is likely to be asymptomatic making early detection difficult. See Promoting a Healthy Lifestyle—Understanding prostate changes in Chapter 24 for more information.

In the ageing male, the amount of pubic hair decreases, and the remaining hair turns grey. Penis size decreases. Due to decreased tone of the dartos muscle, the scrotal contents hang lower, the rugae decrease and the scrotum looks pendulous. The testes decrease in size and are less firm to palpation. Increased connective tissue is present in the tubules, so these become thickened and produce less sperm. As men age their testosterone levels decline slowly, from about the age of 40 years. Some older men will develop very low testosterone levels (androgen deficiency) which will cause symptoms similar to the female menopause such as fatigue, hot flushes, decreased sexual drive and osteoporosis. Although a wide range of individual differences can occur, the older male may find that an erection takes longer to develop and that it is less full or firm. Once obtained, the erection may be maintained for longer periods without ejaculation. Ejaculation is shorter and less forceful, and the volume of seminal fluid is less than when the man was younger. After ejaculation, rapid detumescence (return to the flaccid state) occurs, especially after 60 years of age. This occurs in a few seconds as compared with minutes or hours in the younger male. Erectile dysfunction has been defined as the persistent inability to achieve or maintain an erection sufficient for satisfactory sexual intercourse (European Association of Urology 2018, Healthy Male 2019). The incidence of erectile dysfunction increases with age, occurring in up to 50% of men aged 40 to 70 years (Colson et al 2018). However, lifestyle risk factors such as smoking, alcohol abuse, obesity, lack of physical activity or chronic diseases, for example, diabetes, cardiovascular disease and mental health disorders, are more likely to contribute to erectile dysfunction than chronological age (Colson et al 2018).

CULTURAL AND SOCIAL CONSIDERATIONS

There is a marked inequality in Australian men's health—men have a shorter life expectancy than women and die more often than women from preventable diseases. While men are seeking out healthcare more frequently than in previous years, they often present when a condition or illness is advanced and are unlikely to seek help for mental ill-health (Australian Government, Department of Health 2019). There is a higher rate of risk taking behaviour, suicide, accidents and poorer mental health outcomes including violence, anger, substance and alcohol misuse (AIHW 2019). There is a similar situation for New Zealand men. In an effort to address the specific needs of men's health, the Australian Government has developed a focused health strategy to promote men's health with the goal of 'every man and boy in Australia is supported to live a long, fulfilling and healthy life' (Australian Government, Department of Health 2019). The five priority areas of the strategy are mental health, chronic conditions, sexual and reproductive health and conditions where men are over-represented, injuries and risk taking and healthy ageing.

As has been discussed in previous chapters, a range of determinants influence health, including individual factors, social, economic, environmental, cultural and political contexts (Australian Government, Department of Health 2019). You will also appreciate that there are some population groups which are more at risk than others. The National Men's Health Strategy 2020–2030 is focused on Aboriginal and Torres Strait Islander males, males from socio-economically disadvantaged backgrounds, males living in rural and remote areas of Australia, males with disability including mental illness, males from culturally and linguistically diverse backgrounds, members of the LGBTI+ community, male veterans, socially isolated males and men in the criminal justice system (Australian Government, Department of Health 2019).

Gender identity and sexuality

Gender has been thought of throughout history as a binary—female or male. In the recent past, it has been recognised that not all individuals fall comfortably in this binary, hence a change to vigorous research and lobbying has led to defining gender diversity other than its usual binary. Globally, the legal frameworks have not caught up with correcting gender preference politics such as in birth certificates, marriage certificates or passports, although this is gradually being discussed by governments and organisations. Based on the Australian Bureau of Statistics 2014 General Social Survey, 3% of adults identified as gay, lesbian or as having an 'other' sexual orientation (ABS 2015). In the most recent Australian Census (2016), 35% of sex/gender diverse people indicated they were non-binary or another gender. A further 26% of this sample reported they were trans male, trans female or transgender (ABS 2018). For a list of relevant terminology, see Chapter 26.

The Gay Liberation Movement started in New York with the Stonewall Uprising, as the GLBT+ community set up a series of confrontations against police in the early hours of 28 June 1969. This set off a revolution in cities in Western democracies that had a visible migration of GLBT+ people including Sydney on 24 June 1978. The Gay Rights Movement set about successfully in removing homosexuality as a psychiatric disorder from the DSM in 1974 (APA 2013). GLBT+ rights have since succeeded in acceptance in many social, political and cultural context, including the plebiscite that legalised same sex marriage in 2013 in New Zealand and in 2017 in Australia. However, despite the acceptance of GLBT+ as a norm in sexuality at least in developed nations, there are still significant barriers to health and wellbeing in this group.

While the Trans, Gender Diverse and Non-binary (TGDNB) peoples have been recognised in most Western nations recently, there remains a massive challenge to affirm and create an inclusive global environment in all facets of life—health, education, economics and politics. The Australian Attorney General in amendments to the Sex and Discrimination Act 1984 released Guidelines on the Recognition of Sex and Gender (Attorney General's Department 2015). In affirming their gender, some TGDNB people seek medical or surgical treatments. Hormonal treatments and cosmetic reconstructive surgery might be pursued, and the numbers are unknown, but gender re-assignment surgery is chosen by a minority of TGDNB population. An Australian study (Strauss et al 2017) found that trans young people are at very high risk for poor mental health including self-harm and suicide attempts, anxiety and depression. In addition, trans young people have difficulty accessing healthcare due to a sense of isolation from mainstream services and a lack of respect from health professionals who do not understand or respect their gender identity. They are also more likely to be subjected to bullying, peer rejection, issues with school or other education and lack of family support. There is now an Australian Standard of Care and Treatment Guideline for transgender and gender diverse children and adolescents (Telfer et al 2018). The guideline emphasises the need for individualised care, the use of respectful and affirming language, avoidance of doing harm (in terms of medical or surgical interventions), consideration of socio-cultural factors including fear and stigma and barriers to seeking care, and psychological support.

Treatment as prevention, pre- and post-exposure HIV prophylaxis

The number of newly diagnosed cases of human immunodeficiency virus (HIV) in Australia has declined by 7% over the past five years (Kirby Institute 2018), with 835 diagnoses in 2018 (Kirby Institute 2019). Male-to-male sex continues to be the major HIV risk exposure in Australia, accounting for 63% of diagnoses in 2017, followed by heterosexual sex (25%) (Kirby Institute 2018). In 2017 the notification rate was 1.6 times higher in Indigenous people than in the Australian-born non-Indigenous population (Kirby Institute 2018). Gay, bisexual and other men who have sex with men continue to be the most affected by HIV infection in New Zealand, accounting for 79% of all locally acquired HIV diagnoses in 2018 (University of Otago 2019). There has also been a steady decrease in notifications in recent years. Of the men diagnosed with HIV in 2018, 41% were of European background, 15% were Asian, 10.1% were Māori and 3.9% were Pacific peoples (University of Otago 2019).

In the mid-1990s, highly affective antiretroviral drugs (HAART) reduced the morbidity of AIDS-related diseases and significantly reduced the risk of acquiring AIDS. Recent years have seen a significant improvement in combined antiretroviral treatments (cART) which have not only stopped people from developing AIDS but also, on a population level, reduced the viral load of HIV (Eisinger et al 2019). An undetectable HIV viral load in effect means that the person is no longer infectious (Eisinger et al 2019). Evidence has shown that a person living with HIV on combined antiretroviral treatment, who adheres to the medication regimen will have a close to zero viral load (Altice et al 2019). The use of a two-drug combined antiretroviral therapy has been proven to be effective for individuals to access within 72 hours of a significant sexual or blood-borne exposure (Saag et al 2018). Pre-exposure prophylaxis (PrEP) has an efficacy of 99% if taken every day. However, men need to be reminded that these drugs do not prevent other sexually transmitted infections so condoms should always be used (Saag et al 2018). These drugs are potent, safe with few side effects and convenient with one-pill, once-daily dosing. However, adherence is critical for long-term efficacy. Men using PrEP need regular monitoring for drug side-effects and HIV screening (Gulick et al 2019).

In 2018, there were approximately 37.9 million people living with HIV; of these, approximately 23.3 million were accessing antiretroviral therapy (UNAIDS 2019). Access to sexual health services plays an important role in screening and the provision of pre- and post- (HIV) exposure prophylaxis. This is a significant barrier to people living with HIV in many countries, especially in eastern and southern Africa. Many people living with HIV are not aware of their HIV status, and many still do not have access to anti-retroviral therapies (UNAIDS 2015). Both the World Health Organization (2020a) and UNAIDS (2020) have strategic programs to improve access to healthcare for people living with HIV, HIV prevention programs and ongoing support and education.

Infant male circumcision

Circumcision is a surgical procedure involving the removal of the male foreskin. It is a procedure which has been performed for thousands of years for cultural and religious reasons. There are high rates of male circumcision still practised in some countries; however, in Australia and New Zealand, male circumcision remains a controversial procedure and is not routinely performed. It is estimated that worldwide 37–39% of men are circumcised, with approximately 13% of newborn Australians being circumcised each year (Prabhakaran et al 2018). Male circumcision is still practised in some Aboriginal communities and in some Pacific Islander communities. For some Aboriginal men, circumcision or sub-incision (slitting of the ventral part of the prepuce and urethra) is part of an initiation ceremony which marks the transition from childhood to adulthood (Royal Australasian College of Physicians (RACP) 2010).

The controversy about infant male circumcision has increased in recent years with a number of published papers that strongly support the role of voluntary male circumcision as a means of reducing the spread of human immunodeficiency virus (HIV) in heterosexual men in developing countries especially Africa (Lane et al 2018). There are a number of studies that have found that circumcision in men who have sex with men reduces the risk of HIV and other sexually transmitted diseases (Pintye & Baeten 2019, Yuan et al 2019). Additionally, there is also evidence that male circumcision reduces the prevalence of human papillomavirus (HPV) and other sexually transmitted infections in women (Morris et al 2019). The World Health Organisation (2020b) continues to advocate for voluntary circumcision in 14 countries in southern and eastern Africa in an effort to reduce the transmission of HIV. Male circumcision has also been found to have reduced the risk of urinary tract infection in male infants and children, and the risk of penile cancer in adult males, although these both have very low prevalence (Prabhakaran et al 2018).

The Royal Australasian College of Physicians (RACP 2010) states that routine circumcision as not warranted in an Australian context as it does not provide a therapeutic health role. Circumcision can result in significant complications in 1.5–4% of procedures including infection, haemorrhage and meatal stenosis requiring further surgery (Hung et al 2019, Prabhakaran et al 2018). There are also ethical and moral issues as the foreskin has a functional role and the infant/child is unable to consent. Non-voluntary circumcision has the potential to affect the man's body image, sexuality and sexual function (Bossio & Pukall 2018). The RACP position statement on circumcision (2010) affirms that 'After reviewing the currently available evidence, the RACP believes that the frequency of diseases modifiable by circumcision, the level of protection offered by circumcision and the complication rates of circumcision do not warrant routine infant circumcision in Australia and New Zealand' (p. 1). Clearly this is a complex issue, and in the end it is a decision that is steeped in social, cultural and religious beliefs and parents need to be assisted to make an informed decision.

A foreskin is usually fully retractile by up to age ten years, but this is variable. Genital hygiene needs to be taught in early childhood to help prevent penile problems like balanitis, phimosis and paraphimosis. Genital hygiene includes retracting back and gently stretching the foreskin as well as using soap alternatives for genital skin care (Prabhakaran et al 2018).

Communicating effectively with people about sexuality and sexual function

Discussing sexuality is an important part of health assessment, although many nurses do not feel comfortable in discussing these issues. Please read the section titled 'Communicating effectively with people about sexuality and sexual function' in Chapter 26 before you continue to work through this chapter.

Subjective data

Assessment of male reproductive function is closely linked to assessment of bladder function. Health issues in this area are likely to cause significant distress to the man and his partner and therefore you need to approach the assessment in a tactful and empathic manner. Privacy is of upmost importance and you need to establish a trusting relationship with the person. Detailed questions and physical examination techniques related to urinary and bowel function and the prostate are covered in Chapters 24 and 25.

1. Presenting concern
2. General health history
3. Genitourinary/breast health
4. Sexual health history
5. Health and lifestyle management

Preparation

As you approach the health assessment interview it is important that you:

- Don't make assumptions about the person's gender identity and sexual orientation based on appearance.
- Use open and inclusive questions that are gender neutral and inclusive.
- Make sure that in your approach to the sexual health history the person is encouraged to discuss their sexual orientation, gender identity and relationship status, and that heterosexuality is not assumed.
- A person may choose not to disclose their sexual or gender identity; their choice should be respected.
- Respond positively when the person is prepared to be open about their sexual orientation, gender identity or intersex condition.
- If you are unsure of how to address the person, ask them how they would like to be addressed.
- Begin with open-ended question to assess individual needs.
- Be cautious about recording information about sexual orientation, gender identity or intersex condition in a person's health record. You should seek consent from the person and inform them about why the information is needed and to whom it will be made available

Practice note: Before you commence the assessment, introduce yourself to the person, confirm the person's identity, discuss the purpose and scope of the assessment, clarify any questions the person may have and obtain verbal consent from the person to perform the assessment.

ASSESSMENT GUIDELINES	CLINICAL SIGNIFICANCE AND CLINICAL ALERTS
1. Presenting concern	
It is important to ascertain the person's perception of their sexual and/or reproductive health. From the presenting concern, the person would be able to provide you with some insight into their symptoms and perhaps other health issues. If they do perceive a problem—*how does this impact on their quality of life?* The responses to these questions will guide the sequence of the rest of the subjective data collection. Take the cues from the person. If the person is unable to articulate their health concern, use questions below to assist them to verbalise their health situation. A suggested approach: • I would like to ask you some questions to find out more about how I can help you today. Some of the questions might appear intrusive and personal but will assist me in identifying your healthcare needs. Is it OK with you if I ask these questions? • What brings you here today? Do you have any issues with your sexual and reproductive health?	

ASSESSMENT GUIDELINES	CLINICAL SIGNIFICANCE AND CLINICAL ALERTS
2. General health history	
Recent illness • Have you experienced any recent illness?	
Personal health history • Surgery, medical conditions, allergies, health difficulties (mobility, pain, disability). Ask specifically about genital, prostate, bladder or bowel surgery (see Chapters 23, 24 and 25).	Chronic illness and treatments can contribute to sexual dysfunction.
Family history • Ask about significant family history of diabetes, epilepsy, clotting disorders, hypertension or cardiovascular disease, prostate and testicular cancers, etc.	There is an increased incidence of prostate cancer in men with a first-degree relative who has/had prostate cancer.
Current and past cigarette smoking • How many for how long?	Smoking causes cardiovascular disease which can reduce fertility and cause erectile dysfunction.
Current and past alcohol and illicit substance use • Be specific about how much alcohol, how often and for how long. • Which drugs, how much and how often (including injecting drug use)?	Personal health risks as well as putting the person at risk of unsafe sex or sexual violence.
Current medication • Ask about use of prescribed medications, complementary and traditional therapies and over-the-counter medications.	Broad-spectrum antibiotics alter balance of normal flora which can predispose to candida genital skin infection.
Psychosocial history. (see also Chapter 8: The health history and Chapter 11: Mental health assessment) • What is your highest educational achievement? High school, TAFE or university? • Living arrangements? • Contact and support from family members? Friends? • Hobbies and activities?	
3. Genitourinary/breast health	
Urinary symptoms/lower abdominal pain • Have you experienced any problem with your bladder or voiding? (urinary symptoms such as urgency, slow stream, feeling of incomplete emptying or incontinence) • Have you experienced any problems with bowel function? • Have you experienced any abdominal pain? If the symptom is present ask the person to describe the sign or symptom: • When did it start? • What have they done about it, and did this reduce the symptom?	**Urinary or faecal incontinence** or **lower urinary tract symptoms** can significantly affect a person's sexuality and sexual function and requires further assessment. It is rare for men under the age of 60 years to suffer from a **urinary tract infection.** Unlike in women, the anatomical sites of the male genitalia has no direct contact with the anorectal region. Should an individual present with mild symptoms of urethritis, no high sexual risk, but also urinary frequency including nocturnal frequency, consider a mid-stream urine (MSU) for testing for bacteriuria. For details about assessment of urinary function see Chapter 24; bowel function, see Chapter 25; and assessment of abdominal pain, see Chapter 23.
Genital signs and symptoms • Have you experienced any problem with your penis—foreskin, pain, lesions, itch, redness?	

SUBJECTIVE DATA

SUBJECTIVE DATA

ASSESSMENT GUIDELINES	CLINICAL SIGNIFICANCE AND CLINICAL ALERTS
Urethral discharge • How much (*scant, a lot*)? Has that increased or decreased? • Describe the colour. Any odour? • Discharge associated with pain or with urination?	**Urethral discharge** occurs with infection. Some penile infections will be sexually transmitted. Sexually transmitted infections (STIs) can cause pain on voiding and lower abdominal pain. Individuals with a suspected STI should be referred to a medical or nurse practitioner or sexual health clinic for diagnosis and treatment.
Scrotum and testicles • Have you noticed any difference with your scrotum? Any pain?	**Epididymitis** is an inflammation of the epididymis and caused by pathogens, some of which may be sexually transmitted. **Hydrocoeles and varicocoeles** may cause scrotal enlargement and an ultrasound will confirm whether these lumps might be cancerous.
• Have you noticed any bulge or swelling in the scrotum? For how long? Ever been told you have a hernia? Any dragging, heavy feeling in scrotum?	Possible **hernia**.
• Have you noticed any lump or swelling on testes?	**Testicular cancer** is the second most common cancer in men aged 15–24 years old in Australia. For more information, read 'Promoting a healthy lifestyle' at the end of this chapter. **Testicular torsion** can occur at any age but most commonly in men between the onset of puberty and the mid-20s. The blood supply to the testes is occluded due to twisting of the spermatic cord and can lead to scrotal necrosis. ***Clinical alert:*** Any report of severe pain in the testes or scrotum should be referred to a medical practitioner. It is considered a medical emergency. See also Table 27.5.
Breast symptoms • Have you experienced any pain or other abnormal symptoms in your breasts? If present, ask the person to describe the sign or symptom: • When did it start? • What have they done about it, and did this reduce the symptom?	**Breast cancer** is rare in men; the risk of being diagnosed with breast cancer to age 85 is 1 in 1133. The median age at diagnosis was 69.4 years (AIHW 2019a). Age and a known *BRAC1* or *BRAC2* gene mutation are known risk factors. ***Clinical alert:*** Any unusual change in the breast should be further assessed and/or referred to a medical practitioner. For details about breast assessment see Chapter 28.
4. Sexual health history	
A general statement such as, 'When I conduct a health assessment, I ask people about their sexual health. Is it alright with you if I ask questions about your sexual health?' may help you open up the discussion with the person. Only ask the questions that are relevant to the particular situation.	
Sexual history • Are you currently sexually active? • Age at first sexual contact? • When was the last time that you had sex? • Do you have a regular or casual sexual partner? How long have you been with this person? • Type of sexual contact (oral, vaginal, anal)? • How many sexual partners have you had in the last 12 months? • Have you had sex that you can't remember because of alcohol or substance use? • Any history with partner/s from overseas?	Determining the person's sexual practices will enable you to identify areas for health education or the need for further questioning to identify risk factors for sexually transmitted infections and/or the need for specific physical examination and other investigations.

ASSESSMENT GUIDELINES	CLINICAL SIGNIFICANCE AND CLINICAL ALERTS
Contraception (if relevant) • What do you do to protect your partner from unplanned pregnancy?	
History of sexually transmitted infection • Have you (or your partner) had any current symptoms or past history of STI? For example, gonorrhoea, chlamydia, genital warts (HPV), syphilis? • If so, what symptoms did you experience? How long ago? How was it treated? • Have you ever had a test for HIV or hepatitis B or C? • Screen for knowledge of prevention of STIs—use of condoms.	An **STI** includes all conditions that can be transmitted during intercourse or intimate sexual contact with an infected partner.
Sexual function and satisfaction (if relevant) • Are you satisfied with the sexual relationship you have with your partner/s? • Are you satisfied with the way that you and your partner communicate about sex? • Are you satisfied with your ability to respond sexually?	
Sexual difficulties or dysfunction Ask relevant questions, for example: • Low sexual desire or sexual arousal? • Erectile dysfunction (ability to get an erection, hardness, staying hard) • Difficulty in achieving an orgasm, lack of sexual satisfaction (able to ejaculate (cum), pain or discomfort on ejaculation)? • Loss of urine during sexual activity? • Any other sexual issue? • If you are experiencing any difficulties, how much does this bother you (scale of 1–5; 1 is not bothered at all/5 is extremely bothered)? Erectile dysfunction has been defined as the persistent inability to achieve or maintain an erection sufficient for satisfactory sexual intercourse (McMahon 2019).	There are validated sexual health/satisfaction and erectile function assessment tools available (e.g. the Male Sexual Health Questionnaire (MSHQ)). Men who are concerned about their sexual function should be referred to a medical or nurse practitioner/sexual health clinic for further assessment. There is strong evidence to suggest that erectile dysfunction significantly increases the risk of the man having cardiovascular disease, coronary vessel disease and stroke (Kessler et al 2019). ***Clinical alert:*** All men who have erectile dysfunction should be screened to determine their general cardiovascular health.
Family violence, sexual abuse, assault or unwanted sexual experiences (if relevant): • See questions and approach to assessment described in Chapter 5 for detail on assessment related to screening for family violence and abuse.	May prompt need for follow-up and counselling. See also Chapter 5 for detail on assessment.
5. Health and lifestyle management	
Prostate • For men over 50 years of age or men with a family history of prostate cancer ask: Have you had a discussion with a health professional about prostate health? Please read 'Promoting a healthy lifestyle' in Chapter 24 for further information about prostate health.	
Testicular self-examination • Do you perform testicular self-examination (TSE)? See 'Promoting a healthy lifestyle' in teaching Testicular Awareness below.	
Immunisation • Have you been immunised against human papillomavirus (HPV)? For more information about HPV vaccination see 'Promoting a healthy lifestyle' section of this chapter.	**HPV** can cause cancers of the penis, anus and genital warts. Men can be asymptomatic carriers of the virus and pass it on to sexual partners. For further information about HPV vaccination see the section titled 'Promoting a healthy lifestyle' in Chapter 26.
• Have you been immunised against hepatitis B? Hepatitis B vaccination is part of the Immunisation Schedule in Australia and New Zealand. Most Australians under the age of 30 would have been given the vaccine and the herd immunity is high, >80%, but there are sub-populations that may not have been vaccinated. These include migrants, those whose parents are vaccine conscientious objectors and those who missed out at school.	**Hepatitis B** is a sexually transmissible infection and vertical transmission from mother to baby continues to be the main way of acquiring hepatitis B with long-term sequelae that includes hepatocellular carcinoma.

SUBJECTIVE DATA

ASSESSMENT GUIDELINES	CLINICAL SIGNIFICANCE AND CLINICAL ALERTS
Safer sex practices See points in sexual health history above.	
Activity and exercise Ask about usual activity and exercise patterns.	Part of a general health history. May provide an opportunity to provide more information about the importance of exercise to general health and wellbeing.
Additional subjective data for infants and children (questions for parent or guardian)	
• Does your child have any problem urinating? Does his urine stream look straight? • Have you noticed any evidence of pain with urinating such as crying, holding genitals? • Has your child had a previous urinary tract infection?	If the infant/child has any voiding issues refer to Chapter 24 for specific areas for assessment.
• Has your child experienced any problems with genital area: itching, rash, anal discharge?	Occurs with poor perineal hygiene or insertion of foreign body in the rectum.
• Any problem with child's penis or scrotum: sores, swelling, discolouration?	
• Are you aware if his testes are descended?	
• Has he ever had an inguinal hernia or hydrocoele?	**Hydrocoele**: collection of serous fluid in tunica vaginalis, surrounding testis. See Table 27.5. **Inguinal hernia**: see Table 27.7.
• Have you ever noticed any swelling in his scrotum during crying or coughing?	
• Questions related to suspected child abuse. Please read the important information about the Australian legal requirements about mandatory reporting of suspected child abuse. See Chapter 5 for details and specific approach to screening.	For more information about signs and symptoms related to child abuse refer to Chapter 5.
Additional subjective data for preadolescents and adolescents	
Use the following questions regarding sexual growth and development and sexual behaviour. Use the same principles as discussed in the previous sections related to approach to gender identity and sexual orientation outlined in the sexual health history.	
Ask questions that seem appropriate for the boy's age but be aware that norms vary widely.	
Do not be concerned if a boy will not discuss sexuality with you or respond to offers for information. He may not wish to let on that he needs or wants more information. You do well to 'open the door'. The adolescent may come back at a future time.	
• At about age 12 to 13 years, but sometimes earlier, boys start to change and grow around the penis and scrotum. What changes have you noticed?	
• Have you ever seen charts and pictures of normal growth patterns for boys? Let us go over these now.	
• Who in your family do you talk to about your body changes and about sex information? How do these talks go? Do you think you get enough information? • What about sex education classes at school? Is there a teacher, a nurse, a doctor or a counsellor to whom you can talk?	

SUBJECTIVE DATA

ASSESSMENT GUIDELINES	CLINICAL SIGNIFICANCE AND CLINICAL ALERTS
Boys around age 12 to 13 years have a normal experience of fluid coming out of the penis at night, called nocturnal emissions, or 'wet dreams'. Has this happened to you?	An occasional boy confuses this with a sign of STI or feels guilty.
• Often boys your age have questions about having sex. Do you have questions? If appropriate in the situation, ask further questions about sexual activity (use similar questions to that of the adult outlined in the previous section including questions regarding STI protection and prevention of unplanned pregnancy if relevant).	Determining the young person's sexual practices will enable you to identify areas for health education or the need for further questioning to identify risk factors for sexually transmitted infections and/or the need for specific physical examination and other investigations.
• Questions related to suspected child abuse. Please read the important information about the Australian legal requirements about mandatory reporting of suspected child abuse. See Chapter 5 for details and specific approach to screening.	For more information about signs and symptoms related to child abuse refer to Chapter 5.

Objective data

The techniques and extent of the objective data collection in this area will depend on the presenting signs and symptoms. Nurses working in sexual health clinics and some urological settings may need to develop skill in a more comprehensive assessment of male sexual and reproductive function. For most nurses asking questions about the man's reproductive health will be sufficient for a nursing assessment. **Physical examination, including inspection of the genitalia, is only performed when there is a valid reason to do so.** There needs to be awareness to be mindful that some men may prefer a male clinician and allow for this in your practice. This is particularly so in some cultures and religions, and also Australia's Indigenous populations where 'men's business' and 'women's business' are separated, and gender specific health workers are welcomed.

Preparation

The man's concerns are similar to those experienced by a female during the examination of the genitalia: modesty, fear of pain, cold hands, negative judgement or memory of previously uncomfortable examinations. Additionally, he may fear comparison to others, or fear having an erection during the examination and that this would be misinterpreted by the examiner.

Your demeanour should be *confident* and relaxed, unhurried yet business-like. Use a firm deliberate touch, not a soft, stroking one. If an erection does occur, do *not* stop the examination or leave the room. This only focuses more attention on the erection and increases embarrassment. Reassure the male that this is only a normal physiological response to touch, just as when the pupil constricts in response to bright light. Proceed with the rest of the examination if the man consents. It is preferable not to have a family member or friend present during sexual health history taking and examinations. However, another healthcare professional of the appropriate gender may be present at the person's request.

In the case of a child or adolescent, the parent or guardian normally provides legal consent for assessment and treatment. Young people have the legal right to confidential healthcare unless they cannot be considered a mature minor and/or there is a significant concern or risk, for example harm to self, physical or sexual abuse. It is generally accepted that most young people over the age of 16 years are capable of giving informed consent. Those under 16 years may sometimes be considered mature minors. In some cases, such as adolescents under 16 years, it is legally permissible for a mature adolescent to consent to assessment and treatment (Royal Children's Hospital 2019). The mature minor (Gillick principle) is confirmed in Australian common law that those under 18 years may be able to give informed consent if they have sufficient understanding and intelligence to understand proposed assessment and/or treatment (The Australian Law Reform Commission 2008). However, it is always advisable to obtain verbal consent from a child or adolescent before an examination and this should be documented in the health history.

In addition:

- The bladder should *not* be emptied before a genital examination when the individual has symptoms. Urinating before an examination will flush any discharge and signs on examination. Testing for sexually transmitted infections requires a urine specimen for laboratory testing (first-void urine—that is the urine is voided straight into a sterile urine collection container).
- Allow him to undress in privacy.

For the examination of the external genitalia the man should be assisted to lie down in the supine position with one or two pillows under his head. Ensure privacy before exposing the genital area and cover as much bare skin as possible.

If the man has a chaperone present, ask them to stand at the top (head) of the bed or examination couch to support the man.

- Explain each step in the examination before you do it.
- Assure the man he can stop the examination at any point should he feel any discomfort.
- Communicate throughout the examination. Maintain a dialogue to share information.

Equipment needed

Non-sterile gloves
Appropriate lighting (good examination lighting)
Hand hygiene solution

PROCEDURES AND NORMAL FINDINGS	CLINICAL SIGNIFICANCE AND CLINICAL ALERTS
General inspection	
During collection of subjective data you will have noticed the condition of the person's skin, hair, posture, height to weight ratio, body shape, level of hygiene and grooming and general demeanor. All of these factors provide clues to the man's sexual and reproductive health.	
Inspection of external genitalia	
Penis	
Ask the person to retract the prepuce (foreskin). It should move easily. Inspect the dorsal and the ventral aspect, noting skin colour, erythema, lesions, ulcers or blisters. The glans looks smooth and without lesions. Some cheesy smegma may have collected under the foreskin (this is normal). After inspection, ask the man to slide the foreskin back to the original position. The skin normally looks wrinkled, hairless and without lesions. The dorsal vein may be apparent (Figure 27.4). 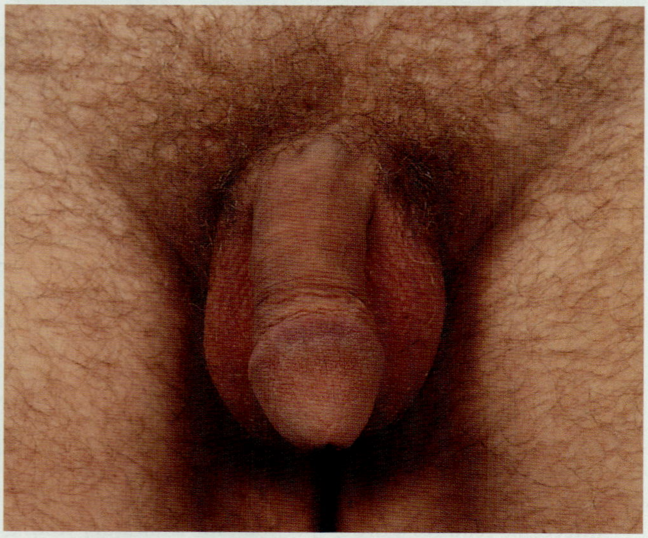 Figure 27.4	**Inflammation.** **Lesions:** nodules, solitary ulcer (chancre), grouped vesicles or superficial ulcers, wart-like papules (see Table 27.2). **Inflammation.** Lesions on glans or corona. Discharge (see Table 27.3) **Phimosis**—unable to retract the foreskin. **Paraphimosis**—unable to return foreskin to original position.
The urethral meatus is positioned just about centrally.	**Hypospadias**—ventral location of meatus. **Epispadias**—dorsal location of meatus (see Table 27.4).
At the base of the penis, pubic hair distribution is consistent with age. Hair is without lice.	**Pubic lice** or nits can be seen with the unaided eye. Excoriated skin usually accompanies.
Scrotum	
Inspect the scrotum skin as male holds the penis out of the way. Alternatively, you hold the penis out of the way with the back of your hand (Figure 27.5). Scrotal size varies with ambient room temperature. Asymmetry is normal, with the left scrotal half usually lower than the right. Inspect the skin of the inner thighs for redness or lesions.	**Scrotal swelling** (oedema) may be taut and pitting. This occurs with heart failure, renal failure or local inflammation. Lesions.

PROCEDURES AND NORMAL FINDINGS	CLINICAL SIGNIFICANCE AND CLINICAL ALERTS
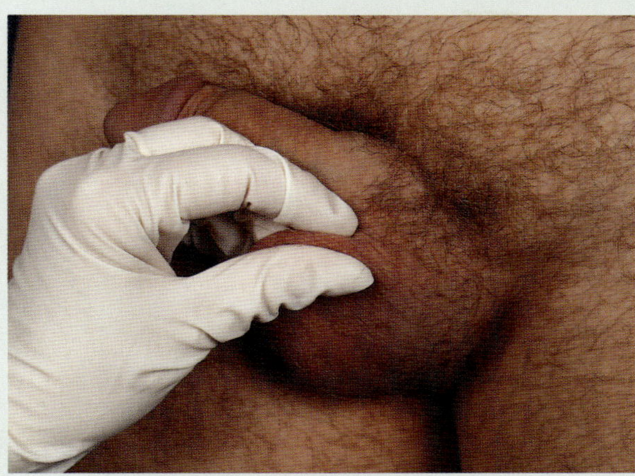 Figure 27.5	
Additional objective data for infants and children	
A parent or guardian should be present. For an infant or toddler, perform this procedure right after the abdominal examination (see Chapter 23). In a preschool-age to young school-age child (3 to 8 years of age), leave underpants on until just before the examination. In an older school-age child or adolescent, offer an extra drape, as with the adult. Reassure child and parents of normal findings.	
Inspect the penis and scrotum. Penis size is usually small in infants (2 to 3 cm) (Figure 27.6) and in young boys until puberty. In the obese boy, the penis looks even smaller because of folds of skin covering the base. 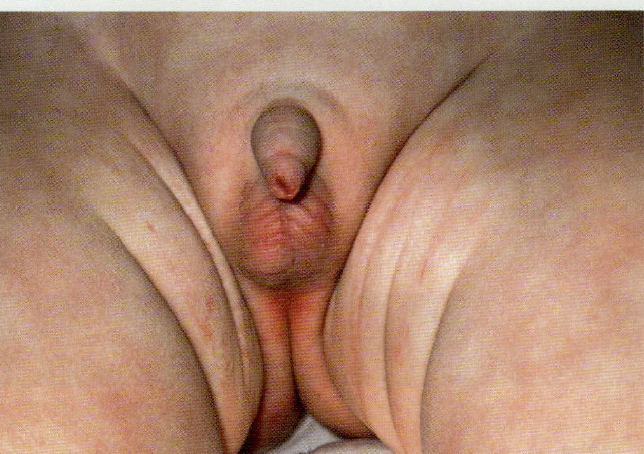 Figure 27.6	Rarely, what appears to be a very small penis may be an enlarged clitoris in a genetically female infant. Enlarged penis—precocious puberty. Redness, swelling, lesions.
The urethral meatus should be located centrally in the tip of the penis.	Discharge (see Table 27.3). Hypospadias, epispadias (see Table 27.4).
The foreskin is normally tight during the first 3 months and should not be retracted because of the risk of tearing the membrane attaching the foreskin to the shaft. This leads to scarring and, possibly, to adhesions later in life. In infants older than 3 months of age, retract the foreskin gently to check the glans and meatus. It should return to its original position easily.	Phimosis—unable to retract the foreskin. Paraphimosis—the foreskin cannot be slipped forward once it is retracted. Dirt and smegma collecting under foreskin.

PROCEDURES AND NORMAL FINDINGS	CLINICAL SIGNIFICANCE AND CLINICAL ALERTS
Scrotal rugae are well formed in the full-term infant. Size varies with ambient temperature, but overall, the infant's scrotum looks large in relation to the penis. No bulges, either constant or intermittent, are present.	
Additional objective data for the adolescent	
The adolescent shows a wide variation in normal development of the genitals. Using the sex maturity charts (Table 27.1), note: (1) enlargement of the testes and scrotum; (2) pubic hair growth; (3) darkening of scrotal colour; (4) roughening of scrotal skin; (5) increase in penis length and width; and (6) axillary hair growth.	
Additional objective data for the adult over 65 years	
In the older male, you may note thinner, greying pubic hair and the decreased size of the penis. The size of the testes may be decreased and may feel less firm. The scrotal sac is pendulous with fewer rugae.	

OBJECTIVE DATA

Further objective assessment for advanced practice

The assessments described in the following sections require advanced skill and scope of practice. Nurse practitioners and nurses working in specialist men's health and sexual health settings, as well as urological and continence nurses, need to develop these skills. Advanced assessment for infants and children is performed by specialist neonatal and paediatric nurses, some midwives and maternal and child health nurses.

Physical examination of male genitals and rectum are intimate invasive assessments and are only performed when there is a valid reason to do so. It is critical that clear communication with the person is maintained throughout the procedure to ensure that the person fully understands the purpose, nature and extent of the assessment. You will have to make a professional judgement about the need for another health professional (a chaperone) to be present during the examination.

Preparation

Position person supine for most of the examination. Cover with sheet or blanket when possible. In addition to the equipment listed previously you will require the following.

Equipment needed

Sterile specimen for specific STI cultures if needed
Penlight torch
Magnifying glass (when the person presents with lesion, warts and skin changes)
Non-sterile gloves and lubricating jelly
Hand hygiene solution

PROCEDURES AND NORMAL FINDINGS	CLINICAL SIGNIFICANCE AND CLINICAL ALERTS
Inspection and palpation of external genitalia	
Penis	
With gloved hands, compress the glans anteroposteriorly between your thumb and forefinger (Figure 27.7). The meatus edge should appear pink, smooth and without discharge.	**Stricture**—narrowed opening. Edges that are red, everted, oedematous, along with purulent discharge, suggest **urethritis** (see Table 27.3).

PROCEDURES AND NORMAL FINDINGS	CLINICAL SIGNIFICANCE AND CLINICAL ALERTS
Figure 27.7	
If you note urethral discharge, collect a smear for microscopic examination and culture. If no discharge shows but the man gives a history of it, ask him to milk the shaft of the penis. This should produce a drop of discharge.	***Clinical alert:*** For men who have sex with men, STIs may be asymptomatic. It is important to collect specimens from appropriate sites to test for STIs. In sexually active men who have sex with men, for those with more than one partner, a screen is recommended at least twice a year. For those with more than five partners, 4–6 monthly screening is recommended. Specimens should include a oropharyngeal swabs, first void urine and an anorectal swab (which can be collected by the person) for gonorrhoea and chlamydia. Blood tests are done to detect HIV and syphillus.
Palpate the shaft of the penis between your thumb and first two fingers. Normally, the penis feels smooth, semi-firm and nontender.	Nodule or induration. Tenderness.
Scrotum and testes	
Spread rugae out between your fingers. Lift the sac to inspect the posterior surface. Normally, no scrotal lesions are present, except for the commonly found sebaceous cysts. These are yellowish, 1-cm nodules and are firm, nontender and often multiple.	**Inflammation.**

OBJECTIVE DATA

PROCEDURES AND NORMAL FINDINGS	CLINICAL SIGNIFICANCE AND CLINICAL ALERTS
Palpate gently each scrotal half between your thumb and first two fingers (Figure 27.8). The scrotal contents should slide easily. Testes normally feel oval, firm and rubbery, smooth and equal bilaterally, and are freely movable and slightly tender to moderate pressure. Each epididymis normally feels discrete, softer than the testis, smooth and nontender. 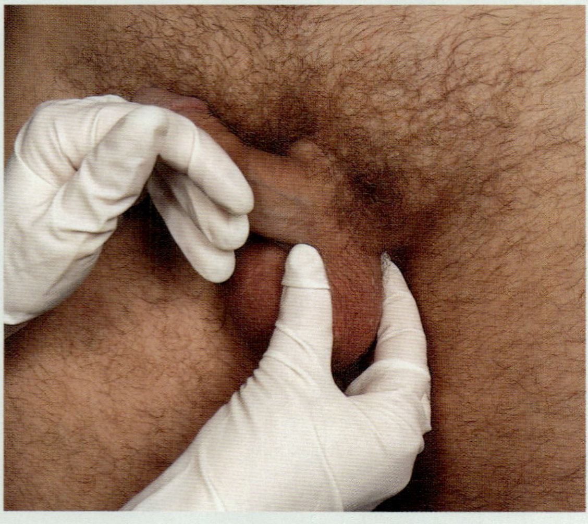 Figure 27.8	**Absent testis**—may be a temporary migration or true cryptorchidism (see Table 27.5). **Atrophied testes**—small and soft. **Fixed testes.** **Nodules** on testes or epididymis. Marked **tenderness**. An indurated, swollen and tender epididymis indicates **epididymitis**. ***Clinical alert:*** Any abnormality of the testis needs referral to a medical practitioner.
Palpate each spermatic cord between your thumb and forefinger, along its length from the epididymis up to the external inguinal ring (Figure 27.9). You should feel a smooth, nontender cord. 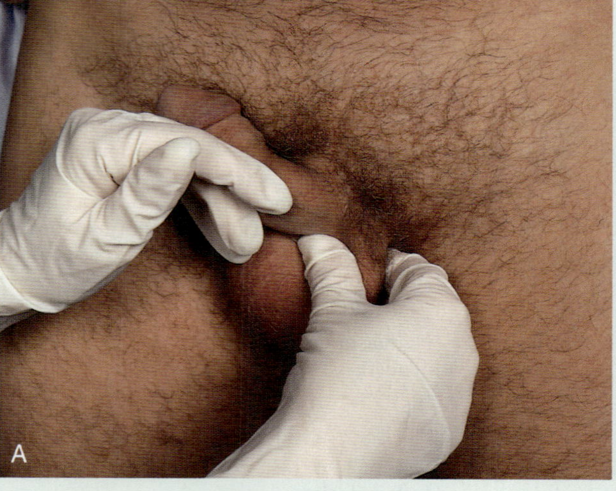 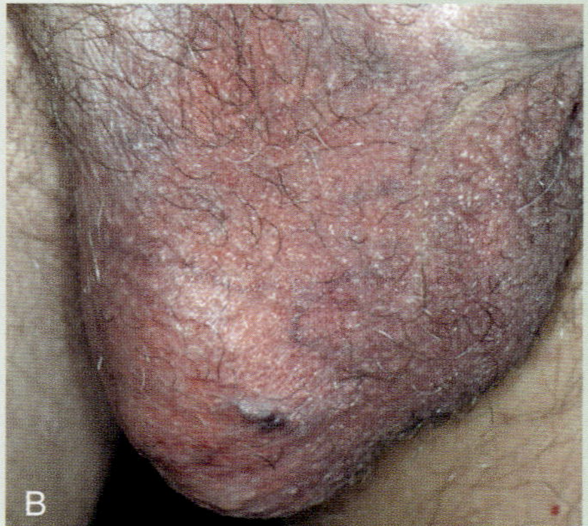 Figure 27.9	Thickened cord. Soft, swollen, and tortuous cord—see the discussion of varicocoele, Table 27.5.
Normally, no other scrotal contents are present. If you do find a mass, note: • Any tenderness? • Is the mass distal or proximal to testis? • Can you place your fingers over it? • Does it reduce when person lies down? • Can you auscultate bowel sounds over it?	Abnormalities in the scrotum: hernia, tumour, orchitis, epididymitis, hydrocoele, spermatocoele, varicocoele (see Table 27.5). ***Clinical alert:*** Any scrotal mass needs referral to a medical practitioner.

PROCEDURES AND NORMAL FINDINGS	CLINICAL SIGNIFICANCE AND CLINICAL ALERTS
Inspect and palpate for hernia	
With the man in a standing position, inspect the inguinal region for a bulge as he strains down. Normally, none is present.	Bulge at external inguinal ring or at femoral canal. (A hernia may be present but easily reduced and may appear only intermittently with an increase in intraabdominal pressure.)
Palpate the inguinal canal (Figure 27.10). For the right side, ask the male to shift his weight onto the left (unexamined) leg. Place your right index finger low on the right scrotal half. Palpate up the length of the spermatic cord, invaginating the scrotal skin as you go, to the external inguinal ring. It feels like a triangular slit-like opening, and it may or may not admit your finger. If it will admit your finger, gently insert it into the canal and ask the person to 'bear down'. Normally, you feel no change. Repeat the procedure on the left side. External inguinal ring **Figure 27.10**	A palpable herniating mass bumps your fingertip or pushes against the side of your finger (see Table 27.7).
Palpate the femoral area for a bulge. Normally you feel none.	
Palpate inguinal lymph nodes	
Palpate the horizontal chain along the groin inferior to the inguinal ligament and the vertical chain along the upper inner thigh.	
It is normal to palpate an isolated node on occasion; it then feels small (less than 1 cm), soft, discrete and movable (Figure 27.11).	Enlarged, hard, matted, fixed nodes.

OBJECTIVE DATA

PROCEDURES AND NORMAL FINDINGS	CLINICAL SIGNIFICANCE AND CLINICAL ALERTS

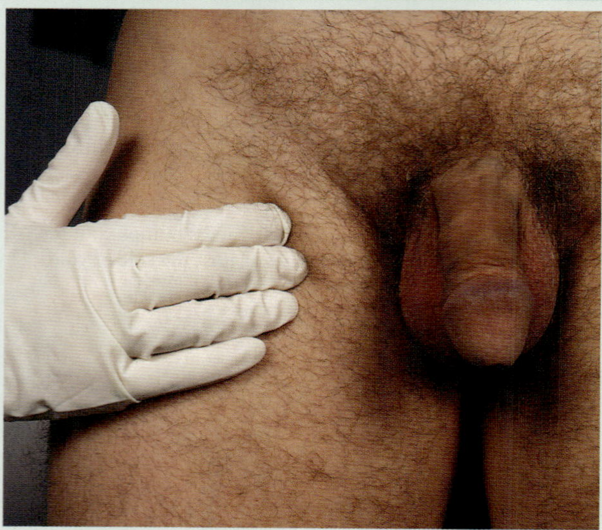

Figure 27.11

Palpate the prostate gland via the rectum

Drop lubricating jelly onto your gloved index finger. Instruct the person that palpation is not painful but may feel like needing to move the bowels. Place the pad of your index finger gently against the anal verge (Figure 27.12). You will feel the sphincter tighten, then relax. As it relaxes, flex the tip of your finger and slowly insert it into the anal canal in a direction towards the umbilicus. *Never* approach the anus at right angles with your index finger extended. Such a jabbing motion does not promote sphincter relaxation and is painful.

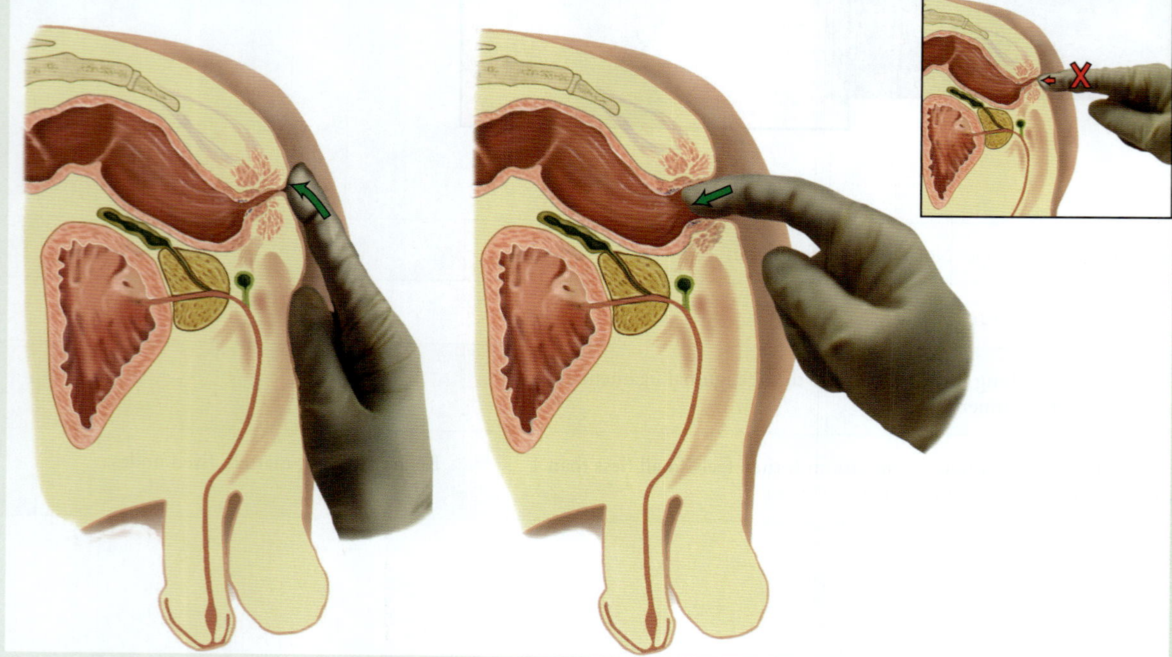

Figure 27.12

PROCEDURES AND NORMAL FINDINGS	CLINICAL SIGNIFICANCE AND CLINICAL ALERTS
Prostate gland. On the anterior wall in the male, note the elastic, bulging prostate gland (Figure 27.13). Palpate the entire prostate in a systematic way, but note that only the superior and part of the lateral surfaces are accessible to examination. Press into the gland at each location, because when a nodule occurs, it will not project *into* the rectal lumen. The surface should feel smooth and muscular; search for any distinct nodule or diffuse firmness. Note these characteristics: 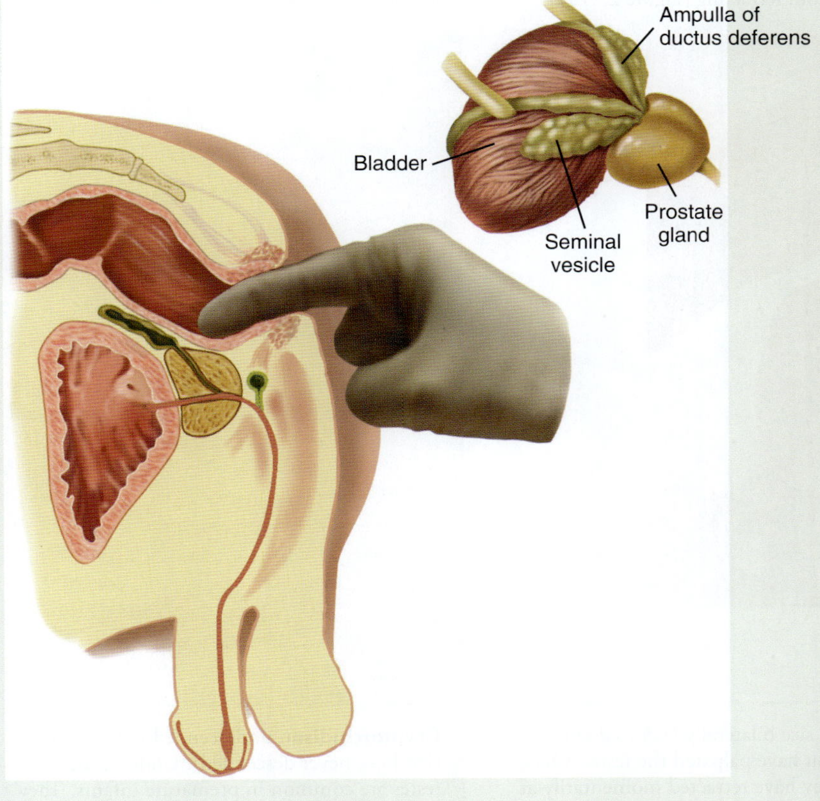 Figure 27.13	Occasionally, digital examination of the prostate can cause a feeling of warmth, flushing, and on occasion a vagal response.
Size—2.5 cm long by 4 cm wide; should not protrude more than 1 cm into the rectum **Shape**—heart shape, with palpable central groove **Surface**—smooth **Consistency**—elastic, rubbery **Mobility**—slightly movable **Sensitivity**—nontender to palpation	Enlarged, or atrophied gland. Flat with no groove. Nodular. Hard; or boggy, soft, fluctuant. Fixed. Tender. Enlarged, firm smooth gland with central groove obliterated suggests benign prostatic hypertrophy. Swollen, exquisitely tender gland accompanies prostatitis. Any stone-hard, irregular, fixed nodule indicates carcinoma—needs referral to medical practitioner (see Table 27.6).

OBJECTIVE DATA

PROCEDURES AND NORMAL FINDINGS	CLINICAL SIGNIFICANCE AND CLINICAL ALERTS
Additional objective data for infants and children	
Palpate the scrotum and testes. The cremasteric reflex is strong in the infant, pulling the testes up into the inguinal canal and abdomen from exposure to cold, touch, exercise or emotion. Take care not to elicit the reflex: (1) keep your hands warm and palpate from the external inguinal ring down; (2) block the inguinal canals with the thumb and forefinger of your other hand to prevent the testes from retracting (Figure 27.14). 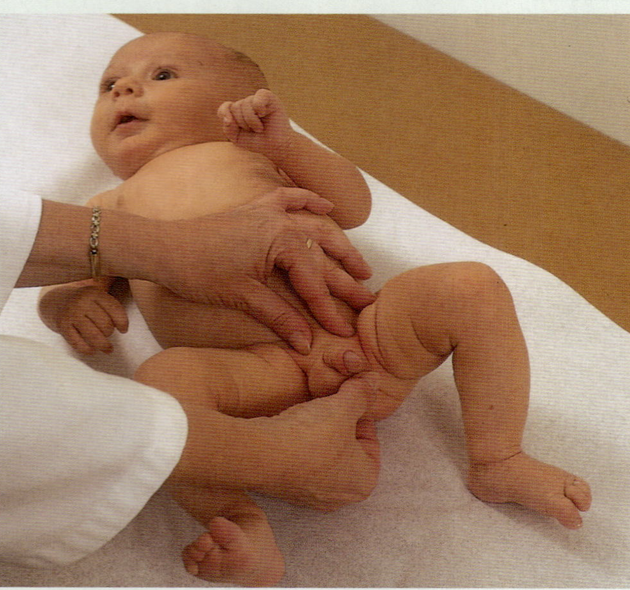 Figure 27.14	
Normally, the testes are descended and are equal in size bilaterally (1.5 to 2 cm until puberty). It is important to document that you have palpated the testes. Once palpated, they are considered descended, even if they have retracted momentarily at the next visit. If the scrotal half feels empty, search for the testes along the inguinal canal and try to milk them down. Ask the toddler or child to squat with the knees flexed up; this pressure may force the testes down. Or, have the young child sit cross-legged to relax the reflex (Figure 27.15).	**Cryptorchidism:** undescended testes (those that have never descended). Undescended testes are common in premature infants. They occur in 3–4% of term infants, although most have descended by 3 months of age. Age at which child should be referred differs among physicians (see Table 27.5).

OBJECTIVE DATA

PROCEDURES AND NORMAL FINDINGS	CLINICAL SIGNIFICANCE AND CLINICAL ALERTS
Figure 27.15	
Migratory testes (physiological cryptorchidism) are common because of the strength of the cremasteric reflex and the small mass of the prepubertal testes. Note that the affected side has a normally developed scrotum (with true cryptorchidism, the scrotum is atrophic) and that the testis can be milked down. These testes descend at puberty and are normal.	
Palpate the epididymis and spermatic cord as described in the adult section. A common scrotal finding in the boy under 2 years of age is a **hydrocoele**, or fluid in the scrotum. It appears as a large scrotum and usually disappears spontaneously.	A **hydrocoele** is a cystic collection of serous fluid in the tunica vaginalis, surrounding the testis (see Table 27.5).
Inspect the inguinal area for a bulge. If you do not see a bulge but the parent gives a positive history of one, try to elicit it by increasing intra-abdominal pressure. Ask the boy to hold his breath and strain down or have him blow up a balloon.	
If a hernia is suspected, palpate the inguinal area. Use your little finger to reach the external inguinal ring.	

Summary Checklist

MALE SEXUAL AND REPRODUCTIVE ASSESSMENT

Subjective data

1. Presenting concern
2. General health history
3. Sexual health history
4. Genitourinary/reproductive health history
5. Health and lifestyle management

Objective data

1. General inspection
2. Inspection of external genitalia

PROMOTING A HEALTHY LIFESTYLE

TESTICULAR SELF-EXAMINATION/TESTICULAR AWARENESS

Testicular cancer accounts for 1.2% of all male cancers. The risk of developing testicular cancer to age 75 years is 1 in 207 for Australian men (Australian Institute of Health and Welfare 2019). And although the prognosis is very good, testicular cancer has the potential to significantly impact on the man's quality of life. In New Zealand, there has been a trend for increasing rates of testicular cancer, especially in Māori men (Gurney 2019, Ministry of Health NZ 2018). It is primarily a disease of young males, with incidence being most frequent in males aged between 15 and 44 years.

Although the pathogenesis of testicular cancer is unclear, several risk factors have been identified including having undescended testis (cryptorchidism), pre-natal exposure to oestrogen, infertility, history of congenital hypospadias (abnormality of the penis and urethra) or inguinal hernia, previous testicular cancer and a family history of testicular cancer (Akers 2018). If identified early almost all testicular cancers are curable.

Men are advised to become aware of the normal size and consistency of their testicles so that they are able to recognise any changes that may occur. Healthy Male (Andrology Australia) recommends that men regularly perform testicular self-examination (TSE) so that they develop a sense of what is normal for them. It only takes a few minutes to perform. Points to include during health teaching are:

- TSE involves feeling the testes, one at a time, using the fingers and thumb.
- It is usually easier after a warm shower or bath (warm water relaxes scrotal sac).
- Advise the man to use the palm of one hand to support the scrotum, then gently roll one testis between the thumb and fingers to feel for any lumps or swelling in or on the surface of the testis (or any changes from the last TSE).
- Normally a testis has a smooth surface and feel firm. It is normal for one testis to feel slightly bigger than the other.
- Using the thumb and fingers continue along the back of the testis to feel the epididymis (a soft coiled tube that carries the sperm from the testis to the ductus deferens).
- If there are any changes to how the testes feel normally, or if the man is concerned, advise them to see their local doctor (GP) as soon as possible.

For more information see the following websites:

Healthy Male (Andrology Australia): www.healthymale.org.au

Testicular Cancer NZ: https://testicular.org.nz

Documentation and critical thinking

DOCUMENTATION AND CRITICAL THINKING

FOCUSED ASSESSMENT: CLINICAL CASE STUDY

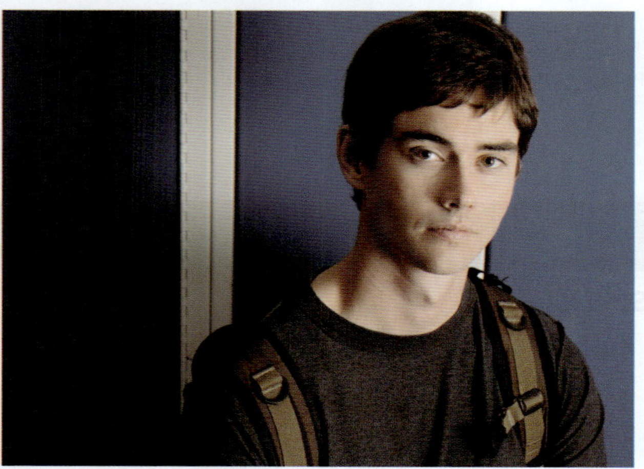

Context

University, student health clinic.

Subjective

Ryan Wilson is a 19-year-old student who noted acute onset of painful urination, frequency and urgency 2 days ago. Noted some thick penile discharge. States has no flank pain, no abdominal pain, no fever or genital skin rash.

Ryan is concerned he has an STI because of an episode of unprotected intercourse with a new female partner 6 days ago. Has no known allergies. Did not use a condom, says he tends not to use condoms. In contact with sexual partner, who says she has no symptoms.

Objective

Temp 37°C; HR 72/min; RR 16/min. No lesions or inflammation around penis or scrotum. Urethral meatus has mild oedema with purulent urethral discharge. No pain on palpation of genitalia. Testes symmetrical with no masses.

Collaborative problem

Urethral discharge—possible STI.

Problem statement/nursing diagnosis

Knowledge deficit about STI and pregnancy prevention.

Abnormal findings for advanced practice

TABLE 27.2 Male genital lesions

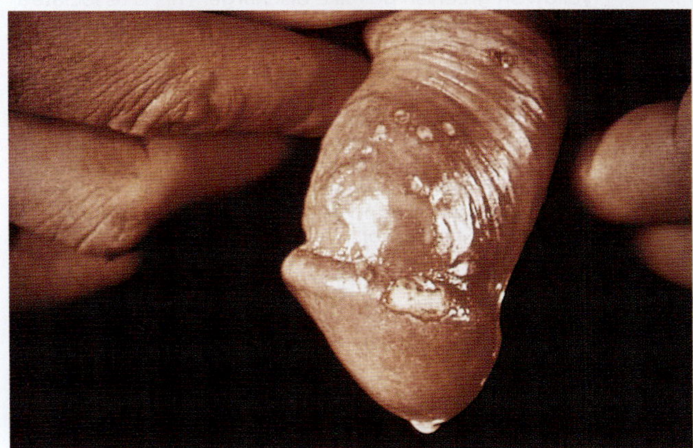

Genital herpes—HSV-2 infection

Clusters of small vesicles with surrounding erythema, which are often painful, erupt on the glans or foreskin. These rupture to form superficial ulcers. A sexually transmitted infection (STI), the initial infection lasts 7–10 days. The virus remains dormant indefinitely; recurrent infections last 3–10 days with milder symptoms.

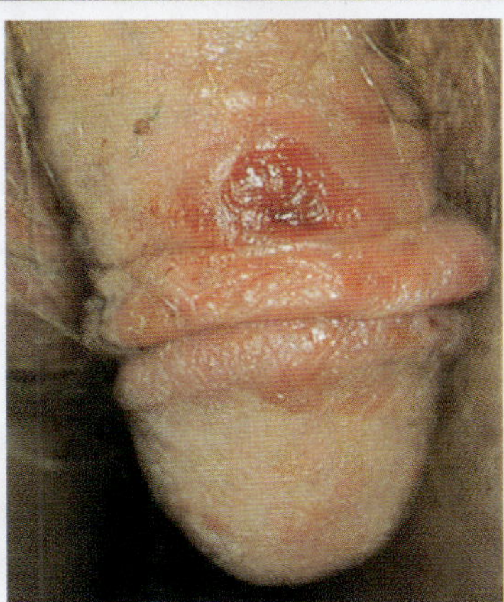

Syphilitic chancre

Begins within 2–4 weeks of infection as a small, solitary, silvery papule that erodes to a red, round or oval, superficial ulcer with a yellowish serous discharge. Palpation reveals a nontender indurated base that can be lifted like a button between the thumb and the finger. Lymph nodes enlarge early but are nontender. This is an STI.

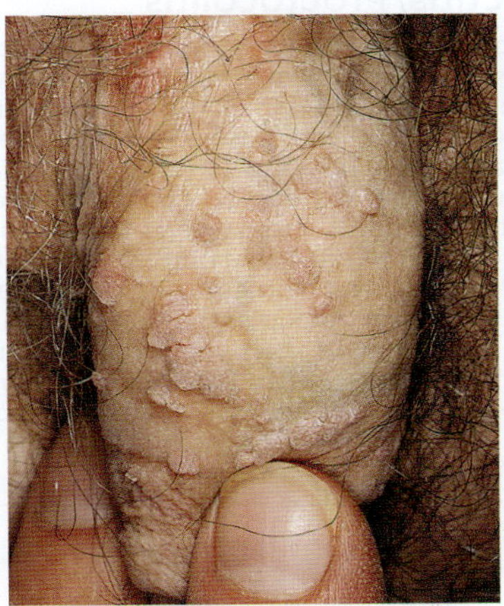

Genital warts

Soft, pointed, moist, fleshy, painless papules may be single or multiple in a cauliflower-like patch. They occur on shaft of penis, behind corona or around the anus where they may grow into large grape-like clusters.

These are caused by the human papillomavirus (HPV) and are one of the most common STIs. The HPV infection is correlated with early onset of sexual activity, infrequent use of condoms and multiple sexual partners.

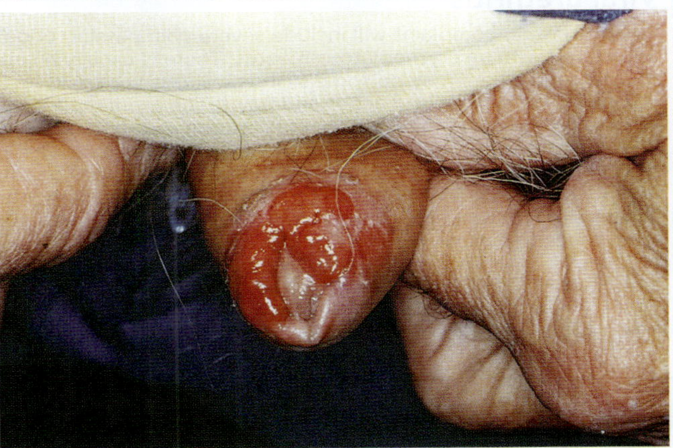

Carcinoma

Begins as red, raised warty growth or as an ulcer, with watery discharge. As it grows, may necrose and slough. Usually painless. Almost always on glans or inner lip of foreskin and following chronic inflammation. Enlarged lymph nodes are common.

TABLE 27.3 Urethritis and proctitis—Sexually transmissible infections

Non-specific urethritis (NSU)/ Non-gonococcal urethritis (NGU)

The history of presenting complaint will include mild non-specific penile symptoms to acute painful symptoms. Penile inflammation caused by a bacteria includes urethral itch and discomfort, burning or tingling passing urine and meatal redness. There may also be a urethral discharge or if any discharge, the patient may complain of the underpants being stained. Symptoms are usually present from 7 to 60 days after sex.

Forty to fifty per cent of all NGU will end up with no aetiological agent identified. Of the common STIs, 30% will test positive for *Chlamydia trachomatis* and 30% *Myocoplasma genitalium* and 1% will test positive for *Neisseria gonorrhoea.*

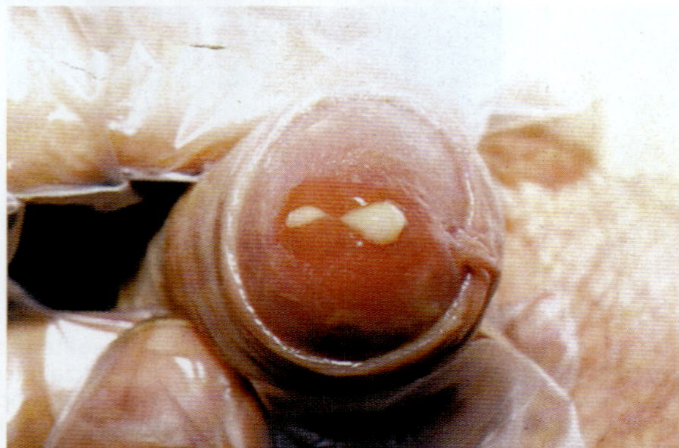

Gonococcal urethritis

Gonococcal urethritis presents with acute obvious urethral symptoms which includes moderate to copious yellowish greenish pus-like discharge. This is associated with pain—moderate to extreme—burning to razor sharp pain, passing urine. This usually occurs 24 hours to 7 days after a sexual encounter.

The physical examination will identify gonococcal urethritis because of its prominent signs. A specimen collected by swab of the discharge (not the meatal or urethral skin) for a Gram stain identifying Gram negative diplococci intracellularly and extracellularly will confirm the diagnosis. However, if there are no facilities for microscopy, a first-void urine is sufficient for a nucleic acid amplification test (NAAT) diagnosis and treatment is syndromic.

Viral urethritis

The presenting complaint will include severe pain passing urine, associated with an erythematous meatus. There is usually an absence of discharge. There may be some systemic illness with mild fevers and complaints of generalised aches and pains. The examination reveals a rather erythematous meatus. The most common aetiological agent is adenovirus. Herpes virus (HSV1 or/and HSV2) will also cause typical symptoms and examination may reveal blisters or lesions on the meatus and adjacent skin. HSV, however, has a shorter natural history than adenovirus. Treatment is conservative measures with push fluids and local anaesthetic cream or gel.

Proctitis/Proctocolitis

The presenting complaint will include mild to severe ano-rectal pain, pruritus ani and an observed mucous discharge on toilet paper. There may be spasms/ pain (tenesmus) with passing motion. The symptoms may appear 24 hours to 3 weeks after an anal sexual encounter. The aetiological agents most related to proctitis include *Neisseria gonorrhoea*, *Chlamydia trachomatis*, *Mycoplasma genitalium* and Herpes simplex virus. Anoscopy may be performed by a clinician who is trained in the procedure and this will yield any abnormal discharge or lesions inferior of the ano-rectal dentate line. Other causes of ano-rectal discomfort include haemorrhoids, where blood on toilet paper after defecating is a common complaint (haemotochezia).

TABLE 27.4 Abnormalities of the penis

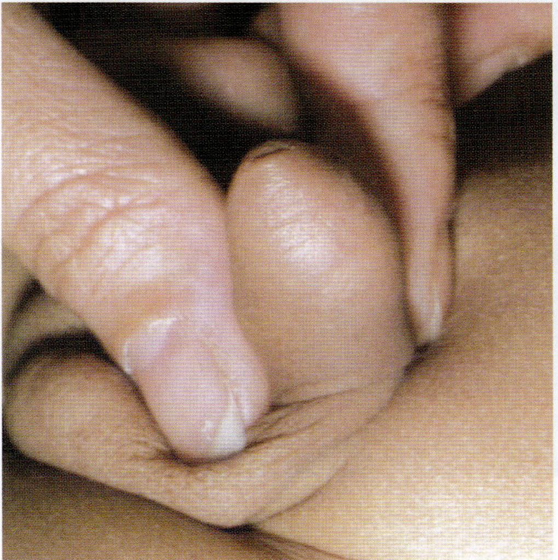

Phimosis

Foreskin is advanced and fixed so tight it is impossible to retract over glans. May be congenital or acquired from adhesions secondary to infection. Poor hygiene leads to retained dirt and smegma, which increases risk of inflammation or calculus formation.

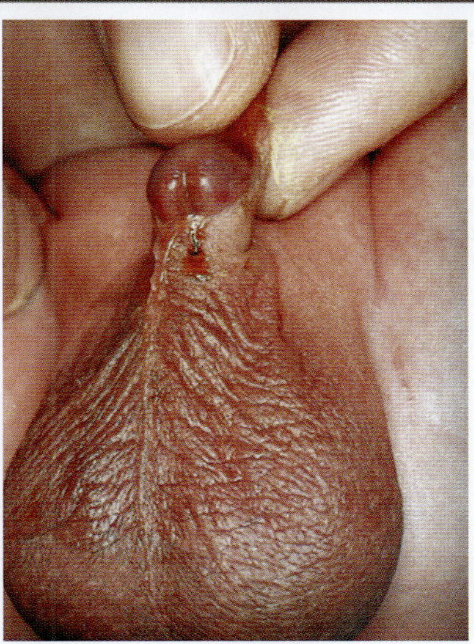

Hypospadias

Urethral meatus opens on the ventral (under) side of glans, shaft, or at the penoscrotal junction. A groove extends from the meatus to the normal location at the tip. This is a congenital defect that is important to recognise at birth. The newborn should not be circumcised because surgical correction may use foreskin tissue to extend urethral length.

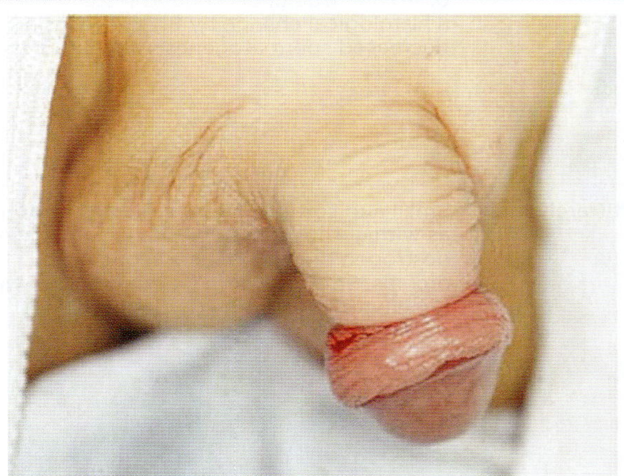

Paraphimosis

Foreskin is retracted and fixed. Once retracted behind glans, a tight or inflamed foreskin cannot return to its original position. Constriction impedes circulation, so glans swells. If untreated, it may compromise arterial circulation. It is important to make sure than the foreskin is placed back to its normal position after urinary catheterisation.

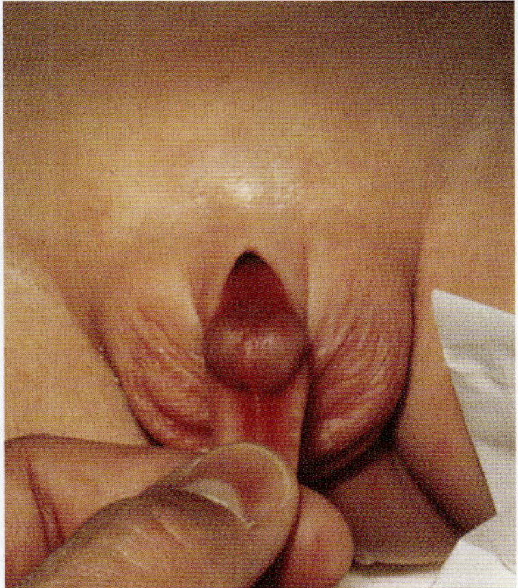

Epispadias

Meatus opens on the dorsal (upper) side of glans or shaft above a broad, spade-like penis. Rare; less common than hypospadias but more disabling because of associated urinary incontinence and separation of pubic bones.

TABLE 27.4 Abnormalities of the penis—cont'd

Peyronie's disease

Hard, nontender, subcutaneous plaques palpated on dorsal or lateral surface of penis. May be single or multiple and asymmetrical. They are associated with painful bending of the penis during erection. Plaques are fibrosis of covering of corpora cavernosa. Usually occurs after 45 years. Its cause is trauma to the erect penis, e.g. unexpected change in angle during intercourse. More common in men with diabetes, gout and Dupuytren's contracture of the palm.

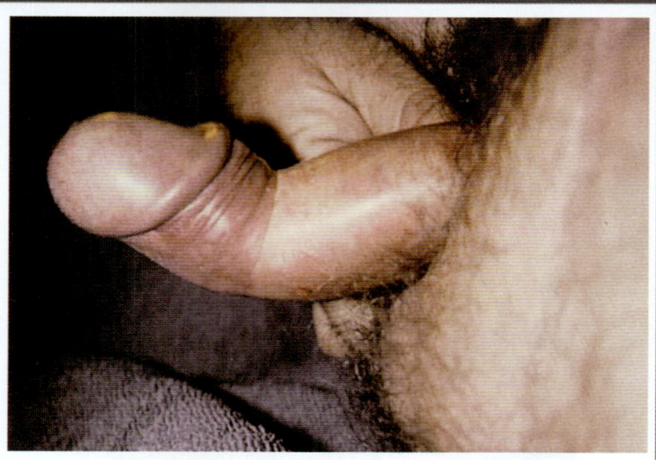

TABLE 27.5 Abnormalities in the scrotum

DISORDER	CLINICAL FINDINGS	DISCUSSION
Absent testis cryptorchidism 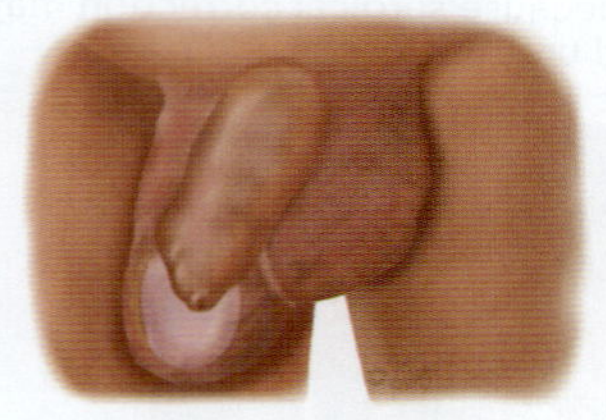	Empty scrotal half Inspection—in true maldescent, atrophic scrotum on affected side Palpation—no testis	True cryptorchidism—testes that have never descended. Incidence at birth is 3–4%; half of these descend in first month. Incidence with premature infants is 30%; in the adult 0.7–0.8%. True undescended testes have a histological change by 6 years, causing decreased spermatogenesis and infertility.
Small testis 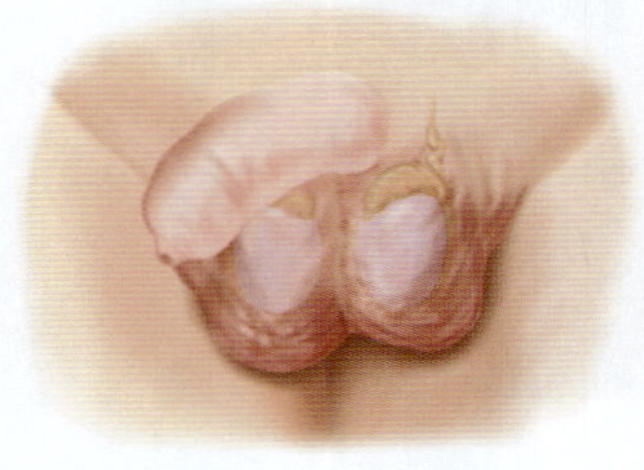	Palpation—small and soft (rarely may be firm) Small testis	Small and soft (<3.5 cm) indicates atrophy as with cirrhosis, hypopituitarism, following oestrogen therapy, or as a sequela of orchitis. Small and firm (<2 cm) occurs with Klinefelter's syndrome (hypogonadism).
Testicular torsion 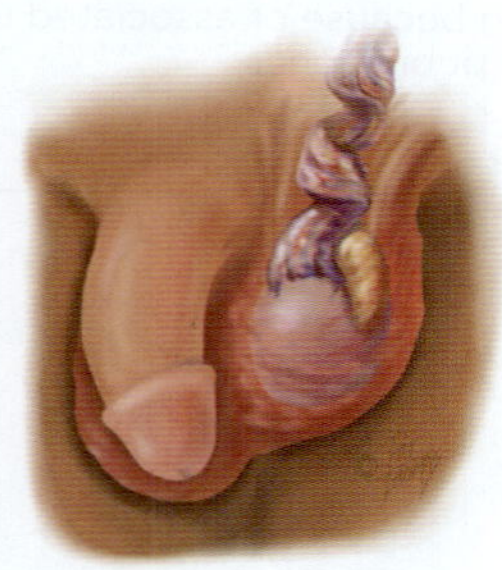	Excruciating pain in testicle of sudden onset, often during sleep or following trauma. May also have lower abdominal pain, nausea and vomiting, no fever. Inspection—red, swollen scrotum, one testis (usually left) higher owing to rotation and shortening. Palpation—cord feels thick, swollen, tender, epididymis may be anterior, cremasteric reflex is absent on side of torsion.	***Clinical alert:*** Sudden twisting of spermatic cord. Occurs in late childhood, early adolescence, rare after age of 20 years. Torsion occurs usually on the left side. Faulty anchoring of testis on wall of scrotum allows testis to rotate. The anterior part of the testis rotates medially towards the other testis. Blood supply is cut off, resulting in ischaemia and engorgement. This is an emergency requiring surgery; testis can become gangrenous in a few hours.

TABLE 27.5 Abnormalities in the scrotum—cont'd

DISORDER	CLINICAL FINDINGS	DISCUSSION
Epididymitis 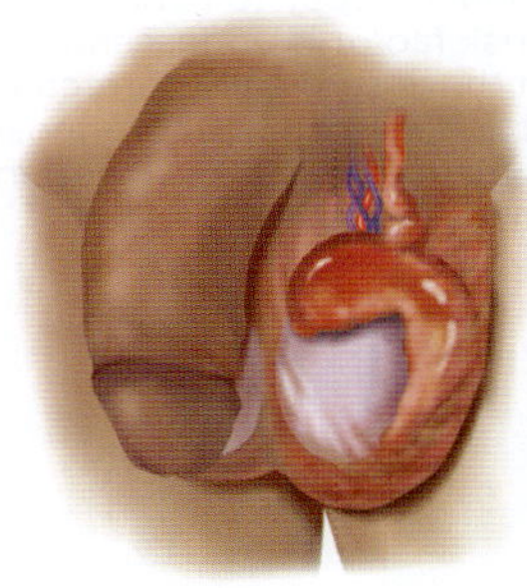	Severe pain of sudden onset in scrotum, somewhat relieved by elevation (a positive Phren's sign); also rapid swelling, fever. Inspection—enlarged scrotum; reddened. Palpation—exquisitely tender; epididymis enlarged, indurated; may be hard to distinguish from testis. Overlying scrotal skin may be thick and oedematous. Laboratory—white blood cells and bacteria in urine.	Acute infection of epididymis commonly caused by prostatitis, after prostatectomy because of trauma of urethral instrumentation or due to chlamydia, gonorrhoea or other bacterial infection. Often difficult to distinguish between epididymitis and testicular torsion.
Spermatic cord varicocoele 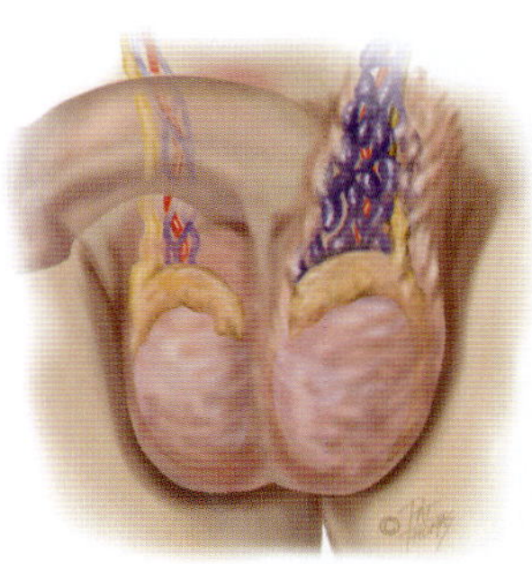	Dull pain; constant pulling or dragging feeling; or may be asymptomatic. Inspection—usually no sign. May show bluish colour through light scrotal skin. Palpation—when standing, feel soft, irregular mass posterior to and above testis; collapses when supine, refills when upright. Feels distinctive, like a 'bag of worms'. The testis on the side of the varicocoele may be smaller owing to impaired circulation.	A varicocoele is dilated, tortuous varicose veins in the spermatic cord due to incompetent valves within the vein, which permit reflux of blood. Most often on left side, perhaps because left spermatic vein is longer and inserts at a right angle into left renal vein. Common in young males. Screen at early adolescence; early treatment is important to prevent potential infertility when an adult.
Spermatocoele 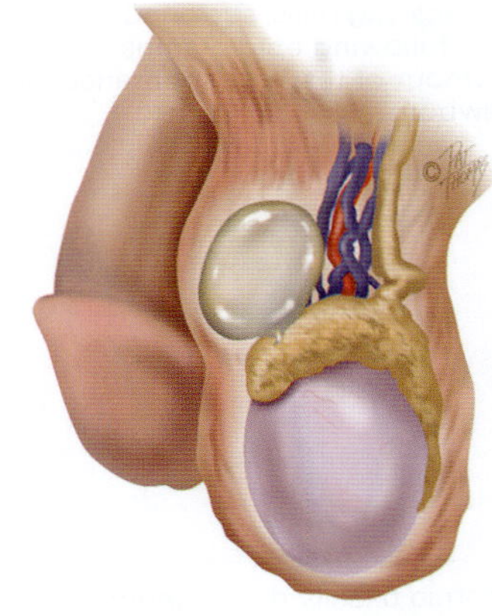	Painless, usually found on examination Palpation—round, freely movable mass lying above and behind testis. If large, feels like a third testis.	Retention cyst in epididymis. Cause unclear but may be obstruction of tubules. Filled with thin, milky fluid that contains sperm. Most spermatocoeles are small (<1 cm); occasionally, they may be larger and then mistaken for hydrocoele.

(Continued)

ABNORMAL FINDINGS FOR ADVANCED PRACTICE

TABLE 27.5 Abnormalities in the scrotum—cont'd

DISORDER	CLINICAL FINDINGS	DISCUSSION
Early testicular tumour 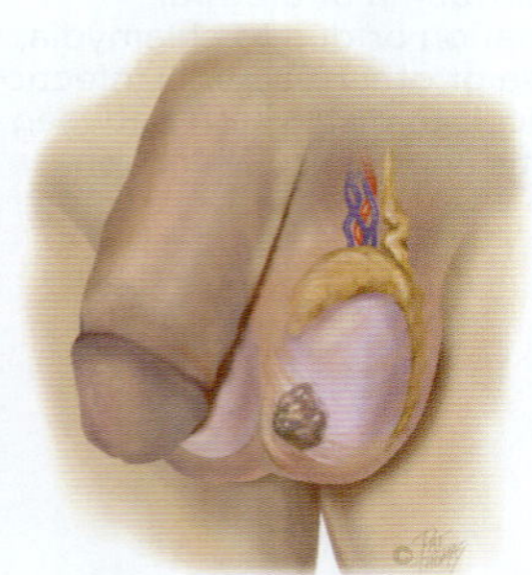	Painless, found on examination. Palpation—firm nodule or harder than normal section of testicle.	Most testicular tumours occur between the ages of 18 and 35. Practically all are malignant. Must biopsy to confirm. Most important risk factor is undescended testis, even those surgically corrected. Early detection important in prognosis, but practice of testicular self-examination is currently low.
Diffuse tumour 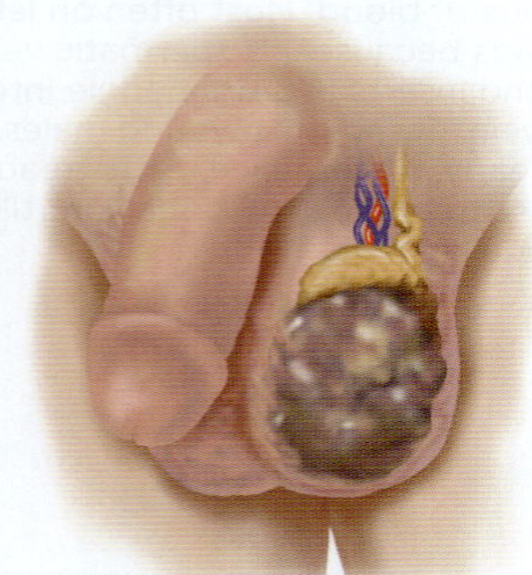	Enlarging testis (most common symptom). When enlarges, has feel of increased weight. Inspection—enlarged. Palpation—enlarged, smooth, ovoid, firm. Important—firm palpation does not cause usual sickening discomfort as with normal testis.	Diffuse tumour maintains shape of testis.
Hydrocoele 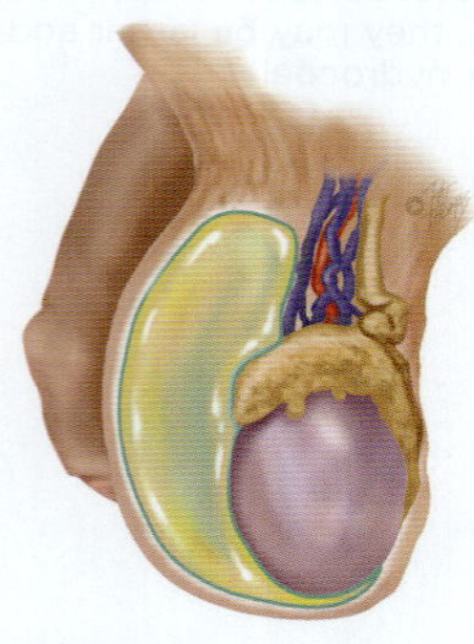	Painless swelling, although person may complain of weight and bulk in scrotum. Inspection—enlarged scrotum. Palpation—nontender mass, able to get fingers above mass (in contrast to scrotal hernia).	Cystic. Circumscribed collection of serous fluid in tunica vaginalis, surrounding testis. May occur following epididymitis, trauma, hernia, tumour of testis or spontaneously in the newborn.
Scrotal hernia 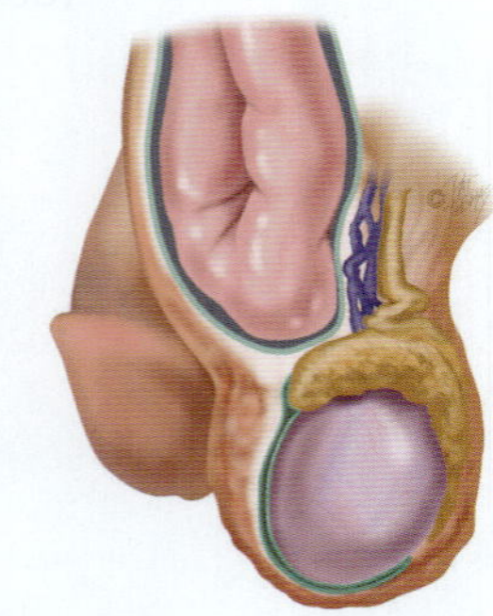	Swelling, may have pain with straining. Inspection—enlarged, may reduce when supine. Palpation—soft mushy mass, palpating fingers cannot get above mass. Mass is distinct from testicle that is normal.	Scrotal hernia usually due to indirect inguinal hernia (see Table 27.7).

TABLE 27.5 Abnormalities in the scrotum—cont'd

DISORDER	CLINICAL FINDINGS	DISCUSSION
Orchitis 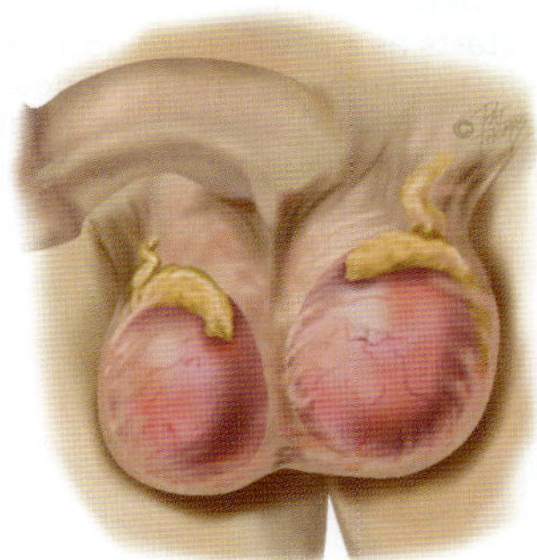	Acute or moderate pain of sudden onset, swollen testis, feeling of weight, fever. Inspection—enlarged, oedematous, reddened. Palpation—swollen, congested, tense and tender; hard to distinguish testis from epididymis.	Acute inflammation of testis. Most common cause is mumps; can occur with any infectious disease. May have associated hydrocoele that does transilluminate.
Scrotal oedema 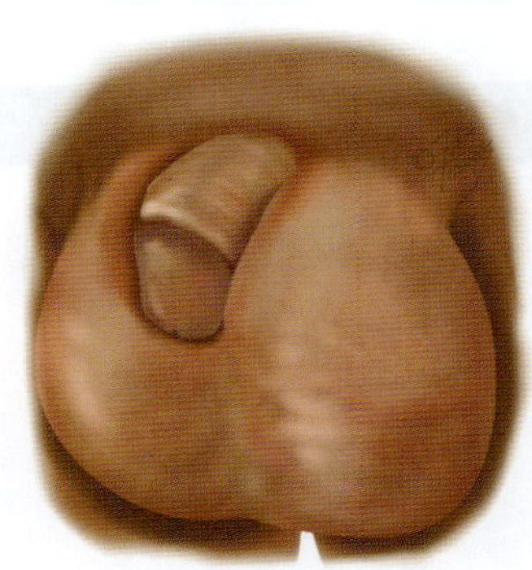	Tenderness Inspection—enlarged, may be reddened (with local irritation). Palpation—taut with pitting. Probably unable to feel scrotal contents.	Accompanies marked oedema in lower half of body, e.g. congestive heart failure, renal failure and portal vein obstruction. Occurs with local inflammation: epididymitis, torsion of spermatic cord. Also obstruction of inguinal lymphatics produces lymphoedema of scrotum.

TABLE 27.6 Abnormalities of the prostate gland

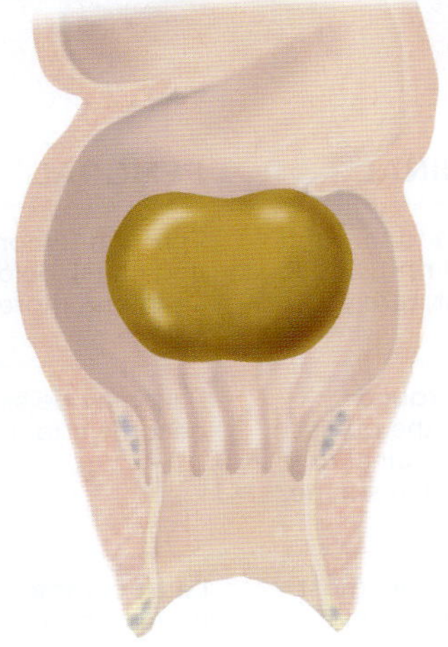 **Benign prostatic hypertrophy (BPH)** Urinary frequency, urgency, hesitancy, straining to urinate, weak stream, intermittent stream, sensation of incomplete emptying, nocturia. A symmetrical nontender enlargement, commonly occurs in males beginning in the middle years. The prostate surface feels smooth, rubbery or firm (like the consistency of the nose), with the median sulcus obliterated.	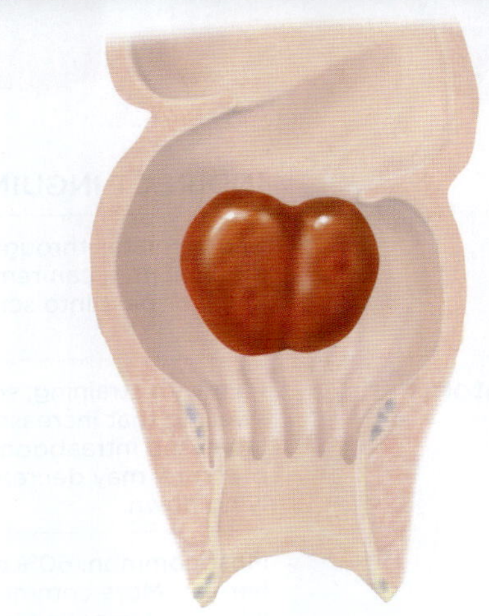 **Prostatitis** Fever, chills, malaise, urinary frequency and urgency, dysuria, urethral discharge, dull, aching pain in perineal and rectal area. An exquisitely tender enlargement is *acute* inflammation of the prostate gland yielding a swollen, slightly asymmetrical gland that is quite tender to palpation. With a chronic inflammation, the signs can vary from tender enlargement with a boggy feel to isolated firm areas due to fibrosis. Or the gland may feel normal.

(Continued)

TABLE 27.6 Abnormalities of the prostate gland—cont'd

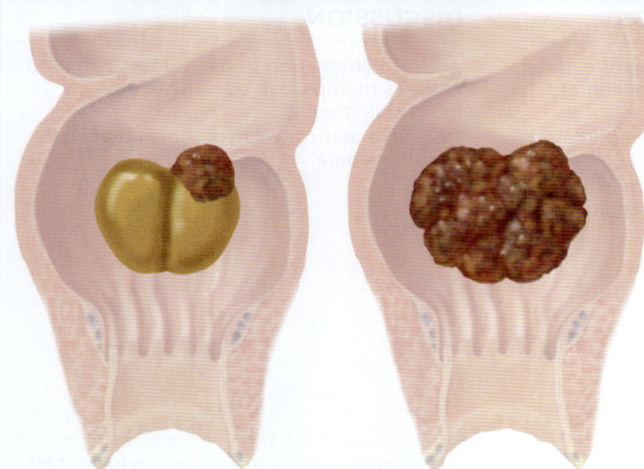

Carcinoma

Asymptomatic until advanced. Frequency, nocturia, haematuria, weak stream, hesitancy, pain or burning on urination, continuous pain in lower back, pelvis, thighs.

A malignant neoplasm often starts as a single hard nodule on the posterior surface, producing asymmetry and a change in consistency. As it invades normal tissue, multiple hard nodules appear, or the entire gland feels stone-hard and fixed. The median sulcus is obliterated.

TABLE 27.7 Inguinal and femoral hernias

	INDIRECT INGUINAL	DIRECT INGUINAL	FEMORAL
Course	Sac herniates through internal inguinal ring; can remain in canal or pass into scrotum.	Directly behind and through external inguinal ring, above inguinal ligament; rarely enters scrotum.	Through femoral ring and canal, below inguinal ligament, more often on right side.
Clinical symptoms and signs	Pain with straining; soft swelling that increases with increased intraabdominal pressure; may decrease when lying down.	Usually painless; round swelling close to the pubis in area of internal inguinal ring; easily reduced when supine.*	Pain may be severe, may become strangulated.
Frequency	Most common; 60% of all hernias. More common in infants <1 year and in males 16–20 years of age.	Less common, occurs most often in men >40, rare in women.	Least common, 4% of all hernias; more common in women.
Cause	Congenital or acquired	Acquired weakness; brought on by heavy lifting, muscle atrophy, obesity, chronic cough or ascites.	Acquired; due to increased abdominal pressure, muscle weakness or frequent stooping.

*__Reducible__—contents will return to abdominal cavity by lying down or gentle pressure. **Incarcerated**—herniated bowel cannot be returned to abdominal cavity. **Strangulated**—blood supply to hernia is shut off. Accompanied by nausea, vomiting and tenderness.

BIBLIOGRAPHY

Akers C. Aetiology, clinical presentation and treatment of testicular cancer. Nurs Stand 2018;32(28):50–61.

Alcohol and Drug Foundation. Anabolic steroids. 2019. Available at: https://adf.org.au/drug-facts/steroids.

Altice F, Evuarherhe O, Shina S, et al. Adherence to HIV treatment regimens: systematic literature review and meta-analysis. Patient Prefer Adherence 2019;13:475–90.

American Psychiatric Association. Diagnostic and Statistical Manual of Mental Disorders: Diagnostic and Statistical Manual of Mental Disorders, Fifth Edition. Arlington, VA: American Psychiatric Association; 2013.

Attorney-General's Department, Australian Government. Australian Government guidelines on the recognition of sex and gender. 2015. Available at: https://www.ag.gov.au/Publications/Pages/AustralianGovernmentGuidelinesontheRecognitionof SexandGender.aspx.

Australian Bureau of Statistics. General social survey: summary results, Australia, 2014. Canbera: ABS; 2015. Available at: https://www.abs.gov.au/Ausstats/abs@.nsf/0/DB1DB47D16CD5848CA257E7000154A7A?OpenDocument.

Australian Bureau of Statistics. Sex and gender diversity in the 2016 census. Canberra: ABS; 2018. Available at: https://www.abs.gov.au/ausstats/abs@.nsf/Lookup/by%20Subject/2071.0~2016~Main%20Features~Sex%20and%20Gender%20Diversity%20in%20the%202016%20Census~100.

Australian Government, Department of Health. National Men's health strategy 2020–2030, Commonwealth of Australia. 2019. Available at: https://www.health.gov.au/internet/main/publishing.nsf/content/86BBADC780E6058CCA257BF000191627/$File/19-0320%20National%20Mens%20Health%20Strategy%20Print%20ready%20accessible1.pdf.

Australian Institute of Health and Welfare. Cancer data in Australia – web report. Cat. no: CAN 122. Canberra: AIHW; 2019a. Available at: www.aihw.gov.au/reports/cancer/cancer-in-australia-2019/contents/table-of-contents.

Australian Institute of Health and Welfare. The health of Australia's males, Web report, Cat. no: PHE 239. Canberra: Australian Institute of Health and Welfare, 2019b [cited 2020 Jun. 16]. Available from: https://www.aihw.gov.au/reports/men-women/male-health

Bossio JA, Pukall CF. Attitude toward one's circumcision status is more important than actual circumcision status for men's body image and sexual functioning. Arch Sex Behav 2018;47(3): 771–81.

Colson MH, Cuzin B, Faix A, et al. Current epidemiology of erectile dysfunction, an update. Sexologies 2018;27(1):e7–13.

Eisinger RW, Dieffenbach CW, Fauci AS. HIV viral load and transmissibility of HIV infection: undetectable equals untransmittable. JAMA 2019;321(5):451–2.

European Association of Urology. Guidelines on male sexual dysfunction. EAU Annual Congress Barcelona, 2019. 2018. Available at: http://uroweb.org/guidelines/compilations-of-all-guidelines/.

Gulick RM, Flexner C. Long-acting HIV drugs for treatment and prevention. Annu Rev Med 2019;70:137–50.

Gurney JK. The puzzling incidence of testicular cancer in New Zealand: what can we learn? Andrology 2019;7(4): 394–401.

Healthy Male. Clinical summary guide - Androgen deficiency: diagnosis and management. Melbourne: Andrology Australia; 2019. Available at: www.healthymale.org.au/files/resources/androgen_deficiency_csg_healthy_male_2019.pdf.

Hedley J. Gay marriage: something old. Something new. In: Modern marriage and the lyric sequence. Cham: Palgrave Macmillan; 2018. p. 211–22.

Hung YC, Chang DC, Westfal ML, et al. A longitudinal population analysis of cumulative risks of circumcision. J Surg Res 2019;233:111–17.

Kessler A, Sollie S, Challacombe B, et al. The global prevalence of erectile dysfunction: a review. BJU Int 2019;124(4):587–99.

Kirby Institute. HIV, viral hepatitis and sexually transmissible infections in Australia: annual surveillance report 2018. Sydney: Kirby Institute, UNSW Sydney; 2018. Available at: https://kirby.unsw.edu.au/sites/default/files/kirby/report/KI_Annual-Surveillance-Report-2018.pdf#page=24.

Kirby Institute. National HIV notifications: Q1 2014-Q4 2018. 2019. Available at: https://kirby.unsw.edu.au/sites/default/files/kirby/report/National-HIV-Quarterly-Report_2018-Q4.pdf.

Lane C, Bailey RC, Luo C, et al. Adolescent male circumcision for HIV prevention in high priority countries: opportunities for improvement. Clin Infect Dis 2018;66(Suppl. 3):S161–5.

Marieb EM, Hoehn K. Human anatomy and physiology. 11th ed. San Francisco: Pearson; 2019.

McMahon CG. Current diagnosis and management of erectile dysfunction. Med J Aust 2019;210(10):469–76.

Ministry of Health, New Zealand. Cancer: historical summary 1948–2015. 2018. Available at: https://www.health.govt.nz/publication/cancer-historical-summary-1948-2015.

Morris BJ, Hankins CA, Banerjee J, et al. Does male circumcision reduce women's risk of sexually transmitted infections, cervical cancer, and associated conditions? Front Public Health 2019;7:4. doi:10.3389/fpubh.2019.00004.

Passos M. Atlas of sexually transmitted diseases: clinical aspects and differential diagnosis. Cham: Springer International Publishing; 2018.

Patel RM, Bariol S. National trends in surgical therapy for benign prostatic hyperplasia in Australia. ANZ J Surg 2019;89(4):345–9.

Pintye J, Baeten JM. Benefits of male circumcision for MSM: evidence for action. Lancet Glob Health 2019;7(4):e388–9.

Power J. Movement, Knowledge, Emotion. Gay activism and HIV/AIDS in Australia. Canberra: ANU Press; 2011.

Prabhakaran S, Ljuhar D, Coleman R, et al. Circumcision in the paediatric patient: a review of indications, technique and complications. J Paediatr Child Health 2018;54(12):1299–307.

Prostate Cancer Foundation, 2019. Available at: https://prostate.org.nz.

Rosen RC, Catania J, Pollack L, et al. Male Sexual Health Questionnaire (MSHQ): scale development and psychometric validation. Urology 2004;64(4):777–82.

Royal Australasian College of Physicians. Position statement – Circumcision of infant males. 2010. Available at: https://www.racp.edu.au/docs/default-source/advocacy-library/circumcision-of-infant-males.pdf.

Royal Children's Hospital. Engaging with and assessing the adolescent patient. 2019. Available at: https://www.rch.org.au/clinicalguide/guideline_index/Engaging_with_and_assessing_the_adolescent_patient.

Saag MS, Benson CA, Gandhi RT, et al. Antiretroviral drugs for treatment and prevention of HIV infection in adults: 2018 recommendations of the International Antiviral Society–USA Panel. JAMA 2018;320(4):379–96.

Strauss P, Cook A, Winter S, et al. Trans Pathways: the mental health experiences and care pathways of trans young people. Summary of results. Perth, Australia: Telethon Kids Institute; 2017. Available at: https://www.telethonkids.org.au/our-research/brain-and-behaviour/mental-health-and-youth/youth-mental-health/trans-pathways/.

Talley NJ, O'Connor S. Clinical examination: a systematic guide to physical diagnosis. 8th ed. Chatswood, NSW: Elsevier; 2018.

Telfer MM, Tollit MA, Pace CC, et al. Australian standards of care and treatment guidelines for transgender and gender diverse children and adolescents. Med J Aust 2018;209(3):132–6.

The Australian Law Reform Commission. For your information: Australian Privacy Law and Practice (ALRC Report 108). Chapter 68: Decision making by and for individuals under the aged of 18: Capacity and Health Information. 2008. Available at: https://www.alrc.gov.au/publications/68.%20Decision%20Making%20by%20and%20for%20Individuals%20Under%20the%20Age%20of%2018/capacity-and-health-info.

Tortora GJ, Derrickson BH. Principles of anatomy and physiology. 2nd Asia Pacific ed. Queensland: John Wiley & Sons; 2019.

UNAIDS. On the fast track to end AIDS—2016–2021 strategy. United Nations, Geneva: UNAIDS; 2015. Available at: https://www.unaids.org/sites/default/files/media_asset/20151027_UNAIDS_PCB37_15_18_EN_rev1.pdf.

UNAIDS. 90-90-90: An ambitious treatment target to help end the AIDS epidemic. Zurich: WHO; 2017. Available at: https://www.unaids.org/en/resources/documents/2017/90-90-90.

UNAIDS. Global HIV & AIDS statistics—2019 fact sheet. 2019. Available at: https://www.unaids.org/en/resources/fact-sheet.

UNAIDS. UNAIDS strategy. 2020. Available at: https://www.unaids.org/en/goals/unaidsstrategy.

University of Otago, AIDS Epidemiology group. AIDS-NZ newsletter—Epidemiological surveillance. 2019. Available at: https://www.otago.ac.nz/aidsepigroup/newsletters/index.html

World Health Organisation. HIV/AIDS. 2020a. Available at: https://www.who.int/health-topics/hiv-aids/#tab=tab_1.

World Health Organisation. Male circumcision for HIV prevention. 2020b. Available at: https://www.who.int/hiv/topics/malecircumcision/en/.

Yuan T, Fitzpatrick T, Ko NY, et al. Circumcision to prevent HIV and other sexually transmitted infections in men who have sex with men: a systematic review and meta-analysis of global data. Lancet Glob Health 2019;7(4):e436–47.

Websites

Andrology Australia: www.andrologyaustralia.org
Australian Lesbian and Gay Archives: http://www.alga.org.au/
Healthy Male (Andrology Australia): www.healthymale.org.au
New Zealand Sexual Health Society (Inc.): www.nzshs.org
Prostate Cancer Foundation of Australia: https://www.prostate.org.au
Prostate Cancer Foundation of New Zealand: https://prostate.org.nz

Chapter Twenty-Eight

Breasts assessment

Written by Carolyn Jarvis
Adapted by Elizabeth Pascoe

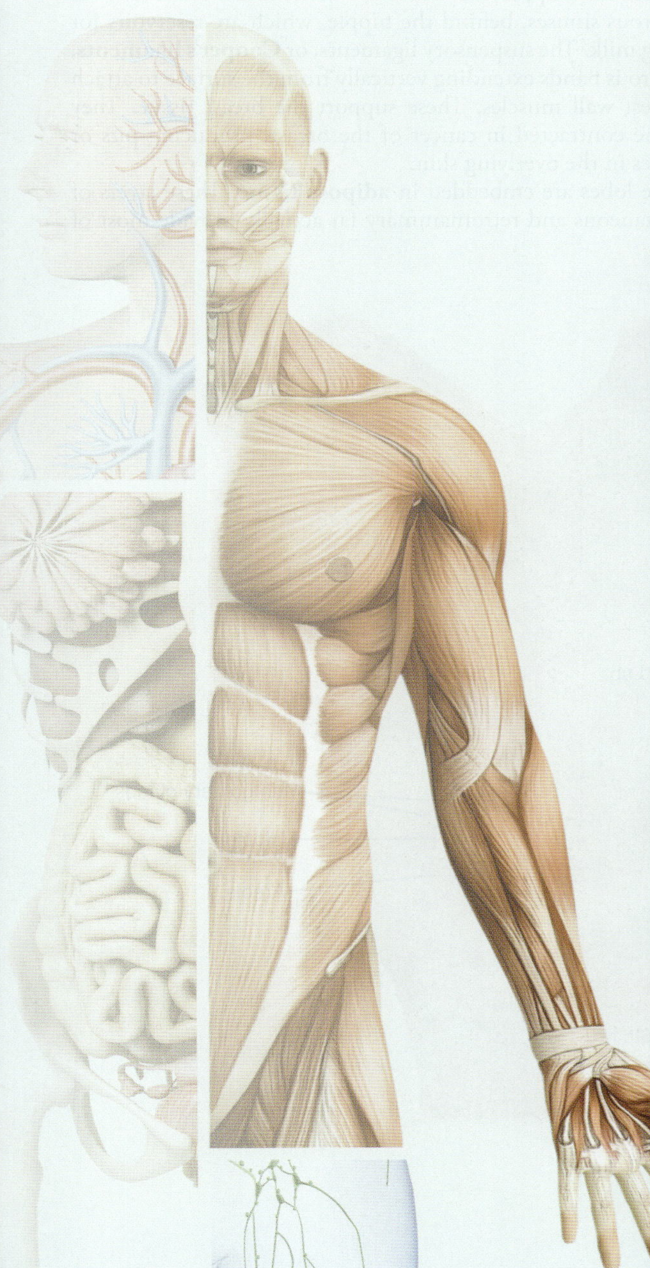

INTRODUCTION

The breasts, or mammary glands, are present in both females and males, although in the male they are rudimentary throughout life. The female breasts are accessory reproductive organs whose function is to produce milk for nourishing the newborn.

Structure and function

SURFACE ANATOMY

The **breasts** lie anterior to the pectoralis major and serratus anterior muscles (Figure 28.1). The breasts are located between the second and sixth ribs, extending from the side of the sternum to the midaxillary line. The superior lateral corner of breast tissue, called the axillary **tail of Spence**, projects up and laterally into the axilla.

The **nipple** is just below the centre of the breast. It is rough, round and usually protuberant; its surface looks wrinkled and indented with tiny milk duct openings. The **areola** surrounds the nipple for a 1- to 2-cm radius. In the areola are small elevated sebaceous glands, called the Montgomery glands. These secrete a protective lipid material during lactation. The areola also has smooth muscle fibres that cause nipple erection when stimulated. Both the nipple and the areola are more darkly pigmented than the rest of the breast surface; the colour varies from pink to brown depending on the person's skin colour and parity.

INTERNAL ANATOMY

The breast is composed of (1) glandular tissue, (2) fibrous tissue including the suspensory ligaments and (3) adipose tissue (Figure 28.2). The **glandular tissue** contains 15 to 20 lobes radiating from the nipple, and these are composed of lobules. Within each lobule are clusters of alveoli that produce milk. Each lobe empties into a lactiferous duct. The 15 to 20 lactiferous ducts form a collecting duct system converging towards the nipple. There, the ducts form ampullae, or lactiferous sinuses, behind the nipple, which are reservoirs for storing milk. The suspensory ligaments, or **Cooper's ligaments**, are fibrous bands extending vertically from the surface to attach on chest wall muscles. These support the breast tissue. They become contracted in cancer of the breast, producing pits or dimples in the overlying skin.

The lobes are embedded in **adipose tissue**. These layers of subcutaneous and retromammary fat actually provide most of

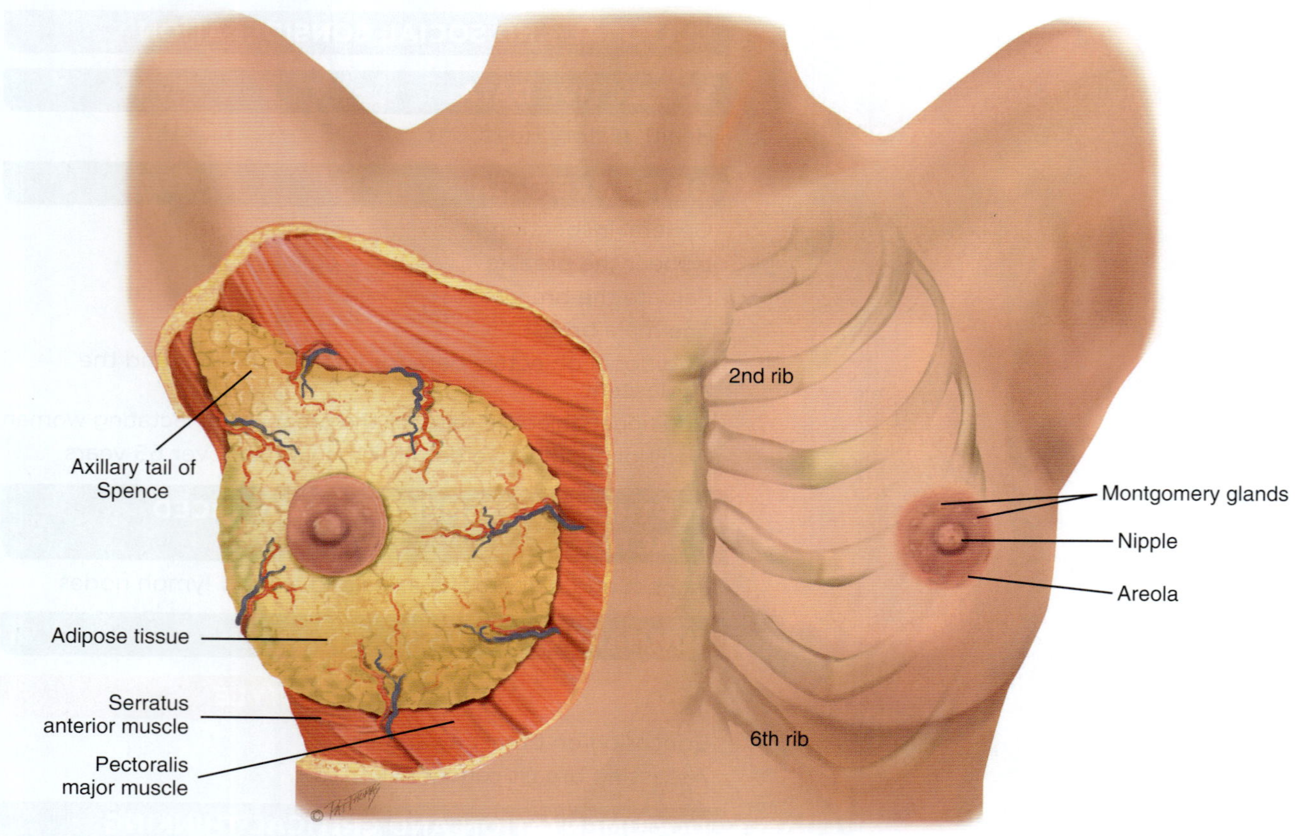

Figure 28.1

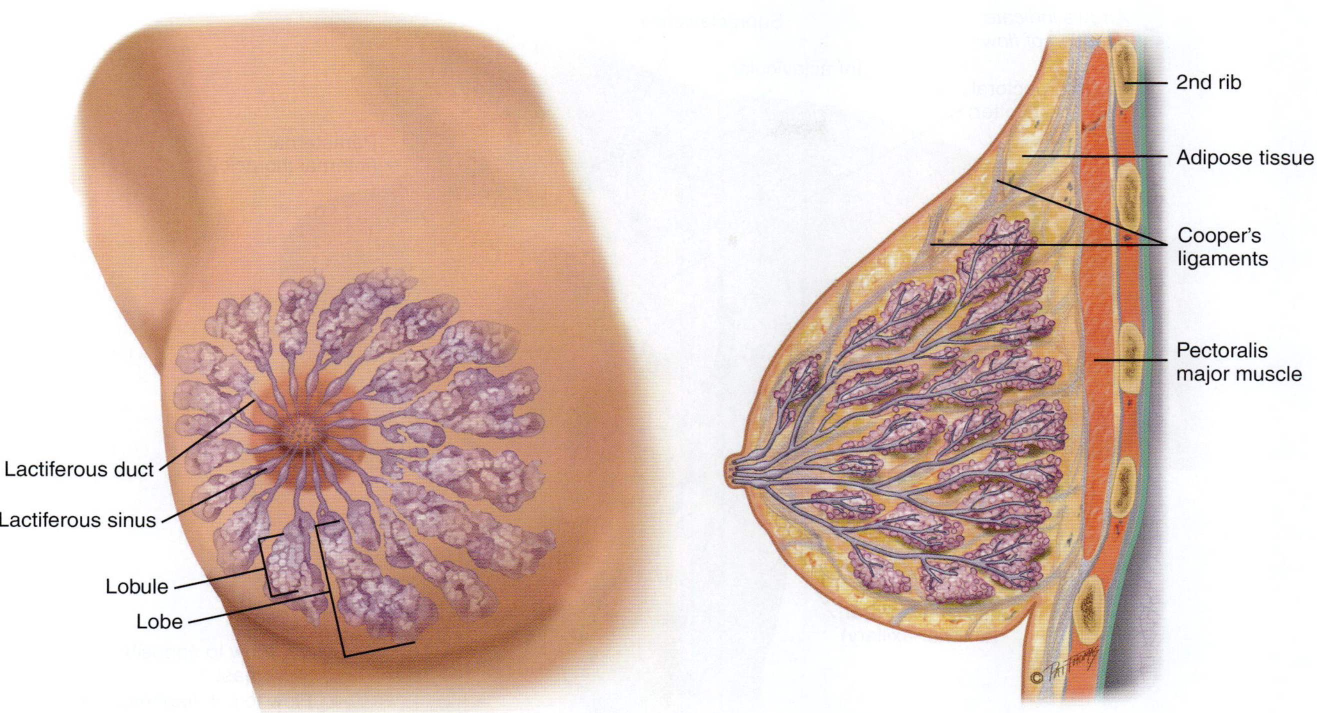

Figure 28.2

the bulk of the breast. The relative proportion of glandular, fibrous and fatty tissue varies depending on age, menstrual cycle, pregnancy, lactation and general nutritional state.

The breast may be divided into four quadrants by imaginary horizontal and vertical lines intersecting at the nipple (Figure 28.3). This makes a convenient map to describe clinical findings. In the upper outer quadrant, note the axillary **tail of Spence**, the cone-shaped breast tissue that projects up into the axilla, close to the pectoral group of axillary lymph nodes. The upper outer quadrant is the site of most breast tumours.

LYMPHATICS

The breast has extensive lymphatic drainage. Most of the lymph, more than 75%, drains into the ipsilateral (same side) axillary nodes. Four groups of axillary nodes are present (Figure 28.4):

1. **Central axillary nodes**—high up in the middle of the axilla, over the ribs and serratus anterior muscle. These receive lymph from the other three groups of nodes.
2. **Pectoral** (anterior)—along the lateral edge of the pectoralis major muscle, just inside the anterior axillary fold.
3. **Subscapular** (posterior)—along the lateral edge of the scapula, deep in the posterior axillary fold.
4. **Lateral**—along the humerus, inside the upper arm.

From the central axillary nodes, drainage flows up to the infraclavicular and supraclavicular nodes.

A smaller amount of lymphatic drainage does not take these channels but flows directly up to the infraclavicular group,

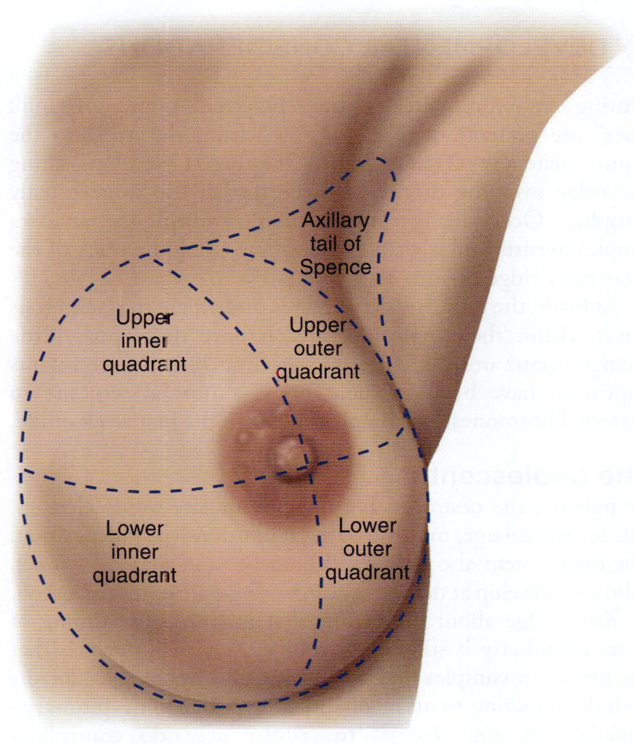

Figure 28.3

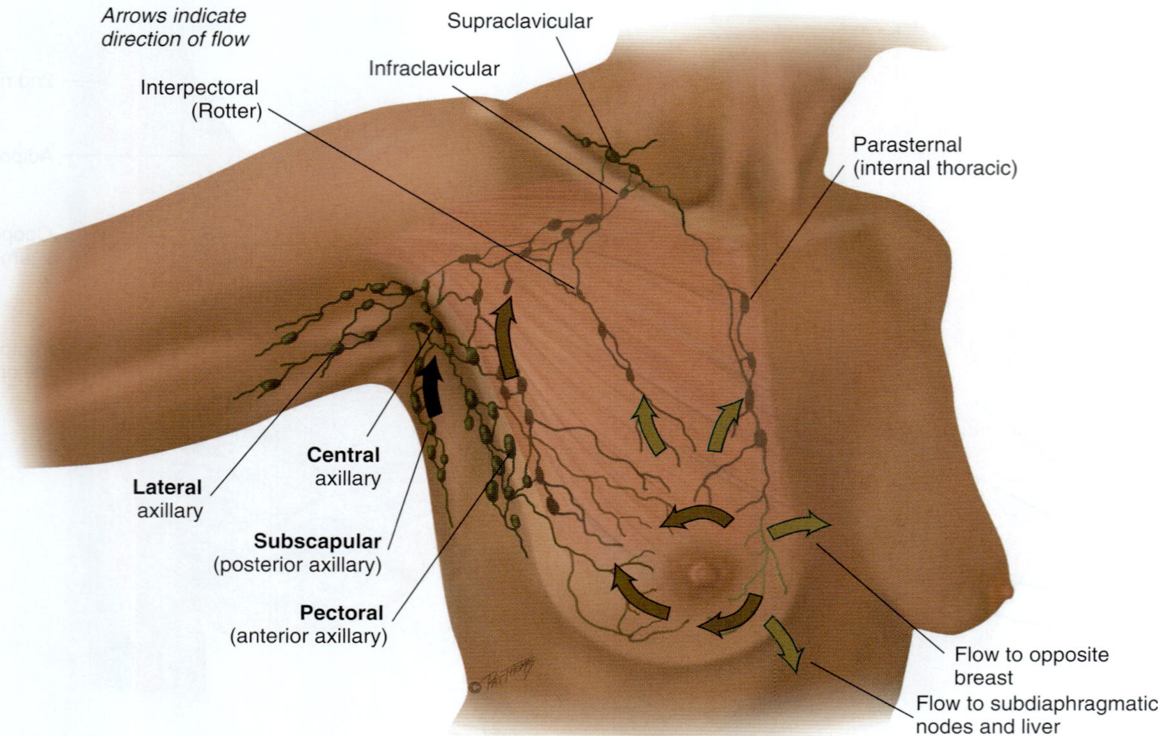

Figure 28.4
© Pat Thomas, 2014.

deep into the chest or into the abdomen or directly across to the opposite breast.

DEVELOPMENTAL CONSIDERATIONS

During embryonic life, ventral epidermal ridges, or 'milk lines', are present; these curve down from the axilla to the groin bilaterally (Figure 28.5). The breast develops along the ridge over the thorax, and the rest of the ridge usually atrophies. Occasionally a **supernumerary nipple** (i.e. an extra nipple) persists and is visible somewhere along the track of the mammary ridge (Figure 28.6).

At birth, the only breast structures present are the lactiferous ducts within the nipple. No alveoli have developed. Little change occurs until puberty. However, at birth, some infants appear to have breast tissue. This is a normal response to maternal hormones and disappears within the first week of life.

The adolescent

At puberty, the oestrogen hormones stimulate breast changes. The breasts enlarge, mostly as a result of extensive fat deposition. The duct system also grows and branches and masses of small, solid cells develop at the duct endings. These are potential alveoli.

Knowledge about the factors that influence the timing of onset of puberty is still being studied. What is known is that the process is complex and multifactorial. Physiological factors include endocrine events involving the hypothalamus–pituitary–gonadal axis and changes to cellular networks controlling gonadotrophin releasing hormone. These mechanisms are likely to be influenced by regulatory gene networks, epigenetic

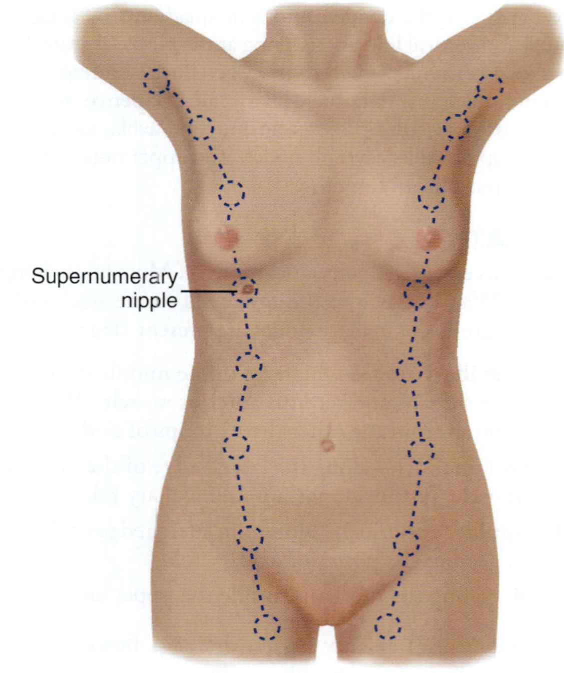

Figure 28.5

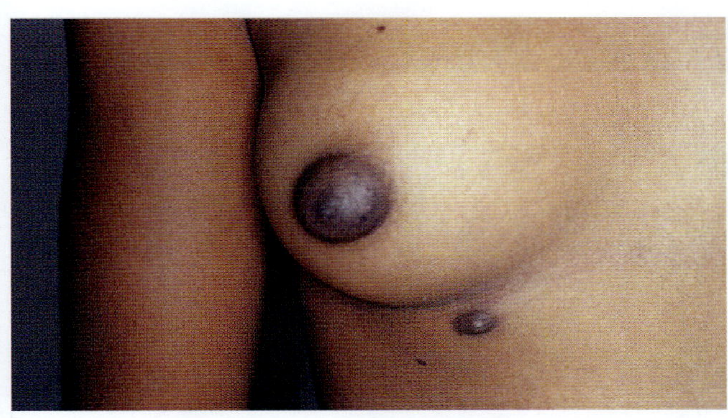

Figure 28.6
Supernumerary nipple and areolar complex.

changes, exposure to endocrine disrupting chemicals, maternal and childhood obesity and low birth weight (Lawn et al 2017, Worthman et al 2019). Social factors such as low socioeconomic status also influence the age of the onset of breast development and onset of menarche (Kelly et al 2017).

Occasionally, one breast may grow faster than the other, producing a temporary asymmetry. This may cause some distress; reassurance is necessary. Tenderness is also common due to the influence of reproductive hormones, particularly oestrogen. Although the age of onset varies widely, the five stages of breast development follow this classic description of sexual maturity rating, or **Tanner staging** (Table 28.1).

Full development from stage 2 to stage 5 takes an average of 3 years, although the range is 1.5 to 6 years. During this time, pubic hair develops and axillary hair appears 2 years after the onset of pubic hair. The beginning of breast development precedes menarche (beginning of menstruation) by about 2 years. Menarche occurs in breast development stage 3 or 4, usually just after the peak of the adolescent growth spurt around age 12 years. This aids in assessing the development of adolescent girls and increases their knowledge about their own development.

Breasts of the nonpregnant woman change with the ebb and flow of hormones during the monthly menstrual cycle. Nodularity increases from midcycle up to menstruation. During the 3 to 4 days before menstruation, the breasts feel full, tight, heavy and occasionally sore. The breast volume is smallest on days 4 to 7 of the menstrual cycle.

The pregnant woman

During pregnancy, breast changes start during the second month and are an early sign of pregnancy for most women. Pregnancy stimulates the expansion of the ductal system and supporting fatty tissue as well as development of the true secretory alveoli. Thus, the breasts enlarge and feel more nodular. The nipples are larger, darker and more erectile. The areolae become larger and grow a darker brown as pregnancy progresses and the tubercles become more prominent. (The brown colour fades after lactation, but the areolae never return to the original colour.) A venous pattern is prominent over the skin surface (see Figure 28.4).

After the fourth month, **colostrum** may be expressed. This thick yellow fluid is the precursor for milk, containing the same amount of protein and lactose but practically no fat. The breasts produce colostrum for the first few days after birth. It is rich with antibodies that protect the newborn against infection, so breastfeeding is important. Milk production (lactation) begins 1 to 3 days postpartum. The whitish colour is from emulsified fat and calcium caseinate.

The woman over 65 years

After menopause, ovarian secretion of oestrogen and progesterone decreases, which causes the breast glandular tissue to atrophy. This is replaced with fibrous connective tissue. The fat envelope atrophies also, beginning in the middle years and becoming marked in the eighth and ninth decades. These changes decrease breast size and elasticity so the breasts droop and sag, looking flattened and flabby. Drooping is accentuated by kyphosis in some older women.

The decreased breast size makes inner structures more prominent. A breast lump may have been present for years but is suddenly palpable. Around the nipple the lactiferous ducts are more palpable and feel firm and stringy because of fibrosis and calcification. The axillary hair decreases.

THE MALE BREAST

The male breast is a rudimentary structure consisting of a thin disc of undeveloped tissue underlying the nipple. The areola is well developed, although the nipple is relatively small. During adolescence, it is common for the breast tissue to temporarily enlarge, producing **gynaecomastia** (see Table 28.8). This condition is usually unilateral and temporary. Reassurance is necessary for the adolescent male, whose attention is riveted on his body image. Gynaecomastia may reappear in the male over 65 years and may be due to testosterone deficiency.

CULTURAL AND SOCIAL CONSIDERATIONS

The mean age at which non-Indigenous Australian women experience their first menstrual period (menarche) is 12.2 years (Mishra et al 2017) and is comparable to findings from studies undertaken in Europe and the United States of America (Biro et al 2018, Lazzeri et al 2018). To date, there is no specific data on age of onset of menarche in Indigenous Australian women.

Breast cancer

Breast cancer is the most common cancer that occurs in Australian and New Zealand women. The risk of developing breast cancer to age 85 years is 1 in 7 for Australian women and 1 in 715 for Australian men (Australian Institute of Health and Welfare (AIHW) 2019). There are similar rates of breast cancer in New Zealand (Ministry of Health 2018).

The incidence of breast cancer varies with different cultural groups. Although the incidence of breast cancer is significantly lower in Indigenous Australian women than in non-Indigenous Australian women, Indigenous Australian women have significantly lower 5-year crude survival rates (81% and 90+% crude survival, respectively) (AIHW 2019). In New Zealand, breast cancer registration among Māori women is 1.4 times more than non-Māori women (Ministry of Health 2018). Further, Māori women are 1.5 times more likely to die from the disease as non-Māori, mainly because they tend to present with late stage breast cancer at the time of diagnosis (Ministry of Health 2018).

In Australia, non-Indigenous women are significantly more likely to have had a mammogram through the BreastScreen Australia Program than are Indigenous Australian women. In

TABLE 28.1 Sexual maturity rating in girls

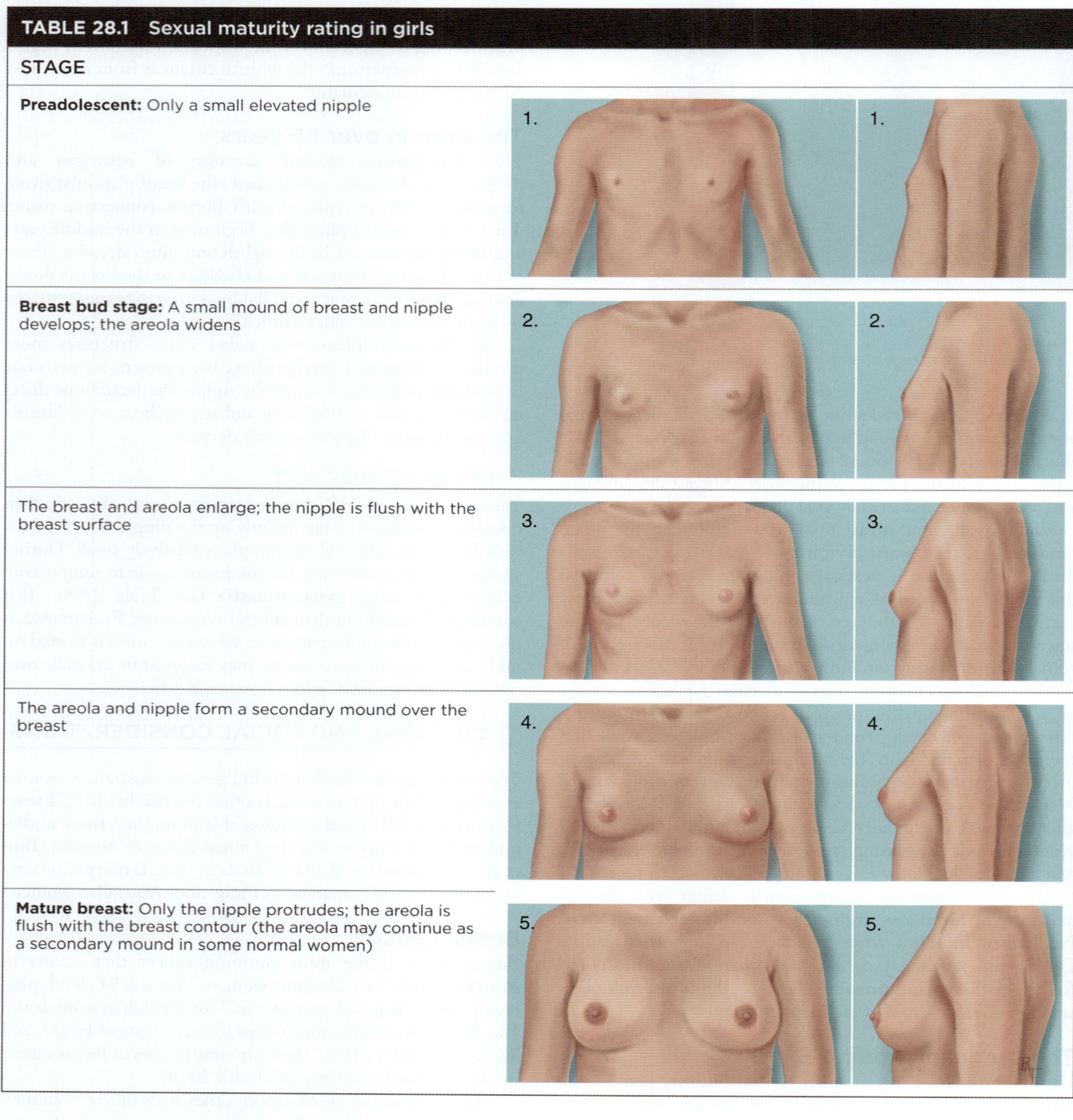

STAGE
Preadolescent: Only a small elevated nipple
Breast bud stage: A small mound of breast and nipple develops; the areola widens
The breast and areola enlarge; the nipple is flush with the breast surface
The areola and nipple form a secondary mound over the breast
Mature breast: Only the nipple protrudes; the areola is flush with the breast contour (the areola may continue as a secondary mound in some normal women)

2015 and 2016, the age-standardised participation rate for non-Indigenous women aged 56–75 years was 54% compared with 39% for Indigenous Australian women in the same age range (AIHW 2018). Although there is no single main factor influencing Indigenous women's decisions to use the BreastScreen Australia Program service, there are historical and culturally related influences. Indigenous distrust of non-Indigenous institutions and beliefs about cancer and western medical treatments are identified as contributing factors (Cunningham et al 2008, Prior 2009). Similarly, there are a range of cultural and social reasons why Māori and Pacific Islander women tend not to have regular screening mammograms (Breast Cancer Foundation NZ 2019).

Cultural and social issues associated with diet and exercise are becoming the focus of increasing attention. Mounting interest in the role that lifestyle factors such as diet, exercise and weight have on breast cancer survival and/or comorbidity and mortality has led researchers to evaluate the effects of these factors on the disease. Current findings point to a possible but inconsistent benefit of a prudent, vegetable rich, low-fat/high vegetable eating pattern on disease-free survival (Harvie et al 2015). Physical activity and weight control are also considered to be lifestyle factors potentially impacting on breast cancer prevention and survival (Lester 2018). At least 150 min of moderate intensity or 75 min of vigorous intensity aerobic exercise (for example, walking, jogging, cycling, swimming) each week, and two to three resistance exercise (i.e. lifting weights) sessions each week, targeting the major muscle groups are recommended (Clinical Oncology Society of Australia 2018). Despite the potential therapeutic effects of lifestyle factors of diet, smoking, alcohol consumption, exercise and weight control on breast cancer prevention, they remain low modifiable breast cancer risk factors (Lester 2018).

Subjective data

In most western cultures, the female breasts signify more than their primary purpose of lactation. Women are surrounded by messages that feminine norms of beauty and desirability are enhanced by and dependent on the size of the breasts and their appearance. More recently, women leaders have tried to refocus this attitude, stressing women's self-worth as individual human beings, not as stereotyped sexual objects. The intense cultural emphasis is gradually changing, yet the breasts are still crucial to a woman's self-concept and her perception of her femininity.

Matters pertaining to the breast affect a woman's body image and generate deep emotional responses. These responses may take strong forms that may be observed as you discuss the woman's history. One woman may be acutely embarrassed talking about her breasts, as evidenced by lack of eye contact, minimal response, nervous gestures or inappropriate humour. Another woman may talk wryly and disparagingly about the size or development of her breasts. A young adolescent is acutely aware of her own development in relation to her peers. Or, a woman who has found a breast lump may come to you with fear, high anxiety and even panic. Although many breast lumps are benign, women initially assume the worst possible outcome—cancer, disfigurement and death. While you are collecting the subjective data, tune in to cues for these behaviours that call for a straightforward and reasoned attitude.

Because of the physiological relationship between the breasts and lymph glands, any assessment of a woman's breast must include an assessment of the axillary lymph glands. Subjective assessment enables you to obtain information directly from the woman about signs and symptoms they are experiencing.

Breast

1. Presenting concern
2. Pain
3. Lump
4. Discharge
5. Rash
6. Swelling
7. Trauma
8. History of breast disease
9. Surgery
10. Heath and lifestyle management

Axilla

1. Tenderness, lump or swelling
2. Rash

Practice note: Before you commence the assessment, introduce yourself to the person, confirm the person's identity, discuss the purpose and scope of the assessment, clarify any questions the person may have and obtain verbal consent from the person to perform the assessment.

ASSESSMENT GUIDELINES	CLINICAL SIGNIFICANCE AND CLINICAL ALERTS
1. Presenting concern	
• Do you feel that you have any problems with your breasts? It is important to ascertain the person's perception of their presenting health concern. • If they do perceive a problem—how does this impact on their quality of life and sexuality?	
2. Pain	
• Any **pain** or tenderness in the breasts? When did you first notice it? • Where is the pain? Localised or all over? Is the painful spot sore to touch? Do you feel a burning or pulling sensation?	***Clinical alert:*** **mastalgia** (pain in the breast) may occur with trauma, inflammation, infection and benign breast disease.
• Is the pain cyclic? Any relation to your menstrual period? • Is pain related to specific cause? Is the pain brought on by strenuous activity, especially involving one arm; a change in activity; touch during sex; part of underwire bra; exercise?	Cyclic pain is common with normal breasts (commonly associated with the menstrual cycle), and benign breast (fibrocystic) disease. Oral contraceptives can also cause breast tenderness.

SUBJECTIVE DATA

ASSESSMENT GUIDELINES	CLINICAL SIGNIFICANCE AND CLINICAL ALERTS
3. Lump	
• Have you ever noticed a **lump** or **thickening** in the breast? Where? • When did you first notice it? Changed at all since then? • Does the lump have any relation to your menstrual period? • Noticed any change in the overlying skin: redness, warmth, dimpling, swelling?	Carefully explore the presence of any lump. A lump present for many years and exhibiting no change may not be serious but still should be explored. Approach any recent change or new lump with suspicion.
4. Discharge	
• Any **discharge** from the nipple? • When did you first notice this? • What colour is the discharge? • Consistency—thick or runny? • Odour?	***Clinical alert:*** **Galactorrhoea** (lactation not associated with childbirth). Note medications that may cause clear nipple discharge: oral contraceptives, phenothiazines, diuretics, digitalis, steroids, methyldopa, calcium channel blockers. Bloody or blood-tinged discharge is always significant. Any discharge with a lump is significant.
5. Rash	
• Any **rash** on the breast? • When did you first notice this? • Where did it start? On the nipple, areola or surrounding skin?	***Clinical alert:*** **Paget's disease of the nipple**. Inflammatory malignant neoplasm of the nipple and areola that is usually associated with carcinoma in deeper breast tissue. Paget's disease starts with a small crust on the nipple apex, then spreads to areola. Eczema (superficial dermatitis) or other dermatitis rarely starts at nipple unless it is due to breastfeeding. It usually starts on the areola or surrounding skin and then spreads to the nipple.
6. Swelling	
• Any **swelling** in the breasts? In one spot or all over? • Related to your menstrual period, pregnancy or breastfeeding? • Any change in bra size?	
7. Trauma	
• Any **trauma** or injury to the breasts? • Did it result in any swelling, lump or break in skin?	A lump from an injury is due to local haematoma or oedema and should resolve shortly. Or, trauma may cause a woman to feel the breast and find a lump that really was there before.
8. History of breast disease	
• Any history of breast disease yourself? • What type? How was this diagnosed? • When did this occur? • How is it being treated?	Past breast cancer increases the risk of recurrent cancer (Table 28.2). The presence of benign breast disease makes the breasts more difficult to examine; the general lumpiness conceals a new lump.
• Any breast cancer in your family? Who? Sister, mother, maternal grandmother, maternal aunts, daughter? • At what age did this relative have breast cancer?	Breast cancer occurring in certain family members increases risk for this woman (Table 28.2).

ASSESSMENT GUIDELINES	CLINICAL SIGNIFICANCE AND CLINICAL ALERTS
9. Surgery	
• Ever had **surgery** on the breasts? Was this a biopsy? What were the biopsy results? • Mastectomy—prophylactic or for treatment of the breast cancer? • Breast reconstruction? • Mammoplasty—augmentation or reduction?	
10. Health and lifestyle management	
• Do you take oral contraceptives? For how long? For post-menopausal women—are you taking hormone replacement therapy? Type? For how long?	**Oral contraceptives** may control symptoms of benign (fibrocystic) breast disease. Combined **menopausal hormone therapy (MHT)** can increase the risk of breast cancer in some women. There is variation in the risk with other variables such as race/ethnicity, body mass index and breast density.
• Do you routinely inspect and feel your breasts? • Are you aware of what you should be looking for? • Do you know when to seek medical advice? Breast awareness and mammograms are complementary screening measures. In the absence of proof that routine systematic breast self-examination (BSE) is effective, Cancer Australia, the National Screening Unit (NSU) New Zealand and the Breast Cancer Foundation New Zealand advocate a less formal Breast Aware approach to encourage women to report unusual breast changes. This approach involves the woman being aware of how her breasts normally look and feel, so that she may be better able to recognise any changes (Breast Cancer Foundation NZ 2019, Cancer Australia 2018, Ministry of Health 2018). No one method a woman uses to check her breasts is recommended over another; however, what is important is that the woman both views and palpates all the breast tissue in both breasts from collarbone to below the bra-line and under the armpit.	A suggested **breast awareness** approach is offered by Cancer Australia (http://canceraustralia.gov.au/publications-and-resources/position-statements/early-detection-breast-cancer). Inform the woman that if she notices any of the following changes in either of her breasts when performing regular breast awareness, she should contact her general practitioner without delay: • A new lump or lumpiness, especially if it is in one breast • A nipple discharge • A change in the size or shape of the breast or nipple • A change in the skin over the breast such as redness or dimpling • An unusual, persistent pain, especially if it is in one breast (Cancer Australia 2018).
• Ever had **mammography**, a screening X-ray examination of the breasts? When was the last X-ray?	**Screening mammograms** are an effective way of detecting early signs of breast cancer in older women, but they are not effective in young women. Younger women's breasts are very dense and appear like white cotton wool on a mammogram. Free screening mammograms are offered to all women over 40 years of age living in Australia. As women become older, their breasts become less dense and so screening mammogram becomes an effective means of revealing cancers too small to be detected by the woman or by the most experienced examiner. In Australia, women aged 50–74 years are recommended to have a free screening mammogram every 2 years. In New Zealand, free screening (National Screening Unit, BreastScreen Aotearoa) is offered biannually to women aged 45–69 years. In Australia, women aged 75 years and older are also offered free screening mammogram every 2 years (AIHW 2018). It is important for women to continue with breast awareness practices as lumps may become palpable between mammograms.

SUBJECTIVE DATA

ASSESSMENT GUIDELINES	CLINICAL SIGNIFICANCE AND CLINICAL ALERTS
11. Axilla	
• **Tenderness, lump or swelling.** Any tenderness or lump in the underarm area? – Where? When did you first notice this? • **Rash. Any axillary rash?** Please describe it. – Seem to be a reaction to deodorant?	Breast tissue extends up into the axilla. Also, the axilla contains many lymph nodes.
Additional subjective data for the preadolescent	
• Have you noticed your breasts changing? – How long has this been happening? • Many girls notice other changes in their bodies, too, that come with growing up. What have you noticed? – What do you think about all this?	Developing breasts are the most obvious sign of puberty and the focus of attention for most girls, especially in comparison to peers. Assess each girl's perception of her own development and provide teaching and reassurance as indicated.
Additional subjective data for the pregnant woman	
• Have you noticed any enlargement or fullness in the breasts? – Is there any tenderness or tingling? – Do you have a history of inverted nipples? • Are you planning to breastfeed your baby? See Chapter 29.	Breast changes are expected and normal during pregnancy. Assess the woman's knowledge and provide reassurance. Inverted nipples may need special care in preparation for breastfeeding. Breastfeeding exclusively for the first 6 months provides the perfect food and antibodies for the baby, decreases risk of ear infections, promotes bonding and provides relaxation. It is also protective against breast cancer.
Additional subjective data for the menopausal woman	
• Have you noticed any change in the breast contour, size or firmness? (**Note:** Change may not be as apparent to obese woman or to the woman whose earlier pregnancies have already produced breast changes.)	Decreased oestrogen level causes decreased firmness. Rapid decrease in oestrogen level causes actual shrinkage.
Risk factor profile for breast cancer	
Breast cancer is the second most common cause of cancer-related death for Australian women (AIHW 2019). However, early detection and improved treatment have increased survival rates. The outcomes for women diagnosed with breast cancer have improved significantly. Nevertheless, notably lower 5-year survival rates persist among Indigenous Australian women (77% compared with 84%) (AIHW 2019). Note the risk factors listed in Table 28.2.	The best way to detect a person's risk for breast cancer is by asking the right history questions. Table 28.2 highlights risk factors for breast cancer, and from these you can fashion your questions. Be aware that most breast cancers occur in women with risk factors classified as nonmodifiable. Just because a woman does not report the cited risk factors does not mean that you or she should fail to consider breast cancer seriously.

TABLE 28.2 Breast cancer risk factors

MODIFIABLE AND NONMODIFIABLE FACTORS THAT MAY INCREASE RISK OF BREAST CANCER		
	RISK FACTOR	RELATIVE RISK
Nonmodifiable	Gender (female greater than male)	High
	Increasing age (higher risk after age 65)	High
	Genetic profile*	
	Family history (2 or more first-degree relatives, younger than at age 50 at diagnosis)	High
	Breast density (including persistent density after menopause)	High
	Abnormal breast biopsy (atypia or lobular carcinoma in situ)	High
	Geographic location (exposure to chemical or ionising radiation)	Moderate (depending on exposure)
	History of chest radiation	Moderate
	Personal history of breast cancer	Moderate
	Endogenous hormone levels high levels of oestrogen or testosterone)	Moderate
	Diethylstilboestrol exposure (secondary to mother's use)	Low
	Personal history of other cancers (endometrium, ovary or colon)	Low
(May be modifiable)	Personal history of increase bone density (signifies increased endogenous oestrogen)	Low
(Modifiable)	Exogenous hormone use (for example, oestrogen, progesterone or testosterone)	Low
	Birth control pills (recent and long-term use)	Low
	Age at menarche (before 12 years of age)	Low
	Age at menopause (after 55 years of age)	Low
	Age at first full-term pregnancy (after 30 years of age)	Low
	Occupational exposure	Low (depending on specific chemicals)
	Lifestyle risks (alcohol, diet, weight, exercise, smoking)	Low
	High socioeconomic status	Low
	Absence of breastfeeding	Low
	Absence of full-term pregnancy	Low
	Ashkenazi Eastern European Jewish descent	Low

*A number of genes have been identified that substantially influence risk of breast cancer (so-called rare, high-penetrant genes), including *BRCA1, BRCA2, TP53, PTEN, CD1* and *STK11* (Wendt & Margolin 2018)
Table adapted from Table 47-1 in Lester 2018.

Objective data

Objective assessment enables you to gather additional information about the person from a direct physical examination. Irrespective of whether the person has had a clinical breast examination performed for the first time or many times, sensitivity to body image, privacy when performing the examination and awareness of cultural norms and practices should be acknowledged and provided. Remember to ensure that the room in which you perform the examination is warm and well lit. Also, warm your hands before you commence.

Preparation

The woman is sitting up and facing you. An alternative draping method is to use a short gown, open at the back, and lift it up to the woman's shoulders during inspection. During palpation when the woman is supine, cover one breast with the gown while examining the other. Be aware that many women are embarrassed to have their breasts examined; use a sensitive but matter-of-fact approach.

After your examination, be prepared to discuss breast awareness techniques.

Equipment needed

Small pillow
Hand hygiene solution

PROCEDURES AND NORMAL FINDINGS	CLINICAL SIGNIFICANCE AND CLINICAL ALERTS
General inspection	
During collection of subjective data you will have noticed the condition of the person's skin, hair, posture, height to weight ratio, body shape, level of hygiene and grooming and general demeanor. All of these factors provide clues to the woman's overall health.	
Inspect the breasts	
Symmetry size and shape	
Note symmetry of size and shape (Figure 28.7). It is common to have a slight asymmetry in size; often the left breast is slightly larger than the right. 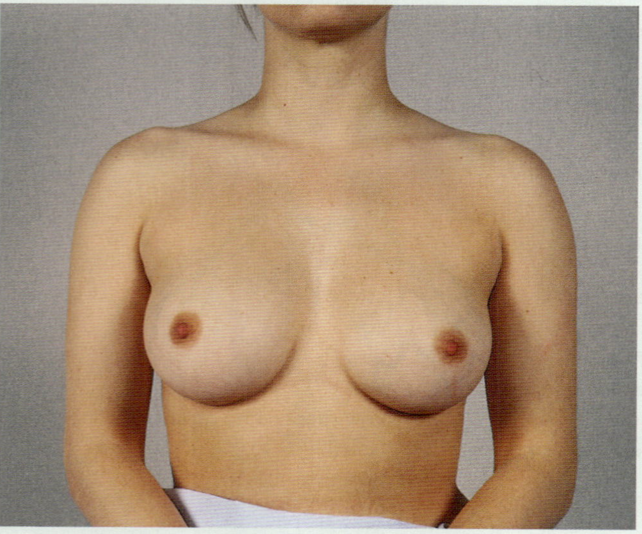 Figure 28.7	A sudden increase in the size of one breast may signify inflammation or new growth.
Skin	
The skin is normally smooth and of even colour. Note any localised areas of redness, bulging or dimpling. Also, note any skin lesions or focal vascular pattern. A fine blue vascular network is visible normally during pregnancy. Pale linear striae, or stretch marks, often follow pregnancy.	**Hyperpigmentation** (darkening of the skin). Redness and heat with inflammation. Unilateral dilated superficial veins in a nonpregnant woman. **Oedema** (see Table 28.3). Normally no oedema is present. Oedema exaggerates the hair follicles, giving a 'pig-skin' or 'orange-peel' look (also called *peau d'orange*).
Lymphatic drainage areas	
Observe the axillary and supraclavicular regions. Note any bulging, discolouration or oedema.	
Nipple	
The nipples should be symmetrically placed on the same plane on the two breasts. Nipples usually protrude, although some are flat and some are inverted. They tend to stay in their original condition. Distinguish a recently retracted nipple from one that has been inverted for many years or since puberty. Normal nipple inversion may be unilateral or bilateral and usually can be pulled out (i.e. it is not fixed).	Deviation in pointing (see Table 28.3). Recent nipple retraction signifies acquired disease (see Table 28.3).

PROCEDURES AND NORMAL FINDINGS	CLINICAL SIGNIFICANCE AND CLINICAL ALERTS
Note any dry scaling, any fissure or ulceration and bleeding or other discharge.	Explore any discharge, especially in the presence of a breast mass.
A **supernumerary nipple** is a normal and common variation (see Figure 28.6). An extra nipple along the embryonic 'milk line' on the thorax or abdomen is a congenital finding. Usually, it is 5 to 6 cm below the breast near the midline and has no associated glandular tissue. It looks like a mole, although a close look reveals a tiny nipple and areola. It is not significant; merely distinguish it from a mole.	Rarely, additional glandular tissue, called a supernumerary breast, is present.

Screen for skin retraction

Direct the woman to change position while you check the breasts for skin retraction signs. First ask her to lift the arms slowly over the head. Both breasts should move up symmetrically (Figure 28.8).

Retraction signs are due to fibrosis in the breast tissue, usually caused by growing neoplasms. The fibrosis shortens with time, causing contrasting signs with the normally loose breast tissue. Note a lag in movement of one breast.

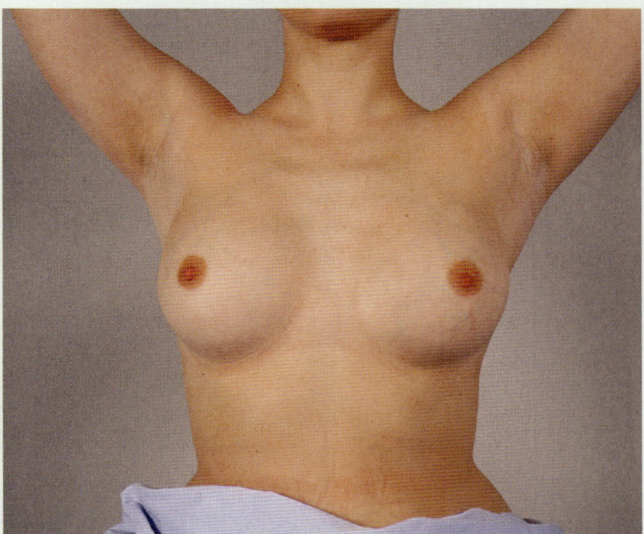

Figure 28.8
Retraction manoeuvre.

Next ask her to push her hands onto her hips (Figure 28.9) and to push her two palms together (Figure 28.10). These manoeuvres contract the pectoralis major muscle. A slight lifting of both breasts will occur.

Note a **dimpling** or a pucker, which indicates skin retraction (see Table 28.3).

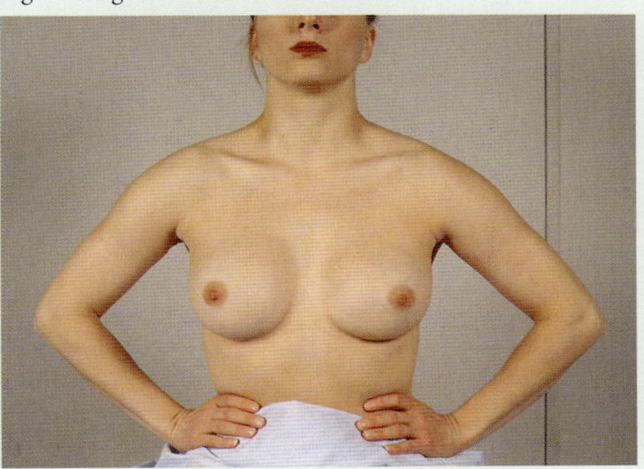

Figure 28.9

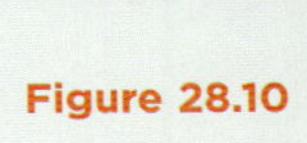

Figure 28.10

OBJECTIVE DATA

PROCEDURES AND NORMAL FINDINGS	CLINICAL SIGNIFICANCE AND CLINICAL ALERTS
Ask the woman with large pendulous breasts to lean forward while you support her forearms. Note the symmetrical free-forward movement of both breasts (Figure 28.11). 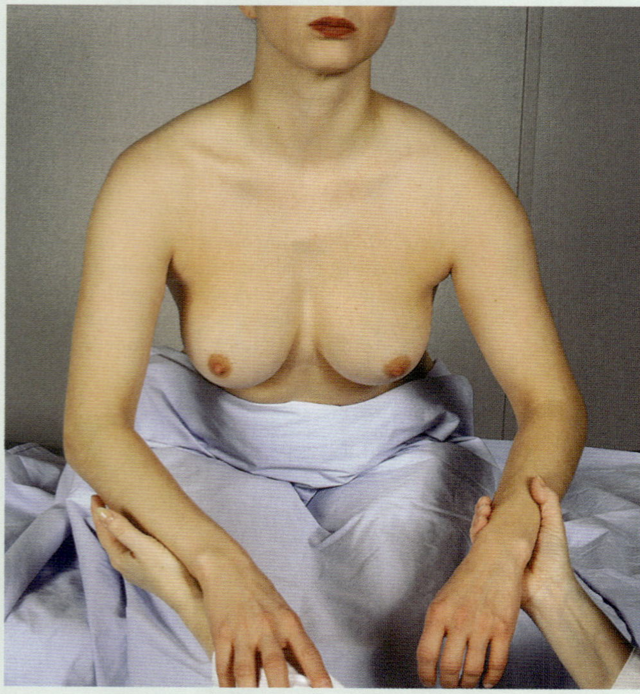 Figure 28.11	Note fixation to chest wall or skin retraction (see Table 28.3).
Palpate the breasts	
Help the woman to a supine position. Tuck a small pad under the side to be palpated and raise her arm over her head. These manoeuvres will flatten the breast tissue and displace it medially. Any significant lumps will then feel more distinct (Figure 28.12). 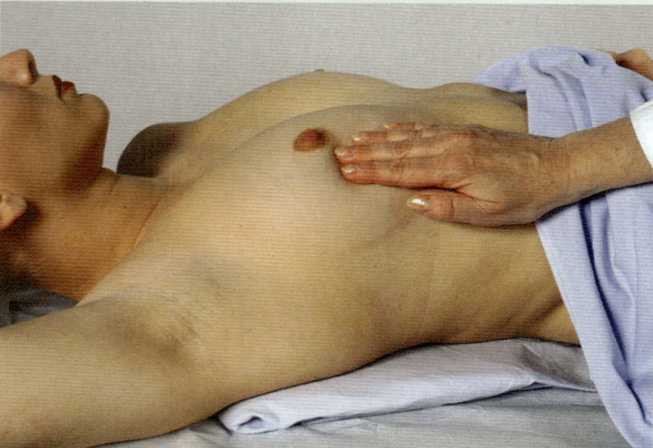 Figure 28.12	

PROCEDURES AND NORMAL FINDINGS	CLINICAL SIGNIFICANCE AND CLINICAL ALERTS
Use the pads of your first three fingers and make a gentle rotary motion on the breast. Vary your pressure so you are palpating light, medium and deep tissue in each location.	
Start high in the axilla and palpate down just lateral to the breast. Proceed in overlapping vertical lines ending at the sternal edge. In every pattern, take care to palpate every square inch of the breast and to examine the tail of Spence high into the axilla. Be consistent and thorough in your approach to each woman.	
In nulliparous women, normal breast tissue feels firm, smooth and elastic. After pregnancy, the tissue feels softer and looser. Premenstrual engorgement is normal from increasing progesterone. This consists of a slight enlargement, a tenderness to palpation and a generalised nodularity; the lobes feel prominent and their margins more distinct.	Heat, redness and swelling in non-lactating and non-postpartum breasts may indicate inflammation.
Also, normally you may feel a firm transverse ridge of compressed tissue in the lower quadrants. This is the inframammary ridge, and it is especially noticeable in large breasts. Do not confuse it with an abnormal lump.	
After palpating over the four breast quadrants, palpate the nipple (Figure 28.13). Note any induration or subareolar mass. With your thumb and forefinger, gently depress the nipple tissue into the well behind the areola. The tissue should move inwards easily. If the woman reports spontaneous nipple discharge, press the areola inwards with your index finger—repeat from a few different directions. If any discharge appears, note its colour and consistency. **Figure 28.13**	Except in pregnancy and lactation, discharge is abnormal (see Table 28.4). Note the number of discharge droplets and the quadrant(s) producing them. Blot the discharge on a white gauze pad to ascertain its colour. Document and report any discharge to a medical practitioner.
For the woman with large pendulous breasts, you may palpate by using a bimanual technique (Figure 28.14). The woman is in a sitting position, leaning forwards. Support the inferior part of the breast with one hand. Use your other hand to palpate the breast tissue against your supporting hand.	

PROCEDURES AND NORMAL FINDINGS	CLINICAL SIGNIFICANCE AND CLINICAL ALERTS
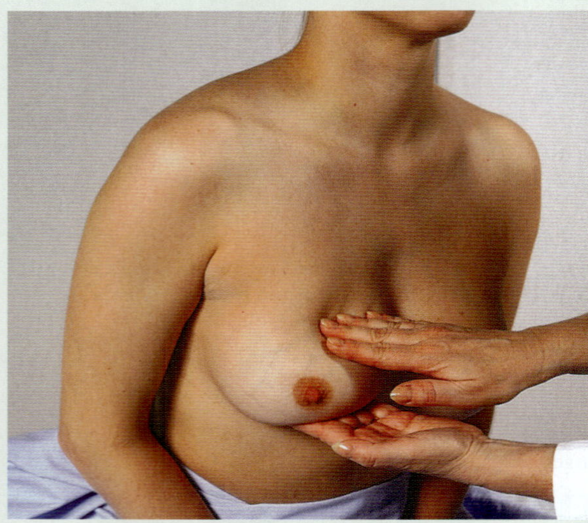 Figure 28.14	
If the woman mentions a breast lump that she has discovered herself, examine the unaffected breast first to learn a baseline of normal consistency for this woman. If you do feel a lump or mass, note these characteristics (Figure 28.15): 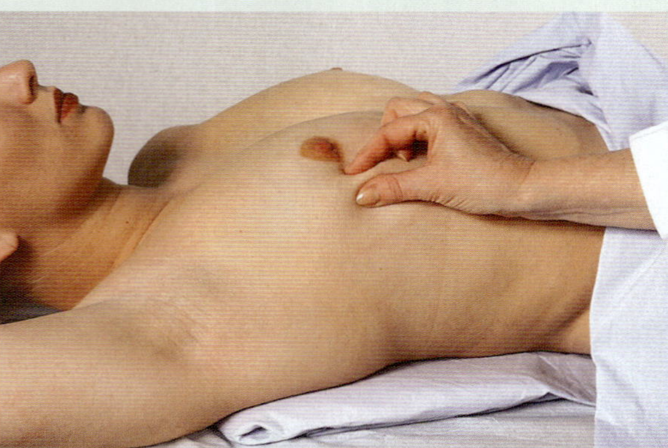 Figure 28.15	
If you detect a lump or change in breast tissue, record as follows: 1. **Location**—using the breast as a clock face, describe the distance in centimetres from the nipple (e.g. '7:00, 2 cm from the nipple'). Or diagram the breast in the woman's record and mark in the location of the lump. 2. **Size**—judge in centimetres in three dimensions: width × length × thickness. 3. **Shape**—state whether the lump is oval, round, lobulated or indistinct. 4. **Consistency**—state whether the lump is soft, firm or hard. 5. **Movable**—is the lump freely movable, or is it fixed when you try to slide it over the chest wall? 6. **Distinctness**—is the lump solitary or multiple? 7. **Nipple**—is it displaced or retracted? 8. **Note the skin over the lump**—is it erythematous, dimpled or retracted? 9. **Tenderness**—is the lump tender to palpation? 10. **Lymphadenopathy**—are any regional lymph nodes palpable?	See Tables 28.5 and 28.6 for description of common breast lumps with these characteristics. ***Clinical alert:*** Any change in breast tissue detected by you or the woman should be reported to medical practitioner for further assessment

OBJECTIVE DATA

PROCEDURES AND NORMAL FINDINGS	CLINICAL SIGNIFICANCE AND CLINICAL ALERTS

The male breast

Your examination of the male breast can be much more abbreviated, but do not omit it. Combine a breast check technique with that of the anterior thorax. Inspect the chest wall, noting the skin surface and any lumps or swelling. Palpate the nipple area for any lump or tissue enlargement (Figure 28.16). It should feel even, with no nodules. Palpate the axillary lymph nodes.

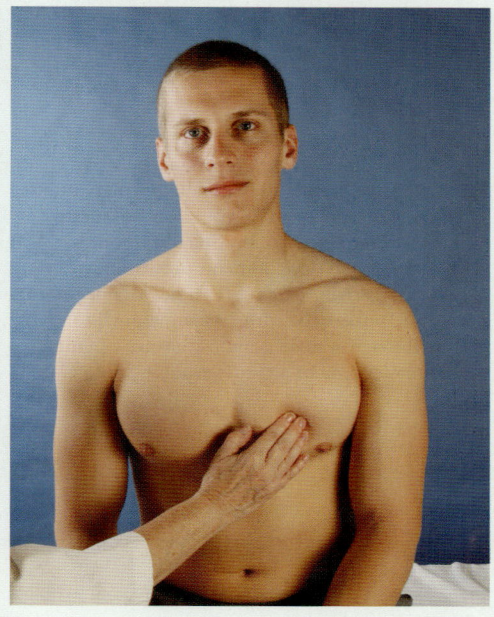

Figure 28.16

The normal male breast has a flat disc of undeveloped breast tissue beneath the nipple. The adolescent is acutely aware of his body image. Reassure him that this change is normal, common and temporary. In contrast, an obese male has an increase of fatty, not glandular, tissue.

Gynaecomastia is an enlargement of this breast tissue, making it clinically distinguishable from the other tissues in the chest wall (Figure 28.17). It feels like a smooth, firm, movable disc. This occurs normally during puberty. It usually affects only one breast and is temporary.
Gynaecomastia also occurs with use of anabolic steroids, some medications and some disease states. See Table 28.8.

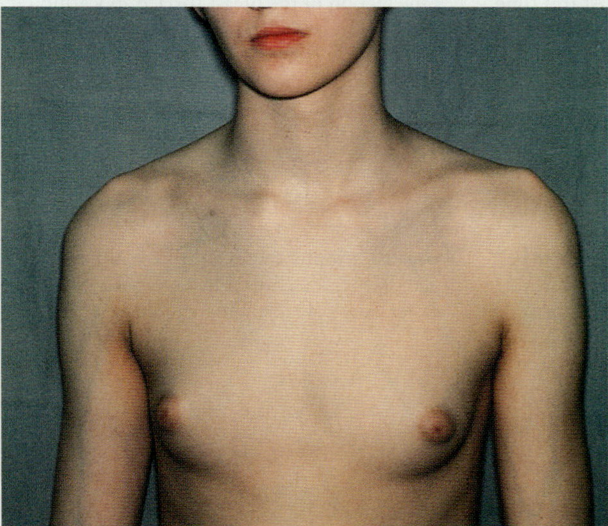

Figure 28.17
Adolescent gynaecomastia.

PROCEDURES AND NORMAL FINDINGS	CLINICAL SIGNIFICANCE AND CLINICAL ALERTS
Additional objective data for infants and children	
In the neonate, the breasts may be enlarged and visible due to maternal oestrogen crossing the placenta. They may secrete a clear or white fluid, called 'witch's milk'. These signs are not significant and are resolved within a few days to a few weeks.	
Note the position of the nipples on the prepubertal child. They should be symmetrical, just lateral to the midclavicular line, between the fourth and fifth ribs. The nipple is flat and the areola is darker pigmented.	**Premature thelarche** is early breast development with no other hormone-dependent signs (pubic hair, menses).
Additional objective data for the adolescent	
Adolescent breast development usually begins on an average between 8 and 10 years of age. Expect some asymmetry during growth. (Distinguish breast development from extra adipose tissue present in obese children.) Record the stage of development using Tanner's staging described in Table 28.1. Use the chart to teach the adolescent normal developmental stages and to assure her of her own normal progress. You should consider BMI when evaluating breast budding before 8 years of age as it may be difficult to distinguish breast budding from adipose tissue. With maturing adolescents, palpate the breasts as you would with the adult. The breasts normally feel firm and uniform. Note any mass. Discuss breast awareness techniques that the young woman can routinely practise. If required, demonstrate how to use finger pads and flats of fingers to feel near the surface and deeper in the breast tissue and under the arm.	Note **precocious development**, occurring before age 8 years. It is usually normal but also occurs with thyroid dysfunction, stilboestrol ingestion or ovarian or adrenal tumour. Note delayed development, occurring with hormonal failure or anorexia nervosa beginning before puberty or with severe malnutrition. At this age, a mass is almost always a benign fibroadenoma or a cyst (see Table 28.4).
Additional objective data for the pregnant woman	
A delicate blue vascular pattern is visible over the breasts. The breasts increase in size, as do the nipples. Jagged linear stretch marks, or striae, may develop if the breasts have a large increase. The nipples also become darker and more erectile. The areolae widen, grow darker and contain the small, scattered, elevated Montgomery glands. On palpation, the breasts feel more nodular, and thick yellow colostrum can be expressed after the first trimester.	
Additional objective data for the lactating woman	
Colostrum changes to milk production around the third postpartum day. At this time, the breasts may become engorged, appearing enlarged, reddened and shiny and feeling warm and hard. Frequent feeding helps drain the ducts and sinuses and stimulate milk production.	One section of the breast surface appearing red and tender indicates a blocked duct (see Table 28.7). A lactating woman who is experiencing nipple soreness or pain should be referred to a midwife or maternal and child health nurse for advice.
Additional objective data for the woman over 65 years	
On inspection, the breasts may look pendulous, flattened and sagging. Nipples may be retracted but can be pulled outwards. On palpation, the breasts feel more granular, and the terminal ducts around the nipple feel more prominent and stringy. Thickening of the inframammary ridge at the lower breast is normal, and it feels more prominent with age. Reinforce the value of breast awareness. Women over 50 years old have an increased risk of breast cancer.	Because atrophy causes shrinkage of normal glandular tissue, cancer detection is somewhat easier. Any palpable lump should be referred.

OBJECTIVE DATA

Further assessment for advanced practice

In addition to previous objective assessment, nurses working in specialist women's health and breast care settings need to develop these advanced skills.

Preparation and communication continue to be important parts of practice to support the woman undergoing this assessment. No additional equipment is required.

PROCEDURES AND NORMAL FINDINGS	CLINICAL SIGNIFICANCE AND CLINICAL ALERTS
Inspect and palpate axillary lymph nodes	
Examine the axillae while the woman is sitting. Inspect the skin, noting any rash or infection. Lift the woman's arm and support it yourself, so that her muscles are loose and relaxed. Use your right hand to palpate the left axilla (Figure 28.18). Reach your fingers high into the axilla. Move them firmly down in four directions: (1) down the chest wall in a line from the middle of the axilla, (2) along the anterior border of the axilla, (3) along the posterior border and (4) along the inner aspect of the upper arm. Move the woman's arm through range-of-motion to increase the surface area you can reach. 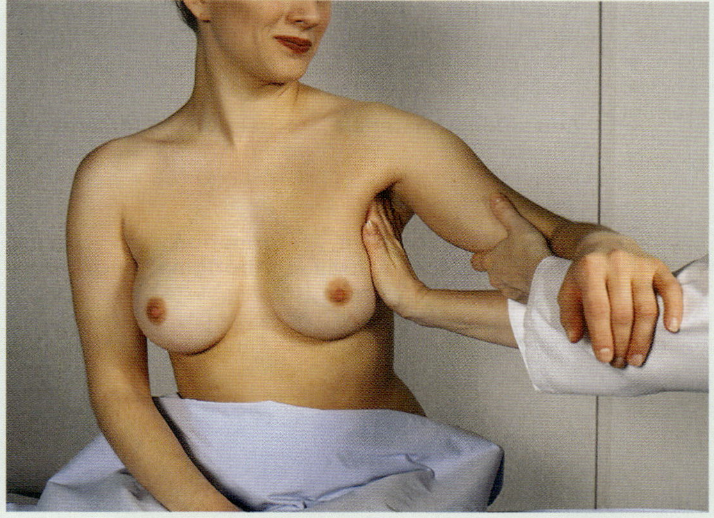 Figure 28.18	
Usually nodes are not palpable, although you may feel a small, soft, nontender node in the central group. Expect some tenderness when palpating high in the axilla. Note any enlarged and tender lymph nodes.	Nodes may enlarge with any local infection of the breast, arm or hand and with breast cancer metastases.

OBJECTIVE DATA

Summary Checklist

BREAST ASSESSMENT

Subjective data

1. Presenting concern
2. Pain
3. Lump
4. Discharge
5. Rash
6. Swelling
7. Trauma to breasts
8. History of breast disease
9. Surgery
10. Heath and lifestyle management
11. Axilla

Objective data

1. General inspection
2. Inspect the breasts
3. Palpate the breasts
4. The male breast

PROMOTING A HEALTHY LIFESTYLE

EDUCATION ON BREAST AWARENESS

Finish your own assessment first, and then take the opportunity to discuss breast awareness strategies. Remember to reinforce that there are no right or wrong breast awareness techniques. If the woman is unsure what she should do, suggest she adopt behaviours that are comfortable to do from time to time. For example, view her breasts in the mirror when dressing or undressing. Feel her breasts while in the shower or bath, lying down or while dressing. Stress that breast awareness will familiarise the woman with her own breasts and their normal variation. Emphasise the absence of lumps (not the presence of them). However, do encourage her to report any unusual finding promptly to her general practitioner.

Focus on the positive aspects of breast awareness; because the woman knows her own breast shape, size and feel, small changes can be detected early.

Knowledge of risk factors and breast awareness techniques should increase confidence in detecting changes and seeking further assessment from a health professional.

Educational materials are helpful reinforcements. Cancer Australia (2018) provides a simple video on breast changes: https://breast-cancer.canceraustralia.gov.au/awareness

Culturally sensitive information on breast awareness for Australian Aboriginal and Torres Strait Islander women is available via the Cancer Australia website: https://canceraustralia.gov.au/affected-cancer/atsi/breast-cancer-awareness

ASSESSING BREAST CANCER RISK

Breast cancer screening tool

During a clinical breast examination, the opportunity often arises to review the individual's breast awareness knowledge and plan for screening mammogram. It is also an opportunity to assess the individual's breast cancer risk, including family history.

The use of breast cancer risk assessment tools in the clinical setting has the potential to improve health substantially by reducing breast cancer incidence through cancer prevention and by more effective early detection programs for high-risk individuals. For clinicians, breast cancer risk assessment tools such as the Gail Model (National Cancer Institute (NCI) Breast Cancer Risk Assessment Tool) has been validated among Australian women to effectively stratify a screened population aged 50–69 years according to the risk of future invasive breast cancer (Nickson et al 2018).

Cancer Australia provides a simple-to-use breast and ovarian cancer screening tool. The user-friendly, interactive calculator is intended for use by women who have not had breast or ovarian cancer. The screening tool helps women to gain a good understanding of their level of risk for breast cancer compared to another woman of a similar age group. The tool is available at: http://canceraustralia.gov.au/affected-cancer/cancer-types/breast-cancer/your-risk/calculate

iPrevent, a new web-based tool developed by the Peter MacCallum Cancer Centre, helps Australian women to understand their personal breast cancer risk and act upon it. The tool is available at: https://www.petermac.org/iprevent

Documentation and critical thinking

FOCUSED ASSESSMENT: CLINICAL CASE STUDY

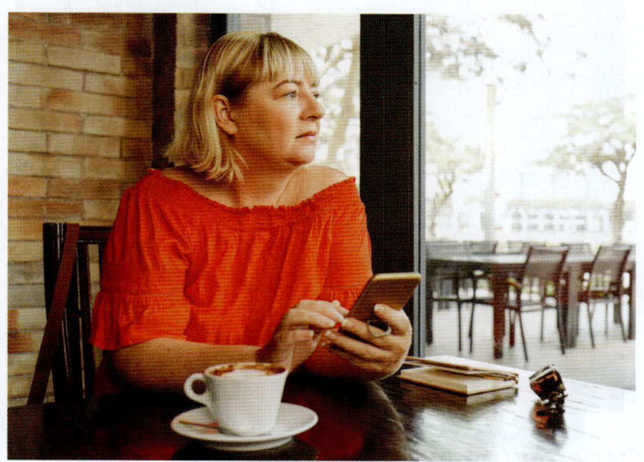

Context

The registered nurse (RN) works in an acute metropolitan hospital accident and emergency department. The patient has been admitted to the accident and emergency department following a minor traffic accident having sustained a mild concussion. Neurological assessment is being conducted at half-hourly intervals and the discharge plan is to continue assessment for 4 hours and after medical reassessment she will be discharged home with GP review in 24 hours. During her admission, the patient informs the RN that she had noticed a lump in her right breast 2 weeks ago.

Subjective data

Ms Jenny Gardner is a 48-year-old female secondary school teacher, married, with two children. She described the lump as a firm, non-movable area 'the size of a pea', in upper outer quadrant of breast, tender on touch only. No skin changes, no nipple discharge. Jenny is not currently taking any medications. She did not notice lump previously. There is no history of breast disease in self or family. Jenny states that she has been feeling very anxious for the past 2 days and has not been able to sleep well or concentrate at work. 'I just know it's cancer.' Jenny reports that her lack of sleep may have contributed to the road traffic accident.

Objective data

Voice trembling and visibly anxious during history. Sitting posture stiff and rigid. B/P 148/78. T 37°C. HR 92/min. RR 16/min.

Breasts symmetrical, nipples everted. No skin lesions, no dimpling, no retraction, no fixation.

On palpation: Left breast firm, no mass, no tenderness, no discharge. Right breast firm, with 2 cm × 2 cm × 1 cm mass at 10 o'clock position, 5 cm from the nipple. Lump is firm, oval, with smooth discrete borders, non-movable, tender to palpation. No other mass. No discharge. No lymphadenopathy.

Collaborative problem

Breast mass requiring further assessment (referral to medical practitioner)

Problem statement/nursing diagnosis

Anxiety related to unknown diagnosis

Abnormal findings

TABLE 28.3 Signs of retraction and inflammation in the breast

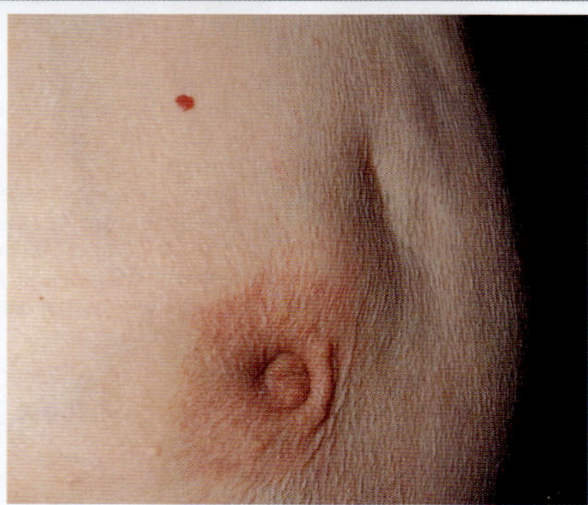 **Dimpling** The shallow dimple (also called a skin tether) shown here is a sign of skin retraction. Cancer causes fibrosis, which contracts the suspensory ligaments. The dimple may be apparent at rest, with compression or with lifting of the arms. Also note the distortion of the areola here as the fibrosis pulls the nipple towards it.	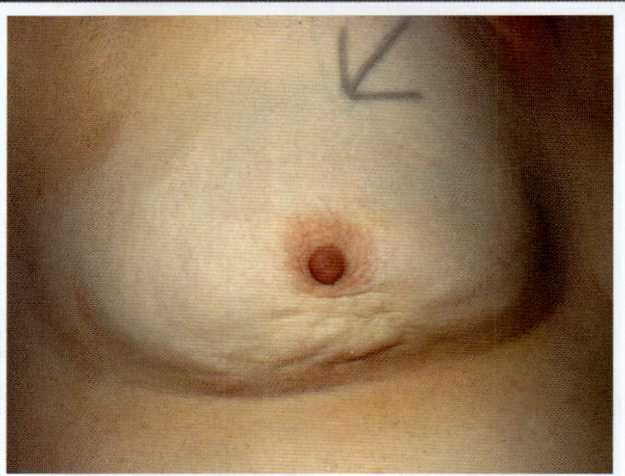 **Oedema (peau d'orange)** Lymphatic obstruction produces oedema. This thickens the skin and exaggerates the hair follicles, giving a pig-skin or orange-peel look. This condition suggests cancer. Oedema usually begins in the skin around and beneath the areola, the most dependent area of the breast. Also note nipple infiltration here.
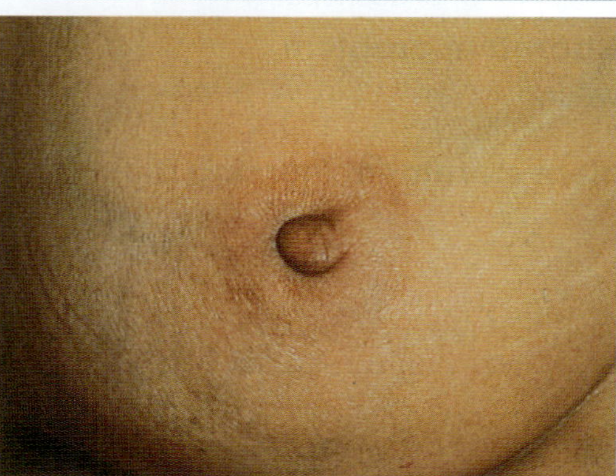 **Deviation in nipple pointing** An underlying cancer causes fibrosis in the mammary ducts, which pulls the nipple angle towards it. Here, note the swelling behind the right nipple and that the nipple tilts laterally.	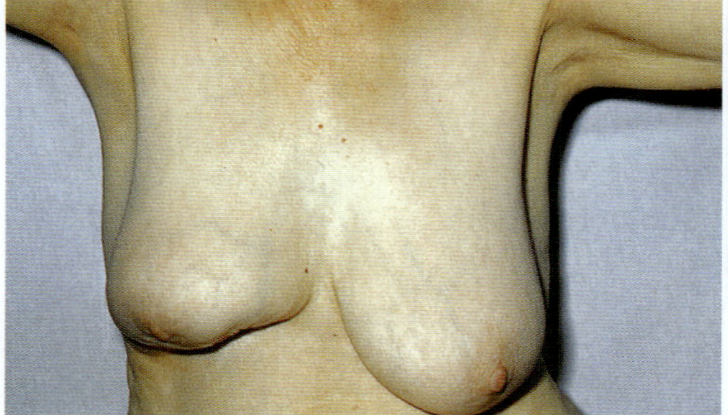 **Fixation** Asymmetry, distortion or decreased mobility with the elevated arm manoeuvre. As cancer becomes invasive, the fibrosis fixes the breast to the underlying pectoral muscles. Here, note the right breast is held against the chest wall.

TABLE 28.4 Breast lump

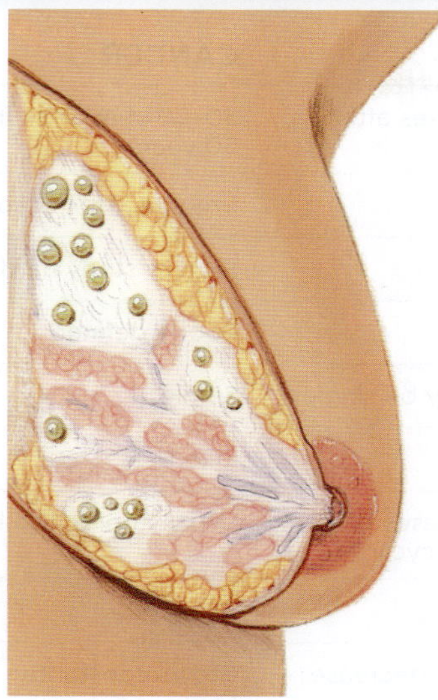

Benign breast disease (formerly fibrocystic breast disease)

Multiple tender masses. 'Fibrocystic disease' is a meaningless term because it covers too many entities. Actually, six diagnostic categories exist, based on symptoms and physical findings:

- Swelling and tenderness (cyclic discomfort)
- Mastalgia (severe pain, both cyclic and noncyclic)
- Nodularity (significant lumpiness, both cyclic and noncyclic)
- Dominant lumps (including cysts and fibroadenomas)
- Nipple discharge (including intraductal papilloma and duct ectasia)
- Infections and inflammations (including subareolar abscess, lactational mastitis, breast abscess and Mondor's disease).

About 50% of all women have some form of benign breast disease. Nodularity occurs bilaterally; regular, firm nodules that are mobile, well demarcated and feel rubbery, like small water balloons. Pain may be dull, heavy and cyclic or just before menses as nodules enlarge. Some women have nodularity but no pain and vice versa. Cysts are discrete, fluid-filled sacs. Dominant lumps and nipple discharge must be investigated carefully and may need biopsy to rule out cancer. Nodularity itself is not premalignant but may produce difficulty in detecting other cancerous lumps.

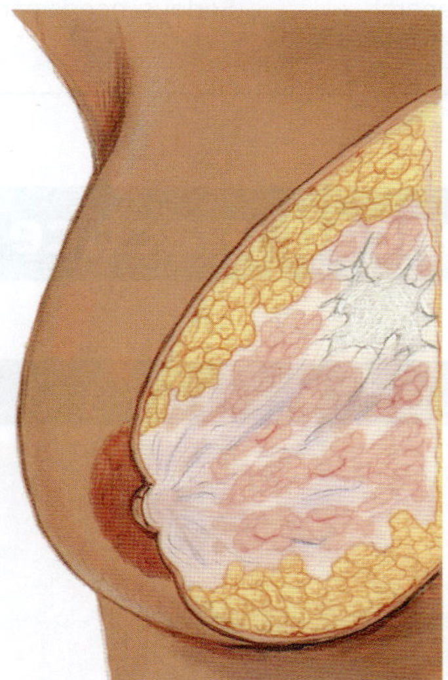

Cancer

Solitary unilateral nontender mass. Single focus in one area, although it may be interspersed with other nodules. Solid, hard, dense and fixed to underlying tissues or skin as cancer becomes invasive. Borders are irregular and poorly delineated. Grows constantly. Often painless, although the person may have pain. Most common in upper outer quadrant. Usually found in women 30 to 80 years of age; increased risk in ages 40 to 44 years and in women older than 50 years. As cancer advances, signs include firm or hard irregular axillary nodes; skin dimpling; nipple retraction, elevation and discharge.

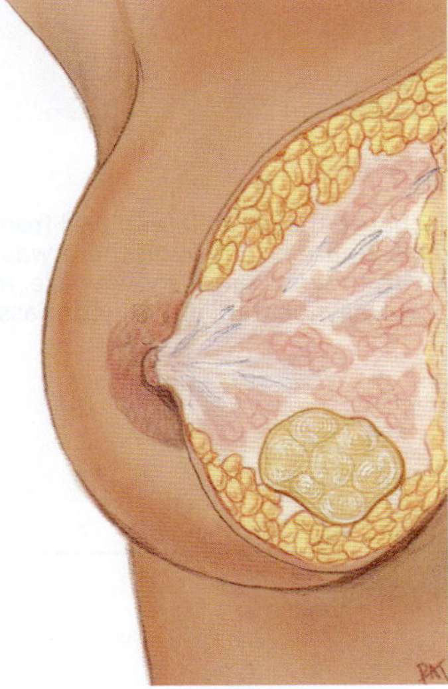

Fibroadenoma

Solitary nontender mass. A category of benign breast disease that deserves mention because of its frequency and characteristic appearance. Solid, firm, rubbery and elastic. Round, oval or lobulated; 1 to 5 cm. Freely movable, slippery; fingers slide it easily through tissue. Most common between 15 and 30 years of age but can occur up to 55 years. Grows quickly and constantly. Benign, although it must be diagnosed by biopsy.

TABLE 28.5 Differentiating breast lumps

	FIBROADENOMA	BENIGN BREAST DISEASE	CANCER
Likely age	15–30 years, can occur up to 55 years	30–55 years, decreases after menopause	30–80 years, risk increases after 50 years
Shape	Round, lobular	Round, lobular	Irregular, star-shaped
Consistency	Usually firm, rubbery	Firm to soft, rubbery	Firm to stony hard
Demarcation	Well demarcated, clear margins	Well demarcated	Poorly defined
Number	Usually single	Usually multiple, may be single	Single
Mobility	Very mobile, slippery	Mobile	Fixed
Tenderness	Usually none	Tender, usually increases before menses, may be noncyclic	Usually none, can be tender
Skin retraction	None	None	Usually
Pattern of growth	Grows quickly and constantly	Size may increase or decrease rapidly	Grows constantly
Risk to health	None; they are benign—must diagnose by biopsy	Benign, although general lumpiness may mask other cancerous lump	Serious, needs early treatment

Abnormal findings for advanced practice

TABLE 28.6 Abnormal nipple discharge

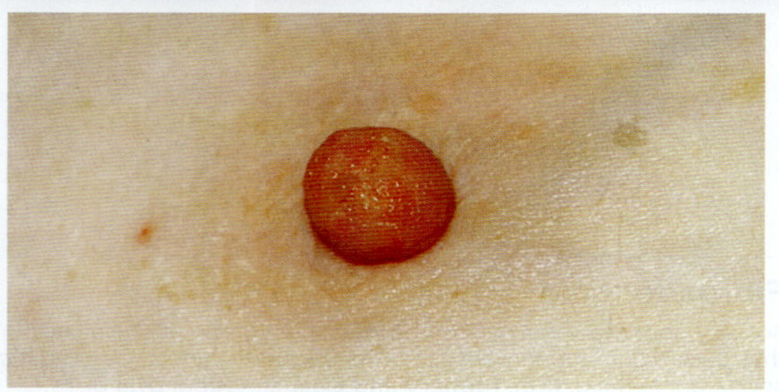

Mammary duct ectasia

Paste-like matter in subareolar ducts produces sticky, purulent discharge that may be white, grey, brown, green or bloody. A light green, single duct discharge is shown here. Caused by stagnation of cellular debris and secretions in the ducts, leading to obstruction, inflammation and infection. Occurs in women who have lactated; usually occurs in perimenopause. Itching, burning or drawing pain occurs around nipple. May have subareolar redness and swelling. Ducts are palpable as rubbery, twisted tubules under areola. May have palpable mass, soft or firm, poorly delineated. Not malignant, but needs biopsy.

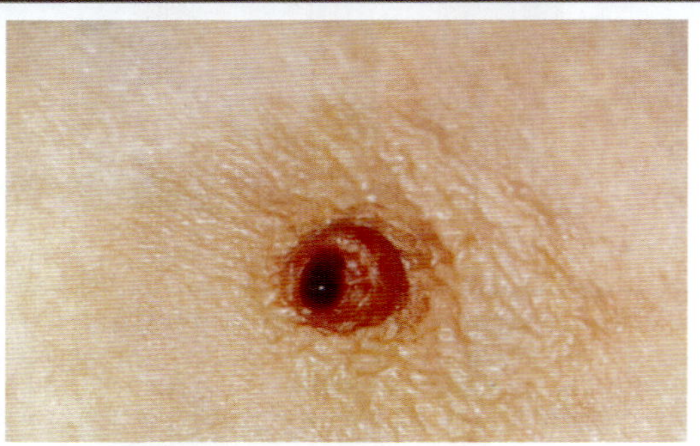

Carcinoma

Bloody nipple discharge that is unilateral and from a single duct requires further investigation. Although there was no palpable lump associated with the discharge shown here, mammography revealed a 1-cm, centrally located, ill-defined mass.

TABLE 28.6 Abnormal nipple discharge—cont'd

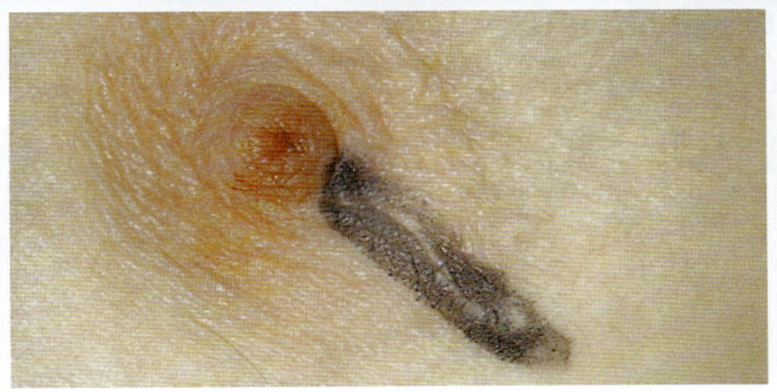

Intraductal papilloma

Serous or serosanguineous discharge, which is spontaneous, unilateral or from a single duct. Lesion consists of tiny tumours, 2–3 mm. Often there is a palpable nodule in the underlying duct (highlighted here). Papillomas affect women 40–60 years of age; most are benign. Refer any bloody discharge for careful evaluation, including biopsy, to rule out cancer.

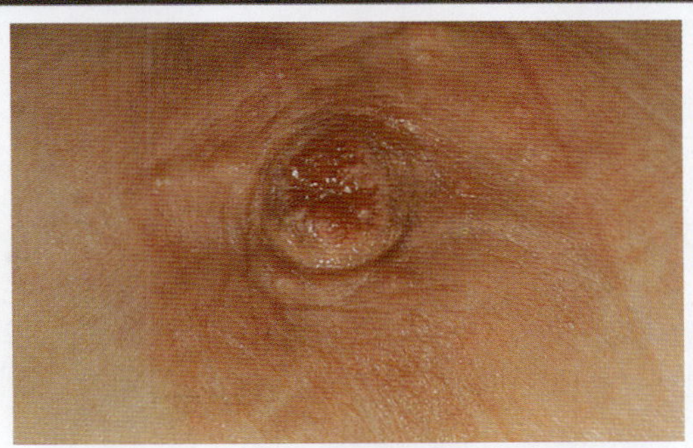

Paget's disease (intraductal carcinoma)

Early lesion has unilateral, clear, yellow discharge and dry, scaling crusts, friable at nipple apex. Spreads outwards to areola with erythematous halo on areola and crusted, eczematous, retracted nipple. Later lesion shows nipple reddened, excoriated, ulcerated, with bloody discharge when surface is eroded, and an erythematous plaque surrounding the nipple. Symptoms include tingling, burning, itching.

Except for the redness and occasional cracking from initial breastfeeding, any dermatitis of the nipple area must be carefully explored and referred immediately.

TABLE 28.7 Disorders occurring during lactation

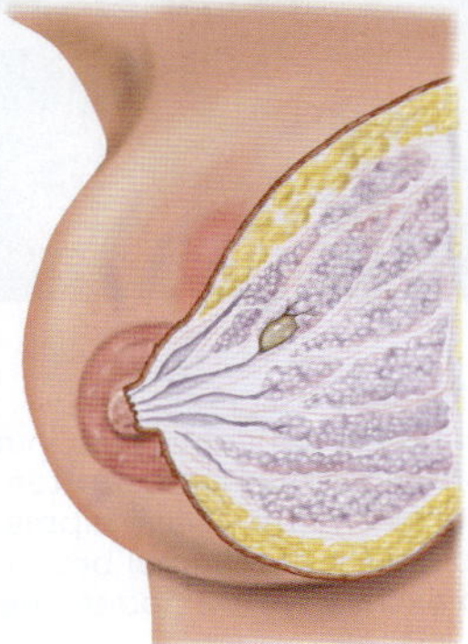

Plugged duct

A fairly common and not serious condition. One milk duct is clogged. One section of the breast is tender; may be reddened. No infection. It is important to keep breast as empty as possible and milk flowing. The woman should nurse her baby frequently, on affected side first to ensure complete emptying, and manually express any remaining milk. A plugged duct usually resolves in less than 1 day.

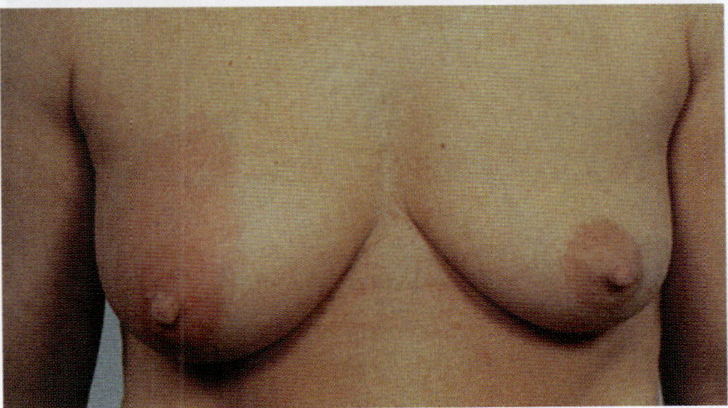

Mastitis

An inflammatory mass before abscess formation. Usually occurs in single quadrant. Area is red, swollen, tender, very hot and hard, here forming outwards from areola upper edge, in right breast. Also the woman has a headache, malaise, fever, chills and sweating, increased pulse, flu-like symptoms. May occur during first 4 months of lactation from infection or from stasis from plugged duct. Treat with rest, local heat to area, antibiotics and frequent nursing to keep breast as empty as possible. Must not wean now or the breast will become engorged and the pain will increase. Mother's antibiotic not harmful to infant. Usually resolves in 2–3 days.

(Continued)

TABLE 28.7 Disorders occurring during lactation—cont'd

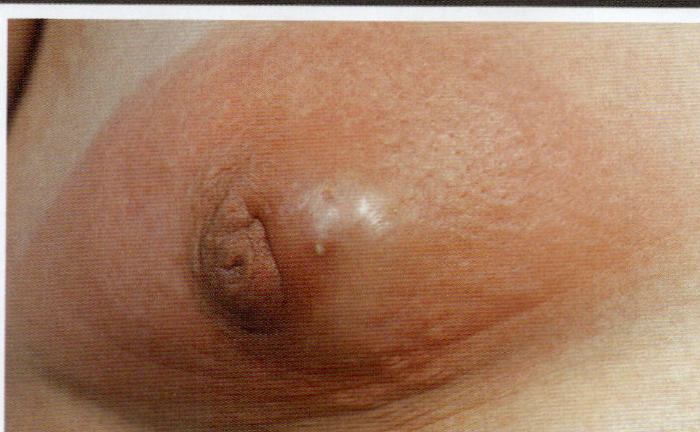

Breast abscess

A rare complication of generalised infection (e.g. mastitis) if untreated. A pocket of pus accumulates in one local area. Here extensive nipple oedema, and abscess is 'pointing' at 3:00 on areolar margin. Must temporarily discontinue nursing on affected breast; manually express milk and discard. Continue to nurse on unaffected side. Treat with antibiotics, surgical incision and drainage.

TABLE 28.8 Abnormalities in the male breast

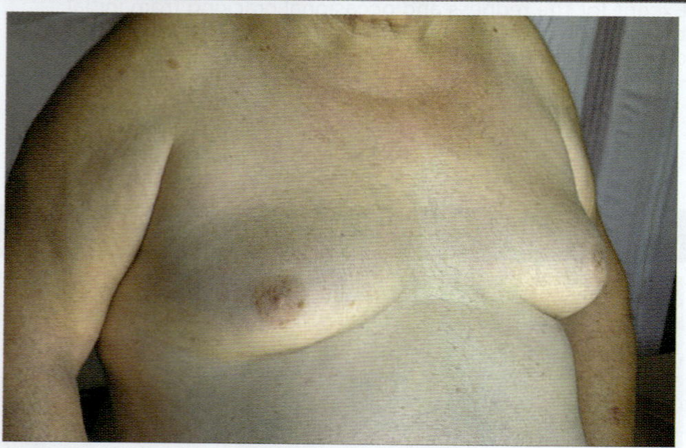

Gynaecomastia

Noninflammatory enlargement of male breast tissue. This is physiological at puberty, unilateral, usually mild and transient. Gynaecomastia occurs commonly in males over 65 years because of changing hormone levels. It is bilateral and may be tender.

It also occurs bilaterally from hormone stimulation (e.g. on oestrogen for cancer of prostate); Cushing's syndrome; cirrhosis of liver as unable to metabolise oestrogen completely; leukaemia occasionally; and sometimes with medication—digitalis, isoniazid, spironolactone and phenothiazines; testicular tumour, lung cancer; adrenal disease; and thyrotoxicosis.

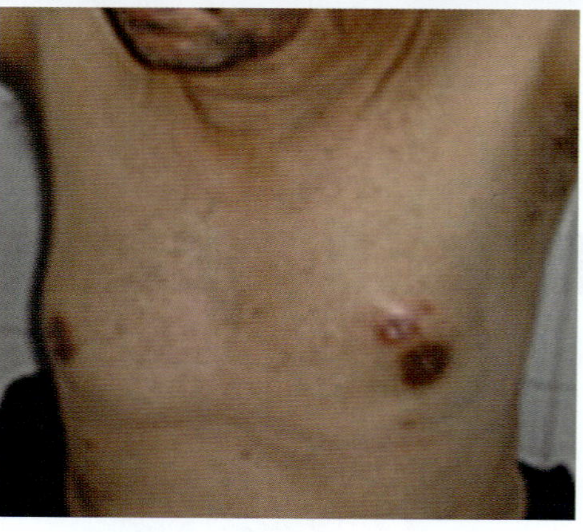

Carcinoma

Fewer than 1% of all breast cancer occurs in men. The lesion is a hard, irregular, nontender mass, most often directly under the areola, fixed to the area and may have nipple retraction. Mass is noticeable early because of minimal breast tissue. There is also early spread to axillary lymph nodes due to minimal breast tissue.

BIBLIOGRAPHY

Australian Institute of Health and Welfare (AIHW). Breast cancer in Australia: An overview. Cancer series no. 71. Cat no. CAN 67. Canberra: AIHW; 2012.

Australian Institute of Health and Welfare (AIHW). BreastScreen Australia monitoring report 2018. Cancer series no. 112. Cat no. CAN 116. Canberra: AIHW; 2018. Available at: https://www.aihw.gov.au/reports/cancer/breastscreen-australia-monitoring-report-2018/contents/table-of-contents.

Australian Institute of Health and Welfare (AIHW). Cancer in Australia 2019. Cancer series no. 119. Cat. No. CAN 123. Canberra: AIHW; 2019. Available at: https://www.aihw.gov.au/reports/cancer/cancer-in-australia-2019/contents/summary.

Biro FM, Pajak A, Wolff MS, et al. Age of menarche in a longitudinal US cohort. J Pediatr Adolesc Gynecol 2018;31(4):339–45.

Breast Cancer Foundation NZ. 2020. Breast awareness. Breast Cancer in NZ. Available at: https://www.breastcancerfoundation.org.nz/breast-awareness/breast-cancer-facts/breast-cancer-in-nz

Cancer Australia. Breast cancer awareness. 2018. Available at: https://breast-cancer.canceraustralia.gov.au/awareness

Clinical Oncology Society of Australia. COSA position statement on exercise in cancer care. Version 1. 2018. Clinical Oncology Society of Australia. Available at: https://www.cosa.org.au/publications/position-statements/

Cunningham J, Rumbold AR, Zhang X, et al. Incidence, aetiology, and outcomes of cancer in Indigenous peoples in Australia. Lancet Oncol 2008;9:585–95.

Harvie M, Howell A, Evans DG. Can diet and lifestyle prevent breast cancer: what is the evidence? Am Soc Clin Oncol Educ Book 2015;35:e66–73.

Kelly Y, Zilanawala A, Sacker A, et al. Early puberty in 11-year-old girls: Millennium Cohort Study findings. Arch Dis Child 2017;102(3):232–7.

Lawn RB, Lawlor DA, Fraser A. Associations between maternal prepregnancy body mass index and gestational weight gain and daughter's age at menarche. Am J Epidemiol 2017;187(4):677–86. doi:10.1093/aje/kwx308.

Lazzeri G, Tosti C, Pammolli A, et al. Overweight and lower age at menarche: evidence from the Italian HBSC cross-sectional survey. BMC Womens Health 2018;18(1):168.

Lester J. Early-stage breast cancer. In: Henke-Yarbro C, Frogge D, Holmes-Gobel B, editors. Cancer nursing: principles and practice. Burlington MA: Jones and Bartlett Learning LLC; 2018, pp. 1279–1334.

Love S, Lindsey K. Dr. Susan Love's Breast Book. Cambridge, MS: Ingram; 2005.

Ministry of Health New Zealand. Breast cancer. 2018. Available at: https://www.health.govt.nz/your-health/conditions-and-treatments/diseases-and-illnesses/breast-cancer.

Mishra GD, Pandeya N, Dobson AJ, et al. Early menarche, nulliparity and the risk for premature and early natural menopause. Hum Reprod 2017;32(3):679–86.

National Cancer Institute [NCI]. Breast cancer risk assessment tool. 2019. Available at: https://bcrisktool.cancer.gov/.

National Screening Unit (NSU). Breast Screening. BreastScreen Aotearoa. 2019. Available at: https://www.timetoscreen.nz/breast-screening/.

Nickson C, Procopio P, Velentzis LS, et al. Prospective validation of the NCI breast cancer risk assessment tool (Gail Model) on 40,000 Australian women. Breast Cancer Res 2018;20:155. doi:10.1186/s13058-018-1084-x.

Prior D. The meaning of cancer for Australian Aboriginal women: changing the focus of cancer nursing. Eur J Oncol Nurs 2009;13:280–6.

Wendt C, Margolin S. Identifying breast cancer susceptibility genes: a review of the genetic background in familial breast cancer. Acta Oncol 2018;58(2):135–46. doi:10.1080/0284186X.2018.1529428.

Worthman CM, Dockray S, Marceau K. Puberty and the evolution of developmental science. J Res Adolesc 2019 29(1):9–31.

Chapter Twenty-Nine
Assessing the pregnant woman

Written by Carolyn Jarvis
Adapted by Nicki Hartney

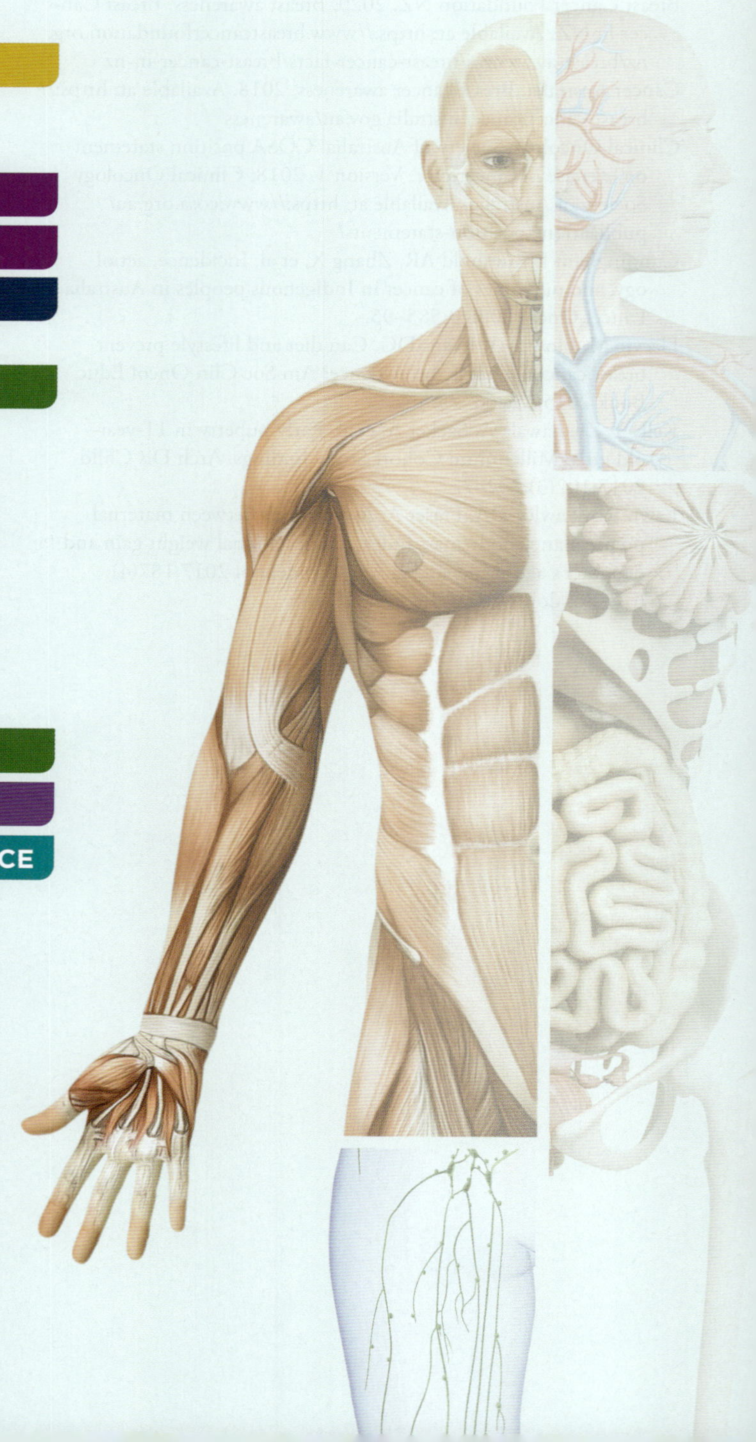

INTRODUCTION

Pregnancy and childbirth result in significant physiological changes in the woman. These changes include the growth of the fetus, placenta and uterus, as well as complex endocrine and circulatory changes. This chapter gives the student a brief overview of the changes to structure and function that occur during normal pregnancy and the approach to routine antenatal assessment. For a detailed description of labour and puerperium you are advised to consult a midwifery textbook.

Structure and function

PREGNANCY AND THE PLACENTA

The first day of the menses is day 1 of the menstrual cycle which is generally referred to as being of 28 days' duration. There is, however, acknowledgement that there are cycle lengths ranging from 15 to 45 days, with length variations primarily occurring in the proliferative phase of the menstrual cycle (Blackburn 2013). During the secretory phase of the menstrual cycle, the corpus luteum secretes a large amount of progesterone to act on the oestrogen-prepared endometrium to convert it into a secretory tissue to prepare for implantation, which occurs 7 days after ovulation. Implantation is completed at 14 days after ovulation when the next menstrual cycle would be due (Rankin 2017).

At the beginning of the menstrual cycle, 15 to 20 primary follicles are stimulated by the follicle stimulating hormone (FSH) but only 6 to 12 enlarge and eventually one follicle becomes dominant and begins to function independently of the FSH. Ovulation is triggered by the mid-cycle action of luteinising hormone (LH), occurring in response to sustained high levels of oestrogen released from the developing follicle (Coad et al 2019). LH secretion increases significantly and precedes ovulation by up to 36 hours (Blackburn 2013). Progesterone production rises immediately after the LH surge and this pre-ovulatory increase may be important in follicular rupture. Fertilisation occurs in the ampulla of the fallopian tube and viability of the sperm is thought to be about 5 days (Coad et al 2019). If the ovum is not fertilised it usually dies within 24 hours (Blackburn 2013).

Although one sperm penetrates the ovum, several hundred are required to support the passage of the spermatozoa through the corona radiata of the ovum. The acrosome reaction with release of enzymes through the acrosomal membrane must occur for successful penetration of the corona radiata and zona pellucida by the sperm. After sperm entry, the sperm–ovum interaction releases a wave of calcium along the zona pellucida resulting in fusion of the cortical granules with the plasma membrane of the ovum, resulting in the release of hydrolytic enzymes, proteases and polysaccharides into the pervillous space. This modifies the zona pellucida glycoproteins thereby preventing entry of other sperm. After entering the cytoplasm of the oocyte, the sperm undergoes rapid morphological changes including sex determination, which is dependent on the X or Y chromosome entering the ovum. The nuclei of the male and female pronuclei fuse and chromatin strands intermingle with inclusion of the diploid number (46) of chromosomes, resulting in the formation of the **zygote** (Blackburn 2013).

The zygote remains in the ampulla for the first 24 hours and is then propelled by ciliary action down the fallopian tube for the next few days while undergoing simultaneous rapid cell division. At the 12 to 16 cell stage (about 3 days after fertilisation), the zygote becomes a solid cluster of cells referred to as the **morula** and by days 3 to 4 reaches the uterine cavity. The series of rapid mitotic cell divisions of the zygote results in the formation of the **blastocyst**, comprising four distinct components (Blackburn 2013, Coad et al 2019). These components include the zona pellucida (a thick glycoprotein membrane); trophoectoderm (to form the placenta and chorion); inner cell mass (to form the embryo); and fluid-filled blastocyst cavity.

Approximately 5 to 6 days after fertilisation (7 to 9 days after ovulation), the blastocyst adheres (implantation) to the endometrium with some bleeding, leading the woman to think that she is experiencing a short but normal menstruation (Rankin 2017). During the secretory phase of the menstrual cycle, the endometrium and, under the control of ovarian steroids, biochemical, physiological and morphological changes have occurred to prepare for implantation. Once implantation has occurred, the blastocyst absorbs nourishment from the decidua and secrete human chorionic gonadotrophin (hCG), to stimulate growth and secretory activity of the corpus luteum to produce steroid hormones for its continued growth as well as that of the decidua (Coad et al 2019). The levels of hCG steadily increase and can first be detected in maternal serum and urine approximately 7 days after ovulation or around the time of implantation. The major function of hCG is to maintain the corpus luteum during early pregnancy to ensure secretion of progesterone and other substances until placental production is adequate by approximately 10 to 12 weeks' gestation (Coad et al 2019).

Pre-embryonic development occurs from the time of fertilisation and zygote formation until 2 weeks' gestation. The embryonic period lasts from 2 weeks after fertilisation until the end of the eighth week, the period of organogenesis, which is a critical time for human development. As they develop, organ systems are susceptible to external influences which may lead to serious congenital abnormalities.

By the end of the eighth week, the embryo, identified as a 'fetus', has already developed a distinct human appearance (Blackburn 2013, Coad et al 2019). During the fetal period, the fetus grows rapidly; tissues and organs differentiate and mature. Calculation of the estimated date of birth (EDB) using Nägele's rule (presented later in this chapter) assists in this calculation.

The placenta and chorion (outer membrane) develop from the trophoblast layer of the blastocyst cells. Other extraembryonic tissues that develop from the inner cell mass include the amnion (inner membrane), the yolk sac, allantois (part of the yolk sac during the embryonic period) and extra-embryonic mesoderm from which the umbilical cord and blood vessels of the placenta are derived (Coad et al 2019). Placental function commences at the end of the third week, and by about 10 to 12 weeks of the pregnancy its function is well established (Blackburn 2013).

The placenta has four major activities including metabolic (nutrient supply), immunological (fetal protection against maternal rejection), transport (i.e. gas exchange, nutrients, waste) and endocrine. Placental endocrine activities are important in maintaining a pregnancy including metabolic adaptations in the mother and fetus. Four major hormones synthesised by the placenta include hCG, human placental lactogen (hPL), steroid hormones including oestrogens and progesterone; and mediators such as proteins and growth factors. Maternal and fetal circulations are separated by layers of tissue referred to as the placental membrane or placental barrier (Blackburn 2013).

A woman who is pregnant for the first time is referred to as a **primigravida** (PG) and after birth she is called a **primipara**. A **multigravida** (MG) is a woman who has previously carried a fetus to the point of viability. The woman is referred to as a **multipara** after birth.

CHANGES DURING NORMAL PREGNANCY

First trimester

The first missed menstrual cycle is a probable sign of pregnancy and is highly suggestive when the second one is also missed. The woman may be led to believe that she has had a cycle but has instead experienced an implantation bleed occurring about the time of the expected menstrual cycle. A feeling of breast fullness may be noticed as early as weeks 3 to 4, increased breast tenderness and tingling around the nipple often occurs from about 4 to 6 weeks; nipples become more erect; and increased breast size and vascularity are usually evident by the end of the second month. In addition, there is enlargement of the sebaceous glands around the nipples (Montgomery's glands), due to hormonal changes. During the first trimester, the ductal system of the woman's breast proliferates under the influence of the hormone oestrogen whereas the lobular formation is enhanced by progesterone. Milk secretion is inhibited by high levels of placental hormones including progesterone (Blackburn 2013).

Uterine hyperplasia begins after implantation and is driven by oestrogen and growth factors. The three layers of the myometrium become more clearly defined as the uterine muscle undergoes hyperplasia and subsequent hypertrophy (increase in length and thickness of existing muscle fibres). Uterine quiescence is mediated by progesterone, relaxin, nitric oxide and prostacyclin (Coad et al 2019). By 12 weeks, the uterine fundus can be located at the brim of the maternal pelvis (see Figure 29.1). Other physical signs of pregnancy in the reproductive system include **Goodell's sign** (softening of the cervix and vagina with increased leucorrhoea discharge); **Hegar's sign** (softening and increased compressibility of the lower uterine segment); and **Chadwick's sign** (bluish purple discolouration of the vaginal mucosa, cervix and vulva) by 8 weeks, but is only useful in assessment of first pregnancies (Blackburn 2013).

Maternal cardiovascular changes begin to occur with stroke volume and cardiac output increasing and systemic vascular resistance decreasing, thereby contributing to increased renal plasma flow and glomerular filtration (Blackburn 2013). Even though there is increased cardiac output and blood volume,

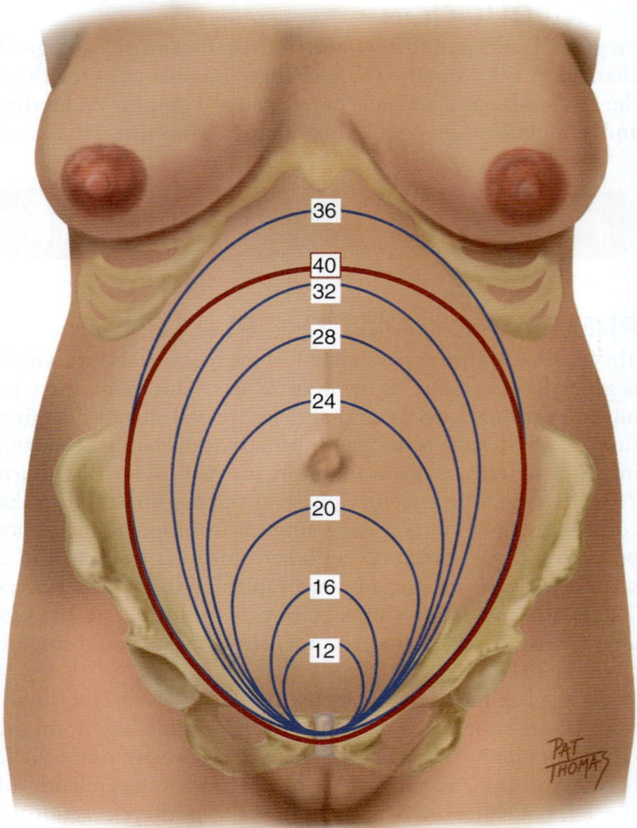

Figure 29.1
Height of fundus at weeks of gestation. ©Pat Thomas

the healthy woman's blood pressure, especially the diastolic pressure, can decrease (Blackburn 2013).

There are a range of symptoms that can be experienced in the first trimester of pregnancy (Figure 29.2). A woman can experience nausea with or without vomiting occurring at any time during the day or night, commencing about 6 weeks after the onset of the last normal menstrual period and continuing for 6 to 12 weeks or even longer for some. The exact cause and function of nausea and vomiting is unknown and the most common hormonal theories are related to rapidly increasing and high levels of oestrogen, hCG and possibly thyroxine (Blackburn 2013, Coad et al 2019) and can be managed through frequent small low-fat content meals. This condition is usually self-limiting and not associated with adverse fetal outcomes. Nausea and vomiting could also be related to emotional health (Rankin 2017). The woman requires ongoing supportive care to manage her symptoms including referral to other health professionals to assist with her emotional wellbeing. A few women develop hyperemesis gravidarum which occurs when there is nausea and excessive vomiting. If this condition is not managed it can result in dehydration and metabolic imbalance and be life threatening for the woman (Rankin 2017).

There can be an increase in frequency of urination (due to pressure of the growing uterus) and excessive fatigue that could be related not only to the hormonal shifts due to pregnancy

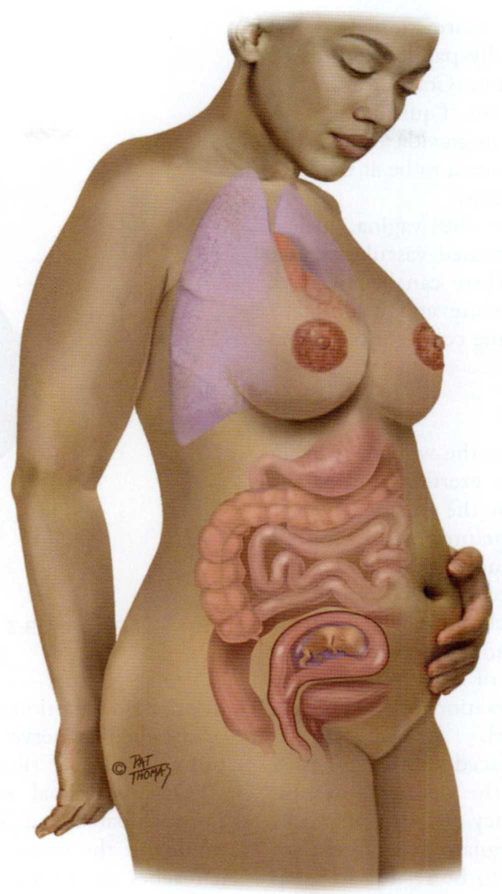

Figure 29.2
First trimester physiological changes. ©Pat Thomas

but also to the impact of nausea, or nausea and vomiting. Minor disorders such as reflux oesophagitis (heartburn) and constipation occur because of maternal physiological adaptations to pregnancy and, in particular, in response to the effect of the hormone progesterone on smooth muscle and connective tissue (Abbott et al 2014, Rankin 2017).

Positive signs of pregnancy include fetal heart sounds, fetal movements and palpation of fetal body parts confirmed through ultrasound (Macdonald & Magill-Cuerdan 2017). By 8 to 10 weeks, a fetal heart rate using, for example, a Doppler can be heard and movements identified in a real-time ultrasound (Blackburn 2013).

Second trimester

By weeks 12 to 16, the nausea, vomiting, fatigue and urinary frequency of the first trimester improve (due to changes in hormone levels). Protein and carbohydrate needs increase, thereby contributing to weight gain.

By the end of the second trimester, the woman can experience heartburn due to the influence of the hormone progesterone that also can cause constipation. There is a need to prevent or care for existing haemorrhoids. Increased oestrogen and progesterone levels can result in increased blood flow causing soft, swollen gums which lead to bleeding gums. Further, there can be fluid retention and there is increased risk of urinary tract infection due to decreased bladder and ureter tone (Blackburn 2013). The maternal blood volume rises and the haemoglobin level begins to fall due to haemodilution; the blood pressure decreases slightly whereas the heart rate increases by 10 to 20 beats per minute and most women develop a systolic murmur during this trimester. Cardiac output usually peaks at 20 to 32 weeks (Macdonald & Magill-Cuerdan 2017).

There is increased skin pigmentation including darkening over the forehead and cheeks—called **chloasma gravidarum**—and a darkened line from the maternal umbilicus to the symphysis pubis referred to as the **linea nigra**. Other cutaneous changes include, for example, the appearance of spider naevi and capillary haemangiomas and the breakdown of connective tissue over the abdomen, breasts or thighs referred to as stretch marks. The fresh tissue breakdown appears as reddish irregular marks (Blackburn 2013) and older ones are faded and silver in appearance.

During the second trimester of pregnancy, there is further lobular growth with formation of new alveoli and ducts and dilation of the lumens of the breast. The breasts become more nodular, the nipples larger and more deeply pigmented and the areolae broadened. Prolactin stimulates production of colostrum which is produced as early as 16 weeks.

The uterus moves into the abdominal cavity to displace the intestines, becoming more ovoid in shape; and the woman will experience tension and stretching of the broad ligament that could be painful for her. Uterine contractions, referred to as Braxton Hicks, are irregular, usually painless and assist in the circulation of blood to the placenta (Coad et al 2019). The woman recognises fetal movement ('quickening') at approximately 18 to 20 weeks (the multigravida earlier). By 20 weeks of pregnancy the uterus is expected to be at the level of the maternal umbilicus (Blackburn 2013).

There is increasing vascularity of the vagina, pelvic viscera and perineal structures and increased vascularity and vasocongestion of the perineal body. There can be increases in vaginal discharge which is thick, white and acidotic to contribute to the inhibition of pathogenic colonisation of the vagina (Blackburn 2013).

Third trimester

During the third trimester of pregnancy, the woman is likely to experience fatigue and dyspnoea on exertion due to the increased weight and pressure exerted by the enlarged uterus. Urinary frequency is increased due to the pressure of the fetal presenting part on the bladder which is pulled up and out of the true pelvis because of the enlarging uterus. This enlargement also displaces the intestines and stomach and a hiatal hernia may develop with associated heartburn and decreased stomach capacity. Haemorrhoids (varicosities of the rectum) are worsened by constipation and the relaxation impact of the hormone progesterone on the large bowel.

The woman's heart is slightly displaced to the left as a consequence of the enlarged uterus. The diastolic pressure reaches its lowest point by mid-pregnancy at 24 to 32 weeks and then gradually returns to non-pregnant baseline values by term of pregnancy. This is thought to be related to a lag in compensation for changes in peripheral resistance. The maternal blood volume peaks at 28 to 34 weeks' gestation and oedema frequently occurs; blood return from the lower extremities is reduced (Blackburn 2013, Rankin 2017).

As pregnancy advances, the fetal placental unit grows and the level of placental hormones, antagonistic to insulin increase, leads to decreased sensitivity or resistance to insulin. This means that insulin is less effective at stimulating glucose uptake. The dominant effect in the second and third trimesters is related to the high levels of human placental lactogen (hPL), but human placental growth hormone, prolactin, and cortisol and progesterone are also involved. Levels of hPL increase markedly after 20 weeks. hPL is a very powerful insulin antagonist and as a consequence there are decreased peripheral tissue responses to insulin with increased levels of circulating glucose and amino acids also available to the fetus (Coad et al 2019).

The woman can experience backache and contributing factors might include postural changes resulting in lumbar lordosis with overstretched abdominal muscles, strained back muscles and broad ligament pain (Figure 29.3). These changes are frequently exacerbated due to the influence of the hormone relaxin in making the intervertebral joints unstable as they try to support the increased weight of pregnancy and in the softening of elastic ligaments of pelvic bones. The increased elasticity of connective and collagen tissue leads to relaxation and hypermobility of the pelvic joints; separation of the symphysis pubis results in instability of the sacroiliac joint and the centre of gravity shifts due to increased cervicodorsal curvature resulting in difficulty in walking (Blackburn 2013). The woman may experience numbness of the arms and hands due to fluid retention of pregnancy which results in compression of the median nerve; this is commonly referred to as 'carpal tunnel syndrome' (Rankin 2017).

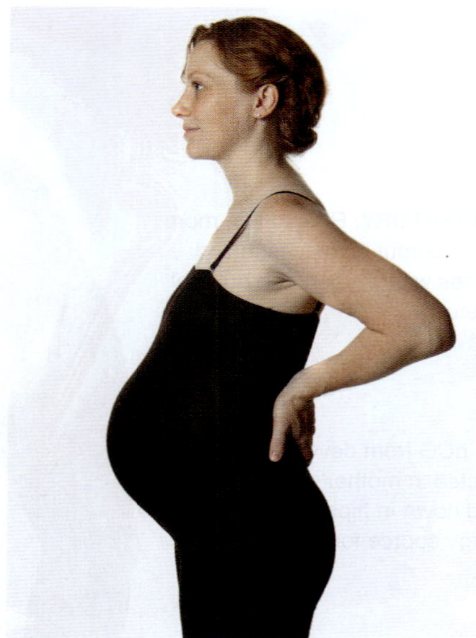

Figure 29.3

On abdominal examination the fetus can usually be easily palpated and movements observed; the growth of the fundus of the uterus continues to rise until 36 weeks when it reaches the level of the maternal xiphisternum. The uterus remains at this level until engagement of the fetal presenting part occurs. Approximately 2 weeks before going into labour, the primigravida woman experiences engagement (also called 'lightening') when the presenting part, normally the fetal head, moves down into the pelvis. Symptoms include a lower-appearing fundus, urinary frequency, increased vaginal secretions from increased pelvic congestion and increased lung capacity. In the multigravida woman, engagement of the presenting part may occur at any time in late pregnancy or, frequently, during labour. The haemodynamic effect of maternal position in late pregnancy can have an impact when the woman is in a supine position and the enlarged uterus may compress the vena cava to reduce venous return to the heart. In turn, this can lead to a decrease in the cardiac output, maternal blood pressure and uterine perfusion (Abbott et al 2014).

The cervix, in preparation for labour, begins to thin (efface) and open (dilate). A thick **mucus plug (operculum)**, formed in the cervix as a mechanical barrier during pregnancy, is expelled at variable times before or during labour. Braxton Hicks contractions are irregular and painless but increase as pregnancy advances. When labour commences, uterine contractions are painful and increase in frequency, intensity and duration to achieve progressive effacement and dilatation of the cervix. Normal labour typically occurs between 37 and 42 weeks (Rankin 2017) and pregnancy is considered to be post term after 42 weeks (Macdonald & Magill-Cuerdan 2017).

Determining weeks of gestation

If fertilisation occurs, according to Nägele's rule (Macdonald & Magill-Cuerdan 2017), the average length of a human gestation is 280 days (40 weeks), measured from the first day of the last normal menstrual period (LNMP), equal to 10 lunar months or just over 9 calendar months (this rule is based on a 28-day cycle; if a longer cycle, for example a 31-day cycle, ten days are added to the due date) (Blackburn 2013). Estimation of the date of birth (EDB) or estimation of the due date (EDD) can be achieved by counting forwards 9 months and adding 7 days from the first day of the LNMP (Macdonald & Magill-Cuerdan 2017). A pregnancy wheel can be used to assist in determining the EDD and weeks of a gestation (Figure 29.4).

Weight gain in pregnancy

Maternal weight gain has traditionally been thought of as a favourable sign applied to assess fetal wellbeing. Factors that influence maternal weight gain include the presence of oedema, maternal metabolic weight, dietary intake, gastrointestinal problems, tobacco smoking and the size of the fetus (Rankin 2017). Weight gain during pregnancy reflects increased maternal stores as well as those of the developing fetus and placenta. Approximately 62% of the gain is water, 30% fat and 8% protein. About 25% of the total weight gain is related to the fetus, 11% to the placenta and amniotic fluid and the remainder to the mother. Optimal weight gain during pregnancy varies with maternal pre-pregnancy weight; greater weight gain is generally recommended for underweight women and a lower weight gain for those who are overweight. Body mass index (BMI) and energy expenditure must also be considered (Blackburn 2013). The woman who has a BMI that is either below or above the healthy range is most likely to require additional care during pregnancy. An underweight woman can have a BMI lower than 18.5 and is at risk of a preterm birth and low birth weight infant, whereas the woman with a BMI greater than 25 can be linked with stillbirth and congenital abnormalities. A woman with a BMI of 30 or more is at increased risk of shoulder dystocia, caesarean birth, difficulty in initiating lactation and is predisposed to postpartum weight retention. The woman with a normal pre-pregnancy BMI would be expected to gain approximately 11.5 to 16 kg (Department of Health 2018).

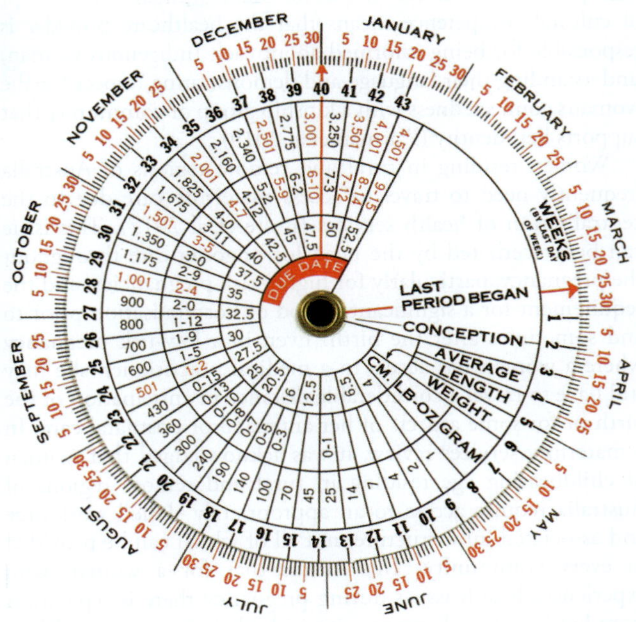

Figure 29.4
Pregnancy Wheel.

DEVELOPMENTAL CONSIDERATIONS

In industrialised countries, the risks for the adolescent who is pregnant are largely psychosocial. The young woman is at risk for the downward cycle of poverty beginning with an incomplete education, failure to limit family size and continuing with failure to establish a vocation and become independent. She may be unprepared emotionally to be a mother. Her social situation may be stressful. She may not have the support of her family, her partner or his family. Medical risks for the pregnant adolescent are generally related to poverty, inadequate nutrition, substance abuse and sometimes sexually transmitted infections (STIs), poor health before pregnancy and emotional and physical abuse from her partner. The proportion of women who gave birth and were teenagers in 2016 varied by place of residence, ranging from a low of 1.1% in the Australian Capital Territory to 6.1% in the Northern Territory. The proportion of Australian teenage mothers (younger than 20) has steadily declined since 2002 (4.9%) to a rate of 2.4% in 2016 (Australian Institute of Health and Welfare (AIHW) 2018a). Teenage fertility rate is approximately 15 births per 1000 women aged between 15 and 19 years. This is a significant decrease from previous statistics (New Zealand Government 2018).

While evidence suggests the adolescent is at risk for pregnancy-induced hypertension, preterm birth and perinatal mortality (Macdonald & Magill-Cuerdan 2017), it is unclear whether these risks are associated with physiological change or social factors. For social reasons, the adolescent often seeks healthcare later, and early antenatal care has been shown to provide optimal management. In 2016 about 1 in 7 (13.6%) Aboriginal and Torres Strait Islander mothers were teenagers, compared with 2.4% of non-Indigenous mothers (AIHW 2018a). Proportionately more Aboriginal and Torres Strait Islander mothers have their babies at a younger age than non-Indigenous mothers (AIHW 2018a). Similarly, in New Zealand, Māori and Pacific Islander birth rates are higher in lower socioeconomic communities (Urale et al 2019).

Since the advent of assisted conception, more women older than age 35 years are now becoming pregnant. In Australia, the proportion of mothers aged 35 and over increased from 19% in 2002 to 23% in 2016 and mothers aged 40 and over made up 4.3% of women giving birth in 2016 compared with 3.4% in 2006 (AIHW 2018a).

Women of 'later maternal age' (over 35 years) are often more prepared emotionally and financially to parent; however, they are more at risk for infertility and age-related anomalies. With reproductive ageing the primary changes occur in the ovary and follicles and particularly the oocytes. Oocytes of the woman over 40 to 45 years have been found to have abnormal chromosomal alignment at metaphase and increased meiotic disjunction (Blackburn 2013). Once conception has occurred, the woman is at increased risk of having a child with congenital abnormalities, particularly Trisomy 21, commonly known as

Down syndrome. Further issues include a decline in fertility, due in part to a decrease in the number and health of eggs to be ovulated; a decrease in ovulation; and other gynaecological conditions such as endometriosis and early onset of menopause.

The woman of later maternal age is also at risk of spontaneous abortions, in part because of the increase in genetically abnormal embryos (Gabbe et al 2017). Since the incidence of chronic medical conditions such as diabetes type 2 and hypertension, for example, increase with age, the pregnant woman over the age of 35 years is considered to be at risk of complications related to these diseases (Bloom et al 2018). The increased incidence of hypertension places the woman at risk of placental abruption and preeclampsia that, in turn, increases the risk of intrauterine growth restriction (IUGR). There are still wide variances in maternal deaths between developed and developing countries. In Australia women aged 40 and over, with higher parity, of Aboriginal and Torres Strait Islander origin or with remote or very remote usual residence were among those at increased risk of maternal death (AIHW 2018a). Maternal deaths worldwide are due to severe bleeding (mostly postpartum), infection (soon after birth), hypertensive disorders of pregnancy and obstructed labour. Indirect causes are diseases that complicate pregnancy such as malaria, AIDS during pregnancy and inadequate skilled healthcare (World Health Organization (WHO) 2018b).

In Australia, the current recommendation is for all women to be offered first trimester screening for fetal genetic abnormality (Department of Health 2018). This screening involves both an ultrasound between 11 and 13 weeks' gestation measuring the fetal nuchal translucency thickness, combined with a maternal blood test that analyses pregnancy-associated placental protein-A (PAPP-A) and beta-human chorionic gonadotrophin (B-hCG). In addition to this, a non-invasive prenatal test (NIPT) is also available from 10 weeks' gestation. This test analyses maternal blood for cell-free deoxyribonucleic acid (cfDNA), with a greater than expected number of relevant chromosome fragments present in genetic fetal abnormality such as Down syndrome. The NIPT test may be offered as a first line test, combined with first trimester screening or in addition to first trimester screening where intermediate risk has been identified (Department of Health 2018). Women who present later in pregnancy (14–20 weeks) are offered second trimester maternal serum screening for fetal chromosomal anomaly. All of these tests are gestation specific, so a known accurate gestation is required and can be determined by early ultrasound, prior to 13 weeks' gestation.

Women who return a high-risk result are offered genetic counselling and diagnostic testing such as **chorionic villus sampling** (CVS) where a small sample of **chorionic villi** is removed, either abdominally or transvaginally, between 11 and 14 weeks or amniocentesis, in which a small amount of amniotic fluid is removed, is performed after 15 weeks under ultrasound guidance (Department of Health 2018).

CULTURAL AND SOCIAL CONSIDERATIONS

In Australia, women are encouraged to make their own decisions about their pregnancy and birth experience supported by a woman-centred approach to maternity care. Key issues include having a safe birth, feeling in control within the birth environment, developing supportive relationships with their carer or carers, and being treated with dignity and respect. The concept of woman-centred care is intended to place the focus on the woman's individual unique needs, expectations and aspirations, rather than the needs of institutions or maternity service professionals. The application of this care is to recognise the woman's right to self-determination in terms of choice, control and continuity of care (Department of Health 2018).

Midwives in their role as primary healthcare providers participate in continuity of care programs and midwifery-led models of care available across Australia with models ranging from caseload/team models to continuity of antenatal and postnatal care. In New Zealand, midwives are expected to work in partnership with women, providing or supporting continuity of midwifery care throughout the woman's experience and work collaboratively with other health professionals when necessary to meet any additional medical, health or social needs of mothers and their babies. Primary maternity care is provided by lead maternity carers (LMCs), selected by women to provide their care. Lead maternity carers can be either midwives, general practitioners with a diploma in obstetrics or obstetricians. LMCs take responsibility for the care provided to women throughout pregnancy and up to 6 weeks following, including the management of labour and birth (New Zealand College of Midwives Inc. 2019).

In promoting woman-centred care there is an increase in the range of maternity care models available to Australian women of diverse cultural and social backgrounds to support improved birth outcomes. Consideration of cultural traditions could include, for example, the traditions of Aboriginal and Torres Strait Islander women, in which the risk of not birthing on country and potentially away from family can result in distress and increase in clinical and medical risk (Department of Health 2019). In New Zealand, Māori culture is integrated in public communications. In the delivery of healthcare 'cultural competence' is promoted and applied in maternity services for Māori women. The concept of cultural competence means that the healthcare provider is responsible for being informed about each Indigenous woman, understanding their language and demonstrating respect for the woman's connectedness with a kinship group or community that supports her identity (Pairman et al 2019).

Women residing in rural and remote regions of Australia frequently need to travel to access maternity care due to the centralisation of health services (Rolfe et al 2017). This issue can be exacerbated by the need for ongoing care throughout the pregnancy, particularly for higher risk pregnancies; and the requirement for a significant period of hospitalisation prior to and sometimes after the birth. Even in a low-risk pregnancy where a woman has access to a medical practitioner, she may still have to travel a considerable distance in anticipation of the birth or for some aspects of her antenatal or postnatal care. In a maternity services review, it was acknowledged that women of childbearing age residing in rural and remote regions of Australia require access to an appropriately skilled workforce and associated infrastructure, not all of which can be provided in every community. This means that for a woman who experiences health issues during pregnancy there is separation from her family and community with likely financial hardship.

Pregnancy is a life event with profound psychological and social meaning for the woman and for her family and community. Pregnancy is a unique period in a woman's life that is surrounded by special customs, traditions, beliefs and spiritual practices. Understanding what role these customs, traditions, beliefs and spiritual practices play in the woman's pregnancy helps the midwife to tailor care to the individual's needs. Understanding what role these beliefs and practices play in the woman's pregnancy helps the healthcare provider to acknowledge individual needs. Pregnancy is intensely personal and involves such charged issues as sexuality, relationships, contraception, nutritional practices, maternal weight gain and abortion. The healthcare provider must be sensitive to these issues. A sensitive approach includes inquiring whether the woman or her significant others have any special requests. This communicates a respectful acknowledgement of individual preferences. A continuing rapport will help enable the woman to discuss issues with the healthcare provider (Pairman et al 2019).

Some complications of pregnancy occur more frequently in certain groups. Women who live in developing countries may not have the advantages of a skilled attendant for pregnancy and birth, let alone technology. Every day 840 women die due to pregnancy or childbirth with 99% of these deaths occurring in developing countries. Common causes of these maternal deaths include infections, hypertension, complications during delivery, unsafe abortion and haemorrhage (WHO 2018b).

Australian demographic data for 2016 show that 310,247 women gave birth to 314,814 babies. This was a 2% decrease in mothers compared to 2015, and a total increase of 11.8% since 2006. The average age of Aboriginal and Torres Strait Islander women who gave birth in 2016 was 25.9 years, compared with 30.5 years for non-Indigenous mothers. In contrast, 9.4% of Aboriginal and Torres Strait Islander mothers were aged 35 and older, compared with 23.4% of non-Indigenous mothers (AIHW 2018a).

From 2006 to 2016 in Australia, there were 281 maternal deaths that occurred within 42 days of the end of pregnancy. The maternal mortality ratio (MMR) was relatively stable between 2006 and 2016 with the MMR for 2016 8.5 per 100,000 women who gave birth. These data should be interpreted with caution due to the rarity of maternal deaths in Australia and associated volatility of small numbers. There were 12 maternal deaths directly related to pregnancy and 11 indirect deaths in 2016. Aboriginal and Torres Strait Islander women were 4.6 times more likely to die than non-Indigenous women, with a maternal mortality ratio of 31.6 deaths per 100,000 Indigenous women giving birth (2012–2016).

In New Zealand in 2016, 3.3 maternal deaths per 100,000 maternities were reported. The three-year maternal mortality ratio for 2014–2016 was 9.4 per 100,000 maternities, occurring during either pregnancy or within 42 days of birth, with 11 being the highest number recorded, for 2015 (Perinatal and Maternal Mortality Review Committee 2018).

Subjective data

The majority of women experience good health during pregnancy. For many women, their care can be managed by a midwife or a medical practitioner or by using a shared model combining the two. As described earlier, the elements of woman-centred care include choice, control and continuity of care; the woman is encouraged to be an active participant in her own care. The midwife is required to practise according to standards of practice and engage in referral and collaboration with other healthcare providers when either maternal or fetal health issues are recognised.

Pregnancy assessment is most commonly conducted by midwives but registered nurses may need to conduct a health assessment if the woman is seeking healthcare for non-pregnancy-related health issues. During pregnancy an extensive health history is obtained at the first antenatal visit. This provides a comprehensive database for establishing an appropriate model of care and for monitoring the progress of both the mother's health and that of her fetus throughout the pregnancy. This approach also provides the opportunity for considerable insight into the mother's needs and concerns that can be addressed through health promotion and education specific to her.

The initial consultation may cause some anxiety as this may be the first time the woman has been pregnant. Conversely, the woman may not be certain she is pregnant and her anxiety may be related to this uncertainty or to what to expect if she is pregnant. It is imperative that this consultation with the woman is conducted in a private room to provide an explanation of the initial history-taking process and the investigations available to her. It is essential that the woman is given information so that she can make informed decisions related to her care.

1. Menstrual history
2. Gynaecological history
3. Obstetric history
4. Current pregnancy
5. Medical history
6. Family history
7. General health history
8. Nutritional history
9. Environment/hazards

Practice note: Before you commence the assessment, introduce yourself to the person, confirm the person's identity, discuss the purpose and scope of the assessment, clarify any questions the person may have and obtain verbal consent from the person to perform the assessment.

SUBJECTIVE DATA

ASSESSMENT GUIDELINES AND NORMAL FINDINGS	CLINICAL SIGNIFICANCE AND CLINICAL ALERTS
1. Menstrual history	
• How old were you at menarche (onset of first menstruation and the commencement of cyclical menstrual function)? • How often do you menstruate and how long for? • Do you experience regularity or irregularity of your menstrual cycle? • Do you experience a heavy loss or intermenstrual bleeding? • Do you experience chronic pelvic pain (CPP)? • When was the first day of your last normal menstrual cycle?	Issues related to the woman's menstrual cycle such as chronic pelvic pain may be due to hormonal conditions such as endometriosis or adenomyosis (Impey & Child 2017). Using **Nägele's rule**, calculate the estimated date of birth (EDB) from the first day of the last normal menstrual cycle by counting forwards 9 months and 7 days for a 28-day regular menstrual cycle.
2. Gynaecological history	
• Have you ever had surgery of the cervix or uterus?	Cervical surgery may affect the integrity of the cervix during pregnancy. During labour it may impede cervical dilation. Uterine surgery increases risk for uterine rupture during pregnancy and labour.
• Do you have any known history of or exposure to herpes simplex virus (HSV types 1 and 2)?	Following the primary episode HSV virions travel to the dorsal root ganglia of the sacral plexus where they remain until reactivation. Recurrent episodes of HSV type 2 spreads back down the sensory neurons to the skin where painful episodes of vulval or cervical infectious lesions can occur. Newborn infants have an impaired immune response to HSV types 1 and 2 and are at increased risk of morbidity (e.g. encephalitis, septicaemia) and mortality if the mother is infectious and experiences a vaginal birth. Management can include use of antiviral agents.
• When was your last cervical screening test ? Have you ever had an abnormal cervical screening test or a colposcopy?	A cervical screening test is done every five years (if normal) and if the woman has not had one previously, suggest that it should be done. An abnormal cervical screening test in the past may have a negative effect on the pregnancy or birth depending on whether there was surgery of the cervix involved.
• Do you have any history of fibroids or uterine abnormalities?	**Fibroids** can increase risk for placental abruption, preterm labour and birth; and postpartum haemorrhage. Uterine abnormalities can include **double uterus, unicornuate or bicornuate uterus; and septate or subseptate uterus.** These can result in abortion.

ASSESSMENT GUIDELINES AND NORMAL FINDINGS	CLINICAL SIGNIFICANCE AND CLINICAL ALERTS
• Have you ever had **sexually transmitted infections** (STIs) such as syphilis, chlamydia, gonorrhoea, pelvic inflammatory disease (PID), trichomoniasis or genital warts? See Chapter 26 for further information about screening for STIs in women.	If untreated, STIs increase the risk of morbidity and mortality of the newborn. **Maternal syphilis** infection results in congenital infection as early as 9–10 weeks of pregnancy and at any subsequent time during pregnancy. **Congenital syphilis** is a serious condition that, if not fatal at a young age, can cause permanent impairment, debilitation and disfigurement. Pancreatitis and inflammation of the gastrointestinal tract are common. **Chlamydia** is caused by the bacterium *Chlamydia trachomatis*. Genital chlamydial infection remains asymptomatic in at least 70% of women and the majority of infections probably clear spontaneously without morbidity. Recent change of sexual partner can place the woman at risk. Complications that may arise for women include chronic pelvic pain, pelvic inflammatory disease, infertility and ectopic pregnancy (Department of Health 2018). **Gonorrhoea**—the causative organism is *Neisseria gonorrhoeae*—transmitted through intimate contact, may initially cause symptoms of mild vaginitis. If untreated it can lead to severe complications of PID, damage to heart valves and joint tissue. For the newborn, the organism can cause severe eye infections. PID is usually due to sexually transmitted pelvic infections and endometritis (Impey & Child 2017). **Trichomoniasis** is a very common STI and the woman can experience vulval itching, dysuria and vaginal discharge that is malodorous. Genital warts, caused by the human papillomavirus (HPV), have been a common STI. A vaccine is now administered to adolescent girls to prevent HPV infection. ***Clinical alert:*** The woman with any of the above infections requires referral to a medical practitioner for further treatment.
• Have you been tested for **human immunodeficiency virus** (HIV)? When? What was the result? Have you ever had a blood transfusion? Used intravenous drugs? Had a sexual partner who had any HIV risk factors?	Address HIV status to promote the health of the woman. Following a complete evaluation, a plan of HIV-related care should be provided taking into account pregnancy-specific maternal or fetal safety issues. Early HIV diagnosis can reduce the risk of mother-to-child transmission and the rate of disease progression in the mother. The woman is to be provided information related to options of healthcare so that she can make an informed choice.
• Are you in a sexual relationship with more than one person?	The number of sexual partners and frequency of partner change increase the risk for STIs.

SUBJECTIVE DATA

ASSESSMENT GUIDELINES AND NORMAL FINDINGS	CLINICAL SIGNIFICANCE AND CLINICAL ALERTS
• Have you had a mammogram, breast biopsy, breast implants, breast augmentation or breast reconstruction (reduction mammoplasty)?	Previous breast surgery may have a significant effect on breastfeeding success. Major issues are loss of sensation in the nipple or areola by nerve injury or compromise of the lactiferous ducts. Large epidemiological studies of infants who have been breastfed by mothers with silicone implants have not shown adverse events (Gabbe et al 2017).
3. Obstetric history	
• Do you have a history of **infertility**? Have you used assisted reproductive technology (ART), for example, sperm or egg donor and/or in vitro fertilisation (IVF)?	There is an increased rate of preterm birth following ART, not only with multiple gestations but with singleton pregnancies as well. Other associated factors include low birth weight and very low birth weight infants and small gestational age infants born following IVF. The reasons for these outcomes are not known (Fitzgerald et al 2018).
• How did you experience **previous pregnancies** and what were your birthing outcomes and the years of each birth? Have you experienced spontaneous miscarriages, elective abortions or ectopic pregnancies and what were the postnatal outcomes?	It is important to obtain from the woman her history of past pregnancy/ies as previous experiences can impact on her emotions regarding the current pregnancy. The woman may require referral to other health professionals for care to term of her current pregnancy.
• What were the **birth weights** of your babies, what sex were they and were they born alive? Were they born at term of pregnancy?	A small infant may indicate prematurity or **intrauterine growth restriction** (IUGR)—complications that may be repeatable. A large infant may indicate gestational diabetes mellitus (GDM). Conversely, birth weights of other children may indicate a 'constitutional size'—e.g. the tendency of a couple to conceive smaller but normal children.
• Have you ever had a **caesarean section** (CS)? If so, what was the indication? At how many centimetres of cervical dilation, if any? What type of uterine incision was made? Have you ever had a **vaginal birth after a caesarean section** (VBAC)?	Although rare, the woman who has a vertical, or 'classical', incision of uterus due to a previous caesarean section carries a higher risk of uterine rupture. This means that all subsequent births will be by caesarean section. The 'low transverse' or horizontal incision carries a low risk and the woman can plan to have a VBAC. Note that the direction of the skin scar does not necessarily tell how the uterus was incised.
• Have you **breastfed** previously? If so, how was that experience for you? How long did you breastfeed for? If you did not breastfeed previously, was this due to your choice or was it unsuccessful? If unsuccessful in breastfeeding, what do you think were the factors?	The woman's experience and knowledge of breastfeeding can influence the level of teaching and support required.
• Did you have any history of breastfeeding problems such as mastitis?	A poor or painful previous breastfeeding experience increases the need for support after this pregnancy. Resources include a lactation consultant or the maternal and child health nurse, general medical practitioner (GP), Australian Breastfeeding Association (ABA) or the New Zealand Breastfeeding Authority.

ASSESSMENT GUIDELINES AND NORMAL FINDINGS	CLINICAL SIGNIFICANCE AND CLINICAL ALERTS
4. Current pregnancy	
The number of weeks of amenorrhoea (absence of menstrual bleeding) for the current pregnancy are elicited when taking the woman's health history at the first antenatal visit.	
• What method of **contraception** did you use most recently, and when did you discontinue it?	Recent use of oral contraception or other hormonal contraceptives may have delayed ovulation and irregular menses—consider when establishing the **estimated date of birth** (EDB). An intrauterine contraceptive device (IUCD) still in place after conception requires removal to reduce the risk of a mid-trimester abortion.
• Is this pregnancy planned? How do you feel about it?	Even a planned pregnancy represents loss for the woman—perhaps a loss of freedom, compromise of goals, loss of time with other children or her partner. This sense of loss can also be influenced by the impact of physiological and physical changes on how she feels about her pregnancy.
• Do you have a partner? How does your partner feel about the pregnancy? How do other family members feel about the pregnancy?	The woman may need assistance with her partner and support group so that they can be more supportive of her. Support strategies include inviting the woman's partner or significant others to attend antenatal visits with her.
• Have you experienced any recent **vaginal bleeding**? When? How much? What colour was the loss (e.g. bright blood loss or dark in colour)? Was it accompanied by any pain?	***Clinical alert:*** Vaginal bleeding may indicate a threatened abortion in early pregnancy; later it could be related to a low-lying placenta. The woman requires referral for further investigation and care.
• Are you experiencing any **nausea and/or vomiting**?	Nausea and vomiting are symptoms of pregnancy that generally occur between 4 and 6 weeks, occasionally at 2 to 3 weeks, peak between weeks 8 and 12 or weeks 14 and 16. Health education and promotion includes advice on small frequent low-fat meals to assist the woman in self-care and to seek medical assistance if vomiting is more serious and unremitting.
• Have you experienced any **abdominal pain**? When? Where in your abdomen? Accompanied by vaginal bleeding?	The most common causes of abdominal pain in early pregnancy are spontaneous abortion, ectopic pregnancy, urinary tract infection (UTI) and round ligament discomfort. Causes of pain later in pregnancy include preterm labour, placental abruption and haemolysis, elevated liver enzymes and low platelet syndrome (HELLP) (see Table 29.1). Also consider other medical and surgical causes for abdominal pain.

SUBJECTIVE DATA

SUBJECTIVE DATA

ASSESSMENT GUIDELINES AND NORMAL FINDINGS	CLINICAL SIGNIFICANCE AND CLINICAL ALERTS
• Have you had any recent unexplained itching, rash or skin infections?	Itching is the most common dermatological symptom of pregnancy. Mild pruritus is common and frequently occurs over the abdomen. The woman requires support and information related to the care of her skin during pregnancy. If there are preexisting skin disorders the woman is encouraged to consult her dermatologist.
• Have you had any X-rays or taken any medication—prescribed, unprescribed or recreational drugs?	Discuss the potential effect of any teratogenic exposure. Refer for expert counselling if necessary.
• Have you experienced any visual changes such as the new onset of blurred vision or spots before your eyes?	In the third trimester, this may be a sign of preeclampsia. Evaluate for other signs and symptoms of preeclampsia (see Table 29.1).
• Have you experienced any oedema? Where and under what circumstances?	In the third trimester, differentiate the normal weight-dependent oedema of pregnancy from that of generalised oedema associated with preeclampsia.
• Have you had any frequency, or burning with urination? Any blood in your urine? Do you void in small amounts? Do you have any history of UTIs, pyelonephritis or kidney stones?	Differentiate the normal urinary frequency of the first and third trimesters from UTI, for which pregnant women are at increased risk. Confirm by urinalysis. UTIs increase the rate of preterm labour.
• Do you have any vaginal burning or itching? Any foul-smelling or coloured discharge?	If symptoms occur, refer to a midwife or medical practitioner.
• Are you feeling your baby move?	Educate the woman to be aware of the normal pattern of her fetal movements each day. Changes in fetal activity may reflect hypoxaemia or placental insufficiency. Advise the woman who has not felt normal fetal movements to contact her healthcare provider immediately.
• Do you have cats in the home?	Explain toxoplasmosis, a teratogenic disease transmitted through raw or undercooked meat, cat faeces and soil. To avoid exposure, ensure careful handwashing following contact with soil and when dealing with cat litter. Ensure thorough cooking of meat and wash hands after handling meat, and fruit and vegetables because of soil contamination.
• Do you plan to breastfeed this baby?	Arrange breastfeeding resources, including classes and other support for the woman who plans to breastfeed. The support will differ for those who are first-time mothers.
5. Medical history	
• Do you have allergies to medications or foods? If so, what type of reaction?	Alerts for health professionals to avoid a prescribing error and to ensure foods causing allergies and for the woman to have specific dietary arrangements when admitted for care during labour, birth and the time following birth.

SUBJECTIVE DATA

ASSESSMENT GUIDELINES AND NORMAL FINDINGS	CLINICAL SIGNIFICANCE AND CLINICAL ALERTS
• Do you have a history of asthma? • Are you aware of your current immunisation status and/or immunity to rubella, chickenpox (varicella), whooping cough (pertussis) or influenza?	Women with asthma have been reported to have higher risks for complications of pregnancy such as preeclampsia, preterm labour and birth, low birth weight or intrauterine growth restriction of the fetus and perinatal mortality. If **rubella** is contracted during the first trimester, it can lead to congenital rubella syndrome. Preventing congenital infection relies on maintaining high levels of immunity to rubella in the general population. There is no treatment to prevent or reduce mother-to-child transmission of rubella once infection has been detected in pregnancy. Rubella vaccination is contraindicated in pregnancy. Rarely, **varicella** causes congenital anomalies. The non-immune woman should avoid exposure. **Whooping Cough** (pertussis) immunisation between 28 and 32 weeks of pregnancy is recommended to provide passive immunity to the fetus which is protective in the first 3 months of life (Halperin et al 2018). **Influenza** in pregnancy has been demonstrated to cause significant complications if contracted during pregnancy. Influenza vaccine can be administered at any time during pregnancy and also provides passive immunity to the infant (Blanchard-Rohner & Eberhardt 2017).
• Have you had any injury to your back or another weight-bearing part of your body?	The localised and overall weight gain of pregnancy and the joint-softening property of progesterone may cause backache and other joint pain.
• Do you smoke cigarettes? How many? For how many years? Have you ever tried to quit? Do you drink alcohol? How many times per week? Do you use any illicit substances such as methamphetamine, cocaine or heroin?	Explain the health risks associated with these substances in pregnancy. Smoking increases the risk of ectopic pregnancy, spontaneous abortion, low birth weight, prematurity, preterm premature rupture of membranes, pregnancy-induced hypertension, placental abruption and sudden infant death syndrome. Alcohol increases the risk to the fetus of **fetal alcohol syndrome** (FAS) (see Table 21.13). Cocaine use during pregnancy is associated with congenital anomalies, a four-fold increased risk for placental abruption and the risk of fetal addiction that after birth can result in developmental delays or behavioural disturbances (Bloom et al 2018). It is recommended that the pregnant woman is referred to drug and alcohol programs for consultation provided by a multidisciplinary team.

SUBJECTIVE DATA

ASSESSMENT GUIDELINES AND NORMAL FINDINGS	CLINICAL SIGNIFICANCE AND CLINICAL ALERTS
• Do you take any prescribed, non-prescribed (over-the-counter) or complementary or traditional medicines?	Screen all medications (prescribed, non-prescribed, complementary and traditional) to establish safety during pregnancy.
• Do you have a regular exercise program? What type of exercise program do you do?	There are many positive physical and psychological benefits of regular exercise in pregnancy for both the woman and the fetus. International pregnancy exercise guidelines agree that pregnant women should undertake at least 30 minutes of exercise across most days of the week. This exercise should be of medium intensity and include aerobic and resistance training elements. Each woman should be evaluated individually by their health care provider in terms of suitability of their current or planned exercise regime in the context of their pregnancy (Savvaki et al 2018). A recent randomised control trial found that women who exercised throughout their pregnancy were at a reduced risk of both excess weight gain and gestational diabetes (GD) (Barakat et al 2018).
6. Family history	
• What is your family medical history?	The woman's family medical history is important in planning her care during pregnancy. Familial diseases such as hypertension and diabetes or congenital abnormalities may require a referral for genetic counselling and diagnostic procedures.
• Do you have anxiety, depression or any other mental illness?	Anxiety and depression can occur during pregnancy and after birth. Assessing the woman for psychosocial risk factors and symptoms of distress during regular pregnancy gives her the opportunity to link with appropriate services. Antenatal screening also seeks to identify whether a woman has experienced, or received treatment for, more severe mental health disorders. If this is affirmed, further understanding of current and future significance is indicated along with collaboration with relevant mental health professionals.
• Is there a history of multiple births in your family?	Approximately two-thirds of twins are **dizygotic** (fraternal), arising from multiple ovulation and one-third **monozygotic** (identical), derived from one fertilised oocyte. The older woman is at risk of spontaneous dizygotic twinning.

ASSESSMENT GUIDELINES AND NORMAL FINDINGS	CLINICAL SIGNIFICANCE AND CLINICAL ALERTS
• Does anyone in your family have congenital anomalies? What is your ethnicity? Does anyone in your partner's family have congenital anomalies? What is the ethnicity of your baby's father?	Some anomalies, such as heart conditions, are familial. Offer a referral to genetic counselling to provide the woman and her family with options such as diagnostic procedures. Establishing ethnicity will indicate any increased risks for known problems such as sickle cell anaemia or thalassaemia.
• Do you have any specific thoughts about how you would like the pregnancy and birth to be managed?	Establishing the woman's preferences will assist healthcare providers in meeting her particular needs.
7. General health history	
• Do you have a preexisting cardiovascular disease, such as vascular disease, a heart murmur or disease of a heart valve?	The woman with cardiac disease who becomes pregnant must be monitored carefully for signs of cardiac compromise. The profound alterations in the cardiorespiratory system and haemodynamics (e.g. blood volume increase of up to 50%) during pregnancy can result in morbidity and mortality for the woman and her fetus. It is recommended that the woman's care is provided within a multidisciplinary team approach (Blackburn 2013).
• Have you ever had anaemia? What kind? When? How was it treated?	Pregnancy worsens any preexisting anaemia because iron is used extensively by the growing fetus. It can be easily managed through iron supplementation. Sickle cell anaemia may worsen during pregnancy thereby placing both the woman and her fetus at risk for complications as a result of the effects of haematological, cardiovascular, renal and respiratory changes. As the plasma volume increases during pregnancy, the woman can become more anaemic. Folic acid can be given during pregnancy and blood transfusions may be required for severe anaemia.
• Have you had thrombophlebitis, pulmonary embolus (PE) or deep venous thrombosis (DVT)?	Pregnancy is an acquired hypercoagulable state due to an increase of blood factors VII, VIII, IX, X and XII in preparation for birth. As a consequence of this increase, there is the risk of thrombosis in pregnancy. These include, for example, venous stasis in the lower extremities and the compression of the inferior vena cava by the enlarging uterus (Gabbe et al 2017).

SUBJECTIVE DATA

ASSESSMENT GUIDELINES AND NORMAL FINDINGS	CLINICAL SIGNIFICANCE AND CLINICAL ALERTS
• Have you had hypertension or renal disease?	Hypertensive (HT) disorders are one of the most common complications of pregnancy and include HT during pregnancy; **chronic HT; preeclampsia (PE); and preeclampsia superimposed on chronic HT and gestational HT.** The woman with renal disease is at increased risk for preeclampsia, preterm birth and fetal growth restriction but in mild disease their renal prognosis is not significantly altered. The woman with moderate to severe renal disease is at risk of worsening renal function (Blackburn 2013).
• Do you have preexisting diabetes mellitus (type 1 or type 2)? If so, when was the onset and how is it managed? Did you experience gestational diabetes (GD) in your previous pregnancies? Is there a family history of diabetes?	A history of **diabetes** indicates that the woman will require increased monitoring and assessment throughout pregnancy. This approach also applies to the woman who has a history of GD and is at risk of developing type 2 diabetes later in life. Diabetes is carefully managed during pregnancy to avoid serious complications, such as fetal macrosomia resulting in interventions during birth and/or operative birth. **Macrosomia** can contribute to maternal morbidity and fetal/infant morbidity and mortality.
• Do you have a history of a thyroid disorder?	Thyroid disorders are the second most common endocrine disorder to gestational diabetes. Close monitoring of women with a history of thyroid dysfunction is required to ensure the woman remains in a euthyroid state, where her thyroid hormones are within normal levels.
• Have you ever had a seizure?	**Seizure disorders** are the most frequent neurological complication in pregnancy including acquired (e.g. trauma, infection, lesions or metabolic disorders) and idiopathic disorders (Gabbe et al 2017). Acquired seizure disorders may result from trauma, infection, space-occupying lesions or metabolic disorders. Idiopathic disorders include tonic-clonic, partial complex with or without generalisation, myoclonic, focal or absence (Gabbe et al 2017).
• Do you have a history of urinary tract infections (UTIs)?	**Urinary tract infection** may occur with increased frequency during pregnancy and is related to anatomical changes in the renal system. Asymptomatic bacteriuria (ASB) can occur in some women and has the potential to develop into pyelonephritis if untreated. If this occurs, the woman can experience a preterm birth of a low birth weight infant. Screening for ASB has been shown to reduce pyelonephritis (Department of Health 2018).

ASSESSMENT GUIDELINES AND NORMAL FINDINGS	CLINICAL SIGNIFICANCE AND CLINICAL ALERTS
• Do you have **hepatitis B virus** (HBV) or **hepatitis C** (HVC)?	Antenatal screening for HBV (transmitted sexually or parenterally) is recommended for all pregnant women. There is risk of transmission of this disease to the fetus. All infants of HBV mothers are routinely prescribed both HBV immunoglobulin and vaccine at birth to prevent infection. HVC is a blood-borne disease that is one of the major causes of liver cirrhosis, hepatocellular carcinoma and liver failure. Perinatal transmission is the main source of hepatitis C in Australian children born to mothers who used intravenous drugs, had invasive procedures overseas or have tattoos. Knowledge of HBC status in pregnancy ensures that interventions that increase the risk of transmission can be avoided. Infants who acquire hepatitis C in utero or at birth do not develop clinically apparent liver problems in early childhood, but most develop chronic hepatitis C and are likely to be at risk of longer term problems related to chronic liver disease, including hepatic fibrosis, cirrhosis and hepatocellular carcinoma (Department of Health 2018).
• Have you been exposed to **tuberculosis** (TB) or had a positive tuberculin skin test (TST)/Mantoux test or chest X-ray? Were your born outside of Australia?	Most new TB cases (90%) occur in people born overseas particularly from geographical areas such as South and South East Asia (Toms et al 2017). Pregnancy does not adversely affect the course of TB, if appropriate therapy is instituted. In the setting of incomplete treatment and advanced or extrapulmonary TB, the chances of perinatal complications such as preeclampsia, intrauterine growth restriction, antepartum haemorrhage, low birth weights, preterm birth and perinatal mortality rates for neonates are increased.
• What was your weight before pregnancy?	The woman's weight baseline is needed to evaluate changes over the course of pregnancy. In the care of the woman who is obese, health professionals should address the issue of obesity but do so in a supportive and positive way to recognise individual needs and expectations. High weight gain in pregnancy increases the risk of large-for-gestational-age babies whereas low weight gain in pregnancy is associated with small-for-gestational-age babies.

ASSESSMENT GUIDELINES AND NORMAL FINDINGS	CLINICAL SIGNIFICANCE AND CLINICAL ALERTS
• When did you last see the dentist? Tell me about your oral care routine.	Gums may be puffy and bleed easily during pregnancy due to the impact of oestrogen on the blood flow and consistency of connective tissue. There is an increase in gingivitis, due to dental plaque, calculus and debris. There may be a transient increase in tooth mobility. Changes in saliva and the nausea and vomiting of pregnancy may increase the risk of caries. Periodontal disease has been associated with intrauterine infection, increased risk of preterm birth and low birth weight risk. The woman needs to take care with brushing her teeth and seek care from her dentist. She needs to advise her dentist of her pregnancy.
• Do you feel safe in your relationship or home environment?	Domestic violence is relatively common during pregnancy. The frequency and severity of violence initiated by a male partner against a woman may be higher during pregnancy. Intimate partner and sexual violence affects a large proportion of the population. The harm caused can last a lifetime, span generations and include serious and adverse effects on the woman's health (AIHW 2018b). Questioning the safety of the woman is part of care. Refer to Chapter 5 for a full discussion of screening for family violence and abuse.
8. Nutritional history	
• What is your vitamin D intake? What is your exposure to natural sunlight?	Vitamin D is essential for bone development in children and skeletal health in adults. It regulates calcium and phosphate absorption and metabolism. Vitamin D is obtained through the direct action of sunlight on the skin (90%) or through dietary nutrients (10%), in particular dairy products, eggs and fish. In the skin, pro-vitamin D is activated by ultraviolet B light to form cholecalciferol (vitamin D_3), which is converted in the liver to 25-hydroxyvitamin D (25-OHD). Reasons for vitamin D deficiency include individuals with darkly pigmented skin, successful skin protection including avoidance of sunlight and sunscreen use, less outdoor activity; and diets lacking in vitamin D. Vitamin D deficiency in pregnancy is very common and linked to several complications such as preeclampsia, gestational diabetes and fetal growth restriction. Vitamin D supplementation during pregnancy is protective of skeletal health of both mother and baby and may improve clinical outcomes for conditions associated with vitamin D deficiency (Pilz et al 2018).

ASSESSMENT GUIDELINES AND NORMAL FINDINGS	CLINICAL SIGNIFICANCE AND CLINICAL ALERTS
• Do you follow a special diet? Are you a vegan?	During pregnancy, growth, development and optimal health rely on good nutrition and adequate quality and quantity of nutrients. For the woman who follows a special diet or is a vegan, encourage and support her to achieve adequate nutrition within the confines of her diet, including carbohydrates, proteins and fats; essential micronutrients, vitamins and minerals as well as water.
• Do you have any food intolerance?	A food intolerance may affect the woman and her fetus's nutrition, such as lactose intolerance limiting calcium intake. It is important the woman informs her healthcare provider of any food intolerances for referral to a dietitian for further support through health education and promotion.
• Do you crave non-foods such as ice, paint chips, dirt or clay? Do you experience food cravings or aversions?	Craving for non-foods is called **'pica'** and is of concern if it prevents the woman from consuming nutrient-rich food. The woman who experiences this condition should be tested for possible iron-deficiency anaemia. Food cravings or aversions during pregnancy are common. For example, the woman may crave highly seasoned foods and develop an aversion to tea, coffee or alcohol. Alcohol consumption is contraindicated during pregnancy.
9. Environment/hazards	
• What is your occupation? What are the physical demands of your work? Are you exposed to any strong odours, chemicals, radiation or other harmful substances?	If the woman's employment is strenuous, physical activity can contribute to fatigue and risk of a diet compromise. If there is heavy lifting or long periods of standing then the woman may need to seek alternative work arrangements. The woman who is a shift worker where there are irregular hours can also experience a compromised diet due to changes in eating patterns. Establish any difficulties that the woman may have at work such as possible teratogenic exposures.
• Do you consider your food and housing adequate?	If appropriate, refer to state and federal programs to assist with food, housing or other needs.
• How do you wear your seat belt when driving?	For maternal and fetal safety, instruct the woman to place the lap belt below the uterus.
• Do you have any other questions or concerns?	Encourage the woman to write down questions between visits or encourage her to have her partner or a support person accompany her to antenatal visits.

SUBJECTIVE DATA

Objective data

The extent of the objective part of a health assessment during pregnancy is dependent on the stage of pregnancy. All procedures are explained to the woman to assist her in informed decision making. Health professionals providing maternity services routinely check the woman's blood pressure, perform an abdominal examination to estimate fundal height, determine fetal position and auscultate the fetal heart rate. The woman's lower limbs need to be checked for the development of oedema, and a urine test needs to be done. Other objective tests and examinations are performed according to the presenting symptoms and signs. When providing antenatal care services, it is also a good opportunity to discuss with the woman and her partner about pregnancy, labour, birth and the time following birth, as well as their expectations and beliefs (cultural and traditional).

Preparation

Ask the woman to empty her bladder (obtain a specimen for analysis) and weigh herself before the following examinations. Assist the woman into a supine position (when the woman is in an advanced stage of pregnancy, she should be positioned in a slight left lateral position to prevent compression of the vena cava).

Equipment needed

Hand hygiene solution
Stethoscope, sphygmomanometer cuff
Centimetre measuring tape
Fetal Doppler
Urine collection containers

PROCEDURES AND NORMAL FINDINGS	ABNORMAL FINDINGS AND CLINICAL ALERTS
General inspection	
Observe the woman's state of nourishment, and her grooming, posture, mood and affect, which reflect her mental state. Throughout the exam, observe her maturity and ability to attend and learn to plan your teaching of the information she needs to successfully complete a healthy pregnancy.	Undernourished or obese. Poor grooming can be a sign of a lack of resources. A slumped posture or flat affect can indicate that the woman is feeling unwell or experiencing depression and is at risk for postpartum depression. A lack of attention may indicate some preoccupation with a concern.
Blood pressure measurement	
Take the blood pressure (BP) when the woman is the most relaxed, in the upright position. Recheck an elevated pressure.	Chronic hypertension is defined when there is a documented history of high BP before pregnancy. Hypertension in pregnancy is defined as a systolic blood pressure greater than or equal to 140 mmHg and/or diastolic blood pressure greater than or equal to 90 mmHg (Korotkoff 5). These measurements should be confirmed by repeated readings over several hours. Elevations of both systolic and diastolic blood pressures are associated with adverse maternal and fetal outcomes (SOMANZ 2015).
Inspection and palpation of skin, mouth, neck, breasts	
Skin	
Note the colour of the skin and any scars (particularly those of previous caesarean delivery). Many women have skin changes during pregnancy that may spontaneously resolve after the pregnancy, or skin lesions present on the upper body. Some women have **chloasma**, known as the 'mask of pregnancy', which is a butterfly-shaped pigmentation of the face. Note the presence of the **linea nigra**, a hyperpigmented line that begins at the sternal notch and extends down the abdomen through the umbilicus to the pubis (Figure 29.5). Also note **striae**, or stretch marks, in areas of weight gain, particularly on the abdomen, breasts and thighs. These marks are bright red when they first form, but they will shrink and lighten to a silvery colour (in the lightly pigmented woman) after the pregnancy (see Figure 29.5).	Multiple bruises may suggest physical abuse and scars (tracks) along easily accessed veins can indicate intravenous drug use. Skin lesions include spider angiomas (also referred to as spider naevi) and palmar erythema usually seen in the first trimester. Skin changes tend to disappear or reduce in size following birth and are thought to be caused by oestrogens.

PROCEDURES AND NORMAL FINDINGS	ABNORMAL FINDINGS AND CLINICAL ALERTS
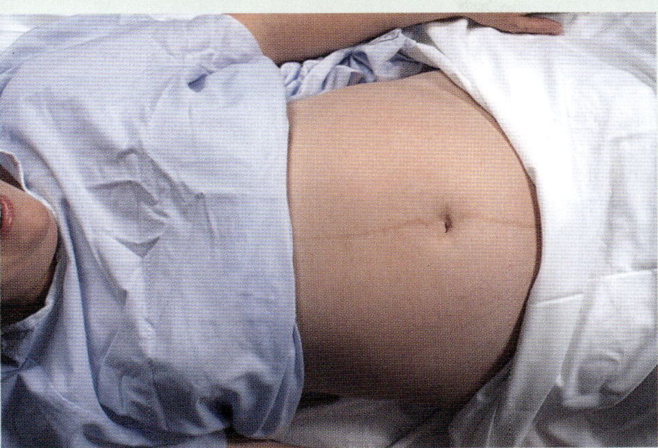 **Figure 29.5** Linea Nigra.	
Mouth	
Mucous membranes should be red and moist. Gingivitis occurs in most women occurring about the second month of pregnancy and peaking in the middle of the third trimester. Oestrogen increases blood flow to the oral cavity and accelerates turnover of gum epithelial lining cells so that they become highly vascularised, hyperplastic and oedematous. The woman can experience bleeding from her gums, particularly after brushing her teeth, discomfort with chewing food, increased periodontal disease and heartburn.	Pale mucous membranes are indicative of anaemia.
Breasts	
The breasts are enlarged (Figure 29.6), perhaps with resulting striae and may be very tender. The areolae and nipples enlarge and darken in pigmentation, the nipples become more erect and 'secondary areolae' (mottling around the areolae) may develop. The blood vessels of the breast enlarge and may shine blue through a seemingly more translucent than usual chest wall. Montgomery's tubercles, located around the areola and responsible for skin integrity of the areola, enlarge. Colostrum, a thick yellow fluid, may be expressed from the nipples. 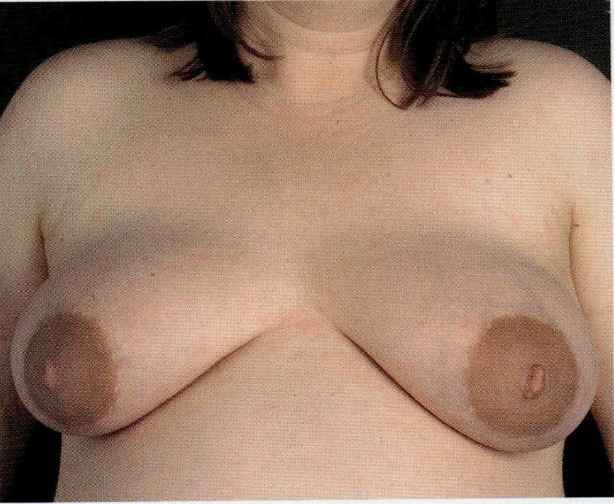 **Figure 29.6** Breasts are enlarged.	

OBJECTIVE DATA

PROCEDURES AND NORMAL FINDINGS	ABNORMAL FINDINGS AND CLINICAL ALERTS
The breast tissue feels nodular as the mammary alveoli increase in size.	Refer any unusual breast changes to other health professionals for further investigation.
Some women have an embryological remnant called a supernumerary nipple, which may or may not have breast tissue beneath it. It could possibly be mistaken previously for a mole. They occur under the arm or in a line directly underneath each nipple on the abdominal wall. This nipple and breast tissue may show the same changes of pregnancy.	
Peripheral vascular assessment (hands, feet, legs)	
The woman may have swelling of her fingers; her legs and feet may show diffuse, bilateral pitting oedema, particularly if the examination is occurring later in the day when she has been on her feet, and especially during the third trimester. Varicose veins in the legs are common in the third trimester. (See also Chapter 14.)	The pregnant woman who has varicosities is at risk for thrombophlebitis. Carefully evaluate any redness or red, hot, tender swelling to rule out phlebitis. It is recommended that the woman not wear restrictive clothing or sit without moving legs for long periods of time. Varicosities will worsen with the weight and volume of pregnancy, and support hosiery is recommended. ***Clinical alert:*** Oedema, together with an increased blood pressure reading and proteinuria, are signs of preeclampsia.
Auscultation of heart and lungs	
Heart	
The woman's heart, due to displacement of the diaphragm and the effect of pregnancy on the shape of the rib cage, is displaced upwards and towards the left, and rotates on its long axis moving the apex laterally. There is enlargement with the greatest change in the left atrium as the blood volume increases in the second and third trimesters. Auscultation of the heart reveals an exaggerated split and loudness of both components of the first heart sounds (mitral and tricuspid valve closure), occurring during second trimester and resolving between 2 and 4 weeks after birth (see Chapter 17: Cardiac assessment).	The woman with preexisting cardiac disease should be managed closely. Alternatively, the woman may be diagnosed with cardiac disease for the first time in pregnancy because of symptoms precipitated by increased demands on the system.
Lungs	
The lungs are clear bilaterally to auscultation with no crackles or wheezing. Shortness of breath is common in the third trimester from pressure of the enlarged uterus on the diaphragm (see Chapter 19: Lower airways assessment).	Changes in lung function during pregnancy related to ventilation, airflow and diffusing capacity. Increased minute volume and tidal volume along with a reduced functional residual capacity all contribute to meeting the increased oxygen requirements of pregnancy and consequently there is minimal effect on respiratory rate. The woman deepens her breathing rather than increasing the rate significantly. The hyperventilation of pregnancy and associated respiratory system alterations are also influenced by the interaction of the acid–base balance changes, increased breathing drive, increased central chemoreflex sensitivity, increased metabolism and decreased cerebral blood flow. When the woman is in labour there is major impact related to muscular and metabolic activity and oxygen consumption (Blackburn 2013). The woman needs to be monitored carefully throughout pregnancy and in particular during labour.

PROCEDURES AND NORMAL FINDINGS	ABNORMAL FINDINGS AND CLINICAL ALERTS
Abdominal examination	
Abdominal examination of the pregnant woman includes inspection, palpation and auscultation of the fetus and is conducted following explanation and informed decision making by the woman—after ensuring the woman's comfort by ensuring she has an empty bladder and privacy. This examination is conducted to observe the signs of pregnancy, assess fetal size, growth, listen to the fetal heart and recognise any deviations from normal.	The uterus is usually non-tender but the examiner should take care to complete an abdominal examination that is gentle. The examiner should be considerate of the risk of possible supine hypotension which can be precipitated by the woman lying flat. The weight of the pregnant uterus compresses the aorta and inferior vena cava which lie slightly to the right of the maternal midline posteriorly. To avoid this, the examination should not be prolonged and the woman encouraged to report any symptoms such as feeling dizzy or lightheaded. Should this occur the woman should be immediately moved into a left lateral position. Following completion, the examiner should give an explanation of findings, health education and promotion to facilitate self-care.
Inspect the abdomen	
Inspect the size, shape and contours of the abdomen to discern fetal position; any incision scars from any previous operations and striae. As the woman lifts her head, **diastasis recti**, the separation of the rectus muscles, may be visible. This separation occurs during pregnancy, is most likely to occur in multiparous women or those with a multiple pregnancy or polyhydramnios. Diastasis recti can take up to 2 years to resolve.	
Palpate the abdomen	
The uterine fundus is usually palpable abdominally from 12 weeks' gestation. In using the ulnar border of the hand that is placed at the uppermost point of the fundus of the uterus, the examiner begins palpating centrally on the abdomen higher than where the uterus is expected to be and continues to palpate down until the fundus (the top of the uterus) is located. This is called fundal palpation and assists in the estimation of gestation in terms of weeks in comparison with the size. Symphyseal fundal (S-F) height measurement is another method of estimating gestational age using a tape measure (described below). The next step for abdominal examination is for the examiner to stand at the woman's right side facing her head (Figure 29.7). The examiner's palm of the right hand is placed on the curve of the uterus in the left lower quadrant, with the left palm on the curve of the uterus in the right lower quadrant. Following the curve of the uterus serves as a guide for the examiner to 'walk' fingers of both hands until they meet centrally at the fundus. This is called lateral palpation and facilitates identification of the fetal back and head. Other palpation manoeuvres used later in pregnancy are presented below.	Palpation of the abdomen should be gently performed and after ensuring the woman's informed consent and physical comfort (i.e. empty bladder and privacy).

PROCEDURES AND NORMAL FINDINGS	ABNORMAL FINDINGS AND CLINICAL ALERTS
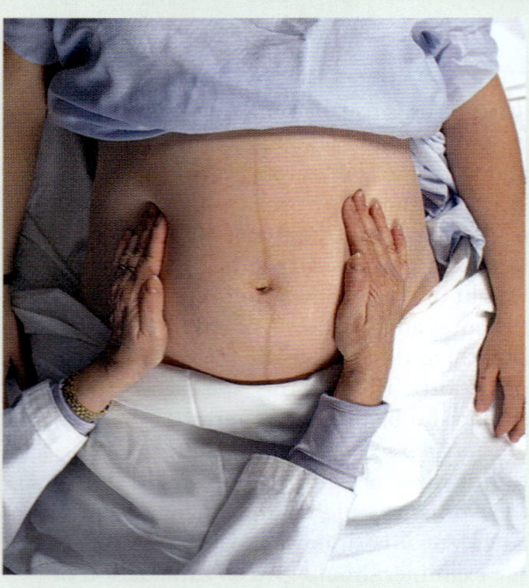 **Figure 29.7** Abdominal examination at the woman's right side facing her head.	
Note the fundal location by referring to landmarks and fingerbreadths, as described in Figure 29.2. Note that individual variations of landmarks and examiner's variations using fingerbreadths make this measurement an inexact but helpful guide. The fundal height measurement should be done with the woman lying flat with her head supported on a single pillow. It is recommended when using the symphyseal fundal (S-F) height assessment, that the tape measure (non-elastic) is used with the scale placed downwards, starting from the fundus of the uterus to the fixed point of the symphysis pubis (Figure 29.8). After 20 weeks, the number of centimetres should approximate the number of weeks of gestation. S-F measurement may provide a degree of reliability and consistency not given by palpation (Department of Health 2018). 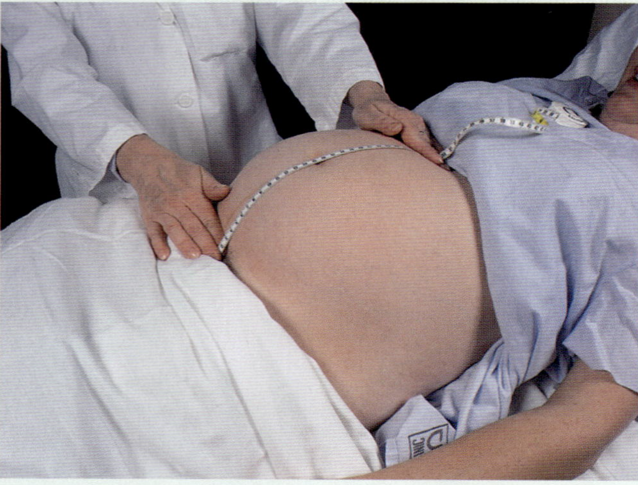 **Figure 29.8** Assessing the fundal height using tape measure.	Ensure the woman's comfort when examining her and be aware of the risk of supine hypotension when in supine position for extended periods. Compare the finding with the previous assessments and measurements.
At approximately 20 weeks' gestation, the examiner may feel fetal movements and the fetal presenting part and from about 25 weeks affirm that fetal growth is consistent with the gestational age. As from 36 weeks' gestation, the presenting part, preferably the fetal head, can be ballotted (moved easily using an external manoeuvre).	

OBJECTIVE DATA

PROCEDURES AND NORMAL FINDINGS	ABNORMAL FINDINGS AND CLINICAL ALERTS
The palpation techniques for identifying the fetal presenting part and other information in the late stages of pregnancy are presented below. In the third trimester, determine fetal size, presentation, lie, attitude, position and whether or not engagement of the presenting part has occurred at approximately 37 weeks in the primigravida woman. This information can be determined from fundal, lateral and pelvic palpations. When performing the fundal palpation, the examiner is facing the woman's head and places both hands on the sides of the fundus of the uterus, with fingers held close together, and gently curving round the upper border of the uterus (Figure 29.9). Gentle but deliberate pressure is applied to determine soft buttocks or a firm fetal head. The purpose of this palpation is to determine fetal size and presentation. The lateral palpation is used to locate the fetal back to assist in determining fetal position and fetal lie, the orientation of the fetal spine to the maternal spine (Figure 29.10). The fetal lie is ideally a longitudinal one. **Presentation** describes the part of the fetus that is entering the pelvis first. **Attitude** refers to the position of fetal parts in relation to each other. Attitudes may include flexed, straight or extended. Ideally the presenting part should be the fetal head with the neck in a well-flexed position so that the smallest diameter passes through the pelvis. **Position** designates the location of a fetal part to the right or left of the maternal pelvis. **Engagement** occurs when the widest diameter of the presenting part has passed through the maternal pelvic brim.	***Clinical alert:*** Fetal size not equivalent to the number of weeks of gestation. If the woman is a primigravida and engagement of the presenting part has not occurred late in her pregnancy, this may require careful assessment and monitoring for possible cephalopelvic disproportion.

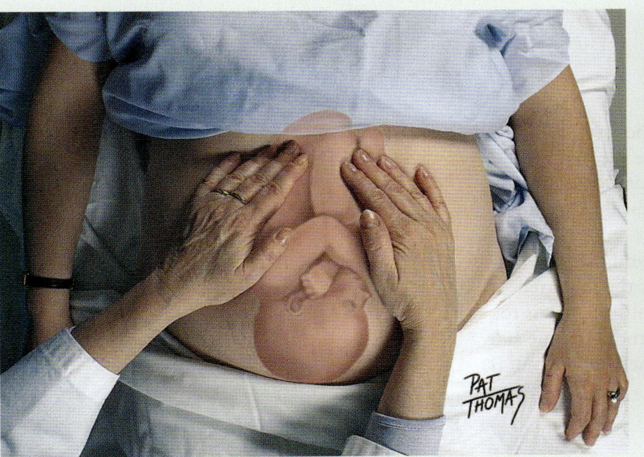

Figure 29.9
Fundal palpation.

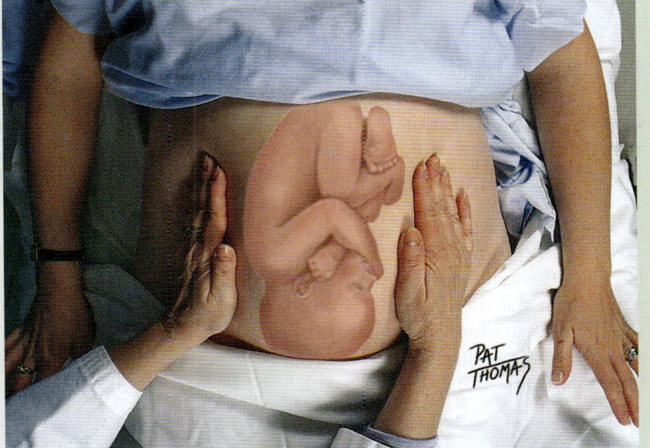

Figure 29.10
Lateral palpation.

Lower abdominal palpation includes **Pawlik's manoeuvre** and deep pelvic palpation. These techniques assess what part of the fetus is presenting at the pelvis and the engagement of the presenting part in late pregnancy. For Pawlik's manoeuvre, the woman is requested to bend her knees up slightly (Figure 29.11) to relax her abdominal muscles and to breathe steadily and slowly to support relaxation. The examiner grasps the lower pole of the uterus between the fingers that are spread sufficiently wide to accommodate a fetal head, to assess mobility of the presenting part. If the presenting part is engaging, it will feel 'fixed'.	

PROCEDURES AND NORMAL FINDINGS	ABNORMAL FINDINGS AND CLINICAL ALERTS

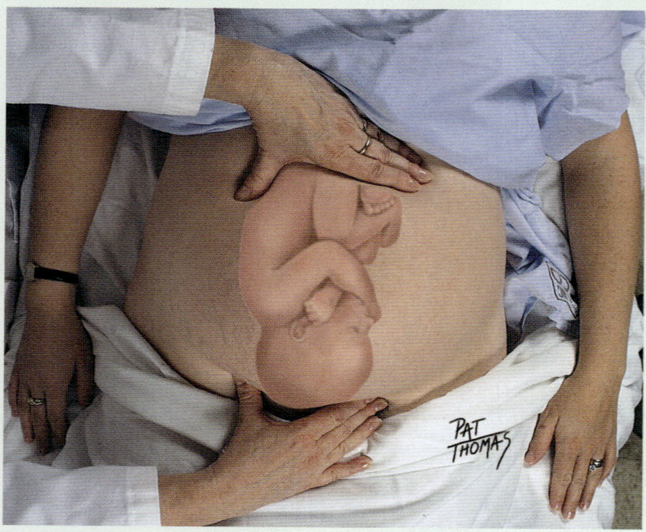

Figure 29.11
Pawlick's Manoeuvre.

Deep pelvic palpation assists in determining fetal presentation and the level of engagement by estimating the amount of the fetal head palpable above the maternal pelvic brim (Figure 29.12). This can be a most uncomfortable procedure for the woman and, once again, request her to bend her knees and breathe steadily and slowly to support relaxation.

To perform this procedure the examiner stands alongside the woman and faces towards her feet. The examiner places one hand on each side of the uterus near the maternal pelvic brim and then carefully sinks the fingers gently and smoothly into the pelvis to feel the presentation. If the finger tips can sink further into the pelvis more on one side than the other, it suggests that the fetal presenting part is flexed and the fetal occiput is on the side opposite to that into which the fingers sink more deeply.

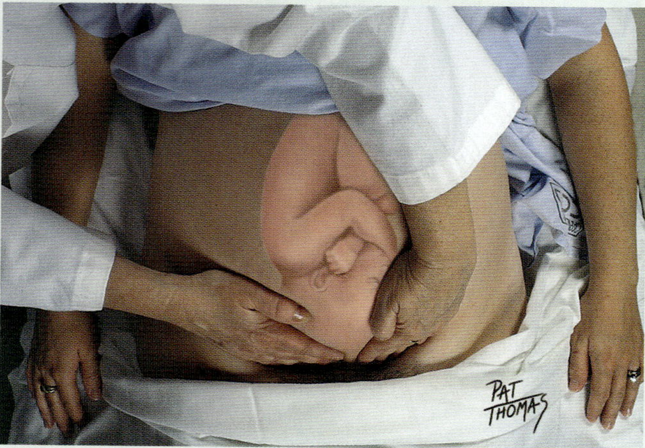

Figure 29.12
Pelvic palpation (fingers are directed inwards and downwards).

OBJECTIVE DATA

PROCEDURES AND NORMAL FINDINGS	ABNORMAL FINDINGS AND CLINICAL ALERTS
See Figure 29.13 for various fetal positions and where to auscultate the fetal heart beats for each. At the end of pregnancy, 97% of fetal presentations are vertex, 2.7% are breech, 0.05% are face and 0.3% are shoulder (Bloom et al 2018).	Most common fetal presentations: Vertex: head first Breech: buttocks first See Table 29.4.

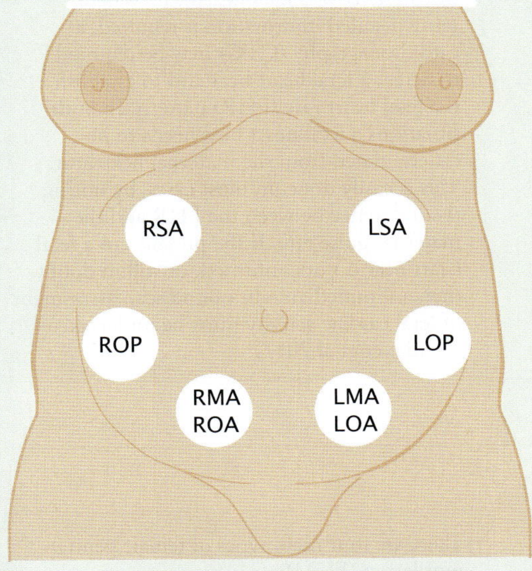

RSA and LSA = right and left sacral anterior (breech)
RMA and LMA = right and left mentum anterior (face)
ROA and LOA = right and left occiput anterior (vertex)
ROP and LOP = right and left occiput posterior (vertex)

Figure 29.13
Fetal positions.

Auscultation of the fetal heart

PROCEDURES AND NORMAL FINDINGS	ABNORMAL FINDINGS AND CLINICAL ALERTS
Identification of the fetal heart rate is a positive sign of pregnancy and can be heard by fetal Doppler from 10 weeks' gestation. The fetal heart rate is best auscultated over the shoulder of the fetus. After identifying the position of the fetus (see Figure 29.13), count the fetal heart beats for a complete minute (Figure 29.14). The normal rate is between 110 and 160 beats per minute. Spontaneous accelerations of fetal heart sounds indicate fetal wellbeing.	A handheld Doppler can immediately confirm the presence of a fetal heart beat so that it can be assessed for rate and rhythm (Bloom et al 2018).

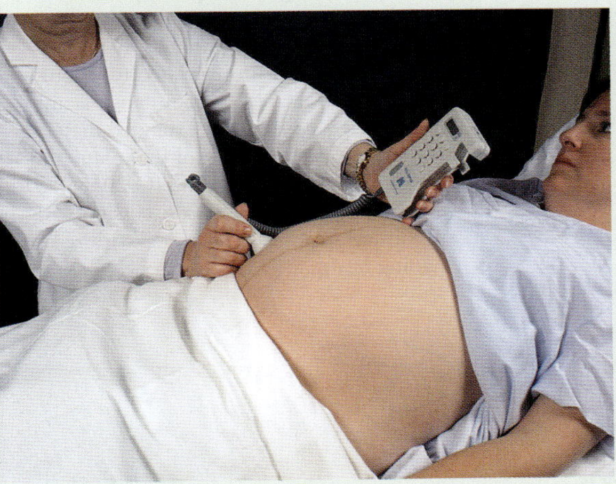

Figure 29.14
Auscultation of the fetal heart using a Doppler.

OBJECTIVE DATA

PROCEDURES AND NORMAL FINDINGS	ABNORMAL FINDINGS AND CLINICAL ALERTS
Sometimes there can be difficulties in locating the fetal heart due to the fetal position (e.g. posterior position) or activity.	Support the woman by an explanation of the fetal movement activity you are noting. A handheld Doppler can immediately confirm the presence of a fetal heartbeat. Where more detailed information is required, a cardiotocography (CTG) may be required to detect a fetal heart beat and to establish the fetal heart rate (FHR) pattern. In both situations a fetal heart beat needs to be differentiated from the maternal heartbeat. This is easily done, in most cases, by noting the difference between the FHR and the maternal pulse rate. If the presence of a fetal heart beat is not confirmed, or still in doubt, then an immediate ultrasound scan assessment of fetal cardiac activity must be undertaken (Gardener et al 2017).
Pelvic examination	
Genitalia	
Use the procedure for the pelvic examination described in Chapter 26 performed following informed consent from the woman. Observe the vulva for the presence of varicosities, oedema and lesions and whether or not there is scarring from a previous perineal injury or episiotomy; and for the presence of haemorrhoids of the rectum. In addition, observe for the presence of female genital mutilation (FGM), particularly for types III and IV. The FGM procedure that seals or narrows a vaginal opening (type III (at right)) needs to be cut open later to allow for sexual intercourse and childbirth. Sometimes the woman goes through repeated opening and closing procedures, further increasing both immediate and long-term risks (WHO 2018a).	There are four main types of female genital mutilation (FGM): *Type I:* Partial or total removal of the clitoris and/or the prepuce (clitoridectomy). *Type II:* Partial or total removal of the clitoris and the labia minora, with or without excision of the labia majora (excision). *Type III:* Narrowing of the vaginal orifice with creation of a covering seal by the cutting of and apposition of the labia minora and/or the labia majora, with or without excision of the clitoris (infibulation). *Type IV:* All other harmful procedures to the female genitalia for non-medical purposes, e.g. pricking, piercing, incising, scraping and cauterisation. Women with FGM are more likely to experience complications related to labour and birth such as caesarean section, postpartum haemorrhage, episiotomy, extended maternal hospital stay, resuscitation of the infant and inpatient perinatal death (WHO 2018a). The woman with FGM requires discussion with appropriate healthcare providers with regard to ongoing health after childbirth.
The maternal and fetal health screening	
Before laboratory tests are carried out, it is essential to explain to the woman and her partner what screening tests are available and that results are confidential. This assists in an informed decision making process. Further, give advice that there are processes for follow-up on positive test results and that the woman who declines testing is offered the opportunity to discuss any concerns without being coerced to reconsider the test (Department of Health 2018).	

OBJECTIVE DATA

PROCEDURES AND NORMAL FINDINGS	ABNORMAL FINDINGS AND CLINICAL ALERTS
Maternal screening tests include blood group, haemoglobin, full blood examination (FBE), ferritin, gestational diabetes (between 24 and 28 weeks' gestation) and screening tests for human immunodeficiency virus (HIV), syphilis, rubella, hepatitis B, hepatitis C, vitamin D.	For a woman with a Rhesus-negative blood group, it is recommended that the presence of Rhesus antibodies is identified. Rhesus antibodies form due to a feto-maternal haemorrhage when fetal Rhesus-positive cells are released into the maternal circulation. This can occur during procedures such as amniocentesis or chorionic villi sampling, antepartum haemorrhage or at the time of birth. When exchange of cells occurs, the administration of anti-D immunoglobin is administered. Anti-D immunoglobin is effective in preventing the production of antibodies and is recommended and administered according to guidelines (Royal Australian and New Zealand College of Obstetricians and Gynaecologists (RANZCOG) 2019). The woman is to be informed that she needs to report any bleeding so that anti-D is administered to protect the fetus from haemolysis. Blood needs to be tested for Rhesus antibody titres prior to administration of anti-D. At 34 weeks, the titre level may be omitted if prophylactic anti-D was given at 28 weeks (RANZCOG 2019). The National Notifiable Diseases Surveillance System (NNDSS) must be advised of notifiable infections. These include HIV, hepatitis B, hepatitis C, rubella, syphilis (Department of Health 2018).
Clean catch specimen of urine. Urinalysis for proteinuria and laboratory microbiology testing for asymptomatic bacteriuria.	Any abnormalities detected on dipstick urine testing should be referred to a medical practitioner for further investigation. The presence of proteinuria is potentially a sign of preeclampsia (a serious multi system pregnancy disorder.)
Vaginal swabs for chlamydia, bacterial vaginosis and group B streptococcal disease (GBS).	Group B streptococcus infection: approximately 25% of women have GBS in their lower genital tract and rectum, but are usually asymptomatic. The aim of this screening test is to prevent neonatal infection through the administration of antibiotic therapy to the woman. Early onset GBS disease (EOGBS) is defined as occurring in infants less than 1 week old and is acquired through vertical transmission from colonised mothers. Clinical presentations include sepsis, pneumonia and meningitis.

PROCEDURES AND NORMAL FINDINGS	ABNORMAL FINDINGS AND CLINICAL ALERTS
Weight and height measure at the first antenatal appointment and the BMI calculation (Department of Health 2018). Cervical screening test is performed if the woman is overdue, having not complied with the recommended screening timeframes.	
Ultrasound screening for chromosomal abnormality must be done between the 11th and 14th weeks of pregnancy (when the fetus has a crown–rump length of 45–84 mm). In addition to this, an NIPT test is also available from 10 weeks' gestation. This test analyses maternal blood for cell-free deoxyribonucleic acid (cfDNA), with a greater than expected number of relevant chromosome fragments present in genetic fetal abnormality such as Down syndrome. The NIPT test may be offered as a first line test, combined with first trimester screening or in addition to first trimester screening where intermediate risk has been identified (Department of Health 2018). Women who present later in pregnancy (14–20 weeks) are offered second trimester maternal serum screening for fetal chromosomal anomaly.	It needs to be explained to the woman what chromosomal abnormalities may be diagnosed, the available tests, the gestation of pregnancy at which these should be undertaken, the process of the procedure and the risks involved. The woman is presented with options to consider if a chromosomal abnormality is identified (e.g. continuation of the pregnancy or termination where this is permitted under jurisdictional legislation) and the need for additional care if the pregnancy continues (e.g. specialist management of the pregnancy and the baby); long-term implications for the woman and her family of having an affected baby and the health and development issues for children with the condition. There needs to be consideration of the impact on a woman and her family of a false negative or false positive result (i.e. anxiety among women receiving false positives may remain) (Department of Health 2018). When fetal abnormalities are detected, the woman requires information and referral to other health professionals for ongoing support.
Ultrasound during the first trimester, usually between 8 and 11 weeks' gestation, is used to confirm gestational age, check the pregnancy when there has been a complication such as bleeding, view the position of the placenta, confirm presence of multiple pregnancy and check fetal growth, physical development and viability. Ultrasound is available to the woman at 18–20 weeks' gestation to obtain information about anatomical structures including internal organs, head, limbs, spine and assessment of fetal growth.	Ultrasound can detect neural tube defects (e.g. anencephaly, an absence of a major portion of the brain; spina bifida, where spinal cord and meninges are exposed through a gap in the vertebrae), cardiac defects, gastrointestinal malformations (gastroschisis, a deficit in the abdominal wall resulting in herniation of gastric organs; exomphalos, herniation of abdominal organs due to a defect around the umbilical cord area), limb defects, central nervous system defects and urinary tract anomalies.

Summary Checklist

THE PREGNANT WOMAN

Subjective data

1. Menstrual history
2. Gynaecological history
3. Obstetric history
4. Current pregnancy
5. Medical history
6. Family history
7. General health history
8. Nutritional history
9. Environment/hazards

Objective data

1. General inspection
2. Measure the blood pressure
3. Inspect and palpate the skin, mouth and breasts
4. Peripheral vascular assessment
5. Auscultate heart and lung sounds
6. Abdominal examination
7. Auscultate the fetal heart
8. Pelvic examination
9. Screen for maternal and fetal health

Documentation and critical thinking

FOCUSED ASSESSMENT: CLINICAL CASE STUDY

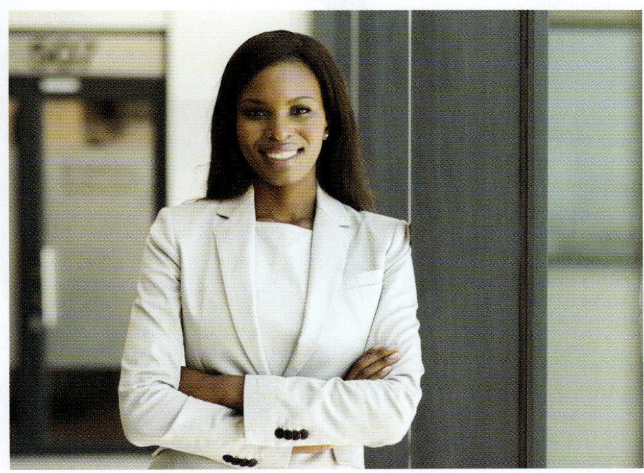

Context

Ms Imani Otieno, a 29-year-old woman, gravida 2 para 1, presents with her husband and daughter for her first antenatal visit to a midwife working in a general practice setting.

Subjective

Imani works full-time as a financial planner. Last normal menstrual period (LNMP) was 4 April of this year (certain of date), with an expected date of birth (EDB) of 11 January of next year, thereby making her 10 weeks' gestation today. Her history includes a normal vaginal birth of a term female infant (Anna) 3 years ago, after a 12-hour-long labour. Imani sustained a small perineal tear that did not require suturing. She breastfed Anna for 1 year. The current pregnancy was planned. Imani is experiencing breast tenderness, and nausea on occasion, which resolves with dry biscuits and ginger tea. No past medical or surgical conditions are present. She has no known allergies. Imani has no significant family history relevant to pregnancy.

Objective

General: Appears well nourished and is carefully groomed.

Skin: Dark skin tone, surface smooth with no lesions.

Mouth: Good dentition and oral hygiene. Oral mucosa pink, no gum hypertrophy.

Chest: Expansion equal, respirations effortless. Lung sounds clear bilaterally with no adventitious sounds.

Heart: Rate 76 bpm, regular rhythm, S_1 and S_2 are identified.

Breasts: Tender, without masses, with supple, everted nipples. Breast awareness discussed.

Abdomen: Bowel sounds present. No masses on palpation. Uterus nonpalpable.

Extremities: No varicosities, redness or oedema. BP 110/68 in semi-recumbent position.

Diagnostics: Dating scan done to reveal a single viable uterine pregnancy, gestation equals last normal menstrual period dates.

Pregnancy health status

Intrauterine pregnancy 10 weeks gestation.

Imani and her husband are happy with the pregnancy; she feels well apart from some breast tenderness and occasional nausea.

Abnormal findings for advanced practice

TABLE 29.1 Preeclampsia

Normal pregnancy is characterised by a slight fall in blood pressure, usually reaching its lowest point in the second trimester and rises to pre-conception levels by term.

Accurate blood pressure measurements are important as levels can impact on the woman's health.

Systolic blood pressure greater than or equal to 140 mmHg and/or diastolic blood pressure greater than or equal to 90 mmHg (Korotkoff 5) after 20 weeks is classified as gestational hypertension.

Accurate blood pressure measurement is important as the level may result in changes in clinical management. It is recommended that the woman should be seated comfortably with her legs resting on a flat surface and her arm resting at the level of her heart. During labour, the woman's blood pressure may be measured while she is in a lateral position to avoid the risk of supine hypotension.

Preeclampsia is a multi-system disorder unique to human pregnancy characterised by hypertension and involvement of one or more other organ systems and/or the fetus when there is an impact on placental perfusion. It is a condition that is unique to human pregnancy with hypertension but this is not always the first manifestation. Proteinuria is the most commonly recognised additional feature after hypertension but should not be considered mandatory to make the clinical diagnosis. Other features of this condition can include central nervous system irritability and possible coagulation or liver function abnormalities. Women with preeclampsia may develop seizures (eclampsia) or a variant with abnormal liver function and thrombocytopenia referred to as HELLP syndrome.

The pathogenesis of preeclampsia is thought to be due to ischaemia or hypoxia of the placenta as a consequence of defective progression of spiral artery remodelling and placental angiogenesis (Blackburn 2013). Preeclampsia places the woman and her fetus at increased risk of morbidity and mortality.

Healthcare providers have an important role in providing the woman with information related to symptoms of preeclampsia such as severe headaches, visual disturbances, epigastric pain or sudden marked generalised oedema (Pairman et al 2019, Department of Health 2018).

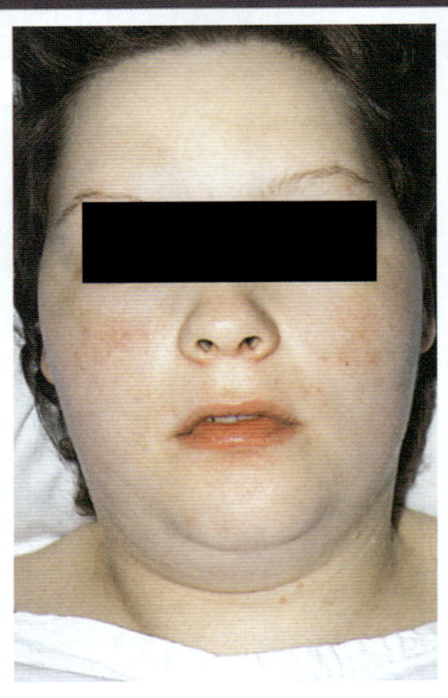

TABLE 29.2 Fetal size inconsistent with dates

SIZE SMALL FOR DATES	Fundal height measures smaller than expected for gestation or not increasing from previous measurements.
Inaccuracy of dates	Conception may have occurred later than originally thought. Reconsider the woman's menstrual history, sexual history, contraceptive use, early pregnancy testing, early sizing of the uterus, ultrasound results, timing of pregnancy symptoms, including the date of quickening, and the fundal height measurements. If, after this review, the EDB is correct, then further investigation is required.
Premature labour	Premature labour occurs before 37 completed weeks of gestation. Possible causes include previous preterm birth; preterm rupture of membranes, multiple pregnancy, antepartum haemorrhage, systemic infections, genital tract infections, cervical insufficiency and congenital uterine abnormalities.
Fetal growth restriction	Fetal growth restriction (FGR) refers to the fetus not reaching the growth potential during pregnancy related to placental insufficiency. FGR is recognised by an estimated fetal weight or serial antenatal ultrasound evidence of growth restriction or growth arrest and is associated with fetal morbidity and mortality (Gardener et al 2017).
Oligohydramnios	Oligohydramnios is a reduction in amniotic fluid volume and is seen in post-term gestations, a fetus diagnosed with fetal growth restriction (FGR) and those with congenital anomalies. A low AFI (0–5 cm) alone or in combination with other findings is a strong predictor of fetal intolerance of labour and Apgar scores less than 7 at 5 min after birth. For women at term, the diagnosis of oligohydramnios is an indication to expedite birth or daily monitoring (Blackburn 2013).
Fetal position	Fetal position varies until about 34 weeks, when the vertex should settle into the pelvis and remain there. The fetus occupying a transverse lie, or shoulder presentation, results in the maternal abdomen widening from side to side and the fundal height diminishing. Fetal malposition may occur with lax maternal abdominal musculature (simply not holding the baby in close), an abnormality in the fetus (e.g. the enlarged head of the hydrocephalic infant), placenta praevia (the placenta being implanted over the cervix, blocking fetal descent) or a restricted maternal pelvis.

TABLE 29.2 Fetal size inconsistent with dates—cont'd	
SIZE LARGE FOR DATES	Fundal height measures larger than expected for dates.
Inaccuracy of dates	Review the same findings as listed above.
Gestational trophoblastic disease	Gestational trophoblastic disease includes hydatidiform mole (complete mole) or molar pregnancy and choriocarcinoma. Hydatidiform mole occurs as a result of degeneration of the chorionic villi at an early age in pregnancy and where the embryo is absent. For this condition, the woman can experience an exacerbation of the minor disorders of pregnancy such as nausea and breast tenderness. Other findings include the uterus larger than for the gestational period and without location of fetal parts. The woman requires careful evacuation of the mole; intensive treatment of this condition may also include chemotherapy. Choriocarcinoma is a malignant, rapidly spreading disease of trophoblastic tissue that is fatal unless it is treated early.
Multiple fetuses	The frequency of multiple fetuses increases with advanced maternal age and is enhanced by the increasing use of fertility drugs. The uterus enlarges where the fundal height may be beyond the calculated/expected gestational age. Ultrasound examination confirms the diagnosis.
Polyhydramnios	Polyhydramnios determined by the amniotic fluid index (AFI) based on the largest amniotic fluid pocket seen on ultrasound (≥ 25 cm at any gestational age or a maximum vertical pocket of ≥ 8 cm depth). The earlier polyhydramnios presents in pregnancy, the greater amount of fluid. This condition can occur gradually during pregnancy or rapidly over a few days or weeks and is usually idiopathic but is associated with maternal disease, multiple gestation, immune and non-immune hydrops, Down syndrome and fetal gastrointestinal, cardiac and neural tube anomalies (Blackburn 2013).
Fibroids (leiomyomata)	Fibroids are preexisting benign tumours of the myometrium of which the woman may be unaware until they are identified during pregnancy. They may be located anywhere in the myometrium and it can be difficult to predict the impact of fibroids on the woman's pregnancy because of their possible number, size and location. During pregnancy fibroid growth is oestrogen- and probably progesterone-dependent and by mid-pregnancy the fibroids may enlarge further. Fibroids with a stalk-like attachment to the uterus occasionally undergo torsion, causing the woman pain. During pregnancy other issues caused by the presence of fibroids include preterm labour, fetal malpresentation such as a transverse lie, obstructed labour and postpartum haemorrhage. Careful assessment supported by ultrasound can assist in a management plan for the childbearing woman. Fibroids stop growing and often calcify after menopause (Impey & Child 2017).
Fetal macrosomia	Macrosomia describes a newborn that is significantly larger than average, e.g. birth weight greater than 4000 to 4500 g in which the birth weight is above the 90th percentile. Fetal macrosomia is more typically associated with women with preexisting diabetes or gestational diabetes where the maternal pancreas has increased insulin secretion to counter the pregnancy-induced insulin resistance. Maternal hyperglycaemia can lead to fetal hyperglycaemia and hyperinsulinaemia resulting in excessive fetal growth. It is therefore important that the woman maintains glycaemic control to reduce the risk of fetal macrosomia. Birth risks to the mother include an increased incidence for caesarean birth, bladder trauma and vaginal tissue trauma. Fetal/neonatal risks include birth trauma such as fractured clavicle and brachial plexus nerve damage from shoulder dystocia, depressed Apgar scores, extended hospitalisations and possible mortality.

ABNORMAL FINDINGS FOR ADVANCED PRACTICE

TABLE 29.3 Disorders of pregnancy

DISORDER/CONDITION	DESCRIPTION
Vaginal bleeding	Some women will have bright red, pink or dark brown spotting at some time during the first trimester. This is not always a sign of pending pregnancy loss but may be from a blighted ovum, friable cervix, ectopic pregnancy, perigestational haemorrhage or cervical lesions. In the second and third trimester, vaginal bleeding may be indicative of placenta abruptio, placenta praevia, uterine rupture, cervical dilation or a friable cervix. Risk factors for placental abruption include increasing parity and maternal age, cigarette smoking, cocaine, trauma (e.g. motor vehicle accident) and preterm pre-labour rupture of membranes (PPROM). This is defined as spontaneous rupture of the membranes before the onset of labour and prior to 37 weeks' gestation. Other possible causes of vaginal bleeding late in pregnancy include rapid uterine decompression associated with multiple gestation or polyhydramnios and maternal hypertensive conditions during pregnancy.
Cervical shortening and insufficiency	Cervical shortening (cervical length of 25 mm or less at 18–20 weeks' gestation) and cervical insufficiency (structural weakness of the cervix). Cervical insufficiency can occur as a consequence of disruption to the complex remodelling process of the cervix during pregnancy. It can result in pregnancy loss or preterm birth that is characterised by recurrent painless dilation of the cervix and is either a congenital or acquired (e.g. by previous surgery) condition. Cervical length is most accurately measured by transvaginal ultrasound and only after the woman has emptied her bladder. The management can include conservative approaches such as vaginal progesterone or cervical surveillance (using transvaginal ultrasound serial scans).
Hyperemesis gravidarum	Hyperemesis gravidarum is a serious and potentially life-threatening form of nausea and vomiting, occurring early in pregnancy, gradually resolving during the middle of the second trimester. If not managed, this condition can interfere with electrolytes, acid-base balance and nutritional status. Dehydration and starvation may ensue and lead to fetal growth restriction. The exact cause of hyperemesis gravidarum is unknown but is believed to be related to the placenta and human chorionic gonadotrophin (hCG); hyperthyroidism may be caused by high levels of hCG. Risk factors include a previous history of hyperemesis, multiple gestation and molar pregnancy. The woman experiencing this condition requires woman-centred care. This care may also include referrals to other health professionals to provide the level of support for her emotional health and wellbeing.
Preterm labour	Preterm labour is labour occurring after 20 weeks' and before completion of 37 weeks' gestation. Preterm labour is a major factor for fetal morbidity and mortality. Risk factors include previous preterm birth, preterm rupture of membranes, multiple pregnancy, obesity, diabetes, systemic infections, urogenital tract infections and cervical insufficiency (Department of Health 2018).
Decreased fetal movement (DFM)	Fetal movement is an indicator of fetal wellbeing and generalised activity usually increases in frequency until approximately 32 weeks' gestation (although fetal movements do not decrease after 32 weeks) (Blackburn 2013). The pregnant woman should be routinely provided with verbal and written information regarding normal fetal movements. This information should include a description of the changing patterns of movement as the fetus develops, normal wake/sleep cycles and factors which may modify the woman's perception of movements such as maternal weight and placental position. The woman who is concerned by decreased or absent fetal movements is advised to make immediate contact with her healthcare provider. This assessment should preferably be undertaken within 2 hours of the woman reporting her concern. Women who report DFM should be assessed for the presence of other risk factors associated with an increased risk of stillbirth (e.g. fetal growth restriction, hypertension, diabetes, advanced maternal age) (Gardener et al 2017).

TABLE 29.4 Malpresentations of the fetus

Malpresentations may be detected by the hands of an experienced examiner, confirmed by the fetal heart beat location and further confirmed by ultrasound. Before 34 weeks' gestation, any position is normal. As assessed via abdominal examination a cephalic presentation is desirable thereafter because spontaneous turning becomes less likely as the fetus grows in proportion to the amount of space and fluid in the uterus and pelvis. Malpresentations of the fetus can include breech, shoulder, face and brow presentations.

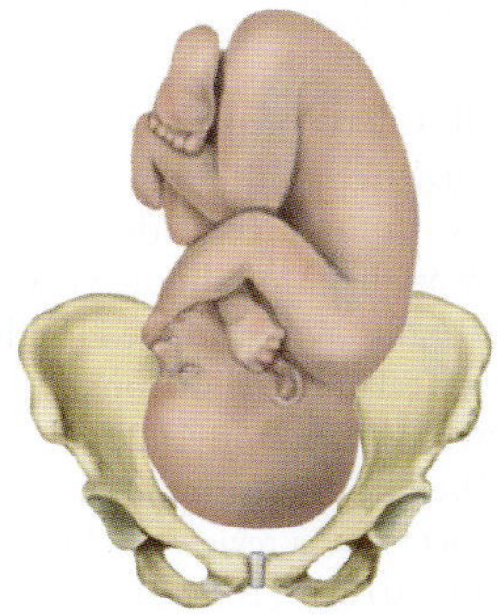
Vertex (for comparison)

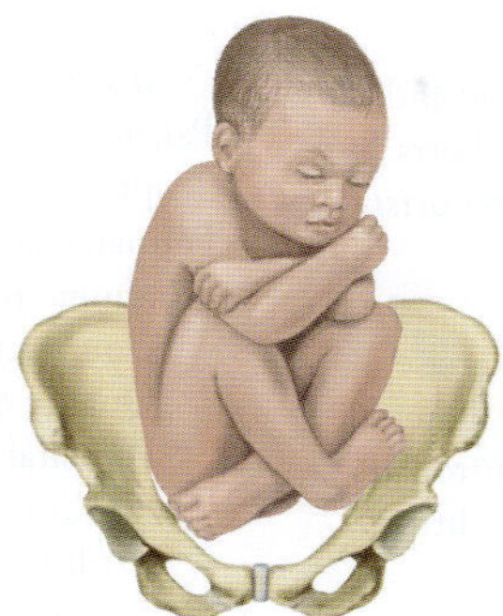
Complete breech

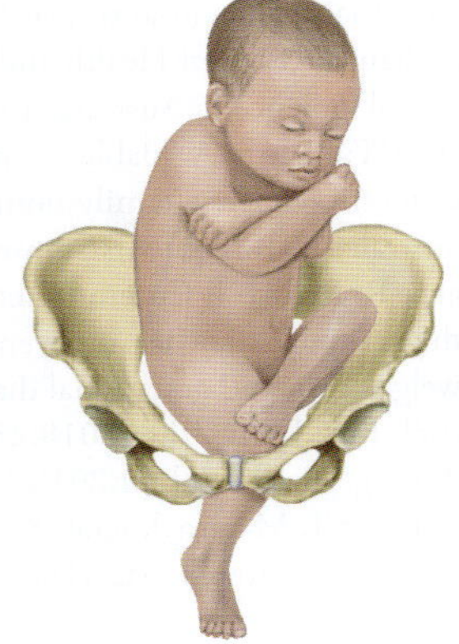
Footling breech

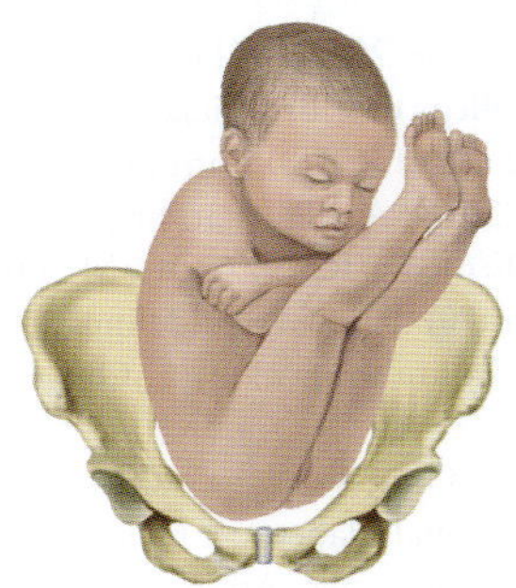
Frank breech

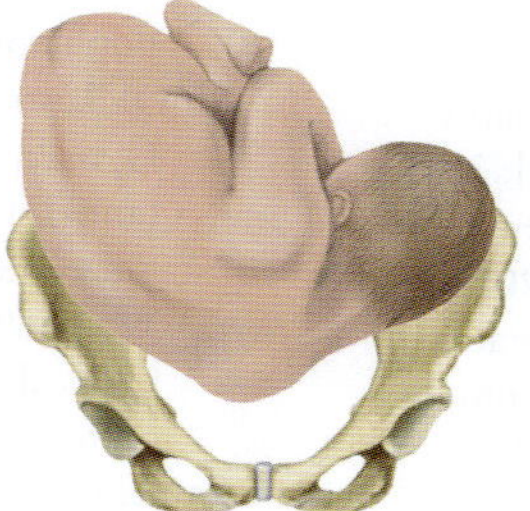
Transverse lie and shoulder presentation

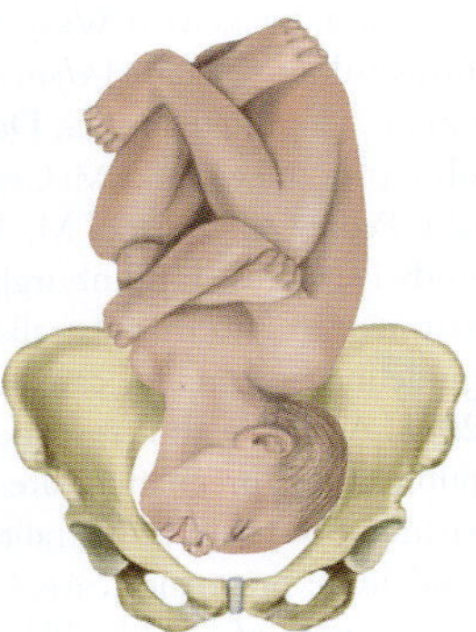
Face presentation

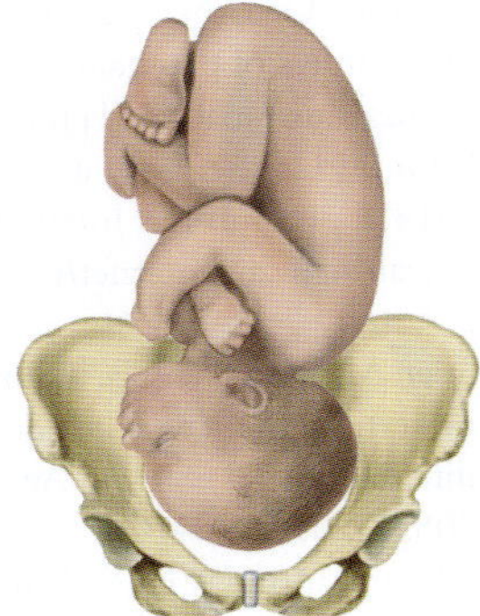
Brow presentation

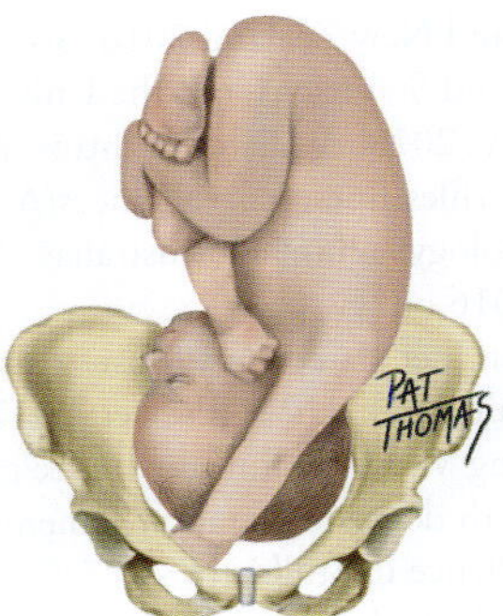

Compound presentation

ABNORMAL FINDINGS FOR ADVANCED PRACTICE

BIBLIOGRAPHY

Abbott J, Bowyer L, Finn M. Obstetrics and gynaecology: an evidence-based guide. 2nd ed. Edinburgh: Churchill Livingstone; 2014.

Australian Institute of Health and Welfare (AIHW). Australia's mothers and babies: Maternal Deaths in Australia 2016. 2018a. Available at: https://www.aihw.gov.au/reports/mothers-babies/maternal-deaths-in-australia-2016/contents/report.

Australian Institute of Health and Welfare. Family, domestic and sexual violence in Australia 2018. Cat. no. FDV 2. Canberra: AIHW; 2018b. Available at: https://www.aihw.gov.au/reports/domestic-violence/family-domestic-sexual-violence-in-australia-2018/contents/summary.

Barakat R, Refoyo I, Coteron J, et al. Original research: Exercise during pregnancy has a preventative effect on excessive maternal weight gain and gestational diabetes. A randomized controlled trial. Braz J Phys Ther 2018;23(2):148–55. Available at: https://doi.org/10.1016/j.bjpt.2018.11.005.

Blackburn ST. Maternal, fetal, & neonatal physiology: a clinical perspective. 4th ed. Maryland Heights, MO: Elsevier Saunders; 2013.

Blanchard-Rohner G, Eberhardt C. Review of maternal immunisation during pregnancy: focus on pertussis and influenza. Swiss Med Wkly 2017;147:w14526. Available at: https://doi.org/10.4414/smw.2017.14526.

Bloom SL, Cunningham FG, Dashe JS, et al., editors. Williams obstetrics. New York: McGraw-Hill Education Medical; 2018.

Coad J, Pedley A, Dunstall M. Anatomy and physiology for midwives. 4th ed. Edinburgh: Churchill Livingstone; 2019.

Department of Health, Australian Government. Clinical practice guidelines: pregnancy care. Canberra: Australian Government; 2018. Available at: https://beta.health.gov.au/resources/publications/pregnancy-care-guidelines.

Department of Health, Australian Government. Clinical practice guidelines: pregnancy care. Canberra: Australian Government Department of Health; 2019. Available at: https://www.health.gov.au/resources/pregnancy-care-guidelines.

Fitzgerald O, Paul RC, Harris K, et al. Assisted reproductive technology in Australia and New Zealand 2016. Sydney: National Perinatal Epidemiology and Statistics Unit, the University of New South Wales Sydney; 2018. Available at: https://npesu.unsw.edu.au/sites/default/files/npesu/surveillances/Assisted%20Reproductive%20Technology%20in%20Australia%20and%20New%20Zealand%202016.pdf.

Gabbe SG, Niebyl J, Simpson J, et al., editors. Obstetrics: normal and problem pregnancies. Philadelphia, PA: Elsevier; 2017.

Gardener G, Daly L, Bowring V, et al. Clinical practice guideline for the care of women with decreased fetal movements. Brisbane: Centre of Research Excellence in Stillbirth; 2017.

Halperin SA, Langley JM, Ye L, et al. A randomized controlled trial of the safety and immunogenicity of tetanus, diphtheria, and acellular pertussis vaccine immunization during pregnancy and subsequent infant immune response. Clin Infect Dis 2018;67(7):1063–71. Available at: https://doi.org/10.1093/cid/ciy244.

Impey L, Child T. Obstetrics and gynaecology. 4th ed. Chichester, West Sussex: John Wiley; 2017.

Macdonald S, Magill-Cuerdan J, editors. Mayes' Midwifery. 15th ed. Edinburgh: Elsevier; 2017.

New Zealand College of Midwives. Midwifery in New Zealand. 2019. Available at: www.midwife.org.nz/in-new-zealand/midwifery-in-new-zealand.

New Zealand Government- NZ Stats. Births and deaths: year ended December 2017. 2018. Available at: https://www.stats.govt.nz/information-releases/births-and-deaths-year-ended-december-2017.

Pairman S, Tracy S, Dahlen G, et al. Midwifery: preparation for practice. 4th ed. Sydney: Elsevier; 2019.

Perinatal and Maternal Mortality Review Committee. 12th annual report of the Perinatal and Maternal Mortality Review Committee: reporting mortality 2016, 8th report to the Health Quality & Safety Commission New Zealand. Wellington: Perinatal and Maternal Mortality Review Committee; 2018.

Pilz S, Zittermann A, Obeid R, et al. The role of vitamin D in fertility and during pregnancy and lactation: a review of clinical data. Int J Environ Res Public Health 2018;15(10):2241. Available at: https://doi.org/10.3390/ijerph15102241.

Rankin J. Physiology in childbearing with anatomy and related biosciences. Edinburgh: Elsevier; 2017.

Rolfe MI, Donoghue DA, Longman JM, et al. The distribution of maternity services across rural and remote Australia: does it reflect population need? BMC Health Serv Res 2017;17(1):163.

Royal Australian and New Zealand College of Obstetricians and Gynaecologists. Guidelines for the use of Rh(D) immunoglobulin (anti-D) in obstetrics in Australia. 2019. Available at: https://ranzcog.edu.au/RANZCOG_SITE/media/RANZCOG-MEDIA/Women%27s%20Health/Statement%20and%20guidelines/Clinical-Obstetrics/Use-of-Rh(D)-Isoimmunisation-(C-Obs-6).pdf?ext=.pdf.

Savvaki D, Taousani E, Goulis DG, et al. Guidelines for exercise during normal pregnancy and gestational diabetes: a review of international recommendations. Hormones (Athens) 2018;17(4):521–9. Available at: https://doi.org/10.1007/s42000-018-0085-6.

Society of Obstetric Medicine of Australia and New Zealand (SOMANZ). The SOMANZ guideline for the management of hypertensive disorders of pregnancy. 2015. Available at: https://www.somanz.org/downloads/HTguidelineupdatedJune2015.pdf.

Toms C, Stapledon R, Coulter C, et al. Tuberculosis notifications in Australia, 2014. Commun Dis Intell 2017;41(3). Available at: http://www.health.gov.au/internet/main/publishing.nsf/Content/cdi4103-k.

Urale PW, O'Brien MA, Fouché CB. The relationship between ethnicity and fertility in New Zealand. Kōtuitui: New Zealand J Soc Sci Online 2019;14(1):80–94. Available at: https://doi.org/10.1080/1177083X.2018.1534746.

World Health Organization (WHO). Female genital mutilation. 2018a. Available at: https://www.who.int/news-room/fact-sheets/detail/female-genital-mutilation.

World Health Organization (WHO). Maternal mortality. Fact sheet no. 348, updated May 2014. 2018b. Available at: https://www.who.int/news-room/fact-sheets/detail/maternal-mortality.

Chapter Thirty

Using health assessment in clinical practice: putting it all together

Written by Helen Forbes and Elizabeth Watt

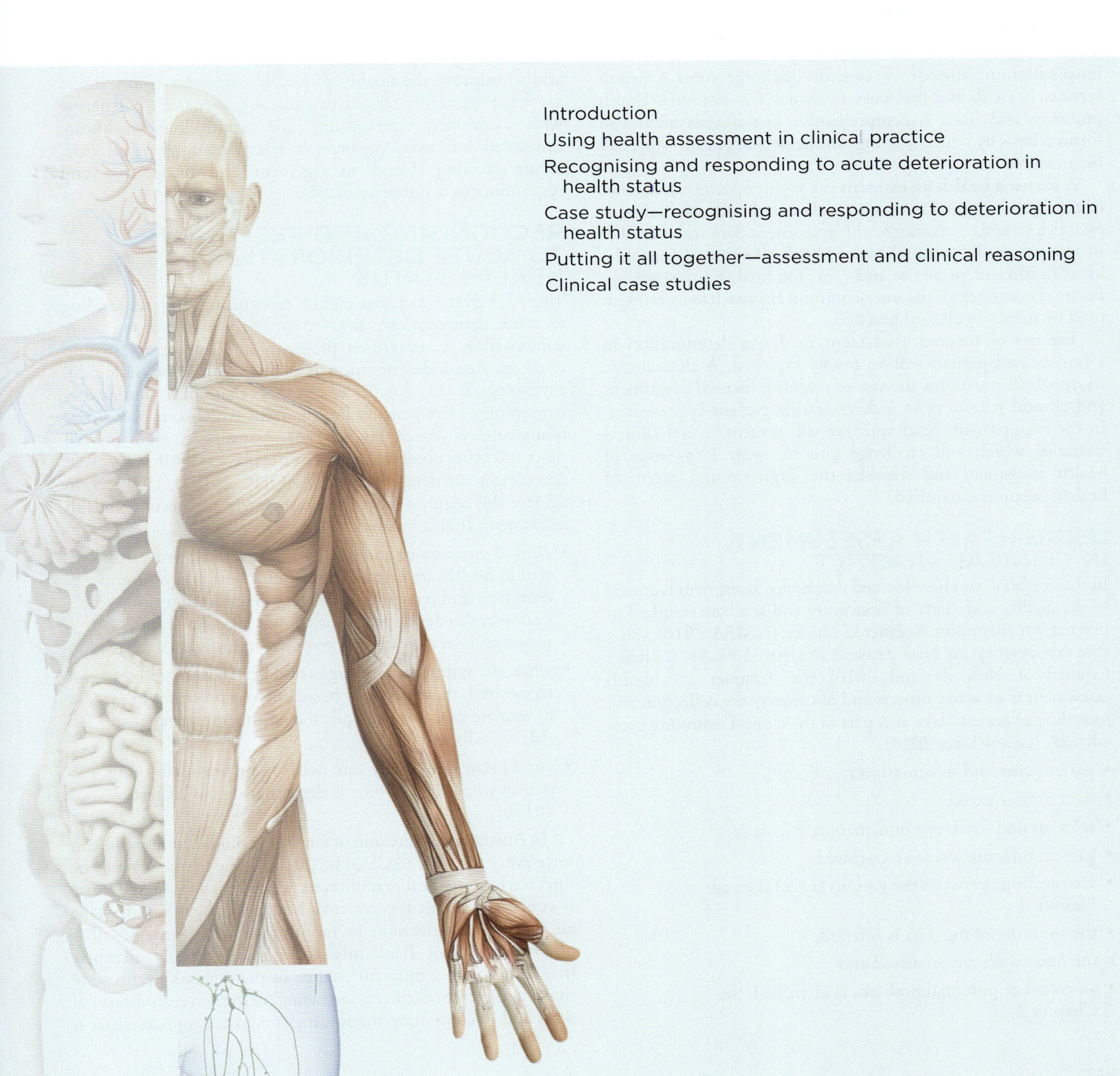

INTRODUCTION

In this final chapter we will further discuss the use of health assessment in nursing practice and its relationship to quality and safety in healthcare. You have learned from a previous chapter (Chapter 1) that a **comprehensive health assessment** is performed at a patient's first entry in an outpatient setting or initial admission to the hospital or other health service. A comprehensive health assessment includes a complete health history (Chapter 8) and relevant physical examination (Chapters 9 and 10). It describes the person's current and past health and forms a baseline against which all future changes can be measured. A comprehensive health assessment includes the person's perception of their health issues or illness, functional ability and the impact of the health issue or illness on activities of daily living and quality of life, health and lifestyle management, coping patterns and health goals.

An important outcome of a comprehensive assessment is to identify potential risk factors that may impact on the person's hospitalisation, episode of care or discharge from a health service. It yields the first cues to actual and potential health problems and risks. A comprehensive health assessment also forms a basis by which a change in the person's health state can be measured.

A **focused health assessment** is a highly specific assessment of a symptom, sign or body system. Focused assessment aims to establish or add to existing health assessment data and is smaller in scope than the comprehensive health assessment. It enables identification of priorities and areas for further investigation. Focused assessment is the most common approach to assessment used by nurses in clinical practice.

The use of focused assessment to detect deterioration in a hospitalised patient will be briefly explored. A clinical case study which illustrates the use of ongoing focused assessment and clinical reasoning in a deteriorating patient is presented. In the final part of the chapter we will present several clinical scenarios which will challenge you to apply knowledge of health assessment and consider the sequence and extent of health assessment required.

USING HEALTH ASSESSMENT IN CLINICAL PRACTICE

In this textbook you have learned that health assessment is critical to the quality and safety of healthcare and is a core standard of practice for Australian Registered Nurses (NMBA 2016) and a core competency for New Zealand Registered Nurses (Nursing Council of New Zealand 2016) (see Chapter 1). Health assessment is an active process and not merely the collection and recording of patient data. It is part of the clinical reasoning cycle whereby (Levett-Jones 2018):

- patient cues and information is collected,
- data is interpreted,
- relevant and irrelevant information is sorted,
- gaps in information are recognised,
- relationships between the various bits of data are identified,
- the meaning of the data is inferred,
- the outcome/s are predicted and
- an actual or potential problem is identified. See Chapter 2.

Important functions of health assessment in any healthcare setting are to:

- gain an understanding of the person's healthcare/illness experience,
- investigate any presenting signs and symptoms (cues),
- monitor the person's response to medical, nursing and allied health treatments and
- identify any indicators of deterioration in the person's physiological, mental and cognitive health status.

Monitoring of patient progress and identifying indicators of deterioration in health status is a core skill for all nurses regardless of the context in which they work. In Australia, the National Safety and Quality in Health Service Standards were developed by the Australian Commission on Safety and Quality in Health Care (ACSQHC 2017a) to set a consistent standard of practice in order to protect patients from harm and to improve the quality of health service provision. There are eight standards related to clinical governance, partnering with consumers, preventing and controlling healthcare associated infection, medication safety, comprehensive care, communicating, blood management and recognising and responding to acute deterioration.

RECOGNISING AND RESPONDING TO ACUTE DETERIORATION IN HEALTH STATUS

The ACSQHC standard eight, 'recognising and responding to acute deterioration', aims to ensure that a person's acute deterioration is recognised promptly and appropriate action is taken. Acute deterioration is defined as the physiological, psychological or cognitive changes that may indicate a worsening of the person's health status which can occur over hours or days (ACSQHC 2017b). Assessing changes in vital signs and other observations over time plays a significant role in detecting acute deterioration (ACSQHC 2017b). However, to achieve this requires more than just timely and accurate health assessment. It also involves:

- clinical governance and quality improvement programs within healthcare organisations to support and promote detection and recognition of acute deterioration (for example, the development of clinical guidelines and processes to review clinical response in individual cases),
- when the symptoms and signs of deterioration are recognised, there needs to be action and processes in place to escalate care (for example, a medical emergency team (MET) call) and
- appropriate and timely care needs to be provided to the person whose health state is deteriorating (ACSQHC 2017b).

In Australia, monitoring of vital signs should be done at least once every 8-h shift (ACSQHC 2017b). The frequency may be directed by a medical practitioner; however, if a registered nurse is concerned about the patient's health status, they can make an independent decision to monitor the vital signs or other observations more frequently. Occasionally, family members may also note a significant change in the person's health state that is a trigger for further assessment. Taking and recording vital signs and documenting the findings on an appropriate chart is only the first part of the assessment process. The ACSQHC (2017b) makes the point that recognising deterioration also requires:

- understanding and interpreting abnormal vital signs and other observations,
- knowledge of the appropriate treatment for the cause of acute deterioration,
- knowledge of when and how to escalate care—for example, initiate a MET call in the specific clinical setting (which may be different depending on the size and location of the healthcare setting) and
- excellent clinical communication skills—to communicate their concern to other healthcare practitioners and to advocate for the patient.

Recognising physiological deterioration

In the acute care hospital environment, patients have a variety of health problems, many of which can lead to unexpected clinical deterioration causing an acute critical illness, cardiac arrest or even death (Chua et al 2019, Massey & Meredith 2010). However, there is significant evidence that clinical deterioration is preceded by changes in the person's physiological status which can be detected in changes to respiratory rate, heart rate, blood pressure and oxygen saturation (Bunkenborg et al 2019, Cretikos et al 2008, Harrison et al 2006). There is also a stepwise increase in mortality with multiple abnormal vital signs as compared to abnormalities in individual vital signs (Andersen et al 2016).

In particular, **tachypnoea** (respiratory rate ≥ 20 breaths/min) has been found to be significantly associated with later deterioration in general ward patients and those in the emergency department (Bunkenborg et al 2019, Churpek et al 2016, Cretikos et al 2008, Harrison et al 2006). Bunkenborg et al make the point that an increased respiratory rate indicates a potential clinical instability which is often anxiety, pain, stress, hypoxia, acidosis or infection related, not necessarily resulting from complications within the respiratory system itself.

Bradycardia (≤ 60 beats/min) or **tachycardia** (≥ 100 beats/min) is associated with clinical deterioration and increased mortality (Andersen et al 2016, Bunkenborg et al 2019). While there are many factors that can increase a person's heart rate—for example, pain, anxiety, a cardiac condition—tachycardia may also reflect a compensatory response to a reduction in circulating volume.

In the study by Bunkenborg et al (2019), **older age** was also found to be significantly associated with clinical deterioration. Ageing is associated with a reduced ability to adapt to significant physiological challenges and Bunkenborg et al advise that close attention to respiratory and heart rate changes in older people and intervening quickly might prevent some patients from severe deterioration.

The **adult deterioration detection system (ADDS) chart** is used throughout Australia (see Chapter 10) (ACSQHC 2017c). It is designed to make it easier to identify trends in changing vital signs and give direction to the nurse (or other health professional) about appropriate action to take when a significant trend or change has been identified. The chart has been designed to make it personalised to the particular patient so that specific modifications to acceptable vital sign changes can be made. For this chart to work effectively, vital signs and other observations need to be assessed and recorded accurately and consistently over time.

Recognising deterioration in mental state

The Australian Commission on Safety and Quality in Health Care (2017d) have released a consensus statement on 'Essential elements for recognising and responding to a deterioration in a person's mental state'. In this statement health professionals are required to be alert for changes in mental and cognitive health in all patients, not just those with an identified risk.

Mental state deterioration is defined as 'a change for the worse in a person's mental state, compared with the most recent information available for that person, which may indicate the need for additional care' (Gaskin & Dagley 2018, p. 6). In addition to validated mental health screening tools (as discussed in Chapter 11), Gaskin & Dagley (2018) have identified five indicators of mental health deterioration:

- **Reported change in mental state**—a person or someone close to the person reporting that there is a change for the worse in their mental state.
- **Distress**—a person shows signs of distress which is evident through observation and conversation.
- **Loss of touch with reality or consequences of behaviours**—a person is losing touch with reality or the consequences of their behaviour.
- **Loss of function**—a person is losing their ability to think clearly, communicate or engage in regular activities.
- **Evaluated risk to self, others or property**—a person's actions indicate an increased risk to self, others or property.

Two other important factors identified by Gaskin and Dagley (2018) are the need for good quality baseline information about the person's usual mental state and the need to ask for and listen closely to the person and their carers' perception of changes in the person's mental state.

An important contribution to potential deterioration in mental state is the development of **delirium**. Delirium can be an indicator of serious underlying illness and can contribute to significant long-term cognitive decline (ACSQHC 2019a, 2019b). Delirium is common in hospitalised patients (see Chapter 12) and nurses need to be alert to the risk of cognitive impairment in patients who (ACSQHC 2019a, p. 6):

- are aged 65 years and over (or aged 45 years and over for Aboriginal and Torres Strait Islander people),
- have known cognitive impairment or a formal diagnosis of dementia,
- have a severe illness or are at risk of dying or
- have a hip fracture.

Typical key signs of delirium to be alert for include your own observations, reports from a family member, carer or support person about changes in a person's cognitive state or previous history of delirium, confusion or dementia (ACSQHC 2019a, p. 10):

- The person cannot answer your questions.
- They are inattentive or easily distracted.
- They have disorganised thinking.
- They have an altered level of consciousness.
- They are agitated.
- They are overly sleepy which may indicate hypoactive delirium.

As with physical health deterioration, when a change in mental state is detected, the nurse needs to initiate a response. This may begin with utilising strategies to calm the person and de-escalate the situation and to mobilise the person's existing supports (ACSQHC 2017c). Escalating care by consulting and/or referring to more experienced or specialist mental healthcare practitioners may be required. In the case of delirium, the person's cognitive state can quickly deteriorate so the person needs further assessment, identification of the cause's delirium and appropriate treatment.

CASE STUDY—RECOGNISING AND RESPONDING TO DETERIORATION IN HEALTH STATUS

The following case study presents an example of a 24-year-old woman who presented to an emergency department with abdominal pain (written by Bucknall, Hewitt & Guinane). Take the time to read through the case study as it illustrates the use of focused assessment over time, clinical decision making, communication, documentation, patient deterioration and responding to patient deterioration (including initiating a MET call).

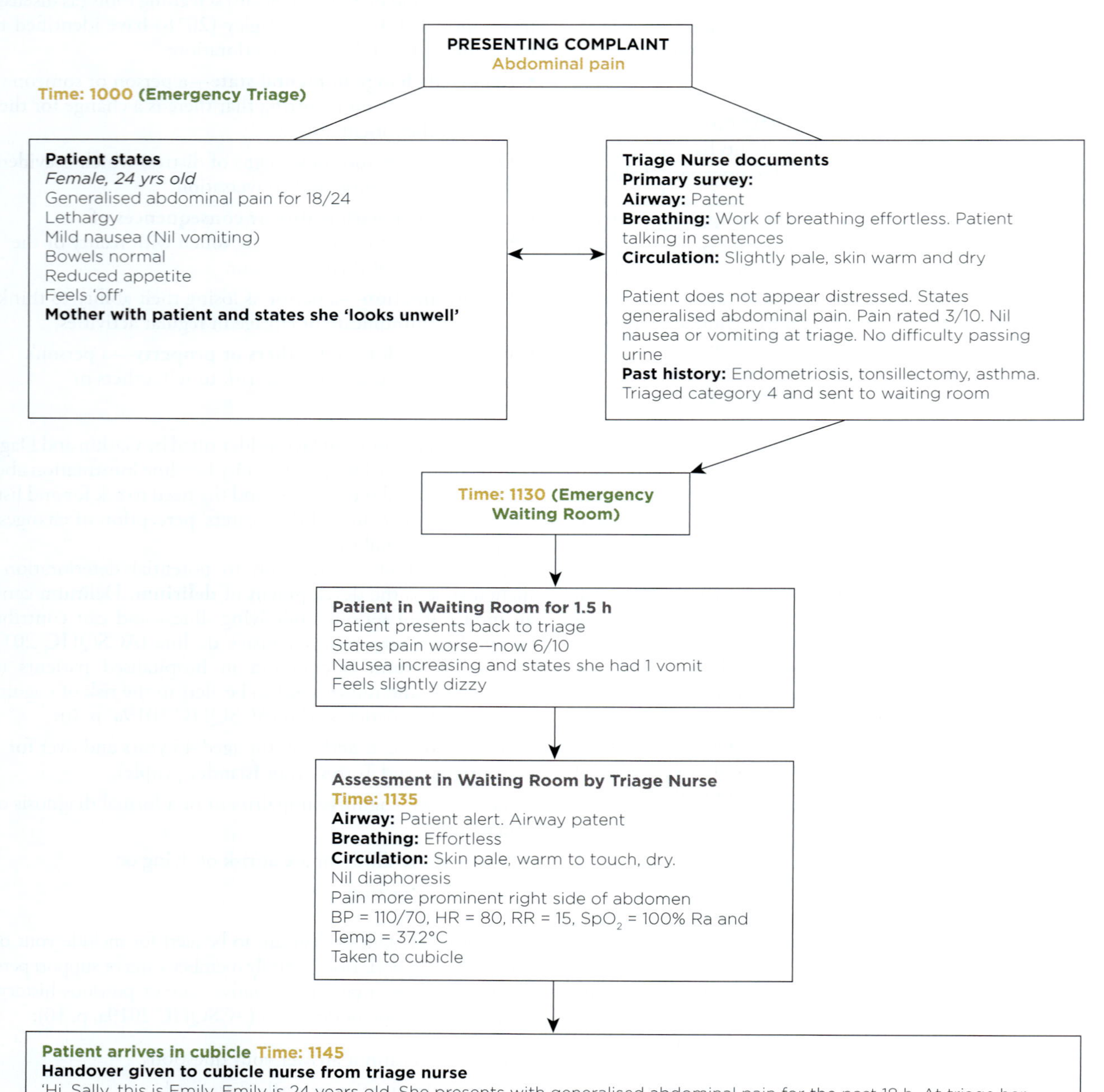

Nursing assessment
Nurse documents:
Time: 1200
Airway: Airway patent. Nil obvious obstruction
Breathing: Slight increased work of breathing (talking in phrases associated with intermittent increases in pain)
Circulation: Skin, pale, warm, slightly sweaty on palpation
Patient appears slightly distressed from pain
Rates pain 6–7/10. More severe to right side of abdomen. Patient asks for analgesia
Mild nausea—no further vomiting since patient arrived in cubicle. Bowels open yesterday—diarrhoea. Bowels opened 0800 and described as normal by the patient. Patient's mother in attendance and states patient looks very pale to her and 'not right'

Medications: Oral contraceptive pill
Past history: Endometriosis, tonsillectomy, asthma
Allergies: None known

Vital signs
BP = 102/55
HR = 92
RR = 17
SpO_2 = 100% Ra
Temp = 37.6°C

IV cannula size 18 inserted. Blood taken and sent to the lab. Await medical review and results

Time: 1225
Nurse gets called away to help with another patient

↓

Time: 1245 Nurse returns to cubicle

Vitals signs re-taken
BP = 95/55
HR = 102
RR = 18
SpO_2 = 100% Ra
Temp = 37.8°C
Pain 8/10

Nurse documents: 'Pt groaning with pain. States pain increased to 8/10. Describes pain as "stabbing" pain to right side of abdomen. Reporting worsening nausea. Patient guarding stomach. Patient's mother expresses concern stating "she is used to pain with her endometriosis but this looks a lot worse". Doctor notified of pt condition and order for morphine 2.5 mg IV and Maxolon 10 mg given.'

Nurse goes to get analgesia and antiemetic—returns to cubicle

Nurse documents: 'Patient pale. Skin hot to touch. Patient is sweaty. Patient holding her abdomen. States pain remains 8/10. Patient had one further vomit. Nil blood or mucus in vomit. Patient given 2.5 mg IV morphine and 10 mg IV Maxolon. Doctor in charge notified of patient condition. Awaits review. Patient's mother becoming anxious and wanting to know how long until a doctor will review patient. Patient's mother notified patient is next to be seen.'

↓

Time: 1310 Nurse goes back to room to check on patient

Doctor is in the room assessing the patient. He states he will review the blood test results and has ordered an ultrasound. He leaves the room.

Nurse documents: 'Patient appears slightly more comfortable after analgesia. Vitals signs re-checked. Patient states pain reduced to 6/10 and requests more morphine for the pain. Nil vomiting. Nausea settled. Patient states pain localised to the right lower quadrant. Patient not voided since arrived to Emergency Department. Pt mother states she "looks so pale". Further morphine 2.5 mg given to patient.

Vital signs
BP = 95/45
HR = 115
RR = 20
SpO_2 = 98% Ra
Temp = 38.1°C

Time: 1320 Nurse documents: 'Patient taken for ultrasound. Doctor notified that patient requests more analgesia and that further 2.5 mg IV morphine was given. Doctor stated he has notified the surgeon of her admission, and request for her to be admitted to the ward. Possible surgery tonight for ? appendicitis. The surgeon will review pt on the ward when he arrives at the hospital at 1500 h. If the ultrasound is normal she will remain in hospital for monitoring overnight.'

Nurse in Charge states: Ward bed ready in 2South. Pt to be transferred to ward on her return from ultrasound.

↓

Time: 1345 Patient returns to cubicle

Nurse documents: 'Patient returns to cubicle following ultrasound. Instructed by doctor and nurse in charge to transfer patient to the ward. Pt pale, skin hot to touch. Slightly sweating. Pt lying in the bed. Currently asleep. Seems comfortable. All belongings taken to ward.'

Time: 1400 Arrives to Ward 2, handover given to ward nurse at nurses' station

Nurse states: 'Hi, Kate, this is Emily. Emily is 24 years old. She has come into hospital today with abdominal pain. She has a past history of endometriosis, tonsillectomy and asthma. She states this pain is different from the pain she gets with endometriosis. The pain started about 18 h before she came into ED. She had one vomit in the waiting room but I gave her Maxolon when she came into the cubicle and has not vomited any more. Just before we transferred her to the ward she went to ultrasound. She was given 2.5 mg of IV morphine for her pain prior to the ultrasound. On return she looked a lot more settled. Before going for the ultrasound she was holding her stomach and groaning. She said the pain was generalised but more severe on her right side. Her mother has been here the whole time, and said to me she was concerned at how much pain she was in and how pale she was. Her last observations before ultrasound were: BP = 95/45, HR = 115, RR = 20, SpO_2 = 98% and Temp = 38.1°C. The plan is for a surgical review this afternoon and most likely theatre tonight for an appendicectomy. Blood tests were taken but I have not seen the results yet. The surgeon will review the ultrasound when he arrives. Her only regular medication is the oral contraceptive pill and she is not allergic to anything.'

↓

Time: 1410 Ward nurse goes in to introduce herself to patient and do an assessment

On arrival to room patient appears to be asleep. RN Kate says hello and gently rubs on her shoulder. Pt groans and opens her eyes. RN Kate notices her skin is very hot to touch and she feels sweaty. RN Kate immediately takes patient's vital signs.

Vital signs
BP = 85/40
HR = 135
RR = 24
SpO_2 = 96% Ra
Temp = 38.9°C

Time: 1420 RN MAKES A MET CALL FOR HYPOTENSION, TACHYCARDIA AND FEVER

↓

Time: 1425 MET arrive and conduct a patient assessment

Primary survey
Airway: Patent. Nil obvious obstruction to airway.
Breathing: Spontaneously breathing. Noted increased work of breathing. Use of accessory muscles. Respiratory rate is 22. Pt able to speak in phrases to sentences depending on pain levels.
Circulation: Skin pale, diaphoretic. Capillary refill is 3 s. Pulse strong, fast and regular.
Disability: GCS is fluctuating between 14 and 15. Pt drowsy but rouses to voice and touch. States pain 9/10 to right side of abdomen.
Exposure: Nil rash noted to limb or torso. Nil obvious abdominal mass. Nil lesions. Nil dilated veins.

Secondary survey (Focused assessment)
Nurse conducts assessment of patient

When did it start?
'I have had this pain now for nearly 24 h.' Patient describes constant dull pain across entire abdomen. But now it is much more severe. It is sharp pain to right lower quadrant. She states 'It is so severe I feel like I can't breathe properly.'

Have you ever had this pain before?
'No. I have endometriosis but the pain is very different. That pain is lower down and is crampy—this feels so much worse.' Patient's mother adds: 'I have had to take my daughter to the GP before when she was in pain caused by her endometriosis, but it was nothing like this. I have never seen her in so much pain.'

What is the quality of the pain (sharp, dull, tender, cramping, burning)?
'It's sharp pain. My entire stomach is aching, it's very sharp and more prominent on the right side.'

Is it intermittent or continuous?
'The aching pain is continuous, and the sharp pain is intermittent.'

Does the pain travel anywhere (radiate) or is it localised?
'As I said my entire abdomen is sore. I can't tell anymore, it's just so painful. It hurts around into my back on the right side.' Patient indicates that pain is most severe in the lower right quadrant.

On a scale of 0 to 10 with 0 being no pain and 10 being the worst pain ever felt, what is your pain level right now?
'Right now, the pain is a 9. But when the severe pain comes it is 10/10.'

Does anything make the pain better or worse?
'No, it just hurts all the time. Well, the morphine took the edge off for a little while, but that only lasted about 45 min. I took Panadeine Forte at home. I usually take that when I get pain from my endometriosis and it works well. But this time, it did nothing. I have never felt this pain before. It didn't even touch the sides.'

Is the pain associated with eating? Has the pain affected your food intake and appetite?
'I'm not sure, I have not eaten since lunch time yesterday. I just have not wanted to eat, I've had no appetite.'

Have you had any recent weight loss? If so, was it planned weight loss or not planned?
'No, I have not lost any weight.'

Have you had any abdominal surgeries? If so, what was the procedure and what was the outcome of the procedure?
'I had a laparoscopy 2 years ago. That is when I found out I had endometriosis. As I said, I just take Panadeine Forte when the pain is bad, but it has been OK now for around 6 months.'

Have you had any menstrual irregularities recently? When was your last period?
'I have not had a period for 2 months. But that is normal for me. The last period was normal.'

Do you have any pain when having intercourse? Any vaginal discharge?
'No'.

Is there any chance you could be pregnant?
'No.'

Are there associated symptoms, such as nausea and vomiting and/or diarrhoea?
'I felt nauseated all night. I had one vomit in emergency. I felt better after I was given Maxolon, but now I feel really nauseated, like I will vomit anytime soon.'

Have you noticed any black stools or blood in your stool? Have your stools been white or chalky?
'No. Yesterday I had one episode of diarrhoea at 2 pm. I did not notice any blood in my stool. This morning I had a normal bowel action.'

Have you noticed blood in your urine? Do you have frequency?
'No, I haven't had any blood. But last time I went to the toilet was around 2 am. It was quite dark at that time. I have not been since then. I don't even feel like I need to go.'

Do you feel as though you have had a fever?
'I don't know. The nurse said I did. I know I have been sweating a lot. But I feel really cold. When I was having the ultrasound I was shaking. I couldn't stop it. I was so freezing.'

Physical examination
Nurse palpates patient's abdomen
Palpation: Involuntary rigidity noted suggestive of peritoneal inflammation. Abdomen is very firm and distended. Pain is reported to be greater with the withdrawal of the hands as compared to palpation itself, thus positive for rebound tenderness. Rebound tenderness could indicate peritoneal inflammation

Listens to patient's bowel sounds
Hypoactive bowel sounds

Listens to patient's chest
Chest clear. Equal air entry to bases. Nil wheeze. Nil crackles. Nil reported cough

↓

The following information is combined:
Subjective data from patient
Discussion with patient's mother
Physical assessment data including patient's visual appearance, assessment of circulation, skin, chest, abdomen and vital signs
Blood test results
Ultrasound report

Medical diagnosis: Peritonitis caused by perforated appendix

Problem statements
Pain related to perforated appendix
Risk for deficient fluid volume related to vomiting and inadequate fluid intake
Fever related to infection

Immediate plan
- Immediate surgery—to remove appendix and wash out blood and pus from the abdominal cavity
- IV antibiotics—tailored to the specific bacteria to kill the infection
- Intravenous fluids—to rehydrate the body and replace lost electrolytes
- Vital signs every 15 min until taken to the operating theatre
- Nil by mouth

PUTTING IT ALL TOGETHER—ASSESSMENT AND CLINICAL REASONING

We have designed the following scenarios to assist you to integrate your assessment and critical thinking knowledge and skills in typical clinical situations. Each will require you to:

- Consider the situation
- Reflect on what you know and what you don't know or are unsure about
- Follow up on these learning issues
- Identify the available cues
- Draw inferences/make predictions related to the information in each scenario
- Decide what additional health assessment data needs to be collected
- Document a detailed assessment plan (both subjective and objective areas for assessment).

Refer to Chapter 2 (Tables 2.1 and 2.2) to refresh your knowledge of the clinical reasoning process.

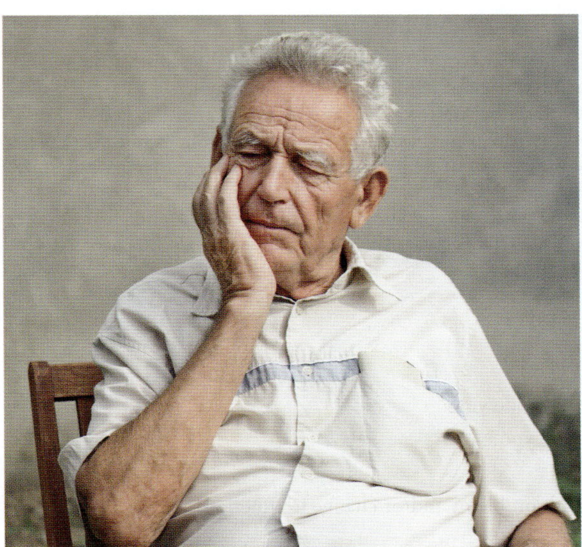

Mr Micha Krawiec

Mr Micha Krawiec, aged 85 years and widowed, is admitted to the rehabilitation centre following a stroke 2 weeks ago.

A summary of the hospital discharge letter notes that Mr Krawiec has left-sided hemiparesis, has lost weight, currently weighs 63 kg (height 184 cm), requires encouragement to eat, and has functional incontinence, impaired mobility and pressure injury on his right hip.

Mr Krawiec's daughter tells you that since the stroke her father seems to have lost the ability to understand and speak English.

Using the information in the case study for Mr Micha Krawiec, complete the following:

1. Identify unfamiliar terminology in the scenario. Use your textbooks to help you.
2. What are the available cues?
3. What inferences/predictions related to symptoms, risks for potential health problems and/or change in function can you make from your knowledge about this situation and the available cues?
4. What additional health assessment data relative to your inferences/predictions will you collect?
5. Document a detailed assessment plan.

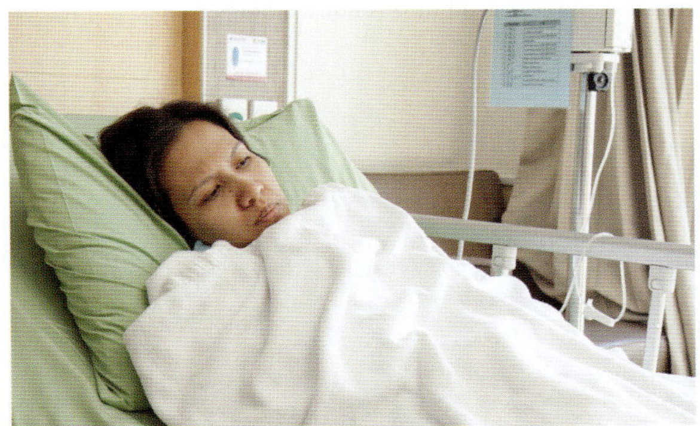

Ms Josephine Magliore

Ms Josephine Magliore, aged 45 years, had a cholecystectomy via laparoscopy this morning. She returned to the day surgical unit 6 hours ago. She tells you that her pain is increasing and is now 8/10 at rest.

She also feels very nauseated.

Using the information in the case study for Ms Joesephine Magliore, complete the following:

1. Identify unfamiliar terminology in the scenario. Use your textbooks to help you.
2. What are the available cues?
3. What inferences/predictions related to symptoms, risks for potential health problems and/or change in function can you make from your knowledge about this situation and the available cues?
4. What additional health assessment data relative to your inferences/predictions will you collect?
5. Document a detailed assessment plan.

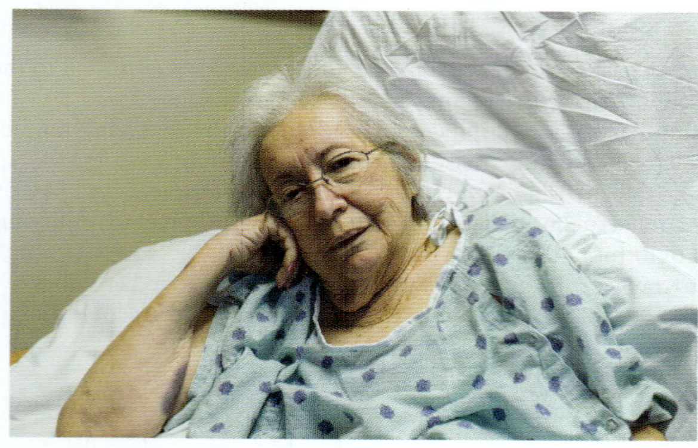

Mrs Jennifer Guyatt

Mrs Jennifer Guyatt, aged 84 years, had a dynamic hip screw for a fractured neck of left femur inserted 3 days ago.
As you set her up for breakfast you notice that her bed is wet and that the urine has a very strong smell. She is not normally incontinent of urine. An indwelling urinary catheter was removed yesterday.
As you go about changing her bed and nightie and cleansing her skin, she tells you that she is ready to go to bed but needs to feed the cat first.

Using the information in the case study for Mrs Jennifer Guyatt, complete the following:

1. Identify unfamiliar terminology in the scenario. Use your textbooks to help you.
2. What are the available cues?
3. What inferences/predictions related to symptoms, risks for potential health problems and/or change in function can you make from your knowledge about this situation and the available cues?
4. What additional health assessment data relative to your inferences/predictions will you collect?
5. Document a detailed assessment plan.

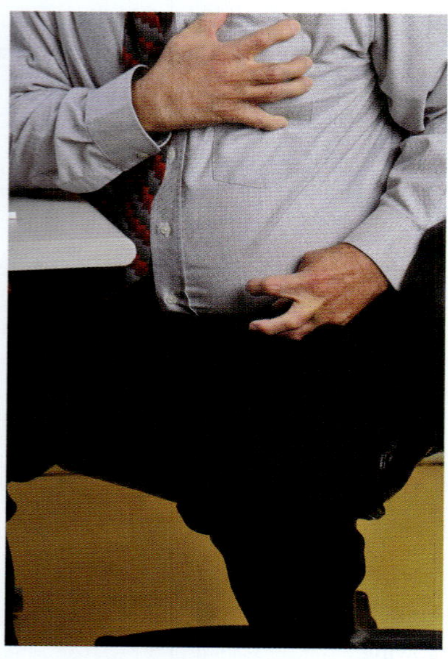

Mr Max Smith

Mr Max Smith, aged 51 years, presents to the Emergency Department reporting severe chest pain.
As the triage nurse you note that Max is morbidly obese and is rubbing his chest and grimacing.
Mr Smith tells you that the GP prescribed esomeprazole for indigestion 3 weeks ago but it is not working.

Using the information in the case study for Mr Max Smith, complete the following:

1. Identify unfamiliar terminology in the scenario. Use your textbooks to help you.
2. What are the available cues?
3. What inferences/predictions related to symptoms, risks for potential health problems and/or change in function can you make from your knowledge about this situation and the available cues?
4. What additional health assessment data relative to your inferences/predictions will you collect?
5. Document a detailed assessment plan.

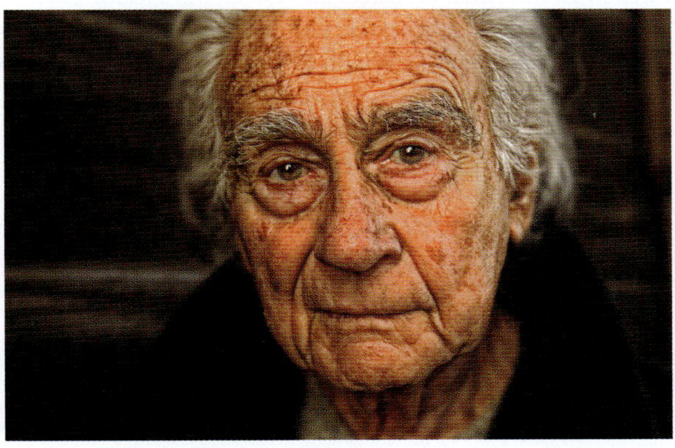

Mr Bill Craven

Mr Bill Craven, aged 86 years, attends his local GP for a postoperative review visit 7 days following an inguinal hernia repair at the local community hospital.

Mr Craven's GP completed his postoperative health check and has referred him to the practice nurse for assessment and advice related to his ongoing constipation.

Mr Craven tells you that he 'goes to the toilet' every 3–4 days and has to strain to empty his bowels nearly every time.

Using the information in the case study for Mr Bill Craven, complete the following:

1. Identify unfamiliar terminology in the scenario. Use your textbooks to help you.
2. What are the available cues?
3. What inferences/predictions related to symptoms, risks for potential health problems and/or change in function can you make from your knowledge about this situation and the available cues?
4. What additional health assessment data relative to your inferences/predictions will you collect?
5. Document a detailed assessment plan.

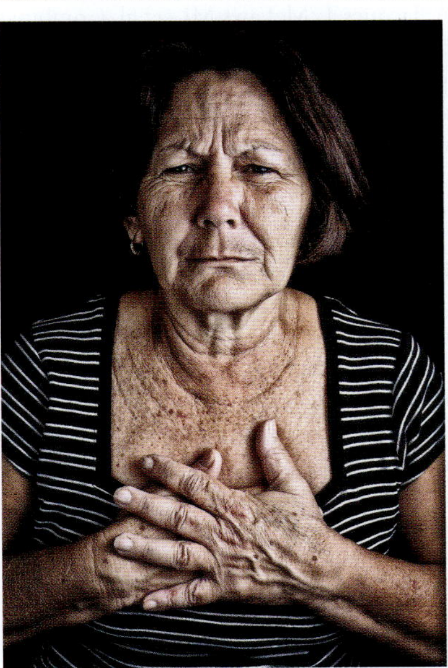

Mrs Christine Thomas

Mrs Christine Thomas, aged 59 years, is admitted to the ward from the Emergency Department with an exacerbation of COPD. When she arrives on the ward you observe that she looks exhausted and anxious, has heavy work of breathing, a rapid respiratory rate and a productive cough.

Using the information in the case study for Mrs Christine Thomas, complete the following:

1. Identify unfamiliar terminology in the scenario. Use your textbooks to help you.
2. What are the available cues?
3. What inferences/predictions related to symptoms, risks for potential health problems and/or change in function can you make from your knowledge about this situation and the available cues?
4. What additional health assessment data relative to your inferences/predictions will you collect?
5. Document a detailed assessment plan.

BIBLIOGRAPHY

Andersen LW, Kim WY, Chase M, et al. The prevalence and significance of abnormal vital signs prior to in-hospital cardiac arrest. Resuscitation 2016;98:112–7.

Australian Commission on Safety and Quality in Health Care. Delirium clinical care standard. Sydney: ACSQHC; 2016. Available at: https://www.safetyandquality.gov.au/our-work/clinical-care-standards/delirium-clinical-care-standard.

Australian Commission on Safety and Quality in Health Care. National safety and quality health service standards. 2nd ed. Sydney: ACSQHC; 2017a. Available at: https://www.safetyandquality.gov.au/sites/default/files/2019-04/National-Safety-and-Quality-Health-Service-Standards-second-edition.pdf.

Australian Commission on Safety and Quality in Health Care. National consensus statement: essential elements for recognising and responding to acute physiological deterioration. 2nd ed. Sydney: ACSQHC; 2017b. Available at: https://www.safetyandquality.gov.au/sites/default/files/migrated/National-Consensus-Statement-clinical-deterioration_2017.pdf.

Australian Commission on Safety and Quality in Health Care. ADDS chart with blood pressure table. Sydney: ACSQHC; 2017c. Available at: https://www.safetyandquality.gov.au/sites/default/files/migrated/ADDS-chart-with-blood-pressure-table-2012.pdf.

Australian Commission on Safety and Quality in Health Care. National consensus statement: Essential elements for recognising and responding to deterioration in a person's mental state. Sydney: ACSQHC; 2017d. Available at: https://www.safetyandquality.gov.au/sites/default/files/2019-06/national-consensus-statement-essential-elements-for-recognising-and-responding-to-deterioration-in-a-persons-mental-state-july-2017.pdf.

Australian Commission on Safety and Quality in Health Care. A better way to care – Safe and high-quality care for patients with cognitive impairment or at risk of delirium in acute health services: actions for clinicians. 2nd ed. Sydney: ACSQHC; 2019a. Available at: https://www.safetyandquality.gov.au/sites/default/files/2019-06/sq19-026_acsqhc_bwtc_d21.sk_june-3_accessible_pdf.pdf.

Australian Commission on Safety and Quality in Health Care. NSQHS Standards user guide for health service organisations providing care for patients with cognitive impairment or at risk of delirium. Sydney: ACSQHC; 2019b. Available at: https://www.safetyandquality.gov.au/sites/default/files/2019-06/sq19-027_acsqhc_cognitive_user_guide_accessible_pdf.pdf.

Bunkenborg G, Poulsen I, Samuelson K, et al. Bedside vital parameters that indicate early deterioration. Int J Health Care Qual Assur 2019;32(1):262–72.

Chua WL, Legido-Quigley H, Ng PY, et al. Seeing the whole picture in enrolled and registered nurses' experiences in recognizing clinical deterioration in general ward patients: a qualitative study. Int J Nurs Stud 2019;95:56–64.

Churpek MM, Adhikari R, Edelson DP. The value of vital sign trends for detecting clinical deterioration on the wards. Resuscitation 2016;102:1–5.

Cretikos MA, Bellomo R, Hillman K, et al. Respiratory rate: the neglected vital sign. Med J Aust 2008;188(11):657–9.

Gaskin C, Dagley G. Recognising signs of deterioration in a person's mental state. Sydney: ACSQHC; 2018. Available at: https://www.safetyandquality.gov.au/sites/default/files/migrated/Recognising-Signs-of-Deterioration-in-a-Persons-Mental-State-Gaskin-Research-Final-Report.pdf.

Harrison GA, Jacques T, McLaws ML, et al. Combinations of early signs of critical illness predict in-hospital death—the SOCCER study (signs of critical conditions and emergency responses). Resuscitation 2006;71(3):327–34.

Levett-Jones T, editor. Clinical reasoning: learning to think like a nurse. 2nd ed. Melbourne: Pearson Australia; 2018.

Massey D, Meredith T. Respiratory assessment 1: why do it and how to do it? Br J Card Nurs 2010;5(11):537–41.

Nursing and Midwifery Board of Australia. Registered nurse standards for practice. 2016. Available at: https://www.nursingmidwiferyboard.gov.au/codes-guidelines-statements/professional-standards.aspx.

Nursing Council of New Zealand. Competencies for registered nurses. 2016. Available at: https://www.nursingcouncil.org.nz/Public/Nursing/Standards_and_guidelines/NCNZ/nursing-section/Standards_and_guidelines_for_nurses.aspx?hkey=9fc06ae7-a853-4d10-b5fe-992cd44ba3de.

Illustration credits

Original illustrations by Pat Thomas, CMI, FAMI
East Troy, Wisconsin
Assessment photographs by Kevin Strandberg
Professor of Art
Illinois Wesleyan University
Bloomington, Illinois

CHAPTER 2

Figure 2.1: Modified from Alfaro-LeFevre R: *Critical thinking and clinical judgement: a practical approach*, 4th edn. Philadelphia, 2008, Saunders.

CHAPTER 3

Figure 3.3: Lissauer T, Clayden G, Craft A: *Illustrated textbook of paediatrics,* 4th edn. 2012, Elsevier.
Figure 3.4: Zitelli BJ, McIntire SC, Nowalk AJ: *Atlas of pediatric physical diagnosis*, 6th edn. Philadelphia, 2012, Elsevier Saunders.
Figure 3.7: CDC/Amanda Mills.
Figures 3.8, 3.9: © Photos.com, 2011.
Figures 3.10, 3.11: CDC/Amanda Mills.
Figure 3.12: CDC/Dawn Arlotta.
Figure 3.13: CDC/Amanda Mills.

CHAPTER 4

Figure 4.1: Shutterstock/JackQ; Shutterstock/sianc; Shutterstock/Tatiana Morozova; Shutterstock/Goodluz; Shutterstock/S L; Flickr/Mark Roy.
Figure 4.2: Courtesy Fuimaono Karl Pulotu-Endemann.
Figure 4.3: Ramsden I: *Kawa Whakaruruhau: guidelines for nursing and midwifery education*. Wellington, 1992, Nursing Council of New Zealand.

CHAPTER 6

Figure 6.1: Australian Government. Department of Health. Standard drinks guide. 2019.
Table 6.2: © John R. Knight, MD, Boston Children's Hospital, 2018. Reproduced with permission from the Center for Adolescent Substance Abuse Research (CeASAR), Boston Children's Hospital. The National Drug and Alcohol Research Centre, UNSW Australia, received funding for the Substance Misuse in Pregnancy Resource. Development Project from the Australian Government

CHAPTER 7

Figure 7.1: iStockphoto.com/Ergin Yalcin
Figure 7.2: Shutterstock/NotarYES.
Figure 7.3: Science Photo Library/Jim Varney.
Figure 7.4: Shutterstock/Photographee.eu.
Figure 7.5: © Newspix/News Ltd/Chloe Erlich.

CHAPTER 8

Figure 8.1: © National Comprehensive Cancer Network 2020. All rights reserved.
Figure 8.2: Adapted from The American Society of Human Genetics. www.ashg.org, 2004.
Figure 8.3: Adapted from Katz S, Down TD, Cash HR et al, The Gerontological Society of America: Progress in the development of the index of ADL, *Gerontologist*, 10:20–30, 1970.
Figure 8.4: Goldenring JM, Rosen DS: Getting into adolescent heads: an essential update, *Contemporary Pediatrics*, 21(1):64–68, 70, 73–74, 2004.

CHAPTER 9

Figure 9.1: Zakus SM: *Mosby's clinical skills for medical assistants*, 4th edn. St Louis, 2001, Mosby.
Figure 9.7: iStockphoto/NormaF.

CHAPTER 10

Figure 10.1: iStockphoto.com/fatcamera.
Figure 10.2: © Commonwealth of Australia 2012.
Figure 10.3: iStockphoto.com/monkeybusinessimages.
Figure 10.5: iStockphoto.com/aldomurillo.
Figure 10.6: iStockphoto.com/tbradford.
Figure 10.7: iStockphoto.com/Image Source.
Figure 10.17: Science Photo Library/BSIP/Astier.

CHAPTER 11

Figure 11.1: Colucci E. et al., (2018). Suicide first aid guidelines for assisting persons from immigrant or refugee background: a Delphi study. Advances in Mental Health, 16(2), 105-116 https://doi.org/10.1080/18387357.2018.1469383
Art for Clinical Case Study: Shutterstock/Irina Borsuchenko.

CHAPTER 12

Figure 12.9: © Pat Thomas, 2014.
Figure 12.13: Adapted from Institute of Neurological Sciences, 2015.
Figures 12.51, 12.52: Murray SS, McKinney ES: *Foundations of maternal-newborn and women's health nursing*, 5th edn. St Louis, 2010, Saunders.
Figure 12.63B: Fenichel GM: *Clinical pediatric neurology*, Philadelphia, 1988, Saunders.
Art for Table 12.12: © Pat Thomas, 2010.
Art for Table 12.14: (Decorticate rigidity) © Pat Thomas, 2006; (Decerebrate rigidity) © Pat Thomas, 2006; (Flaccid quadriplegia) © Pat Thomas, 2006; (Opisthotonos) © Pat Thomas, 2006.
Art for Table 12.16: (Snout) © Pat Thomas, 2006; (Sucking) © Pat Thomas, 2006; (Grasp) © Pat Thomas, 2006.
Art for Table 12.17: (Parkinson's syndrome) Glynn M, Drake WM: *Hutchison's clinical methods: an integrated approach to*

clinical practice, 23rd edn. Philadelphia, 2012, Elsevier Saunders; (Bell's palsy [right side]) Swartz MH: *Textbook of physical diagnosis: history and examination*, 5th edn. Philadelphia, 2006, Saunders; (Stroke) Nolte J, Sundsten J: *The Human brain: an introduction to its functional anatomy,* 6th edn. Philadelphia, 2009, Elsevier Mosby.
Art for Clinical Case Study: iStockphoto.com/RAUL RODRIGUEZ.

CHAPTER 13

Figure 13.4: (Reflexive sympathetic dystrophy) © Pat Thomas, 2010.
Figure 13.5: © Pat Thomas, 2018.
Figures 13.6, 13.7: McAffery M, Pasero C: *Pain: clinical manual,* 2nd edn. St Louis, 1999, Mosby.
Figure 13.8: Acute Pain Management Guideline Panel, 1992.
Figure 13.9: Abbey J, De Bellis A, Piller N et al: Funded by the JH & JD Gunn Medical Research Foundation 1998–2002.
Figure 13.10: Warden, V., Hurley, A. C., & Voticer, L. (2003). Development and psychometric evaluation of the Pain Assessment in Advanced Dementia (PAINAD) Scale. *J Am Med Dir Assoc. 4*(1), 9-15.
Figure 13.11: Hicks CL, von Baeyer CL, Spafford P et al: Faces Pain Scale—Revised: toward a common metric in pediatric pain measurement, *Pain*, 93:173–183, 2001. Copyright 2001 the International Association for the Study of Pain (IASP). From Hockenberry MJ, Wilson D, Winkelstein ML: Wong's essentials of pediatric nursing, 7th edn. St. Louis, 2005, p. 1259. Used with permission. Copyright, Mosby.
Figure 13.12: Krechel SW, Bildner J: CRIES: a neonatal postoperative pain measurement score: initial testing of validity and reliability, *Pediatric Anesthesia*, 5:53–61, 1995.
Figure 13.13: Voepel-Lewis, T., Zanotti, J., Dammeyer, J. A., et al. (2010). Reliability and validity of the face, legs, activity, cry, consolability behavioral tool in assessing acute pain in critically ill patients. *Am J Crit Care*, 19(1), 55-61.
Art for Clinical Case Study 1: Shutterstock.com/De Visu.
Art for Clinical Case Study 2: Shutterstock.com/AJP.

CHAPTER 14

Figure 14.1: © Pat Thomas, 2006.
Figure 14.3: © Pat Thomas, 2006.
Figure 14.4: © Pat Thomas, 2006.
Figure 14.10: Lemmi and Lemmi, 2011.
Figure 14.11: Kidd DP, Newman NJ, Biousse V: *Neuro-ophthalmology*. Copyright © 2008 by Butterworth–Heinemann, an imprint of Elsevier Inc.
Figure 14.14: Zitelli BJ, Davis HW: *Atlas of pediatric physical diagnosis*, 5th edn. St Louis, 2007, Mosby.
Figure 14.15: Albert DM, Jakobiec FA: *Principles and practice of ophthalmology*, Philadelphia, 1994, Saunders.
Figure 14.16: Swartz MH: *Textbook of physical diagnosis: history and examination*, 5th edn. Philadelphia, 2005, Saunders.
Figure 14.29: Heather Boyd-Monk and Wills Eye Hospital, Philadelphia.
Figures 14.30, 14.31: Lemmi and Lemmi, 2011.
Figure 14.32: Douglas G, Nicol F, Robertson C: *Macleod's clinical examination*, 13th edn. Elsevier Churchill Livingstone, 2013.
Figure 14.33: Friedman N, Kaiser PK, Pineda R: *The Massachusetts Eye and Ear Infirmary illustrated manual of ophthalmology*, 4th edn. Philadelphia, 2014, Saunders.
Art for Table 14.1: (Left esotropia) Zitelli BJ, Davis HW: *Atlas of pediatric physical diagnosis*, 5th edn. St Louis, 2007, Mosby; (Exotropia) Zitelli BJ, Davis HW: *Atlas of pediatric physical diagnosis*, 5th edn. St Louis, 2007, Mosby.
Art for Table 14.2: (Periorbital oedema) Ibsen OAC, Phelan JA: *Oral pathology for the dental hygienist,* 2nd edn. Philadelphia, 1992, Saunders; (Orbital cellulitis) Uddin JM, Scawn RL: *Pediatric ophthalmology and strabismus*, 4th edn. Elsevier, 2013; (Exophthalmos [protruding eyes]) Lemmi and Lemmi, 2011; (Ptosis [drooping upper lid]) Lemmi and Lemmi, 2011; (Upward palpebral slant) Hockenberry MJ, Wilson D: *Wong's essentials of pediatric nursing*, 9th edn. St Louis, 2013, Mosby; (Ectropion) Albert DM, Jakobiec FA: *Principles and practice of ophthalmology*, Philadelphia, 1994, Saunders; (Entropion) Albert DM, Jakobiec FA: *Principles and practice of ophthalmology*, Philadelphia, 1994, Saunders.
Art for Table 14.3: (Blepharitis [inflammation of the eyelids]) Friedman N, Kaiser PK, Pineda R: *The Massachusetts Eye and Ear Infirmary illustrated manual of ophthalmology*, 4th edn. Philadelphia, 2014, Saunders; (Chalazion) Heather Boyd-Monk and Wills Eye Hospital, Philadelphia; (Hordeolum [stye]) Lemmi and Lemmi, 2011; (Basal cell carcinoma) Friedman NJ, Kaiser PK, Pineda R: *The Massachusetts Eye and Ear Infirmary illustrated manual of ophthalmology,* 4th edn. Philadelphia, 2014, Saunders Elsevier; (Squamous cell carcinoma) Krachmer JH: *Cornea atlas*, 3rd edn. Elsevier, 2014.
Art for Table 14.6: (Conjunctivitis) Lemmi and Lemmi, 2011; (Subconjunctival haemorrhage) Lemmi and Lemmi, 2011; (Iritis [circumcorneal redness]) Scheie HG, Albert DM: *Textbook of ophthalmology*, 9th edn. Philadelphia, 1977, Saunders; (Primary angle-closure glaucoma) Atkinson P, Kendall R, Resnburg LV: *Emergency medicine: an illustrated color text.* Philadelphia, 2011, Churchill Livingstone; (Herpes simplex virus) Friedman NJ, Kaiser PK, Pineda R: *The Massachusetts Eye and Ear Infirmary Illustrated Manual of Ophthalmology*, 4th edn. Philadelphia, 2014, Saunders Elsevier.
Art for Table 14.7: (Pterygium) Lemmi and Lemmi, 2011; (Corneal abrasion) Heather Boyd-Monk and Wills Eye Hospital, Philadelphia; (Hyphaema) Lemmi and Lemmi, 2011; (Hypopyon) Scheie HG, Albert DM: *Textbook of ophthalmology*, 9th edn. Philadelphia, 1977, Saunders.
Art for Table 14.8: (Central grey opacity—nuclear cataract) Friedman N, Pineda R: *The Massachusetts Eye and Ear Infirmary illustrated manual of ophthalmology*. Philadelphia, 1998, Saunders; (Star-shaped opacity—cortical cataract) Friedman N, Pineda R: *The Massachusetts Eye and Ear Infirmary illustrated manual of ophthalmology*. Philadelphia, 1998, Saunders.
Art for Table 14.9: (Optic atrophy [disc pallor]) Friedman NJ, Kaiser PK, Pineda R: *The Massachusetts Eye and Ear Infirmary illustrated manual of ophthalmology*, 4th edn. Philadelphia, 2014, Saunders Elsevier; (Papilloedema) Friedman NJ, Kaiser PK, Pineda R: *The Massachusetts Eye and Ear Infirmary illustrated manual of ophthalmology*, 4th edn. Philadelphia, 2014, Saunders Elsevier; (Excessive cup–disc ratio) Friedman NJ, Kaiser PK, Pineda R: *The Massachusetts Eye and Ear Infirmary illustrated manual of ophthalmology*, 4th edn. Philadelphia, 2014, Saunders Elsevier.
Art for Table 14.10: (Arteriovenous crossing [nicking]) Friedman N, Kaiser PK, Pineda R: *The Massachusetts eye and*

ear infirmary illustrated manual of ophthalmology, 4th edn. Philadelphia, 2014, Saunders; (Narrow [attenuated] arteries) Lemmi and Lemmi, 2011; (Diabetic retinopathy) Friedman N, Kaiser PK, Pineda R: *The Massachusetts eye and ear infirmary illustrated manual of ophthalmology*, 4th edn. Philadelphia, 2014, Saunders.
Art for Clinical Case Study: iStockphoto.com/seb_ra.

CHAPTER 15

Figure 15.4: Hreib KK, Choi E, Catalano PJ: 'Cranial Nerve VIII: Auditory and Vestibular' in Jones HR et al: *Netter's Neurology*, 2nd edn. Philadelphia, 2012, Saunders.
Figure 15.8: Lemmi and Lemmi, 2011.
Figure 15.13: Casey JR, Bluestone CD: 'Otitis Media' in Cherry J, Demmler-Harrison GJ, Kaplan SL et al: *Feigin and Cherry's Textbook of Pediatric Infectious Diseases*. Philadelphia, 2019, Elsevier.
Art for Table 15.1: (Frostbite) Science Photo Library/Custom Medical Stock; (Otitis externa [swimmer's ear]) Lemmi and Lemmi, 2011; (Branchial remnant and ear deformity) Liebert PS: *Color atlas of pediatric surgery,* 2nd edn. Philadelphia, 1996, Saunders.
Art for Table 15.2: (Sebaceous cyst) Liebert PS: *Color atlas of pediatric surgery,* 2nd edn. Philadelphia, 1996, Saunders; (Tophi) Science Photo Library; (Chondrodermatitis nodularis helicus) Habif TP, Campbell JL, Dinulos JGH et al: *Skin disease: diagnosis and treatment,* 2nd edn. St Louis, 2005, Mosby; (Keloid) Lemmi and Lemmi, 2011; (Carcinoma) Ameerally PJ, Colver GB: Cutaneous cryotherapy in maxillofacial surgery, *Journal of Oral and Maxillofacial Surgery*, 65(9):1785–1792, 2007.
Art for Table 15.3: (Excessive cerumen) © Pat Thomas, 2010; (Otitis externa) Lim EKS, Thompson AM, Loke YK: *Medicine & surgery: an integrated textbook.* New York, 2007, Churchill Livingstone; (Osteoma) © Pat Thomas, 2010; (Foreign body) Swartz MH: *Textbook of physical diagnosis*, 2nd edn. Philadelphia, 2014, Elsevier; (Exostosis) © Pat Thomas, 2010; (Furuncle) © Pat Thomas, 2010; (Polyp) © Pat Thomas, 2010.
Art for Table 15.4: (Retracted drum) Adams GL, Boies LR Jr, Hilger PA: *Boies fundamentals of otolaryngology: a textbook of ear, nose and throat diseases*, 6th edn. Philadelphia, 1989, Saunders; (Otitis media with effusion [OME]) Swartz MH: *Textbook of physical diagnosis: history and examination*, 5th edn. Philadelphia, 2005, Saunders; (Acute [purulent] otitis media) Adams GL, Boies LR Jr, Hilger PA: *Boies fundamentals of otolaryngology: a textbook of ear, nose and throat disease,* 6th edn. Philadelphia, 1989, Saunders; (Perforation) Dhillon RS, East CA: *Ear, nose and throat and head and neck surgery*, 4th edn. Philadelphia, 2013, Churchill Livingstone; (Insertion of tubes [grommets]) Fireman P: *Atlas of allergies*, 2nd edn. London, 1996, Mosby; (Cholesteatoma) Swartz MH: *Textbook of physical diagnosis: history and examination,* 5th edn. Philadelphia, 2005, Saunders; (Scarred drum) Lim EKS, Thompson AM, Loke YK: *Medicine & surgery: an integrated textbook.* New York, 2007, Churchill Livingstone; (Blue drum [haemotympanum]) Dhillon RS, East CA: *Ear, nose and throat and head and neck surgery*, 4th edn. Philadelphia, 2013, Churchill Livingstone; (Bullous myringitis) Swartz MH: *Textbook of physical diagnosis: history and examination*, 5th edn. Philadelphia, 2005, Saunders; (Fungal infection [otomycosis]) © Pat Thomas, 2010.
Art for Clinical Case Study 1: iStockphoto.com/Techin24
Art for Clinical Case Study 2: iStockphoto.com/RichLegg

CHAPTER 16

Figures 16.1–16.4, 16.6: © Pat Thomas, 2010.
Figure 16.5: © Pat Thomas, 2014.
Figure 16.18B: Bloom A, Watkins, PH, Ireland J: *Color atlas of diabetes*, 2nd edn. St Louis, 1992, Mosby.
Figure 16.20B: Lemmi and Lemmi, 2011.
Art for Table 16.2: (Arteriosclerosis—ischaemic ulcer) Dockery GL: *Cutaneous disorders of the lower extremity*. Philadelphia, 1997, Saunders; (Venous [stasis] ulcer) Lookingbill DP, Marks JG: *Principles of dermatology*, 2nd edn. Philadelphia, 1993, Saunders; (Diabetic [neuropathic] related foot ulcer) Lemmi and Lemmi, 2011; (Superficial varicose veins) Lemmi and Lemmi, 2011; (Deep vein thrombophlebitis) Cronenwett JL, Johnston KW: *Rutherford's vascular surgery*, 8th edn, 2014, Saunders.
Art for Table 16.4: (Raynaud's phenomenon) Lemmi and Lemmi, 2011; (Lymphoedema) Walsh TD, Caraceni AT, Fainsinger R et al: *Palliative medicine*. Philadelphia, 2009, Saunders.
Art for Table 16.5: © Pat Thomas, 2010.
Art for Clinical Case Study: iStockphoto.com/Grigorev_Vladimir.

CHAPTER 17

Figures 17.3–17.5, 17.8–17.10, 17.13: © Pat Thomas, 2006.
Figure 17.15: Lakatta EG: Cardiovascular function in later life, *Cardiovascular Medicine*, 10:37–40, 1985.
Art for Table 17.2: Adapted from Zitkus BS: Take chest pain to heart, *Nurse Practitioner*, 35(9):41–47, 2010.
Art for Tables 17.9–17.11: © Pat Thomas, 2006.
Art for Clinical Case Study: Shutterstock.com/Pablo Rogat.

CHAPTER 18

Figures 18.2, 18.3: © Pat Thomas.
Figure 18.6B: Fireman P: *Atlas of allergies*, 2nd edn. London, 1996, Mosby.
Figure 18.11: Zitelli BJ, Davis HW: *Atlas of pediatric physical diagnosis,* 5th edn. St Louis, 2007, Mosby.
Figure 18.17: © Burghart Messtechnik GmbH.
Figure 18.18: © Amy Johnston.
Art for Table 18.1: (Foreign body) Fireman P: *Atlas of allergies*, 2nd edn. London, 1996, Mosby; (Perforated septum) Science Photo Library/Dr P Marazzi; (Acute rhinitis) Fireman P: *Atlas of allergies*, 2nd edn. London, 1996, Mosby; (Allergic rhinitis) Fireman P: *Atlas of allergies*, 2nd edn. London, 1996, Mosby; (Nasal polyps) Fireman P: *Atlas of allergies*, 2nd edn. London, 1996, Mosby; (Carcinoma) Rosai J: *Rosai & Ackerman's surgical pathology*, 10th edn. 2011, Elsevier.
Art for Table 18.2: (Cleft palate) Zitelli BJ, Davis HW: *Atlas of pediatric physical diagnosis*, 4th edn. St Louis, 2002, Mosby, Courtesy of Dr Michael Sherlock; (Bifid uvula) Neville BW, Damm DD, Allen CM et al: *Oral and maxillofacial pathology*, 2009, Elsevier Saunders; (Oral Kaposi's sarcoma) Flint PW, Haughey BH, Lund VJ et al: *Otolaryngology head & neck surgery*, 5th edn. Philadelphia, 2010, Saunders; (Acute tonsillitis and pharyngitis) Science Photo Library/Dr P Marazzi.
Art for Clinical Case Study: iStockphoto.com/romrodinka.

CHAPTER 19

Figures 19.1, 19.2, 19.10: © Pat Thomas, 2010.
Figure 19.11: © Pat Thomas, 2006.
Figure 19.12: Nichols FH, Zwelling E: *Maternal-newborn nursing: theory and practice*. Philadelphia, 1997, Saunders.
Figure 19.13: © Copyright 2013 GSK. All rights reserved.
Art for Table 19.7: Wahls SA: Causes and evaluation of chronic dyspnea, *American family physician*, 86(2): 173–180, 2012.
Art for Clinical Case Study: Shutterstock.com/Lopolo.

CHAPTER 20

Figures 20.2–20.4, 20.7–20.14: © Pat Thomas, 2006.
Figure 20.15: Douglas G, Nicol F, Robertson C: *Macleod's clinical examination*, 13th edn. Elsevier Churchill Livingstone, 2013.
Figures 20.34C, 20.35B: Dieppe PA, Cooper C, McGill N: *Arthritis and rheumatism in practice*, London, 1991, Gower Medical Publishing.
Figure 20.44: © Pat Thomas, 2006.
Figure 20.50: Zitelli BJ, Davis HW: *Atlas of pediatric physical diagnosis*, 4th edn. St Louis, 2002, Mosby.
Art for Table 20.2: (Atrophy) Science Photo Library/Dr P Mazarri; (Dislocated shoulder) Roberts JR: *Roberts and Hedges' Clinical Procedures in Emergency Medicine*, 6th edn. 2014, Elsevier Saunders; (Joint effusion) Science Photo Library/Dr P Mazarri; (Tear of rotator cuff) Waldman SD: *Physical diagnosis of pain: an atlas of signs and symptoms,* 2nd edn. Philadelphia, 2010, Saunders; (Frozen shoulder—adhesive capsulitis) Peñas CF, Cleland JA, Huijbregts PAL: *Neck and arm pain syndromes: evidence-informed screening, diagnosis and management*. Philadelphia, 2011, Churchill Livingstone.
Art for Table 20.3: (Olecranon bursitis) Stanley D, Trail IA: *Operative elbow surgery*. 2012, Elsevier Churchill Livingstone; (Gouty arthritis) Polley HF, Hunder GG: *Physical examination of the joints*, 2nd edn. Philadelphia, 1978, Saunders; (Subcutaneous nodules) Callen JP et al. *Color atlas of dermatology*. Philadelphia, 1993, Saunders; (Epicondylitis—tennis elbow) Skirven TM, Osterman AL, Fedorczyk JM et al: *Rehabilitation of the hand and upper extremity,* 6th edn. St Louis, 2011, Mosby.
Art for Table 20.4: (Ganglion cyst) Callen JP et al. *Color atlas of dermatology*. Philadelphia, 1993, Saunders; (Carpal tunnel syndrome with atrophy of thenar eminence) Science Photo Library/Mike Devlin; (Ankylosis) Slutsky DJ: *Principles and practice of wrist surgery*. Philadelphia, 2010, Saunders; (Dupuytren's contracture) Canale ST, Beaty JH: *Campbell's operative orthopaedics,* 12th edn. St Louis, 2013, Mosby; (Swan-neck and boutonnière deformity) Reprinted from the Clinical Slide Collection on the Rheumatic Diseases. Copyright © 1991, 1995, 1997. Used by permission of the American College of Rheumatology; (Ulnar deviation or drift) Walker JM, Helewa A: *Physical therapy in arthritis*. Philadelphia, 1996, Saunders; (Degenerative joint disease or osteoarthritis) Walker JM, Helewa A: *Physical therapy in arthritis*. Philadelphia, 1996, Saunders; (Syndactyly) Liebert PS: *Color atlas of pediatric surgery*, 2nd edn. Philadelphia, 1996, Saunders; (Polydactyly) Liebert PS: *Color atlas of pediatric surgery*, 2nd edn. Philadelphia, 1996, Saunders.
Art for Table 20.5: (Mild synovitis) Dieppe PA, Cooper C, McGill N: *Arthritis and rheumatism in practice*. London, 1991, Gower Medical Publishing; (Prepatellar bursitis) Science Photo Library/Dr P Marazzi; (Swelling of menisci) Jones A, Owen R: *Color atlas of clinical orthopaedics*, 2nd edn. London, 1995, Mosby; (Osgood-Schlatter disease) Zitelli BJ, Davis HW: *Atlas of pediatric physical diagnosis*, 4th edn. St Louis, 2002, Mosby.
Art for Table 20.6: (Achilles tenosynovitis) Science Photo Library/CMSP/Dr P Marazzi; (Tophi with chronic gout) Dockery GL: *Cutaneous disorders of the lower extremity*. Philadelphia, 1997, Saunders; (Acute gout) Science Photo Library/Dr P Marazzi; (Hallux valgus with bunion and hammertoes) Walker JM, Helewa A: *Physical therapy in arthritis*. Philadelphia, 1996, Saunders.
Art for Table 20.7: (Scoliosis) Zitelli BJ, Davis HW: *Atlas of pediatric physical diagnosis*, 4th edn. St Louis, 2002, Mosby; (Herniated nucleus pulposus) Polley HF, Hunder GG: *Physical examination of the joints*, 2nd edn. Philadelphia, 1978, Saunders.
Art for Table 20.8: (Developmental hip dysplasia) Zitelli BJ, Davis HW: *Atlas of pediatric physical diagnosis*, 4th edn. St Louis, 2002, Mosby; (Talipes equinovarus [clubfoot]) Dr AE Chudley, MD; (Spina bifida) Thompson DNP: Spinal dysraphic anomalies; classification, presentation and management, *Paediatrics and Child Health*, 20(9):397–403, 2010.
Art for Clinical Case Study: Shutterstock.com/Phovoir.

CHAPTER 21

Figure 21.1: © Pat Thomas, 2010.
Figure 21.3: © Pat Thomas, 2006.
Figure 21.5: © Commonwealth of Australia 2014, Creative Commons Attribution 3.0 Australia License.
Figure 21.6: *Food and Nutritional Health for Adults, Risk Screening and Monitoring Outline*, Department of Health & Human Services, State Government of Victoria, 2012.
Figure 21.10: Ibsen OAC, Phelan JA: *Oral pathology for the dental hygienist*, 2nd edn. Philadelphia, 1996, Saunders.
Figures 21.11, 21.16B: Lemmi and Lemmi, 2011.
Figure 21.12: © Pat Thomas, 2006.
Art for Table 21.4: (Starved appearance) Hall R, Evered DC: *Color atlas of endocrinology*, 2nd edn. London, 1990, Mosby.
Art for Table 21.5: (Pellagra) Latham MC et al: *Scope manual on nutrition*. Kalamazoo, 1980, The Upjohn Company, copyright Thomas Spies, MD; (Follicular hyperkeratosis) Taylor KB, Anthony LE: *Clinical nutrition*. New York, 1983, McGraw-Hill, copyright by Harold H Sandstead; (Scorbutic gums) Taylor KB, Anthony LE: *Clinical nutrition*. New York, 1983, McGraw-Hill, copyright by The Upjohn Company; (Bitot's spots) Taylor KB, Anthony LE: *Clinical nutrition*. New York, 1983, McGraw-Hill, copyright by Helen Keller International, Inc; (Rickets) Nunn T, Rollinson P, Scott B: Blount's disease, *Orthopaedics and Trauma*, 25(6):454–461, 2011; (Magenta tongue) McLaren DS: *Color atlas of nutritional disorders*. London, 1981, Wolfe Medical, copyright by CE Butterworth, Jr.
Art for Table 21.6: (Cleft lip) Ibsen OAC, Phelan JA: *Oral pathology for the dental hygienist*, 2nd edn. Philadelphia, 1996, Saunders; (Herpes simplex 1) Callen JP et al: *Color atlas of dermatology*. Philadelphia, 1993, Saunders; (Angular cheilitis [stomatitis, perlèche]) Callen JP et al: *Color atlas of dermatology*.

Philadelphia, 1993, Saunders; (Carcinoma) Science Photo Library/Dr P Marazzi; (Retention 'cyst' [mucocoele]) Zitelli BJ, McIntire SC, Nowalk AJ: *Atlas of pediatric physical diagnosis*, 6th edn. Philadelphia, 2012, Elsevier Saunders.

Art for Table 21.7: (Baby bottle tooth decay) Courtesy of F Ferguson, Department of Children's Dentistry, School of Dental Medicine, SUNY at Stony Brook, Stony Brook, NY 11733; (Dental caries) Courtesy of A McWhorter, Pediatric Dentistry, Baylor College of Dentistry, The Texas A & M University System, Dallas, TX; (Epulis) Ibsen OAC, Phelan JA: *Oral pathology for the dental hygienist*, 2nd edn. Philadelphia, 1996, Saunders; (Gingival hyperplasia) Ibsen OAC, Phelan JA: *Oral pathology for the dental hygienist*, 2nd edn. Philadelphia, 1996, Saunders; (Gingivitis) Callen JP et al: *Color atlas of dermatology*. Philadelphia, 1993, Saunders; (Meth mouth) Neville BW et al: *Oral and maxillofacial pathology*, 3rd edn. St Louis, 2009, Saunders.

Art for Table 21.8: (Ankyloglossia) Ibsen OAC, Phelan JA: *Oral pathology for the dental hygienist*, 2nd edn. Philadelphia, 1996, Saunders; (Fissured or scrotal tongue) Lemmi and Lemmi, 2011; (Geographic tongue [migratory glossitis]) Lemmi and Lemmi, 2011; (Smooth, glossy tongue [atrophic glossitis]) Adams GL, Bois LR, Hilger PA: *Boies fundamentals of otolaryngology: a textbook of ear, nose, and throat diseases*, 6th edn. Philadelphia, 1989, Saunders; (Black hairy tongue) Callen JP et al: *Color atlas of dermatology*. Philadelphia, 1993, Saunders; (Enlarged tongue [macroglossia]) Zitelli BJ, Davis HW: *Atlas of pediatric physical diagnosis*, 4th edn. St Louis, 2002, Mosby, courtesy of Dr Christine Williams; (Carcinoma) Wenig BM, Heffess CS, Adair CF: *Atlas of endocrine pathology*. Philadelphia, 1997, Saunders.

Art for Table 21.9: (Aphthous ulcers) Lemmi and Lemmi, 2011; (Koplik's spots) Feigin RD, Cherry JD: *Textbook of pediatric infectious diseases*, 4th edn. Philadelphia, 1998, Saunders; (Leucoplakia) Sleisinger MH, Fordtran JS: *Gastrointestinal diseases: pathophysiology, diagnosis, and management*, vol 1, 5th edn. Philadelphia, 1993, Saunders; (Candidiasis or monilial infection) Callen JP et al: *Color atlas of dermatology*. Philadelphia, 1993, Saunders.

Art for Table 21.10: (Metabolic syndrome [MetS]) Ford ES, Li C, Zhao G et al: Prevalence of the metabolic syndrome among U.S. adolescents using the definition from the International Diabetes Federation, *Diabetes Care*, 31(3):587–589, 2008 and Mozumdar A, Liguori G: Persistent increase in prevalence of metabolic syndrome among U.S. adults: NHANES III to NHANES 1999–2006, *Diabetes Care*, 34(1):216–219, 2011.

Art for Table 21.12: (Thyroid—multiple nodules) Swartz MH: *Textbook of physical diagnosis: history and examination*, 5th edn. Philadelphia, 2006, Saunders; (Parotid gland enlargement) Swartz MH: *Textbook of physical diagnosis: history and examination*, 5th edn. Philadelphia, 2006, Saunders; (Fetal alcohol syndrome) © Pat Thomas, 2006; (Congenital hypothyroidism) Zitelli BJ, Davis HW: *Atlas of pediatric physical diagnosis*, 4th edn. St Louis, 2002, Mosby, courtesy of Dr Thomas P Foley Jr; (Hyperthyroidism) Swartz MH: *Textbook of physical diagnosis: history and examination*, 5th edn. Philadelphia, 2006, Saunders; Myxoedema [hypothyroidism]) Hall R, Evered DC: *Color atlas of endocrinology*, 2nd edn. London, 1990, Mosby.

Art for Clinical Case Study: Shutterstock.com/Zurijeta.

CHAPTER 22

Figure 22.3AB: Lookingbill DP, Marks JG: *Principles of dermatology*, 2nd edn. Philadelphia, 1993, Saunders.

Figures 22.4A, 22.4B: Hurwitz S: *Clinical pediatric dermatology: a textbook of skin disorders of childhood and adolescence*, 2nd edn. Philadelphia, 1993, Saunders.

Figure 22.4C: Lookingbill DP, Marks JG: *Principles of dermatology*, 2nd edn. Philadelphia, 1993, Saunders.

Figure 22.5: Patton KT, Thibodeau GA, Douglas MM: *Essentials of anatomy & physiology*. St Louis, 2012, Mosby.

Figures 22.7–22.12: Lemmi and Lemmi, 2011.

Figure 22.13: Bowden VR, Dickey SB, Greenburg CS: *Children and their families: the continuum of care*, Philadelphia, 1998, Saunders.

Figures 22.14, 22.15: Hurwitz S: *Clinical pediatric dermatology: a textbook of skin disorders of childhood and adolescence*, 2nd edn. Philadelphia, 1993, Saunders.

Figure 22.16: Lemmi and Lemmi, 2011.

Figure 22.17: Hurwitz S: *Clinical pediatric dermatology: a textbook of skin disorders of childhood and adolescence*, 2nd edn. Philadelphia, 1993, Saunders.

Figure 22.18: Murray SS, McKinney ES: *Foundations of maternal-newborn and women's health nursing*, 5th edn. Philadelphia, 2010, Saunders.

Figures 22.19A, B: Habif TP, Campbell JL, Dinulos JGH et al: *Skin disease: diagnosis and treatment,* 2nd edn. St Louis, 2005, Mosby.

Figure 22.20: Lookingbill DP, Marks JG: *Principles of dermatology*, 2nd edn. Philadelphia, 1993, Saunders.

Figure 22.21: Lemmi and Lemmi, 2011.

Figure 22.22: Habif TP, Campbell JL, Dinulos JGH et al: *Skin disease: diagnosis and treatment,* 2nd edn. St Louis, 2005, Mosby.

Figure 22.23: Lookingbill DP, Marks JG: *Principles of dermatology*, 2nd edn. Philadelphia, 1993, Saunders.

Figure 22.24: Callen JP et al: *Color atlas of dermatology*. Philadelphia, 1993, Saunders.

Art for Table 22.4: (Macule and patch) © Pat Thomas, 2010. Photos courtesy Lemmi and Lemmi, 2011; (Papule and plaque) Pat Thomas, 2010. Photos courtesy Lemmi and Lemmi, 2011; (Nodule tumour and Wheal) © Pat Thomas, 2010. Photos courtesy Lemmi and Lemmi, 2011; (Urticaria [hives]) © Pat Thomas, 2010. Fireman P: *Atlas of allergies*, 2nd edn. St Louis, 1996, Mosby; (Vesicle and bulla) © Pat Thomas, 2010. Photos courtesy Lemmi and Lemmi, 2011; (Cyst) © Pat Thomas, 2010. Photos courtesy Lemmi and Lemmi, 2011; (Pustule) © Pat Thomas, 2010. Photos courtesy Lemmi and Lemmi, 2011.

Art for Table 22.5: (Crust) © Pat Thomas, 2010. Photo courtesy Lemmi and Lemmi, 2011; (Scale) © Pat Thomas, 2010. Photo courtesy Lemmi and Lemmi, 2011; (Fissure) © Pat Thomas, 2010. Photo courtesy Lemmi and Lemmi, 2011; (Erosion) © Pat Thomas, 2010. Photo courtesy Lemmi and Lemmi, 2011; (Ulcer) © Pat Thomas, 2010. Photo courtesy Lemmi and Lemmi, 2011; (Excoriation) © Pat Thomas, 2010. Photo courtesy Lemmi and Lemmi, 2011; (Scar) © Pat Thomas, 2010. Photo courtesy Lemmi and Lemmi, 2011; (Atrophic scar) © Pat Thomas, 2010. Photo courtesy Lemmi and Lemmi, 2011; (Lichenification) © Pat Thomas, 2010. Photo courtesy Lemmi and Lemmi, 2011; (Keloid) © Pat

Thomas, 2010. Photo courtesy Lemmi and Lemmi, 2011.
Art for Table 22.6: (Pressure injury [decubitus ulcer] Stage I) Potter PA, Perry AG: *Fundamentals of nursing*, 7th edn. St Louis, 2009, Mosby; (Pressure injury [decubitus ulcer] Stage II) Potter PA, Perry AG: *Fundamentals of nursing*, 7th edn. St Louis, 2009, Mosby; (Pressure injury [decubitus ulcer] Stage III) Potter PA, Perry AG: *Fundamentals of nursing*, 7th edn. St Louis, 2009, Mosby; (Pressure injury [decubitus ulcer] Stage IV) Potter PA, Perry AG: *Fundamentals of nursing*, 7th edn. St Louis, 2009, Mosby.
Art for Table 22.8: (Port-wine stain [naevus flammeus]) Paller AS, Mancini AJ: *Hurwitz clinical pediatric dermatology: a textbook of skin disorders of childhood and adolescence*, 4th edn. Philadelphia, 2011, Saunders; (Strawberry mark [immature haemangioma]) Lookingbill DP, Marks JG: *Principles of dermatology*, 2nd edn. Philadelphia, 1993, Saunders; (Cavernous haemangioma [mature]) Habif TP, Campbell JL, Dinulos JGH et al: *Skin disease: diagnosis and treatment,* 2nd edn. St Louis, 2005, Mosby; (Telangiectasia) Lemmi and Lemmi, 2011; (Spider or star angioma) Lemmi and Lemmi, 2011; (Venous lake) Habif TP, Campbell JL, Dinulos JGH et al: *Skin disease: diagnosis and treatment,* 2nd edn. St Louis, 2005, Mosby; (Petechiae) Dockery GL: *Cutaneous disorders of the lower extremity*, Philadelphia, 1997, Saunders; (Ecchymosis) Lemmi and Lemmi, 2011; (Purpura) Paller AS, Mancini AJ: *Hurwitz clinical pediatric dermatology: a textbook of skin disorders of childhood and adolescence*, 4th edn. Philadelphia, 2011, Saunders.
Art for Table 22.9: (Nappy dermatitis) Paller AS, Mancini AJ: *Hurwitz clinical pediatric dermatology: a textbook of skin disorders of childhood and adolescence*, 4th edn. Philadelphia, 2011, Saunders; (Intertrigo [candidiasis]) Lemmi and Lemmi, 2011; (Impetigo) Lemmi and Lemmi, 2011; (Atopic dermatitis [eczema]) Paller AS, Mancini AJ: *Hurwitz clinical pediatric dermatology: a textbook of skin disorders of childhood and adolescence*, 4th edn. Philadelphia, 2011, Saunders; (Measles [rubeola] in dark skin) Feigin RD, Cherry JD: *Textbook of pediatric infectious diseases*, 4th edn. Philadelphia, 1998, Saunders; (Measles [rubeola] in light skin) Lemmi and Lemmi, 2011; (German measles [rubella]) Paller AS, Mancini AJ: *Hurwitz clinical pediatric dermatology: a textbook of skin disorders of childhood and adolescence*, 4th edn. Philadelphia, 2011, Saunders; (Chickenpox [varicella]) Callen JP et al: *Color atlas of dermatology*. Philadelphia, 1993, Saunders.
Art for Table 22.10: (Primary contact dermatitis) Lookingbill DP, Marks JG: *Principles of dermatology*, 2nd edn. Philadelphia, 1993, Saunders; (Allergic drug reaction) Lookingbill DP, Marks JG: *Principles of dermatology*, 2nd edn. Philadelphia, 1993, Saunders; (Tinea corporis [ringworm of the body]) Paller AS, Mancini AJ: *Hurwitz clinical pediatric dermatology: a textbook of skin disorders of childhood and adolescence*, 4th edn. Philadelphia, 2011, Saunders; (Tinea pedis [ringworm of the foot]) Lemmi and Lemmi, 2011; (Psoriasis) Lookingbill DP, Marks JG: *Principles of dermatology*, 2nd edn. Philadelphia, 1993, Saunders; (Tinea versicolor) Lemmi and Lemmi, 2011; (Labial herpes simplex [cold sores]) Lemmi and Lemmi, 2011; (Herpes zoster [shingles]) Lemmi and Lemmi, 2011; (Lyme disease) Swartz MH: *Textbook of physical diagnosis: history and examination,* 5th edn. Philadelphia, 2005, Saunders.
Art for Table 22.11: (Basal cell carcinoma) Lookingbill DP, Marks JG: *Principles of dermatology*, 2nd edn. Philadelphia, 1993, Saunders; (Squamous cell carcinoma) Habif TP, Campbell JL, Dinulos JGH et al: *Skin disease: diagnosis and treatment,* 2nd edn. St Louis, 2005, Mosby; (Malignant melanoma) Lookingbill DP, Marks JG: *Principles of dermatology*, 2nd edn. Philadelphia, 1993, Saunders.
Art for Table 22.12: (AIDS-related Kaposi's sarcoma: patch stage) Friedman-Kien AE: *Color atlas of AIDS*. Philadelphia, 1989, Saunders.
Art for Table 22.13: (Seborrhoeic dermatitis [cradle cap]) Hurwitz S: *Clinical pediatric dermatology: a textbook of skin disorders of childhood and adolescence*, 2nd edn. Philadelphia, 1993, Saunders; (Tinea capitis [scalp ringworm]) Lookingbill DP, Marks JG: *Principles of dermatology*, 2nd edn. Philadelphia, 1993, Saunders; (Toxic alopecia) Hurwitz S: *Clinical pediatric dermatology: a textbook of skin disorders of childhood and adolescence*, 2nd edn. Philadelphia, 1993, Saunders; (Alopecia areata) Hurwitz S: *Clinical pediatric dermatology: a textbook of skin disorders of childhood and adolescence*, 2nd edn. Philadelphia, 1993, Saunders; (Traumatic alopecia: traction alopecia) Hurwitz S: *Clinical pediatric dermatology: a textbook of skin disorders of childhood and adolescence*, 2nd edn. Philadelphia, 1993, Saunders; (Trichotillomania) Callen JP et al: *Color atlas of dermatology*. Philadelphia, 1993, Saunders; (Pediculosis capitis [head lice]) Callen JP et al: *Color atlas of dermatology*, Philadelphia, 1993, Saunders; (Furuncle and abscess) Lookingbill DP, Marks JG: *Principles of dermatology*, 2nd edn. Philadelphia, 1993, Saunders.
Art for Table 22.14: (Scabies) Lemmi and Lemmi, 2011; (Paronychia) Lemmi and Lemmi, 2011; (Beau's line) Callen JP et al: *Color atlas of dermatology*. Philadelphia, 1993, Saunders; (Splinter haemorrhages) Callen JP et al: *Color atlas of dermatology*. Philadelphia, 1993, Saunders; (Late clubbing) Reprinted from the Clinical Slide Collection on the Rheumatic Diseases. Copyright © 1991, 1995, 1997. Used by permission of the American College of Rheumatology; (Onycholysis) Lemmi and Lemmi, 2011; (Pitting) Lemmi and Lemmi, 2011; (Habit–tic dystrophy) Lemmi and Lemmi, 2011.
Art for Clinical Case Study 1: Shutterstock.com/Steve Buckley
Art for Clinical Case Study 2: iStock Image ID 77021236

CHAPTER 23

Figures 23.1–23.6: © Pat Thomas, 2006.
Art for Table 23.2: © Pat Thomas, 2014.
Art for Table 23.4: (Umbilical hernia) Zitelli BJ, Davis HW: *Atlas of pediatric physical diagnosis*, 4th edn. St Louis, 2002, Mosby, courtesy of Dr Thomas P Foley, Jr; (Epigastric hernia) Conroy K, Malata CM: Epigastric hernia following DIEP flap breast reconstruction: Complication or coincidence? *Journal of Plastic, Reconstructive & Aesthetic Surgery*, 65(3):387–391, 2012; (Incisional hernia) Lemmi and Lemmi, 2011; (Diastasis recti) Clark DA: *Atlas of neonatology*, 7th edn. Philadelphia, 2000, Saunders.
Art for Tables 23.5–23.7: © Pat Thomas.
Art for Clinical Case Study: iStockphoto.com/Juanmonino.

CHAPTER 24

Figures 24.1, 24.2: © Pat Thomas, 2006.
Figure 24.3: Brown D, Edwards H: *Lewis's medical–surgical nursing*, 3rd edn. Chatswood NSW, 2011, Elsevier.
Figure 24.4: © Pat Thomas.

Figure 24.5: © Pat Thomas, 2010.
Table 24.1: Courtesy Connie Cooper.
Art for Table 24.2: © Pat Thomas.
Art for Clinical Case Study: iStockphoto.com/torwai.

CHAPTER 25

Figures 25.1, 25.2: © Pat Thomas.
Figure 25.3: Bristol Stool Scale, CC BY SA 3.0, Wikipedia/Kyle Thompson. Based on the Bristol Stool Scale developed by Dr Ken Heaton at the University of Bristol.
Art for Table 25.2: © Pat Thomas.
Art for Clinical Case Study: iStockphoto.com/SilviaJansen.

CHAPTER 26

Figures 26.1, 26.2: © Pat Thomas.
Figure 26.3: Adapted from Figure 47-8 in Brown D, Edwards H, Buckley T: *Lewis's medical surgical nursing*, 4th edn. Sydney, 2014, Mosby Elsevier.
Figures 26.11, 26.12, 26.17, 26.22: © Pat Thomas.
Figure 26.14: © 2017 Victorian Cytology Service Limited (ACN 609 597 408). These materials are subject to copyright and are protected by the Copyright Laws of Australia. All rights are reserved. Any copying or distribution of these materials without the written permission of the copyright owner is not authorized.
Art for Table 26.1: Adapted from Tanner JM: *Growth at adolescence*. Oxford, England, 1962, Blackwell Scientific.
Art for Table 26.2: (Pediculosis pubis [crab lice]) from Callen JP et al: *Color atlas of dermatology*. Philadelphia, 1993, Saunders; (Herpes simplex virus—type 2 [herpes genitalis]) Lemmi and Lemmi, 2011; (Syphilitic chancre) Reprinted from Emond R, Rowland HAK, Welsby P: *Colour atlas of infectious diseases,* 3rd edn. London, 1995, Mosby; (Red rash—contact dermatitis) Courtesy of Pfizer Laboratories Division, Pfizer Inc, New York. From *A close look at VD*: a slide presentation produced as a public service; (Human papillomavirus [HPV] genital warts) Habif TP, Campbell JL, Chapman JS et al: *Skin disease: diagnosis and treatment*. St Louis, 2001, Mosby; (Abscess of Bartholin's gland) Reprinted from Emond R, Rowland HAK, Welsby P: *Colour atlas of infectious diseases*, 3rd edn. London, 1995, Mosby; (Urethral caruncle) Rimsza ME: An illustrated guide to adolescent gynecology, *Pediatric Clinics of North America*, 36(3):641, 1989.
Art for Table 26.3: (Cystocele) Lemmi and Lemmi, 2011; (Uterine prolapse) Symonds EM, McPherson MBA: *Diagnosis in color: obstetrics and gynecology*. London, 1997, Mosby-Wolfe.
Art for Table 26.4: (Human papillomavirus [HPV, condylomata]) Symonds EM, McPherson MBA: *Diagnosis in color: obstetrics and gynecology*. London, 1997, Mosby-Wolfe; (Polyp) Lemmi and Lemmi, 2011; (Cervical cancer) Symonds EM, McPherson MBA: *Diagnosis in color: obstetrics and gynecology*. London, 1997, Mosby-Wolfe.
Art for Table 26.5: (Candidiasis (moniliasis)] Lemmi and Lemmi, 2011; (Gonorrhoea) Courtesy of Pfizer Laboratories Division, Pfizer Inc, New York. From *A close look at VD*: a slide presentation produced as a public service.
Art for Table 26.8: (Ambiguous genitalia) Moore KL, Persaud TN: *Before we are born: essentials of embryology and birth defects*, 5th edn. Philadelphia, 1998, Saunders; (Vulvovaginitis in child) Muram D, Simmons KJ: Pattern recognition in pediatric and adolescent gynecology—a case for formal education, *Journal of Pediatric and Adolescent Gynecology*, (21)2:103–108, 2008.
Art for Clinical Case Study: iStockphoto.com/FatCamera.

CHAPTER 27

Figures 27.1–27.3, 27.15: © Pat Thomas.
Figure 27.6: Science Photo Library/Dr P. Marazzi.
Figure 27.9B: Lemmi and Lemmi, 2011.
Art for Table 27.1: Adapted from Tanner JM: *Growth at adolescence*, Oxford, 1962, Blackwell Scientific Publications.
Art for Table 27.2: (Genital herpes—HSV-2 infection) Lemmi and Lemmi, 2011; (Syphilitic chancre) Reprinted from Emond R, Rowland HAK, Welsby P: *Colour atlas of infectious diseases*, 3rd edn. London, 1995, Mosby; (Genital warts) Habif TP, Campbell JL, Dinulos JGH et al: *Skin disease: diagnosis and treatment,* 2nd edn. St Louis, 2005, Mosby; (Carcinoma) Callen JP et al: *Color atlas of dermatology*. Philadelphia, 1993, Saunders; (Urethritis [urethral discharge and dysuria]) Reprinted from Emond R, Rowland, HAK, Welsby P: *Colour atlas of infectious diseases*, 3rd edn. London, 1995, Mosby.
Art for Table 27.3: (Phimosis) Liebert PS: *Color atlas of pediatric surgery*, 2nd edn. Philadelphia, 1996, Saunders; (Paraphimosis) Keys C, Lam JPH: Foreskin and penile problems in childhood, *Surgery* (Oxford) 31(3):130–134, 2013; (Hypospadias) Liebert PS: *Color atlas of pediatric surgery*, 2nd edn. Philadelphia, 1996, Saunders; (Epispadias) Zitelli BJ, Davis HW: *Atlas of pediatric physical diagnosis*, 4th edn. St Louis, 2002, Mosby; (Peyronie's disease) Courtesy of Dr Hans Stricker, Department of Urology, Henry Ford Hospital, Detroit, MI.
Art for Tables 27.4–27.5: © Pat Thomas, 2006.
Art for Clinical Case Study: iStockphoto.com/stray_cat.

CHAPTER 28

Figures 28.1, 28.2: © Pat Thomas, 2010.
Figure 28.4: © Pat Thomas, 2014.
Figure 28.6: From Callen JP et al: *Color atlas of dermatology*. Philadelphia, 1993, Saunders.
Figure 28.17: Moore KL, Persaud TVN: *Before we are born: essentials of embryology and birth defects*, 7th edn. Philadelphia, 2008, Saunders.
Art for Table 28.1: © Pat Thomas.
Art for Table 28.3: (Dimpling) Evans AJ et al: *Atlas of breast disease management: 50 illustrative cases*. Philadelphia, 1998, Saunders; (Oedema [peau d'orange]) Mansel R: *Color atlas of breast diseases*. London, 1995, Mosby; (Deviation in nipple pointing) Mansel R: *Color atlas of breast diseases*. London, 1995, Mosby; (Fixation) Mansel R: *Color atlas of breast diseases*. London, 1995, Mosby.
Art for Table 28.4: © Pat Thomas.
Art for Table 28.6: (Mammary duct ectasia) Mansel R: *Color atlas of breast diseases*. London, 1995, Mosby; (Intraductal papilloma) Mansel R: *Color atlas of breast diseases*. London, 1995, Mosby; (Carcinoma) Evans AJ et al: *Atlas of breast disease management: 50 illustrative cases*. Philadelphia, 1998, Saunders; (Paget's disease [intraductal carcinoma]) Mansel R: *Color atlas of breast diseases*. London, 1995, Mosby.
Art for Table 28.7: (Breast abscess) Mansel R: *Color atlas of breast diseases*. London, 1995, Mosby; (Mastitis) Mansel R: *Color atlas of breast diseases*. London, 1995, Mosby.

Art for Table 28.8: (Gynaecomastia) Lorenzo GD, Autorino R, Perdonà S et al: Management of gynaecomastia in patients with prostate cancer: a systematic review, *Lancet* 6(12): 972–979, 2005; (Carcinoma) Elshafieya ME, Zeeneldinb AA, Elsebaia HI et al: Epidemiology and management of breast carcinoma in Egyptian males: experience of a single Cancer Institute, *Journal of the Egyptian National Cancer Institute*, 23(3):115–122, 2011.
Art for Clinical Case Study: iStockphoto.com/JohnnyGreig.

CHAPTER 29

Figures 29.1, 29.2: © Pat Thomas, 2018.
Figure 29.4: Black M, Ambros-Rudolph CM, Edwards L et al: *Obstetric and gynecologic dermatology*, 3rd edn. St Louis, 2008, Mosby.
Figures 29.9–29.12: © Pat Thomas, 2018.
Art for Table 29.1: Symonds EM, McPherson MBA: *Diagnosis in color: obstetrics and gynecology*. London, 1997, Mosby-Wolfe.
Art for Table 29.2: Meur S, Mann NP: Infant outcomes following diabetic pregnancies, *Paediatrics and Child Health*, (17)6:217–222, 2007.
Art for Table 29.4: © Pat Thomas.
Art for Clinical Case Study: iStockphoto.com/michaeljung.

CHAPTER 30

Art for scenarios: (1. Mr Micha Krawiec) Shutterstock/Budimir Jevtic; (2. Ms Josephine Magliore) Shutterstock/jeep5d; (3. Mrs Jennifer Guyatt) Shutterstock/Fotoluminate LLC; (4. Mr Max Smith) Shutterstock/A Master Image; (5. Mr Bill Craven) Shutterstock/Laurin Rinder; (6. Mrs Christine Thomas) Shutterstock/Kamira.

Index

b = box, f = figure, t = table

B

C

E

F

G

H

J

K

L

M

N

S

U

V

W

X

Z